FOURTH EDITION

FUNDAMENTAL ORTHOPEDIC MANAGEMENT

for the Physical Therapist Assistant

ELSEVIER

3251 Riverport Lane
St. Louis, Missouri 63043

FUNDAMENTAL ORTHOPEDIC MANAGEMENT FOR THE PHYSICAL THERAPIST ASSISTANT, FOURTH EDITION

ISBN: 978-0-323-11347-2

Details on how to seek permission, further information about the Publisher's permissions policies and our arrangements with organizations such as the Copyright Clearance Center and the Copyright Licensing Agency, can be found at our website: www.elsevier.com/permissions.

This book and the individual contributions contained in it are protected under copyright by the Publisher (other than as may be noted herein).

International Standard Book Number: 978-0-323-11347-2

Vice President and Publisher: Loren Wilson
Content Strategy Director: Penny Rudolph
Executive Content Strategist: Kathy Falk
Content Development Manager: Jolynn Gower
Associate Content Development Specialist: Laurel Berkel
Publishing Services Manager: Julie Eddy
Senior Project Manager: Celeste Clingan
Design Direction: Maggie Reid

Printed in The United States of America

Last digit is the print number: 9 8 7 6 5 4 3 2 1

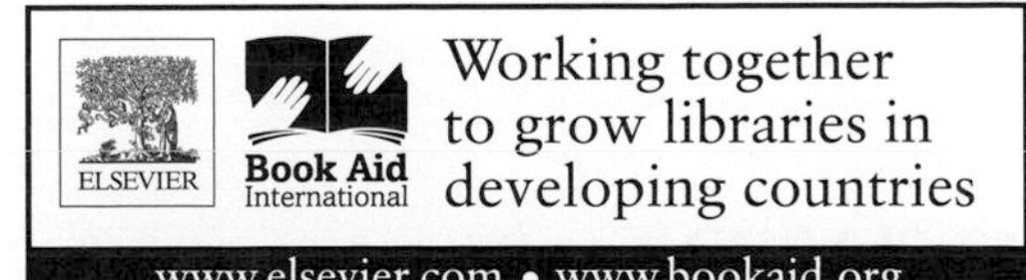

FOURTH EDITION

FUNDAMENTAL ORTHOPEDIC MANAGEMENT *for the* Physical Therapist Assistant

Robert C. Manske, PT, DPT, MEd, SCS, ATC, CSCS
Professor and Chair
Wichita State University
Department of Physical Therapy
Via Christi Health Physical Therapy
Wichita, Kansas

ELSEVIER

To my new friend,
Gary Shankman, for writing the first 3 editions
of this incredibly valuable text!
I am honored to continue your vision! I hope that you continue to enjoy
your "second" journey, which is probably even more valuable than your first!

To my many physical therapy mentors, who include both PTs and PTAs.
You know who you are. There are too many of you to list here. Rest assured,
I fully understand—without YOU this text would not be possible!

To my three exceptional children,
Rachael, Halle, and Tyler

To my amazing wife,
Julie

—Robert C. Manske

Contributors

Candy Bahner, PT, DPT, MS
Professor and Chair
Stefani Doctor of Physical Therapy Program
University of Saint Mary
Leavenworth, Kansas

Jason Brumitt, PT, PhD, ATC, CSCS
George Fox University
Doctor of Physical Therapy Program
Newberg, Oregon

Marc Campolo, PT, PhD, SCS, ATC, CSCS
Chair
Department of Physical Therapy
Samson College of Health Sciences
University of the Sciences in Philadelphia
Philadelphia, Pennsylvania

John T. Cavanaugh, PT, MEd, ATC, SCS
Clinical Supervisor
Hospital for Special Surgery
Sports Rehabilitation & Performance Center
New York, New York

Jennifer E. Celso, PT, MPT, DPT, WCS
Doctor of Physical Therapy and ABPTS Board Certified Women's Health Specialist
Director of Clinical Education
Department of Physical Therapy
Wichita State University
Wichita, Kansas

Terry Cox, PT, DPT, OCS, FAAOMPT
Professor
Department of Physical Therapy
Southwest Baptist University
Bolivar, Missouri

Jamie Dehan, PT, DPT, MS
DPT Director of Clinical Education
Assistant Professor
Stefani Doctor of Physical Therapy Program
University of Saint Mary
Leavenworth, Kansas

John DeWitt, DPT, SCS, ATC
Assistant Clinical Professor
Division of Physical Therapy
The Ohio State University
Columbus, Ohio

Steven Elliott
Benchmark Physical Therapy
Knoxville, Tennessee

LaDonna S. Hale, PharmD
Professor
Wichita State University
Wichita, Kansas

Michael Hales, PhD, CSCS
Assistant Professor and Director of Applied Kinesiology Laboratory
Department of Health & Physical Education
Kennesaw State University
Kennesaw, Georgia

Amy Hassen, PT, DPT, OCS, MTC
Clinical Assistant Professor
Physical Therapy Program
Walsh University
North Canton, Ohio

Charles Hazle, PT, PhD
Associate Professor
Department of Rehabilitation Sciences
University of Kentucky
Center of Excellence in Rural Health
Hazard, Kentucky

Jessica Hettler, PT, MSPT, ATC Cert, MDT, SCS
Board Certified Clinical Specialist Sports Physical Therapy
Sports Rehabilitation and Performance Center
Hospital for Special Surgery
New York, New York

Walter L. Jenkins PT, DHS, LATC, ATC
Professor and Chair
Department of Physical Therapy
College of Allied Health Services
Health Sciences Building
East Carolina University
Greenville, North Carolina

Jeromy Jones, PT, DPT, OCS, ATC, CSCS
Physical Therapist
Stillwater Medical Center
Stillwater, Oklahoma

Joseph Kelly, MSPT
Assistant Professor
Department of Physical Therapy and Health Science
Bradley University
Peoria, Illinois

Thomas W. Kernozek, PhD, FACSM
Professor and Director of the La Crosse Institute for Movement Science
University of Wisconsin-La Crosse
Department of Health Professions
Physical Therapy Program
La Crosse, Wisconsin

Leslie K. King, CPO
Practice Manager
Hanger Prosthetics and Orthotics
Knoxville, Tennessee

Marsha Lawrence, PT, CHT
Handworx, LLC
Stilwell, Kansas

B. J. Lehecka, DPT
Assistant Professor
Wichita State University
Wichita, Kansas

Adriaan Louw, PhD, PT
Senior Faculty
International Spine and Pain Institute
Story City, Iowa

Lenny Macrina MSPT, SCS, CSCS
Co-Founder
Director of Physical Therapy
Champion PT & Performance
Waltham, Massachusetts

Terry Malone, PT, EdD, ATC, FAPTA
Professor
Department of Rehabilitation Sciences
University of Kentucky
Lexington, Kentucky

Erik P. Meira, PT, DPT, SCS, CSCS
Black Diamond Physical Therapy
Portland, Oregon

Daryl L. Menke, PT, DPT, MCMT
Normal, Illinois

Victoria Moran, PT, DPT
Certified Schroth Therapist
New York, New York

Jaime C. Paz, PT, DPT, MS
Clinical Associate Professor
Division of Physical Therapy
Walsh University
North Canton, Ohio

Michael P. Reiman, PT, DPT, OCS, SCS, ATC, FAAOMPT, CSCS
Assistant Professor
Duke University Medical Center
Department of Orthopaedic Surgery
Division of Physical Therapy
Durham, North Carolina

Bryan L. Riemann, PhD, ATC, FNATA
Professor, Sports Medicine
Director, Biodynamics and Human Performance Center
Armstrong State University
Savannah, Georgia

Justin Rohrberg, DPT, ATC
Department of Physical Therapy
Wichita State University
Wichita, Kansas

Gary A. Shankman, PTA
Heritage Healthcare
Knoxville, Tennessee
Hillcrest South
Knoxville, Tennessee

Barbara Smith, PhD, PT
Wichita State University
Department of Physical Therapy
Wichita, Kansas

Cheryl Sparks, PT, DPT
Assistant Professor
Department of Physical Therapy and Health Science
Bradley University
Peoria, Illinois

Terry L. Trundle, ATC, LAT, PTA
Owner
Athletic Rehab Institute
Acworth, Georgia

Harvey W. Wallmann, PT, DSc, SCS, ATC, CSCS
Director and Professor
Western Kentucky University
Doctor of Physical Therapy Program
Bowling Green, Kentucky

Pawel Wawrzyniak, PT, DPT, SCS
Physical Therapist
Hospital for Special Surgery
New York, New York

D. S. Blaise Williams III, PhD, MPT
Director, VCU RUN LAB
Department of Physical Therapy
Department of Kinesiology and Health Sciences
Virginia Commonwealth University
Richmond, Virginia

John Willson, PT, PhD
Associate Professor, Department of Physical Therapy
Director, Human Movement Analysis Lab
East Carolina University
Greenville, North Carolina

Preface

As it has been 5 years since the last edition of *Fundamental Orthopedic Management for the Physical Therapist Assistant*, I hope the fourth edition is exactly what you wanted! This text never seems to be finished, rather it continues to be more in evolution. This evolution comes from the requirements of educational programs and the needs of both student and practicing physical therapists assistants (PTAs).

The field of orthopedic physical rehabilitation continues to change, and the new fourth edition is committed to bringing those "Fundamental Orthopedic Management" changes to PTA education. The focus of this latest edition continues to be on the critical thinking and application of the physical therapy examination, development of treatment plans, and interventions that can be used by PTAs during clinical practice. Although an ability to thoroughly evaluate the orthopedic patient is not within the scope of the PTA's practice, we feel that it is necessary for the PTA to understand basic evaluation components and tests and measures that are used in the evaluation and differential diagnosis process. Each chapter in the fourth edition of *Fundamental Orthopedic Management for the Physical Therapist Assistant* has been extensively updated to reflect changes in practice patterns. This includes the use and descriptions of evidence-based treatments wherever available. Therefore, the fourth edition of *Fundamental Orthopedic Management for the Physical Therapist Assistant* continues to be the "one stop" for all things orthopedic and should be used by both PTA students and the practicing PTAs as their resource for physical therapy practice.

Regional experts have continued to greatly enhance this new fourth edition of *Fundamental Orthopedic Management for the Physical Therapist Assistant.* Regional experts in various subject areas again contributed as authors, which has significantly elevated the depth and breadth of the entire text. Although numerous authors have helped us reach this goal, I would like to highlight just a few. To begin, Daryl Menke and Jeromy Jones have written a chapter that clearly and systematically describes the important process of differential diagnosis, which will help the PTA understand the importance of this examination and evaluation concept. This will allow the PTA to better appreciate which forms of injury could mimic others that will need to be ruled out by the referring physical therapist. The ability of the PTA to pick up some of the subtle differences in patient history or during examination will allow a greater amount of teamwork to pick up potentially disabling problems that could be otherwise referred to more appropriate healthcare providers. Terry Malone and Charles Hazle have written a chapter that describes the basics of orthopedic imaging. Although not yet in the scope of practice for most physical therapists, with the increased amount of autonomy with direct referral privileges, it is imperative that physical therapists and PTAs understand the common uses and instances when a referral to a radiologist may be needed. Terry and Charles have written an easy-to-read, very informative chapter to teach the PTA the basics of orthopedic imaging. Jennifer Celso has provided this edition with a chapter on women's health. As it is more than likely that half of the patients we may ever see in our career will be women, we should all understand the differences that may be needed to treat females. Treatment of women's issues is becoming a huge niche market in rehabilitation, and this chapter is a great resource for those wanting to work in a specialized practice or for those just wanting to understand our better half! This is just a brief sampling of the excitement that awaits you inside the fourth edition of *Fundamental Orthopedic Management for the Physical Therapist Assistant.*

Additional changes will specifically help PTA educators and the PTA students who use the educational resources. In this fourth edition, we have provided new testing and quiz materials and resources. Each chapter has ample number of multiple-choice questions, true/false questions, short answer and fill-in-the-blank–type learning strategies to help in test and quiz preparation. Furthermore, new material has been incorporated to the Evolve website for the fourth edition. Throughout each chapter, I have also included important concepts that contain some of the "meat of the chapter" content in which these new highlighted areas are more easily seen and remembered by the student while reading this text. It is my hope that these educational-type additions will not only give the educator more ease and variety for use with teaching but also allow the student to better understand and to learn the valuable concepts of each chapter. As this text continues to evolve, we will continue to add these special valuable educational strategies.

I am sure that you will continue to rely on the fourth edition as you have the past editions for your fundamental orthopedic management needs. I want to graciously thank the few who have emailed suggested changes. I greatly appreciate any feedback you may have regarding this text. Constructive criticism is what allows me to develop the exact textbook that fits your educational needs. If you have recommendations or additions that you think we should consider in the fifth edition, please feel free to email me at: Robert.Manske@wichita.edu. I promise all emails will be accepted and given the highest priority. This textbook is for you and I will be happy to entertain your educational requests.

Robert C. Manske

Acknowledgments

Three editions ago, Gary Shankman had a vision to write a text, *Fundamental Orthopedic Management for the Physical Therapist Assistant*. The concept was to write a textbook specifically focusing on the needs of the physical therapist assistant (PTA) that addressed basic, foundational information on orthopedic management. He felt that there was a need for a condensed, yet not simplified, text to equip entry-level PTA students with essential and practical information concerning orthopedics written from the perspective, training, and experience of a PTA for PTAs. This became the seminal textbook for orthopedics in PTA programs and ever hard-working clinicians over the years.

As the years have passed, this textbook has evolved. And like a great wine, it gets better every year. I was fortunate enough to be asked by Gary to help with the third edition of this text. We addressed more issues and added respected and very qualified educators and clinicians to help with various chapters. The third edition became a multi-authored unity of various orthopedic topics, addressing a wide range of issues and pathologies with substantial depth to challenge the student and practicing clinician alike. Without these contributors, the book would have remained unidimensional, as it is extremely hard for a single author to be an expert in all areas of rehabilitation. With the addition of new authors in each section, richness was developed that continues today with the fourth edition.

To begin with, I have to thank Gary Shankman for developing this unbelievable text. Gary, your vision has educated thousands upon thousands of PTAs throughout the years! To each and every contributor, I say thank you for your time, expertise, and willingness to share your wisdom, talents, and gifts. To the contributors of the three new chapters—Daryl Menke, Jeromy Jones, Terry Malone, Charles Hazle, and Jennifer Celso—I offer a deep and personal thank you for your time and effort in creating totally new chapters that will help continue the tradition of excellence for this state-of-the-art text.

Naturally, there are numerous individuals at Elsevier who enabled a project of this magnitude to take shape. To each of these, I say thank you. The leadership team on this project started with Megan Fennell and finished with Laurel Berkel. Thank you both for all the time and effort put forth to get this book on track and finished. To Kathy Falk and Jolynn Gower, thank you so much for continuing to put your never-ending faith in me to tackle these big projects. Without your support I would not be "living the dream!"

Hopefully this book will honor all of the patients, therapists, physicians, and educators that both Gary and I have had the privilege to learn from and work with. From the words of Gary himself: "It is with great delight, humility, deep appreciation, and profound gratitude that I say thank you for this remarkable journey of learning and sharing."

Robert C. Manske

Contents

Part I

Basic Concepts of Orthopedic Management

The foundations for the appropriate application of skills and therapeutic techniques related to orthopedic physical therapy are based on the interdependence of basic science principles and the relationships between the patient, the supervising physical therapist (PT), and the physical therapist assistant (PTA). The PTA, although responsible for proper patient supervision and clinical observation during treatment, is frequently guided and directed to modify or adjust selected interventions in consultation with the supervising PT based on specific physiologic responses from the patient. Keen observation skills, properly directed patient supervision techniques, and a thorough understanding of physiologic and therapeutic adaptations to exercise techniques help the PTA to apply selected interventions effectively and skillfully under the direction and supervision of the supervising PT.

Therefore, this section introduces basic orthopedic physical therapy concepts of patient supervision; the role of the PTA in physical assessment and problem solving with specific reference to the *Guide to Physical Therapist Practice 3.0,*[1] the problem-solving algorithm used by PTAs in patient or client intervention, and related key elements of systems review and a systems approach to physical assessment; unique characteristics of strength and adaptation in young and elderly patients; closed kinetic chain exercise; neuromuscular fatigue; and balance, coordination, and the enhancement of the afferent neural input system related to orthopedic physical therapy management.

The focus and specific intent of this section is to provide a sound, practical, and purposeful introduction to the principles of basic orthopedic management as well as the therapeutic application of these critical components related to specific tissue healing constraints, immobilization, and postsurgical recovery after orthopedic injury or surgery.

---

[1]American Physical Therapy Association. *Guide to physical therapist practice 3.0,* Alexandria, VA, 2014, APTA.

Chapter 1

Patient Supervision and Observation During Treatment

Candy Bahner

CHAPTER OUTLINE

LEARNING OBJECTIVES

1. Discuss the "Problem-Solving Algorithm Utilized by PTAs in Patient/Client Intervention."
2. Identify and discuss the rationale for clear and concise communication among all members of the rehabilitation team.
3. Discuss the skills necessary to provide patient supervision.
4. Define objective scales of measurement used to communicate changes in a patient's status to the supervising physical therapist.
5. Apply proactive listening skills and objective scales of measurement to provide appropriate, accountable, and responsible observation and supervision of the patient during treatment.
6. Define open-ended and closed-ended questioning.
7. Define the quadrants of the basic dimensional model.
8. Discuss the four categories of behavior of the physical therapist assistant: dominance, submission, hostility, and warmth.
9. Describe the differences between prompting and cueing.

KEY TERMS

Accountability
Basic dimensional model
Clinical decision making
Closed-ended questions
Communication
Cueing
Dominance
Hostility
Interpersonal communication
Interventions
Listening
Open-ended questions
Proactive
Probing questions
Prompting
Responsibility
Submission
Warmth

SUPERVISING THE PATIENT DURING TREATMENT

Among the many challenges for the physical therapist assistant (PTA) are supervising the patient during selected **interventions**, solving problems effectively, and making appropriate decisions. The PTA must recognize that **interpersonal communication** skills, patient supervision methods, data collection skills, effective problem solving, and responsive **clinical decision making** must be learned, practiced, and demonstrated to function efficiently and effectively.

Initial contact with a patient establishes a framework of rapport and sets the stage for all future interactions with that individual. The PTA has the opportunity to convey confidence, capability, and sensitivity during the initial introductions by the supervising physical therapist (PT). This leads the patient to trust the PTA and minimizes fear and anxiety.

Important Concepts

"Physical therapist assistants provide physical therapy services under the direction and supervision of the physical therapist. They implement selected components of patient/client interventions and obtain data related to that intervention; make modifications in selected interventions either to progress the patient/client as directed by the physical therapist or to ensure patient/client safety and comfort; educate and interact with physical therapist assistant students, aides, technicians, volunteers, patients/clients families, caregivers; and respond to patient/client and environmental emergency situations."[1]

The PTA is responsible for carrying out prescribed selected interventions, patient supervision, data collection, and appropriate problem solving and clinical decision making. The Department of Education, Accreditation, and Practice of the American Physical Therapy Association developed the "Problem-Solving Algorithm Utilized by PTAs in Patient/Client Intervention,"[1] which reflects current policies and positions on the problem-solving processes to be used by PTAs in the provision of selected interventions (Fig. 1-1). For proper care to be given, the PTA must monitor the patient's response to selected interventions and accurately and swiftly report changes to the supervising PT. This involves constant patient interaction, observation, data collection, reassessment of initial data, problem solving, and responsive action to clarify and enhance the effectiveness of prescribed selected interventions. Positive and negative changes in the patient's status can occur throughout the treatment program, whether during a single treatment or over the span of multiple treatments. Some of these changes are subtle and require keen awareness of the initial objective data and acute sensitivity to the patient's subjective reports. Other changes are profound and sudden. In either situation, the PTA observes the patient and collects appropriate data, such as range of motion, strength, pain, balance, coordination, swelling, endurance, or gait deviations. When reported to the supervising PT, these changes dictate and can significantly affect the course of treatment.

COMPONENTS OF PATIENT SUPERVISION

Clinical patient supervision can be viewed as a process with the following purposes:

- To gather relevant information and data
- To establish and enhance rapport, trust, and confidence
- To facilitate understanding of the PTA's concept of the patient's problem as outlined, described, and initially determined by the supervising PT
- To assist in the management of the patient
- To provide a conduit or therapeutic outlet for the patient to voice concerns about his or her problem

Clearly gathering information from the patient and interpreting the data during the initial evaluation are the responsibility of the PT. However, the PTA may need to assist the PT in helping the patient understand the problem throughout the course of rehabilitation. The PTA must recognize how difficult it is for patients to grasp all the components of their condition well enough to appreciate fully the rationale for the prescribed treatment. The PTA may be asked, when appropriate, to help the patient understand the disorder being treated, the supervising PT's plan of care, and the selected interventions to be provided. During this patient interaction, the PTA must be keenly aware of and sensitive to subtle or apparent signs of patient apprehension, fear, and anxiety.

Although direct patient supervision is frequently the task of one individual, responsibility for the patient's care is shared by the entire rehabilitation team. In addition, the patient must be actively involved in the treatment and accept shared responsibility for his or her own care.

While providing selected interventions, the PTA makes observations of the patient, collects relevant data, and develops an objective assessment using appropriate scales of measurement (Box 1-1). Using applicable questioning techniques ensures that the patient is actively involved. This interactive approach to supervision as well as the skills of the PTA to seek, understand, and relay accurately information related to the patient's status distinguishes the PTA from an aide who is trained on the job.[5]

PATIENT SUPERVISION BY THE REHABILITATION TEAM

The PTA must be aware of the key members of the rehabilitation team. The PT and PTA are involved with direct patient care on a daily basis and may be assisted by supportive personnel, such as physical therapy aides or technicians. Occupational therapists and occupational therapy assistants, speech language pathologists, audiologists, rehabilitation counselors, nurses, respiratory therapists, psychologists, and dietitians all play significant roles in daily patient care. These rehabilitation specialists seek to maximize recovery for each patient and always must be regarded as resources to meet specific patient needs as they are identified by any member of the team. The PTA charged with direct patient care and supervision is only one vital member of the team, and he or she can take comfort in knowing that every member of the team is prepared to provide appropriate skills so that the patient can achieve the highest functional gains in recovery. Developing a team mindset helps the PTA to be responsible and accountable to the other members of the team for his or her own contribution and to reach out to others when their expertise is needed.[7]

Effective **communication** is the hallmark of a great team and should be maximized. To supervise effectively and provide the best care for the patient, the PTA must learn to communicate openly and freely with honesty and respect and in a professional manner with every member of the team.[7] He or she must differentiate between the language used for communicating among peers and language used to define and explain injury, disease, and physical therapy interventions to a patient. The PTA must employ appropriate and professional medical terminology to outline and describe an orthopedic problem to a PT and must be able to use familiar terms to describe the same pathologic condition to a patient or family member. If the PTA uses medical jargon inappropriately, the patient or family member might perceive the PTA as insensitive, aloof, and impersonal. Use of language appropriate to the patient's comprehension generally conveys understanding, sensitivity, **warmth,** and reassurance and removes uncomfortable and unnecessary barriers to communication.[2]

Important Concepts

Use of language appropriate to the patient's comprehension conveys understanding, sensitivity, warmth, and reassurance and removes uncomfortable and unnecessary barriers to communication.

The PTA also must be aware that **listening** is an effective communication tool. Listening demonstrates interest and provides the opportunity for a better understanding of the patient's concept of the problem.[4] Through active listening, the PTA is better able to integrate verbal and nonverbal messages that the patient may have received.[4] In addition, patients may be more comfortable and

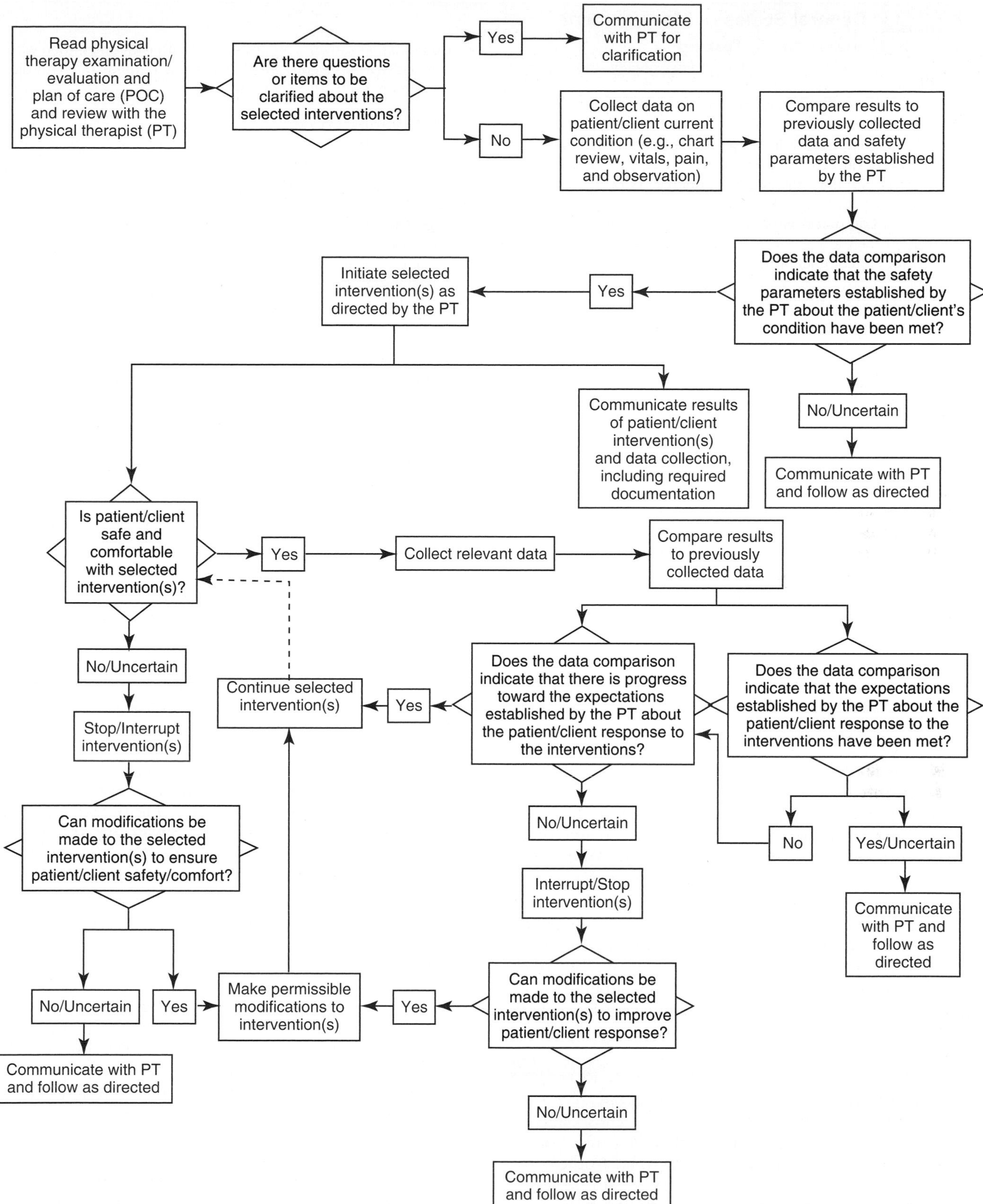

FIG 1-1 Problem-solving algorithm utilized by PTAs in patient/client intervention. *(Adapted from* A normative model of physical therapist assistant education, *version 2007, with permission of the American Physical Therapy Association. Copyright © 2007 American Physical Therapy Association.)*

BOX 1-1 General Scales of Measurement

Strength: Manual Muscle Testing
- 5/5 Normal: Holds test position against gravity and maximal resistance
- 4/5 Good: Holds test position against gravity and moderate resistance
- 3/5 Fair: Completes full range of motion against only the resistance of gravity
- 2/5 Poor: Completes full range of motion in a gravity minimized position
- 1/5 Trace: Can detect visually or by palpation some contractile activity in the muscle
- 0/5 Zero: No contraction felt in the muscle

Pain: Analog Scale
- Graded from 0 to 10 (0 absent, 10 severe)

Swelling: Generally Measured by
- Circumferential measurement
- Water displacement

Vital Signs
- Blood pressure: Less than 120/80 mm Hg normal; use sphygmomanometer and stethoscope
- Pulse: Between 60 and 100 bpm; average 72 bpm; pulse can be lower (e.g., 55) for trained athletes
- Respirations: Average 12 to 16 breaths per minute
- Temperature: Normal range 97° F to 99° F
- Oxygen saturation: Normal ranges from 95% to 100%

Coordination
- Tapping foot or hand
- Finger to nose
- Heel to shin
- Coordination activities are tested first with eyes open, then with eyes closed. All events are described as degrees of rhythmic, symmetric, even, and consistent.

Stretch Reflex (DTR)
- 0 = Areflexia
- 1 to 3 = Average
- 3+ to 4 = Hyperreflexia

Range of Motion: Standard Goniometry
- Shoulder
  - Flexion 1° to 180°
  - Extension 0° to 60°
  - Abduction 0° to 180°
  - Internal rotation 0° to 70°
  - External rotation 0° to 90°
- Hip
  - Flexion 0° to 120°
  - Extension 0° to 30°
  - Abduction 0° to 45°
  - Adduction 0° to 30°
  - External rotation 0° to 45°
  - Internal rotation 0° to 45°
- Ankle
  - Dorsiflexion 0° to 20°
  - Plantar flexion 0° to 50°
  - Inversion 0° to 35°
  - Eversion 0° to 15°
- Knee
  - Flexion 0° to 135°
- Elbow
  - Flexion 0° to 150°

DTR, deep tendon reflex.

trusting with a good listener and be more willing to provide information.[4]

Supervision of patients by the PTA must be done systematically and reliably with an emphasis on **accountability** and effective and efficient patient care. Appropriate and responsible investigative questioning of the patient during selected interventions helps the PTA focus on the areas to probe, findings to quantify, and objective changes to assess. As indicated in the "Problem-Solving Algorithm Utilized by PTAs in Patient/Client Intervention,"[1] PTAs are responsible for reporting all findings to the supervising PT so that modifications can be made in accordance with changes in patient status.

Important Concepts

The PT is responsible for the five elements of patient/client management (examination, evaluation, diagnosis, prognosis, and intervention) and the direction and supervision of all selected interventions provided by the PTA.

BASIC PATIENT SUPERVISION SKILLS

Communication Skills

The PTA can be most effective if he or she develops an understanding of human behavior and adopts a **proactive** role in supervising patients. In a proactive role, the PTA does not wait to be placed in a reactive position. Use of appropriate **probing questions** is a proactive method to use during patient supervision. Questioning patients during treatment can be insightful, rewarding, and helpful for both the supervising PT and the PTA. The format of asking probing questions is critical and strongly influences the responses received (Fig. 1-2). Using **open-ended questions** invites the patient to share feelings, thoughts, concerns, and opinions.[9] Examples are as follows:
- "Tell me about your pain."
- "How does that feel?"
- "What do you think about this exercise?"

These types of questions are generally not answered by "yes" or "no." They open discussions and prompt the patient to express a wide range of views and opinions.[9] Open-ended questions for patients have been described as "a good medium for facilitating rapport and, as such, are particularly useful. ..."[4] Using open-ended questions promotes personal interactions between the PTA and patient, may allow the patient to give a more in-depth explanation of the problem, and may lead to discussions of what the patient identifies as important. Although this type of questioning does not enable the patient to give precise, clear answers, it is appropriate in situations that require compassion and empathy from the PTA and shared feelings between the PTA and patient.

Probe	Definition	Objectives	Characteristics	Examples
Open-ended questions	A question or statement that invites a wide-ranging response, often asks for ideas, opinions, or views.	• Open up discussion • Invite broad response • Give other freedom to talk • Gets involvement	• Can't be answered "yes" or "no" • Gets at feelings, opinions, thoughts	• "What do you think about...?" • "Tell me about..." • "Why do you feel...?" • "What's your opinion?"
Pause	An intentional, purposeful period of silence.	• Give other a chance to think and respond • Slow down pace • Draw out other	• Usually follows open-ended question • Deliberate	• "Why do you say that?" (silence) • "Tell me more." (silence)
Reflective	A statement that describes and reflects a feeling or emotion (without implying agreement or disagreement).	• Identify emotions • Show you understand • Vent interfering emotions	• Names a feeling or emotion • Usually uses the word "you" or "you're" • May state cause of the emotion	• "You're pretty mad about it." • "You seem reluctant to talk about it." • "Sounds like you're excited."
Neutral phrase or question	A question or statement that encourages other to elaborate.	• Get other to tell more about a subject	• Few words • About subject under discussion	• "Tell me more." • "Please elaborate." • "Explain that." • "Amplify on that."
Brief assertion	A short statement, sound, or gesture, which shows involvement.	• Encourage other to continue • Increase receptivity	• Elicits additional information • Occurs automatically	• "Oh, okay." • "Yes, sure." • "I see." • Nodding your head.
Summary statements	A brief statement, in your own words, of the content of what was said.	• Check understanding • Prove you're listening • Give structure and direction • Help other clarify thinking • Invite other to comment or expand	• Summarizes content, not feelings • Restatement of essential ideas • In own words	• "So you disagree about..." • "The way you see it is..." • "You prefer working overtime..." • "Let me summarize how I..."
Closed-ended questions	A question that limits the answer by requesting specific facts, or a "yes" or "no" answer.	• Find out details, specifics • Check understanding • Direct the discussion • Get other to take a stand	• Often starts with "Who," "Which," "When," "Where," "How many," etc. • Can sometimes be answered with a simple "yes" or "no"	• "Who is...?" • "Which order...?" • "When will you...?" • "Do you think...?"
Leading questions	A question that implies only one answer, or a rhetorical question—no answer is needed.	• Pin down positions or agreements • Can verify assumptions • Can be threatening	• The question gives the answer • No answer is required	• "Shouldn't we discuss...?" • "This is the best way to go, isn't it?"

FIG 1-2 Probes and probing questions: The use of questions, statements, and pauses to elicit information, thoughts, and opinions. The type of question used elicits a characteristic response. *(From Buzzotta VR, Lefton RE.* Dimensional management training, *St Louis, 1989, Psychological Associates.)*

Closed-ended questions are directed toward finding facts, obtaining specific responses, and filling in details. They can be very helpful in focusing and clarifying essential details of the patient's condition.[9] By asking the patient questions such as, "Where is your pain?" "When does your knee feel unstable?" or "Does your back hurt when you bend forward?" the PTA proactively directs the discussion and sequence of questions instead of sifting out pertinent information from among all the data gathered in open-ended questioning.

Summary-type statements check understanding, help the patient clarify thinking, and provide direction for the PTA. Examples include the following: "So your back hurts only at night?" and "Then your knee doesn't hurt with this exercise." Using precise closed-ended questions with summary statements elicits information that can lead to an objective assessment of the patient. The approach the PTA takes influences the balance of questioning between open-ended and closed-ended questions.

Important Concepts

Open-ended questions: Invite the patient to share feelings, thoughts, concerns, and opinions.
Closed-ended questions: Are directed toward finding facts, obtaining specific responses, and filling in details.
Summary-type statements: Check understanding, help the patient clarify thinking, and provide direction for the PTA.

Behavior

The behavior of the PTA during patient supervision can either reassure the patient and demonstrate appropriate responsive professional care or create a sense of indifference. Four broad categories of behavior are **dominance**, **submission**, **hostility**, and warmth.[2] Buzzotta and Lefton[2] define these four categories as follows:

Dominance. Dominance can be defined as exercising control or influence. People who show dominant behavior are forceful, dynamic, and assertive. They push their ideas forward or try to sway the way other people think or behave. They take charge, guide, lead, and move other people to action.

Submission. Submission can be defined as being passive. People who show submissive behavior are willing to take a back seat. They are ready to comply, quick to give in, and reluctant to try to exert influence.

Hostility. Hostility can be defined as being unresponsive or insensitive to others and their needs. People showing hostile behavior tend to care only about themselves; they lack regard for other people's feelings and ideas. Although anger is a form of hostility, people can be hostile while showing no open anger.

Warmth. Warmth can be defined as being responsive and sensitive to others and their needs. People who show warm behavior are open and caring and have a high regard for other people's ideas and feelings. This does not mean they automatically gush with affection. A person can be warm without being openly affectionate.

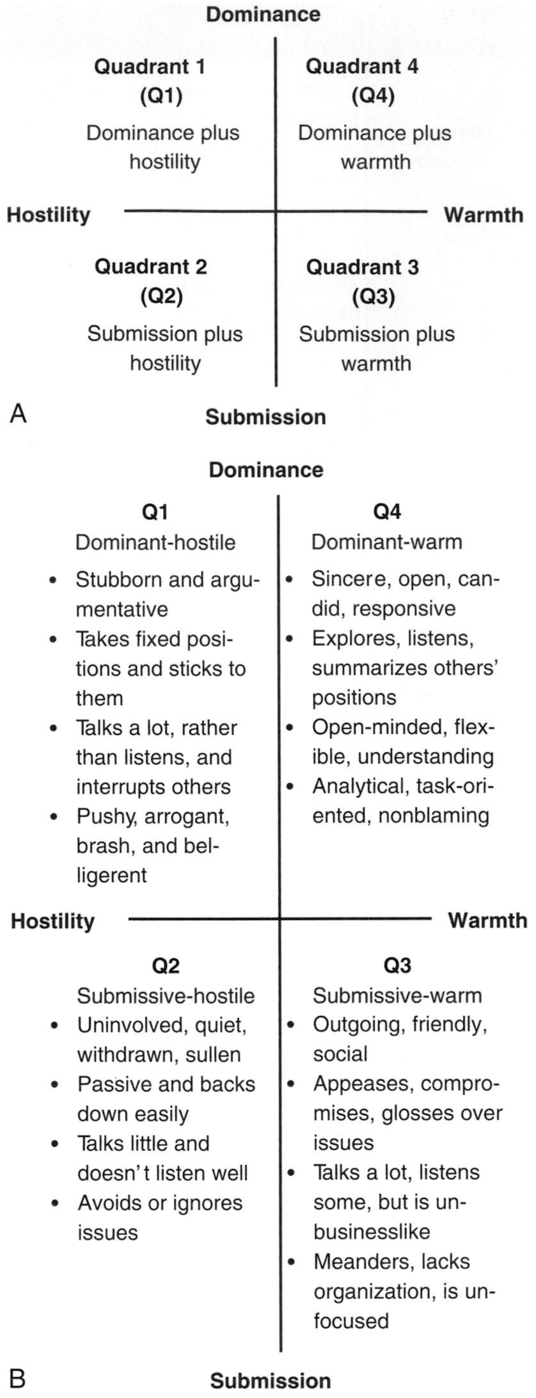

FIG 1-3 **A,** The dimensional model is a tool to size up behavior. The model applies to subordinates, peers, and superiors. Quadrants are formed among dominance, submission, hostility, and warmth that create certain patterns of behavior. **B,** Four distinct patterns and characteristics are formed between the four quadrants. *(From Buzzotta VR, Lefton RE.* Dimensional management training, *St Louis, 1989, Psychological Associates.)*

These four categories of behavior are used to describe the extremes of the **basic dimensional model** (Fig. 1-3, *A*). Quadrants (Q) are formed and certain patterns of behavior exist when two dimensions are combined:

- Q1: Dominant hostile
- Q2: Submissive hostile
- Q3: Submissive warm
- Q4: Dominant warm

Four patterns, or types, of human behavior come from this (Fig. 1-3, *B*).

Dominance	Active behavior—leading, controlling, making things happen
Submission	Passive behavior—following, letting things happen, reacting
Hostility	A lack of concern or regard and unresponsiveness for other people and their position/ideas
Warmth	Concern, regard, and responsiveness for other people and their position/ideas

Applying this model when asking open-ended and closed-ended questions shows such questions to be equally balanced within Quadrant 4 (Q4). The goal of the PTA during supervision of the patient is to demonstrate consistently the qualities found in Q4—for example, being appropriately friendly, attentive, responsive, involved, exploring, analytical, and task oriented.

While supervising patients according to the Q4 model, the PTA must understand the differences between **prompting** and **cueing** a patient to perform a specific task. Prompting a patient to perform a task can be viewed as the presentation of a question. For example, when instructing a patient to ambulate with a standard walker, the assistant should prompt the patient by asking, "After you move the walker, what foot do you move next?" Prompting allows patients to decipher information, solve problems, and provide solutions to activities they must overcome during recovery. Cueing can be viewed as a direction. An example is, "After you move the walker, move your injured leg." Although the solution is provided for the patient, he or she must still demonstrate appropriate follow-through and proper understanding of the command.

Important Concepts

Prompting: The presentation of a question. Allows patients to decipher information, solve problems, and provide solutions to activities they must overcome during recovery.

Cueing: Viewed as a direction. Although the solution is provided for the patient, he or she must still demonstrate appropriate follow-through and proper understanding of the command.

MODIFICATIONS DURING TREATMENT

Using attentive Q4 behavior with balanced open-ended and closed-ended questioning of the patient helps the PTA identify and quantify changes in the patient's condition. After consulting the supervising PT and receiving direction, the PTA can effectively modify a specific intervention in accordance with changes in patient status.

The following example helps to clarify the scope of treatment modifications during postoperative rehabilitation after anterior cruciate ligament reconstruction.

Swelling (joint effusion) after knee surgery is common and occurs in about 13% of cases after knee ligament surgery.[8] Usually the effusion is a hemarthrosis (blood within the joint, which can impair voluntary muscle contraction). In such a case, the supervising PT provides baseline evaluation data about the degree of swelling present by making comparative circumferential measurements at midpatella, 2 inches superior to the midpatella, and 2 inches inferior to the midpatella. The PTA maintains daily records of the three comparative circumferential measurements. Because re-education and strengthening of muscle is influenced negatively by postoperative swelling, any increase or decrease in swelling necessitates a modification in the initial program outlined by the supervising PT. The degree of swelling documented influences the adjustment made in the exercise prescription.

As the PTA identifies objective changes in the patient's status each day, the concept of visual, nonresponsive, and noninteractive supervision is altered to one of appropriate, responsive, and accountable supervision.

Isometric exercises generally are used early in the rehabilitation of acute postoperative knee injuries. Concentric and eccentric exercises are introduced as rehabilitation proceeds. Concentric and eccentric exercises are defined as dynamic, producing work, and creating changes in joint angles and muscle length.[6] The progression from isometric to dynamic exercise produces an increase in force generated, increases muscle soreness, and causes greater articular stresses.[3] If swelling and pain increase as the patient progresses from isometric to concentric and eccentric contractions, the PTA, with direction and input from the supervising PT, can adjust or modify the program back to isometrics or reduce the amount of resistance, joint angle of exercise, volume of exercise, or velocity of movement. The specific sequence or combination of these modifications depends on the patient's specific needs, the surgical procedure, and the patient's tolerance to exercise. Usually it is prudent to begin with the least drastic change in exercise prescription and then progress (Box 1-2).

The clinical decision-making process used by the PTA involves recognizing that a problem exists, then taking orderly and specific steps to notify the supervising PT and adjust the program accordingly. The PTA takes an active, participatory role while supervising patients, using his or her training and skills to the fullest extent.

Important Concepts

Clinical decision making by the PTA involves observation, information processing, critical thinking, evaluation of evidence, application of relevant knowledge, problem solving, reflection, and clinical judgment to select the best course of action that would benefit the patient.

The recognition of changes in patient status does not imply interpretation of objective, measurable data by the PTA. The task of the PTA is to provide information to the supervising PT on a daily basis, keep the supervising PT

BOX 1-2 Knee Extension: Isotonic Exercise Modifications

If pain and swelling develop during full range of motion isotonic knee extension:

- Adjust the resistance. Reduce the amount of weight being used.
- Adjust the range of motion to limit full knee flexion: Example: Begin knee extension exercises from 45° of flexion or less instead of 90° or greater. Note: Some acute, chronic, and postsurgical conditions prohibit terminal knee extension (0°). In this case, limit full extension to −10° or greater.
- Adjust the speed or velocity of the performance of the exercise. Closely observe the speed of the exercise. Perform slow, controlled, nonballistic exercise.
- Adjust the volume of exercise.
  - Reduce the number of repetitions being performed.
  - Reduce the number of sets being performed.
  - Reduce the number of days per week performing the exercise.
- Change the performance of exercise.
  - Perform only isometric holds followed by eccentric loads. No concentric lifting.

informed concerning patient status, and provide insightful and meaningful suggestions for modifications.

The objective data supplied to the supervising PT by the PTA may include, but is not limited to, goniometric measurements, circumferential measurements, manual muscle testing, endurance grading, heart rate, blood pressure, respirations, dynamic balance, and coordination measurements, according to the scope of the assistant's training.

UNDERSTANDING DIFFERENT PHILOSOPHIES OF PHYSICAL THERAPISTS

Fundamental differences exist among PTs concerning the methods, protocols, and directives they use to treat patients. In addition, just as the PTA is directed by the supervising PT, the PT may sometimes be directed by the physician. Within a hospital physical therapy department, the PTA may have contact with many supervising PTs, each with different backgrounds, experiences, and education. The PTA sees PTs use various protocols to manage the same pathologic condition. It is not the role of the PTA to change or modify treatment plans or protocols without the direction and approval of the supervising PT. Opinions and controversies exist concerning how best to manage various orthopedic pathologic conditions. Changes in surgery and physical therapy occur because of advanced technology and rigorous research in rehabilitation medicine and orthopedic surgery. New procedures in arthroscopic anterior cruciate ligament surgery allow a more rapid return to function, motion, and strength than ever before. Although ideally we presume all surgical procedures and rehabilitation techniques to be universally accepted, the specialties of orthopedics and physical therapy are both art and science; therefore diversity is accepted.

The PTA can be placed in frustrating and confusing situations when dealing with various supervising PTs with different backgrounds and opinions concerning the management of patients. To minimize the confusing array of treatment protocols, the PTA must communicate effectively and efficiently with the supervising PT to clarify differences in patient care, always remembering that the PT has ultimate **responsibility** for the physical therapy interventions provided. The PTA does not divest interest in the care of any patient because of a disagreement in strategy with the supervising PT. The PTA's role requires a broader perspective and understanding that there are many ways to manage effectively the same pathology.

Having strong opinions on how to care for patients with orthopedic conditions is appropriate and shows passion, interest, and confidence in a certain method or protocol that has demonstrated good results. However, particular experience with the successful management of patients by one supervising PT may conflict with the course of treatment prescribed by another. On the surface, this situation may seem particularly frustrating and stressful. To understand this difference better, the PTA must identify the key elements of disagreement and seek an appropriate explanation from the supervising PT. This situation gives the supervising PT the opportunity to teach and explain the rationale for the particular treatment and exposes the PTA to new information. The PTA then can observe and learn new methods that may prove equally or more successful than the previous plan of care.

Fully understanding the rationale and purpose of each selected intervention allows for improved delivery of service to the patient. During direct patient supervision, the PTA can provide any selected interventions the supervising PT directs him or her to perform so long as allowed by law, and the safety and welfare of the patient are not compromised.

A well-adapted PTA views any apparent roadblocks as learning opportunities. The PTA is advised to take advantage of the broad knowledge and experience of many PTs, constantly inquire about the rationale and scientific basis for a particular program, and establish himself or herself as an eager learning participant who is open to innovative ways of managing various pathologic conditions.

GLOSSARY

Accountability: Systematic, reliable, and appropriate investigative questioning, listening, and active participation at all levels of patient care.

Basic dimensional model: Two-dimensional model that consists of four behaviors (dominance, submission, hostility, and warmth), which fall into four quadrants: Q1 = dominance-hostility; Q2 = submission-hostility; Q3 = submission-warmth; Q4 = dominance-warmth.

Clinical decision making: Complex process that involves observation, information processing, critical thinking, evaluation of evidence, application of relevant knowledge, problem solving, reflection, and clinical judgment to select the best course of action that would benefit the patient.

Closed-ended questions: Communication technique that requires a "yes" or "no" answer. This method effectively directs specific responses aimed at details of the patient's condition.

Communication: The exchange of information between people. In health care, to gather information relevant to the patient's problem; to establish rapport and to provide confidence; to facilitate understanding of the patient's problem to assist in comprehensive patient management.

Cueing: Can be viewed as a direction; although a solution is provided, appropriate follow-through and proper understanding of the direction(s) must be demonstrated.

Dominance: Exercising control or influence; being assertive; putting one's idea forward.

Hostility: Defined as self-centered, unresponsive, and insensitive.

Interpersonal communication: Selective, systemic, individual, ongoing transactions that allow people to reflect and build personal knowledge and insight about one another and create shared meanings.

Interventions: Purposeful and skilled interactions with the patient and other individuals involved in the patient's care, using various physical therapy procedures and techniques to produce a change in the patient's condition.

Listening: An effective communication tool that demonstrates interest and concern for the patient and his or her individual needs.

Open-ended questions: A communication technique to facilitate rapport and let the patient see that the PTA is effectively listening that allows patients the opportunity to provide substantial information concerning their care.

Proactive: By using probing questions and appropriate communications skills, accountability, listening, and responsibility, the patient avoids being placed in a reactive position.

Probing questions: Technique of questioning patients that leads to insightful, rewarding, and responsive care.

Prompting: The presentation of a question; allows patients to decipher information, solve problems, and provide solutions to activities.

Responsibility: A component of active involvement of all areas of patient care.

Submission: Defined as following the lead of others, being passive and quick to comply.

Warmth: Defined as open-minded, responsive, and sensitive.

REFERENCES

1. American Physical Therapy Association: *A normative model of physical therapist assistant education: version 2007*, Alexandria, VA, 2007, American Physical Therapy Association.
2. Buzzotta VR, Lefton RE: *Dimensional management training*, St Louis, 1989, Psychological Associates.
3. Kisner C, Colby LA: *Therapeutic exercise foundations and techniques*, ed 6, Philadelphia, 2012, FA Davis.
4. Lombardo P, Stolberg S: Interviewing and communication skills. In Ballweg R, Stolberg S, Sullivan EM, editors: *Physician assistant: a guide to clinical practice*, ed 4, Philadelphia, 2008, Saunders, pp 258–274.
5. Lupi-Williams FA: The PTA, role and function: an analysis in three parts. Part I. Education. *Clin Manage Phys Ther* 3(3):35–38, 1983.
6. Nordin M, Frankel V: *Basic biomechanics of the musculoskeletal system*, ed 4, Baltimore, 2012, Lippincott Williams & Wilkins.
7. Payne M: *Teamwork in multiprofessional care*, Chicago, 2000, Lyceum.
8. Sacks RA, et al: Complications of knee ligament surgery. In Daniel D, Akeson W, O'Connor J, editors: *Knee ligaments: structure, function, surgery and repair*, New York, 1990, Raven Press.
9. Servellen GV: *Communication skills for the health care professional: concepts, practice, and evidence*, ed 2, Sudbury, MA, 2009, Jones & Bartlett.

REVIEW QUESTIONS

Multiple Choice

1. Which of the following require a "yes" or "no" answer?
   a. Closed-ended questions
   b. Open-ended questions
   c. Probing questions
   d. None of the above
2. Which of the following is defined as self-centered, unresponsive, and insensitive?
   a. Dominance
   b. Hostility
   c. Submission
   d. Accountability
3. Applying the dimensional model to the use of open-ended and closed-ended probing questions, which quadrant represents the behavioral goal of the PTA during patient supervision?
   a. Quadrant 1
   b. Quadrant 2
   c. Quadrant 3
   d. Quadrant 4
4. Which type of questioning allows the patient the opportunity to provide substantial information concerning his or her care and is a technique to facilitate rapport between the patient and the PTA?
   a. Open-ended questions
   b. Closed-ended questions
   c. Probing questions
   d. Prompting questions
5. Which of the following is an example of "cueing"?
   a. "After you move the walker and right leg, move your left leg."
   b. "After you move forward in your chair, what do you do next?"
   c. "After you move your cane, what leg do you move next?"
   d. None of the above
6. A person who is willing to take a back seat, is ready to comply, is quick to give in, and is reluctant to try to exert influence is said to be:
   a. Dominant.
   b. Hostile.
   c. Submissive.
   d. Warm and caring.
7. All of the following are examples of "summary-type" statements except which one?
   a. "So your knee hurts only when you run?"
   b. "Your back doesn't hurt when you do your home exercise program?"

   c. "Tell me about your work environment."
   d. "Your neck only bothers you when you work at your desk?"
8. In general, use of language appropriate to the patient's comprehension conveys:
   a. Understanding.
   b. Sensitivity.
   c. Warmth.
   d. All the above.
9. Components of patient supervision by the PTA includes all of the following except:
   a. Gathering of relevant information and data about the patient.
   b. Assisting in the management of the patient.
   c. Determining the plan of care for the patient.
   d. Establishing rapport with the patient.
10. The PTA is responsible for carrying out all of the following except:
    a. Appropriate problem solving.
    b. Patient supervision.
    c. Data collection.
    d. Prescribing and selecting interventions.
11. All of the following are key members of the rehabilitation team except:
    a. PT and PTA.
    b. OT and OTA.
    c. Nurse.
    d. Housekeeping staff member.
12. According to the "Problem-Solving Algorithm Utilized by PTAs in Patient/Client Intervention," PTAs are responsible for reporting all findings to:
    a. The patient's medical doctor.
    b. The patient's nurse.
    c. The supervising PT.
    d. The patient's discharge planner.
13. All of the following are true statements except which one?
    a. The PTA has ultimate responsibility for the physical therapy interventions provided.
    b. To minimize confusion, the PTA must effectively and efficiently communicate with the supervising PT to clarify differences in patient care.
    c. A well-adapted PTA views any apparent roadblocks as learning opportunities.
    d. Having strong opinions on how to care for various diagnoses is appropriate and shows passion, interest, and confidence in a certain method or protocol that has demonstrated good results.
14. Clinical decision making involves which of the following?
    a. Observation and information processing
    b. Application of relevant knowledge and problem solving
    c. Critical thinking and evaluation of evidence
    d. All the above
15. In describing "prompting," which of the following is true?
    a. Can be viewed as a direction
    b. Allows patients to decipher information and solve problems
    c. Is the presentation of a question
    d. Both b and c

Short Answer

16. Give three examples of open-ended probing questions that may be appropriate during the course of patient observation and interactive supervision.
17. Give three examples of closed-ended probing questions that may be appropriate during the course of patient observation and interactive supervision.
18. Draw the dimensional model and label the various parts.
19. Give an example of prompting a patient to attempt a specific task.
20. Give an example of cueing a patient to attempt a specific task.

Fill in the Blank

21. The five components of patient supervision are ________, ________, ________, ________, and ________.
22. Effective ________ is the hallmark of a great team and should be maximized.
23. Appropriate medical language used with the patient and his or her family helps to convey ________, ________, ________, and ________.
24. The PTA also must be aware that ________ is an effective communication tool.
25. The ________ is a tool to size up behavior and can be applied to subordinates, peers, and superiors.

True/False

26. As the PTA identifies objective changes in the patient's status each day, the concept of appropriate, responsive, and accountable supervision should be altered to one of visual, nonresponsive, and noninteractive supervision.
27. The clinical decision-making process used by the PTA involves recognizing that a problem exists, then taking orderly and specific steps to notify the supervising PT and adjust the patient's treatment.
28. The objective data supplied to the supervising PT by the PTA should be limited to goniometric measurements, manual muscle testing, heart rate, blood pressure, and respirations.
29. According to the "Problem-Solving Algorithm Utilized by PTAs in Patient/Client Intervention," it is the role of the PTA to change and/or modify treatment plans and/or protocols.
30. The Basic Dimensional Model consists of four behaviors: dominance-hostility, submission-hostility, submission-caring, and dominance-caring.

Chapter 2

The Role of the Physical Therapist Assistant in Physical Assessment

Candy Bahner, Jamie Dehan

CHAPTER OUTLINE

LEARNING OBJECTIVES

1. Apply the language of the *Guide to Physical Therapist Practice* to physical assessment procedures.
2. Identify the common elements of examination, evaluation, and assessment.
3. Describe the role of the physical therapist assistant in the performance of physical assessment based on the physical therapy plan of care.
4. Discuss the role of the physical therapist assistant in data collection.
5. Explain methods of modifying the physical therapy plan of care or actions to be taken in response to physical assessment of the patient.
6. Identify critical elements to include with documentation of physical assessment.
7. Relate physical assessment to goals and outcomes of a physical therapy plan of care.

KEY TERMS

Assessment
Centralization
Evaluation
Examination
Peripheralization
Referred pain
Trigger points
Visceral pain

As any prospective or current student in the field of physical therapy is aware, changes in the profession are emerging rapidly. In an effort to bring physical therapy professionals to the "health care table" for discussion of legislative, regulatory, and reimbursement issues, the leaders of our profession are striving for standardization of terminology and recognition and application of evidence-based practice.[2] Needless to say, controversy or at least animated debate occurs among interested parties any time such an in-depth self-scrutiny of a profession takes place. One significant element of this debate in physical therapy revolves around the role of the physical therapist assistant (PTA) in the profession, including how the PTA participates in the administration of the physical therapy plan of care, including selected interventions, data collection techniques, and the terminology associated with the PTA's role. The purpose of this chapter is to summarize available standards and guidelines associated with the PTA's role in physical therapy treatments and to discuss techniques and implications of selected interventions and their associated data collection techniques to be used for patients with musculoskeletal conditions.

AMERICAN PHYSICAL THERAPY ASSOCIATION GUIDING DOCUMENTS

GUIDE TO PHYSICAL THERAPIST PRACTICE, SECOND EDITION

The *Guide to Physical Therapist Practice,* second edition (the *Guide*) is a tool that was developed by the American Physical Therapy Association (APTA) in part to "… describe physical therapist practice in general; … standardize terminology used in and related to physical therapist practice; … delineate preferred practice patterns that will help physical therapists … promote appropriate utilization of health care services; [and] increase efficiency and reduce unwarranted variation in the provision of services. …"[2] The stated purpose of the *Guide* reads, in part, that it is "… a resource not only for physical therapist clinicians, educators, researchers, and students, but [for] health care policy makers, administrators, managed care providers, third-party payers, and other professionals."[2] According to the *Guide,* the definition of the PTA is: "A technically educated health care provider who assists the physical therapist in the provision of selected physical therapy interventions."[2] **Assessment** is defined as: "The measurement or quantification of a variable or the placement of a value on something."[2] The *Guide* further states: "Assessment should not be confused with examination or evaluation."[2] **Examination** involves preliminary gathering of data and performing various screens, tests, and measures to obtain a comprehensive base from which to make decisions about physical therapy needs for each individual patient, including the possibility of referral to another health care provider. **Evaluation** is the specific process reserved solely for the physical therapist (PT), in which clinical judgments are made from this base of data obtained during the examination.[2]

STANDARDS OF ETHICAL CONDUCT FOR THE PHYSICAL THERAPIST ASSISTANT

The Standards of Ethical Conduct for the Physical Therapist Assistant is a tool developed by the APTA to delineate the ethical obligations of all PTAs.[7] There are eight standards of ethical conduct for the PTA, and they can be found in the "Practice & Patient Care" section under "Ethics & Professionalism" on the APTA website (www.apta.org).

PROFESSIONALISM IN PHYSICAL THERAPY: CORE VALUES

The APTA has also developed a list of values, known as *core values,* which reflect what one would call a professional in physical therapy. The core values include accountability, altruism, compassion/caring, excellence, integrity, professional duty, and social responsibility.[5] Each core value, along with its corresponding definition as provided by the APTA, can be found in the "Practice" section on the APTA website.

THE PHYSICAL THERAPIST ASSISTANT CLINICAL PERFORMANCE INSTRUMENT

The Physical Therapist Assistant Clinical Performance Instrument, a uniform clinical education grading tool developed by the APTA,[4] includes the following essential skills related to the PTA's role in clinical problem solving (criterion #7):

- "Presents sound rationale for clinical problem solving, including review of data collected and ethical and legal arguments."
- "Seeks clarification of plan of care and selected interventions from clinical instructor and/or supervising physical therapist."
- "Collects and compares data from multiple sources (e.g., chart review, patient caregivers, team members, observation) to determine patient's readiness before initiating interventions."
- "Demonstrates sound clinical decisions within the plan of care to assess and maximize patient safety and comfort while performing selected interventions."
- "Demonstrates sound clinical decisions within the plan of care to assess and maximize intervention outcomes, including patient progress and/or intervention modifications."
- "Demonstrates the ability to determine when the clinical instructor and/or supervising physical therapist needs to be notified of changes in patient status, changes or lack of change in intervention outcomes, and completion of intervention expectations (i.e., goals have been met)."
- "Demonstrates the ability to perform appropriately during an emergency situation to include notification of appropriate staff."

A NORMATIVE MODEL OF PHYSICAL THERAPIST ASSISTANT EDUCATION: VERSION 2007

A Normative Model of Physical Therapist Assistant Education: Version 2007[3] (the *Model*) is a consensus-based document developed by the APTA. Briefly, the *Model* was designed to provide a representation of all of the elements that provide the foundation for the development and evaluation of educational programs preparing PTAs.[3] According to the *Model,* PTAs "… implement selected components of patient/client interventions and obtain data related to that intervention; make modifications in selected interventions either to progress the patient/client as directed by the physical therapist or to ensure patient/client safety and comfort."[3]

The *Model* includes the following five physical therapy performance expectation themes:

1. Interventions
2. Communication
3. Education
4. Resource Management
5. Career Development[3]

The Interventions physical therapy performance expectation theme is subdivided into the following seven sections:

- Plan of Care Review
- Provision of Procedural Interventions
- Patient/Client Instruction
- Patient/Client Progression
- Data Collection
- Documentation
- Emergency Response[3]

Each performance expectation theme includes educational outcomes, terminal behavioral objectives, and instructional objectives to be achieved in the classroom and clinic.

Important Concepts

Only a physical therapist may perform any of the following:

- Interpretation of a referral
- Performance and documentation of an initial examination, testing, evaluation, diagnosis, and prognosis
- Development or modification of a plan of care that is based on a re-examination of the patient or client that includes the physical therapy goals for intervention
- Timely review of documentation, re-examination of the patient or client, and revision of the plan of care when indicated
- Establishment and documentation of the discharge plan and discharge summary
- Spinal and peripheral joint mobilization techniques[3]

Frequently, the response to the question about the difference between PTs and PTAs is simply, "PTAs don't do evaluations." Considering the elements of judgment and decision making involved with evaluation and from the preceding discussion, does this imply that the PTA does not exercise judgment or make decisions? Of course not. However, the judgments and subsequent decisions of the PTA are made within the context of the existing physical therapy plan of care, established by the supervising PT through the examination and evaluation process. This process occurs on an ongoing basis.[23] Without effective data collection and reporting by the PTA, the PT would lack key information on which this data management process relies.[23]

It may be helpful to consider the functions of data collection and patient management as integral parts of managing a patient's physical therapy case, which is a dynamic process as illustrated in the APTA's "Problem-Solving Algorithm Utilized by PTAs in Patient/Client Intervention" (see Fig. 1-1).[3]

This discussion of specific assessment techniques and issues begins with two conditions frequently encountered among patients with musculoskeletal involvement: inflammation and pain.

INFLAMMATION

WHAT IS INFLAMMATION?

Inflammation is the first response of a living organism to injury or disruption of normal processes. It is a normal response and can be considered the body's immediate trigger for healing. Inflammation involves the responses of several body constituents, including vascular components, fluid and semifluid (humoral) substances, and neurologic and cellular reactions. Inflammation that does not resolve within expected time frames may develop into a chronic state (as a result of either abnormality in the individual's immune or inflammatory response or prolonged, continuous, or repeated exposure to the injurious agent). Chronic inflammation (considered a pathologic condition) may result in secondary complications or permanent changes in the makeup of the involved tissue, including scarring or granulomatosis. Two important factors must be kept in mind: (1) inflammation is a normal and necessary response to trigger tissue healing, and (2) unresolved (chronic) inflammation may lead to permanent and undesired tissue changes. It is imperative for the PTA to monitor changes in the inflammatory response of the area being treated. In addition, extreme changes in the appearance of inflammation may signal the onset of serious complications, necessitating further evaluation by the PT or, in some cases, referral to the physician for immediate medical evaluation.

Physical agents are employed to control (but not eliminate) the acute inflammatory response or accelerate it, moving the healing process along. Depending on the degree of inflammation present, certain physical agents may be contraindicated. How does the PTA differentiate between normal inflammation and an inflammatory reaction indicating the potential for contraindicated procedures or serious complications?

The commonly accepted and normal (cardinal) signs and symptoms of inflammation are localized heat, redness, swelling, and pain with a resultant loss of function in the injured area. Temperature and redness are discussed here in relation to the PTA's role in collecting data and communicating concerns appropriately to the PT. The assessments of edema and pain are discussed in separate sections.

Important Concepts

Cardinal Signs and Symptoms of Inflammation

- Localized heat
- Redness
- Swelling
- Pain

GENERAL CONTRAINDICATIONS AND PRECAUTIONS CONCERNING INFLAMMATION

In general, remember that inflammation is a reaction to tissue trauma or injury; the increased inflammatory reactions after exercise or other interventions may indicate that the intervention is too aggressive or contraindicated, resulting in new trauma or injury to healing tissues. Responses to interventions between visits must also be assessed; if a patient experiences joint pain or muscle soreness lasting longer than 24 hours after application of exercise or stretching techniques, the techniques were too intense.[19]

ACUTE VERSUS CHRONIC

Under normal circumstances, signs of acute inflammation persist for 4 to 6 days, assuming the precipitating condition, agent, or event is removed. In the initial 48 hours after tissue injury, the observable signs of inflammation are associated with the normal inflammatory vascular response to trauma.[19] An important distinction to make is the definition of acute versus chronic in relation to the actual cause of injury or trauma. It is common for sources to refer to these tissue states in terms of time frames only, with the acute phase lasting 4 to 6 days and the chronic phase lasting 6 months to 1 year.[19] A more useful way to consider inflammation incorporates the concept of whether there is real or impending tissue damage present. The significance of this designation relates to the PTA's role in determining whether, based on the stage of inflammation present, certain interventions may be implemented or are contraindicated.[29] If an intervention normally results in an inflammatory reaction, it is contraindicated when the tissue is in an acute inflammatory state that indicates ongoing tissue damage. For example, in the presence of acute inflammation (indicating an active state of injury, tissue damage, or early tissue healing), dynamic resistance exercises are contraindicated.[19] However, the PTA also may proceed with interventions included in the plan of care that accelerate the inflammatory process if it has been determined that the original causal agent or condition no longer results in ongoing tissue damage. Contraindications related to specific diagnoses are discussed elsewhere in this book.

During interventions involving range of motion (ROM) activities, the PTA also may note that the patient reports pain before tissue resistance is felt (before end ROM); this is an indication of acute inflammation.[19] Pain reported at the same time end ROM is reached is indicative of a subacute inflammatory state, and pain reported as a stretching sensation at the limit of ROM is a sign of inflammation in the chronic state.[19] If the PTA determines that the established plan of care includes interventions that are not appropriate for the apparent stage of inflammation, the PT must be consulted to adjust goals, time frames, or possibly the plan itself to ensure that the treatment does not contribute to a prolonged or abnormal state of inflammation.

TEMPERATURE

The PTA must be able to differentiate between expected temperature responses in a normal inflammatory response and abnormal responses. A normal increase in temperature is local and initially mild to moderate (compared with the contralateral anatomic region) versus a more pervasive change, which may manifest as significant compared with the contralateral side or as a systemic increase in temperature (fever). In the former case, joint effusion may be present; the latter may represent a systemic response to the injury (e.g., infection) or an unrelated condition, such as an acute disease process (e.g., flu). Either of these situations warrants action on the part of the PTA. In the presence of systemic infection, the patient's ability to participate in the physical therapy plan is affected. Because of the exclusive one-on-one time traditionally associated with physical therapy care, it is common for the PTA to be the member of the health care team who provides important pieces to the puzzle of the patient's total health or illness picture.

Both the degree of temperature elevation and the duration of fever are relevant to diagnostic processes when elevated body temperature is evident. During the initial examination and evaluation, any abnormality in temperature, either locally or systemically, should be noted. The PTA's role is to note deviations from the examination findings; determine the length of time the fever has been present (through patient interview); and note other possible related signs and symptoms, such as rash, cough, and complaints of sore throat. Also, it should be noted if the patient reports any pattern of temperature changes because this may have diagnostic implications for the PT or physician. Immediate implications include whether or not exercise or other interventions may be contraindicated and to what extent infection control issues must be addressed. Normal adult body temperature (oral measurement) ranges from 96.8° F to 99.5° F (36° C to 37.5° C).[14] Temperature is affected by factors including age, time of day, emotions and stress, exercise, menstrual cycle, pregnancy, external environment, measurement site, and ingestion of warm or cold foods.[27] Clinical signs and symptoms of fever vary based on the underlying cause and stage and may include general malaise, headache, increased pulse and respiratory rates, general chills, shivering, piloerection, loss of appetite, pale skin, nausea, irritability, restlessness, constipation, sweating, thirst, coated tongue, decreased urinary output, insomnia, and weakness.[27] In the case of the presence of fever, the PTA must gather the related data, document it, and report it to the supervising PT. The data and report should include adequate information to enable the PT to respond appropriately, with either immediate modification to the physical therapy plan of care or consultation with the medical team.

FEVER AND INFECTION CONTROL

As always, the PTA must attend to his or her responsibility of exercising appropriate precautions for both the patient and himself or herself. The importance of hand washing by the caregiver and patient cannot be overstated as an effective means of controlling the transmission of infectious agents. In addition, treatment areas should be properly cleaned and disinfected as a routine procedure, not only in the case of patients with obvious infectious conditions. (Detailed information and guidelines for hand washing in the health care setting can be found on the website of the U.S. Centers for Disease Control and Prevention).

FEVER AND EXERCISE

In terms of exercise precautions, discretionary caution should be applied with any patient with a fever because of stresses on the cardiopulmonary and immune systems and the possible further complications related to dehydration.[14] The PTA must be familiar with specific exercise techniques (e.g., aquatic exercise) contraindicated in the presence of diseases transmitted via water or air.

FEVER AND LYMPH NODES

Another condition that may become readily apparent to the PTA in the course of carrying out elements of the physical therapy plan of care is tenderness or exquisite pain in particular regions of the body. The presence of tender or enlarged lymph nodes is of particular concern to the PTA who is performing soft tissue interventions on a patient with an elevated body temperature (or otherwise). Figure 2-1 provides a visual reference for the location of lymph nodes. PTAs using hands-on techniques such as soft tissue massage and manual stretching are incidentally afforded the opportunity during the course of treatment to assess for the presence of unusual conditions in areas of lymph node clusters (e.g., in the neck and axilla). Because symptoms of pain, tenderness, or enlargement of lymph nodes can signify the presence of potentially serious pathologic conditions, the presence of these symptoms represents a situation in which the PTA must consult with the supervising PT to pursue medical follow-up for definitive diagnosis.[14] In addition, certain interventions are considered contraindicated if the patient has an underlying pathology related to changes in the lymph nodes.

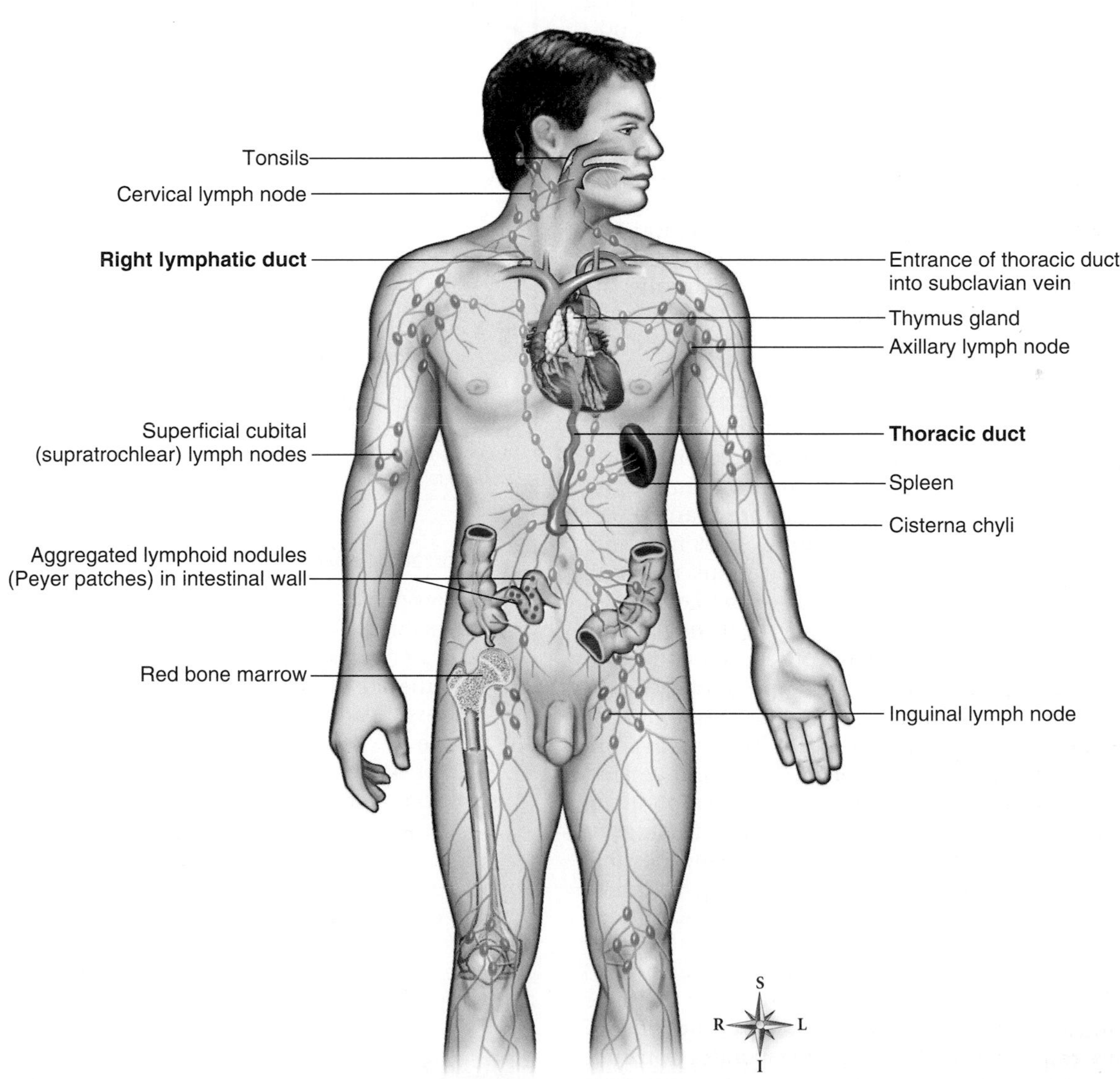

FIG 2-1 Location of lymph vessels and nodes. Note clusters of nodes in axillae and groin areas. *(From Patton KT, Thibodeau GA.* Anatomy and physiology, *ed 7, St Louis, 2010, Mosby.)*

REDNESS AND SKIN COLOR CHANGES

Redness (erythema) is a normal component of the inflammatory reaction. The PTA must be alert to abnormal or unexpected changes in skin color, which may indicate the presence of secondary complications or underlying pathologies. Redness may be considered normal when it is noted in the immediate area of injury and is associated with local temperature changes. Depending on the patient's pigmentation, color changes may appear in tones other than red.

Unexpected findings in terms of changes in skin color should be reported to the supervising PT for further evaluation. These changes include rashes or redness that appear as a streak originating from the site of injury. Red streaks may indicate an acute inflammation secondary to a bacterial infection (streptococci, staphylococci, or both), resulting in acute inflammation of the lymph vessels.[14] Redness along with superficial tenderness and hardness (induration) of the area may be a sign of superficial thrombophlebitis.[14] These findings should be reported to the supervising PT because they may be a precursor to more serious conditions. A loss of skin color (paleness or pallor) associated with temperature changes, edema, or pain may be indicative of an occlusion in a blood vessel and warrants immediate medical referral. Homans' sign is a commonly used quick assessment technique to rule out the presence of a deep vein thrombosis (DVT) that is performed by gentle passive stretching of the ankle into full dorsiflexion and assessing for pain in the calf. Some clinicians also incorporate a gentle squeezing of calf musculature during the passive dorsiflexion to assess for tenderness. Other structures that are stretched during this test include the calf muscles and the Achilles tendon; a positive Homans' sign may be noted in error if a patient has tightness or inflammation of these structures. Although Homans' sign is still commonly assessed, it is considered an insensitive and nonspecific test; it is present in less than one third of all patients with a documented DVT, and more than 50% of patients with a positive Homans' sign do not have evidence of venous thrombosis.[14] Also, a serious potential complication of a DVT is that a piece of the coagulated blood (the clot) may break free from the inside of the vessel wall as a result of the test (or otherwise) and travel through the bloodstream, lodging in a pulmonary artery and causing a life-threatening condition (pulmonary embolism). It is recommended that the PTA refrain from performing the assessment for Homans' sign and be alert to the risk factors and the clinical signs and symptoms of a DVT as outlined in Box 2-1 and report these findings to the supervising PT for further investigation and possible immediate medical referral.

The PTA should be aware of differences in superficial skin changes based on the patient's skin color. In other words, these findings in individuals with darkly pigmented skin may be less obvious and do not manifest as the same changes in skin tones as in light-skinned individuals. A critical element to be included in the laboratory practice and skill development of the PTA student is exposure to numerous normal subjects of different body types and skin tones (often represented within a classroom population of adult learners). By observing and practicing on different subjects, the PTA student develops an awareness of normal variations, which will subsequently enhance his or her ability to recognize differences or abnormalities in patients.

BOX 2-1 Risk Factors and Clinical Signs and Symptoms for Deep Venous Thrombosis

Risk Factors

- Previous personal/family history of thromboembolism
- Congestive heart failure
- Age older than 50 years
- Oral contraceptive use

Blood Stasis

- Immobilization or inactivity
  - Burns
  - Obstetric/gynecologic conditions
  - Obesity
  - Spinal cord injury, stroke

Endothelial Injury

- Neoplasm
- Recent surgical procedures
- Trauma or fracture of the legs or pelvis
- Blood disorders (e.g., hypercoagulable state, clotting abnormalities)
- History of infection, diabetes mellitus
- Oral contraceptive use

Clinical Signs and Symptoms

Superficial Venous Thrombosis

- Subcutaneous venous distention
- Palpable cord
- Warmth, redness
- Indurated (hard)

Deep Venous Thrombosis

- Unilateral tenderness or leg pain
- Unilateral swelling (difference in leg circumference)
- Warmth
- Discoloration
- Pain with placement of blood pressure cuff around calf inflated to 160 to 180 mm Hg

From Goodman CC, Snyder TE. *Differential diagnosis for physical therapists screening for referral,* ed 4, St Louis, 2007, Saunders, p 312.

Important Concepts

The following changes in skin color should be reported to the supervising PT:

- Rashes or redness that appear as a streak originating from the site of injury
- Redness along with superficial tenderness and hardness
- Loss of skin color (paleness or pallor) associated with temperature changes, edema, or pain

EDEMA

Because edema and its management have significant implications in the practice of physical therapy, the

TABLE 2-1 Sample Format for Documenting Edema

UE	Right	Left
Axilla	_______ inches	_______ inches
4 inches above elbow	_______ inches	_______ inches
2 inches above elbow	_______ inches	_______ inches
Elbow*	_______ inches	_______ inches
2 inches below elbow	_______ inches	_______ inches
4 inches below elbow	_______ inches	_______ inches
Wrist*	_______ inches	_______ inches

*A standard for elbow could be from the cubital fossa around the elbow, crossing the olecranon process; a standard for wrist could be just distal to the radial and ulnar styloid processes.
UE, upper extremity.

entry-level PTA should develop the ability to recognize the signs and symptoms of edema and to measure and document it effectively and efficiently. For purposes of this text, the focus is on localized edema, resulting from injury or trauma to musculoskeletal tissue or structures. Other terms and conditions are defined and discussed in relation to the PTA's responsibility in the event unrelated or unexpected conditions are discovered.

Edema refers to excessive pooling of fluid in the spaces between tissues (interstitial spaces).[14] In relation to patients with orthopedic injuries or conditions, the main consideration for assessment by the PTA is measurement of the edematous part or extremity. Typically, the technique used to measure edema in an extremity is straightforward—use of a tape measure to obtain circumferential dimensions of the involved part. The data must be reliable, and the measurement must be reproducible, regardless of who is conducting the assessment. To ensure this level of consistency, the PTA must use precisely the same landmarks as the evaluating PT. Specifically, palpable bony landmarks must be used as the starting standard reference point; then circumferential measurements can be taken at determined distances from that point. For example, to measure the lower leg, circumference measured with the tape measure at the inferior pole of the patella may be used as a reference point, with measurements taken every 2 inches distally and at the ankle. One note of caution: the PTA must be careful to not pull the tape measure too tight when performing this skill. The skin should not have an indention if the skill is performed correctly. An example of a flow chart for recording circumferential measurements of the upper extremity is provided in Table 2-1.

A figure-of-eight technique may be used at the ankle to ascertain a gross estimate of generalized ankle edema.[11,22,32] Refer to Box 2-2 for the steps involved in this procedure.

Another technique used to obtain a quantitative measure of edema in a limb involves immersing the limb into a specially designed container of fluid (a volumeter) and measuring the amount of water displaced.[20] Karges and colleagues[17] established correlations between different techniques of volumetric measurement but also emphasized the importance of ensuring reliability of the data for a given patient, in terms of employing a consistent technique for edema measurement of the same patient. In other words, as stated, the PTA must use the same method of measurement, employing the same technique chosen by the evaluating PT.[17,20]

BOX 2-2 Technique for Figure-of-Eight Edema Measurement of Ankle

1. Position the patient in a long sitting position so that the lower leg is supported and the ankle is in a neutral position.
2. Mark the following landmarks with a skin pencil: tuberosity of the navicular (palpable projection on the anteromedial aspect of the hindfoot), base of the fifth metatarsal, distal tip of the medial malleolus, distal tip of the lateral malleolus, and tibialis anterior tendon.
3. Place the (0) edge of the tape measure midway between the tibialis anterior tendon and the lateral malleolus.
4. Wrap the tape medially across the instep (bottom surface of the foot), and place just distal to the navicular tuberosity.
5. Draw the tape across the arch of the foot, winding it back to the dorsum of the foot just proximal to the tuberosity (base) of the fifth metatarsal.
6. Cross back over the tibialis anterior tendon.
7. Wrap the tape measure around the ankle, drawing it just distal to the tip of the medial malleolus, crossing the calcaneal (Achilles) tendon and drawing the tape measure just distal to the lateral malleolus, back to the starting point.
8. For consistency, it is recommended that this process be repeated three times, with the average of the three measurements recorded.

Adapted from Magee DJ. *Orthopedic physical assessment,* ed 5, St Louis, 2008, Saunders; Tatro-Adams D, McGann S, Carbone W. Reliability of the figure-of-eight method of ankle measurement, *J Orthop Sports Phys Ther* 1995; 22(4):161-163; and Esterson PS. Measurement of ankle joint swelling using a figure of 8, *J Orthop Sports Phys Ther* 1979; 1(1):51-52.

In addition to a quantitative measurement of edema through circumferential measurement or volumetrics, data relating to the quality of edema should be collected and documented by the PTA. Characteristics of edema that may be observed are described as *brawny* or *pitting*. Brawny edema refers to edema that feels hard, tough, or thick and leathery. This indurated quality is frequently associated with chronic inflammation or systemic pathologies involving fluid shift abnormalities (e.g., congestive heart failure [CHF]). Pitting edema is characterized by the formation of a sustained indentation when the swollen area is compressed.[9,16] Pitting edema may be further quantified according to the scale in Figure 2-2.

In contrast to transient inflammatory reactions that may normally occur in response to certain physical therapy interventions, a significant increase in edema should be regarded as abnormal and reported accordingly. On first noticing edema in the extremity being treated, the PTA must determine if the swelling is confined to the involved extremity or if the contralateral extremity is also involved. If the opposite extremity is also edematous, this finding could indicate a systemic pathologic condition.[14] For example, bilateral pitting edema of the distal lower extremities is a common manifestation in CHF, which is a relatively common diagnosis encountered among individuals with cardiac disease and individuals older than 65 years of age. Because CHF is common and it develops gradually, the PTA may play an important role in the

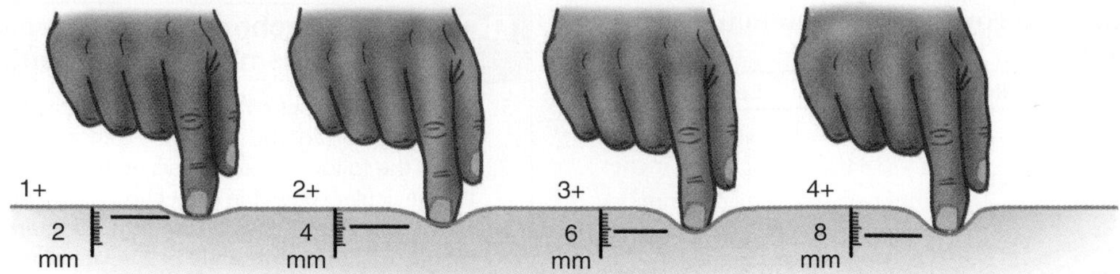

FIG 2-2 Pitting edema scale. 1+: Mild edema; 2-mm depression that disappears rapidly. 2+: Moderate pitting edema; 4-mm depression that disappears in 10 to 15 seconds. 3+: Moderately severe pitting edema; 6-mm depression that may last more than 1 minute. 4+: Severe pitting edema; 8-mm depression that can last more than 2 minutes. *(From Potter P, Perry A.* Fundamentals of nursing, *ed 7, St Louis, 2009, Mosby.)*

diagnostic process via astute recognition of signs and symptoms associated with the onset of this pathology. In addition to bilateral lower extremity pitting edema, the PTA may note a decrease in tolerance to exercise (fatigue, shortness of breath, and dizziness).[14] The presence of this clinical response necessitates prompt consultation with the supervising PT for medical diagnostic work-up and possible subsequent modifications to the physical therapy plan of care.

Important Concepts

"Red Flag" Symptoms of Congestive Heart Failure

Weight gain of 3 pounds or greater or gradual, continuous gain over several days that results in swelling of the ankles, abdomen, and hands combined with shortness of breath, fatigue, and dizziness.[14]

Compartment syndrome is a potentially serious condition involving edema. This condition occurs in anatomic compartments (of the calf or, less frequently, the antebrachium) as a result of increased fluids in an area tightly bound by fascia. Because fascia does not "give" to allow more space to accommodate this fluid buildup, this edema can compress nerves and blood vessels as they course through the compartment, leading to ischemia and possible nerve damage. Because the edema is contained within the compartment, the PTA should be alert to other associated signs and symptoms, such as history of blunt trauma, crush injury, or unaccustomed exercise; severe, persistent leg pain that is intensified when a stretch is applied to the involved muscles; swelling, severe tenderness, and palpable tension of the involved structures; and paresthesia, paresis, and pulselessness.[8] Immediate consultation with the supervising PT and possibly immediate medical referral are warranted if the signs and symptoms are noted.

PAIN

An important skill that novice clinicians must develop along the path to entry-level competence is to attend to the patient as a whole being, with the various elements being assessed working together to produce full function. It is crucial for the PTA to collect data about the patient's pain responses and behaviors throughout each patient interaction. A common behavior of a novice clinician performing basic assessment and data collection skills is to focus only on the involved body part and overlook the overall response of the patient to specific procedures. For example, a patient may exhibit strength of the quadriceps muscle group that measures 4+/5. However, if the student PTA performing the assessment of strength fails to observe that the patient is grimacing in pain during the resisted isometric test, he or she is overlooking an important determinant of true function of the muscle group. Likewise, other components of function, such as ROM and flexibility, must include pain-free performance to be wholly functional. Ideally, the PTA student will make the transition from focusing only on the involved body part during assessment procedures and interventions to performing assessments that include comprehensive observation of the patient's responses and behaviors.

Pain is considered subjective, but because there are multiple internal factors that determine a patient's perception of pain, complaints of pain always should be addressed as legitimate or "real." The PTA's role in assessing pain is to gather data that present a clear picture of the following:

- Changes in pain since last physical therapy visit or examination
- Responses of the patient in terms of how interventions to date or at present affect pain
- Patterns of pain (e.g., physical or temporal)
- Modalities, types, or characteristics of pain (e.g., sharp or burning)

Several standardized instruments are available to record findings of pain assessment. As with all assessment and data collection techniques, the PTA must use the same instrument or same technique for recording data related to a patient's pain complaints as was used by the supervising PT during the initial examination. Simple and commonly used tools are pain rating scales and visual analog scales as shown in Figures 2-3, 2-4, and 2-5.

During the course of carrying out elements of the supervising PT's plan of care, the PTA may notice a change in the quality of a patient's pain from more acute to chronic pain. As described in the section on inflammation, a chronic state is one in which the symptoms (pain in this case) persist for a period of time longer than expected, based on physiologic principles of tissue healing.

McGill-Melzack
Pain Questionnaire

Patient's name____________________ Age____________________
File No.___________________________ Date____________________
Clinical category (e.g., cardiac, neurologic)
Diagnosis: _______________
____
____

Analgesic (if already administered):
1. Type____
2. Dosage______________________________________
3. Time given in relation to this test_______________

Patient's intelligence: circle number that represents best estimate.

1 (low) 2 3 4 5 (high)

This questionnaire has been designed to tell us more about your pain. Four major questions we ask are:

1. Where is your pain?
2. What does it feel like?
3. How does it change with time?
4. How strong is it?

It is important that you tell us how your pain feels now. Please follow the instructions at the beginning of each part.

Part 1. Where Is Your Pain?

Please mark on the drawing below the areas where you feel pain. Put E if external, or I if internal, near the areas you mark. Put EI if both external and internal.

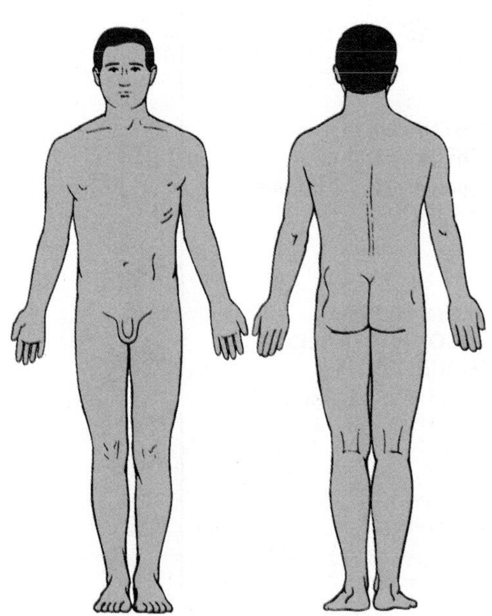

Part 2. What Does Your Pain Feel Like?

Some of the words below describe your present pain. Circle *ONLY* those words that best describe it. Leave out any category that is not suitable. Use only a single word in each appropriate category—the one that best applies.

1
Flickering
Quivering
Pulsing
Throbbing
Beating
Pounding

2
Jumping
Flashing
Shooting

3
Pricking
Boring
Drilling
Stabbing
Lancinating

4
Sharp
Cutting
Lacerating

5
Pinching
Pressing
Gnawing
Cramping
Crushing

6
Tugging
Pulling
Wrenching

7
Hot
Burning
Scalding
Searing

8
Tingling
Itchy
Smarting
Stinging

9
Dull
Sore
Hurting
Aching
Heavy

10
Tender
Taut
Rasping
Splitting

11
Tiring
Exhausting

12
Sickening
Suffocating

13
Fearful
Frightful
Terrifying

14
Punishing
Grueling
Cruel
Vicious
Killing

15
Wretched
Blinding

16
Annoying
Troublesome
Miserable
Intense
Unbearable

17
Spreading
Radiating
Penetrating
Piercing

18
Tight
Numb
Drawing
Squeezing
Tearing

19
Cool
Cold
Freezing

20
Nagging
Nauseating
Agonizing
Dreadful
Torturing

Part 3. How Does Your Pain Change with Time?

1. Which word or words would you use to describe the *pattern* of your pain?

1	2	3
Continuous	Rhythmic	Brief
Steady	Periodic	Momentary
Constant	Intermittent	Transient

2. What kind of things *relieve* your pain?
3. What kind of things *increase* your pain?

Part 4. How Strong Is Your Pain?

People agree that the following 5 words represent pain of increasing intensity. They are:

1	2	3	4	5
Mild	Discomforting	Distressing	Horrible	Excruciating

To answer each question below, write the number of the most appropriate word in the space beside the question.

1. Which word describes your pain right now? ______
2. Which word describes it at its worst? ______
3. Which word describes it when it is least? ______
4. Which word describes the worst toothache you ever had? ______
5. Which word describes the worst headache you ever had? ______
6. Which word describes the worst stomachache you ever had? ______

FIG 2-3 McGill-Melzack Pain Questionnaire. *(Redrawn from Melzack R. The McGill Pain Questionnaire: major properties and scoring methods,* Pain *1:277, 1975. In Clayton BD.* Basic pharmacology for nurses, *ed 15, St Louis, 2010, Mosby.)*

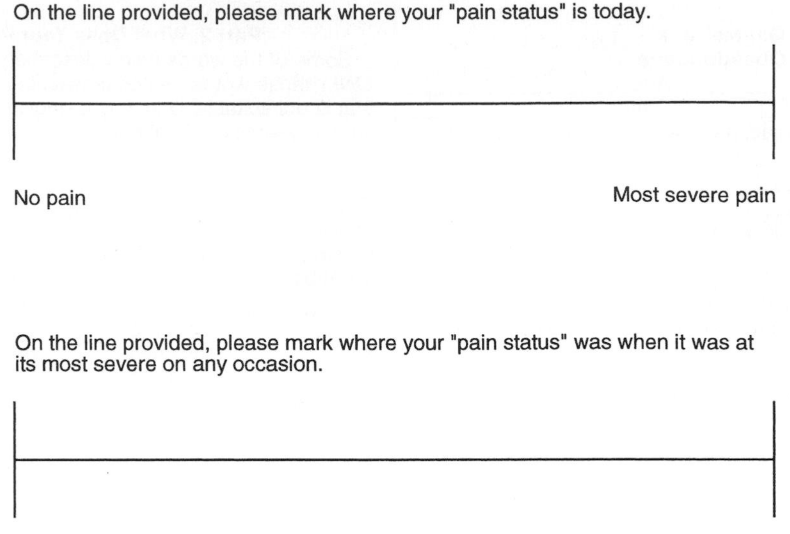

FIG 2-4 Visual analog scales for pain. *(From Magee DJ.* Orthopedic physical assessment, *ed 4, Philadelphia, 2002, Saunders.)*

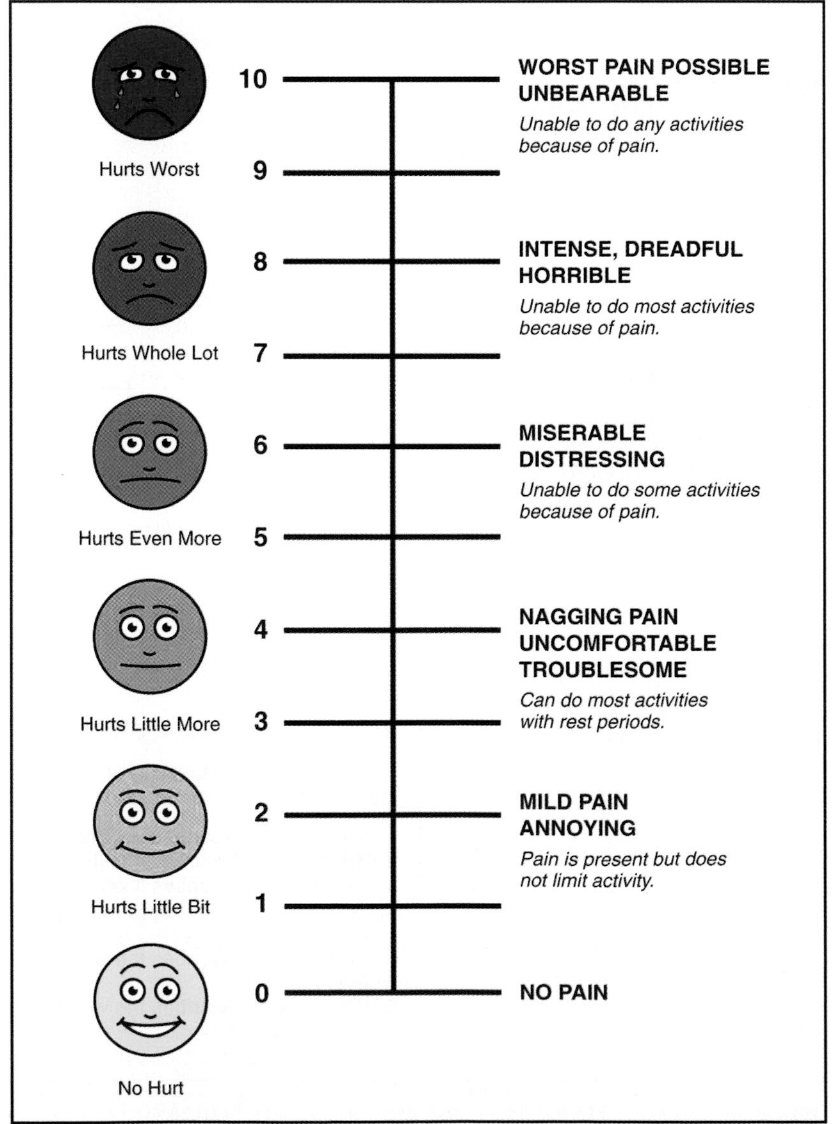

FIG 2-5 Wong-Baker FACES Pain Rating Scale. *(From Hockenberry MJ, Wilson D.* Wong's essentials of pediatric nursing, *ed 8, St Louis, 2009, Mosby.)*

Chronic pain has been described as pain that lasts more than 3 months.[24] Recall also that one descriptive feature of a chronic condition relates to the lack of real, ongoing, or pending tissue damage. In regard to pain, this circumstance also often coincides with complaints of pain that are nonspecific, diffuse, or indirectly proportional to the physical appearance or presentation of the patient.

In this case, the PTA's documentation or other interaction with the supervising PT may assist the therapist in making appropriate changes in the goals and plan of care to address the pain by incorporating interventions that will attend to the more complex issues involved with chronic pain. Specifically, depression and a cycle involving decreased activity levels and associated decreased tolerance to activity often ensue with chronic pain. The PTA may ask the supervising PT about the possible inclusion of relaxation exercises and a comprehensive gradual conditioning program in this case. When the PTA notices that a patient is exhibiting signs and symptoms of chronic pain, further diagnostic work-up may be indicated by the supervising PT because the presence of chronic pain may signal involvement of systems or factors other than musculoskeletal structures (e.g., depression).

Certain changes that occur in complaints of pain in response to therapeutic interventions are expected. **Peripheralization** may indicate a worsening or progressive condition. A typical example of this occurs with a progressively herniating spinal disk, indicating increasing compression of the associated nerve root. **Centralization** of pain symptoms may indicate improvement of the condition, such as in the case of decreasing compression on a nerve root as a disk herniation is reduced.

The PTA must establish the location of pain when the patient reports changes in pain symptoms associated with certain positions or movements. For example, a patient with a primary diagnosis of low-back pain secondary to herniated nucleus pulposus may complain of pain when lying prone. The PTA must not assume that the pain is in the area of the disk lesion, which is a positive indication of centralization and a desired response. If, on further questioning, it is determined that the pain is referred to the lower extremity along the neural distribution for the involved spinal segment, this is a sign of peripheralization of the symptoms, indicating that the prone position is not appropriate at this time. The importance of understanding neuromuscular anatomy and function cannot be overlooked. The PTA student must become familiar with these anatomic relationships to understand fully the implications of data collected during pain assessment.

"RED FLAG" PAIN SYMPTOMS

The PTA must also be keenly aware of pain that sends a "red flag" signal. In this case, the PTA should not proceed with any interventions or data collection techniques that are potentially contraindicated and should immediately report the findings to the supervising PT. Table 2-2 presents a summary of "red flag" or potentially serious pain conditions and the possible associated pathology or body system.

In addition to knowing the "red flag" symptoms described here, the PTA working with any client must be

TABLE 2-2 "Red Flag" Pain Symptoms

Pathology or Body System	Pain Complaint or Symptom
Cardiovascular	Pain or feeling of heaviness in the chest Pulsating pain anywhere in the body Constant and severe pain in lower leg (calf) or arm Discolored or painful feet
Cancer	Persistent pain at night Constant pain anywhere in the body
Gastrointestinal	Frequent or severe abdominal pain
Neurologic	Frequent or severe headaches with no history of injury

Adapted from Magee DJ. *Orthopedic physical assessment,* ed 6, St Louis, 2014, Saunders; and Stith JS, Sahrmann SA, Dixon KK, et al. Curriculum to prepare diagnosticians in physical therapy, *J Phys Ther Educ* 1995; 9:50.

alert to signs and symptoms of myocardial infarction (MI), or heart attack. Certain patterns of pain have been identified as early warning signs of a heart attack (Fig. 2-6). The PTA working with a patient exhibiting any of these patterns of pain should consult with the supervising PT right away for possible immediate medical referral. Concurrent symptoms of MI may include nausea, pallor, and profuse perspiration. MI may occur over a period of time and may be experienced while the patient is undergoing exertion or even at rest.

INTERMITTENT CLAUDICATION

Intermittent claudication is another distinct pattern or type of pain that may manifest coincidentally with musculoskeletal symptoms or conditions; the term *intermittent claudication* is used to describe activity-related discomfort associated with peripheral arterial disease (PAD). Intermittent claudication of vascular origin is typically described as a "burning," "cramping," or "sharp" pain that is localized in the region affected by the impaired circulation.[14] Because it involves a systemic condition, it typically manifests bilaterally and usually involves the calves, thighs, hips, buttocks, or feet, areas that are often symptomatic with musculoskeletal pathologies.[14] When the aggravating activity is discontinued, it is characteristic for the symptoms of claudication (burning, cramping, or sharp pain) to improve rapidly.

The assessment for intermittent claudication consists of determining what is referred to as *claudication time.* The basic protocols involve assessing maximal treadmill walking time, pain-free walking time, and walking time to severe claudication.[10] As with other standardized tests and measures, the data collection technique employed by the PTA must be the same technique used by the supervising PT.

The PTA may be the first clinician to recognize the symptoms associated with undiagnosed peripheral arterial occlusive vascular disease in terms of the nature, characteristics, and location of symptoms as described. Other signs and symptoms that are consistent with PAD include pallor, decrease in peripheral pulses, sensory changes, and weakness of the involved area (distal to the site of blocked circulation).[14] Diabetes mellitus and nonhealing wounds

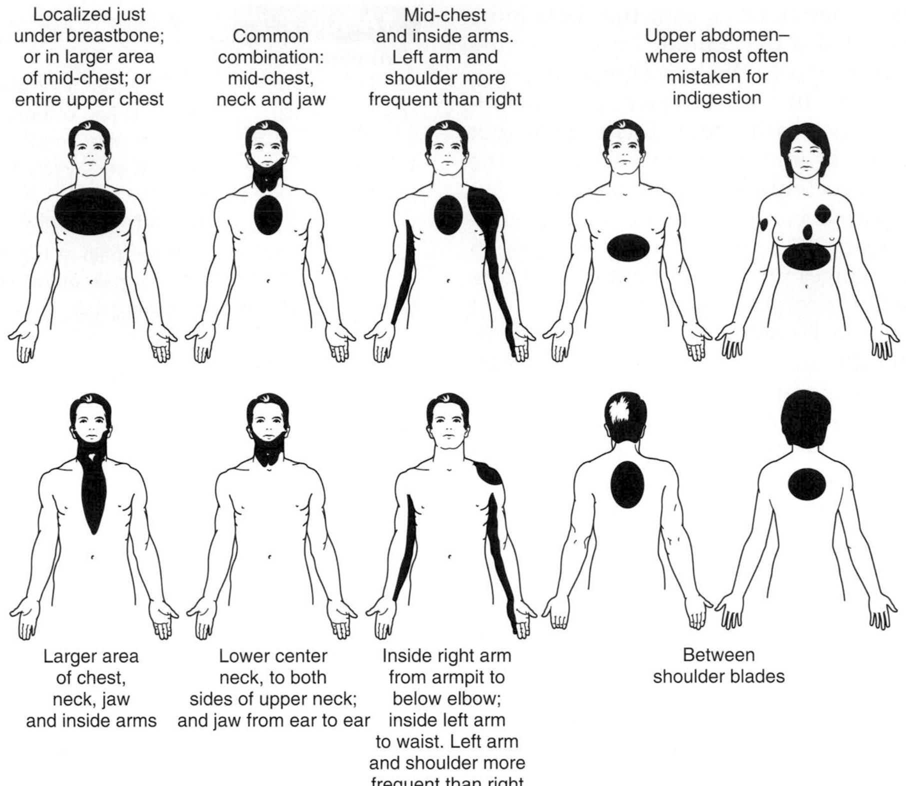

FIG 2-6 Early warning signs of a heart attack. *(From Goodman CC, Fuller K.* Pathology: implications for the physical therapist, *ed 3, St Louis, 2009, Saunders.)*

on the feet also are frequently associated with PAD.[14] Observation of the signs of undiagnosed PAD should be reported to the supervising PT immediately.

REFERRED PAIN

Referred pain is defined as pain that is "felt in an area far from the site of the lesion, but supplied by the same or adjacent neural segments."[14] Referred pain can originate from any cutaneous, somatic, or visceral source and is commonly associated with problems of the musculoskeletal system. It is usually well localized but with indistinct boundaries, tends to be felt deeply, and radiates segmentally without crossing the midline.[22] No objective sensory deficits (paresthesia, numbness, or weakness) are associated with referred pain.[14,22]

VISCERAL PAIN

The term **visceral pain** refers to pain that originates from a body organ. The primary concerns for the PTA related to this type of pain are for the PTA to be aware of how visceral pain may manifest and to report suspicious pain symptoms to the supervising PT. Often disease processes involving specific or multiple organs reveal themselves through various symptoms and not just pain. However, it is possible for a patient to have more than one pathologic condition at the same time. In other words, a patient with a confirmed diagnosis of herniated disk in the lumbar spine also could have some type of developing abdominal pathology. Pain of a visceral origin may manifest as musculoskeletal symptoms because of the innervation pattern of the involved organ. Visceral pain is not well localized secondary to viscera innervation being multisegmental. Additionally, isolation of visceral pain is difficult because of its correspondence to dermatomes from which the problem organ receives its innervation. Figure 2-7 provides a visual representation of innervation to major internal organs in terms of spinal levels of nerve supply. The organs are supplied via plexuses or ganglia, resulting in innervation from multiple segmental levels. For this reason, organ pain may be diffuse and difficult for the patient to localize, appearing as nonspecific musculoskeletal discomfort. Figure 2-8 illustrates common visceral pain referral sites to aid the PTA further in recognizing the challenges in differentiating between visceral and nonspecific musculoskeletal pain. In the case of disease processes that develop over time, the PTA must be alert to changes in the patient's complaints of pain and reports from the patient of patterns that are not consistent with musculoskeletal conditions.

TRIGGER POINTS

"**Trigger points** are small, localized tender areas found within skeletal muscles, fascia, tendons, ligaments, periosteum, and pericapsular areas."[31] Trigger points are associated with musculoskeletal conditions such as temporomandibular joint dysfunction, cervical strain, fibromyalgia, and myofascial pain syndrome. The pain produced by trigger points is characterized by tenderness

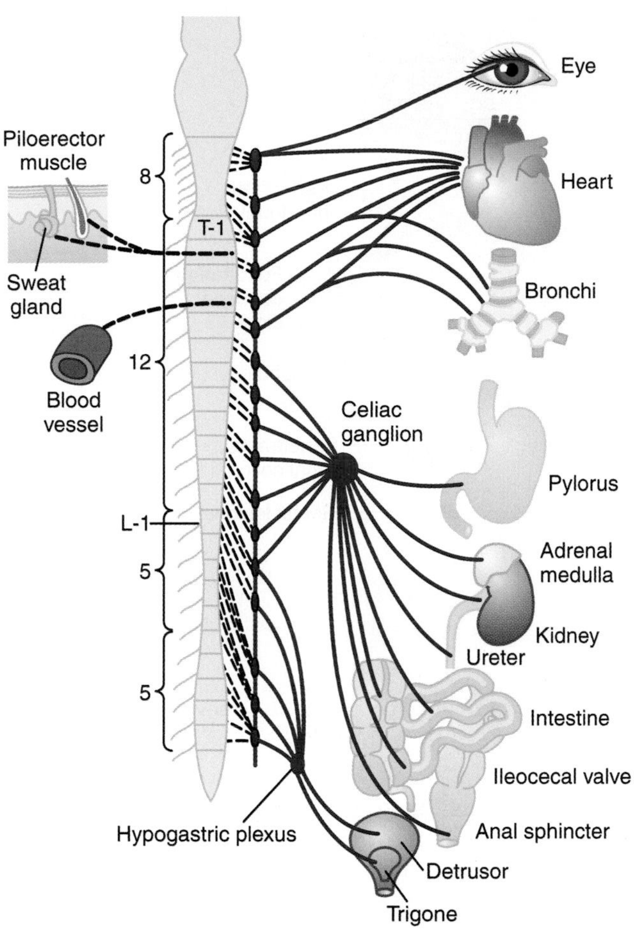

FIG 2-7 Diagram of the autonomic nervous system. The visceral afferent fibers mediating pain travel with the sympathetic nerves except for the fibers from the pelvic organs, which follow the parasympathetics of the pelvic nerve. *(From Guyton AC, Hall JE.* Textbook of medical physiology, *ed 9, Philadelphia, 1996, Saunders.)*

and a referred pattern of pain to palpation, usually in upper quarter or pelvic girdle muscles. According to an article in *American Family Physician,*[1] "Palpation of a hypersensitive bundle or nodule of muscle fiber of harder than normal consistency is the physical finding typically associated with a trigger point. Palpation of the trigger point will elicit pain directly over the affected area or cause radiation of pain toward a zone of reference and a local twitch response." During the process of applying hands-on soft tissue interventions or passive exercises, if the PTA notices signs and symptoms of possible trigger points that have not been previously documented, these findings should be documented and reported to the supervising PT.

PAIN: A FINAL NOTE

The PTA occasionally may encounter a patient whose complaints of pain do not match observed behaviors of the patient. In this case, it is not the role of the PTA to judge the patient and conclude that the patient is malingering or "faking" the condition. Instead the PTA should objectively document his or her observations and discuss them with the supervising PT.

VITAL SIGNS

An objective measure of physiologic status, particularly as related to cardiopulmonary function, can be obtained quickly through measurement and assessment of vital signs. Body temperature is discussed in the section on inflammation; heart rate, blood pressure, respiration, and pulse oximetry are discussed here. It may be observed that vital signs are not routinely assessed in the outpatient clinic that serves mainly patients with orthopedic diagnoses. However, as the profession of physical therapy strives toward achieving the status of a recognized point of entry for the health care consumer, we must shift our perception of routine procedures to include a more thorough and comprehensive assessment of the patient's overall health status and responses to our treatments.

The PTA student is encouraged to become proficient with effective assessment of vital signs through repeated practice on a variety of subjects and on subjects in different positions (supine, sitting, and standing) and performing different activities (e.g., activities of daily living and exercise).

Important Concepts

The PTA should employ the same technique the PT uses during the initial evaluation for assessment procedures to enhance consistency and determine better any deviation from the baseline measure.

It is not within the scope of this text to discuss or review detailed physiology related to cardiopulmonary function or pathology. General guidelines for collecting vital sign data and determining when modification to planned interventions is warranted are discussed.

PULSE (HEART RATE)

Heart rate should be measured at the time of evaluation to establish a baseline rate and subsequently when beginning any exercise program or new activity. There are eight possible sites (Fig. 2-9) from which heart rate can be measured, but the most common and easily accessible sites are the radial and carotid arteries.[12] Accepted values for normal heart rate in adults range from 60 to 100 beats per minute (bpm).[14,25,27] Factors that influence heart rate include age, gender, emotional state, medications, exercise or conditioning level, and systemic or local heat.[27]

In addition to the quantitative measure, the quality of the pulse should be noted. Often in a setting where the PTA is working primarily with healthy clients (e.g., trained or conditioned athletes), it may be sufficient to perform a 10-second beat count and multiply by 6 to determine quickly the cardiovascular response to an activity. However, it is important to consider that the margin of error is plus or minus each multiplied value, meaning that if the pulse is counted for 10 seconds and multiplied by 6, the margin of error for the data collected is ± 6 bpm.[12] Ultimately, if the PTA perceives any abnormal quality to the pulse, such as an irregular rhythm, the heart rate should be monitored for a full minute.[27] In such a case, if the abnormality has not previously been noted, this finding should be reported to the supervising PT immediately. Otherwise, as in the

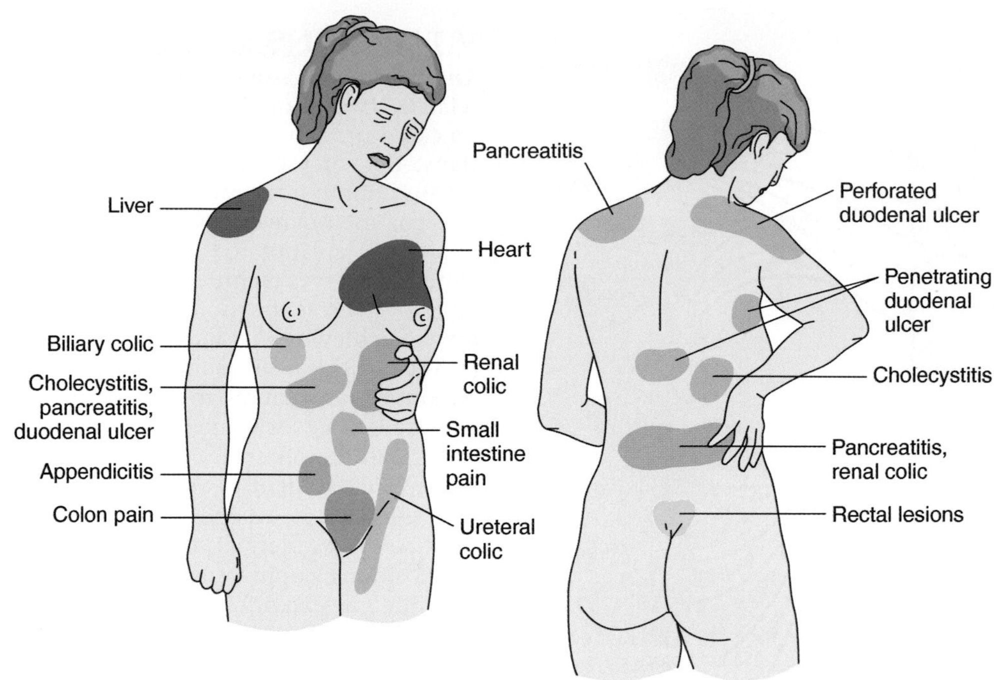

FIG 2-8 Diagram of common sites of visceral referred pain. *(From Saxton D, Green J, et al.* Mosby's comprehensive review of nursing for NCLEX-RN® Examination, *ed 19, St Louis, 2009, Mosby.)*

case with other assessment procedures, the PTA should employ the same technique the PT uses during the initial evaluation to enhance consistency and determine any deviation from the baseline measure.

Textbooks commonly used by PTA educational programs offer specific guidelines for setting exercise intensity using heart rate as a determinant.[19,25,27] An increase in the pulse of more than 20 bpm with activity that lasts for more than 3 minutes after rest or after changing positions should be reported to the supervising PT.[14]

RESPIRATION

As with pulse, respirations should be assessed for both rate and quality. In a healthy adult, normal respiratory rate ranges from 12 to 20 breaths per minute.[14,27] Variations in the range of normal respiration rate are expected among age groups. Other factors influencing respirations include age, body size, stature, exercise, body position, environment, emotions and stress, and pharmacologic agents.[27]

At rest, respiration should be smooth and steady, with uniform chest movement. Observe for excessive use of accessory breathing muscles (anterior upper quarter, anterolateral shoulder, and cervical muscles), which may indicate ventilatory compromise (e.g., chronic obstructive pulmonary disease, asthma, chronic bronchitis caused by smoking, or other pathologic conditions). Also observe to ensure that chest expansion is symmetric bilaterally. Because respiration includes voluntary control, it is best to assess respiration discreetly in conjunction with heart rate to avoid the patient inadvertently altering breathing pattern or rate in response to feeling self-conscious if he or she is aware that the PTA is observing the rise and fall of the chest. The rate is counted for 30 seconds and multiplied by 2; if irregularities are noted, a full 60-second count is preferred. Refer to the section of this chapter on fatigue for information relating specifically to the assessment of pulmonary response to exercise and activity.

BLOOD PRESSURE

Assessment of blood pressure provides an objective measurement of vascular resistance to blood flow at a given time. In a healthy adult, the normal blood pressure systolic value should be less than 120 millimeters of mercury (mm Hg), and the normal diastolic value should be less than 80 mm Hg.[27] The pressure exerted by blood is influenced by various factors and conditions, including age and cardiac output, both of which are directly proportional to systolic blood pressure.[27] Age is a nonmodifiable factor, so an increase in systolic blood pressure of elderly patients may not indicate an active pathologic process. As always, these findings should be noted in relation to the baseline measurement obtained by the supervising PT during the initial examination.

The PTA working with patients who have musculoskeletal dysfunction or impairment is most concerned with noting responses in blood pressure as new therapeutic activities are introduced or advanced during the course of progression through the established plan of care. Most notably, blood pressure is affected by exercise and activity level in the following ways. Cardiac output increases proportionally to increased physical activity.[16] An even greater and potentially dangerous increase in blood pressure also may occur if the patient holds his or her breath during periods of exertion with exercise. Patients may do this subconsciously in an effort to increase the weight-bearing function of the abdominal cavity, which becomes more stable with an attempt at strong exhalation against a closed glottis, nose, and mouth.[27] As noted in the

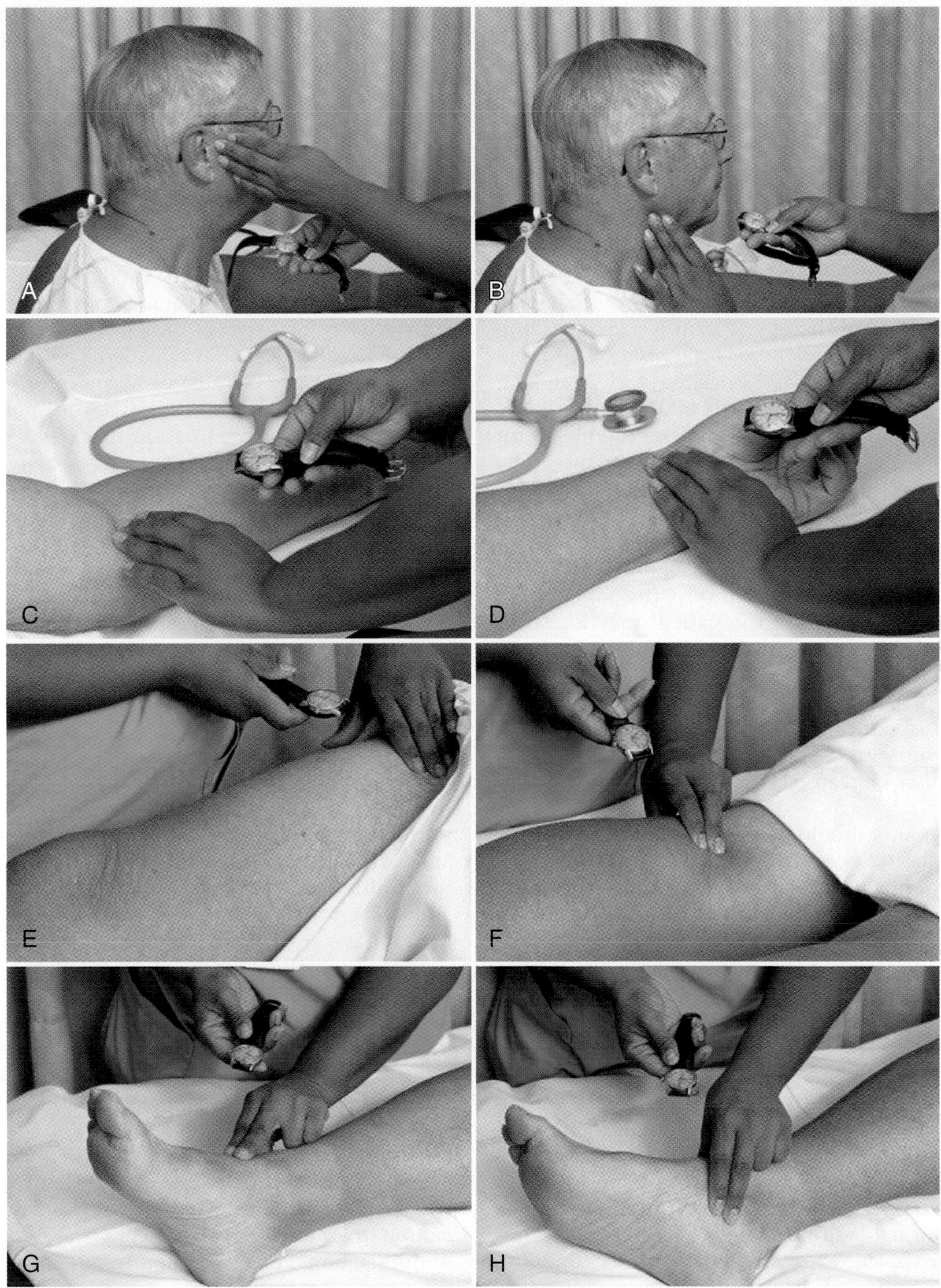

FIG 2-9 Pulse measurement sites. **A,** Temporal. **B,** Carotid. **C,** Brachial. **D,** Radial. **E,** Femoral. **F,** Popliteal. **G,** Dorsal pedal. **H,** Posterior tibial. *(From Fairchild S.* Pierson and Fairchild's principles and techniques of patient care, *ed 5, St Louis, 2013, Saunders.)*

discussion about pain, the PTA must be alert to the patient's total response to interventions and data collection techniques. When the observant PTA notices that the patient is holding his or her breath during exertion, the patient should be educated in techniques to avoid this behavior. The PTA also may want to reassess blood pressure at this time, although the effect on blood pressure from this activity, known as the *Valsalva maneuver,* is transient. It is particularly critical that the Valsalva maneuver be avoided by patients with a known history of hypertension or cardiac disease.[16]

Another important blood pressure response that may occur during a physical therapy session is a sudden drop in blood pressure, called *orthostatic hypotension*. This rapid decrease in blood pressure is associated with a sudden change in the patient's position. It is most frequently the result of the patient being immobile or recumbent for prolonged periods, and baseline measurements should be determined before the initiation of upright activities. Signs of orthostatic hypotension include a decrease in blood pressure, increase in pulse, lightheadedness, weakness, dizziness, syncope, mental or visual blurring, or diaphoresis.[14] If not addressed (by returning the patient to at least a semireclined position), the patient may lose consciousness. Because of the rapid change in blood pressure, the PTA must be prepared to assess the blood pressure immediately on the change in position. The blood pressure response is critical to obtain, record, and report because the symptoms associated with orthostatic hypotension can also be caused by other serious medical conditions.

Three final points should be noted by the student PTA. First, the PTA should check to be sure of any precautions or contraindications for the assessment of blood pressure that may be present. If the patient has a history of circulatory or lymphatic drainage compromise in one upper extremity, blood pressure must be assessed in the contralateral upper extremity, and if both upper extremities are compromised, blood pressure should be taken from the femoral artery.[27] Second, as mentioned in relation to assessment of other vital signs, the PTA student should practice taking and monitoring blood pressure on a variety of healthy individuals to reinforce a sense of values and ranges considered normal. To prevent unnecessary pressure from being applied, the safest technique to use is inflating the cuff only 15 to 20 mm Hg above the patient's documented normal systolic value.[12] Finally, the psychomotor skills involved with applying and securing the blood pressure cuff and attached sphygmomanometer, applying and holding the stethoscope diaphragm, pumping air into the bulb, releasing pressure from the cuff, and reading the meter while listening for the blood pressure sounds (called *Korotkoff sounds*) take coordination and skill. Although the process is basic and consistent, practice reinforces efficient application in actual patient care situations.

PULSE OXIMETRY

In addition to the measurement of vital signs described, pulse oximetry is a tool used to provide instant information about a subject's cardiopulmonary status. Specifically, the pulse oximeter is a noninvasive probe (in the form of a clip-on device placed on the ear, finger, foot, or nose) that provides a digital readout of oxyhemoglobin saturation. Most commonly, this device is used to identify hypoxemia, to monitor the patient's tolerance to activity, and to evaluate patient response to treatment.[27] However, for a patient in the hospital setting who has coexisting cardiopulmonary and musculoskeletal involvement, pulse oximetry is a viable tool for establishing goals to address tolerance to progressive activities.

The standard normal value for oxygen saturation ranges from 95% to 100%; this value is not expected to change with activity or exercise in a healthy individual.[14] This level noticeably decreases in patients with chronic respiratory disease; the PTA must be aware of normal ranges for a given individual in this case. Caution should be taken if the value of oxygen saturation drops below 90% during activity, and if it drops below 88%, activity should be discontinued.[16] If the referring physician has indicated any other specific level of oxygen saturation to use as a guideline for a given patient, the PTA must be aware of this level so that exercise tolerance is not exceeded. PTAs should also assess other vital signs, skin and nail bed color, tissue perfusion, mental status, breath sounds, and respiratory pattern in patients with whom they use pulse oximetry.[14] As a general rule, if your patient cannot talk easily while at rest, his or her oxygen saturation level is likely to be inadequate.

VITAL SIGNS AND EXERCISE

As the profession of physical therapy evolves, with the pursuit of uniform direct access throughout the United States, PTs will more often be the "point of entry" for the health care consumer. With this increased autonomy and recognition, physical therapy providers, including PTAs, have increased responsibilities to assess and monitor the patient's general health status, making decisions and judgments accordingly. For the PTA working with orthopedically involved patients, this responsibility includes being aware of normal and expected vital signs, values, and responses and monitoring for the unexpected.

Certain responses in vital signs are expected with exercise. In a "Scientific Statement" published by the American Heart Association,[13] detailed guidelines for exercise testing and training are provided, taking into consideration the cardiovascular health status of the patient. Abnormal blood pressure responses include the absence of an increase in systolic pressure or a decrease in systolic pressure with exercise; a normal response is an increase that correlates to the rate and intensity of exercise initiation.[19] If the patient's systolic blood pressure exceeds 200 mm Hg or if the diastolic pressure exceeds 100 mm Hg during exercise, the activity should be reduced or discontinued.[14] The systolic pressure should not increase more than 20 mm Hg with minimal to moderate exercise or more than 40 to 50 mm Hg with intensive exercise.[14] Diastolic blood pressure is not expected to increase or decrease more than 10 mm Hg with exercise in a healthy adult.[14] Box 2-3 summarizes abnormal responses of vital signs to exercise.

BOX 2-3 Abnormal Responses to Exercise

- Heart rate increases more than 20 to 30 bpm above resting heart rate
- Heart rate decreases below resting heart rate
- Systolic blood pressure increases more than 20 to 30 mm Hg above resting level
- Systolic blood pressure decreases more than 10 mm Hg below resting level
- Oxygen saturation drops below prescribed level
- Patient becomes short of breath or respiratory rate increases to level not tolerated by the patient
- Electrocardiogram changes

From Hillegass EA. *Essentials of cardiopulmonary physical therapy,* ed 3, St Louis, 2011, Saunders, p 586.

FATIGUE

In general, the PTA is expected to be competent in performing data collection techniques and selected interventions such that they can make appropriate modifications based on patient responses.[3] In relation to fatigue, this competency may involve observing and reporting abnormal responses to activity and making modifications to the interventions within the context of the PT's plan of care. Fatigue may be specific to an individual muscle or muscle group, or it may affect the entire body, manifesting as cardiopulmonary (also called *cardiorespiratory* or *general*) fatigue.[19] Frequently, associated symptoms such as dyspnea, chest pain, palpitations, or headache are associated with cardiopulmonary fatigue.[14]

A muscle in a state of fatigue is unable to generate a normal contraction, which may manifest by decreased force, ROM, or quality of the contraction. The patient may complain of discomfort or cramping in the muscle being exercised.[19] When a muscle is fatigued, the patient may compensate by consciously or subconsciously substituting with another muscle or muscle group that performs the same or similar action. For this reason, it is important for the PTA to be particularly familiar with muscle actions and potential substitutions and observe patients during exercise activities. In terms of quality of motion, fatigue may result in tremulous or jerky motions, instead of a smooth contraction through the ROM.[19]

Generalized fatigue is apparent when the patient is experiencing dyspnea or inability to breathe normally with activity, indicating a decreased ability of the body to use oxygen efficiently.[19] One tool that has been determined to be a good indicator of a patient's pulmonary tolerance to exercise is a standardized scale referred to as the *Borg scale,* or the *Rate of Perceived Exertion scale.*[16] This instrument calls for the patient to place an objective grade on the amount of exertion he or she perceives with exertion, making a subjective report more measurable. A similar instrument, the Dyspnea Scale, is used for rating the level of shortness of breath, or dyspnea.[16] As with all standardized instruments, the PTA uses the form, instrument, or technique consistent with that of the supervising PT. If the PT chose to use a standardized instrument to document examination data related to the patient's tolerance to activity, it is likely that a goal addressing that impairment is included in the plan of care, with the outcome to be measured using the same instrument.

TABLE 2-3 Normal and Abnormal End-Feels

	End-Feel	Example
Normal	Bone to bone	Elbow extension
	Soft tissue approximation	Knee flexion
	Tissue stretch	Ankle dorsiflexion, shoulder lateral rotation, finger extension
Abnormal	Early muscle spasm	Protective spasm after injury
	Late muscle spasm	Spasm owing to instability or pain
	"Mushy" tissue stretch	Tight muscle
	Spasticity	Upper motor neuron lesion
	Hard capsular	Frozen shoulder
	Soft capsular	Synovitis, soft tissue edema
	Bone to bone	Osteophyte formation
	Empty	Acute subacromial bursitis, limitation owing to pain
	Springy block	Meniscus tear

From Magee DJ. *Orthopedic physical assessment,* ed 6, St Louis, 2014, Saunders, p 35.

ASSESSMENT OF MUSCULOSKELETAL STRUCTURES

Detailed reviews of anatomy and function of specific structures are not presented here because the scope of this chapter is limited to the PTA's role in assessment. This section provides information relating to entry-level data collection techniques and assessment procedures pertaining to structures involved with musculoskeletal diagnoses commonly encountered by the PTA.

END-FEEL

The term *end-feel* describes the barrier encountered that prevents further motion at the end of passive ROM in a joint. Because different types of tissue have different characteristics and qualities to their constituency, there are associated normal (physiologic) and abnormal (pathologic) end-feels for each tissue. Normal end-feels are described simply as soft, firm, or hard.[26] Other terms used to denote normal end-feels include *soft tissue approximation,* such as occurs with knee flexion; *muscular stretch,* such as occurs with hip flexion with the knee straight; *capsular stretch,* as denoted in extension of metacarpophalangeal joints of the fingers; *ligamentous stretch,* as found in forearm supination; or *bone contacting bone,* such as occurs with elbow extension.[26] Table 2-3 summarizes these end-feels. These terms are descriptive of the specific anatomic relationships of structures that normally limit the motion of each joint. The PTA student is encouraged to practice assessing the different normal end-feels on a variety of subjects because the exact perception varies depending on the structure and build of each individual tested.

When one of the end-feels is noted in a joint that normally exhibits a different end-feel, it is considered to be an abnormal or pathologic end-feel. Abnormal end-feels may be classified as soft, firm, hard, or empty. A soft end-feel occurs sooner or later in the ROM than is usual for a joint or in a joint that normally has a firm or hard end-feel and is described as feeling "boggy." A firm end-feel occurs sooner or later in the ROM than is usual, or it may be noted in a joint that normally would have a soft or hard end-feel. Hard end-feels occur sooner or later in the ROM than is normal for a joint or in a joint that normally has a soft or firm end-feel in which a bony grating or bony block is noted. When no real end-feel is noted because pain prevents the examiner from reaching the end of ROM, this is known as an empty end-feel.[26] Resistance is not noted with an empty end-feel other than protective muscle splinting or spasm of the patient or client.[26] As always, when the PTA recognizes these abnormal circumstances, these findings must be documented and reported to the evaluating PT.

SKELETAL MUSCLE TISSUE

Skeletal muscle tissue has various characteristics that allow it to function as it does. Three such characteristics are excitability, contractility, and extensibility. Excitability (or irritability) refers to the ability of skeletal muscle tissue to be stimulated; contractility is the ability of skeletal muscle tissue to contract or shorten; and extensibility is the ability of skeletal muscle to extend or stretch and to return to its resting length after having contracted.[33]

Strength Testing

It is beyond the scope of this text to provide detailed instruction in the performance of techniques used to measure strength of specific muscles. However, because specific strength increases are frequently included as physical therapy goals, the PTA must be competent with measuring strength through use of both specific and gross testing techniques. Procedures for assessing muscle strength to determine changes or unexpected findings are discussed here.

When the plan of care includes goals related to increase in specific muscle grades, the PTA must use the same technique for assessing the muscle strength as the evaluating PT used at the time of the initial examination and evaluation. In general, specific manual muscle testing takes into account the precise attachments, action, and position of a muscle during movements or isometric contractions against gravity. Scales for specific muscle grades are also precise, based on word/letter or number scales with strict definitions for each. A table is an organized and convenient way to record data relating to muscle strength testing; an example of a table format is provided in Table 2-4.

In contrast to specific manual muscle testing, gross manual muscle testing techniques are used to determine quickly a nonprecise, yet objective measurement of functional strength. This technique might be used as an efficient method to determine a patient's readiness to progress with exercise or gait activities. This method also may be used to gather data about any changes in the patient's status since the initial examination or last therapy session. In general, movements should be resisted bilaterally and, when possible, simultaneously on both sides for easy comparison. Positions or test movements do not take gravity into account but focus more on functional positions and movements, such as shaking hands, grasping the therapist's fingers, or lowering and rising to and from a squatting position. In addition to gross strength, the PTA should be alert for any signs of pain or discomfort with resisted muscle testing. When conducting gross manual muscle tests, the PTA is not attempting to obtain a precise measurement of strength, but rather is gathering data relevant to the patient's progress toward goals, readiness to progress through the established plan of care, and status in terms of changes in condition. The PTA must document and report any unexpected changes or previously undocumented data related to muscle strength to the supervising PT.

TABLE 2-4 Sample Format for Recording Muscle Strength

Joint/Motion Shoulder	Muscle Test Grade*		Other Responses†
	Right	Left	
Flexion	4–/5	2+/5	
Extension	4/5	3/5	
Internal rotation	4/5	3–/5	
External rotation	4+/5	3–/5	

*Measurements represent example of ascending 0-to-5 scale.
†Other responses could include notation regarding the presence of pain.

If the PTA observes signs of pain with resisted movements during strength testing, he or she must make certain that the test is being performed in such a way as to avoid causing active insufficiency of muscles being tested. Kendall and associates[18] defined active insufficiency as follows: "The inability of a Class III or IV two-joint (or multijoint) muscle to generate an effective force when placed in a fully shortened position." Active insufficiency can result from improper positioning of a two-joint or multijoint muscle and causes a cramping type of pain. Pain experienced with muscle testing during a properly performed technique could be indicative of an inflammatory state or strain of the tissues being stressed. Because the musculotendinous tissue is responsible for sustaining joint position during resistance, the presence of pain with muscle testing, even if the result indicates intact strength, points to involvement of the muscle or tendon. Again, if these data represent a change from the initial examination or evaluation data, they should be documented and reported to the evaluating PT.

Another indication of muscle weakness or the possibility of undiagnosed musculoskeletal or neuromuscular pathology is change in muscle mass or tone. Changes in mass may manifest as either atrophy (muscle wasting) or hypertrophy (excessive mass). The PTA should be able to recognize changes in mass as well as make observations about any pattern of these manifestations, such as the involvement of a specific muscle versus a muscle group;

the involvement of muscles innervated by common peripheral or spinal nerve segments; and the involvement of unilateral, asymmetric muscles or groups versus bilateral, symmetric involvement.

Tone refers to the resistance of muscle tissue to passive elongation or stretch and is determined through observation of movements for quality of motion and control of motion (including grading and coordination) and through palpation.[27] True changes in muscle tone should also be noted in the context of patterns of involvement such as previously described and should be differentiated from a local muscle guarding or splinting response.

Stretching and Palpation

The stage of inflammation generally determines when pain is felt with movement. During the acute stage of inflammation, pain is usually encountered before tissue resistance; during the subacute stage, pain is usually synchronous with tissue resistance; and during the chronic stage, pain usually occurs after tissue resistance is encountered.[27] If the patient reports an increase in pain with stretching, it could be that a previous stretching or strengthening exercise program was performed too vigorously or aggressively, and appropriate modifications to therapy activities should be made within the scope of the established plan of care.

In addition to pain at end range, muscle and tendon tissue that is in a state of inflammation or injury is tender to palpation over the involved area. Trigger points also may be noted on palpation (see previous discussion of trigger points).

Muscle tenderness or soreness to palpation is not by itself an accurate indicator of the tissues involved because referred pain can also manifest as tenderness. However, the PTA should note and document the location and degree of tenderness or soreness for purposes of comparison with initial examination findings and possibly as a measure of progress toward goals, if the supervising PT addressed this area in the plan of care. A previously unnoticed pattern of tenderness revealed while the PTA is working with the patient should also be documented and reported to the supervising PT because patterns of the distribution of tender points represent the hallmark characteristic of conditions such as fibromyalgia. The core features of fibromyalgia syndrome include widespread pain lasting more than 3 months and widespread local tender points that are described as painful on palpation.[14]

As with pain on stretching contractile tissue to end range, palpable tightness or spasm also may occur after exercise or other activity that is too vigorous or aggressive. A muscle may respond to overwork by subconscious splinting or guarding, which results in a feeling of tightness or increased tension to palpation. When increased tightness or spasm is noted on palpation, modifications to the level of activity or exercise could be warranted within the parameters of the established plan of care.

Flexibility

The loss of the ability of the muscle or tendon unit to obtain full length results in decreased flexibility. Decreased flexibility may be differentiated from decreased joint ROM or loss of accessory motions, which may result from involvement of intra-articular structures (discussed in the section on joints).

The end-feel associated with a loss of muscle or tendon flexibility secondary to increased tension in a muscle is described as *muscular* end-feel, and *muscle-spasm* end-feel relates to when joint movement is stopped abruptly with some rebound secondary to muscles contracting reflexively to prevent further joint movement.[15]

In terms of assessment, the PTA should use a technique consistent with that used by the evaluating PT. Because a loss of flexibility is a problem that may have a significant impact on function, it is an area frequently addressed in the physical therapy plan of care. Examination techniques and subsequent goals may be addressed in terms of specific quantitative outcomes or be more functionally based. An example of a quantitative measurement is the use of goniometric measurements. As with manual muscle testing, detailed instruction in goniometry techniques is beyond the scope of this text. The most important elements of goniometric measurement are accuracy and consistency among testers and testing techniques. PTA educational programs are organized to allow the student to establish a solid foundation in human anatomy, typically including specific emphasis on the musculoskeletal system and structures. To be effective with the application of assessment or data collection techniques such as goniometry, the student is strongly encouraged to ensure that he or she possesses this critical knowledge base. In addition to a solid grasp of skeletal and superficial anatomic landmarks, the student must learn other principles associated with goniometric testing, such as the differences among passive, active, and active-assisted ROM. It is common for the novice to document goniometric measurements as an indicator of flexibility, failing to indicate whether the data represent the patient's ability to actively move through the range or whether passive overpressure was applied to obtain the measurement. The functional implications relating to this concept are significant.

Another technique that may be used to obtain and document information related to flexibility is a functional measurement, such as measuring the distance between the patient's fingertips and the floor during forward flexion (e.g., to measure hamstring flexibility). Although this technique may have specific functional implications, many factors may confound the results and make it less specific to the area of focus. For example, forward trunk flexion performed in this manner may be limited by loss of mobility in the lumbar spine, not the hamstring group. For purposes of data collection for accurate assessment of the patient's progress, the PTA must employ the same technique as the supervising PT for each patient case. There should be consistency among PTs and PTAs within a practice setting to ensure continuity of care for the patient and valid outcome measurements.

Overuse

As in the case with overuse caused by overaggressive or vigorous exercise (active strengthening or passive stretching), the PTA must be alert for signs of overuse or cumulative stress to contractile tissue, particularly tendons. Signs of tendinitis (an inflammatory condition that results from overuse) include painful but strong resisted isometric contraction (e.g., with manual muscle testing techniques) and possibly pain at end range with stretching as well as tenderness to palpation over the site of irritation, often near or at the tendinous insertion of the involved muscle. The PTA must not dismiss the possibility that a patient progressing through an exercise program may develop signs and symptoms of tendinitis, even if this is not the original reason for referral. As discussed earlier, the long-term effects of inflammation can have serious implications. It is imperative for the PTA to present this information to the supervising PT so that modifications to the plan of care can be made to avoid further excessive stresses to these tissues.

BONES

Of primary importance to the physical therapy clinician is the need to rule out conditions or disease processes that are beyond the professional scope of physical therapy, warranting medical diagnosis and treatment. Even without the advent of direct access to physical therapy care, it is possible that a patient may be referred to physical therapy in error for treatment of a condition that requires strict medical attention. The main consideration with bone tissue is fracture. The potential exists for the fracture to be missed on initial examination (medical or physical therapy). An existing fracture also may progress, in terms of malalignment, in the case of a hairline or crack fracture, in which case referral for immobilization may be indicated. It is critical for the PTA to have an understanding of the signs and symptoms of fracture (Box 2-4), regardless of the severity. Common signs and symptoms include pain and local tenderness, deformity, edema, ecchymosis, and a loss of overall function and mobility.[8]

If the patient exhibits exquisite point tenderness over a localized site other than a ligament or other supportive structure, a fracture may be indicated versus other musculoskeletal involvement (e.g., a ligamentous sprain).[14] The PTA should also be aware that fractures can occur as a result of relatively minor trauma, such as sneezing, coughing, or leaning over to tie one's shoe. Fractures from minor trauma can occur in patients who have osteoporosis.[8] Because of the high prevalence and risk of osteoporosis, the astute PTA must recognize the possibility of vertebral compression fractures in a patient with complaints of mid-back or low-back pain. Although sudden impact fractures are the most common type of fracture, the PTA must also be aware of the possibility of stress and pathologic fractures. A stress fracture is a microscopic disruption or break in a bone that is not displaced and produces pain that is described as a localized tenderness or deep aching pain that increases with activity and improves with rest.[14] Pathologic fractures occur in bones that are weakened by disease or tumors and frequently occur spontaneously with very little or no stress. They can be local to the cause, such as with infections, cysts, or tumors, or generalized, as in osteoporosis, Paget's disease, or disseminated tumors.[28]

BOX 2-4 Signs and Symptoms of Bone Fractures

- Pain and localized tenderness
- Deformity
- Edema
- Ecchymosis
- Loss of overall function and mobility

Adapted from Boissonnault WG. *Primary care for the physical therapist examination and triage,* ed 2, St Louis, 2011, Saunders.

JOINTS AND LIGAMENTS

Accessory Joint Motions

As a component of evaluation, the PT assesses ligamentous integrity and accessory joint motions for the purposes of differential diagnosis and making decisions on which to base the plan of care. It is the position of the APTA that spinal and peripheral joint mobilization techniques are interventions performed exclusively by the PT.[6] Although the PTA is not responsible for these elements of physical therapy patient care, it is nonetheless important that he or she understands the implications of assessment procedures that may reveal problems with structures that contribute to joint integrity.

The term *accessory joint motions* refers to "motions between adjacent joint surfaces that occur when a bone moves through a range of motion; includes slides (glides), distractions, compressions, rolls, and spins."[27] Accessory joint motions are also described as motions that occur during active motion but are not under voluntary control.[19] Another term used to describe these motions is arthrokinematics. For the accessory motions of roll, slide, and spin to occur in a joint, there must be adequate capsule laxity.[19] Roll occurs when one bone within a joint rolls on another bone within the joint. It always occurs in the same direction as bone motion, and new points on one bone meet new points on the other bone.[19] The slide accessory motion relates to the concave-convex rule. If the surface of the moving bone segment is convex, sliding is in the direction opposite of the angular movement of the bone; if the surface of the moving bone is concave, sliding is in the same direction as the angular movement of the bone.[19] Spin occurs when there is rotation around a stationary axis, and a point on the moving surface creates an arc as it spins. Abnormal findings that may be noted in the presence of impaired accessory motions include decreased joint ROM, a capsular end-feel during stretching techniques, and substitution or compensatory attempts by the patient to obtain full motion.

Distraction and Compression

Distraction (a manual separating of adjacent joint surfaces) and *compression* (a manual approximation of joint surfaces) are assessment techniques that can provide information about the involvement of tissues or structures that serve to provide support to the joint (ligaments), that lie between the joint surfaces (cartilage), or that are directly affected by joint mechanics (bursae). In the presence of mechanical or structural problems that result in impingement on structures located within or near a joint, distracting the joint may produce a relief of symptoms such as pain (radiating or local) or dysesthesia. The PTA's role in this case is to report and document any previously undocumented findings that may provide information regarding the nature of the patient's problem.

Likewise, if the PTA notices an increase in the patient's symptoms such as pain or signs such as crepitus (joint noise resulting from changes—usually increased coarseness or roughening—of the joint surfaces) during approximation or weight-bearing activities, he or she should suspect degenerative or inflammatory conditions and should document these findings and report them to the supervising PT.

Bursae are fluid-filled sacs that are located near tendinous insertions to reduce friction with motion. Bursae also may develop as an adaptive mechanism in the presence of excessive friction. An inflamed bursa sometimes is visible near a joint as a small, soft, encapsulated protrusion that is tender to touch. With bursitis, movement of the nearby joint is painful or motion may be restricted in a noncapsular pattern.[15] Any signs of a pathologic or inflamed bursa should be documented and reported to the supervising PT. Changes in exercise programs or functional activities should be incorporated into the plan of care. If a patient presents with a lump under the skin, joint pain and swelling, fever, chills, malaise, and redness, the patient may be exhibiting signs of gout and requires referral for further medical work-up if this condition has not been diagnosed previously.[14]

Ligamentous Integrity

During the course of administering components of the physical therapy plan of care for a patient with a history or diagnosis of ligament sprain, the PTA must be able to assess the patient's readiness to progress with interventions that will increase stresses to the healing tissue. Ligamentous laxity or improper healing results in decreased joint stability, which may manifest as complaints from the patient that the joint or weight-bearing extremity feels as if it may "give." In this case, the PTA should consult with the supervising PT before initiating progressive activities; failure to modify interventions in this case may result in impaired healing, regression of healing, or permanent tissue damage.

If the PTA notices the sudden onset of increased edema, heat to touch, and extremely painful and limited mobility during the course of treatment of a patient with a ligament sprain, the supervising PT must be consulted to seek medical referral to rule out hemarthrosis (bleeding inside the joint capsule).[19]

GAIT

For the PTA to be proficient with assessment of gait, he or she must first have a solid understanding of the normal mechanics of walking. When this underlying knowledge is present, the PTA observes the patient walking, compares the pattern against the normal gait pattern, and notes the deviations. As with all assessment procedures, the PTA must ensure that the techniques he or she employs are consistent with techniques used by the supervising PT. Gait assessment should be performed on flat surfaces as well as uneven surfaces when indicated and with the patient wearing and not wearing shoes. The shoes also can be examined for signs of abnormal wear, such as scuff marks on the toe of one shoe or flattening of one side of the shoe sole.

Deviations in gait primarily occur as a result of pain, weakness, or other imbalance between muscle strength and flexibility. Typically, the short-term goals in the plan of care address the specific cause of the deviation, with the long-term goal or outcome addressing the overall quality or function of gait. The PTA is responsible for assessing the components of gait that have been specifically addressed in the plan of care. For example, a patient exhibiting an uncompensated Trendelenburg gait during the initial evaluation may have a goal addressing increased gluteus medius strength on the involved side. In this case, the PTA observes the patient's gait to assess for changes in the Trendelenburg pattern and measure strength of the gluteus medius for comparison with initial evaluation data.

The PTA also has a role in determining if a patient is ready to progress to gait training activities with a lesser assistive device. To make appropriate recommendations, the PTA must be familiar with advantages and disadvantages of various assistive devices and must understand purposes and limitations of each. The PTA should keep in mind that ultimately the patient will be best served by the assistive device that allows for maximum safety, independence, and the most normal gait pattern.

BALANCE

According to the Normative Model,[3] the PTA is to be competent in performing balance, coordination, and agility training. Three physiologic systems linked to balance control include somatosensory (musculoskeletal and neuromuscular components), visual, and vestibular. The vestibular system involves the structures and organs of the inner ear, which play a key role in maintaining upright posture, equilibrium, and orientation, which are all components of balance. Although the application of interventions designed to correct vestibular problems is beyond the skill level of an entry-level PTA, he or she must be aware that patients who report symptoms of vertigo, dizziness, balance problems, coordination problems, trouble focusing or tracking objects, hearing loss, tinnitus, nausea, vomiting, motion sickness, ear pain, headaches, or a sensation of fullness in the ears may need further physical therapy or medical assessment to rule out or confirm involvement of vestibular conditions. (Detailed information about vestibular disorders can be found on the website of the Vestibular Disorders Association at www.vestibular.org.)

Important Concepts

Three physiologic systems are linked to balance control:

- Somatosensory (musculoskeletal and neuromuscular components)
- Visual
- Vestibular

A patient who constantly or frequently looks at the floor during ambulation or other activities that challenge balance is likely depending excessively on visual input to compensate for somatosensory impairment (e.g., weakness, loss of sensation, or limited joint mobility). In this case, ongoing assessment should include these components or musculoskeletal or neuromuscular integrity according to the plan of care as established by the evaluating PT. Data collection and documentation must relate changes in the patient's musculoskeletal and neuromuscular function (e.g., ROM, loss of sensation, or weakness) to balance.

Likewise, a patient with visual impairment may depend heavily on musculoskeletal and neuromuscular control to compensate for this deficit. In this case, the PTA may notice that the patient reaches for props or ambulates with a wide base of support.

DOCUMENTATION

Documentation is a critical element of the patient's physical therapy experience. In the present health care environment, the focus of documentation often emphasizes reimbursement for services at the cost of cutting short other very important purposes of effective record keeping. In addition to serving as a permanent record of the patient's physical therapy episode of care, documentation is used as a communication tool among members of the health care team; it also may be an effective tool for quality assurance or management within a service or department to measure consistency between providers, set standards for assessment and interventions, and measure effectiveness of outcomes.

The *Physical Therapist Assistant Clinical Performance Instrument*[6] lists the following essential skills associated with documentation (criterion #13):

- "Selects relevant information to document the delivery of physical therapy care."
- "Documents all aspects of physical therapy care provided, including interventions, patient response to interventions (e.g., vital signs, pain, observation), selected data collection measurements, and communication with family and others involved in the delivery of care."
- "Produces documentation that is accurate, concise, timely, legible, grammatically and technically correct (e.g., abbreviations, terminology, etc.)."
- "Produces documentation (e.g., electronic, dictation, chart) consistent with guidelines, format, and requirements of the facility, regulatory agencies, and third-party payers."[4]

This discussion focuses on the PTA's role in documenting assessment. Early in his or her educational experience, the PTA student learns to recognize the standard elements of the subjective objective assessment plan (SOAP) format of documentation; this format is effective as a tool to organize one's thoughts and the content of a treatment note, even if it is not the standard format used by a given facility.

In the subjective section of the note, the PTA would document any patient reports related to functional status or disability, including patient reports of pain. In the objective section of the SOAP note, the PTA would document treatment performed, including frequency, duration, and intensity; patient education; equipment provided; and changes in patient's status including observed changes during or after treatment and any measurements taken during the treatment.[30] In the plan section of the SOAP note, the PTA would indicate the intervention or interventions for the next patient visit, what the patient is to be doing between treatments, and steps that will be taken to reach the established goals.[21]

How does assessment fit into the PTA's documentation? The assessment is the key portion of documentation that links subjective and objective data to the physical therapy goals, outcomes, and plan. The assessment justifies or explains "why" the patient exhibits the subjective and objective facts. In the assessment section of the note, "... the PTA summarizes the information in the S and O sections and reports the progress being made toward accomplishing the goals."[21] Box 2-5 provides a sample SOAP note that is an example of an effectively documented assessment by a PTA.

BOX 2-5 Sample SOAP Document

S: Pt. c/o UEs feeling tired with parallel bars and pregait activities. Pt. reports 6/10 pain in UEs.

O: Before gait training, GMMT reveals overall strength WFL, with the exception of poor hip clearance with wc. push-up. 50% of attempts, pt. required specific instructions and tactile guidance with proper hand placement with sit-to-stand and stand-to-sit; otherwise carries out this task properly. In parallel bars, pt. took 3 steps forward and back + mod. assist; stand with trunk and (L) LE flexed and does not push adequately with UEs.

A: Concerns re: difficulty maintaining NWB status (R) LE with pre-amb. activities because of insufficient shoulder depression strength; as a result, pt. is not ready to begin gait training with walker. Pt. will benefit from ex. to increase shoulder depression strength to enhance use of assistive device for NWB (R) LE.

P: Include push-up blocks with ther. ex. next visit; progress with gait training with walker, NWB (R) LE as indicated.

Signature, PTA.

SUMMARY

This chapter began with reference to the rapid changes occurring in the physical therapy profession today. It is imperative for PTAs just entering the profession to possess an awareness and understanding of the issues surrounding the dynamics of this evolution. As PTA students gain an understanding of the foundational principles and core documents that affect their clinical and professional roles and function, they will be better equipped to be active participants in these discussions. This chapter was designed with this outcome in mind and focused on the PTA's role in the performance and documentation of assessment procedures used in the care of patients with musculoskeletal disorders.

GLOSSARY

Assessment: "The measurement or quantification of a variable or the placement of a value on something."[2]

Centralization: The increase of signs and symptoms in the immediate area of the lesion.

Evaluation: The specific process reserved solely for the PT, in which clinical judgments are made based on the data obtained during the examination.

Examination: The preliminary gathering of data and performing various screens, tests, and measures to obtain a comprehensive base from which to make decisions about physical therapy needs for each individual patient, including the possibility of referral to another health care provider.

Peripheralization: The spread of pain to areas outside of or distant from the immediate area of involvement.

Referred pain: Pain that is "felt in an area far from the site of the lesion, but supplied by the same or adjacent neural segments."[14]

Trigger points: "Small, localized tender areas found within skeletal muscles, fascia, tendons, ligaments, periosteum, and pericapsular areas."[31]

Visceral pain: Pain that originates from a body organ.

REFERENCES

1. Alvarez DJ, Rockwell PG: Trigger points: diagnosis and management. *Am Fam Physician* 65(4):653–660, 2002.
2. American Physical Therapy Association: *Guide to physical therapist practice*, ed 2, Alexandria, VA, 2001, American Physical Therapy Association.
3. American Physical Therapy Association: *A normative model of physical therapist assistant education: version 2007*, Alexandria, VA, 2007, American Physical Therapy Association.
4. American Physical Therapy Association: *Physical therapist assistant clinical performance instrument*, April 2008 Revised ed. Alexandria, VA, 2008, American Physical Therapy Association.
5. American Physical Therapy Association Board of Directors: *Professionalism in physical therapy: core values*, Alexandria, VA, 2004, American Physical Therapy Association.
6. American Physical Therapy Association House of Delegates: *Procedural interventions exclusively performed by physical therapists*, Alexandria, VA, 2000, American Physical Therapy Association.
7. American Physical Therapy Association House of Delegates: *Standards of ethical conduct for the physical therapist assistant*, Alexandria, VA, 2009, American Physical Therapy Association.
8. Boissonnault WG: *Primary care for the physical therapist examination and triage*, ed 2, St Louis, 2011, Saunders.
9. Crowley LV: *An introduction to human disease pathology and pathophysiology correlations*, ed 9, Burlington, MA, 2013, Jones & Bartlett.
10. Ehrman JK, Gordon P, Visich PS, et al: *Clinical exercise physiology*, Champaign, IL, 2003, Human Kinetics.
11. Esterson PS: Measurement of ankle joint swelling using a figure of 8. *J Orthop Sports Phys Ther* 1(1):51–52, 1979.
12. Fairchild S: *Pierson and Fairchild's principles and techniques of patient care*, ed 5, St Louis, 2013, Saunders.
13. Fletcher GF, Balady GJ, Amsterdam EA, et al: Exercise standards for testing and training: a statement for health care professionals from the American Heart Association. *Circulation* 104:1694–1740, 2001.
14. Goodman CC, Snyder TK: *Differential diagnosis for physical therapists: screening for referral*, St Louis, 2007, Saunders.
15. Hertling D, Kessler RM: *Management of common musculoskeletal disorders: physical therapy principles and methods*, ed 4, Philadelphia, 2006, Lippincott Williams & Wilkins.
16. Hillegas EA: *Essentials of cardiopulmonary physical therapy*, ed 3, St Louis, 2011, Saunders.
17. Karges JR, Mark BE, Strikeleather SJ, et al: Concurrent validity of upper-extremity volume estimates: comparison of calculated volume derived from girth measurements and water displacement volume. *Phys Ther* 83(2):134–145, 2003.
18. Kendall FP, McCreary EK, Provance PG: *Muscles: testing and function*, Baltimore, 1993, Lippincott Williams & Wilkins.
19. Kisner C, Colby LA: *Therapeutic exercise foundations and techniques*, ed 6, Philadelphia, 2013, FA Davis.
20. Kloth LC, McCulloch JM: *Wound healing: alternatives in management*, ed 3, Philadelphia, 2002, FA Davis.
21. Lukan M: *Documentation for physical therapist assistants*, ed 2, Philadelphia, 2001, FA Davis.
22. Magee DJ: *Orthopedic physical assessment*, ed 6, St Louis, 2014, Saunders.
23. May BJ: *Home health and rehabilitation: concepts of care*, Philadelphia, 1999, FA Davis.
24. Merskey H, Bogduk N: *Classification of chronic pain: descriptions of chronic pain syndromes and definitions of pain terms*, ed 2, Seattle, WA, 1994, International Association for the Study of Pain.
25. Minor SD, Minor MA: *Patient care skills*, ed 7, Upper Saddle River, NJ, 2013, Pearson.
26. Norkin CC, White DJ: *Measurement of joint motion: a guide to goniometry*, ed 4, Philadelphia, 2009, FA Davis.
27. O'Sullivan SB, Schmitz TJ: *Physical rehabilitation*, ed 6, Philadelphia, 2014, FA Davis.
28. Porth CM: *Essentials of pathophysiology: concepts of altered health states*, ed 2, Philadelphia, 2007, Lippincott Williams & Wilkins.
29. Prentice WE, Voight ML: *Techniques in musculoskeletal rehabilitation*, New York, 2001, McGraw-Hill.
30. Quinn L, Gordon J: *Functional outcomes documentation for rehabilitation*, St Louis, 2003, Saunders.
31. Tan JC: *Practical manual of physical medicine and rehabilitation*, ed 2, St Louis, 2005, Mosby.
32. Tatro-Adams D, McGann S, Carbone W: Reliability of the figure-of-eight method of ankle measurement. *J Orthop Sports Phys Ther* 22(4):161–163, 1995.
33. Thibodeau GA, Patton KT: *Anatomy and physiology*, ed 2, St Louis, 1993, Mosby.

REVIEW QUESTIONS

Multiple Choice

1. Signs of a deep venous thrombosis include:
   a. Pale skin, increased local temperature, edema, and pain.
   b. Pale skin, increased heart rate, increased respiratory rate, and pain.
   c. Venous distention, palpable cord, increased local temperature, and redness.
   d. Redness, decreased local temperature, edema, and pain.
2. Which of the following motions is the best example of a "hard" end-feel?
   a. Elbow flexion
   b. Elbow extension
   c. Shoulder external rotation
   d. Hip flexion with the knee bent
3. When a PTA identifies a "red flag" symptom in a patient during treatment, the PTA should:
   a. Immediately call 911.
   b. Continue with interventions or data collection techniques and be sure to document the symptoms and notify the supervising PT.
   c. Not proceed with any interventions or data collection techniques and should immediately report the findings to the supervising PT.
   d. Continue with current plan of care, but tell the patient to be sure to follow up with his or her physician.

4. A 57-year-old man with a diagnosis of chronic low-back pain reports dizziness and a lightheaded feeling during exercise treatment. The patient is instructed to sit down, and his vital signs are measured. Respiration rate is 14 breaths per minute, pulse rate is 88 bpm, and blood pressure is 152/92 mm Hg. Which of the following statements is most accurate regarding these results?
   a. His pulse rate and blood pressure are above normal limits.
   b. His vital signs are within normal limits.
   c. His blood pressure and respiration rate are below normal limits.
   d. His pulse rate and respiration rate are below normal limits.
5. While gathering subjective data from a patient, you determine that his or her pain is referred to the lower extremity along a neural distribution for a specific spinal segment. This is an indication of:
   a. Trigger points.
   b. Centralization of pain.
   c. Visceral pain.
   d. Peripheralization of pain.
6. When collecting data about a patient's edema, to ensure the data are reliable and reproducible and that there is a level of consistency:
   a. Only bony landmarks should be used.
   b. The tape measure should be pulled as taut as possible around the limb.
   c. Only the affected limb should be measured.
   d. Precisely identifiable landmarks should be documented with data measurements.
7. When edema is identified in a patient's bilateral lower extremities, this typically indicates:
   a. The patient is experiencing sympathetic pain symptoms in the noninjured lower extremity.
   b. A systemic pathologic condition such as CHF.
   c. The patient did not tolerate the therapy activity progression well and activities should be modified.
   d. A musculoskeletal pathologic condition affecting the synovial joints.
8. Which of the following is a potentially serious condition involving edema that is a result of increased fluids in an area tightly bound by fascia?
   a. Compartment syndrome
   b. CHF
   c. Pitting edema
   d. Intermittent claudication
9. It is important for the PTA to be able to recognize potential muscular substitutions and to identify when this occurs during patient exercise activities to detect the onset of which of the following?
   a. Intermittent claudication
   b. Muscle fatigue
   c. Abnormal vital signs
   d. Overuse syndrome
10. When the PTA needs to assess a patient's readiness to progress through the established plan of care, he or she might perform what type of strength testing?
   a. Gross manual muscle testing
   b. Specific manual muscle testing
   c. Unilateral manual muscle testing
   d. Gradual manual muscle testing
11. The loss of the ability of the muscle or tendon unit to obtain full length results in decreased:
   a. Pain.
   b. Strength.
   c. Flexibility.
   d. Circulation.
12. What is the term used to describe increasing pain symptoms in the immediate area of the lesion (as opposed to spreading pain)?
   a. Trigger point
   b. Centralization of pain
   c. Visceral pain
   d. Peripheralization of pain
13. What are the three systems linked with balance control?
   a. Heart rate, respiratory rate, and blood pressure
   b. Somatosensory, visual, and vestibular
   c. Range of motion, strength, and gait
   d. Central, peripheral, and autonomic
14. The assessment portion of documentation is crucial because it links subjective and objective data to:
   a. The physical therapy goals.
   b. The outcomes.
   c. The plan.
   d. All of the above.
15. What is a distinct pattern or type of pain that may manifest simultaneously with musculoskeletal symptoms that is caused by activity-related discomfort and typically reported by patients as aching or cramping in a localized region bilaterally?
   a. Compartment syndrome
   b. CHF
   c. Pitting edema
   d. Intermittent claudication

Short Answer

16. List typical signs and symptoms of MI (heart attack) that may occur concurrently with the pattern of pain identified as early warning signs of a heart attack.
17. What technique should be employed by the PTA when performing standardized tests and measures and data collection?
18. List five factors that affect respiration rate.
19. What is the term used to describe joint noise that results from degenerative joint changes?
20. What are two potential long-term complications of chronic, unresolved inflammation?

Fill in the Blank

21. Enlarged and tender lymph nodes represent a __________ localized response to __________.
22. Examination of a patient's shoes may provide information about deviations in the patient's __________.
23. Inflammation is typically a reaction to tissue __________ or __________.
24. Fractures associated with osteoporosis may be __________ and diagnosed after healing during medical work-up for subsequent fractures.

25. A manual separating of adjacent joint surfaces is _________, whereas a manual approximation of joint surfaces is _________.

True/False

26. Assessment of patients' vital signs is unnecessary on a routine basis in the outpatient orthopedic clinical setting.
27. Fractures can occur as a result of relatively minor trauma, and they can occur spontaneously with little or no stress.
28. For accurate data collection related to gait, assessment should be performed only on level surfaces and only while the patient ambulates with shoes on.
29. It is the role of the PTA to judge the patient and conclude that the patient is malingering or "faking" the condition.
30. The patient does not play an active role in establishing the severity of general fatigue he or she may experience during activity.

Chapter 3

Differential Diagnosis and Emergent Conditions

Daryl Menke, Jeromy Jones, Robert C. Manske

CHAPTER OUTLINE

LEARNING OBJECTIVE

1. Define and distinguish the purpose and process of differential diagnosis as it relates to the provision of physical therapy.
2. Discuss the indirect role of the physical therapist assistant as it relates to differential diagnosis.
3. Identify and assimilate key communication strategies and techniques used in client management.
4. Explain common potential complications and identifiers related to the musculoskeletal, neuromuscular, cardiopulmonary, integumentary, and other systems.
5. Identify critical elements to communicate to the primary physical therapist and appropriate documentation of findings.

KEY TERMS

Assessment
Diagnosis
Differentiate
Evaluation
Examination
Infection
Intervention
Prognosis
Understanding

As evidenced by the continued growth patterns of the physical therapy profession and legislative and regulatory changes at the national and local levels, the physical therapist (PT) is emerging as a health care practitioner of choice for individuals who experience dysfunction with the interrelated movement systems of the body. In 2000, the American Physical Therapy Association (APTA) introduced the current vision of the physical therapy profession entitled Vision 2020, which includes the following sentence:

> By 2020, physical therapy will be provided by physical therapists who are doctors of physical therapy, recognized by consumers and other health care professionals as the practitioners of choice to whom consumers have direct access for the diagnosis of, interventions for, and prevention of impairments, activity limitations, participation restrictions, and environmental barriers related to movement, function, and health.[6]

An integral aspect of the physical therapy profession's vision is the scope of practice that involves **diagnosis.** Multiple sources have defined the term *diagnosis* as that which includes the commonalities of providing a label for the recognition of specific signs and symptoms and correlating this to an identifiable disease or disorder.[8,16,17,33] The process of diagnosis is far more complex than this simplistic overview implies. The methods used to determine an appropriate diagnosis must involve the practice of differentiating the multitude of often similar signs and symptoms into a specific pattern that guides the practitioner's choice of **intervention** and the eventual outcome of the episode of care.

Important Concepts

An integral aspect of the physical therapy profession's vision is the scope of practice that involves diagnosis.

Differential diagnosis is the process of carefully comparing and contrasting patient data points with the goal of appropriate exclusion and inclusion that terminates with the development of intervention strategies. This is a dynamic process that may result in minor alterations or significant shifts and revisions in the patient plan of care (POC).

> **Important Concepts**
>
> Differential diagnosis is the process of carefully comparing and contrasting patient data points with the goal of appropriate exclusion and inclusion that terminates with the development of intervention strategies.

Diagnosis is within the scope of practice for the PT and not the physical therapist assistant (PTA). However, the PTA must have an identifiable role in this activity to fulfill the requirements of the patient POC.[2,4] The purpose of this chapter is to provide the PTA with information that explains the process of differential diagnosis, the role of the PTA in this process, and definitive identifiers the PTA can use when determining the need for referral to the PT.

PATIENT CARE MANAGEMENT

Physical therapy is a unique body of knowledge that is provided only by qualified, trained, and credentialed PTs and PTAs under the direction and supervision of a PT. Although some legal jurisdictions and payer sources continue to require proof of collaboration between the PT and medical practitioner using a referral, PTs are rapidly progressing as autonomous health care practitioners. The basis for the roles and responsibilities of a PT and PTA related to patient care is contained within the core documents of the APTA, including, but not limited to, documents on standards of practice for physical therapy, criteria for standards of practice for physical therapy, code of ethics for PTs, and standards of ethical conduct for PTAs.

> **Important Concepts**
>
> Physical therapy is a unique body of knowledge that is provided only by qualified, trained, and credentialed PTs and PTAs under the direction and supervision of a PT.

The practice of physical therapy encompasses various aspects of acute, rehabilitative, and chronic phases of patient care with the focus primarily on the musculoskeletal, neuromuscular, cardiopulmonary, and integumentary systems. The PT and PTA have an integral role in primary, secondary, and tertiary care and prevention and the promotion of health, wellness, and fitness. The process of patient management has been outlined in the APTA *Guide to Physical Therapist Practice* (Fig. 3-1). The ultimate objective is a positive outcome that affects not only the individual but also the public as a whole.

The process of patient management begins with the **examination,** which has been described as a comprehensive screening that includes specific tests and measures.[8] The PT obtains a history using a communication

> **Important Concepts**
>
> The practice of physical therapy encompasses various aspects of acute, rehabilitative, and chronic phases of patient care with the focus primarily on the musculoskeletal, neuromuscular, cardiopulmonary, and integumentary systems.

cycle that attempts to procure data. The data collected lead the PT to formulate a postulate about the patient's potential impairment or functional deficit. A systems review follows that includes a screening of the anatomy and physiology of the appropriate systems and an **assessment** of the patient's communication abilities and certain mental capacities. The hands-on aspect of the examination involves specific tests and measures that are designed to assist in ruling in or ruling out the cause of the impairment or functional deficit. There are 26 common test and measure categories that have been identified in the *Guide to Physical Therapy Practice* (Box 3-1). It is imperative that the use of any tests or measures meets certain standards including high levels of reliability, validity, specificity, and sensitivity.

After the data have been collected, the PT must synthesize the information obtained during the examination and begin to develop clinical decisions in a process referred to as **evaluation.** During this procedure, the PT accounts for influencing factors that include, but are not limited to, the following:

BOX 3-1 Common Tests and Measures

- Aerobic capacity/endurance
- Anthropometric characteristics
- Assistive technology
- Balance
- Circulation (arterial, venous, lymphatic)
- Community, social, and civic life
- Cranial and peripheral nerve integrity
- Education life
- Environmental factors
- Gait
- Integumentary integrity
- Joint integrity and mobility
- Mental functions
- Mobility (including locomotion)
- Motor function
- Muscle performance (including strength, power, endurance, and length)
- Neuromotor development and sensory processing
- Pain
- Posture
- Range of motion
- Reflex integrity
- Self-care and domestic life
- Sensory integrity
- Skeletal integrity
- Ventilation and respiration
- Work life

Adapted from *Guide to physical therapist practice*, ed 2, with permission of the American Physical Therapy Association.

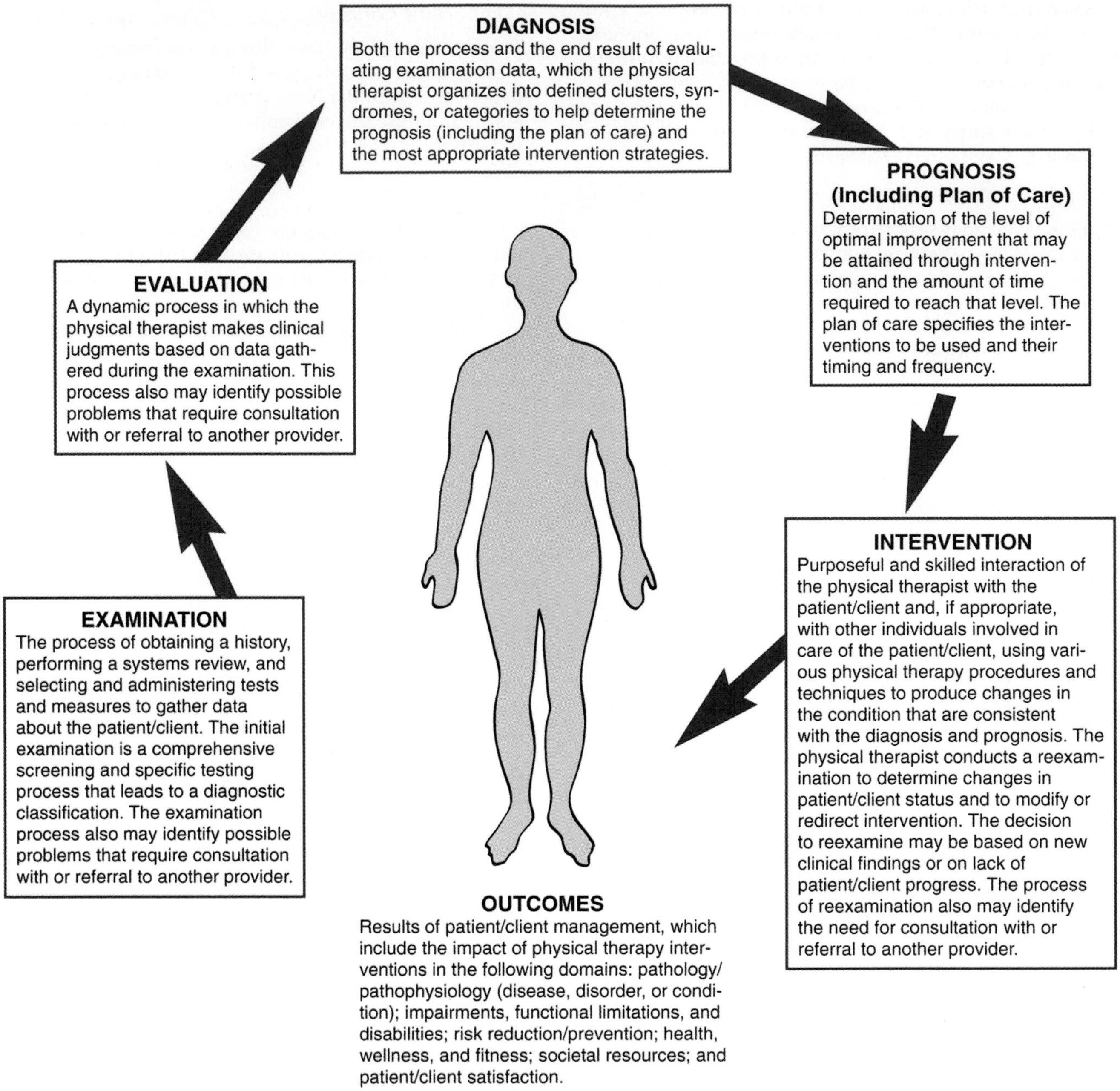

DIAGNOSIS
Both the process and the end result of evaluating examination data, which the physical therapist organizes into defined clusters, syndromes, or categories to help determine the prognosis (including the plan of care) and the most appropriate intervention strategies.

PROGNOSIS (Including Plan of Care)
Determination of the level of optimal improvement that may be attained through intervention and the amount of time required to reach that level. The plan of care specifies the interventions to be used and their timing and frequency.

EVALUATION
A dynamic process in which the physical therapist makes clinical judgments based on data gathered during the examination. This process also may identify possible problems that require consultation with or referral to another provider.

INTERVENTION
Purposeful and skilled interaction of the physical therapist with the patient/client and, if appropriate, with other individuals involved in care of the patient/client, using various physical therapy procedures and techniques to produce changes in the condition that are consistent with the diagnosis and prognosis. The physical therapist conducts a reexamination to determine changes in patient/client status and to modify or redirect intervention. The decision to reexamine may be based on new clinical findings or on lack of patient/client progress. The process of reexamination also may identify the need for consultation with or referral to another provider.

EXAMINATION
The process of obtaining a history, performing a systems review, and selecting and administering tests and measures to gather data about the patient/client. The initial examination is a comprehensive screening and specific testing process that leads to a diagnostic classification. The examination process also may identify possible problems that require consultation with or referral to another provider.

OUTCOMES
Results of patient/client management, which include the impact of physical therapy interventions in the following domains: pathology/pathophysiology (disease, disorder, or condition); impairments, functional limitations, and disabilities; risk reduction/prevention; health, wellness, and fitness; societal resources; and patient/client satisfaction.

FIG 3-1 The five elements of client management. *(Reprinted from* Guide to physical therapist practice, *ed 2 [revised], with permission of the American Physical Therapy Association. Copyright © 2003 American Physical Therapy Association.)*

1. Overall physical and mental health status
2. Specific phase of healing (acute, subacute, or chronic)
3. Severity of pathology
4. Involvement of singular or multiple sites or systems
5. Preexisting conditions or comorbidities

The PT must also consider information and data from additional sources, such as laboratory reports, radiologic reports, and referral sources (advanced nurse practitioners, chiropractors, dentists, physicians, physician assistants, allied health professionals, and employers). This type of information often is not provided to PTs who practice in non–institution-based facilities (i.e., private practices, school systems, or industrial settings).

The end result of the examination and evaluation process is the determination of a diagnosis. As previously stated, this process involves providing a label for the recognition of specific signs and symptoms and correlating this to an identifiable disease or disorder. There is a distinct difference between a medical diagnosis and the diagnosis determined by the PT. Medical practitioners provide a diagnosis that labels a disease or disorder at the cellular, tissue, organ, or system level. Examples of medical diagnoses with which patients present to PTs include low-back pain, shoulder pain, rotator cuff tear, fracture, and cerebrovascular accident. The difficulty with this type of diagnostic labeling is that it is often nonspecific and provides no information related to a patient's overall functional status. The physical therapy diagnosis focuses on the influences of the disease or disorder on the patient's functional status at the system level and the interrelationship between the systems and the person as a whole.[23]

The basis of developing an accurate diagnosis targets the ability of the PT to **differentiate** the data into a specific pattern that guides the practitioner's choice of intervention. Differential diagnosis requires a global **understanding** of the functions of all systems and how each interacts with and influences the others. This understanding requires critical thinking skills that culminate in a calculated intervention decision. Delaune[23] stated, "Very simply, it is problem solving." Problem solving involves data collection, formulation of a solution, application of the intervention, and assessment of the outcome. If the desired outcome is achieved, the problem is often considered solved. However, if the desired outcome is not achieved, the process of problem solving must be repeated. The ability to problem solve successfully involves the recognition of the need for a different solution or acknowledgment that the practitioner should reassess to determine if a different problem exists. The end result of the diagnostic procedure includes three potential solutions, as follows:

1. Specific evidence-based interventions for specific identified problems
2. Short-term interventions to reduce symptoms to allow reexamination that produces a more definitive diagnosis
3. Referral to an appropriate health care provider or alternative sources

Important Concepts

Differential diagnosis requires a global understanding of the functions of all systems and how each system interacts with and influences the others.

The classification schemes that result in a physical therapy diagnosis are called Preferred Practice Patterns and can be found in the APTA *Guide to Physical Therapist Practice*. Several resources agree that the development of this classification scheme is ongoing and requires research to assist with validating and ensuring the reliability and sensitivity of the diagnostic categories.[8,17,33] The APTA Guide explains that the development of a diagnostic classification system must meet certain standards and criteria, which include schemes that meet the intention of all laws, rules, and regulations for a profession; examination techniques that are allowable by statute; and interventions that meet the legal scope of practice. The Preferred Practice Patterns are based on the four systems most commonly addressed in physical therapy: musculoskeletal, neuromuscular, cardiovascular/pulmonary, and integumentary. The content of each pattern includes six sections covering the following:[7]

1. Client diagnostic classification—inclusion and exclusion diagnostic criteria
2. *International Classification of Diseases, Ninth Revision, Clinical Modification* codes—medical diagnostic codes that may relate to practice pattern
3. Examination descriptions
4. Evaluation, diagnosis, and prognosis descriptions
5. Intervention recommendations
6. Reexamination, outcome, and discharge descriptions

BOX 3-2 Typical Physical Therapy Interventions

- Coordination, communication, and documentation
- Client-related instruction
- Procedural interventions
  - Therapeutic exercise
  - Functional training in self-care and home management (including ADL and independent ADL)
  - Functional training in work (job/school/play), community, and leisure integration and reintegration (including independent ADL, work hardening, and work conditioning)
  - Manual therapy techniques (including mobilization/manipulation)
  - Prescription, application, and, as appropriate, fabrication of devices and equipment (assistive, adaptive, orthotic, protective, supportive, and prosthetic)
  - Airway clearance techniques
  - Integumentary repair and protection techniques
  - Electrotherapeutic modalities
  - Physical agents and mechanical modalities

ADL, activities of daily living.
Adapted from *Guide to physical therapist practice*, ed 2, with permission of the American Physical Therapy Association. Copyright © 2001 American Physical Therapy Association.

The therapist assimilates all of the information from the patient history, objective tests and measures, and diagnosis into a prediction of the outcome. The fourth element of patient management is known as **prognosis,** which involves the prediction of the outcome of the physical therapy episode of care with the establishment of the POC. The POC is initiated with the development of patient-based goals that address the problems exposed during the examination and evaluation. Each goal concentrates on a specific problem, provides a prediction of the desired outcome, is objective and measurable, and contains a definitive time frame. Interventions are then chosen.

Interventions are actions taken by the PT or PTA under the direction and supervision of the PT to facilitate improvement or resolution of the specified problems. Application of these activities requires skillful integration of physical and mental processes used to achieve the predicted and desired outcome. Typical physical therapy interventions from the APTA Guide are listed in Box 3-2.[8]

The intervention may involve collaboration with other health care providers or referral to a different health care provider or alternative sources. Consistent with all other processes of patient care management, interventions are dynamic in nature and require timely reexamination. Periodic reexaminations are performed to assess the changes produced by the interventions and the need to modify or redirect the POC. This process may reveal progress toward the predicted outcome, new clinical findings, or lack of progress that may require consultation with or referral to a different health care provider or alternative sources.

PHYSICAL THERAPIST ASSISTANT

Although the development of a physical therapy differential diagnosis is solely within the scope of practice of the PT, the PTA must possess a working knowledge of the methods and procedures of the diagnostic process and how this process directs the chosen interventions. Other chapters of this text discuss the basic role of the PTA in patient care that includes the provision of delegated interventions and monitoring the patient's responses. This role requires assessment skills that involve problem solving and clinical decision making that may result in appropriate immediate adaptations during a treatment session or collection of data that are reported to the primary PT resulting in the need for changes of the POC.

The definition of assessment includes the concepts of determination of an amount, size, or value.[37] The health care field definitions of assessment also include the methods of appraising the patient's condition, performing an interview, collection of objective data, and effectively communicating the information verbally and in writing. These skills are essential components of education and clinical training of the PTA and are outlined in several documents. *A Normative Model of Physical Therapist Assistant Education: Version 2007* profiles performance expectations that include data collection, formulation of a judgment or decision, and effective communication.[9] The APTA Guideline on minimum required skills of PTA graduates at entry level was developed in collaboration with physical therapy clinicians, educators, and policymakers.[10] This document clearly delineates the assessment skills the PTA must possess at entry level and how these skills directly and indirectly contribute to the differential diagnosis of the patient. A brief summary of the minimum required skills of PTA graduates at entry level is contained in Table 3-1. The APTA Standard on ethical conduct for the PTA further confirms the importance of assessment skills, as evidenced by Standard No. 3: "Physical therapist assistants

TABLE 3-1 Minimum Required Skills of Physical Therapist Assistant Graduates at Entry Level

PTA Skill Category	Description of Minimum Skills for PTA
Plan of care review	• Note indications, contraindications, precautions, and safety considerations for patient. • Monitor medical record for changes in medical status and medical procedures. • Collect data on patient's current condition, compare results with previously collected data and safety parameters established by PT, and determine if safety parameters have been met. • Communicate to PT when there are significant changes in patient's medical status; when there is physician referral; or when the criticality and complexity of patient are beyond the knowledge, skills, and abilities of PTA.

Provision of procedural interventions	• Ensure safety of patient and self throughout patient care:
	  • Identify need for and take action when safety of patient or self may be at risk or has been compromised.
	• Determine patient's response to intervention:
	  • Interview patient and interpret verbal and nonverbal responses accurately.
	  • Identify secondary effects or complications caused by intervention.
	  • Determine outcome of intervention (positive or negative), including data collection and functional measures.
	• Use clinical problem solving skills in patient care:
	  • Determine if patient is safe and comfortable with intervention and, if not, determine appropriate modifications.
	  • Compare results of intervention with previously collected data and determine if there is progress toward expectations established by PT or if expectations have been met.
	  • Determine if modifications to interventions are needed to improve patient response.
	• Modify interventions to improve patient response:
	  • Determine modifications that can be made to intervention within plan of care.
	  • Communicate with PT when modifications are outside scope of work or personal scope of work of PTA.
	  • Select and implement modification.
	  • Determine patient outcomes from modification.

Patient progression	• Identify changes in patient response as a result of intervention. • Recognize when other variables (e.g., psychological, social, cultural) appear to be affecting patient's progression with intervention.
Data collection	• Provide accurate, reproducible, safe, valid, and timely collection and documentation of data to measure patient's medical status and progress within intervention as indicated. • Provide timely communication to PT regarding findings of data collection techniques. • Recognize when intervention should not be provided or should be modified because of change in patient status.

PT, physical therapist; *PTA,* physical therapist assistant.
Adapted from *Guideline: minimum required skills of physical therapist assistant graduates at entry-level,* with permission of the American Physical Therapy Association.

shall make sound decisions in collaboration with the physical therapist and within the boundaries established by laws and regulations."[1]

The APTA Practice and Education Unit and PTA Services department have developed three algorithms that can be used as generalized guidelines that assist the PT with decisions on delegation of services to the PTA and the decision process for the PTA in referring the patient back to the PT (see Figs. 1-1 and 3-2).

Basic Assessment Skills

The basic skills required to begin the practice of assessment include observation, listening, manual proficiencies (range of motion [ROM], manual muscle testing [MMT], anthropometric measurements, and motor and sensory screening), and communication. Observation is the ability to incorporate visually all activities and events in a given environment and filter the information to incorporate the correct data as they relate to the task of assessment. This skill requires the discipline of avoiding "tunnel vision" or developing a preconceived notion or idea of what one expects to see or "thinks" he or she sees. A simple demonstration of this phenomenon is holding an object such as an ink pen in your hand at arm's length and describing all that you observe. If you simply answer "ink pen" you significantly narrowed and limited your observation skills. Successful observation with the assessment process requires a global viewpoint that can be isolated as needed to gather and direct the individual's decisions on what should be included and excluded. The PTA must develop the ability to filter properly distractions or data that do not pertain or are not essential to the task at hand.

Important Concepts

The basic skills required to begin the practice of assessment include observation, listening, manual proficiencies (ROM, MMT, anthropometric measurements, and motor and sensory screening), and communication.

Listening is a dynamic endeavor that requires dedication and effort. Listening is more than recognizing the "noise"; it involves interpreting the sounds carefully and accurately. Active listening requires mental and physical attributes that include, but are not limited to, the physiologic ability to hear sounds without dysfunction or disruption, the willingness to perform listening, interest in the person, and the knowledge to interpret the sounds accurately. A simple appraisal of active listening during a communication cycle with a patient is as follows: if the PTA hears his or her own voice more than the patient's voice, active listening is likely not being practiced or accomplished. The skills involved in active listening are listed in Box 3-3.

The PTA is educated and trained in a multitude of assessment skills that require manual proficiency and competence in activities including, but not limited to, ROM, MMT, anthropometric measurements, motor and sensory screening, and palpation. Mastery of these skills requires a comprehensive knowledge and understanding of the human anatomy and the ability to locate and isolate specified tissues accurately. It also requires the ability to differentiate tissue types and determine if changes have occurred. The PTA must develop an innate and enhanced awareness of the sensations encountered during palpation and integrate the information obtained with the other basic assessment skills to formulate a judgment regarding normality or abnormality. Although these manual skills require obvious physical capabilities, the mental aspects such as visualization, discrimination, accurate interpretation, and assimilation into a decision are equally critical to the process. These mental aptitudes are the cornerstone to the idea behind differential diagnosis.

BOX 3-3 Active Listening Skills

- Attentiveness (face patient, eye contact, open posture)
- Duplicate or restate (verify and express your understanding)
- Clarify
- Perception (correct interpretation)
- Summarize
- Interested (responsiveness)

Communication is the nucleus of effective, efficient, and quality patient care and includes verbal, nonverbal, and written exchanges. The algorithms featured in Figure 3-2 include communication as a keystone. The outcome of communication must be understanding. Without understanding, confusion ensues leading to potential harm to the patient and public. Communication involves an exchange that occurs between two or more sources and is cyclical in nature, meaning it must be a bilateral and not unilateral exchange (Fig. 3-3).

The communication sources must possess a level of affinity and reality to produce an exchange that results in understanding. The concepts of the definitions of affinity that are applied in this analogy include the view that the communication sources must possess a level of willingness to enter into and reciprocate an exchange. Examples of this concept are spouses, teachers and students, PTs/PTAs and patients, and PTs and PTAs. The success of communication significantly diminishes if the sources cannot or will not allow sufficient flow for the exchange to occur. Biases, fears, and dislikes are a few of the many human experiences and characteristics that interfere with the development of an appropriate level of affinity that allows successful communication. In addition, factors such as gender, culture, religious beliefs and values, political views, age, and education can positively or negatively affect the concepts of affinity and reality.

Reality involves the communication sources possessing a certain agreement on the topic with the exchange resulting in an understanding or additional exchange that ultimately ends with understanding. A common communication cycle in a physical therapy clinic that demonstrates a deficiency in the principle of reality involves patients seen for pain symptoms that occur in the posterior thigh. The physical therapy examination and evaluation process may lead to the determination of lumbar pathology as the basis for the symptoms. If the patient's reality of the symptoms is a problem with the hamstrings, the communication cycle between the patient and the therapist will not result in understanding.

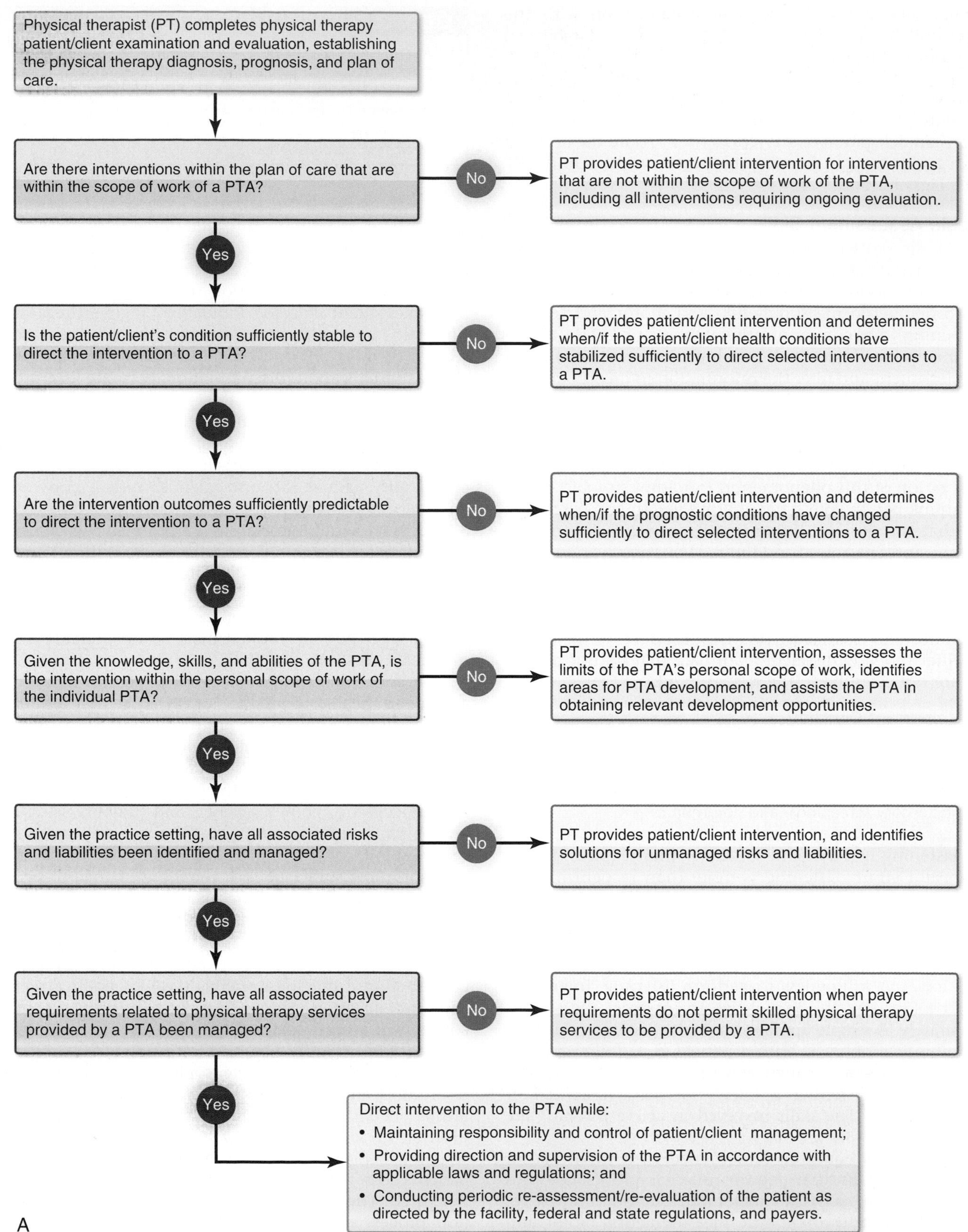

FIG 3-2 Algorithms charting the thinking process used by PTs to determine the appropriate direction and supervision of the PTA for optimal care. **A,** PTA direction algorithm. *(Modified from* PTinM. *2010;2(8):47-50, with permission of the American Physical Therapy Association.)*

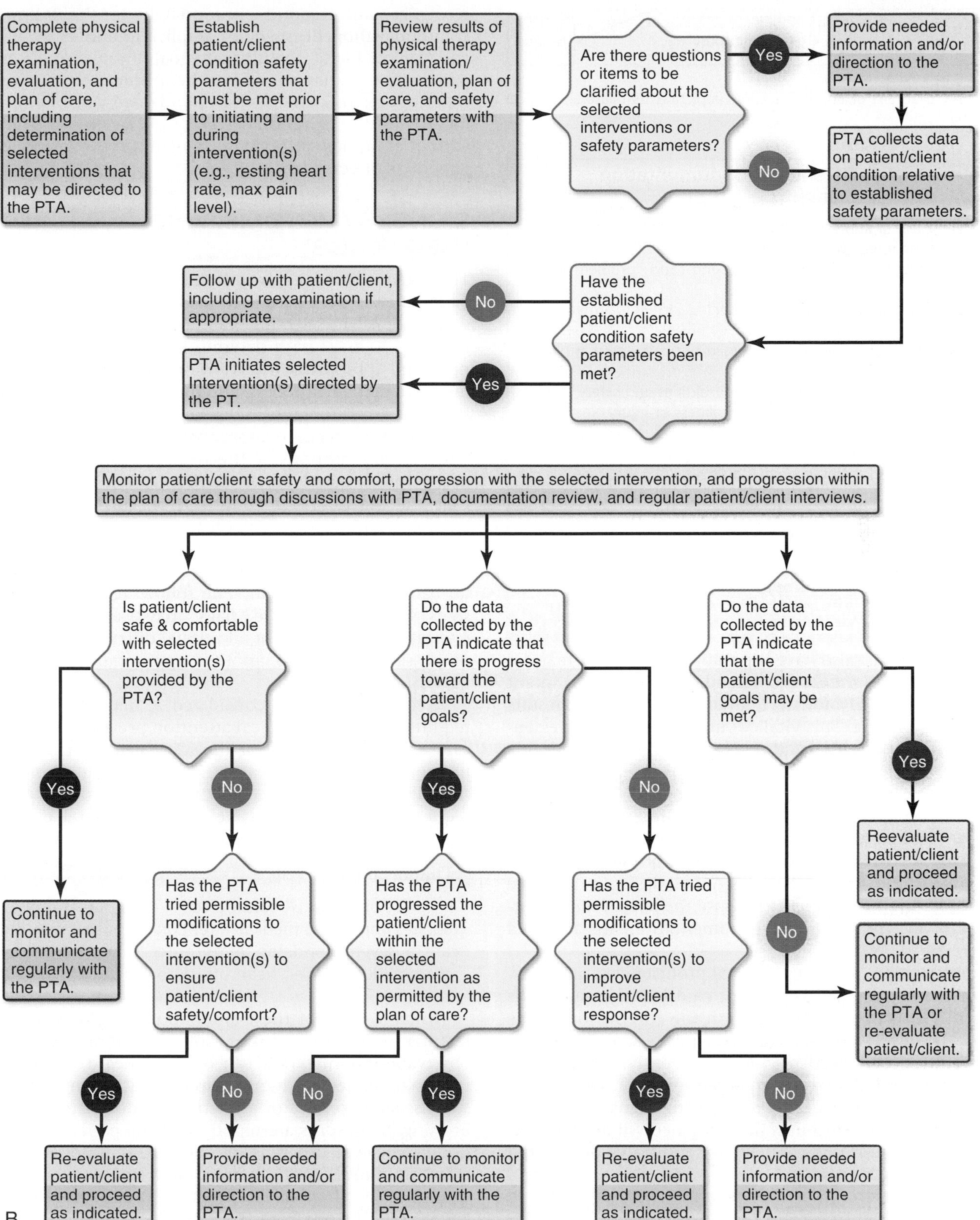

FIG 3-2, cont'd **B,** PTA supervision algorithm. *(Modified from Crosier J: PTA direction and supervision algorithms.* PT in Motion *9(2):47–50, 2010.)*

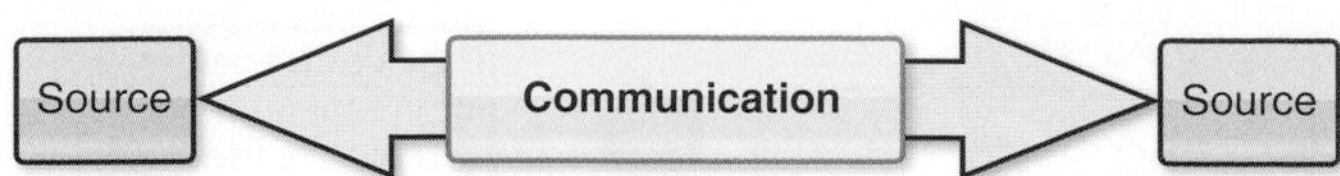

FIG 3-3 Diagram of communication depicting its bilateral, cyclical nature.

BOX 3-4 Defensible Documentation Elements

- Limit use of abbreviations
- Document legibly
- Document clinical decision-making and problem-solving process
- Document interventions connected to impairment and functional limitation
- Document interventions connected to goals stated in plan of care
- Document complications of comorbidities and safety issues
- Document nature and severity of illness or injury
- Document valid and reliable tests and measures as appropriate
- Document standardized tests and measures
- Document changes in client status
- Document factors that modify frequency and intensity of intervention and progression of goals

Adapted from *Defensible documentation for patient/client management* with permission of the American Physical Therapy Association. Copyright © 2012 American Physical Therapy Association.

The PTA must also have the ability to write in a manner that documents the data obtained during the assessment process completely and accurately in a format that results in understanding. This vital communication tool is essential for recording information that will be used from one session of care to another as well as for future episodes of care including the potential revision of the physical therapy diagnosis by the PT. In many clinical settings, this is the main communication that occurs between the health care team (PT and PTA, PT and physician, PT/PTA and nursing staff).[22,38] The APTA has designed multiple resources the PTA can use to ensure the appropriate information and procedure of documentation are achieved (Box 3-4).[3,5,8,11]

Observation, listening, manual proficiencies, and communication are essential patient care management skills the PTA uses to assist the PT with the completion of the POC. The PTA must possess the requisite knowledge and capabilities of effectively and efficiently reading the medical record, discerning and appropriately applying the correct interventions, and recognizing signs and symptoms or physical attributes that may necessitate the referral of the patient back to the PT for additional differential diagnostic interventions.

The purpose of this chapter and textbook is not to educate and train the PTA in the application of every differential diagnosis; rather, the intention is to provide the PTA with information in a general format that explains what types of potential complications may arise including any "red flags" or "yellow flags" related to the cardiopulmonary, neuromuscular, integumentary, musculoskeletal, and other systems. By virtue of having the ability to recognize and respond appropriately to the following common orthopedic specific complications and "red flags" and "yellow flags," the ultimate goal of safe and effective patient care management may be achieved. It is beyond the scope of this chapter to include every scenario; the focus is on the common scenarios a PTA may encounter with the fundamental management of the orthopedic patient as directed by the PT.

SIGNS, SYMPTOMS, AND "RED FLAGS"

The diagnostic process is initiated by obtaining a detailed patient history. The information garnered from the history guides the PT in selecting the most appropriate tests and measures to assist with determining the differential diagnosis and appropriate interventions. Health care management is a dynamic process, and the patient is in a constant state of flux. Some of these changes are predictable, whereas others seem to appear without warning or reason. The primary purpose of the examination process is to determine if, based on presenting signs and symptoms, the intervention is appropriate or consultation with another health care provider is warranted; if the intervention is not applicable, it is determined if the patient should be treated by another medical provider or requires a referral back to the physician. The following illustrations of signs, symptoms, and "red flags" may warrant immediate referral back to the PT for additional differential diagnosis or possible referral to another appropriate health care professional.

A condition that is considered a "red flag" problem requires immediate medical attention because it may indicate a severe condition or disorder, such as **infection,** inflammation, cancer, heart attack, or fracture (Table 3-2). A "yellow flag" condition identifies a disorder that may require caution with treatment but in general is not as serious as a "red flag" problem.

Important Concepts

A condition that is considered a "red flag" problem requires immediate medical attention because it may indicate a severe condition or disorder such as infection, inflammation, cancer, heart attack, or fracture.

A major focus of the examination should be the differentiation between signs and symptoms. Signs are observable findings that can be seen, heard, smelled, or shown to someone. Signs include swelling in a joint or soft tissue, deformity of a fracture, or discoloration from bruising. Symptoms are reported by the patient and may not be perceived otherwise by the PTA. Symptoms include pain, numbness and tingling, and fatigue. Symptoms cannot be seen by the PTA, and the examiner is reliant on an accurate history from the patient.

CONSTITUTIONAL AND SYSTEMIC SYMPTOMS

Constitutional symptoms are symptoms that affect the whole body and imply there is a possibility that a systemic disease or illness process exists.[31,41] Unchecked, these

TABLE 3-2 "Red Flags" = Immediate Need for Referral to Physician

Condition	Symptom
Cancer	• Bone pain with weight bearing • Constant pain anywhere in the body not relieved by change in position or activity • Loss of appetite • Persistent pain at night or pain that awakens patient • Unexplained weight loss (4.5-6.8 kg [10-15 pounds] in ≤2 weeks) • Unusual lumps or growths • Unwarranted fatigue
Cardiovascular (heart attack)	• Angina not relieved by rest or nitroglycerin • Diaphoresis (heavy sweating) • Dyspnea (shortness of breath) • High pulse rate that does not diminish with rest • Indigestion, nausea, vomiting, or sweating with chest symptoms • Pain or a feeling of heaviness or squeezing in the chest • Pain in the jaw, left shoulder, or arm or deep pain in between scapulae • Patient has doubts about condition • Persistent increase or decrease in blood pressure • Sensation of flutter, palpitations, irregular heart beat • Weakness, numbness, feeling faint
Diabetic	• Blurred vision • Change in mental alertness and function • Confusion • Fatigue and weakness • Fruity odor to breath • Lethargy • Muscle and abdominal cramping • Polydipsia (excessive thirst) • Polyphagia (excessive appetite) • Polyuria (excessive urination, especially at night) • Unstable blood sugars (normal = 80-120 mg/dL; safe = 100-250 mg/dL) • Weight loss with polyphagia
Gastrointestinal/genitourinary	• Blood in urine or stool • Change in or problems with bowel or bladder function • Frequent heartburn or indigestion • Frequent nausea or vomiting • Frequent or severe abdominal pain • Unusual menstrual irregularities
Neurologic (stroke or TIA)	• Changes in hearing • Changes in vision (e.g., blurriness or loss of sight) • Faint spells (drop attacks) • Frequent or severe headaches with no history of injury • Problems with balance, coordination, or falling • Problems with swallowing • Slurred speech • Sudden weakness in one arm or one leg
Miscellaneous	• Fever or night sweats • Recent severe emotional disturbances • Suspicion of pregnancy • Swelling or redness in any joint with no history of injury

TIA, transient ischemic attack.
Adapted from Goodman CC, Snyder TEC: *Differential diagnosis in physical therapy,* ed 4, St Louis, 2007, Saunders; Magee DJ: *Orthopedic physical assessment,* ed 6, St Louis, 2014, Saunders; and Stith JS, Sahrmann SA, Dixon KK, et al: Curriculum to prepare diagnosticians in physical therapy. *J Phys Ther Educ* 9:50, 1995.

symptoms can affect the general well-being of the patient and impede the progress of the physical therapy POC (Box 3-5). If any of these symptoms are noticed by the PTA, he or she should refer the patient directly back to the PT because the symptoms could indicate a condition outside the scope of physical therapy practice that requires timely referral to another medical provider.

Important Concepts

Constitutional symptoms are defined as symptoms that affect the whole body and imply there is a possibility that a systemic disease or illness process exists.

BOX 3-5 Constitutional Symptoms

- Diaphoresis (unexplained sweating)
- Diarrhea
- Dizziness/syncope (fainting)
- Fatigue (unexplained/unusual)
- Fever
- Malaise (feeling of discomfort, lack of health)
- Nausea
- Night sweats (can occur during the day)
- Pallor (paleness or lack of healthy color)
- Vomiting
- Weight loss (unexplained)

When certain signs and symptoms are present, the PTA must take immediate action for the safety of the patient. These signs and symptoms may be a prelude to or identify life-threatening situations such as myocardial infarction (heart attack), cerebrovascular accident (stroke), or transient ischemic attack (ministroke). If the PT is immediately available, he or she should evaluate the patient for referral to an appropriate health care provider. If the PT is not immediately available and the judgment is made that the patient must see a physician, the PTA should contact the patient's physician of choice or refer the patient to the nearest emergency department. Life-threatening situations should be handled by using local emergency services (call 911). "Red flag" symptoms for myocardial infarction, cerebrovascular accident, and transient ischemic attack include chest pain or discomfort; presence of irregular heartbeats such as arrhythmia or dysrhythmia; breathlessness or dyspnea; fainting (syncope); or unusual recent fatigue, cough, cyanosis, or edema.

Many systemic pathologies can mimic musculoskeletal pain. Although these symptoms sometimes seem similar, there are commonly small clues that can direct the PT or PTA to the correct diagnosis of the source of symptoms and pain. Care should be taken to attempt to delineate the subtle differences between systematic versus musculoskeletal pain patterns. For example, systemic conditions such as cancer would most likely not be altered, provoked, alleviated, or eliminated with movements of the body. However, musculoskeletal pain patterns can almost always be altered by movement (Table 3-3).

Important Concepts

"Red flag" symptoms for myocardial infarction, cerebrovascular accident, and transient ischemic attack include chest pain or discomfort; presence of irregular heartbeats such as arrhythmia or dysrhythmia; breathlessness or dyspnea; fainting (syncope); or unusual recent fatigue, cough, cyanosis, or edema.

VITAL SIGNS

A basic assessment method used by most health care professionals is monitoring vital signs. Vital signs provide an objective overview of the patient's cardiopulmonary function and body temperature. Factors that may influence vital signs include exercise, disease processes, infection, stress or emotional instability, environment, and age. Baseline data should always be obtained before the initiation of a POC and then monitored during the episode of care as indicated. Altered readings may precede an adverse response, and the underlying cause must be identified (Table 3-4).[12,43]

The normal reaction of the body to any injury or trauma is the development of an inflammatory response. Under normal conditions, the inflammatory response is well organized and follows a distinct pattern and timeline. In addition to the inflammatory response, if the individual's inherent defense systems are overtly stressed or overwhelmed, the opportunities for developing an infection become exponential. Individuals who have undergone surgical intervention for correction of a musculoskeletal pathology may be at risk. In 2% to 5% of patients undergoing orthopedic surgery, infection develops.[42] Some signs and symptoms of infection often mimic the signs and symptoms of inflammation, such as redness, edema, pain, and increased skin temperature (Box 3-6). It is imperative that visual observation of the involved area along with specific screening questions occur at each visit.

DEEP VEIN THROMBOSIS AND PULMONARY EMBOLISM

Another complication of a musculoskeletal injury, trauma, or surgical intervention is the potential for the development of a venous thrombosis. During the early inflammatory phase, an immediate vascular response results in constriction of the involved vessels. Within 1 hour of the injury, the clotting mechanism is facilitated to reduce and eliminate blood loss.[30] An abnormal response to this process involves the excessive collection of red and white blood cells along with fibrin resulting in a partial or complete occlusion of the vessel.[30,32] Superficial or deep veins may be affected, with the involvement of the deep veins being more common and producing a greater health risk (Box 3-7). Deep vein thrombosis (DVT) is the third most common cardiovascular disease process, occurring in 30% to 60% of all people who have undergone major surgery, with 90% of DVT occurring in the lower extremities (Box 3-8).[30] The major concern with all cases of DVT is the potential for a piece of the clot to break free and eventually travel to the small vessels of the heart resulting in a myocardial infarction, the pulmonary arteries resulting in reduced pulmonary function (pulmonary embolism) (Box 3-9), or the brain resulting in a cerebrovascular accident.

BOX 3-6 Signs and Symptoms of Infection

- Malaise
- Fever (temperature >100° F)
- Expanding redness or radiating streaks
- Increasing skin temperature
- Drainage (colored and smells)
- Increasing pain despite pain interventions
- Increased edema or joint effusion
- Loss of appetite, nausea, and vomiting
- Chills
- Night sweats
- Unexplained rashes

TABLE 3-3 Comparison of Systemic versus Musculoskeletal Pain Patterns

	Systemic Pain	Musculoskeletal Pain

Onset	• Recent, sudden
	• Does not manifest as observed for years without progression of symptoms
		• May be sudden or gradual, depending on history
		  • Sudden—usually associated with acute overload stress, traumatic event, repetitive motion; can occur as a side effect of some medications (e.g., statins)
		  • Gradual—secondary to chronic overload of affected part; may be present off and on for years

Description	• Knifelike quality of stabbing from the inside out, boring, deep aching • Cutting, gnawing • Throbbing • Bone pain • Unilateral or bilateral	• Usually unilateral • May be stiff after prolonged rest, but pain • Achy, cramping pain level decreases • Local tenderness to pressure is present
Intensity	• Related to degree of noxious stimuli; usually unrelated to presence of anxiety • Mild to severe • Dull to severe	• May be mild to severe • May depend on person's anxiety level—level of pain may increase in a client fearful of a "serious" condition
Duration	• Constant, no change, awakens person at night	• Duration can be modified by rest or change in position • May be constant but is more likely to be intermittent, depending on activity or position
Pattern	• Although constant, may come in waves • Gradually progressive, cyclic • Night pain • Location—chest/shoulder • Accompanied by shortness of breath, wheezing • Eating alters symptoms • Sitting up relieves symptoms (decreases venous return to heart—possible pulmonary or cardiovascular etiology) • Symptoms unrelieved by rest or change in position • Migratory arthralgias—pain/symptoms last for 1 week in one joint, then resolve and appear in another joint	• Restriction of active, passive, and accessory movements observed • One or more particular movements "catch" client and aggravate pain

Aggravating factors	• Cannot alter, provoke, alleviate, eliminate, or aggravate symptoms
	• Organ dependent (examples):
	  • Esophagus—eating or swallowing affects symptoms
	  • Heart—cold, exertion, stress, and heavy meal, especially when combined, bring on symptoms
	  • Gastrointestinal—peristalsis (eating) affects symptoms
		• Altered by movement; pain may become worse with movement, or some myalgia decreases with movement

Relieving factors	• Organ dependent (examples):
	  • Gallbladder—leaning forward may reduce symptoms
	  • Kidney—leaning to affected side may reduce symptoms
	  • Pancreas—sitting upright or leaning forward
		• Symptoms reduced or relieved by rest or change in position
		• Muscle pain relieved by short periods of rest without resulting stiffness except in the case of fibromyalgia; stiffness may be present in older adults
		• Stretching
		• Heat, cold

Continued

TABLE 3-3 Comparison of Systemic versus Musculoskeletal Pain Patterns—cont'd

	Systemic Pain	Musculoskeletal Pain

Associated signs and symptoms	• Fever, chills
	• Sweats (at any time day or night)
	• Unusual vital signs
	• Warning signs of cancer
	• GI symptoms—nausea, vomiting, anorexia, unexplained weight loss, diarrhea, constipation
	• Early satiety (feeling full after eating)
	• Bilateral symptoms (e.g., paresthesias, weakness, edema, nail bed changes, skin rash)
	• Painless weakness of muscles—more often proximal but may occur distally
	• Dyspnea (breathlessness at rest or after mild exertion)
	• Diaphoresis (excessive perspiration)
	• Headaches, dizziness, fainting
	• Visual disturbances
	• Skin lesions, rashes, or itching that client may not associate with musculoskeletal symptoms
	• Bowel/bladder symptoms
	  • Hematuria (blood in urine)
	  • Nocturia
	  • Urgency (sudden need to urinate)
	  • Frequency
	  • Melena (blood in feces)
	  • Fecal or urinary incontinence
	  • Bowel smears
		• Usually none, although stimulation of trigger points may cause sweating, nausea, blanching

From Goodman CC, Marshall C: *Recognizing and reporting red flags for the physical therapist assistant,* St Louis, 2015, Saunders.

TABLE 3-4 Vital Signs

Vital Sign	Resting Norms	Precaution with PT
Pulse	Adult = 60-100 bpm Child (1-7 years old) = 80-120 bpm Newborns (1-12 months old) = 100-130 bpm	• Slow or no increase during active exercise • Slow or no decline when activity intensity declines or ceases • Rhythm becomes irregular • Increase exceeds expected level • Resting heart rate >130 bpm • Resting heart rate <40 bpm • Increase in heart rate >220 – age
Blood pressure	Adult systolic = 90-139 mm Hg Adult diastolic = 60-89 mm Hg Infant systolic = 70-90 mm Hg Infant diastolic = 50-70 mm Hg	• Systolic should gradually increase with exercise • Systolic should return to normal 5-7 minutes after exercise ceases • Resting systolic 180-200 mm Hg • Increase in systolic >240 mm Hg • Decrease in systolic >20 mm Hg • Resting diastolic 105-110 mm Hg • Diastolic should remain unchanged • Diastolic change of 10-15 mm Hg is a concern
Respirations	Adults = 12-20 breaths/minute Infants (≤12 months) = 40-60 breaths/minute	• Dizziness • Dyspnea • Fatigue
Body temperature	Adults = 96.8° F-99.5° F	• >100° F • Stresses on cardiopulmonary system • Dehydration

From Meadows JT: *Orthopedic differential diagnosis in physical therapy—a case study approach,* New York, 1999, McGraw-Hill, p. 100. In Magee DJ: *Orthopedic physical assessment,* ed 6, St Louis, 2014, Saunders.

BOX 3-7 Signs and Symptoms of Superficial Vein Thrombosis

- Palpable cord (vein is hardened along its length)
- Redness
- Subcutaneous vein distention
- Warmth

Adapted from Goodman CC, Snyder TEC: *Differential diagnosis in physical therapy,* ed 4, St Louis, 2007, Saunders.

BOX 3-8 Signs and Symptoms of Deep Vein Thrombosis

- Discoloration or cyanosis (bluish hue)
- Pain or tenderness of affected area
- Pain with placement of blood pressure cuff around calf inflated to 160 to 180 mm Hg
- Positive Homans's sign (pain with gentle forced dorsiflexion)
- Unilateral tenderness or leg pain usually in calf
- Unilateral swelling (difference in leg circumference)
- Warmth of skin

Adapted from Goodman CC, Snyder TEC: *Differential diagnosis in physical therapy,* ed 4, St Louis, 2007, Saunders.

BOX 3-9 Signs and Symptoms of Pulmonary Embolism

- Anxiety, restlessness, apprehension
- Diffuse chest pain
- Dyspnea (shortness of breath)
- Fever
- Hemoptysis (bloody sputum)
- Persistent cough
- Pleuritic chest pain (sharp, localized)
- Possible sudden death
- Tachycardia (rapid pulse)
- Tachypnea (rapid, short breathing)

Data from Goodman CC, Snyder TEC: *Differential diagnosis in physical therapy,* ed 4, St Louis, 2007, Saunders. In Goodman CC, Fuller KS: *Pathology for the physical therapist assistant,* St Louis, 2012, Saunders.

Important Concepts

DVT is the third most common cardiovascular disease process, occurring in 30% to 60% of all people who have undergone major surgery, with 90% of DVT occurring in the lower extremities.

LYMPHEDEMA

Patients may develop chronic swelling of an area that leads to involvement of the entire extremity. This relatively benign process is referred to as lymphedema (Box 3-10). Accumulation of protein-enriched fluids may be secondary to a developmental disorder of the lymphatic system, known as primary lymphedema.[40] The more common type of this disorder is known as secondary lymphedema and is a direct result of obstruction or damage to the lymphatic system (nodes, vessels, and organs).[17,40]

BOX 3-10 Signs and Symptoms of Lymphedema

- Edema of an entire extremity (usually unilateral)
- Pain may or may not be present
- Paresthesias
- Skin is taut and shiny
- Stemmer's sign (taut skin on dorsum of foot)
- Worse with dependent positions

Data from Goodman CC, Snyder TEC: *Differential diagnosis in physical therapy,* ed 4, St Louis, 2007, Saunders. In Cameron MH, Monroe LG: *Physical rehabilitation for the physical therapist assistant,* St Louis, 2011, Saunders.

BOX 3-11 Signs and Symptoms of Orthostatic Hypotension

- Blurred vision
- Disorientation or confusion
- Fatigue
- Lightheadedness
- Loss balance
- Mental or visual blurring
- Nausea
- Sense of weakness or "rubbery" legs
- Syncope (faintness)

Adapted from Goodman CC, Snyder TEC: *Differential diagnosis in physical therapy,* ed 4, St Louis, 2007, Saunders. Adapted from Cleveland Clinic: Diseases and Conditions: Orthostatic hypotension. Available at: http://my.clevelandclinic.org/disorders/orthostatic_hypotension/hic_orthostatic_hypotension.aspx. Accessed July 24, 2012.

ORTHOSTATIC HYPERTENSION

Elderly patients or patients who have been on prolonged bed rest taking nitrates, hypertensives, diuretics, or antidepressants may exhibit symptoms of orthostatic hypotension (Box 3-11). Orthostatic hypotension is defined as a fall in systolic blood pressure of 20 mm Hg or more or a fall in diastolic blood pressure of 10 mm Hg when a patient moves from a lying position to an erect sitting or standing position or from sitting to standing.[19,33,36] This aberration in blood pressure is a deviation in the patient's ability to regulate blood pressure normally with these positional changes. When orthostatic hypotension is suspected, the PTA must obtain baseline blood pressure readings taken with the patient supine, sitting, and standing. Pulse rate, respirations, and oxygen saturations should also be obtained as well as observing and listening to the patient's responses. Appropriate safety precautions, including the use of a gait belt, additional assistance, and alerting others to the situation, should be followed.

Important Concepts

Orthostatic hypotension is defined as a fall in systolic blood pressure of 20 mm Hg or more or a fall in diastolic blood pressure of 10 mm Hg when the patient moves from a lying position to an erect sitting or standing position or from sitting to standing.

BOX 3-12 Signs and Symptoms of Anemia

- Dyspnea with exertion
- Fatigue
- Heart palpitations
- Listlessness
- Pallor (palms, nail beds)
- Rapid pulse

Data from Goodman CC, Snyder TEC: *Differential diagnosis in physical therapy,* ed 4, St Louis, 2007, Saunders.

Individuals who have undergone surgical correction of an orthopedic condition may experience changes in blood serum levels including abnormalities with oxygen-enriched erythrocytes (red blood cells). Anemia is a dysfunction that is a direct result of a reduction in the quality or quantity of erythrocytes. The resultant oxygen deficiency can lead to multiple tissue and organ disturbances that further impair an individual's healing capacity and overall functional capabilities (Box 3-12).

PULMONARY

The signs and symptoms outlined to this point have primarily involved the cardiovascular system. Elderly individuals and individuals in poor general health who have had a reduction in activity and mobility secondary to a musculoskeletal disorder or dysfunction may also become susceptible to pulmonary dysfunction or disease. Humans typically manage a certain level of bacteria, viruses, or fungi in the respiratory and digestive systems that present no danger to the individual's health. Immobility may lead to a reduction in the ability of the immune system to maintain healthy levels of these potentially infectious agents resulting in a pulmonary disorder or disease. A common insult to the pulmonary system is pneumonia, which is an inflammation of the lung tissues that creates excessive fluids resulting in difficulty breathing (Box 3-13). Patients may develop pneumonia secondary to increased levels of bacteria, viruses, or fungi.[30] Patients who have mobility compromise and weakness are also susceptible to aspiration of food, liquids, or regurgitated stomach contents, which may lead to pneumonia.[33]

BOX 3-13 Signs and Symptoms of Pneumonia

- Chills and fever
- Cyanosis
- Dyspnea
- Hacking cough
- Headache
- Malaise
- Productive cough (rust-colored or green sputum)
- Sudden and sharp pleuritic pain
- Tachypnea

Important Concepts

A common insult to the pulmonary system is pneumonia, which is an inflammation of the lung tissues that creates excessive fluids resulting in difficulty breathing.

Another pulmonary pathology that PTAs may encounter with children and athletic individuals is asthma. Asthma occurs when the bronchial airways become inflamed in response to allergens, infectious agents, pollutants, aspirin, and exercise.[30] The bronchi spasm or abnormally constrict resulting in the accumulation of excessive fluids and mucus. The patient develops a "panting"-type breathing pattern with a nonproductive, hacking cough. Paying close attention to the details of the patient history and asking specific questions related to this dysfunction can often prevent or reduce the severity of an asthma attack (Box 3-14).

BOX 3-14 Signs and Symptoms of Asthma

- Abnormal fatigue
- Cough (hacking, nonproductive)
- Cyanosis of fingernail and toenail beds
- Dyspnea (shortness of breath)
- Lips may be dark red
- Pale
- Prolonged expiration
- Speaks with short and panting phrases
- Wheezing (inspiration or expiration)

Adapted from Goodman CC, Fuller KS: *Pathology for the physical therapist assistant,* St Louis, 2012, Saunders.

Important Concepts

Asthma occurs when the bronchial airways become inflamed in response to allergens, infectious agents, pollutants, aspirin, and exercise.

BOWEL AND BLADDER

Appropriate management of a patient being seen in physical therapy after orthopedic surgery must include obtaining information about the bowel and bladder habits and function of the patient. Any complaints of pain in the lower back; pelvic region; or lower anterior, lateral, or posterior aspects of the abdominal area must be thoroughly investigated. Questions must be included about volume, color, consistency, odor, and symptoms the patient experiences during defecation or urination. Early detection and appropriate medical intervention assist in avoiding complications that may result in the need for additional hospitalizations (Box 3-15).

PSYCHOLOGICAL PROBLEMS

The PTA not only must possess the requisite knowledge and skills to recognize and acknowledge signs and symptoms of biologic or physiologic dysfunctions but also must develop the ability to recognize and acknowledge psychological characteristics that could enhance or impede the patient's progress. The key to having a patient provide adequate disclosure is the development of a trusting patient–health care provider relationship based on pure interest and devoid of evaluation. When interviewing the patient, questions related to sleep, fears, anxieties, stressors, and

BOX 3-15 Signs and Symptoms of Urinary Tract Infection

- Dyspareunia (pain during intercourse)
- Dysuria (painful urination)
- Fever and chills
- Flank pain
- Hematuria (blood in urine)
- Low-back pain
- Pelvic/lower abdominal pain
- Pyuria (pus in urine)
- Urinary frequency
- Urinary urgency

Adapted from Goodman CC, Fuller KS: *Pathology for the physical therapist assistant,* St Louis, 2012, Saunders.

BOX 3-16 Signs and Symptoms of Depression

- A sense of hopelessness
- Appetite loss (or overeating)
- Difficulty in concentrating, remembering, and making decisions
- Fatigue or decreased energy
- Feelings of guilt
- Frequent or unexplained crying spells
- Loss of interest or pleasure in ordinary activities
- Persistent sadness or feelings of emptiness
- Problems sleeping

Data from Goodman CC, Snyder TEC: *Differential diagnosis in physical therapy,* ed 4, St Louis, 2007, Saunders.

changes in personal behaviors or habits should be included (Box 3-16).

TABLE 3-5 "Red Flags" for the Low-Back Region

Condition	"Red Flags"
Back-related tumor	• Age >50 years • History of cancer • Unexplained weight loss • Failure of conservative therapy
Back-related infection (spinal osteomyelitis)	• Recent infection (e.g., urinary tract or skin infection) • Intravenous drug user/abuser • Concurrent immunosuppressive disorder
Cauda equina syndrome	• Urine retention or incontinence • Fecal incontinence • Saddle anesthesia • Global or progressive weakness in lower extremities • Sensory deficits in the feet (i.e., L4, L5, S1 areas) • Ankle dorsiflexion, toe extension, and ankle plantar flexion weakness
Spinal fracture	• History of trauma (including minor falls or heavy lifts for osteoporotic or elderly individuals) • Prolonged use of steroids • Age >70 years

Data from Deyo RA, Diehl AK: Cancer as a cause of back pain: frequency, clinical presentation, and diagnostic strategies. *J Gen Intern Med* 3:230–238, 1988; Deyo RA, Rainville J, Kent DL: What can the history and physical examination tell us about lower back pain? *JAMA* 268:760–765, 1992; Vanharanta H, Sachs BI, Spivey M, et al: A comparison of CT/discography, pain response and radiographic disc height. *Spine* 13:321–324, 1988; and Bigos S, Bowyer O, Braen G, et al: *Acute lower back problems in adults. Clinical practice guideline no 14*. AHCPR Publication No. 95-0642, Rockville, MD, 1994, Agency for Health Care Policy and Research, Public Health Service, U.S. Department of Health and Human Services. From Boissonnault WG: *Primary care for the physical therapist: examination and triage,* St Louis, 2005, Saunders.

MUSCULOSKELETAL

Low-Back Pain

Many patients present with a medical diagnosis of either spinal or peripheral joint musculoskeletal pathology. These conditions may be masking a deeper, more severe problem, and an astute PTA should pick up on the often subtle clues that the condition is a more serious medical condition mimicking a musculoskeletal condition. Serious conditions such as tumors, spinal infections, vertebral fractures, and cauda equina syndrome commonly manifest as typical low-back pain.[14] Significant "red flags" for patients presenting with low-back pain can be determined by obtaining a standard medical history and performing an adequate clinical examination (Table 3-5). Suspicion of a back-related tumor should be elevated as a patient ages. Incidences of back tumors are rare in younger patients; however, when one reaches age 50 years, the odds are increased that a back tumor may be the pathology. As with many tumors, a previous history of cancer, especially one that is metastatic, should arouse suspicion. In the presence of unexplained recent weight loss, pain at night, and inability to obtain a comfortable position, tumor or cancer type of pathology needs to be ruled out.[24] Infectious problems of the spine such as osteomyelitis are considered if the patient has had any other recent form of infection (e.g., postsurgical, cutaneous, urinary tract). Additionally, patients who have used intravenous drugs or have a concomitant immunosuppressive disorder that has caused a weakened immune system should be screened for infections.[14] Cauda equina syndrome is a serious condition that requires immediate medical attention.[24] Any injury to the lumbar spine that results in disk injury can result in pressure onto the cauda equina leading to a lumbar myelopathy. Saddle anesthesia (sensory deficits in the regions of L4-S1) (Fig. 3-4) and bowel or bladder dysfunction result.[45] Other "red flags" include a progressive weakness in the lower extremities including ankle dorsiflexors, plantar flexors, and toe extensors. Sensory deficits in the regions of L4-S1 also are common. Spinal compression fractures occur at a rate of 1.5 million per year in the United States.[13] Spinal fractures are usually the result of trauma; however, in individuals older than 70 years, the amount of trauma is relative and sometimes may be minimal. The higher the level of osteoporosis, the less trauma that is needed to fracture the spine. In elderly individuals with low levels of bone stock, injury can result from a very small fall or

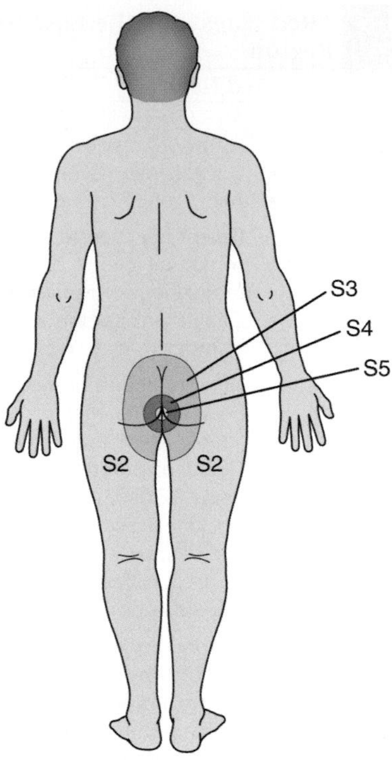

FIG 3-4 Saddle anesthesia. The S3, S4, and S5 nerves provide sensory innervation to the inner thigh, perineum, and rectum. *(From Magee DJ:* Orthopedic physical assessment, *ed 6, St Louis, 2014, Saunders.)*

from lifting or coughing. Additionally, prolonged use of steroids increases the risk of injury because of the weakening effect this medication has on inert tissues.

Important Concepts

In the presence of unexplained recent weight loss, pain at night, and inability to obtain a comfortable position, tumor or cancer type of pathology needs to be ruled out.

Pelvis, Hip, and Thigh

Serious medical conditions can be associated with the pelvis, hip, and thigh. Some conditions that need to be considered are colon cancer, femoral neck fractures, osteonecrosis of the femoral head, Legg-Calvé-Perthes disease, and slipped capital femoral epiphysis (Table 3-6). Cancer of the colon is common in men and women. It is more common in people older than 50 and who have a family history. Risk factors for colon cancer include obesity,[44] eating red meat,[20] cigarette smoking,[29] and alcohol consumption.[26] As with other cancers, a history of recent unexplained weight loss or the inability to alter hip pain via position or movement of the hip can be present. Other symptoms are changes in bowel movements including rectal bleeding or black stools. The stool is red if the lesion is near the rectum and black if the lesion is in the proximal colon.

Important Concepts

Risk factors for colon cancer include obesity, eating red meat, cigarette smoking, and alcohol consumption.

TABLE 3-6 "Red Flags" for the Pelvis, Hip, and Thigh Region

Condition	"Red Flags"
Colon cancer	• Age >50 years • Bowel disturbances (e.g., rectal bleeding, black stools) • Unexplained weight loss • History of colon cancer in immediate family • Pain unchanged by positions or movement
Pathologic fractures of femoral neck	• Older women (>70 years old) with hip, groin, or thigh pain • History of a fall from a standing position • Severe, constant pain worse with movement • Shortened and externally rotated lower extremity
Osteonecrosis of femoral head (also known as AVN)	• History of long-term corticosteroid use (e.g., in patients with RA, SLE, asthma) • History of AVN of contralateral hip • Trauma
Legg-Calvé-Perthes disease	• 5- to 8-year-old boys with groin/thigh pain • Antalgic gait • Pain symptoms aggravated with hip movement, especially hip abduction and IR
Slipped capital femoral epiphysis	• Overweight adolescent • History of recent growth spurt or trauma • Groin aching exacerbated with weight bearing • Involved leg held in external rotation • ROM limitations of hip IR and abduction

AVN, avascular necrosis; *IR,* internal rotation; *RA,* rheumatoid arthritis; *ROM,* range of motion; *SLE,* systemic lupus erythematosus.
Data from Busch MT, Morrissy RT: Slipped capital femoral epiphysis. *Orthop Clin North Am* 18:637–647, 1987; Stulberg BN, Bauer TW, Belhobek GH, et al: A diagnostic algorithm for osteonecrosis of the femoral head. *Clin Orthop Relat Res* 249:176–182, 1989; Suadicani P, Hein, HO, Gyntelberg F: Height, weight, and risk of colorectal cancer. An 18-year follow-up in cohort of 5249 men. *Scand J Gastroenterol* 28:285–288, 1993; Tronzo RG: Femoral neck fractures. In Steinburg ME, editor: *The hip and its disorders,* Philadelphia, 1991, Saunders, pp. 247–279; and Weinstein JN, McLain RF: Primary tumors of the spine. *Spine* 12:843–851, 1987. From Boissonnault WG: *Primary care for the physical therapist: examination and triage,* St Louis, 2005, Saunders.

Multiple problems can occur at the proximal femur. Of great concern is the fact that hip fracture in elderly adults is expected to increase by 50% by 2025 with the increasing elderly population in North America, Europe, and other industrialized regions.[18] Fractures of the femoral neck can occur in older patients, and is especially likely in patients older than 70 with hip, groin, or thigh pain. In contrast to cancers, a proximal hip fracture causes severe pain that is worse with movement or activity. The history for this injury is usually traumatic, such as from a fall. In elderly patients, a minor fall can result in fracture, and in some

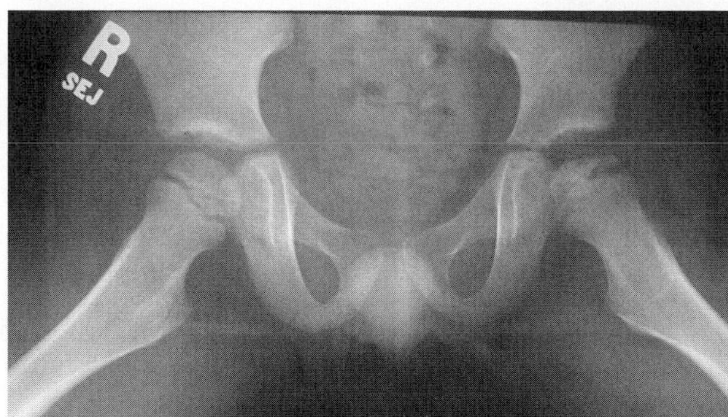

FIG 3-5 Legg-Calvé-Perthes disease of the left hip. *(From Cummings NH, Stanley-Green S, Higgs P:* Perspectives in athletic training, *St Louis, 2009, Mosby.)*

instances the fracture itself may have been what caused the fall. In this instance, the fracture is probably due to some disease process that has weakened the bone around the femur such as osteoporosis.

Another condition of the proximal femur is avascular necrosis of the femoral head. This condition is caused by a lack of blood flow to the femoral head. Avascular necrosis can be posttraumatic in nature following hip fractures or a dislocation or due to long-term use of corticosteroids in patients with rheumatoid arthritis or systemic lupus erythematosis. In a 58-year-old man with hip, pelvis, groin, or knee pain, this condition should be immediately ruled out. Pain is worse with hip movements, especially abduction and internal rotation. A similar condition that occurs in younger children is called Legg-Calvé-Perthes disease (Fig. 3-5). Affected children typically have limited hip ROM, especially abduction and internal rotation.[21] Weight bearing may or may not be painful. In adolescents, a common proximal hip condition is termed *slipped capital femoral epiphysis*. One typical clue to this diagnosis is that bilateral involvement almost always demonstrates hips to be in different stages of the disease.[21] This condition typically occurs in male patients more often than female patients and has a greater propensity to affect individuals who are overweight. Slipped capital femoral epiphysis is caused by a progressive displacement of the femoral head relative to the femoral neck secondary to a disruption of the growth plate. Groin and hip discomfort is more pronounced in weight bearing. Similar to Legg-Calvé-Perthes disease, slipped capital femoral epiphysis may also refer pain distally to the knee. Because the leg is held in an externally rotated position, the ROM of hip internal rotation is generally limited.

Knee, Leg, Ankle, and Foot

Potentially devastating injuries, such as arterial occlusive problems, DVT, compartment syndrome, sepsis, or cellulitis, can affect the knee, leg, ankle, and foot (Table 3-7). Arterial occlusive disease usually occurs secondary to atherosclerosis in the peripheral arteries. Risk factors for this condition are similar to the risk factors for heart disease and include smoking, type 2 diabetes, and a sedentary lifestyle. Arterial occlusive disease is typically not a problem of younger individuals and more commonly affects individuals older than 50. When the condition is severe, the patient may exhibit a cool distal extremity on the affected side. Additionally, the clinician may be able to observe decreased pedal pulses of the posterior tibial artery and dorsalis pedis artery. Care should be taken because these pulses are hard to find in many people. Finally, a prolonged arterial filling time may be observed

TABLE 3-7 "Red Flags" for the Knee, Leg, Ankle, or Foot Region

Condition	"Red Flags"
Peripheral arterial occlusive disease	• Age >60 years • History of type 2 diabetes • History of ischemic heart disease • Smoking history • Sedentary lifestyle • Concurrent intermittent claudication • Unilaterally cool extremity • Decreased pedal pulses—posterior tibial artery, dorsalis pedis artery • Prolonged venous filling time • Abnormal ankle-to-arm systolic pressure
Deep vein thrombosis	• Calf pain, edema, tenderness, and warmth • Calf pain that is intensified with standing or walking and relieved by rest and elevation • Recent surgery, malignancy, pregnancy, trauma, or leg immobilization
Compartment syndrome	• History of blunt trauma, crush injury, or unaccustomed exercise • Severe, persistent leg pain that is intensified with stretch applied to involved muscles • Swelling, exquisite tenderness, and palpable tension (hardness) of involved compartment • Paresthesia, paresis, and pulselessness
Septic arthritis	• Constant aching or throbbing pain, joint swelling, tenderness, warmth • History of recent infection, surgery, or injection • Coexisting immunosuppressive disorder
Cellulitis	• Pain, skin swelling, warmth, and advancing irregular margin of erythema/reddish streaks • Fever, chills, malaise, and weakness • History of recent skin ulceration or abrasion, venous insufficiency, CHF, or cirrhosis

CHF, Congestive heart failure.
Data from Boyko EJ, Ahroni JH, Davignon D, et al: Diagnostic utility of the history and physical examination for peripheral vascular disease among patients with diabetes mellitus. *J Clin Epidemiol* 50:659–668, 1997; McGee SR, Boyko EJ: Physical examination and chronic lower-extremity ischemia: a critical review. *Arch Intern Med* 158:1357–1364, 1998; and Wells K: Nephrolithiasis with unusual initial symptoms. *J Manipulative Physiol Ther* 23:196–205, 2000. From Boissonnault WG: *Primary care for the physical therapist: examination and triage,* St Louis, 2005, Saunders.

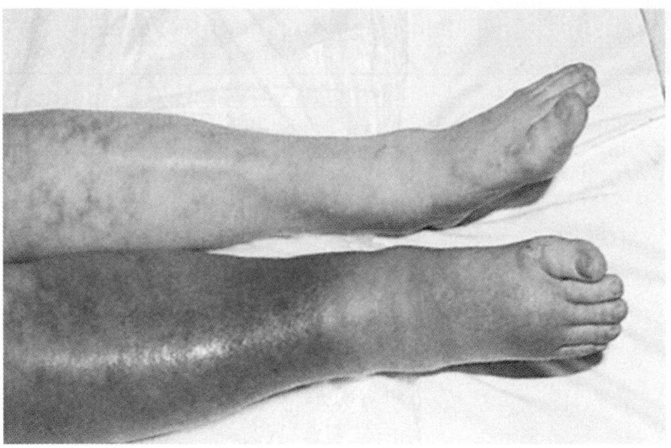

FIG 3-6 Deep vein thrombosis. *(From Moser D, Riegel B:* Cardiac nursing, *Philadelphia, 2007, Saunders.)*

when assessing revascularization. Revascularization is assessed by pressing the nail bed of one of the toes and visually watching how long it takes for the nail to go from whitened to become reperfused with blood. A normal capillary filling time is within 3 seconds.

A DVT should always be taken seriously, and the PTA should always err on the side of caution in assessment. This occlusive venous condition is commonly caused by immobilization from recent surgery or trauma. However, pregnancy and malignancy may also cause a thrombosis. DVT manifests with pain in the posterior calf that increases with the dependent position and weight bearing and is relieved with rest and elevation. Pain in the calf is also accompanied by swelling, edema, tenderness, warmth, and sometimes discoloration (Fig. 3-6). In 50% of people who have a DVT, no pain is noted. The primary concern with DVT is that the thrombosis may dislodge and move proximal to the lungs to create a pulmonary embolism.

Compartment syndrome usually occurs after significant trauma to the leg or following repetitive exercise. Compartment syndrome following blunt trauma or crushing-type injuries is more serious than the exercise-induced form. In the context of trauma, this is usually a medical emergency, and treatment with fasciotomy should be performed as soon as possible to save the limb. The swelling that occurs is usually extreme with significant persistent pain. The involved compartment is generally very hard or firm to palpate. If swelling is severe enough, loss of sensation, paresis, and loss of peripheral pulse can occur.

Athletes can develop chronic exertional compartment syndrome secondary to accumulation of fluid within the interstitial space of skeletal muscle, especially during repetitive stressful activities. This increase of interstitial fluid combined with a limited ability to expand the fascial compartments can lead to elevated intramuscular pressures, causing capillary occlusion.[43] The decreased blood flow owing to occlusion can result in eventual cell death if left untreated. Although risk factors are inconclusive, it is thought that landing mechanics, muscle composition, and capillary density all may play a role in exercise-induced exertional compartment syndrome.[27]

Septic arthritis and cellulitis are disorders associated with infections. Septic arthritis is a serious bacterial infection of the joint. The joint is usually swollen, warm, reddish in color, and tender to palpate. This infection most commonly occurs in larger joints such as the knees and hips, although other smaller joints, including the temporomandibular joint, can be affected.[28] Cellulitis is an infection of skin and superficial tissues usually caused by an infection following bacterial inhabitation of a wound. This infection is observed by signs and symptoms including localized pain, swelling, reddish discoloration, and warmth of tissues. Affected individuals may also have fever, chills, malaise, and weakness.

Thoracic Spine

Because of the close proximity of the thoracic spine to the internal organs of the body, many problems can create spinal symptoms. These problems can occur in the heart, lungs, stomach, and kidneys (Table 3-8).

A heart attack or myocardial infarction caused by a blockage of the coronary arteries resulting in the death of heart muscle can cause symptoms such as pain in the left chest or arm. Other symptoms can be pressure, tightness, or squeezing in the neck or jaw. These symptoms are classically referred to as angina or heart pain. Risk factors for cardiac arrest include history of previous heart attack, diabetes, increased age, female sex, smoking, high blood pressure, and history of congestive heart failure or stroke. Angina or chest pain can be described as either unstable or stable. Unstable angina does not occur in a predictable pattern and is not as responsive to nitroglycerin, whereas stable angina does occur with predictable patterns and is responsive to medication.

> **Important Concepts**
>
> Because of the close proximity of the thoracic spine to the internal organs of the body, many problems can create spinal symptoms. These problems can occur in the heart, lungs, stomach, and kidneys.

The pericardium is the sac or covering over the heart, and when this becomes inflamed it is called pericarditis. When the pericardium is inflamed secondary to disease or other conditions, the heart is unable to work at optimal levels resulting in less blood able to leave the heart. Oxygenation of tissues is decreased because of less blood leaving the heart. This condition usually results in emergency treatment to remove pressure on the heart. Causes of pericarditis include inflammation by bacterial, viral, or systemic disease such as kidney failure, systemic lupus, and rheumatoid disease or any other problem causing increased fluid around the heart.

A pulmonary embolism can result from a dislodged blood clot from the calf or lower leg (Fig. 3-7). The pulmonary embolism causes chest pain similar to a myocardial infarction as well as shoulder pain and upper abdominal pain. The patient presents with a loss of breath, dyspnea, wheezing, and a decrease in blood pressure. Pulmonary embolism is also a medical emergency.

TABLE 3-8 "Red Flags" for the Thoracic Spine and Rib Cage Region

Condition	"Red Flags"
Myocardial infarction	• Chest pain • Pallor, sweating, dyspnea, nausea, and palpitations • Presence of risk factors: previous history of coronary artery disease, hypertension, smoking, diabetes, elevated blood serum cholesterol (>240 mg/dL) • Men >40 years old, women >50 years old • Symptoms lasting >30 minutes and not relieved with sublingual nitroglycerin
Unstable angina pectoris	• Chest pain that occurs outside of a predictable pattern • Not responsive to nitroglycerin
Stable angina pectoris	• Chest pain/pressure that occurs with predictable levels of exertion • Symptoms are predictably alleviated with rest or sublingual nitroglycerin
Pericarditis	• Sharp/stabbing chest pain that may be referred to lateral neck or either shoulder • Increased pain with left-side lying • Relieved with forward lean while sitting (supporting arms on knees or a table)
Pulmonary embolus	• Chest, shoulder, or upper abdominal pain • Dyspnea • History of or risk factors for developing deep vein thrombosis
Pleurisy	• Severe, sharp, knifelike pain with inspiration • Dyspnea, decreased chest wall excursion • History of recent or concurrent respiratory disease (e.g., infection, pneumonia, tumor, tuberculosis)
Pneumothorax	• Chest pain, intensified with inspiration • Difficulty ventilating or expanding rib cage • Recent bout of coughing or strenuous exercise or trauma • Hyperresonance on percussion • Decreased breath sounds
Pneumonia	• Pleuritic pain, may be referred to shoulder • Fever, chills, headaches, malaise, and nausea • Productive cough
Cholecystitis	• Colicky pain in right upper abdominal quadrant with accompanying right scapular pain • Symptoms may worsen with ingestion of fatty foods • Symptoms not increased by activity or relieved by rest
Peptic ulcer	• Dull or gnawing pain or "burning" sensation in epigastrium, mid-back, or supraclavicular regions • Symptoms relieved with food • Localized tenderness at right epigastrium • Constipation, bleeding, vomiting, tarry stools, and coffee-ground emesis
Pyelonephritis	• Recent or coexisting urinary tract infection • Enlarged prostate • Kidney stone or past episode of kidney stone
Nephrolithiasis (kidney stones)	• Sudden, severe back or flank pain • Chills, fever, nausea, and vomiting • Renal colic • Symptoms of urinary tract infection • Residence in hot and humid environment • Past episodes of kidney stone; 50% of patients experience recurrence

From Boissonnault WG: *Primary care for the physical therapist: examination and triage,* St Louis, 2005, Saunders.

Important Concepts

Unstable angina does not occur in a predictable pattern and is not as responsive to nitroglycerin, whereas stable angina does occur with predictable patterns and is responsive to medication.

Another lung problem termed *pleurisy* is due to an inflammation of the lining of the lungs. A deep inspiration creates a knifelike sharp pain in the chest. Another lung condition is a pneumothorax, in which air is brought into the lungs by a rupture in the lung lining wall. In elderly individuals, pneumothorax can occur spontaneously after a cough or strenuous physical activity. Factors that predispose one to a pneumothorax include menstruation, asthma, chronic obstructive lung disease, cystic fibrosis, and lung cancer. Finally, pneumonia is common, especially in younger and older populations, and is due to a bacterial or viral infection of the lungs. Symptoms of pneumonia include chest pain and cough with sputum that may have varied colors from light green to dark brown. Patients with pneumonia are also likely to exhibit chills, fever, nausea, or vomiting.

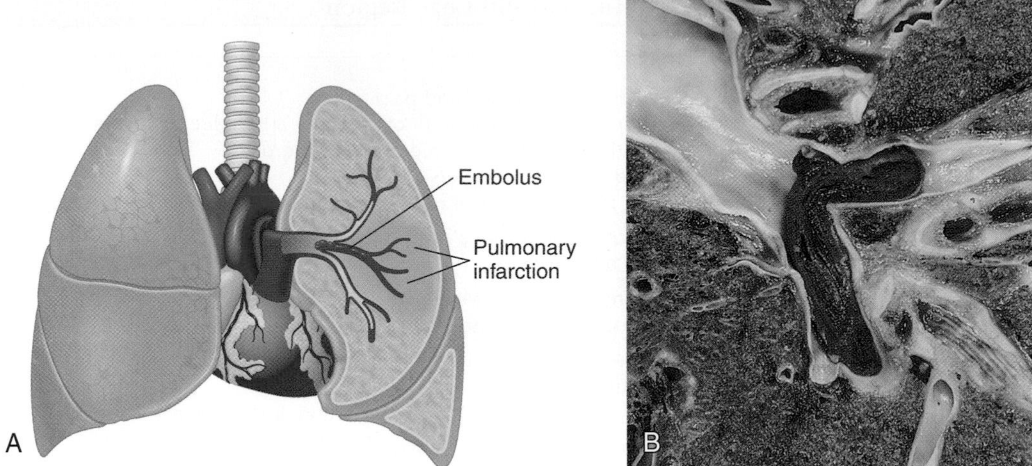

FIG 3-7 **A** and **B,** Pulmonary embolism. *(From Chabner D:* The language of medicine, *ed 8, St Louis, 2007, Saunders.)*

Several forms of gastrointestinal disorders can cause spinal pain, including ulcers and cholecystitis. Ulcers are lesions in the stomach or intestinal tract lining. These generally occur as a result of excessive digestive acids that eat away at the lining of the tract. Ulcers cause dull, aching, or burning pain. Relief is usually temporary and best when eating. Pain is worse with an empty stomach. Cholecystitis is an inflammation of the gallbladder. This condition causes pain in the right upper abdominal quadrant or the interscapular or right scapular region. Pain can be severe and is not relieved with traditional therapy.

Kidney problems include pyelonephritis and nephrolithiasis. All kidney problems may create pain in the posterior upper lumbar or lower thoracic region. This area includes what a therapist may call the flank area. Pyelonephritis is caused by an infection in the kidney and can occur in patients with recent urinary tract infections. Nephrolithiasis refers to the formation of kidney stones. Kidney stones are hard masses of salt precipitate that comes from urine. Risk factors for stones include certain foods, caffeine, and diseases that cause high cell turnover.

Shoulder and Neck

Patients with pain in the shoulder and neck area constitute a huge proportion of patients with general musculoskeletal conditions seen by PTs.[15,25,34] Conditions to assess for "red flags" in the shoulder and cervical spine include central cord syndromes, ligamentous instability, brachial plexus neuropathies, and tumors (Table 3-9). Just as in the thorax region, a myocardial infarction can refer symptoms to the shoulder and jaw area. These similar symptoms and causes were described previously.

Cervical spine ligamentous instability may cause neck pain secondary to possible cord compromise. These injuries are usually higher level traumatic injuries such as falls or motor vehicle accidents. However, some individuals may be prone to cervical ligamentous instability, such as individuals with rheumatoid arthritis, Down syndrome, or ankylosing spondylitis. If unsure, the PTA should have the supervising PT rule out instability of the alar and transverse ligaments via special physical examination tests. The symptoms caused by cervical instability include tingling, numbness, weakness, and burning pain in one or more extremities. Dizziness, vertigo, and nystagmus associated with head or neck movements may also be present in an individual affected with instability.

Important Concepts

Conditions to assess for "red flags" in the shoulder and cervical spine include central cord syndromes, ligamentous instability, brachial plexus neuropathies, and tumors.

Upper extremity peripheral neuropathy secondary to peripheral nerve entrapment can be difficult to identify. Initially, an ordinary overuse problem may appear to be present. These entrapments can affect sensory, motor, or mixed nerve distributions. The pain caused by these entrapments is not always well localized, is usually present at rest and with activity, and may have a retrograde distribution. There may or may not be atrophy of the affected muscles depending on the chronicity of the entrapment. However, the affected muscle may be very tender to palpate giving the illusion that this is a purely muscular strain. The main upper extremity nerves that can become affected include the spinal accessory nerve, axillary nerve, long thoracic nerve, and suprascapular nerve.

A spinal accessory nerve injury should be suspected in patients who present with weakness in shoulder abduction and scapular elevation. The patient may appear to have a drooped shoulder and present with dull aching shoulder pain (Fig. 3-8). This injury can occur as a result of direct trauma to the neck or head or neck cancer.[35] A common mechanism in athletes is a traction injury that can occur during tackling; this can occur as a physical stress depresses the shoulder while laterally flexing the neck toward the opposite side which can create enough traction to cause injury.

TABLE 3-9 "Red Flags" for the Cervical Spine and Shoulder Region

Condition	"Red Flags"
Myocardial infarction	• Chest pain • Pallor, sweating, dyspnea, nausea, and palpitations • Presence of risk factors: previous history of coronary artery disease, hypertension, smoking, diabetes, elevated blood serum cholesterol (>240 mg/dL) • Men >40 years old, women >50 years old
Cervical ligamentous instabilities with possible cord compromise	• Major trauma such as a motor vehicle accident or a fall from a height • Rheumatoid arthritis or ankylosing spondylitis • Oral contraceptive use • Long tract neurologic signs especially present in more than one extremity, dizziness, nystagmus, vertigo with head/neck movements and positions, clonus, and positive Babinski's sign
Cervical and shoulder girdle peripheral entrapment neuropathies	• Paresthesias • Pain present at rest and possibly with retrograde distribution • Muscles innervated can be tender to palpate • Muscles and sensory distribution follow specific nerve pattern
Spinal accessory nerve	• Weakness of shoulder abduction • Inability to shrug shoulders • Dull pain, weakness, and drooping of shoulder • Lack of scapular stabilization
Axillary nerve	• Weakness of shoulder abduction and flexion • Lack of sensation of lateral aspect of upper arm
Long thoracic nerve	• Serratus anterior weakness with scapular winging • Loss of scapulohumeral rhythm
Suprascapular nerve	• Presentation similar to rotator cuff tear because of wasting of supraspinatus or infraspinatus muscles • Loss of strength in abduction and external rotation of shoulder • Pain is deep and poorly localized
Pancoast's tumor* (superior sulcus lung tumor)	• Men >50 years old with history of cigarette smoking • "Nagging"-type pain in shoulder and along the vertebral border of scapula • Pain that has progressed from nagging to burning in nature, often extending down arm and into ulnar nerve distribution

*Data from Spengler D, Kirsh M, Kaufer H: Orthopaedic aspects and early diagnosis of superior sulcus lung tumor. *J Bone Joint Surg Am* 55:1645–1650, 1973.
From Boissonnault WG: *Primary care for the physical therapist: examination and triage,* St Louis, 2005, Saunders.

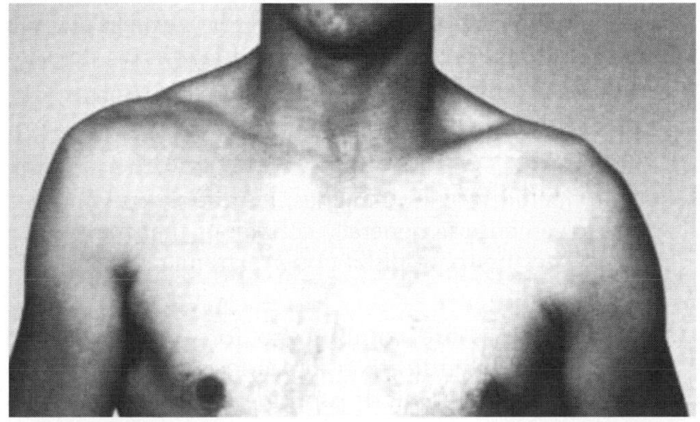

FIG 3-8 Atrophy of the left trapezius muscle secondary to spinal accessory nerve injury. *(From Skirven TM, Osterman AL, Fedorczyk JM, et al:* Rehabilitation of the hand and upper extremity, *ed 6, Philadelphia, 2011, Mosby.)*

Important Concepts

A spinal accessory nerve injury should be suspected in patients who present with weakness in shoulder abduction and scapular elevation.

A patient with axillary nerve damage presents with weakness of shoulder abduction and flexion. This injury is common after a glenohumeral dislocation because there is traction placed on the nerve during the dislocation. In some instances, there may also be a loss of light touch sensation in the area of the upper lateral shoulder. A long thoracic nerve injury can create a dramatic loss of shoulder strength because the patient presents with significant serratus anterior weakness, which causes scapulothoracic winging and a loss of normal overhead kinematics. These injuries are also generally due to traction of the upper extremity or from trauma to the lateral chest wall where the nerve is more superficial in location. In other cases, the injury occurs secondary to an asynchronous motion of the arm and scapula during athletics while missing a shot in golf, tennis, or handball. The scapular winging and altered scapulohumeral rhythm are observed during overhead lifting or during a physical test such as a wall push-up, which elicits high electromyographic activity of the serratus anterior.

Important Concepts

A patient with axillary nerve damage presents with weakness of shoulder abduction and flexion.

The suprascapular nerve can be injured as a result of trauma or compression or traction (Fig. 3-9). This injury is very hard to diagnose because it mimics a standard rotator cuff injury as a result of weakness and, if chronic, wasting of the supraspinatus or infraspinatus muscles. Pain is poorly localized because this nerve is a motor nerve that is located deep in the shoulder. The nerve runs through the suprascapular notch that is roofed by the transverse scapular ligament and gives off innervation for the supraspinatus muscle. It continues around the lateral border of the spine of the scapula and passes through the spinoglenoid notch to reach the infraspinatus. If the nerve is compressed or injured at the suprascapular foramen, the supraspinatus and the infraspinatus are affected. However, if the injury occurs at the spinoglenoid notch, only the infraspinatus is affected.

Pancoast's tumor is a malignant tumor that is located in the upper apices of the lung. This tumor is more common in men older than 50. Despite the tumor being in such close proximity to the lung, patients usually complain of pain more than pulmonary symptoms.[46]

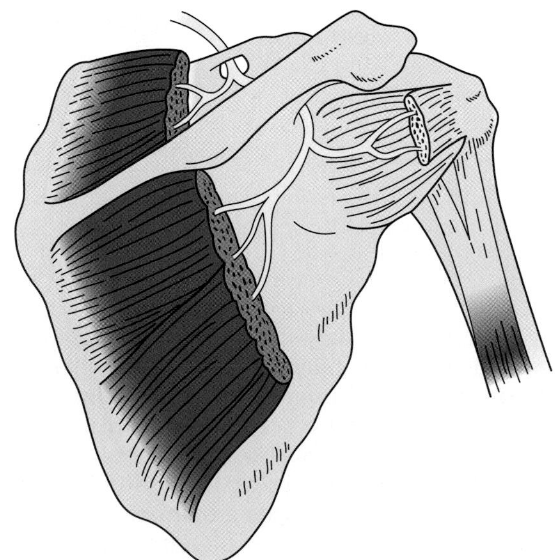

FIG 3-9 Mechanism of injury in compression of the suprascapular nerve. *(Modified from Raj PP, Lou L, Erdine S, et al:* Interventional pain management: image-guided procedures, *ed 2, Philadelphia, 2008, Saunders.)*

Important Concepts

A long thoracic nerve injury can create a dramatic loss of shoulder strength because the patient presents with significant serratus anterior weakness, which causes scapulothoracic winging and a loss of normal overhead kinematics.

Elbow, Forearm, and Hand

While performing a differential diagnosis screening for the elbow, forearm, and hand, one does not usually find conditions as serious as those found in more proximal areas of the body. Multiple fractures, tendon injuries, infections, and neurologic involvement are generally conditions that may elicit "red flags" in the more distal upper extremities (Table 3-10).

Most fractures in the upper extremities are due to injuries resulting from falls on an outstretched hand (FOOSH). One must always keep fractures in mind after a FOOSH injury because they are not always displaced fractures that are more easily picked up by simple visual inspection. These injuries are often nondisplaced and require radiographs to rule in or out. These injuries can happen to anyone, but they are more common in elderly individuals secondary to osteoporosis. An individual susceptible to injury is anyone with a history of repetitive steroid use or any pathology caused by slow bone repair. After a FOOSH injury, if the patient is unable to supinate or pronate the forearm without proximal elbow pain, a radial head fracture or dislocation should be suspected. After the injury, the patient holds the arm and hand near the body in a protected position. Colles' fracture is a fracture of the distal radius that has localized distal swelling with pain during active wrist movements in most directions but especially flexion and extension. A scaphoid fracture is another injury that is easily missed because of its location and proximity to other wrist bones and ligaments and tendons. A distinguishing feature of a scaphoid fracture is tenderness to palpation in the anatomical snuff-box. Because of the risk of avascular necrosis after this injury, patients should be referred for imaging if at all in doubt. Even if the radiograph is reported negative initially, the injury should be casted or splinted for 2 weeks with a follow-up radiograph ordered, which may better demonstrate this potentially devastating fracture.

Important Concepts

Multiple fractures, tendon injuries, infections, and neurologic involvement are generally conditions that may elicit "red flags" in the more distal upper extremities.

Tendon injuries are common to forearm flexor and extensor muscles. Tendinitis or tendinosis injuries are less of a concern than a grade III rupture of the tendons. This injury causes immediate pain followed by weakness, dull aching, or cramping sensations in the affected muscles. Usually there is a palpable defect in the tendon; there is a loss of strength of the given digit and most often edema, ecchymosis, and tenderness associated with the rupture.

TABLE 3-10 "Red Flags" for the Elbow, Wrist, and Hand Regions

Condition	"Red Flags"
Fractures	• Recent fall or trauma • Pain, tenderness, swelling, and ecchymosis • History of osteoporosis • Extended use of steroids (e.g., respiratory problems) • Pathologies with improper bone remodeling
Radial head fracture	• Fall onto outstretched arm that is supinated • Anterolateral pain and tenderness at elbow • Inability to supinate and pronate forearm • Elbow held against the side with 70° of flexion and slightly supinated
Distal radius (Colles' fracture)	• Fall onto outstretched arm with forceful wrist extension • Wrist held in neutral resting position • Wrist swelling • Movements into wrist extension are painful
Scaphoid fracture	• Fall onto outstretched arm • Wrist swelling • Wrist held in neutral position • Pain in anatomical snuff-box
Lunate fracture or dislocation	• Diffuse synovitis • Generalized wrist swelling and pain • Decreased motion • Decreased grip strength (rule out capitate fracture)
Long flexor tendon rupture	• Grade I and II muscle tear—local tenderness, swelling, muscle spasms, hematoma, and pain with motion and with passive stretch • Grade III muscle rupture—total loss of motion and palpable defect in muscle, swelling, tenderness, and ecchymosis of overlying skin
Space infection of the hand	• Recent puncture of skin • Presence of an abscess • Purulent tenosynovitis of tendons that go through a space • Typical signs of inflammation—swelling in palm, dorsum of hand, or fingertips • Pain, tenderness, warmth, and erythema • Signs of long-standing infection: high fever, chills, weakness, and malaise
Raynaud's phenomenon or Raynaud's disease	• Hands or feet that blanch, become cyanotic, and then become red when exposed to cold or emotional stress • Pain and tingling in hands or feet when they turn red • Past medical history significant for rheumatoid arthritis, occlusive vascular disease, smoking, or use of beta blockers
Complex regional pain syndrome (reflex sympathetic dystrophy)	• Trauma including fracture, dislocation, or surgery • Severe aching, stinging, cutting, or boring pain that is not typical of injury; hypersensitivity • Area swollen (pitting edema), warm, and erythematous • Pain does not respond to typical analgesics

From Boissonnault WG: *Primary care for the physical therapist: examination and triage,* St Louis, 2005, Saunders.

Trauma, cuts, scrapes, and puncture wounds of the hands all can cause localized infections. Infections in the hands, similar to any other location of the body, manifest with pain, tenderness, warmth, and erythema. The case becomes a serious "red flag" and of much greater concern when high fever, chills, weakness, and malaise are present. Because of the lack of deep subcutaneous tissue in the hands, an infection is usually readily seen as an unusual swelling, especially on the dorsum of the hand.

Raynaud's disease or Raynaud's syndrome is a disorder that affects either the hands or the feet (Fig. 3-10). A progressive redness, blanching, or cyanosis occurs in the extremities when the patient is exposed to cold or emotional stress. This condition is not life-threatening; however, the symptoms can become very disabling. This condition is more common in people who smoke; people with rheumatoid arthritis; and people taking beta-adrenergic blocking medications for other problems, such as angina, hypertension, or migraines. Complex regional pain syndrome can occur after trauma such as fractures, sprains, dislocations, crush injury, or any surgical procedure to the hand or wrist; this condition was historically known as reflex sympathetic dystrophy. Symptoms following these injuries do not respond as normally expected and seem to worsen as time progresses. There is occasionally a lag time between initial insult and symptom progression. Symptoms can be severe and create aching, burning, stinging, cutting, or boring pain that is usually completely out of proportion to the injury that caused the pain.

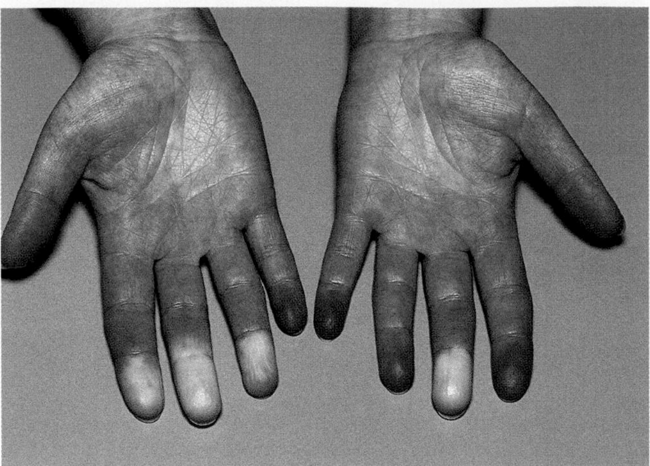

FIG 3-10 Severe Raynaud's syndrome. *(From Hallett JW, Mills JL, Earnshaw JJ, et al:* Comprehensive vascular and endovascular surgery, *ed 2, Philadelphia, 2009, Mosby Ltd.)*

SUMMARY

As the physical therapy profession progresses toward autonomous practice, PTs and PTAs under the direction and supervision of a PT must continue to develop and enhance the skills of identifying and distinguishing signs and symptoms that require further investigation or referral to another health care provider. This chapter provided an overview of the elements of client management that culminate in the differentiation of the data into a specific pattern that guides the practitioner's choice of interventions. The basic role of the PTA in patient care includes the provision of delegated interventions and monitoring patients' responses. Assessment skills involve problem solving and clinical decision making that may result in appropriate immediate adaptations during a treatment session or collection of data that are reported to the primary PT resulting in the need for changes of the POC. The basic skills of assessment as outlined in this chapter include observation, listening, manual proficiencies (e.g., ROM, MMT, anthropometric measurements, motor and sensory screening), and communication. A review of the common orthopedic "red flags" a PT uses in aiding the determination of a patient's differential physical therapy diagnosis provided the PTA with information that explains the pathology and the interventions chosen. The chapter concluded with a brief review of common signs, symptoms, and "red flags" a PTA may encounter while handling orthopedic patients resulting in the need for immediate referral back to the PT for additional differential diagnosis or possible referral to another appropriate health care professional.

GLOSSARY

Assessment: A judgment about something based on an understanding of the situation.

Diagnosis: The identification of an illness or disorder in a patient based on physical examination, medical tests, or other procedures.

Differentiate: To see or show the differences between two or more things.

Evaluation: The act of considering or examining something to judge its value, quality, importance, extent, or condition.

Examination: The process of looking at and considering something carefully with the idea of learning something.

Infection: The reproduction and proliferation of microorganisms within the body.

Intervention: The act of intervening, especially a deliberate entry into a situation or dispute to influence events or prevent undesirable consequences.

Prognosis: A medical opinion regarding the likely course and outcome of a disease.

Understanding: The ability to perceive and explain the meaning or the nature of somebody or something.

REFERENCES

1. American Physical Therapy Association: Standard: Standards of ethical conduct for the physical therapist assistant. HOD S06-09-20-18; Amended HOD S06-00-13-24; HOD 06-91-06-07; Initial HOD 06-82-04-08. 1982. Available at: http://www.apta.org/uploadedFiles/APTAorg/About_Us/Policies/HOD/Ethics/Standards.pdf. Accessed June 5, 2012.
2. American Physical Therapy Association: Position Statement: *Diagnosis by Physical Therapist.* HOD 06-84–19-78. 1984. Available at: http://www.apta.org/Policies/ Open Link: Positions, Standards, Guidelines, Policies & Procedures—Full Packet (.pdf) pg. 528. Accessed February 22, 2015.
3. American Physical Therapy Association: Guideline: *Physical Therapy Documentation of Patient /Client Management.* Amended BOD 02-02-16-20; BOD 11-01-06-10; BOD 03-01-16-51; BOD 03-00-22-54; BOD 03-99-14-41; BOD 11-98-19-69; BOD 03-97-27-69; BOD 03-95-23-61; BOD 11-94-33-107; BOD 06-93-09-13; Initial BOD 03-93-21-55]. 1993, American Physical Therapy Association. Available at: http://www.apta.org/Policies/CoreDocuments/ Open link: Guidelines: Physical Therapy Documentation of Patient / Client Management. Accessed February 22, 2015.
4. American Physical Therapy Association: Position Statement: *Distinction Between the Physical Therapist and the Physical Therapist Assistant in Physical Therapy.* HOD P06-96-24-39. 1996. Available at: http://www.apta.org/Policies/ Open Link: Positions, Standards, Guidelines, Policies & Procedures—Full Packet (.pdf) pg. 670. Accessed February 22, 2015.
5. American Physical Therapy Association: *Physical therapist assistant clinical performance instrument,* Alexandria, VA, 1998, American Physical Therapy Association.
6. American Physical Therapy Association: Position statement: Vision 2020. HOD P06-00-24-35. 2000. Available at: http://www.apta.org/Vision2020/. Accessed May 26, 2012.
7. American Physical Therapy Association: *Preferred practice pattern—guide to physical therapist practice,* ed 2, Alexandria, VA, 2001, American Physical Therapy Association.
8. American Physical Therapy Association: *Guide to physical therapist practice,* ed 2, Alexandria, VA, 2001, American Physical Therapy Association.
9. American Physical Therapy Association: *A normative model of physical therapist education: version 2007,* Alexandria, VA, 2007, American Physical Therapy Association.
10. American Physical Therapy Association: Guideline: Minimum required skills of physical therapist assistant graduates at entry-level. BOD G11-08-09-18. 2008. Available at: http://www.apta.org/uploadedFiles/APTAorg/About_Us/Policies/BOD/Education/MinReqSkillsPTAGrad.pdf. Accessed June 5, 2012.
11. American Physical Therapy Association: Defensible documentation for patient/client management. 2012. Available at: http://www.apta.org/Documentation/DefensibleDocumentation/. Accessed June 10, 2012.

12. Auerbach AD: Prevention of surgical site infections. Available at: http://www.ahrq.gov/clinic/ptsafety/chap20a.htm. Accessed July 22, 2012.
13. Barr JD, Barr MS, Lemley TJ, McCann RM: Percutaneous vertebroplasty for pain relief and spinal stabilization. *Spine* 25:923–928, 2000.
14. Bigos S, Bowyer O, Braen G, et al: *Acute lower back problems in adults. Clinical practice guideline no 14. AHCPR Publication No. 95-0642*, Rockville, MD, 1994, Agency for Health Care Policy and Research, Public Health Service, U.S. Department of Health and Human Services.
15. Boissonnault W: Prevalence of comorbid conditions, surgeries, and medication use in a physical outpatient population: a multicentered study. *J Orthop Sports Phys Ther* 29:506–519, 1999.
16. Boissonnault WG: *Primary Care for the Physical Therapist—Examination and Triage*, St Louis, 2005, Saunders.
17. Brody LT, Hall CM: *Therapeutic Exercise—Moving Toward Function*, ed 3, Philadelphia, 2011, Lippincott Williams & Wilkins.
18. Burge R, Dawson-Hughes B, Solomon DH, et al: Incidence and economic burden of osteoporosis-related fracture sin the United States, 2005-2025. *J Bone Miner Res* 22:465–475, 2007.
19. Cameron MH, Monroe LG: *Physical Rehabilitation for the Physical Therapist Assistant*, St Louis, 2011, Mosby.
20. Chan DS, Lau R, Aune D, et al: Red and processed meat and colorectal cancer incidence: meta-analysis of prospective studies. *PLoS ONE* 6:e20456, 2011.
21. Chaudhry S, Phillips D, Feldman D: Legg-Calve-Perthes disease. An overview with recent literature. *Bull Hosp Jt Dis* 72:18–27, 2014.
22. Crosier J: PTA direction and supervision algorithms: step-by-step problem-solving diagrams to guide PTs and PTAs. *PT in Motion* 9:47–50, 2010.
23. Delaune MF: Moving from mystery diagnosis to diagnosis in physical therapist practice. *PT in Motion* 10:58–59, 2009.
24. Deyo RA, Diehl AK: Cancer as a cause of back pain: frequency, clinical presentation, and diagnostic strategies. *J Gen Intern Med* 3:230–238, 1988.
25. DiFabio R, Boissonnault W: Physical therapy and health-related outcomes for patients with common orthopaedic diagnoses. *J Orthop Sports Phys Ther* 27:219–230, 1998.
26. Fedirko V, Tramacere I, Bagnardi V, et al: Alcohol drinking and colorectal cancer risk: an overall and dose-response meta-analysis of published studies. *Ann Oncol* 22:1958–1972, 2011.
27. Gallo RA, Plakke M, Silvis L: Common leg injuries of long-distance runners. *Sports Health* 4:485–495, 2012.
28. Gayle EA, Young SM, McNaughton CD: Septic arthritis of the temporomandibular joint: case reports and review of the literature. *J Emerg Med* 45:674–678, 2013.
29. Gong J, Hutter C, Baron JA, et al: A pooled analysis of smoking and colorectal cancer: timing of exposure and interactions with environmental factors. *Cancer Epidemiol Biomarkers Prev* 21:1974–1985, 2012.
30. Goodman CC, Fuller KS, Boissonnault WG: *Pathology implications for the physical therapist*, ed 2, Philadelphia, 2003, Saunders.
31. Goodman CC, Fuller KS: *Pathology implications for the physical therapist*, ed 3, St Louis, 2009, Saunders.
32. Goodman CC, Fuller KS: *Pathology for the physical therapist assistant*, St Louis, 2012, Saunders.
33. Goodman CC, Snyder TEC: *Differential diagnosis in physical therapy*, ed 2, Philadelphia, 1995, Saunders.
34. Jette AM, Davis KD: A comparison of hospital-based and private outpatient physical therapy practices. *Phys Ther* 71:366–375, 1991.
35. Lorei M, Herhsman E: Peripheral nerve injuries in athletes. *Sports Med* 16:130–147, 1993.
36. Mayo Clinic: Orthostatic hypotension (postural hypotension). Available at: http://www.mayoclinic.com/health/orthostatic-hypotension/ds00997/dsection=tests-and-diagnosis. Accessed July 24, 2012.
37. Merriam-Webster. Available at: http://www.merriam-webster.com/dictionary/assess. Accessed June 7, 2012.
38. Mineyama S, Tsutsumi A, Takao S, et al: Supervisors' attitudes and skills for active listening with regard to work conditions and psychological stress reactions among subordinate workers. *J Occup Health* 49:81–87, 2007.
39. Minor S, Minor MD: *Patient Care Skills*, ed 6, Upper Saddle River, NJ, 2009, Prentice Hall.
40. O'Brien JG, Chennubhotla SA, Chennubhotla RV: Treatment of edema. *Am Fam Physician* 71:2111–2117, 2005.
41. Pierson F: *Principles and techniques of patient care*, ed 3, Philadelphia, 2003, Saunders.
42. Pryde JA: Inflammation and tissue repair. In Cameron M, editor: *Physical agents in rehabilitation: from research to practice*, ed 3, St Louis, 2009, Saunders.
43. Qvarfordt P, Christenson JT, Eklof B, et al: Intramuscular pressure, muscle bold flow, and skeletal muscle metabolism in chronic anterior tibial compartment syndrome. *Clin Orthop Rel Res* 179:284–290, 1983.
44. Renehan AG, Flood A, Adams KF, et al: Body mass index at different adult ages, weight change, and colorectal cancer risk in the National Institutes of Health-AARP Cohort. *Am J Epidemiol* 176:1130–1140, 2012.
45. Spector LR, Madigan L, Rhyme A, et al: Cauda equina syndrome. *J Am Acad Orthop Surg* 16:471–479, 2008.
46. Spengler D, Kirsh M, Daufer H: Orthopedic aspects and early diagnosis of superior sulcus lung tumor. *J Bone Joint Surg Am* 55:1645–1650, 1973.

REVIEW QUESTIONS

Multiple Choice

1. Which of the following terms is defined as providing a label for the recognition of specific signs and symptoms and correlating this to an identifiable disorder?
   a. Examination
   b. Diagnosis
   c. Intervention
   d. Prognosis
2. The practice of physical therapy encompasses various phases of patient care focusing on what types of conditions?
   a. Musculoskeletal
   b. Neuromuscular
   c. Cardiopulmonary
   d. All of the above
3. Which of the following terms is defined as a comprehensive screening that includes specific tests and measures?
   a. Examination
   b. Diagnosis
   c. Intervention
   d. Prognosis
4. Which of the following terms is defined as the synthesization of data collected during an examination that is used to develop clinical decisions regarding treatment?
   a. Assessment
   b. Diagnosis
   c. Evaluation
   d. Prognosis
5. Low-back pain is an example of what type of diagnosis?
   a. Medical diagnosis
   b. Physical diagnosis
   c. Rehabilitation diagnosis
   d. Physical therapy diagnosis
6. Which of the following is considered a physical therapy diagnosis?
   a. Impaired mobility
   b. Cerebrovascular accident

c. Rotator cuff tear
d. Femur fracture

7. Which of the following terms describes a medical opinion predicting a given outcome for a specific disease or pathology?
   a. Assessment
   b. Diagnosis
   c. Evaluation
   d. Prognosis
8. Which of the following is not a basic skill that can be used by PTAs to assess a patient with a musculoskeletal condition?
   a. Diagnosing disorders
   b. Sensory screening
   c. MMT
   d. ROM
9. Essential patient care management skills required of a PTA include:
   a. Observation.
   b. Listening.
   c. Manual proficiencies.
   d. All of the above
10. Which of the following would not be considered a "red flag" symptom?
   a. Loss of appetite with loss of weight
   b. Unusual bumps or growths
   c. Redness
   d. Blood in urine
11. Blood in urine would indicate which type of "red flag"?
   a. Cancer
   b. Diabetic
   c. Gastrointestinal
   d. Neurologic
12. Which of the following symptoms would lead the clinician to suspect pain is musculoskeletal in origin versus being systemic?
   a. Pain lessens at night
   b. Pain usually decreases with activity
   c. Pain is intermittent in nature
   d. All of the above
13. Which of the following symptoms would lead the clinician to suspect pain is musculoskeletal in origin versus being systemic?
   a. Aggravated by mechanical stress
   b. Reduced by pressure
   c. Constant waves of pain or spasm
   d. Disturbs sleep
14. What is the normal pulse rate for a man?
   a. 50 to 75 beats per minute (bpm)
   b. 60 to 100 bpm
   c. 70 to 110 bpm
   d. None of the above
15. Which of the following is a sign of pulmonary embolism?
   a. Discoloration
   b. Diffuse chest pain
   c. Unilateral leg tenderness
   d. Warmth of skin

Short Answer

16. What is the difference between diagnosis and prognosis?
17. Describe several forms of pathology from each of the four practice patterns.
18. Why is communication to the supervising PT important for continuity between therapy sessions?
19. Why is the ability to determine "red flag" conditions important during treatment of musculoskeletal conditions?
20. Describe several constitutional symptoms that may affect the entire body and indicate a need for referral back to a physician or appropriate health care provider?

Fill in the Blank

21. Malaise, fever, redness, and increased temperature are all common signs of ____________ in a joint.
22. ____________ is the process of comprehensive screening that includes tests and measures.
23. Pain in the jaw, left shoulder, or arm or deep pain between the scapulae may indicate a ____________ attack.
24. A ____________ causes symptoms such as redness, subcutaneous vein distention, and warmth.
25. ____________ causes unilateral swelling and tight shiny skin that may be worse when the limb is placed in a dependent position.

True/False

26. Diagnosis is within the function and scope of practice for a PTA.
27. Communication is vital to ensure accurate recording of information about patients from one session of care to another.
28. Differential diagnosis is the process of carefully comparing and contrasting patient data points with the goal of developing appropriate intervention strategies.
29. Examination of patients with musculoskeletal complaints typically requires a hands-on approach to perform tests and measures.
30. Prognosis is used to help determine and establish a basic POC.

Chapter 4

Muscle Flexibility and Range of Motion

Harvey W. Wallmann

CHAPTER OUTLINE

LEARNING OBJECTIVES

1. Describe viscoelasticity and the properties associated with collagen.
2. Explain the stress-strain curve and factors that influence change.
3. Discuss Golgi tendon organs and muscle spindles.
4. Discuss how temperature affects connective tissue.
5. Define and discuss range of motion, flexibility, and stretching.
6. Outline various methods used to measure flexibility.
7. Identify and describe various stretching techniques.
8. Discuss precautions and essential components of stretching program development.
9. Discuss at least two proposed benefits of stretching.
10. Explain how stretching might negatively impact activity performance.
11. Describe the clinical applications for stretching soft tissue contractures.
12. Describe and contrast the differences and similarities between scar tissue and adhesions.

KEY TERMS

Adhesion
Collagen
Contracture
Creep phenomenon
Deformation
Golgi tendon organs
Load
Muscle spindles
Remodeling
Strain
Stress
Viscoelasticity

Enhancing flexibility is an important component of a fitness program[7] and is useful not only for sport-specific activities but also for activities of daily living (ADLs). Flexibility is particularly necessary if mobility has been impaired, resulting in compromised range of motion (ROM). ROM is the amount of movement available to a joint moving within its anatomic range. Muscular imbalances resulting from shortened muscles may lead to faulty postural alignment, which may lead to injury and joint dysfunction. The ability to restore ROM is crucial when implementing or following a rehabilitation program; consequently, incorporating stretching exercises to restore flexibility as well as normal ROM and function becomes a primary goal for the physical therapist assistant (PTA).

Important Concepts

Muscular imbalances resulting from shortened muscles may lead to faulty postural alignment, which may lead to injury and joint dysfunction.

Many clinicians emphasize that a more flexible body is more efficient, improves muscle balance, and more easily undergoes strength and endurance training. Overall purported benefits of flexibility resulting from stretching include injury prevention, quicker recovery from workouts, a reduction in soreness after exercise, and facilitation of relaxation.[2,133] However, the effects of stretching on performance are more controversial. Some literature shows that it may potentially help improve performance,[49] whereas other literature and research reveal potential detrimental effects on maximal performance of activities after stretching.[68,116,128,135] Research into flexibility and stretching is ongoing in an attempt to determine the effects of stretching on the body. Consequently, some of the long-held beliefs about stretching, especially regarding performance, are being challenged.

PROPERTIES OF CONNECTIVE TISSUE

Before discussing the concepts of flexibility and stretching, a general review of several biomechanical concepts is presented to help form a foundation for later material. Specifically, concepts of **viscoelasticity**, **stress**, and **strain** and associated variables related to tensile load are discussed in relation to **collagen**.

Just as amino acids are the building blocks of protein, tropocollagen is the building block of collagen (Fig. 4-1). Collagen fibers are made of short subunits (fibrils) and are found in varying amounts within the different connective tissues including bone, tendon, muscle, skin, hyaline cartilage, and joint capsule.[20,41,123] Collagen is a protein building block of connective tissue, and it provides the strength needed to withstand high levels of tension and force during movement and exercise. There are more than 20 types of collagen, but most of the collagen in the body consists of types I, II, and III.[38] Of these, type I collagen is the most abundant in the body.

Type I collagen fibers are thick fibers gathered into bundles and display very little elongation when placed under tension (they have an ability to resist pulling). Type II collagen fibers are thinner and possess slightly less tensile strength. These fibers are observed primarily in tissues such as articular cartilage (found at the end of long bones) and the nucleus pulposus (located within the vertebral disk). Type III collagen serves mainly in a structural support capacity and is found in expansible organs (e.g., arteries, liver, lungs).[60] It is also common in fast-growing or healing tissue and is often seen at the early stages (phase 1) of wound repair. It is later replaced by the tougher type I collagen.[93]

Elastin is a structural protein present in tendons in amounts of less than 1%.[35,139] Tissues with greater amounts of elastin usually demonstrate greater degrees of flexibility. Elastin assists collagen in the recovery of tissues after stress (initial loading of the tissue).

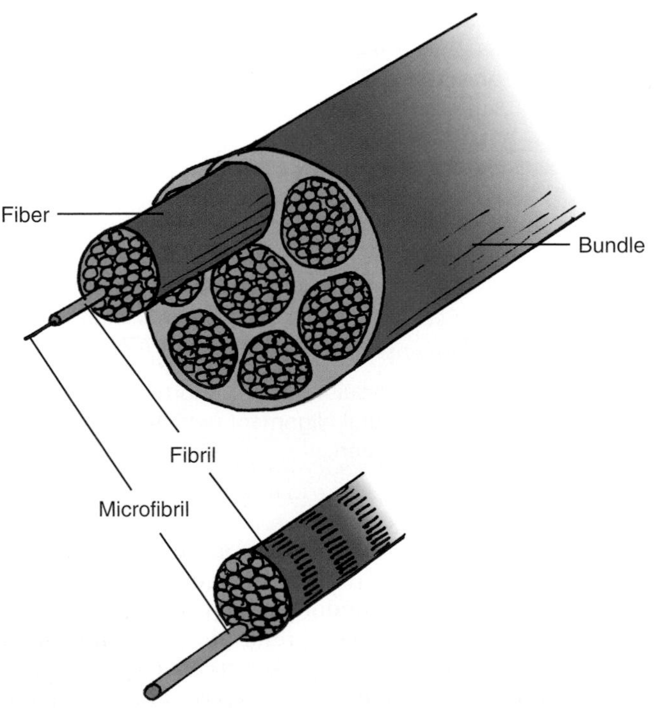

FIG 4-1 Collagen bundle.

STRESS AND STRAIN

Stress or **load** is given in units of force/area, where the units may be pounds per square inch or Newtons per square centimeter.[99] Stress is directly related to the magnitude of force and inversely related to the unit area but is independent of the amount of a material.[100] The complementary measure related to stress is strain or **deformation**. Strain is usually dimensionless because the units of measure cancel each other out, but units are often provided (e.g., inches/inch) to give a perspective of scale applied to the loads.[99]

The relationship of stress and strain depends on several factors, including the material properties used, the magnitude of the stresses, and the rate of stress application. Subsequently, the graphical representation of stress and strain is different for each type of material discussed. This representation is known as the *stress-strain* or *load-deformation curve*.[95] Figure 4-2 demonstrates the various regions within the stress-strain curve, with each region demonstrating a biomechanical property of a tissue.

The *toe region* represents how a slightly pulled tissue (i.e., a ligament) produces only a small amount of tension within the tissue; it indicates that the collagen fibers within the tissue must first be pulled taut before a stretch can be induced. This minimal amount of tension simply results in the slack of the tissue being taken up with no stretch being encountered. The *elastic region* represents a linear change in strain, which occurs if the tissue continues to be pulled at higher stress levels. The mechanical behavior of the tissue is directly proportional to the stress imposed. A good example of this linear relationship is a stretched rubber band. The greater the load on the rubber band, the more the rubber band stretches. As the tension on the rubber band is removed, the band shortens, nearing its original length. Given this behavior, it is referred to as the *elastic zone*. The stretch (strain or deformation) applied to the tissue in this zone is generally experienced during many body movements. The slope (the angle of the curve) in this zone is indicative of the relative *stiffness* of the tissue. Stiffness is defined as the change in force per unit change in length.[41] The stiffer the tissue, the steeper (more vertical) the slope. Tissues such as ligaments change length at higher levels of stress compared with tissues of less stiffness, such as loose connective tissue. Tissues with less stiffness are considered more *compliant*. Stretching of a

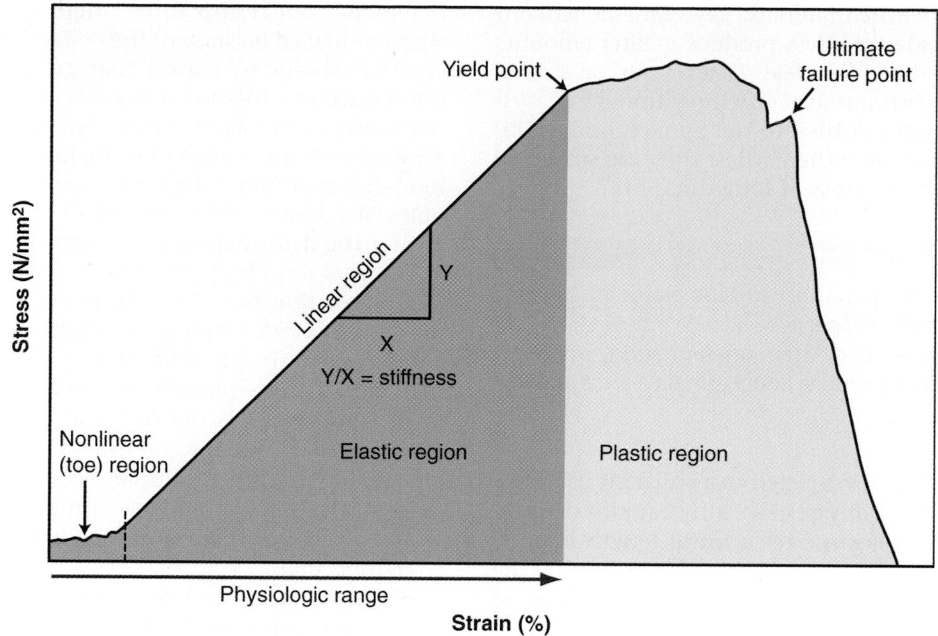

FIG 4-2 The stress-strain relationship of an excised ligament that has been stretched to a point of mechanical failure (disruption). *(From Neumann DA:* Kinesiology of the musculoskeletal system: foundations for rehabilitation, *ed 2, St Louis, 2010, Mosby.)*

tissue with increased compliance would result in a more horizontal slope.

The upper level of the elastic region marks a transition from the linear slope to one where the slope begins to flatten. This is called the *plastic region* and is a point where an increasing level of stress on the tissue results in proportionately increased changes in tissue length, probably as a result of microscopic failure of the tissue. This is termed the *plastic zone* because of the tissue damage resulting in permanent deformation (plastic deformation). In contrast to the elastic region, the plastic energy is not recoverable in its entirety when the load is removed; additionally, there is a change in its resting length. Continued stretch in the plastic region would result in additional deformation of the tissue and would occur until it reached its initial point of failure. The toe region can include strains up to 3%; the elastic region, from 6% to 10%; and the plastic region, from 10% to 15%.[41,115]

VISCOELASTICITY

All connective tissue exhibits the property of *viscoelasticity,* which is simply a combination of the behavior of the properties of *elasticity* and *viscosity*.[76,79] Elasticity refers to the ability of a material to return to its original state following strain or deformation (i.e., change in length or shape) after a removal of the stress or load. This mutable change is termed *elastic deformation* and is similar to the changes that occur in a rubber band under high rates of strain. The rubber band rapidly conforms to a new length and is able to return to its original resting length when the stress is removed. However, the rubber band breaks if the degree of stress exceeds the strain capabilities (Fig. 4-3). Viscosity refers to the ability of a material to resist a change in form or to dampen shearing forces (think of slow pouring molasses). Tissues exhibiting viscosity have time-dependent and rate-dependent properties when forces are applied to them.

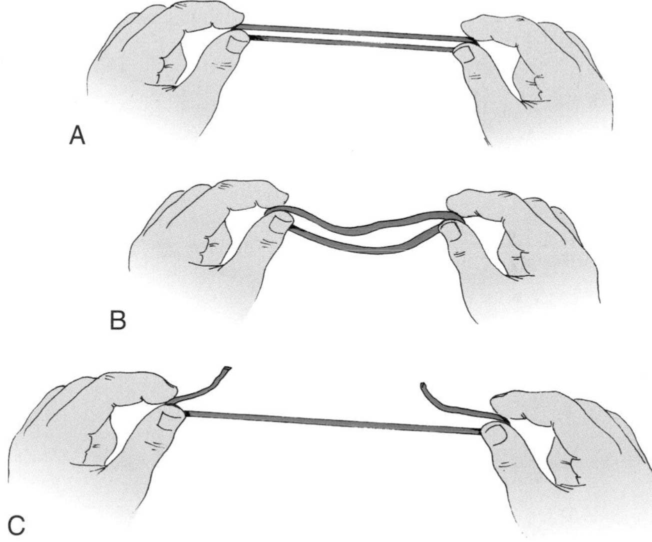

FIG 4-3 Elastic deformation. **A,** Stress applied to a rubber band. **B,** When stress is removed, the rubber band returns to its original length. **C,** If the stress exceeds the strain capabilities of the band, it can break.

The rate at which tissues are stretched has a profound effect on the degree or percent of strain. As mentioned, tensile (distractive) or compressive forces produce deformation on viscoelastic materials but allow return to their original state after removal of the force. However, given normal conditions, viscoelastic materials do not immediately return to their original state. Viscoelastic materials, in contrast to pure elastic materials, have time-dependent properties. Slower rates of stress produce greater amounts of strain or elongation, whereas faster rates of stretch produce much smaller amounts of elongation.[29,35,123] Viscoelastic materials are sensitive to the applied force duration. Tissues gradually lengthen when they are subjected to constant or repeated stress of long duration.

Important Concepts

Viscoelastic materials, in contrast to pure elastic materials, have time-dependent properties. Slower rates of stress produce greater amounts of strain or elongation, whereas faster rates of stretch produce much smaller amounts of elongation.

A viscoelastic material subjected to a constant compressive or tensile load initially responds by rapidly deforming; it continues to deform over a finite length of time even if the load remains constant. This deformation of the tissue continues until a state of equilibrium is reached when the load is balanced. This is called the ***creep** phenomenon* (Fig. 4-4),[79] which simply means the gradual increase in tissue length that occurs when maintaining a constant stress (or force). For example, if one uses a constant force against the muscle with slow and passive stretching, the muscle eventually elongates. However, the tissue does not return to its original length immediately when unloaded because of the collagen's viscoelastic property.[76] It stands to reason that creep changes are more pronounced during slow-velocity rather than high-velocity stretching. High-force, short-duration stretching favors primarily elastic tissue deformation, whereas low-force, long-duration stretching favors plastic deformation. Essentially, the longer the duration of the applied force, the greater the deformation or stretching of the tissue.

Another term frequently used is **stress-relaxation,** or force-relaxation (see Fig. 4-4). In contrast to creep, stress-relaxation occurs when a viscoelastic material experiences a constant strain (no deformation occurs). In this case, a high initial stress placed on a tissue decreases over time until equilibrium is reached and the stress equals zero, resulting in relaxation of the tissue. Consequently, no change in length is produced. For example, if a muscle is held at a certain length over time, a reduction in stress would occur, but there would be no change in length (no stretch occurs).

The loading and unloading of tissue is influenced by its viscoelastic properties. This loading and unloading is quantified by measuring the *hysteresis* area (Fig. 4-5). The loading (*solid line* in Fig. 4-5) and unloading (*dashed line* in Fig. 4-5) phases represent a measurement of the stress and strain that is applied to a tissue and then released. The hysteresis area lies between the two lines and represents

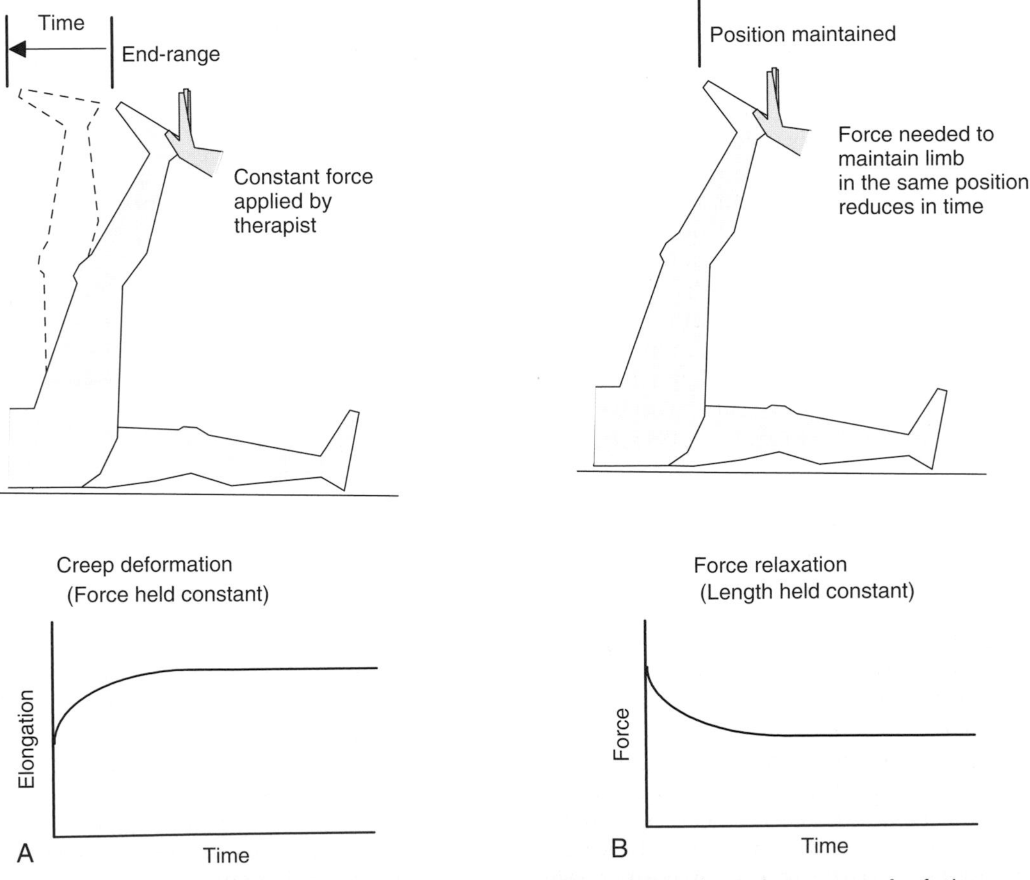

FIG 4-4 Creep deformation **(A)** and force relaxation **(B)** are biomechanical responses of soft tissue that are not neurologically mediated. *(From Lederman E:* Fundamentals of manual therapy: physiology, neurology, and psychology, *New York, 1997, Churchill Livingstone.)*

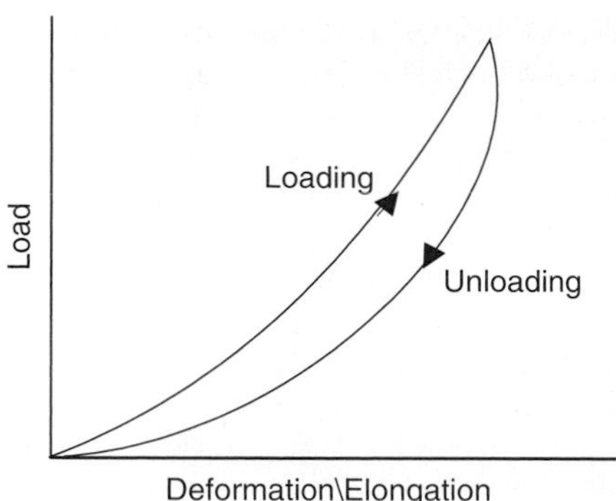

FIG 4-5 Hysteresis is the discrepancy between the mechanical energy used to perform tissue stretch and the energy needed to return the tissue to its original shape. *(From Lederman E:* Fundamentals of manual therapy: physiology, neurology, and psychology, *New York, 1997, Churchill Livingstone.)*

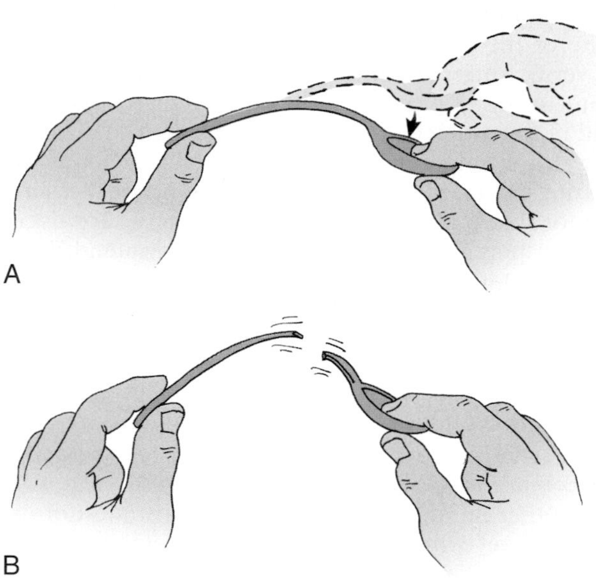

FIG 4-6 Plastic deformation. **A,** A low degree of stress is applied to a plastic spoon. The spoon will deform slowly and accommodate to a new shape. **B,** If stress is applied suddenly and with great force, the spoon will break.

the amount of energy dissipated in the loading and unloading process.[41,76]

The ability of tissues to recover after stress is extremely important in relation to flexibility. Woo and colleagues[140] showed that increasing the levels of stress produces an increase in collagen within ligaments and tendons, whereas reducing the levels of stress causes weakening in connective tissues. Recovery is the ability of tissues to return to their previous resting state. However, it does not imply that permanent elongation or microscopic damage has not occurred. Plastic deformation is force dependent on slow rates of stress and is used to describe permanent change in a tissue. For example, when a low degree of stress is applied to a plastic spoon, the spoon slowly deforms to a new shape. The spoon breaks if the stress is applied too fast (Fig. 4-6). Lehmann and colleagues[77] and Warren and co-workers[130] demonstrated that recovery of the tissue's resting length had occurred after microscopic failure had begun.

In addition to stress and the rate of stress applied to tissues, temperature affects connective tissue extensibility and the rate of creep. High temperatures of 37° C to 40° C (98.6° F to 104° F) affect the viscoelastic properties of connective tissue and increase the rate of creep.[29,76] The higher the temperature (approximately 45° C [113° F] is the therapeutic upper limit), the greater the degree of deformation before tissue failure.[111] Because viscoelastic and plastic changes in connective tissue occur at higher temperatures, there is less microscopic damage under stress at these temperatures. Studies by Warren and colleagues[131] demonstrated that a temperature of 45° C is needed to reduce tissue damage during strains of 2.6% or less. To stretch out a connective tissue structure, one should heat it and use a large load over a long period of time to produce creep.[99] Low temperatures decrease the rate of creep—hence the need for an initial warm-up period before stretching the tissue.

Important Concepts

To stretch out a connective tissue structure, one should heat it and use a large load over a long period of time to produce creep. Low temperatures decrease the rate of creep—hence the need for an initial warm-up period before stretching the tissue.

Muscle or contractile tissue responds to stretch by elastic and plastic deformation properties in ways similar to connective tissue. The contractile properties of muscle allow for the greatest degree of freedom of movement around a joint. Although connective tissue is considered a passive resistant to joint motion, muscle tissue is considered an active restraint to joint motion by virtue of its elastic and contractile elements. Active exercise (muscular contractions) affects intramuscular temperature. Increases to approximately 39° C are observed in exercised muscle.[6] Commonly used passive thermal agents that increase tissue temperature are moist heat and ultrasound. The judicious use of active exercise and passive thermal agents before and during stretching programs enhances the effectiveness of the prescribed program.

FLEXIBILITY

Kisner and Colby[66] defined flexibility as the ability of a muscle to relax and yield to a stretch force. Others have defined flexibility as the ability to move muscles and joints through a full ROM.[12,105] In essence, flexibility refers to the degree of normal ROM available. Flexibility can refer to various measurable components of joint motion. Muscles, tendons, ligaments, skin, joint capsule, and bone geometry all influence the degree of movement in joints. For example, a muscle can stretch or elongate, creating a measurable effect on the joint or joints on which it acts. If a muscle becomes damaged by trauma or disease or becomes shortened because of immobilization, its ability to stretch and allow freedom of joint motion is affected. Flexibility diminishes over time if tissues are not stretched or exercised using regular and proper stretching regimens.[2] This diminished flexibility results quite often in the hip flexor and hamstring muscles in individuals who sit a

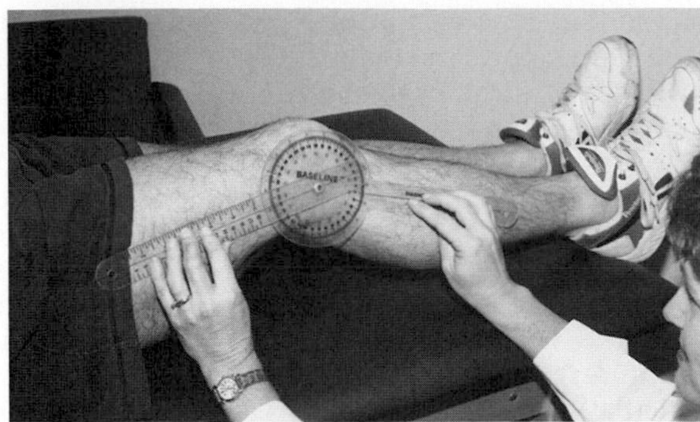

FIG 4-7 Measuring joint motion with a goniometer.

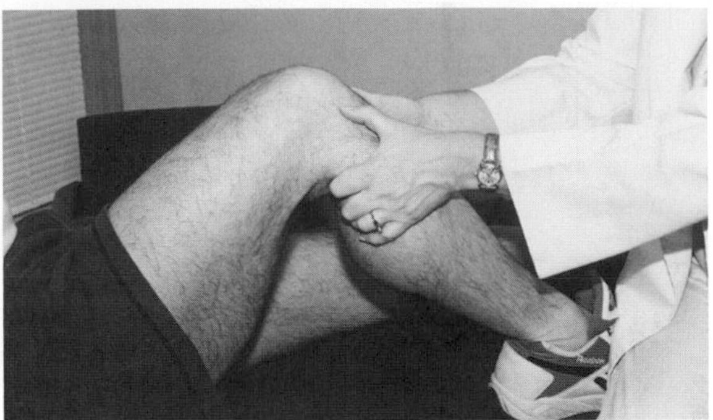

FIG 4-8 Joint stability is measured by manually applied clinical tests. Anterior drawer test of the knee is shown.

good portion of the day because we adapt to the way we function. The goal of any flexibility program would be to improve or maintain ROM at all joints.

Different classifications of flexibility currently exist, depending on how the tissue is stretched. For example, static flexibility occurs as a result of static stretching, whereas dynamic flexibility relates to moving through a ROM with normal or rapid velocity.[2] However, evidence does not support the existence of flexibility as a single general characteristic of the whole body. Instead, it is specific to particular joints, joint actions, or movements and is highly variable among different individuals.[55] For example, an individual may have good shoulder ROM or flexibility in the shoulder musculature but lack good hamstring flexibility. An understanding of the properties and components of various connective tissues is fundamental in delivery of various stretching and flexibility regimens.

Important Concepts

Evidence does not support the existence of flexibility as a single general characteristic of the whole body. Instead, it is specific to particular joints, joint actions, or movements and is highly variable among different individuals.

MEASURING FLEXIBILITY

It is important to assess overall flexibility by measuring ROM at specific joints because no specific composite test provides an index of an individual's overall flexibility characteristics.[55,56] Subsequently, some measurements of overall flexibility are difficult because they involve a complexity of movements over several joints (e.g., sit and reach test).

Measuring joint ROM is accomplished by using standard goniometric instruments. The measuring device most commonly used to measure ROM is the universal goniometer (Fig. 4-7), which is a protractor with degree measurements. The goniometer arms are placed along the proximal and distal components of a joint with the axis centered over the joint axis and are moved in accordance with the body part being measured. The goniometer can be used to measure joint position and ROM at almost all joints of the body.[98] Other types of goniometers used less frequently in the clinical setting are the inclinometer, the pendulum goniometer, and the fluid goniometer.

Consistency in measurement is crucial, so it is important to use the same type of goniometer for a specific patient each time the patient is measured. Additionally, to increase assessment or testing reliability further, it would be apropos for the same clinician to remeasure the patient because of the increased reliability observed with intrarater versus interrater measurements. Because different goniometers may provide slightly different results, they should not be interchangeable in their use in the clinical setting. For example, when using an inclinometer as the measuring device, it should be used for all future measurements for that patient to ensure consistency.[99] For documentation purposes, most authorities recommend using goniometry rather than visual estimates because of its increased accuracy and reliability of measurement.[132,141]

Joint stability differs from joint ROM in that the ligaments and surface geometry of joint articulations dictate static joint integrity (stability). On one hand, a patient may demonstrate limited ROM in knee flexion and extension (by goniometry); however, anterior and posterior joint mobility may be excessive and unstable (Fig. 4-8). On the other hand, a patient may demonstrate normal joint ROM, yet when tested statically the joint may be very stable, tight, and unyielding to pressure.

The sit and reach test (Fig. 4-9, *A* and *B*), standing toe touch for back and hamstring flexibility (Fig. 4-9, *C*), seated hip external rotation test (Fig. 4-9, *D*), and standing knee recurvatum test generally are less specific flexibility tests. These tests and others are used to provide very general assessment of multijoint flexibility. Such tests also can be used as stretching techniques to improve limitations in movement. However, objective clinical documentation of joint ROM is accomplished by joint goniometry.

FACTORS AFFECTING FLEXIBILITY

In addition to muscles, tendons, and their surrounding fascia, other structures, such as bone, fat, connective tissue lesions, skin, and postural problems, may lead to flexibility and joint ROM limitations.[5] Age and gender are other factors that may affect flexibility.[14,25]

The physiologic changes that occur with aging beyond adolescence can be responsible for the decrease in overall musculoskeletal flexibility, especially in elderly individuals. The loss of muscle function, along with the increase in intramuscular connective tissue stiffness, results in decreased ROM and a gradual decline in the efficiency of performance of ADLs.

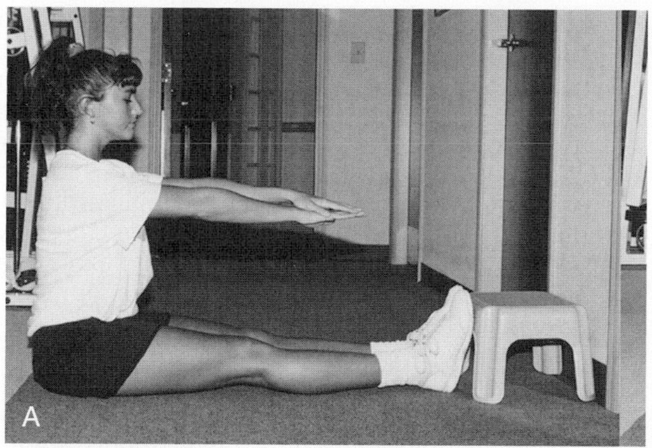

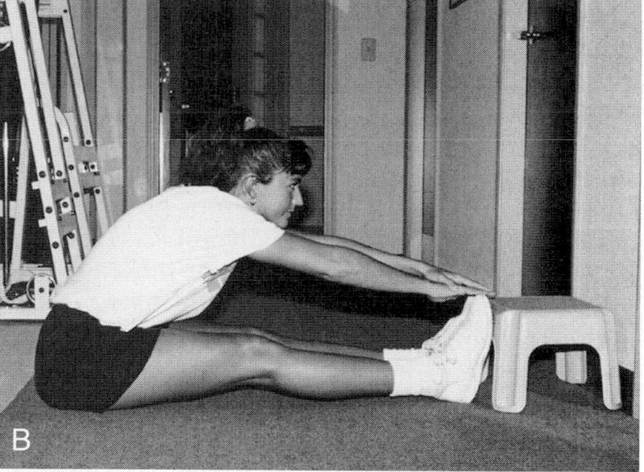

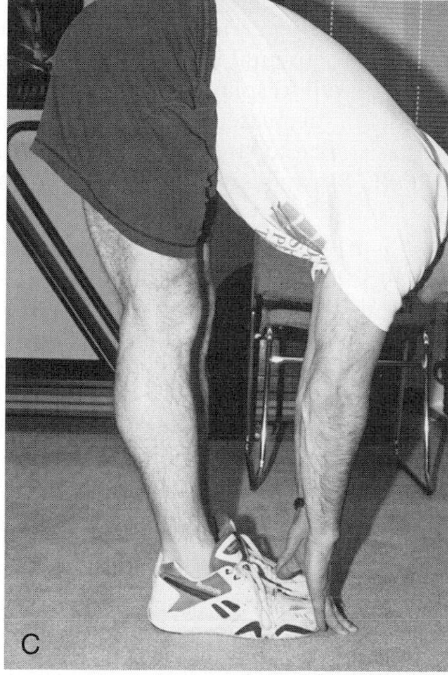

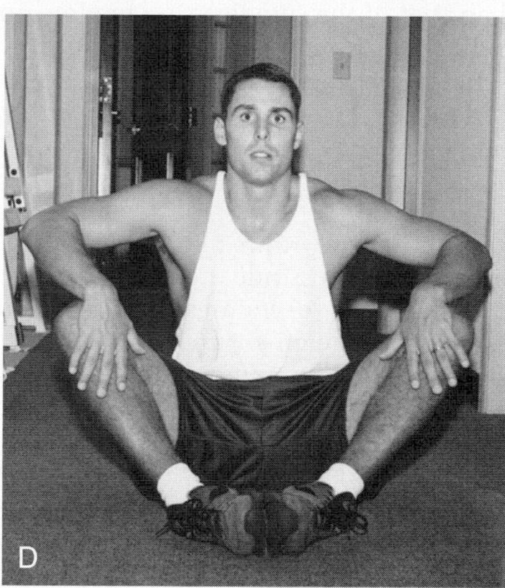

FIG 4-9 General, nonspecific flexibility test. **A,** Sit and reach test for hamstrings and low-back flexibility, starting position. **B,** End position of sit and reach test. **C,** General, nonspecific standing toe-touch flexibility test for the hamstring and lower back. **D,** Seated hip external rotation butterfly stretch.

Women are generally more flexible than men.[2] This may be due to physiologic and anatomic differences. For example, pregnancy affects flexibility, making the pelvic joints and ligaments relaxed and capable of greater movement. Some of the differences in flexibility may be due to the gender-specific nature of different regular and social activities. Additionally, although no firm conclusions can be drawn, hormonal fluctuations may play a role in ligamentous laxity of certain joints, potentially predisposing women to greater ROM differences than men.

INFLUENCE OF SENSORY AND MOTOR SYSTEMS ON FLEXIBILITY AND STRETCHING

Short-term or long-term changes in biologic tissues depend on more than just the biomechanical properties of tissue. The activation or relaxation of muscle may be a critical component of many flexibility programs. Many flexibility strategies are influenced by the contractile component of muscle. For example, a clinical technique designed to improve hamstring flexibility may have different results depending on the level of relaxation of the hamstring muscles during the stretching technique. The sensory and motor components of the nervous system can have a significant impact on the efficacy of flexibility programs.

Two sensory receptors that monitor muscle activity, **muscle spindles** and **Golgi tendon organs** (GTOs), can activate both spinal reflexes and long-loop pathways involving supraspinal centers. Muscle spindles, which are distributed throughout the belly of the muscle, have two types of *intrafusal* muscle fibers (nuclear bag and nuclear chain fibers) that send information to the central nervous system to monitor overall *muscle length* and the *rate of change* in the muscle.[53]

The purpose of the muscle spindle is to compare the length of the spindle with the length of the muscle that surrounds it. The muscle spindle can be stimulated in two different ways: (1) by stretching the whole muscle, which stretches the midportion of the spindle and excites the receptor, and (2) by contracting only the end portion of the intrafusal fibers, exciting the receptor (even if muscle length does not change). Additionally, muscles are innervated by the *alpha motor neurons,* whereas muscle spindles have their own motor supply—*gamma motor neurons*. As alpha motor neurons stimulate contraction of the *extrafusal fibers,* gamma motor neurons cause contraction of the intrafusal fibers at the ends.[46] In short, the intrafusal fiber contraction serves as a sensitivity meter for the changing lengths of the muscle. If the length of the muscle surrounding the spindle is less than that of the spindle, a decrease in intrafusal fiber *afferent* activity occurs. If the central portion of the intrafusal fiber is stretched secondary to gamma *efferent* activity, its sensory receptors discharge more impulses, which stimulate the alpha motor neurons to activate the extrafusal muscle fibers to contract.

Changes in length in the intrafusal fibers within the muscle spindle (i.e., via extrafusal fiber stretch) stimulate primary (Ia) and secondary (II) sensory nerve endings (afferent), sending information about the stretch to the higher brain centers and to the alpha motor neurons of the same muscle, activating the muscle to contract. Shortening of the muscle relieves the stretch on the spindles, temporarily removing the stimulus on the intrafusal fibers. Gamma motor neuron (efferent) activity adjusts for the new muscle length.

In contrast to the muscle spindle, the GTO is a relatively simple sensory receptor: it has a single afferent (Ib) and no efferent connections. It is not a stretch receptor. The function of the GTO is to monitor muscle contraction. Muscle spindles are arranged parallel with extrafusal fibers, whereas GTOs are situated in series with the muscle fibers.[46] Few GTOs are located in the tendon proper, where most of the organs are grouped around a few extrafusal muscle fibers near the aponeurosis of the attachment.[41] When a muscle and its connective tissue attachments are actively contracted or stretched, the group Ib afferent nerve endings fire.

Passive stretching of the muscle activates both the muscle spindles and the GTOs, increasing the afferent output of both receptors. However, these two receptors act differently with active muscle contraction. GTOs are activated by muscle contraction, whereas the muscle spindles are deactivated. As can be seen, GTOs sense muscle tension more directly; the muscle spindles sense increasing muscle length.

STRETCHING

Stretching involves elongating the muscles and tendons to the end of the available ROM. Applying a tensile force to a muscle results in a transient deformation, which elongates the musculotendinous unit, resulting in a stretch.[2,40] Given that the mechanical behavior of connective tissue is primarily influenced by the amount of collagen available,[76,123] the amount of stretching that occurs depends on the type of connective tissue present (i.e., skin, fascia, ligaments, tendons, joint capsules, and muscle fascia).

Although gradually increasing flexibility to increase ROM is the main goal, other adaptations occur from a regular stretching program. For example, research has shown that as a result of training, the stretch reflex may be reset to a different level.[137,138] Several types of stretching exercises have been detailed in the literature and are described in this section.

STRETCHING PRINCIPLES

Stretching is effective primarily because of its mechanical and neurophysiologic effects.[72,123] As mentioned, the muscle-tendon unit responds viscoelastically during stretching, displaying a mechanical effect. However, some stretching exercises are based on the neural inhibition of the muscle undergoing stretch as well, displaying a neurophysiologic effect. In this case, a decreased reflex activity would result in reduced resistance to stretch, resulting in further gains of joint ROM. Most likely, both mechanisms are responsible.

Stiffness relates to a tissue's ability to resist stretch and indicates the amount of deformation proportional to the load applied.[84] The stiffer the tissue, the less compliance it has, and the less likely it is to stretch; conversely, less stiffness means greater compliance. It stands to reason that flexibility training is designed to decrease the stiffness of the muscle-tendon unit.[72,123] Also, a rapidly applied stretch (e.g., ballistic stretching) results in a greater resistance to that stretch.

Important Concepts

Stiffness relates to a tissue's ability to resist stretch and indicates the amount of deformation proportional to the load applied. The stiffer the tissue, the less compliance it has, and the less likely it is to stretch; conversely, less stiffness means greater compliance.

Both mechanical and neurophysiologic components are inherent within muscular flexibility.[43,51,108,121,123] However, some researchers believe that the ability of stretching to produce greater flexibility is primarily a result of the viscoelastic nature of muscle and connective tissue.[87,123] The most resistance to stretching probably is due to the connective tissue framework and sheathing from within and around the muscle and not the muscle itself (because the muscle itself can be stretched to 150% of its resting length); this includes the epimysium, perimysium, and endomysium and may include the sarcolemma.[110,112,119,120]

Many researchers suggest that the immediate result of stretching is attributed to neurophysiologic phenomena.[72] They categorize these phenomena as either a *stretch tolerance* or active contractile responses and claim that the limiting factor during stretching is the muscular resistance secondary to reflex activity. A stretch tolerance simply means an accommodation to the discomfort of stretching over time. With this philosophy, the aim of stretching is to inhibit the reflex activity, subsequently decreasing the

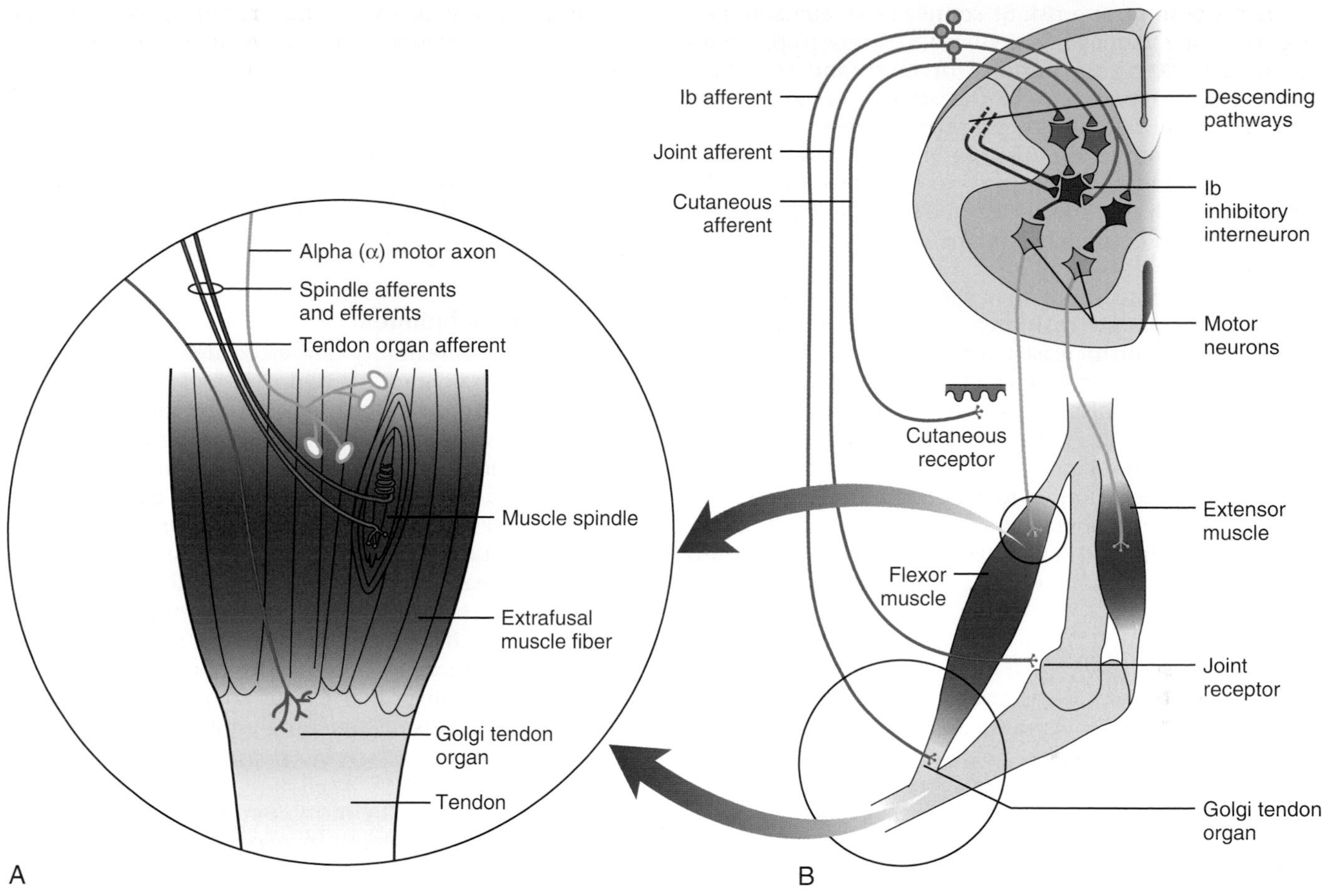

FIG 4-10 **A,** Muscle spindle and Golgi tendon organ (GTO). Fibers of the muscle spindle (intrafusal fibers) are activated by stretch. Type Ia and II sensory afferents of the spindle send information about stretch and the stretch velocity to the spinal cord. Nerve impulses return to the muscle (extrafusal fibers) through the efferent alpha motor neurons that cause the muscle to contract and resist the stretch. The GTOs exist in series as the junction between extrafusal muscle fibers and tendons. The sensory afferents of the GTO are known as *type Ib* and are sensitive to changes in tendon tension that occur with either muscle stretch or contraction. **B,** Reflex action of type Ib afferent fibers from GTO. Type Ib inhibitory neurons receive input from GTO, spindles, joint cutaneous receptors, and descending pathways. *(**A,** Redrawn from Kandel E, Schwartz J, and Jessell T, editors:* Principles of neural sciences, *ed 3, East Norwalk, CT, 1991, McGraw-Hill. **B,** Modified from Kandel E, Schwartz J, and Jessell T, editors:* Principles of neural sciences, *ed 4, New York, 2000, McGraw-Hill.)*

resistance and improving ROM. Several other researchers agree and recommend certain types of stretching for its reduction in reflex activity.[3,43,51] Muscle spindles and GTOs are the mechanoreceptors responsible for the contractile responses (Fig. 4-10).

Important Concepts

A stretch tolerance simply means an accommodation to the discomfort of stretching over time. With this philosophy, the aim of stretching is to inhibit the reflex activity, subsequently decreasing the resistance and improving ROM.

Warm-Up

Warm-up is necessary to help prepare the tissue for activity. Stretching only before exercise is not recommended by most researchers and health professionals.[68,69,114,128] The purpose of warm-up exercises, including stretching, is to prepare the body for the stresses it will encounter during an activity or sport and is necessary for increasing the core body temperature. Heat is produced with muscle contraction, increasing the intramuscular temperature.[23] ROM increases as a result of warmed tissue.[110] A warmed muscle will be able to contract more forcefully and relax more quickly,[15] enhancing work production for the muscles used.[16] In training, a general body warm-up is needed first. The beneficial effects of a warm-up before strenuous activities include the following:

- Blood flow to working muscles is increased.
- Temperature in working muscles is increased.
- Cardiovascular response to sudden, dynamic exercise is improved.
- Breakdown of oxyhemoglobin for the delivery of oxygen to the working muscles is increased.

With warm-up, the risk of connective tissue and contractile tissue damage is reduced. Warm-up protocols usually last 10 to 25 minutes or more and may vary depending on the nature of the activity or event.[8] The warm-up should be intense enough to cause an increase in body temperature but not so intense as to cause fatigue. One should taper the warm-up 5 to 10 minutes before the actual event.[3] It is clinically assumed that a more compliant muscle can be stretched further and is less susceptible to injury.[49]

However, some think that the warm-up period may not be the best time to stretch for increasing ROM, primarily because of increased tissue stiffness. Because the concept of stretching to prevent injury has come under question, benefits of stretching only before activity may be incorrect. Activity of gradually increasing intensity (dynamic stretching) may be more appropriate than static stretching as a warm-up activity.[99] Some researchers have examined the combination of stretching and active warm-up and have shown that the decrease in stiffness mainly results from increased muscle temperature and not stretching.[88,107]

Important Concepts

Some researchers have examined the combination of stretching and active warm-up and have shown that the decrease in stiffness mainly results from increased muscle temperature and not stretching.

Increasing intramuscular temperature to help increase ROM may also be achieved through external means.[113] Henricson and colleagues[59] reported on results that followed the application of heat to the hip. Heat alone did not improve hip ROM; stretching without heat increased hip ROM; and stretching with heat combined resulted in the greatest increase in ROM, maintaining it for 30 minutes. These results are consistent with the research of others,[64,77,131] who reported that collagen extensibility increases and musculotendinous stiffness decreases with heat. However, most authors recommend using exercise as the primary way of increasing intramuscular temperature.[99] It has not been definitively shown whether a general warm-up serves to improve sports performance.[17,18,21,47] However, research investigating the effects of various types of stretching on the 40-yard dash revealed that a warm-up only (no stretching) before a baseline 40-yard run resulted in decreased run times (improved performance) compared with a warm-up only (no stretching) before a baseline run followed by the different types of stretching.[127]

Stretching Techniques

In discussion of flexibility and associated stretching programs, the stretching of nonpathologic muscle must be separated from stretching noncontractile connective tissue. Improving muscle extensibility in nonpathologic conditions and in adaptive muscle shortening after injury or immobilization requires a complement of active exercise techniques and thermal agents. Types of stretching exercises are static stretching (active and passive), ballistic stretching, dynamic stretching, and proprioceptive neuromuscular facilitation (PNF) techniques (contract-relax, contract-relax with agonist contraction, and hold-relax). All four techniques have been shown to increase flexibility.[31,58,63,83,85,108] The proper execution of the exercises is essential to a successful stretching program for improving flexibility.

Static Stretching. The most common form of stretching exercise that is used to increase the ROM in a joint safely is static stretching. This form of stretching allows one to sustain a controlled stretch by placing a muscle in a fully elongated position and holding that position for a period of time (Fig. 4-11). A passive static stretch implies that the force is applied externally (i.e., with a partner or gravity-assisted) (Fig. 4-12). If an opposing muscle action is used to aid the stretch, the stretch is called an *active static stretch*. However, to obtain optimal passive stretching, all voluntary and reflex muscular resistance must be eliminated.

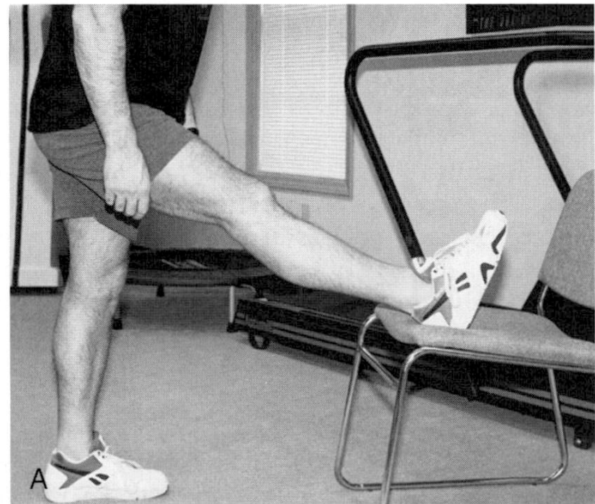

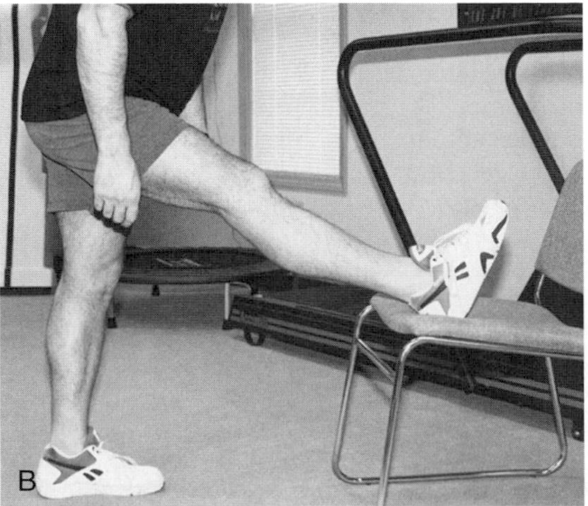

FIG 4-11 **A,** Static stretching. Initial starting position for standing hamstring stretch. **B,** Ending position for standing hamstring stretch (note trunk flexion). The muscle will slowly conform to an elongated position by maintaining stress on the tissue for a period of time.

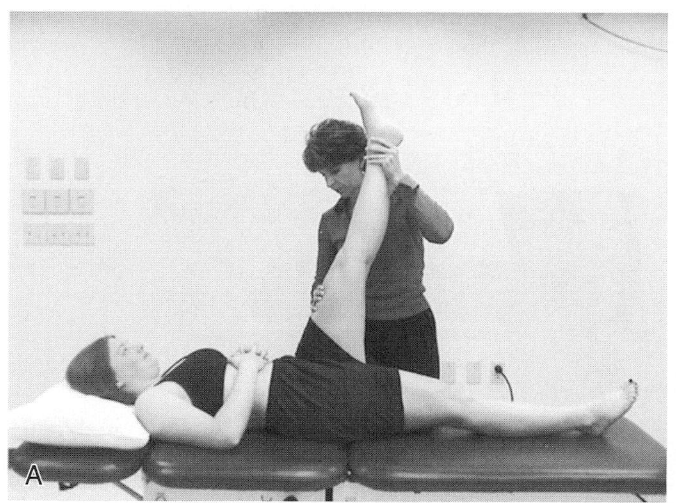

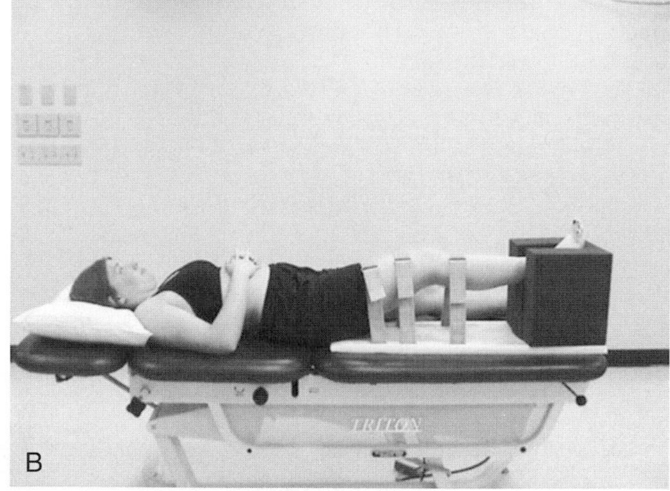

FIG 4-12 **A,** Partner assisted passive stretch for hamstrings; **B,** External device providing passive stretch to knee extension. *(From Mancinelli CA, Davis DS: Range of motion and stretching. In Huber FE, Wells CL (eds.):* Therapeutic exercise: treatment planning for progression, *St Louis, 2006, Saunders.)*

Research supports that slow passive stretching through the ROM will not induce muscle activity in normal relaxed subjects.[13,110] The muscle should be slowly and passively stretched to a new length so that the stretch reflex is not elicited. Additionally, the stretch should not elicit pain, although some discomfort with stretching may be noted.[3,108] As is described later, the stretch is maintained for an extended period of time before the muscle is returned to its starting position. Subsequently, a lengthening of the muscle is accomplished.

Athletes use static stretching before sports activities as part of a warm-up before a workout and as part of a cooldown after a workout. Because intramuscular temperature increases to approximately 39° C during exercise,[6] active general body movements can improve muscle temperature before stretching is done. Most warm-up programs use primarily active static stretches, using gravity to assist the stretch.

Studies on rat tail tendons[77] demonstrated that ruptures occurred with 31% of normal loads when temperatures were at 25° C, whereas increasing temperatures to 45° C delayed tendon rupture until 102% of normal load. This research demonstrates that excessive stretching at normal body temperatures may damage tissue,[131] but elevating tissue temperature before and during prolonged stretch is less damaging.[130,131]

Static stretching has distinct advantages, such as reduced chance of exceeding strain limits of tissues, reduced energy requirements compared with other forms of stretching, and reduced potential for muscle soreness.[29,111,139] The ease and practicality of teaching patients to perform static stretching is another advantage. For example, hamstring stretches can be taught with the patient in various positions (Fig. 4-13). The general goals of static stretching are to prevent or minimize the risk of soft tissue injury from participation in sports or physical activities (although research has not demonstrated that this actually occurs), improve movement and increase flexibility, and prevent contracture.[8,66]

Ballistic Stretching. Another technique used often by athletes is ballistic stretching (Fig. 4-14). Many researchers believe that this is the least desirable technique because it potentially places the tissue at risk secondary to the use of jerking or bouncing movements at the end of the ROM to stretch the muscles.[74] Athletes use dynamic, high-velocity, and even violent motions during sporting events and require extraordinary flexibility to prevent or reduce the risk of potential musculoskeletal injury. Relatively high-velocity or quick bouncing may not be appropriate for many patients. The potential for tissue damage exists in all forms of exercise, but ballistic stretching may increase the risk of connective tissue and contractile tissue trauma, although a narrow segment of patients may benefit.

The reason ballistic stretches are considered undesirable is that they stimulate the muscle spindles during the stretch. This results in a continuous resistance to further stretch, which causes a high rate of tension strong enough potentially to injure the musculotendinous unit.[69,110,126] Ballistic stretching does not imply aggressive, violent, high-velocity stretches throughout the ROM; instead it involves a slight but progressively greater bounce at the end of the range achieved through static stretching.

Important Concepts

The reason ballistic stretches are considered undesirable is that they stimulate the muscle spindles during the stretch. This results in a continuous resistance to further stretch, which causes a high rate of tension strong enough potentially to injure the musculotendinous unit.

Dynamic Stretching. A type of stretching technique that has become increasingly popular is dynamic stretching. With dynamic stretching, muscular contraction is used to stretch a muscle; the effect is to increase or decrease the joint angle where the muscle crosses, elongating the musculotendinous unit as the end ROM is obtained.[11] What sets dynamic stretching apart is that it uses

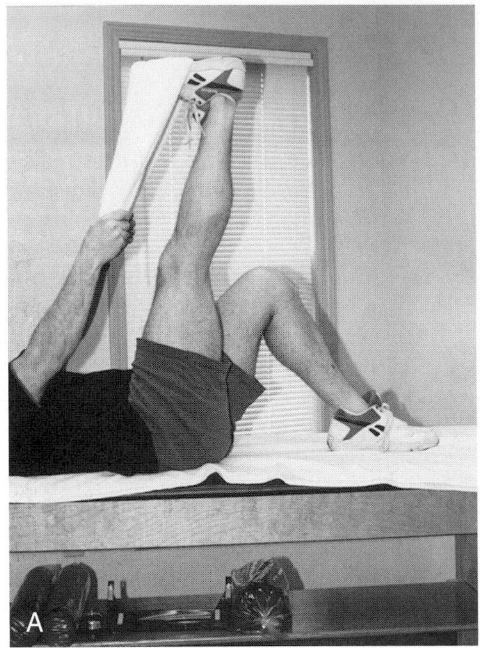

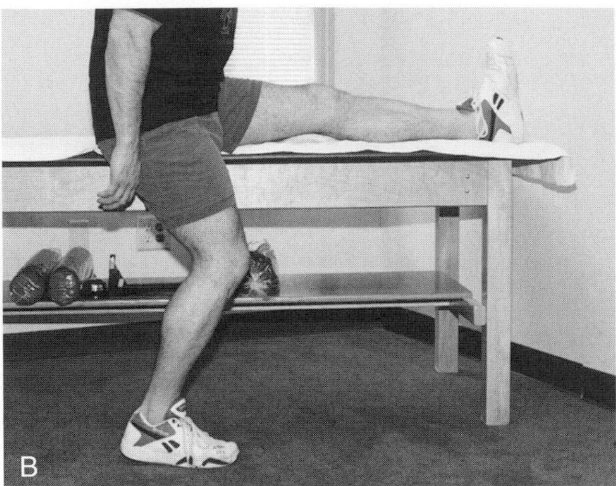

FIG 4-13 **A,** Supine static hamstring stretch using a towel. **B,** Sitting hamstring stretch.

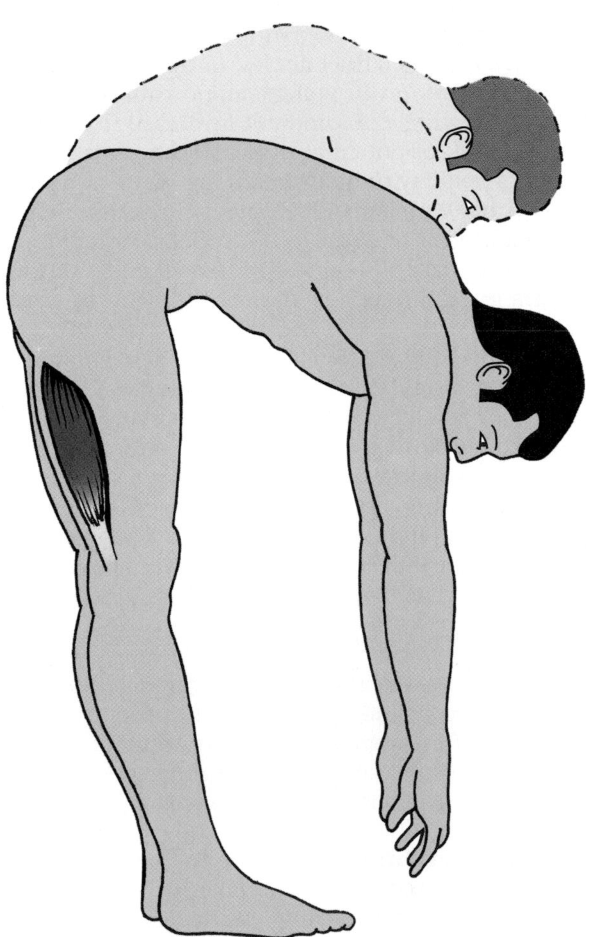

FIG 4-14 Ballistic stretching requires a relatively high-velocity bounce at the end-range of motion. Typically ballistic stretching techniques are reserved for an athletic population in preparation for high-velocity, ballistic, and sometimes violent physical activity.

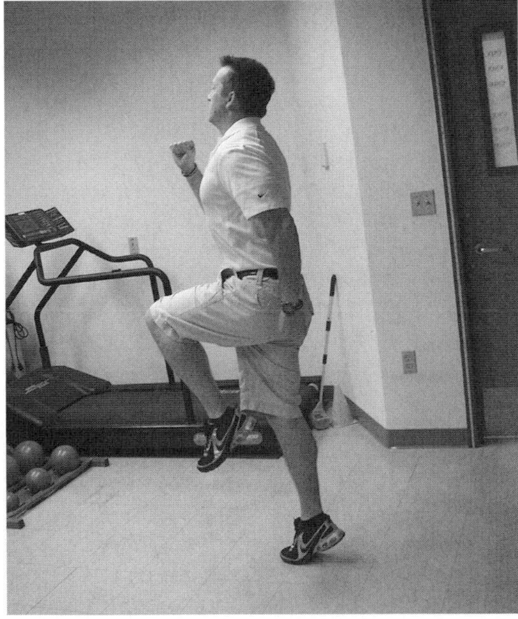

FIG 4-15 Dynamic stretching.

activity-specific movements, preparing the muscles by taking them through the movements used in a particular sport. An example would be a sprinter who walks using exaggerated long strides, emphasizing hip flexion and extension (Fig. 4-15); this subsequently actively contracts and stretches the muscles used by the sprinter—the hip flexors and extensors.[62] Dynamic stretching does not incorporate end-range ballistic movements that are bouncy or jerky in nature. Rather, all movements are under control.[99]

Proprioceptive Neuromuscular Facilitation. PNF is another technique used to facilitate ROM increases via stretching. PNF is a system of therapy that uses different techniques designed to promote neuromuscular responses via stimulation of the proprioceptive system.[125] These techniques use volitional contractions to increase ROM by decreasing the resistance caused by the spinal reflex pathways.[24] PNF stretching uses movements in diagonal patterns along with an isometric contraction before the stretch; this allows greater gains in ROM than stretching alone. However, depending on the clinical setting, many clinicians have modified the various PNF patterns, deviating from the proposed diagonal patterns originally described by Knott and Voss[67] to straight plane patterns. As a result, it is difficult to determine if the effects of PNF treatment are consistent among practitioners and in the research literature.

PNF stretching techniques, which are based on the stretch reflex, appear to increase ROM through the stimulation of the proprioceptors[2] and, in some cases, have been found to produce greater increases in ROM than static stretching.[94,104] Two neurophysiologic sensory receptors involved with the stretch reflex are GTOs and muscle spindles. The GTOs are inhibitory sensory receptors located within the musculotendinous junction that signal tension in a muscle (see Fig. 4-10, *B*). Stimulation of the GTO results in self-inhibition of that muscle, termed *autogenic inhibition*. They also signal minute changes in muscle tension, providing information about muscle contraction.[65]

Muscle spindles are excitatory specialized fibers within the muscle (see Fig. 4-10, *A*) that are sensitive to changes in muscle length as well as maintenance of that length. When a muscle is stretched, the spindles send messages to the spinal cord, which signals the muscle to contract. The classic clinical demonstration of the stretch reflex is produced by tapping the relaxed patellar tendon, which causes the reflexive contraction of the quadriceps. The muscle spindles within the quadriceps are activated by the quick stretch of the patellar tendon, causing the quadriceps to contract reflexively (Fig. 4-16).[65]

Despite the advantages, PNF stretching has some disadvantages as well. For example, it is more time-consuming than other methods, requires skillful application by trained professionals to be effective, and may lead to mild complaints of patient discomfort.[111] Some of the more commonly used techniques are contract-relax, contract-relax with agonist contraction, and hold-relax.

The *contract-relax* technique involves instructing the patient to relax the affected muscle while the therapist passively moves the limb to the limit of motion (until the person feels a stretch). The patient is instructed to actively contract the restricted muscle (antagonist) against the manually applied resistance of the therapist for 5 to 8 seconds.[1] The patient is then instructed to relax while the therapist passively moves the limb to the new limits of motion, at which point the clinician holds the stretch for 10 seconds (Fig. 4-17). This relaxation of the antagonist muscle during contraction is an example of *autogenic inhibition*. The process is repeated by continuing from the new limit of pain-free motion until the required number of repetitions is performed or until no more range is gained.[1]

In the *contract-relax with agonist contraction* technique, there is a contraction of the opposite (agonist) muscles instead of the shortened or restricted muscles.[1] In this case, the limb is taken to the point of stretch while the

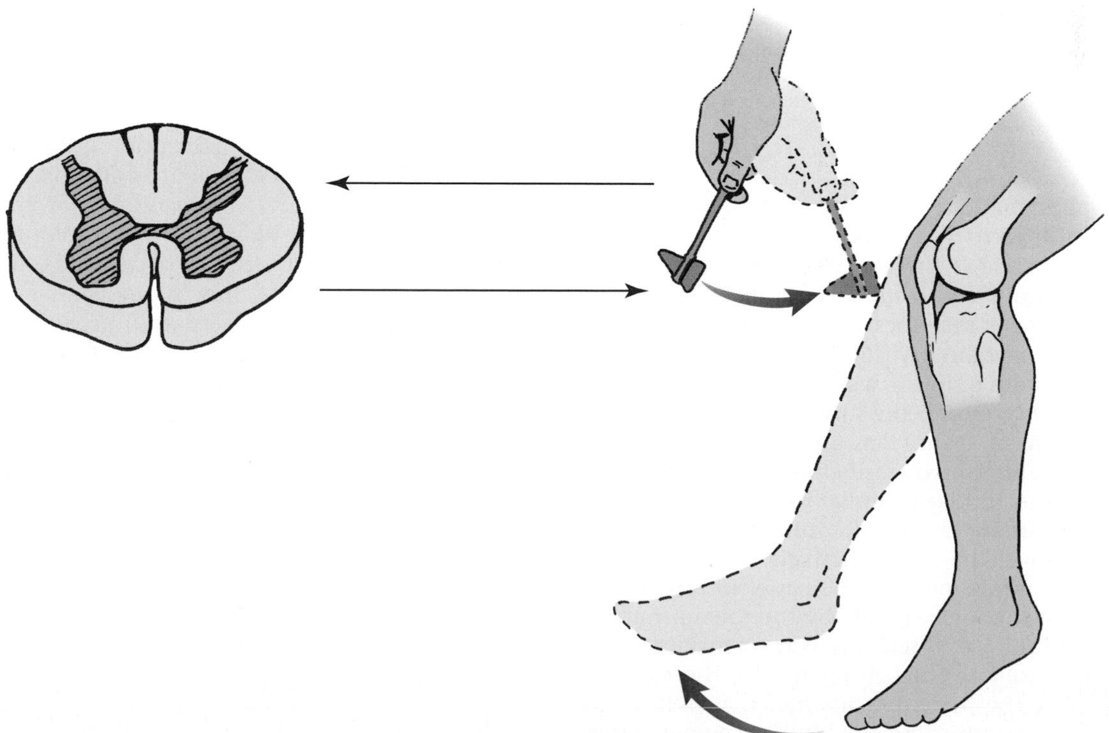

FIG 4-16 Muscle spindle activation by quick stretch-reflex between the spinal cord and quadriceps.

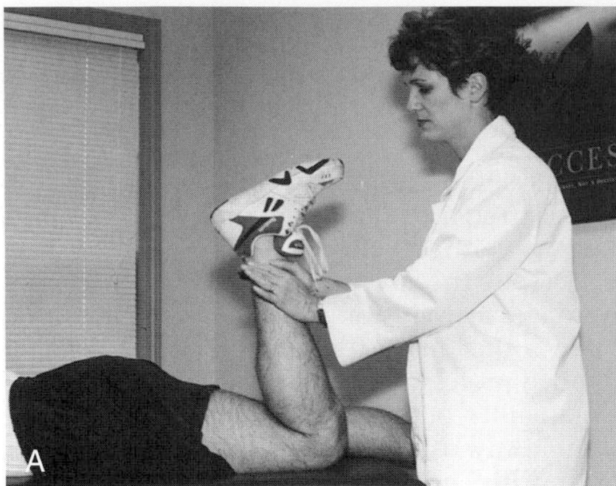

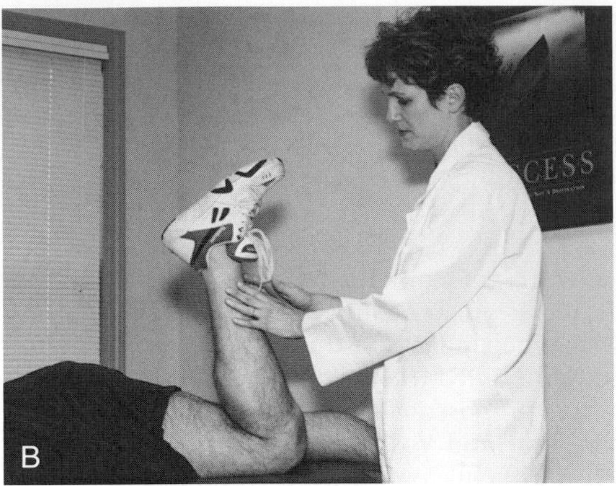

FIG 4-17 Proprioceptive neuromuscular facilitation, contract-relax technique. **A,** The patient actively contracts against manually applied resistance for 5 to 8 seconds. **B,** The patient relaxes while the therapist passively moves the limb to the new limits of motion.

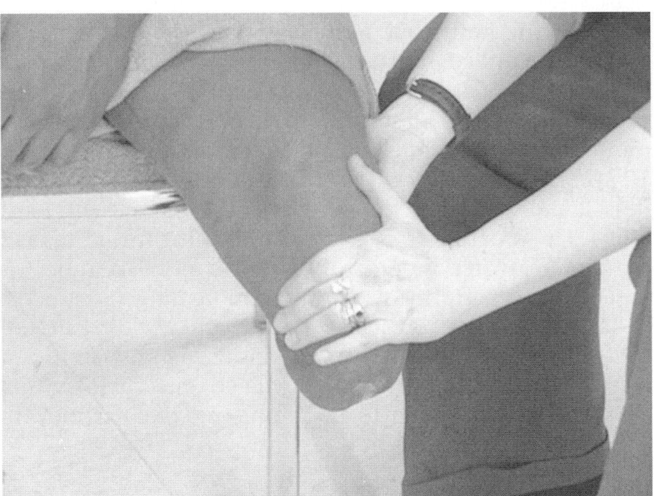

FIG 4-18 Proprioceptive neuromuscular facilitation, contract-relax technique. *(From Mancinelli CA, Davis DS: Range of motion and stretching. In Huber FE, Wells CL (eds.):* Therapeutic exercise: treatment planning for progression, *St Louis, 2006, Saunders.)*

clinician applies manual resistance against the muscle being stretched for 5 to 8 seconds (as in the contract-relax method). The muscle is then relaxed while the agonist muscle concentrically contracts; this facilitates the stretch using the principle of reciprocal inhibition (Fig. 4-18). In *reciprocal inhibition,* voluntary isometric contraction of the agonist muscle group results in a subsequent reflex inhibition on the muscle groups being stretched (reciprocal inhibition). The clinician again takes up any slack and holds the new position for 10 seconds before continuing.

The *hold-relax* technique is similar to contract-relax and consequently initiates autogenic inhibition. However, with this technique, the patient actively moves the limb to the end of pain-free motion. The patient isometrically contracts against the force applied by the therapist at the end of the ROM for 5 to 8 seconds as resistance is slowly increased. After holding the contraction for the requisite amount of time, the patient is instructed to relax. The patient then actively stretches the limb to the new limits of motion (Fig. 4-19).[1]

Duration, Frequency, and Intensity of Stretching

Recommendations in the literature regarding the specific duration, frequency, intensity, and number of stretching repetitions vary. Stretch duration depends on the joint targeted, the flexibility goal, and the type of stretching technique used. Generally, static stretches may be held in a fully elongated position for 10 to 60 seconds, with most research recommending that stretches be held between 15 and 30 seconds.[8-11,84,106,125] An attempt is then made to extend the stretched position farther within tolerable limits (Fig. 4-20). When the muscle-tendon unit is cyclically stretched to a fixed tension or length, the properties of creep and stress relaxation occur with each cycle. Researchers have reported that 80% of the length changes occurred in the first four stretches of 30 seconds each.[122] However, because of the structural diversity of tissue, predicting the duration of stretch for each tissue becomes very difficult.[76] Current American College of Sports Medicine guidelines recommend three to five repetitions for each stretching exercise.[101]

The limits of motion achieved during a stretching program depend on the patient's tolerance, age, pathologic condition (if any), motivation, and commitment. The muscle's ability to adapt is a prolonged process. Patients must be cautioned not to exceed their pain limits and must receive counseling about the fact that many sessions of stretching are needed to produce change and lasting improvement. Approximately 6 weeks of stretching are necessary to demonstrate significant increases in muscular flexibility.[37] An individual must stretch at least three times per week to improve flexibility. An individual must stretch at least 1 day per week to maintain the flexibility gained during the program.[111]

Important Concepts

An individual must stretch at least three times per week to improve flexibility. An individual must stretch at least 1 day per week to maintain the flexibility gained during the program.

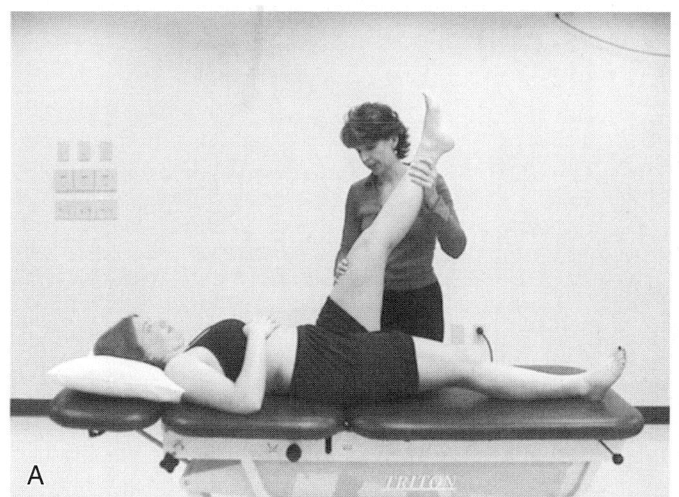

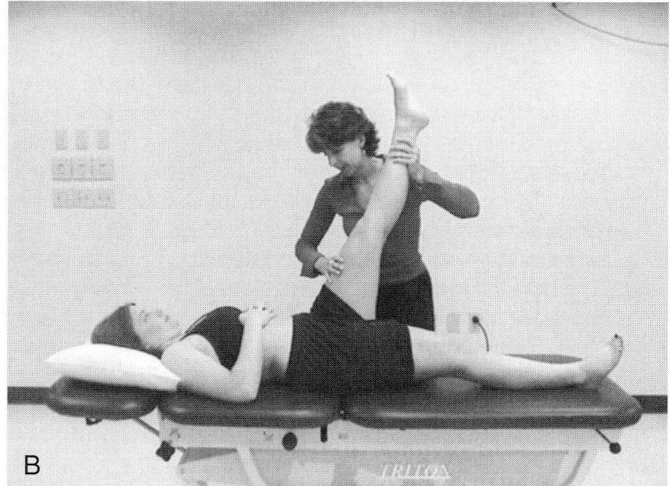

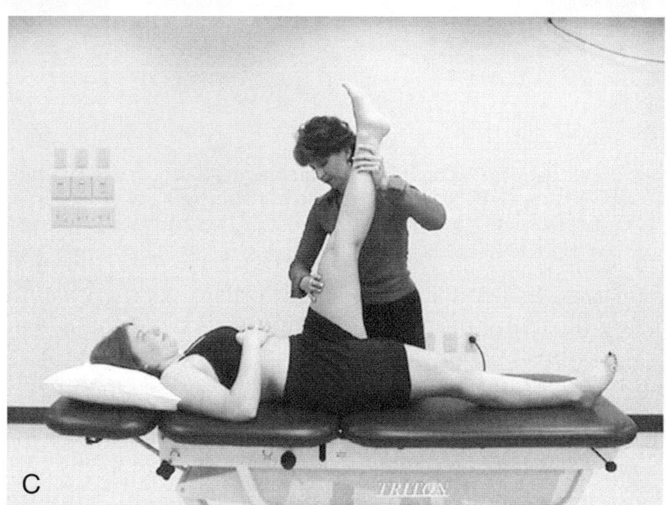

FIG 4-19 Proprioceptive neuromuscular facilitation hold-relax technique. **A,** Patient actively moves limb to end of available motion. **B,** Patient isometrically contracts against force applied by therapist at end of ROM. **C,** After brief relaxation, patient then actively stretches limb to new limits of available motion. *(From Mancinelli CA, Davis DS: Range of motion and stretching. In Huber FE, Wells CL (eds.):* Therapeutic exercise: treatment planning for progression, *St Louis, 2006, Saunders.)*

Intensity. Increases in ROM can be significantly affected by the intensity of the stretch.[110,129] Structural damage subsequent to stretching could result with increased levels of force and may result in structural weakening of the muscle-tendon unit, increasing the risk of injury.[97,122] The appropriate intensity for static stretching is to stretch slowly and hold the position at low force levels. This is most often communicated to the individual as pain-free or mild discomfort.

How Long Does It Last? Little has been reported on the long-lasting effects of stretching. Some researchers reported that stretching techniques using cyclic and sustained stretching for 15 minutes on 5 consecutive days increased hamstring muscle length with a significant percentage of the increased length being retained 1 week after treatment.[118] Some researchers reported that the knee ROM was able to be maintained for 3 minutes but had returned to prestretched levels in 6 minutes,[36] whereas other researchers reported that increased ROM from stretching remained for up to 90 minutes.[45,92] These differences have been explained by variations in warm-up, stretching position, stretching force, and stretching duration.[142] Some research has shown that stretching at least once a week after a 30-day training program will maintain the gained flexibility.[126]

COMPARISONS OF DIFFERENT STRETCHING TECHNIQUES

All stretching techniques previously discussed have been shown to increase flexibility and ROM.[48,50,82] However, the appropriate stretching frequency and duration for long-lasting changes in flexibility has not been adequately defined in the literature.[103] It is also not completely evident which stretching technique increases flexibility most effectively. Ballistic stretching and static stretching appear to be similar in their effects on flexibility,[58,63,108] yet existing research indicates that dynamic stretching may produce about the same flexibility gains as static and ballistic stretching.[11]

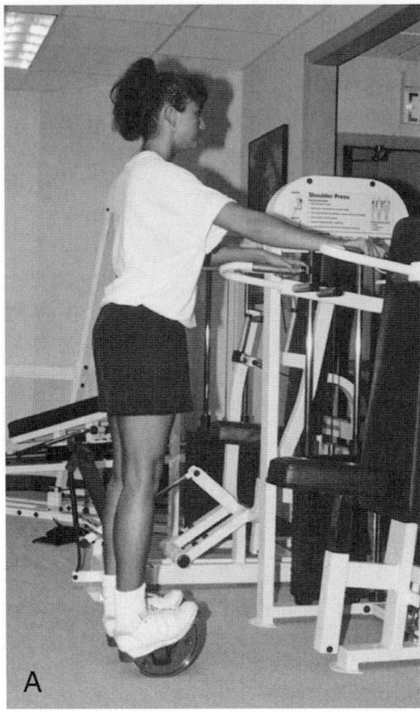

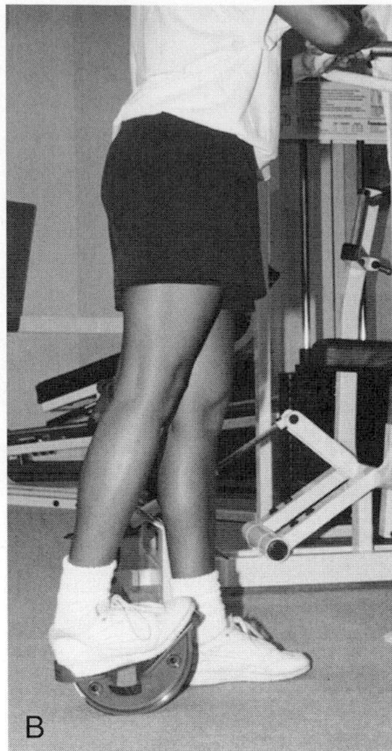

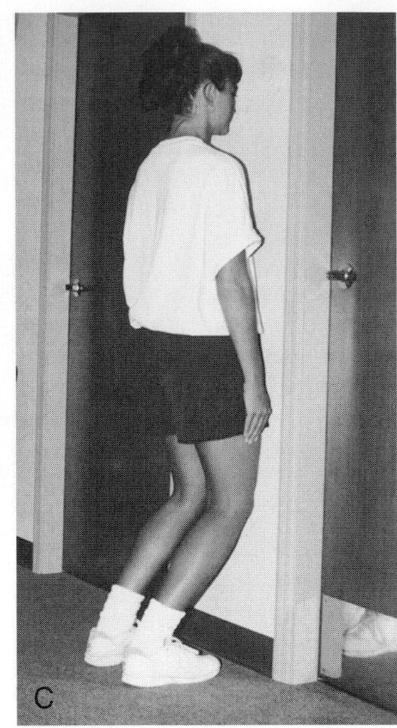

FIG 4-20 Examples of static stretching positions and techniques for the gastrocnemius-soleus complex. **A,** Standing bilateral calf stretch. **B,** Single limb static calf stretch. **C,** Gastrocnemius-soleus stretch.

Although many studies have revealed that PNF may be the preferred method for increasing flexibility over static and ballistic stretching,[27,42,54,104,121] direct comparison between methods is very difficult to determine because of the differences in methodology, experimental design, procedures, and measurement instruments and the use of inadequate control groups.[99] Additionally, some studies found no significant differences between techniques.[58,82,89,94] Some authors have reviewed stretching studies and reported conflicting evidence regarding the efficacy of these methods[44,54]; they reported that most of the differences between studies were probably due to variations in training methods, measuring instruments, and confounding variables.

PROPOSED STRETCHING BENEFITS

Enhanced Flexibility

Research has shown that a long-term, routine stretching program can result in increased long-term flexibility, whereas a short-term stretching program does not.[11,68] Wiktorsson-Moller and colleagues[134] reported that stretching significantly increased hip ROM for flexion/extension, hip abduction, knee flexion, and ankle dorsiflexion. The effect was significantly greater than that obtained by massage and warming up, separately or combined. Similarly, Williford and associates[136] showed that increases in flexibility could occur as a result of a static stretching training program.

Relief of Muscular Soreness

Previous research has indicated that slow stretching exercises were able to reduce postexercise muscular soreness,[30,32] but other research, examining the effect of static stretching on soreness, revealed no significant effect on perceived pain compared with a control group.[86] Later research showed that stretching had no effects on decreasing exercise soreness over the postexercise period or immediately after an acute bout of stretching.[22,52] Some research has demonstrated that stretching may cause muscle soreness. In a study investigating the effects of static and ballistic stretching on delayed-onset muscle soreness (DOMS), researchers found that similar bouts of static and ballistic stretching induced significant increases in DOMS in subjects unaccustomed to such exercise.[117]

Muscle Relaxation

The literature has shown that chronic increased muscular tension can result in negative side effects, such as high blood pressure, headaches, ulcers, and muscle and joint pain.[75] Subsequently, many individuals use certain types of stretching as a way to facilitate muscle relaxation. An example of this type of flexibility training is used in yoga.[2] The belief is that chronic tension affects muscles so that they become less strong, less supple, and not as capable of absorbing the shock and stress of various types of movements. Stretching may be implemented to facilitate muscular relaxation, decreasing stress and muscular tension.[33,34] A possible explanation may be that, with stretching, the muscle spindles may adapt to the stretch, or while held at a constant length, force relaxation may occur, which would decrease the tension on the muscle. In examining electromyograms before and after warm-up, Mohr and colleagues[91] found that muscle activity during static stretching of the gastrocnemius muscle for about 30 seconds was significantly lower and sufficient to attain muscle relaxation.

Injury Prevention

Evidence is unclear as to whether stretching before or after exercise decreases the chance of injury. On one hand, some research has shown that stretching may decrease the rate of injury.[28,57,90,109] Researchers also stated that stretching, as part of a warm-up or a rehabilitation program, decreased the percentage or recurrence of injuries.[39] On the other hand, research has also shown that stretching is not effective in preventing injury.[124] A 12-week training study of 1538 male army recruits revealed that stretching had little influence on injuries associated with weight-bearing physical training such as running, marching, and walking.[102]

Performance Enhancement

Many assume that performance is enhanced by stretching before the activity and usually point to sports that require extreme ROM at particular joints (e.g., gymnastics and pitching). However, no conclusive data support a correlation between flexibility or stretching and performance. It is generally agreed that a warm-up is necessary before exercising to perform an activity safely and successfully.[69] Stretching is widely accepted as an important part of the warm-up. Also, many have traditionally believed that performing stretching immediately before physical activity improves performance.[49] Although it is plausible that increased flexibility may potentially improve performance in many activities where ROM is necessary to perform certain skills, whether stretching beforehand can improve performance is questionable.[68,116,135] Some studies have reported that stretching beforehand neither helps nor inhibits performance,[50,70] whereas other studies have revealed negative performance effects.[45,71,128]

Important Concepts

Although it is plausible that increased flexibility may potentially improve performance in many activities where ROM is necessary to perform certain skills, whether stretching beforehand can actually improve performance is questionable.

The reason for these negative effects, according to some researchers, is probably that the muscle-tendon unit becomes weaker after acute stretching and is less able to produce high-intensity force. Consequently, there is a period of time during which the muscle-tendon unit stays stretched (lag period), in which it may need to "take up the slack" before peak tension is reached. Stretching immediately before a performance task may cause a strength deficit, resulting in impeded performance.[128] Because of this possibility, it has been suggested that low-intensity muscle contractions should be performed immediately before sport performance (i.e., dynamic stretching).[19]

WHEN TO STRETCH

Very little literature is available to determine when stretching should occur in an exercise program. Some clinicians believe that stretching should be part of the warm-up to enhance musculotendinous extensibility but should not constitute the entire warm-up.[73] Wiktorsson-Moller and associates[134] showed that warm-up before stretching resulted in significant changes in joint ROM. Some authors think that stretching should not be performed at the beginning of a warm-up routine.[73,110] They believe that the tissue temperatures may be too low for optimal muscle-tendon function, subsequently leading to a less compliant tissue, which may not adequately prepare the tissue for activity. Many authors recommend at least 5 minutes of light progressive exercise before stretching.[110] Conversely, some discourage exercise before stretching, stating that muscle tissue after warm-up does not stretch better and is not less likely to be injured.[96]

Some researchers found that stretching should be performed after an exercise session because of the improved joint ROM.[88] However, Cornelius and colleagues[26] revealed that performing static stretching before, after, and both before and after each workout in a 6-week program did not make a difference in increasing ROM. Significant increases in ROM were produced with all protocols.

STRETCHING OF SOFT TISSUE CONTRACTURES

The stretching of soft tissue contractures involves muscle, capsule, tendon, ligament, bursa, and skin. Many options exist for the therapist when prescribing stretching exercises for patients after immobilization or injury, which differ from static, ballistic, or PNF stretching. Long-duration, low-load static stretching has been an effective technique that produces long-lasting connective tissue changes.[29,77,130,131] The PTA must recognize adaptive changes that occur in various soft tissues after injury or immobility.

Initially, scar tissue is formed, which may result in the development of a scar contracture if the tissue is not adequately mobilized. A **contracture** in this case is defined as a permanent or transient limitation of movement or shortening of muscle or other soft tissues; in other words, a contracture is the result of healed tissue that forms a fixed, rigid scar and causes cosmetic deformity or functional deficits.[60] Scar tissue formation may be the result of **adhesions** and other tissue damage (Fig. 4-21, *A*). An adhesion involves a limitation of function resulting from scar tissue that forms between structures. For example, when scar tissue forms after knee surgery, it can bind down and cross-link collagen tissue, resulting in adhesions around the patella, suprapatellar pouch, and quadriceps tendon (Fig. 4-21, *B*).

Generally, immature scar is defined as adaptable for up to 8 weeks and becomes progressively less changeable for up to 14 weeks. Scar becomes quite inextensible at 14 weeks and is termed *inadaptable,* or mature scar.[4] Adaptable scar is highly vascular, with many cells (including myofibrocytes) that give the scar the ability to contract. Immature scar tissue also has a high rate of **remodeling,**[4] which is the process of tissue restructuring in response to stress or immobilization.[29]

As new scar tissue is formed, the collagen fibers become highly unorganized and arranged randomly, creating an immobile structure.[81] Adaptable or immature scar tissue becomes increasingly organized and oriented, with

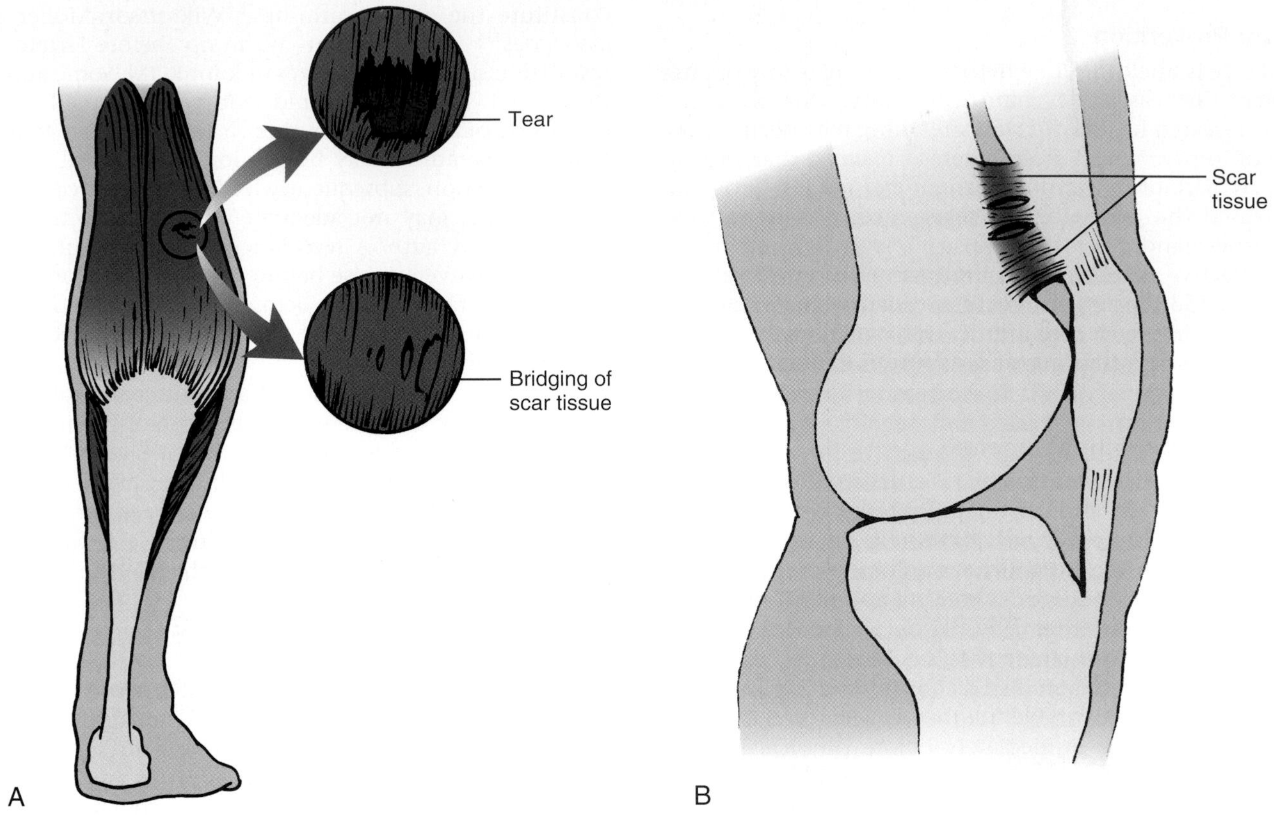

FIG 4-21 Scar tissue. **A,** Scar tissue formation. **B,** Adhesions formed between the quadriceps tendon and underlying bone result in a limitation of function.

specific directional lines of stress. The formation of collagen fibers is in response to stress imposed from mechanical loads.[60] Where stretching is concerned, the PTA must be attentive to the following critical components:

- The nature of scar tissue is time dependent and stress reactive.
- Immature, adaptable scar tissue is fragile.
  - At 5 days, new scar is only 10% of its maximum potential strength.
  - At 40 days, new scar is 40% of its maximum strength.
  - At 60 days, new scar is 70% of its maximum strength.
  - At 12 months, new scar is approximately 100% of its maximum strength.
- New scar tissue organizes and aligns itself along lines of stress; appropriately applied stress helps to remodel unorganized scar.
- Low-load, long-duration stretching of joint contractures in combination with thermal agents to preheat extensible connective tissue has proved effective in the treatment of soft tissue contracture.[61,78,80] Long-duration stretching means stretching over a period of 20 to 60 minutes.

Clinically, the following areas are involved in a low-load, prolonged stretch technique:

1. Preheat the involved structures with moist heat or ultrasound.[29]
2. Place the involved structures in a position of comfort, not maximum stretch. This is an extremely important point. To elicit relaxation, the involved structures must be placed in a supported and comfortable gravity-assisted position.
3. Maintain moist heat application during the entire course of treatment (20 to 60 minutes).
4. Apply stress or load gradually and minimally. With new immature scar, gravity alone may be enough to effect change clinically. With mature scar, only slightly greater loads should be used. This is a critical point. Lentell and colleagues[78] found that the magnitude of force used in their study (0.5% of body weight) to create a significant long-lasting change in motion fostered such relaxation that many subjects were not even aware of stretching taking place during the procedure. For example, in an effort to gain knee extension after surgery, it would behoove one to use this technique to avoid reflexive splinting or muscle guarding (Fig. 4-22).
5. Allow the patient to rest or recover for a few minutes during the course of treatment if the sensation of stretch becomes too uncomfortable.
6. Maintain heat application for 5 to 10 minutes after removal of the loads. Some researchers[110] have advocated the use of ice packs after stretch in this protocol. Lentell and colleagues[78] did not find cooling to be effective in their study. However, cooling the involved structures after stress may be effective in selected cases where pain and an inflammatory response are present.
7. Initiate isometric contractions after the application of heat and passive stretching to enhance strength gains at the new end of ROM.

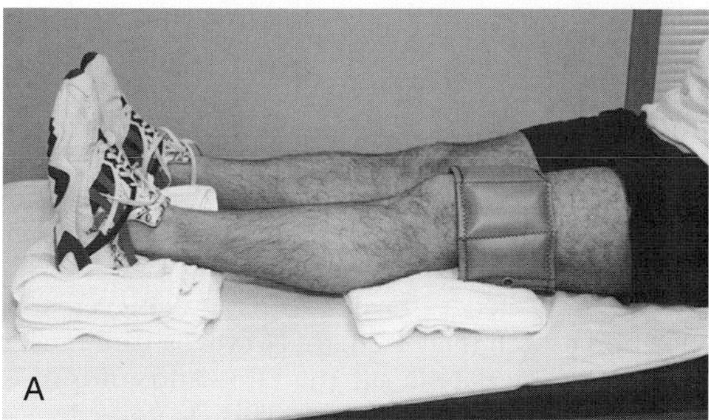

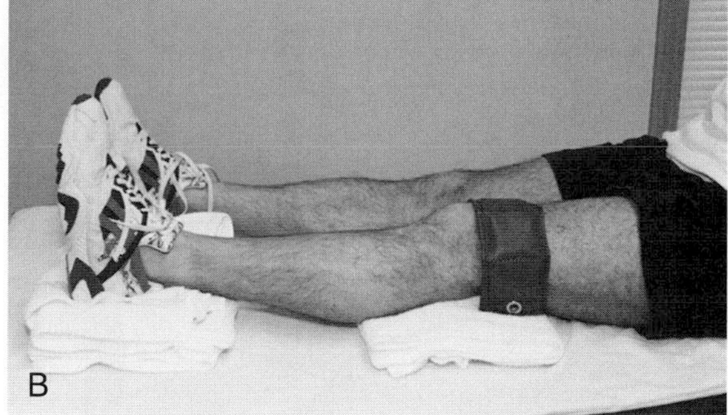

FIG 4-22 External force is applied to enhance passive low-load prolonged stretch. **A,** Excessive weight causes reflexive muscle splinting and guarding. **B,** Only very light resistance is necessary to elicit appropriate relaxation.

Lentell and colleagues[78] demonstrated the effectiveness of applying heat before and during low-load, prolonged stretching and external rotation of nonpathologically involved shoulders. Heat application before and during such stretching was clinically superior to bouts of stretching alone, stretching plus ice, and a heat-stretch-ice protocol. Clinically, few contraindications exist when attempting to gain motion after specific surgical procedures.

Adhesions are desirable and are a surgical goal in selected cases. Desirable permanent shortening of connective tissue is needed to prevent a functional loss of movement in some knee surgeries and surgical correction of some shoulder instabilities. If an attempt is made to regain external shoulder rotation fully after surgery to correct recurrent dislocation, the intent to scar down and protect the joint from further dislocation may be derailed. In this case, it is wise to gain functional motion very slowly to allow enough time for a mature scar to form (14 weeks).

The clinical application of low-load, prolonged stretch can be modified to varying degrees depending on the surgical procedure, time constraints of healing, and goals of the rehabilitation program. For example, supine wall slides are a modified technique that uses some of the points of low-load, prolonged stretch (Fig. 4-23). When attempting to gain knee flexion range, it is wise to preheat the quadriceps muscles and suprapatellar pouch before stretching. Next, the patient is placed in a supine position, and the foot of the involved limb is put on a towel against a wall. To reduce friction against the wall, the contact surface of the towel is lightly coated with baby powder so that it slides more easily against the wall. As the patient relaxes, gravity assists in knee flexion, and the foot slides down the wall.

This concept can be modified further. In keeping with the example of gaining knee flexion range, the use of isotonic exercise equipment can be helpful. With the patient in a seated position on a knee extension machine, moist heat or ultrasound can be used before and during the stretch (Fig. 4-24). Many knee extension machines are manufactured with an adjustable range-limiting device that allows the patient to adjust the starting and stopping angle of the exercise. Before the stretch is begun, the patient's hips are secured with straps to keep them from rising during the treatment. An angle is selected that is comfortable to the patient. As the tissues are continually heated, a very gradual increase in the flexion angle is initiated. The angle does not have to be excessive to be effective. The protocol remains essentially the same, but the equipment and the position of the patient are changed.

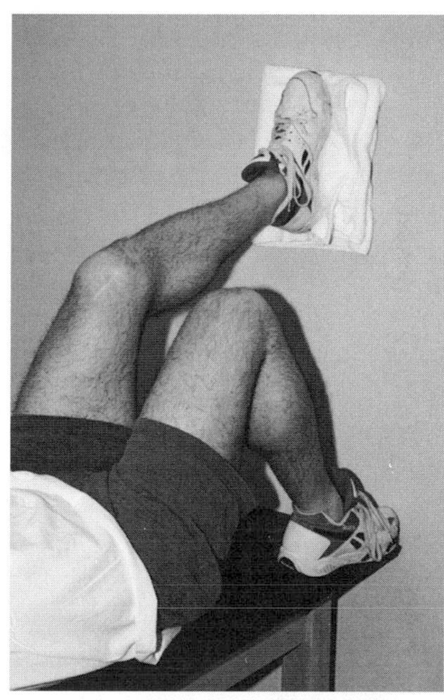

FIG 4-23 Supine wall slides to gain knee flexion motion.

The knee serves as an excellent example to describe and clarify further methods to improve ROM by prolonged static stretching. To gain knee extension range, the patient can be supine with moist heat applied behind the knee (popliteal fossa) and on the hamstring and quadriceps. The heel of the involved limb is placed on a small folded towel (Fig. 4-25, *A*). For example, if the knee is contracted to −20°, towels are added under the hot packs under the knee to ensure a very comfortable starting position. During the course of treatment, small layers of towel can be removed gradually to allow for improved range of knee extension. As a progression to this technique, a small vertical force can be applied on the knee. Care should be taken to ensure that this force is sufficiently small (1 to 2 lb or lighter) and that it is applied superior to the patella

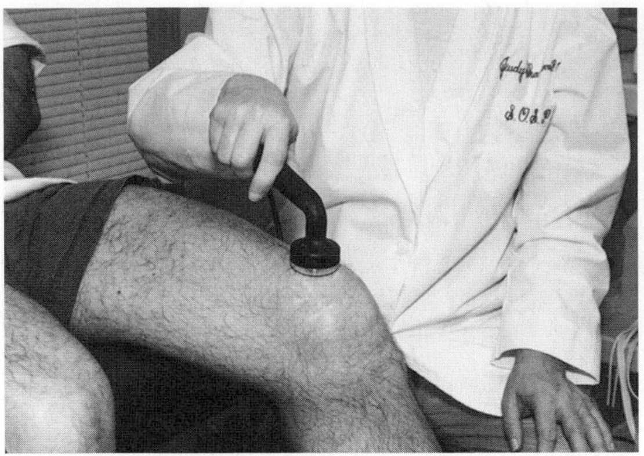

FIG 4-24 Thermal agents of moist heat and ultrasound applied before passive stretching techniques help elevate tissue temperature and aid in soft tissue extensibility and patient relaxation.

to avoid compressive forces between the patella and femur (Fig. 4-25, *B-C*).

The patient is brought to a sitting position to enhance this stretch further. A towel is used to dorsiflex the involved foot, and the patient is instructed to lean forward slowly to stretch the hamstrings (Fig. 4-26, *A*). Simultaneous isometric quadriceps sets also are used to improve strength at the new limits of knee extension.

Gaining knee extension can be achieved in a prone position as well (Fig. 4-26, *B*). However, care must be taken to elevate the patella off the table and prevent excessive patellofemoral compression. This is done by placing a small folded towel superior to the patella. This position works well when only slight degrees of motion are needed (5° to 10° of knee extension). This procedure also can be done on an isotonic exercise apparatus following the same

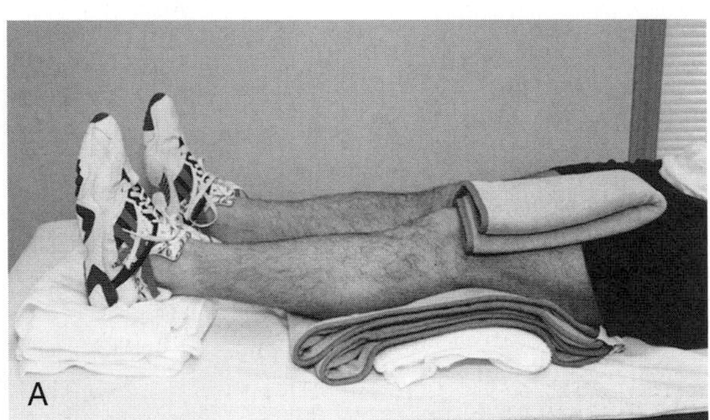

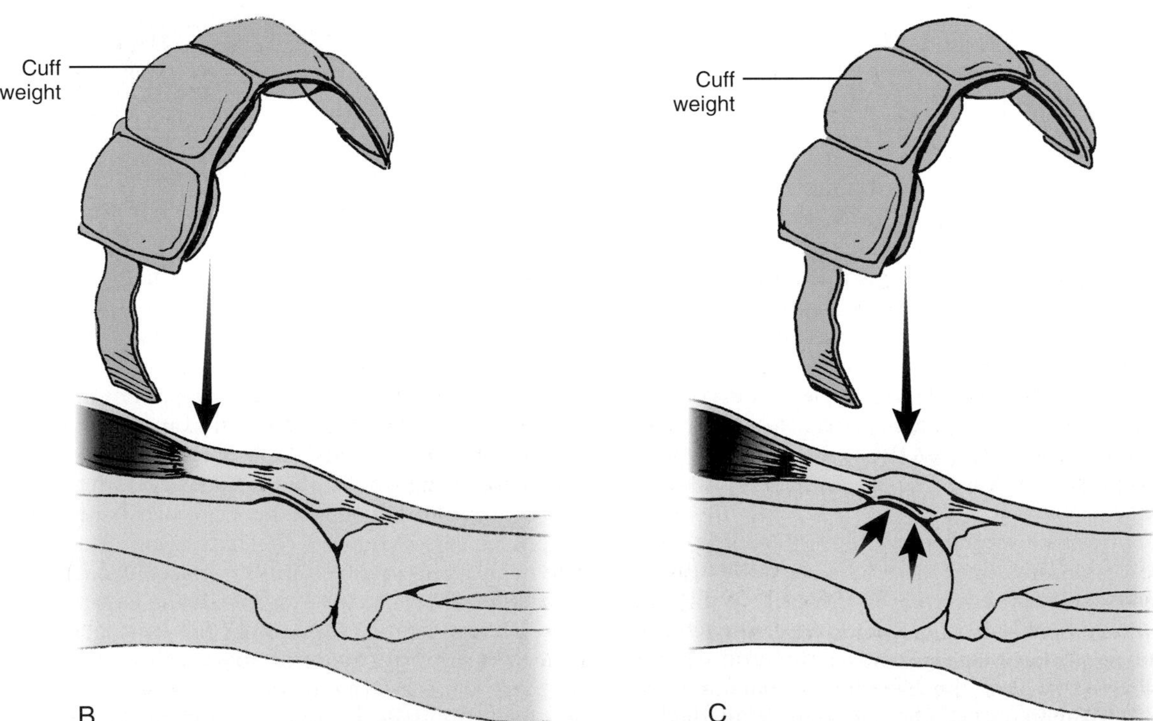

FIG 4-25 **A,** Gaining knee extension using thermal agents (moist heat) and low-load, prolonged stretch. **B,** When applying resistance on the knee to gain extension, it is essential that the resistance be placed superior to the patella. **C,** If resistance is placed directly on the patella, there is a sharp concentration of force, which increases patellofemoral compression.

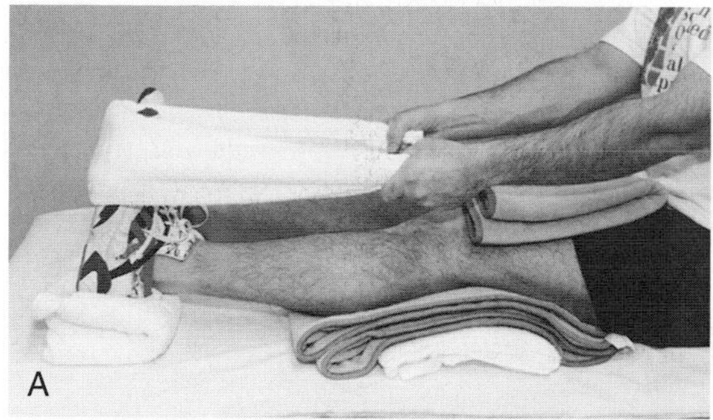

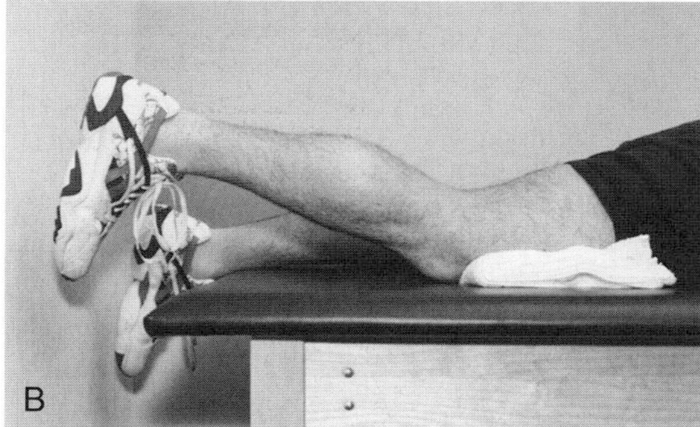

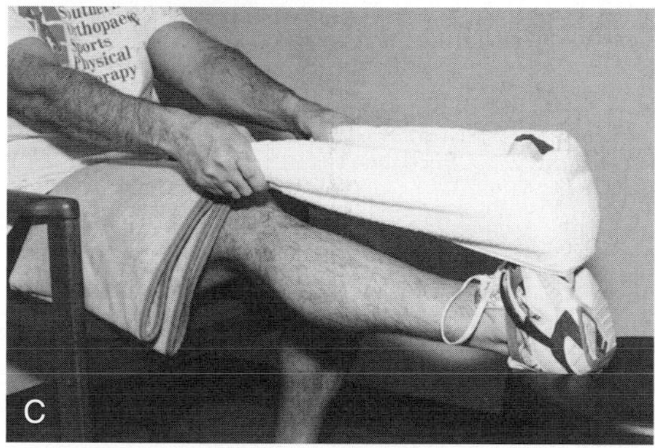

FIG 4-26 **A,** Seated passive towel stretch. **B,** Passive prone knee extension stretch. Note the use of towels placed under the quadriceps to elevate the patella off the table to reduce patellofemoral compression. **C,** Stretch is enhanced by using a towel to dorsiflex the foot of the involved limbs. Instruct the patient to flex the trunk forward.

process as described with gaining knee flexion on an isotonic exercise machine. Knee extension range also can be improved in a sitting position, with or without the aid of isotonic exercise equipment (Fig. 4-26, *C*).

There are many commercially available tools that use the concept of low-load, prolonged stretch. Dynasplint (Dynasplint Systems, Inc.) and Pro-glide (DeRoyal Medical Products) are two examples of dynamic splints used for progressive loading of selected joints to gain motion (Fig. 4-27). An arrangement of pivot points and incrementally adjustable degrees of tension provides the levels of stress needed to effect change in joint motion. The selection of patients for use of one of these splints must be made carefully. Skin integrity is an issue that must be addressed in the elderly population. Metal hinges and spring-loaded tension flanges may not be appropriate for elderly patients because of the weight of the devices and the potential for skin breakdown in patients.

Simple tools for dynamic stretching can be used at home. A wand, cane, or shortened broomstick can be used for general shoulder flexibility (Fig. 4-28, *A*). Increased mobility can be gained by using the unaffected arm to assist the affected extremity (Fig. 4-28, *B*).

Codman's pendulum exercises are effective for gaining relaxation and small degrees of motion in the shoulder. Relaxation is paramount to the effectiveness of this exercise. In one exercise technique, the patient is placed prone on a treatment table, and a very light weight is held in the hand of the affected extremity. This light distraction force is used in conjunction with gradual, light oscillations in various directions (Fig. 4-29). Relaxation is enhanced by applying moist heat followed by ultrasound to the affected joint before pendulum exercise. When one is teaching the oscillation component of this exercise, it must be made clear that muscular contractions must not be used to initiate and maintain the prescribed motions. The oscillation movements can be initiated by gently swinging the upper body or torso.

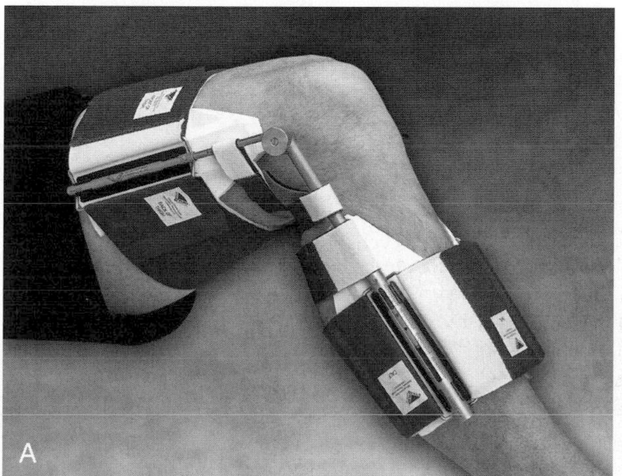

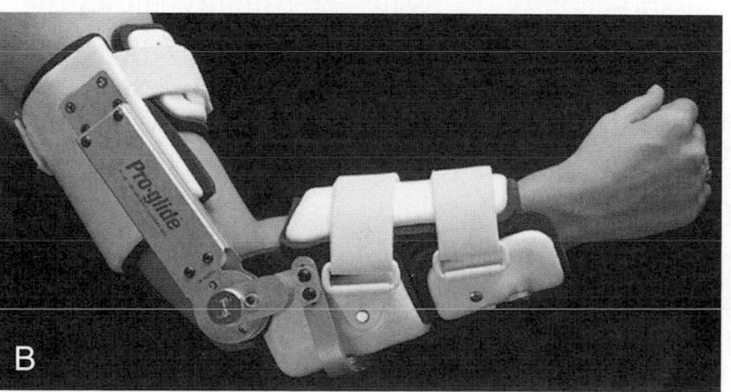

FIG 4-27 **A,** Dynasplint commercial appliance for low-load prolonged stretch. **B,** Pro-glide appliance. *(**A,** Courtesy Dynasplint Systems, Inc., Severna Park, MD. **B,** Courtesy DeRoyal Medical Products, Powell, TN.)*

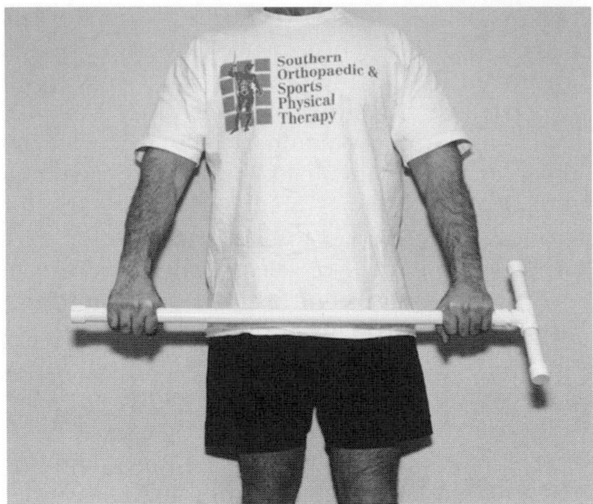

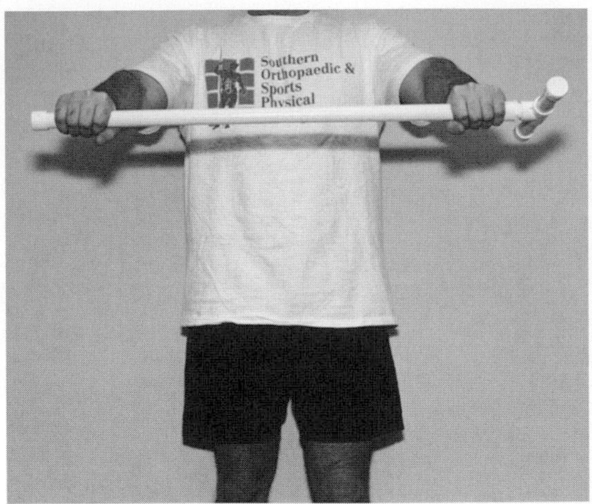

FIG 4-28 A wand can be used to enhance motion of the shoulder.

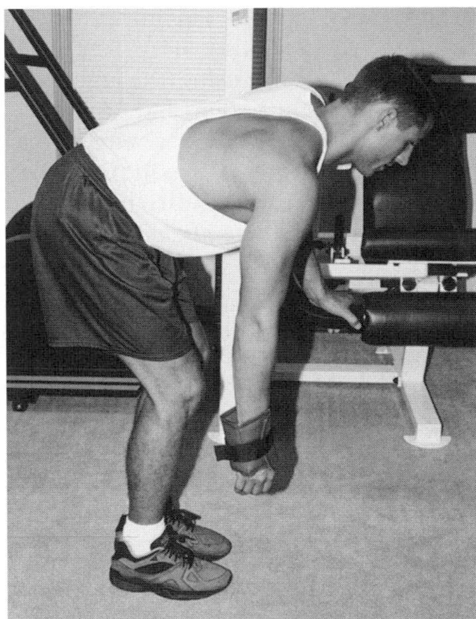

FIG 4-29 Codman's pendulum exercise. For the exercise to be effective, the patient must relax completely and allow the affected arm to hang and gently oscillate in various directions.

SUMMARY

It is necessary to have knowledge of the basic biomechanical and physiologic properties of tissues supporting human movement. Understanding these properties and the effects of exercise and activity on tissue extensibility allows the clinician to modulate appropriate variables to recommend patient-specific therapeutic exercise programs that have an impact on strength, coordination, endurance, and flexibility.

GLOSSARY

Adhesion: A limitation of function resulting from scar tissue that forms between individual structures.

Collagen: A fibrous building block of connective tissue that provides strength during movement and exercise.

Contracture: A permanent or transient limitation of movement or shortening of muscle or other soft tissues.

Creep: A viscoelastic property in which there is a change in the shape (deformation) of tissue without actual loss of continuity.

Deformation: Temporary deformations display transient elastic properties. Permanent deformations display plastic properties. Change in loads results in change in deformations.

Golgi tendon organ: A proprioceptive sensory receptor organ that is located at the insertion of skeletal muscle fibers into the tendons of skeletal muscle.

Load: The force sustained by the body. Types of loads include compression, tension, shear, and torsion.

Muscle spindles: Sensory receptors within the belly of a muscle, which primarily detect changes in the length of the muscle.

Remodeling: A process that alters the structure of connective tissue in response to stress.

Strain: The relative measure of the deformation of a body as a result of loading. Strain equals the change in length or original length of a tissue.

Stress: Intensity of internal force. Stress equals force divided by area. It can be compressive, tensile, or shear.

Viscoelasticity: Stress or strain behavior that is time rate dependent.

REFERENCES

1. Adler SS, Beckers D, Buck M: *PNF in practice: an illustrated guide*, ed 2, Berlin, 2000, Springer.
2. Alter MJ: *Science of flexibility*, ed 2, Champaign, IL, 1996, Human Kinetics.
3. Anderson B, Burke ER: Scientific, medical, and practical aspects of stretching. *Clin Sports Med* 10:63–86, 1991.
4. Arem AJ, Madden JW: Effects of stress on healing wounds: I. Intermittent noncyclical tension. *J Surg Res* 20:93–102, 1976.
5. Arnheim DD, Prentice WE: *Principles of athletic training*, Madison, WI, 1997, Brown & Benchmark.
6. Asmussen E, Boje O: Body temperature and capacity to work. *Acta Physiol Scand* 10:1–21, 1945.
7. Aten D, Knight K: Therapeutic exercise in athletic training: principles and overview, *Athl Train* 13:123–126, 1978.
8. Baechle TR, Earle RW, National Strength, & Conditioning Association (U.S.): *Essentials of strength training and conditioning*, ed 2, Champaign, IL, 2000, Human Kinetics.

9. Bandy WD, Irion JM: The effect of time on static stretch on the flexibility of the hamstring muscles. *Phys Ther* 74:845–850, 1994.
10. Bandy WD, Irion JM, Briggler M: The effect of time and frequency of static stretching on flexibility of the hamstring muscles. *Phys Ther* 77:1090–1096, 1997.
11. Bandy WD, Irion JM, Briggler M: The effect of static stretch and dynamic range of motion training on the flexibility of the hamstring muscles. *J Orthop Sports Phys Ther* 27:295–300, 1998.
12. Bandy WD, Sanders B: *Therapeutic exercise: techniques for intervention*, Baltimore, 2001, Lippincott Williams & Wilkins.
13. Becker RO: The electrical response of human skeletal muscle to passive stretch. *Surg Forum* 10:828–831, 1960.
14. Bell RD, Hoshizaki TB: Relationships of age and sex with range of motion of seventeen joint actions in humans. *Can J Appl Sport Sci* 6:202–206, 1981.
15. Bergh U: Human power at subnormal body temperatures. *Acta Physiol Scand Suppl* 478:1–39, 1980.
16. Bergh U, Ekblom B: Influence of muscle temperature on maximal muscle strength and power output in human skeletal muscles. *Acta Physiol Scand* 107:33–37, 1979.
17. Bishop D: Warm up I: potential mechanisms and the effects of passive warm up on exercise performance. *Sports Med* 33:439–454, 2003.
18. Bishop D: Warm up II: performance changes following active warm up and how to structure the warm up. *Sports Med* 33:483–498, 2003.
19. Bracko MR: Can stretching prior to exercise and sports improve performance and prevent injury? *ACSMs Health Fit J* 6:17–22, 2002.
20. Burgeson RE, Nimni ME: Collagen types. Molecular structure and tissue distribution. *Clin Orthop Relat Res* 282:250–272, 1992.
21. Burnley M, Doust JH, Jones AM: Effects of prior warm-up regime on severe-intensity cycling performance. *Med Sci Sports Exerc* 37:838–845, 2005.
22. Buroker K, Schwane J: Does postexercise static stretching alleviate delayed muscle soreness? *Phys Sports Med* 17:65–83, 1989.
23. Ciullo JV, Zarins B: Biomechanics of the musculotendinous unit: relation to athletic performance and injury. *Clin Sports Med* 2:71–86, 1983.
24. Condon SM, Hutton RS: Soleus muscle electromyographic activity and ankle dorsiflexion range of motion during four stretching procedures. *Phys Ther* 67:24–30, 1987.
25. Corbin CB, Noble L: Flexibility: a major component of physical fitness. *J Phys Educ Rec* 51:23–24, 1980.
26. Cornelius WL, Hagemann RW, Jr, Jackson AW: A study on placement of stretching within a workout. *J Sports Med Phys Fitness* 28:234–236, 1988.
27. Cornelius WL, Hinson MM: The relationship between isometric contractions of hip extensors and subsequent flexibility in males. *J Sports Med Phys Fitness* 20:75–80, 1980.
28. Cross KM, Worrell TW: Effects of a static stretching program on the incidence of lower extremity musculotendinous strains. *J Athl Train* 34:11–14, 1999.
29. Currier DP, Nelson RM: *Dynamics of human biologic tissues*, Philadelphia, 1992, FA Davis.
30. de Vries HA: Electromyographic observations of the effects of static stretching upon muscular distress. *Res Q* 32:468–479, 1961.
31. de Vries HA: Evaluation of static stretching procedures for improvement of flexibility. *Res Q* 33:222–229, 1962.
32. de Vries HA: Quantitative electromyographic investigation of the spasm theory of muscle pain. *Am J Phys Med* 45:119–134, 1966.
33. de Vries HA: Physical fitness programs: does physical activity promote relaxation. *J Phys Educ Rec* 46:52–53, 1975.
34. de Vries HA, Wiswell RA, Bulbulian R, et al: Tranquilizer effect of exercise. Acute effects of moderate aerobic exercise on spinal reflex activation level. *Am J Phys Med* 60:57–66, 1981.
35. DeLee J, Drez D, Stanitski CL: *Orthopaedic sports medicine: principles and practice*, Philadelphia, 1994, Saunders.
36. DePino G, Webright W, Arnold B: Duration of maintained hamstring flexibility after cessation of an acute static stretching protocol. *J Athlet Train* 35:56–59, 2000.
37. Dotson CO, Humphrey JH: *Exercise physiology: current selected research*, New York, 1985, AMS Press.
38. Dutton M: *Orthopaedic examination, evaluation, and intervention*, New York, 2004, McGraw-Hill.
39. Ekstrand J, Gillquist J: The avoidability of soccer injuries. *Int J Sports Med* 4:124–128, 1983.
40. Enoka R: *Neuromechanical basis of kinesiology*, ed 2, Champaign, IL, 1994, Human Kinetics.
41. Enoka RM: *Neuromechanics of human movement*, Champaign, IL, 2002, Human Kinetics.
42. Etnyre BR, Abraham LD: Antagonist muscle activity during stretching: a paradox re-assessed. *Med Sci Sports Exerc* 20:285–289, 1988.
43. Etnyre BR, Abraham LD: H-reflex changes during static stretching and two variations of proprioceptive neuromuscular facilitation techniques. *Electroencephalogr Clin Neurophysiol* 63:174–179, 1986.
44. Etnyre BR, Lee EJ: Comments on proprioceptive neuromuscular facilitation techniques. *Res Q Exerc Sport* 58:184–188, 1987.
45. Fowles JR, Sale DG, MacDougall JD: Reduced strength after passive stretch of the human plantarflexors. *J Appl Physiol* 89:1179–1188, 2000.
46. Fredericks CM, Saladin LK: *Pathophysiology of the Motor Systems: Principles and Clinical Presentations*, Philadelphia, 1996, FA Davis.
47. Genovely H, Stamford BA: Effects of prolonged warm-up exercise above and below anaerobic threshold on maximal performance. *Eur J Appl Physiol Occup Physiol* 48:323–330, 1982.
48. Gibble P, Guskiewicz K, Prentice W, et al: Effects of static and hold-relax stretching on hamstring range of motion using the flexibility LE1000. *J Sport Rehabil* 8:195–208, 1999.
49. Gleim GW, McHugh MP: Flexibility and its effects on sports injury and performance. *Sports Med* 24:289–299, 1997.
50. Godges JJ, MacRae H, Longdon C, et al: The effects of two stretching procedures on hip range of motion and gait economy. *J Orthop Sports Phys Ther* 7:350–357, 1989.
51. Guissard N, Duchateau J, Hainaut K: Muscle stretching and motoneuron excitability. *Eur J Appl Physiol Occup Physiol* 58:47–52, 1988.
52. Gulick DT, Kimura IF, Sitler M, et al: Various treatment techniques on signs and symptoms of delayed onset muscle soreness. *J Athlet Train* 31:145–152, 1996.
53. Guyton AC: *Textbook of Medical Physiology*, ed 7, Philadelphia, 1986, Saunders.
54. Hardy L: Improving active range of hip flexion. *Res Q Exerc Sport* 56:111–114, 1985.
55. Harris M: A factor analytic study of flexibility. *Res Q Exerc Sport* 40:62–70, 1969.
56. Harris ML: Flexibility. *Phys Ther* 49:591–601, 1969.
57. Hartig DE, Henderson JM: Increasing hamstring flexibility decreases lower extremity overuse injuries in military basic trainees. *Am J Sports Med* 27:173–176, 1999.
58. Hartley-O'Brien SJ: Six mobilization exercises for active range of hip flexion. *Res Q Exerc Sport* 51:625–635, 1980.
59. Henricson A, Fredriksson K, Persson I, et al: The effect of heat and stretching on range of hip motion. *J Orthop Sports Phys Ther* 6:110–115, 1984.
60. Hertling D, Kessler RM: *Management of common musculoskeletal disorders: physical therapy principles and methods*, ed 4, Philadelphia, 2006, Lippincott Williams & Wilkins.
61. Hettinga DL: II. Normal joint structures and their reaction to injury. *J Orthop Sports Phys Ther* 1:83–88, 1979.
62. Holcomb W: Stretching and warm-up. In Baechle T, Earle R, editors: *Essentials of strength training and conditioning*, ed 2, Champaign, IL, 2000, Human Kinetics.
63. Holt LE, Travis TM, Okita T: Comparative study of three stretching techniques. *Percept Mot Skills* 31:611–616, 1970.
64. Hunter SK, Enoka RM: Sex differences in the fatigability of arm muscles depends on absolute force during isometric contractions. *J Appl Physiol* 91:2686–2694, 2001.
65. Kandel ER, Schwartz JH, Jessell TM: *Principles of neural science*, ed 4, New York, 2000, McGraw-Hill.
66. Kisner C, Colby LA: *Therapeutic exercise: foundations and techniques*, ed 5, Philadelphia, 2007, FA Davis.

67. Knott M, Voss P: *Proprioceptive neuromuscular facilitation*, ed 3, New York, 1985, Harper & Row.
68. Knudson D: Stretching: from science to practice. *J Phys Ed Rec Dance* 69:38–45, 1998.
69. Knudson D: Stretching during warm-up: do we have enough evidence? *J Phys Educ Rec Dance* 70:24–32, 1999.
70. Knudson D, Bennett K, Corn R, et al: Acute effects of stretching are not evident in the kinematics of the vertical jump. *J Strength Cond Res* 15:98–101, 2001.
71. Kokkonen J, Nelson AG, Cornwell A: Acute muscle stretching inhibits maximal strength performance. *Res Q Exerc Sport* 69:411–415, 1998.
72. Komi PV, IOC Medical Commission, International Federation of Sports Medicine: *Strength and power in sport*, Oxford, UK, 1992, Blackwell Scientific.
73. Kulund DN, Tottossy M: Warm-up, strength, and power. *Orthop Clin North Am* 14:427–448, 1983.
74. Lamontagne A, Malouin F, Richards CL: Viscoelastic behavior of plantar flexor muscle-tendon unit at rest. *J Orthop Sports Phys Ther* 26:244–252, 1997.
75. Larson LA, Michelman H: *International guide to fitness and health*, New York, 1973, Crown.
76. Lederman E: *Fundamentals of manual therapy: physiology, neurology, and psychology*, New York, 1997, Churchill Livingstone.
77. Lehmann JF, Masock AJ, Warren CG, et al: Effect of therapeutic temperatures on tendon extensibility. *Arch Phys Med Rehabil* 51:481–487, 1970.
78. Lentell G, Hetherington T, Eagan J, et al: The use of thermal agents to influence the effectiveness of a low-load prolonged stretch. *J Orthop Sports Phys Ther* 16:200–207, 1992.
79. Levangie PK, Norkin CC: *Joint structure and function: a comprehensive analysis*, ed 3, Philadelphia, 2001, FA Davis.
80. Light KE, Nuzik S, Personius W, et al: Low-load prolonged stretch vs. high-load brief stretch in treating knee contractures. *Phys Ther* 64:330–333, 1984.
81. Longacre JJ, Children's Hospital (Cincinnati Ohio), Research Institute, Research Group for the Facially Crippled: The ultrastructure of collagen: its relation to the healing of wounds and to the management of hypertrophic scar. In *Proceedings, May 30-31, 1973, Research Institute of Children's Hospital*, Springfield, IL, 1976, Thomas.
82. Lucas RC, Koslow R: Comparative study of static, dynamic, and proprioceptive neuromuscular facilitation stretching techniques on flexibility. *Percept Mot Skills* 58:615–618, 1984.
83. Madding S, Wong J, Medeiros J: Effect of duration of passive stretch on hip abduction range of motion. *J Orthop Sports Phys Ther* 8:409–416, 1987.
84. Magnusson SP, Simonsen EB, Aagaard P, et al: Mechanical and physical responses to stretching with and without preisometric contraction in human skeletal muscle. *Arch Phys Med Rehabil* 77:373–378, 1996.
85. Markos PD: Ipsilateral and contralateral effects of proprioceptive neuromuscular facilitation techniques on hip motion and electromyographic activity. *Phys Ther* 59:1366–1373, 1979.
86. McGlynn GH, Laughlin NT, Rowe V: Effect of electromyographic feedback and static stretching on artificially induced muscle soreness. *Am J Phys Med* 58:139–148, 1979.
87. McHugh MP, Magnusson SP, Gleim GW, et al: Viscoelastic stress relaxation in human skeletal muscle. *Med Sci Sports Exerc* 24:1375–1382, 1992.
88. McNair PJ, Stanley SN: Effect of passive stretching and jogging on the series elastic muscle stiffness and range of motion of the ankle joint. *Br J Sports Med* 30:313–317, 1996.
89. Medeiros JM, Smidt GL, Burmeister LF, et al: The influence of isometric exercise and passive stretch on hip joint motion. *Phys Ther* 57:518–523, 1977.
90. Millar AP: An early stretching routine for calf muscle strains. *Med Sci Sports* 8:39–42, 1976.
91. Mohr KJ, Pink MM, Elsner C, et al: Electromyographic investigation of stretching: the effect of warm-up. *Clin J Sport Med* 8:215–220, 1998.
92. Moller M, Ekstrand J, Oberg B, et al: Duration of stretching effect on range of motion in lower extremities. *Arch Phys Med Rehabil* 66:171–173, 1985.
93. Monaco JL, Lawrence WT: Acute wound healing an overview. *Clin Plast Surg* 30:1–12, 2003.
94. Moore MA, Hutton RS: Electromyographic investigation of muscle stretching techniques. *Med Sci Sports Exerc* 12:322–329, 1980.
95. Neumann DA: *Kinesiology of the musculoskeletal system: foundations for physical rehabilitation*, ed 1, St Louis, 2002, Mosby.
96. Noakes T: *Lore of running*, ed 3, Champaign, IL, 1991, Leisure Press.
97. Noonan TJ, Best TM, Seaber AV, et al: Identification of a threshold for skeletal muscle injury. *Am J Sports Med* 22:257–261, 1994.
98. Norkin CC, White DJ: *Measurement of joint motion: a guide to goniometry*, ed 2, Philadelphia, 1995, FA Davis.
99. Nyland J: *Clinical decisions in therapeutic exercise: planning and implementation*, Upper Saddle River, NJ, 2006, Pearson Prentice Hall.
100. Oatis CA: *Kinesiology: the mechanics and pathomechanics of human movement*, ed 1, Philadelphia, 2004, Lippincott Williams & Wilkins.
101. Pollock ML, Gaesser GA, Butcher JD, et al: American College of Sports Medicine Position Stand. The recommended quantity and quality of exercise for developing and maintaining cardiorespiratory and muscular fitness, and flexibility in healthy adults. *Med Sci Sports Exerc* 30:975–991, 1998.
102. Pope RP, Herbert RD, Kirwan JD, et al: A randomized trial of preexercise stretching for prevention of lower-limb injury. *Med Sci Sports Exerc* 32:271–277, 2000.
103. Pratt K, Bohannon R: Effects of a 3-minute standing stretch on ankle-dorsiflexion range of motion. *J Sport Rehabil* 12:162–173, 2003.
104. Prentice WE: A comparison of static stretching and PNF stretching for improving hip joint flexibility. *Athl Train* 18:56–59, 1983.
105. Prentice WE, Voight ML: *Techniques in musculoskeletal rehabilitation*, New York, 2001, McGraw-Hill.
106. Roberts JM, Wilson K: Effect of stretching duration on active and passive range of motion in the lower extremity. *Br J Sports Med* 33:259–263, 1999.
107. Rosenbaum D, Hennig EM: The influence of stretching and warm-up exercises on Achilles tendon reflex activity. *J Sports Sci* 13:481–490, 1995.
108. Sady SP, Wortman M, Blanke D: Flexibility training: ballistic, static or proprioceptive neuromuscular facilitation? *Arch Phys Med Rehabil* 63:261–263, 1982.
109. Safran MR, Garrett WE, Jr, Seaber AV, et al: The role of warmup in muscular injury prevention. *Am J Sports Med* 16:123–129, 1988.
110. Sapega AA, Quedenfeld RA, Moyer RA, et al: Biophysical factors in range of motion exercise. *Phys Sports Med* 9:57–65, 1981.
111. Scully RM, Barnes MR: *Physical therapy*, Philadelphia, 1989, Lippincott.
112. Shear CR, Bloch RJ: Vinculin in subsarcolemmal densities in chicken skeletal muscle: localization and relationship to intracellular and extracellular structures. *J Cell Biol* 101:240–256, 1985.
113. Shellock FG, Prentice WE: Warming-up and stretching for improved physical performance and prevention of sports-related injuries. *Sports Med* 2:267–278, 1985.
114. Shrier I: Stretching before exercise does not reduce the risk of local muscle injury: a critical review of the clinical and basic science literature. *Clin J Sport Med* 9:221–227, 1999.
115. Simon SR: *American Academy of Orthopaedic Surgeons: Orthopaedic basic science*, Rosemont, IL, 1994, American Academy of Orthopaedic Surgeons.
116. Smith CA: The warm-up procedure: to stretch or not to stretch. A brief review. *J Orthop Sports Phys Ther* 19:12–17, 1994.
117. Smith LL, Brunetz MH, Chenier TC, et al: The effects of static and ballistic stretching on delayed onset muscle soreness and creatine kinase. *Res Q Exerc Sport* 64:103–107, 1993.
118. Starring DT, Gossman MR, Nicholson GG, Jr, et al: Comparison of cyclic and sustained passive stretching using a mechanical device to increase resting length of hamstring muscles. *Phys Ther* 68:314–320, 1988.

119. Stolov WC, Weilepp TG, Jr: Passive length-tension relationship of intact muscle, epimysium, and tendon in normal and denervated gastrocnemius of the rat. *Arch Phys Med Rehabil* 47:612–620, 1966.
120. Street SF: Lateral transmission of tension in frog myofibers: a myofibrillar network and transverse cytoskeletal connections are possible transmitters. *J Cell Physiol* 114:346–364, 1983.
121. Tanigawa MC: Comparison of the hold-relax procedure and passive mobilization on increasing muscle length. *Phys Ther* 52:725–735, 1972.
122. Taylor DC, Dalton JD, Seaber AV, et al: Viscoelastic properties of muscle-tendon units. The biomechanical effects of stretching. *Am J Sports Med* 18:300–309, 1990.
123. Taylor DC, Dalton JD, Jr, Seaber AV, et al: Experimental muscle strain injury. Early functional and structural deficits and the increased risk for reinjury. *Am J Sports Med* 21:190–194, 1993.
124. van Mechelen W, Hlobil H, Kemper HC, et al: Prevention of running injuries by warm-up, cool-down, and stretching exercises. *Am J Sports Med* 21:711–719, 1993.
125. Voss DE, Ionta MK, Myers BJ, et al: *Proprioceptive neuromuscular facilitation: patterns and techniques*, ed 3, Philadelphia, 1985, Harper & Row.
126. Wallin D, Ekblom B, Grahn R, et al: Improvement of muscle flexibility. A comparison between two techniques. *Am J Sports Med* 13:263–268, 1985.
127. Wallmann HW, Christensen SD, Perry C, Hoover DL: The acute effects of various types of stretching static, dynamic, ballistic, and no stretch of the iliopsoas on 40 yard sprint times in recreational runners. *Int J Sports Phys Ther* 7:540–547, 2012.
128. Wallmann HW, Mercer JA, McWhorter JW: Surface electromyographic assessment of the effect of static stretching of the gastrocnemius on vertical jump performance. *J Strength Cond Res* 19:684–688, 2005.
129. Walter J, Figoni SF, Andres FF, et al: Training intensity and duration in flexibility. *Clin Kinesiol* 50:40–45, 1996.
130. Warren CG, Lehmann JF, Koblanski JN: Elongation of rat tail tendon: effect of load and temperature. *Arch Phys Med Rehabil* 52:465–474, 1971.
131. Warren CG, Lehmann JF, Koblanski JN: Heat and stretch procedures: an evaluation using rat tail tendon. *Arch Phys Med Rehabil* 57:122–126, 1976.
132. Watkins MA, Riddle DL, Lamb RL, et al: Reliability of goniometric measurements and visual estimates of knee range of motion obtained in a clinical setting. *Phys Ther* 71:90–96, 1991.
133. Wharton J, Wharton P: *The Wharton's stretch book*, New York, 1996, Three Rivers Press.
134. Wiktorsson-Moller M, Oberg B, Ekstrand J, et al: Effects of warming up, massage, and stretching on range of motion and muscle strength in the lower extremity. *Am J Sports Med* 11:249–252, 1983.
135. Wilkinson A: Stretching the truth. A review of the literature on muscle stretching. *Aust J Physiother* 38:283–287, 1992.
136. Williford HN, East JB, Smith FH, et al: Evaluation of warm-up for improvement in flexibility. *Am J Sports Med* 14:316–319, 1986.
137. Wolpaw JR: Acquisition and maintenance of the simplest motor skill: investigation of CNS mechanisms. *Med Sci Sports Exerc* 26:1475–1479, 1994.
138. Wolpaw JR, Carp JS: Memory traces in spinal cord. *Trends Neurosci* 13:137–142, 1990.
139. Woo SL, Buckwalter JA, American Academy of Orthopaedic Surgeons, et al: *Injury and repair of the musculoskeletal soft tissues: workshop, Savannah, GA, June 1987*, Park Ridge, IL, 1988, American Academy of Orthopaedic Surgeons.
140. Woo SL, Matthews JV, Akeson WH, et al: Connective tissue response to immobility. Correlative study of biomechanical and biochemical measurements of normal and immobilized rabbit knees. *Arthritis Rheum* 18:257–264, 1975.
141. Youdas JW, Carey JR, Garrett TR: Reliability of measurements of cervical spine range of motion-comparison of three methods. *Phys Ther* 71:98–104, 1991.
142. Zito M, Driver D, Parker C, et al: Lasting effects of one bout of two 15-second passive stretches on ankle dorsiflexion range of motion. *J Orthop Sports Phys Ther* 26:214–221, 1997.

REVIEW QUESTIONS

Multiple Choice

1. Which of the following represents the mechanical behavior of connective tissue within the elastic region of the stress-strain curve?
   a. It is directly proportional to the stress imposed
   b. The tissue has a wavy configuration
   c. The curve consists of a horizontal slope
   d. Permanent tissue deformation occurs
2. The stiffer the tissue, the:
   a. Greater the proportion of elastin.
   b. Longer the toe region.
   c. More vertical the curve.
   d. More compliant it is.
3. Under normal conditions, a viscoelastic tissue:
   a. Immediately returns to its original shape.
   b. Has time dependent mechanical properties.
   c. Does not undergo deformation.
   d. Is unable to be compressed.
4. High forces of short duration favor which of the following?
   a. Creep deformation
   b. Static stretching
   c. Tissue relaxation
   d. Elastic tissue deformation
5. When the central portion of the muscle spindle is stretched secondary to gamma activity, which of the following is directly stimulated to change the muscle length?
   a. Alpha motor neurons
   b. Secondary endings
   c. Golgi tendon organs
   d. Primary endings
6. Which of the following factors is responsible for ROM loss in elderly adults?
   a. Increased muscle function
   b. Increased connective tissue stiffness
   c. Increased efficiency of ADL performance
   d. Increased activity
7. Women may be more flexible than men because:
   a. Women stretch more than men.
   b. Women have a greater inherent flexibility.
   c. Women have hormonal fluctuations that contribute to more lax joints.
   d. Men are less active in general than women.
8. Static stretching is useful if the clinician is looking for a technique that:
   a. Requires more skill than other techniques.
   b. Has decreased energy requirements.
   c. Requires a partner.
   d. Does not require a warm-up.
9. Which of the following metabolic effects results from increased muscle temperature?
   a. Increased muscle viscosity
   b. Decreased tissue compliance
   c. Increased ROM
   d. Decreased metabolic rate
10. According to the research, when performing cyclical stretching, 80% of the length changes occur during the first:

a. Stretch.
b. Two stretches.
c. Three stretches.
d. Four stretches.

11. Which of the following is defined as stretch tolerance?
    a. Ballistically stretching a muscle repeatedly
    b. Stretching a muscle to 150% of its resting length
    c. Accommodating to the discomfort of stretching
    d. Increase in tissue length when maintaining a constant stress
12. Which of the following most likely provides the greatest resistance to stretching?
    a. The muscle
    b. Reflex activity
    c. Rate of application
    d. Connective tissue
13. Which of the following techniques would stimulate the muscle spindles during the stretch causing a high rate of tension?
    a. Static stretching
    b. Ballistic stretching
    c. Contract-relax
    d. Dynamic stretching
14. Which of the following techniques is the most common form of stretching exercise?
    a. Static stretching
    b. Ballistic stretching
    c. Contract-relax
    d. Dynamic stretching
15. According to some researchers, how might stretching immediately before a performance task impede dynamic muscle performance?
    a. Stretching may weaken the muscle-tendon unit
    b. Stretching may increase muscle-tendon unit stiffness
    c. Stretching may increase motor unit activation
    d. Stretching may enhance the length-tension relationship

Short Answer

16. Is muscle tissue considered to be an active or passive restraint to joint motion?
17. Name three types of stretching techniques.
18. What are some advantages and disadvantages of PNF stretching techniques?
19. Why should the muscle be slowly and passively stretched to a new length?
20. Describe the research and findings on when stretching should take place in an exercise program.

Fill in the Blank

21. The building block of collagen is ________________.
22. Tissues exhibiting viscosity have ________-dependent and ________________-dependent properties when forces are applied to them.
23. A(n) ________________ is an inhibitory neurophysiologic sensory receptor involved with the stretch reflex.
24. The ________________ is an excitatory specialized fiber found in muscle.
25. At 60 days, new scar is ________________ percent of its maximum strength.

True/False

26. Stress is the amount of tension or load placed on tissues.
27. Tissue temperature does not affect connective tissue extensibility.
28. Active exercise has an effect on intramuscular temperature and tissue extensibility.
29. Research has shown that performing static stretching before or after a workout does not make a difference in increasing ROM.
30. Research has shown that an acute stretching program can result in increased long-term flexibility.

Chapter 5

Muscle Strength

Marc Campolo

CHAPTER OUTLINE

LEARNING OBJECTIVES

1. Name the noncontractile and contractile elements of muscle tissue.
2. Give examples of concentric and eccentric contractions.
3. State two definitions of strength.
4. List methods used to measure strength.
5. Compare muscle contraction types related to tension produced and energy liberated.
6. Identify clinical features of delayed onset muscle soreness.
7. List three clinically relevant exercise programs to enhance strength.
8. Explain open kinetic chain and closed kinetic chain exercise.
9. Identify goals and applications of strength training programs for elderly adults.

KEY TERMS

Actin
Atrophy
Closed kinetic chain (CKC) exercise
Concentric
Delayed onset muscle soreness (DOMS)
Eccentric
Endomysium
Epimysium
Fasciculi
Fast-twitch (type II, white glycolytic) muscle fiber
Hypertrophy
Isometric
Myofibrils
Myosin
Open kinetic chain (OKC) exercise
Perimysium
Plyometrics
Power
Progressive resistance exercise (PRE)
Specific adaptations to imposed demands (SAID) principle
Slow-twitch (type I, red oxidative) muscle fiber
Strength
Tension
Work

Strength training is physical activity intended to increase muscle strength and mass.[47] Adults who engage in strength training are less likely to experience loss of muscle mass and functional decline.[64]

Maintaining, enhancing, and regaining strength are critical for improving body function during all phases of recovery after surgery, injury, or disease affecting the musculoskeletal system. The terms *strength training, resistance training,* and *weight training* are synonymous and refer to physical conditioning that uses **isometric,** isotonic, or isokinetic exercise to develop muscle.[28] Resistance exercise is any form of active exercise in which a dynamic or static muscle contraction is resisted by an outside force, applied either manually or mechanically. Therapeutic exercise is resistance training that is applied in a systematic and individualized manner designed to improve, restore, or enhance physical function. The physical therapist assistant (PTA) must understand the basic foundations of strength development and, more importantly, how to apply principles of strength gaining during recovery after immobilization, surgery, or musculoskeletal injury. This chapter introduces basic concepts and universally accepted principles that can be applied in numerous clinical situations with various orthopedic pathologies.

Important Concepts

The terms *strength training, resistance training,* and *weight training* are synonymous and refer to physical conditioning that uses isometric, isotonic, or isokinetic exercise to develop muscle.[28]

The strength or **tension**-generating capacity of a muscle is determined by many diverse but interrelated factors, including neural control (motor unit recruitment and rate coding; the number and rate at which the motor units are fired), cross-sectional area (muscle fiber number and size), muscle fiber arrangement (angle of pennation or how fibers are aligned in relation to an imaginary line between the muscle's origin and insertion), muscle length (length-tension ratio; muscle produces the greatest tension when it is near or at the physiologic resting position at the time of contraction), angle of pull (muscle's tension-generating capacity is increased when the tendon is perpendicular to the bone), and fiber type distribution (high percent of type I, low force production, fatigue resistant; type IIA and IIB, high force production, rapid fatigue).[6,42] One also has to consider other factors that may affect tension generation, such as energy stores of the muscle, recovery from exercise, fatigue, age, gender, and state of health of the muscle.

A basic understanding of muscular composition and gross structure helps clarify concepts of therapeutic exercise and provides a foundation for developing advanced principles and applications of strength.

GENERAL MUSCLE BIOLOGY

The body of an individual muscle is surrounded by noncontractile connective tissue called the **epimysium.** Within the muscle are bundles of fibers called **fasciculi,** which are surrounded by another noncontractile connective tissue called the **perimysium.** The **endomysium** is a noncontractile connective tissue that surrounds each individual muscle fiber. The individual muscle fibers are composed of **myofibrils** that lie parallel to each other and the muscle fiber itself (Fig. 5-1, *A*). The structural components of the myofibrils are called myofilaments, and they comprise two predominant proteins, **actin** and **myosin.** The functional, or contractile, unit of a muscle fiber cell is called the sarcomere (Fig. 5-1, *B*). Myosin (a thick protein) and actin (a thin protein) are actively involved with the mechanics of muscular contraction, which involves a complex and highly structured series of chemical and mechanical events.

The extraordinarily complex biochemical excitation-contraction coupling and mechanical actions of muscular contraction are described in physiology textbooks. In simple terms, the neurologic stimulus to contract a muscle causes the release of acetylcholine, which initiates the release of calcium. The calcium ions bond with troponin and tropomyosin, two proteins within the actin filaments. This allows actin–adenosine triphosphate (ATP) to react with myosin–adenosine triphosphatase (ATPase), producing energy so that the thick myosin and thin actin filaments can "slide" past each other, generating tension and producing contraction of the muscle.

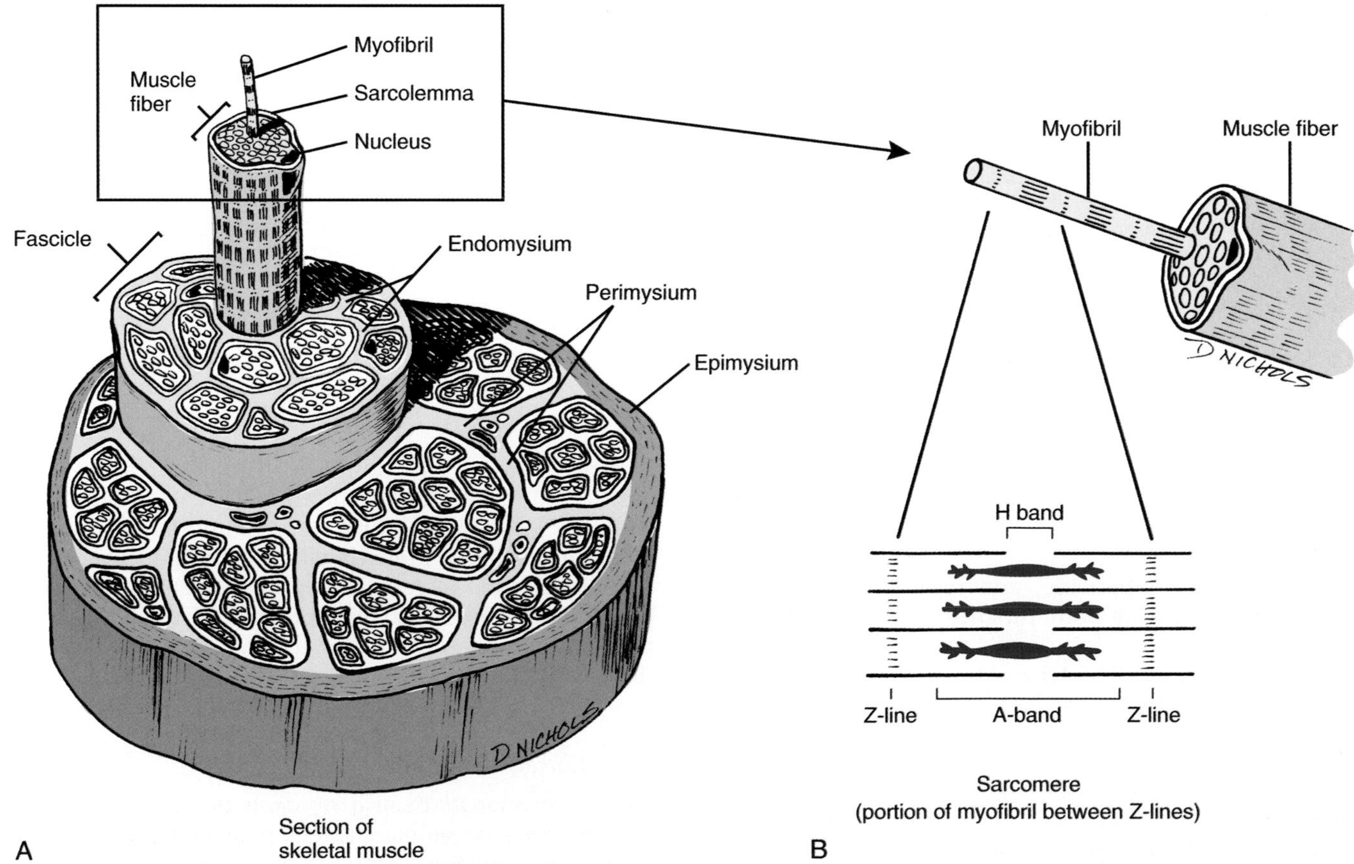

FIG 5-1 **A,** Section of skeletal muscle with contractile and noncontractile connective tissue. **B,** Functional or contractile unit of skeletal muscle fiber cell.

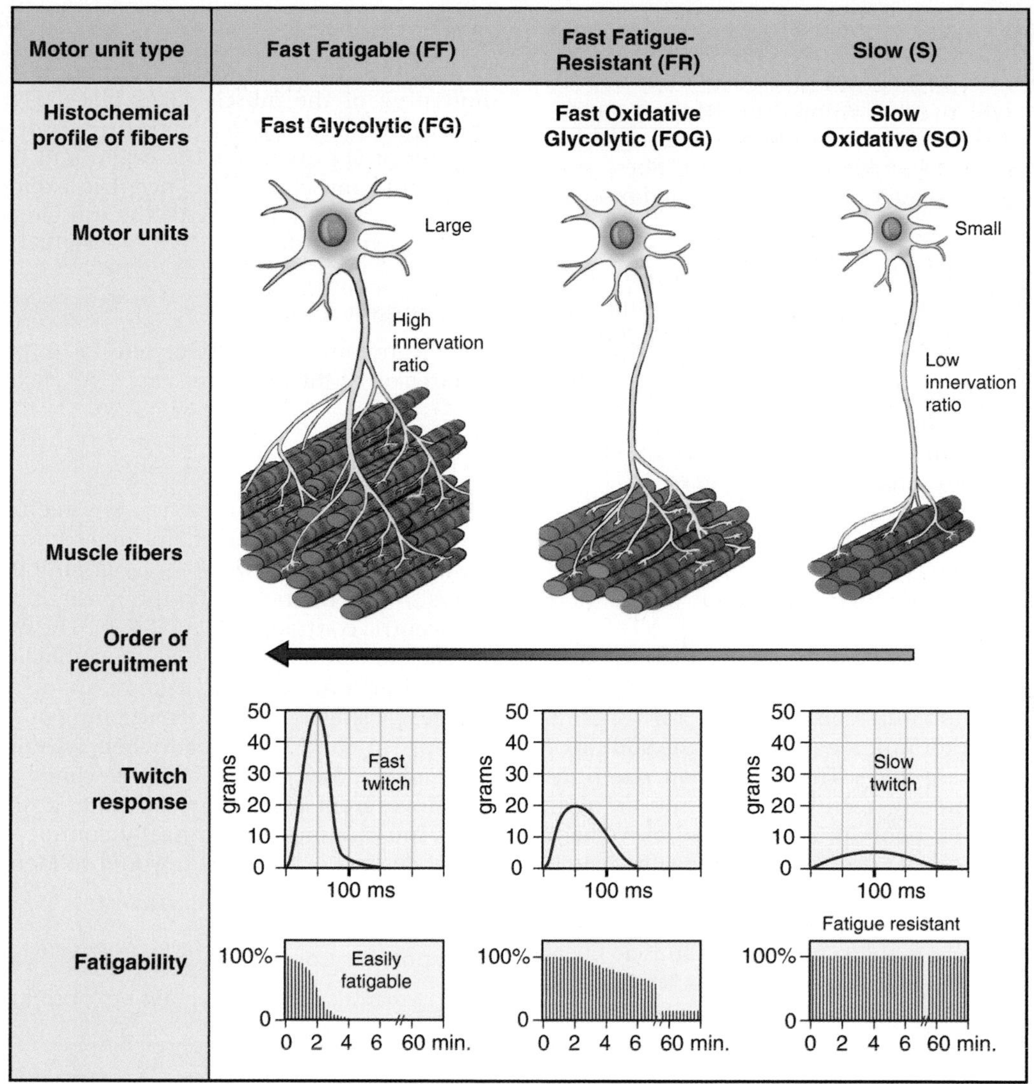

FIG 5-2 Classification of motor unit types from muscle fibers based on histochemical profile, size, and twitch (contractile) characteristics. A theoretical continuum of differing contractile and morphologic characteristics is shown for each of the three motor unit types. The range of any single characteristic may vary considerably within any given motor unit (either within or between whole muscles). *(From Neumann DA:* Kinesiology of the musculoskeletal system: foundations for rehabilitation, *ed 2, St Louis, 2010, Mosby.)*

MUSCLE FIBER TYPES

Generally, two distinct types of muscle fibers have been identified in humans. These fibers are classified by their contractile and metabolic characteristics (Fig. 5-2).

Slow-twitch (type I, red oxidative) muscle fibers possess relatively large and numerous mitochondria, triglycerides, and oxidative enzymes (succinic dehydrogenase), which allow for aerobic work. They also have relatively low myosin-ATPase and glycolytic activity as well as slower calcium handling ability and shortening speed. This type of fiber is specialized for muscular endurance activities. These fatigue-resistant fibers contract slowly but are highly efficient for prolonged aerobic events.

Fast-twitch (type II, white glycolytic) muscle fibers are anaerobic. These fibers are not as vascular as type I fibers, but they fire, or contract, at a higher speed than type I fibers and with more force. These fibers have a very high level of myosin-ATPase, which provides energy for speed of contraction and tension; they also have low myoglobin content and very few mitochondria. However, they are larger in diameter than red fibers. These fibers are used mainly in activities that require speed, strength, and power.

Important Concepts

Slow-twitch fibers are type I fibers that are red oxidative fibers that have large and numerous mitochondria and oxidative enzymes that allow for aerobic work. These muscle fibers are specialized for muscular endurance activities because they are very fatigue resistant.

Important Concepts

Fast-twitch fibers are type II fibers that are white oxidative fibers that are not as vascular but contract at a much higher speed with more force. They have low myoglobin content and few mitochondria. These muscle fibers are used for activities that require speed, strength, and power.

Type II fibers can be further broken down into three distinct subclassifications: type IIA; type IIAB; and type IIB.[50,74] These fiber types differ mainly in terms of contraction velocity and endurance and are classified as intermediate fiber types with aerobic and anaerobic capacities.

- The type IIA (fast-oxidative-glycolytic) fiber has a fast contraction speed and a moderate capacity for energy transfer from aerobic and anaerobic sources.
- The type IIB (fast-glycolytic) fiber possesses the greatest anaerobic capacity and the fastest shortening speed.
- The type IIAB fiber is rare and undifferentiated and may contribute to reinnervation and motor unit transformation.

The motor unit is the basic unit of movement. It consists of the anterior motor neuron and all the muscle fibers it innervates. A motor unit contains only one specific muscle fiber type. Motor unit recruitment is the adding of motor units to increase force. The Henneman size principle proposes an orderly recruitment of motor units within a motor neuron pool during a defined movement task.[37] When a low force is needed, only the slow-twitch motor units (type I) are activated; with increasing force requirements, larger and faster motor units (type IIA, type IIB) are recruited. The orderly recruitment of muscle fibers during contraction proceeds according to increased force requirements, as shown in Fig. 5-3.

Important Concepts

The Henneman size principle proposes an orderly recruitment of motor units within a motor neuron pool during a defined movement task.[37] When a low force is needed, only the slow-twitch motor units (type I) are activated; with increasing force requirements, larger and faster motor units (type IIA, type IIB) are recruited.

TYPES OF MUSCLE CONTRACTIONS

The three true types of muscle contractions are **concentric, eccentric,** and isometric. Two other terms have been used to describe muscle contractions: *isotonic* and *isokinetic*. These are not types of contractions but rather terms used to describe events.

CONCENTRIC

In a concentric contraction, tension is produced, and shortening of the muscle takes place (Fig. 5-4, *A*). The action produced by a concentric contraction brings together or approximates the origin and insertion of the contracting muscle. In a concentric exercise, tension is developed, and shortening of the muscle occurs to overcome an external force, such as a weight.

Important Concepts

In a concentric contraction, tension is produced, and shortening of the muscle occurs.

ECCENTRIC

An eccentric muscle contraction is sometimes referred to as a *lengthening contraction*. In an eccentric contraction, tension is produced; however, lengthening of the muscle occurs so that the net action is opposite that produced by a concentric contraction (Fig. 5-4, *B*). The origin and insertion of the contracting muscle move farther apart during the contraction. Eccentric exercise involves loading of a muscle, causing a physical lengthening of the muscle as it attempts to control the load when lowering the weight. For example, as a person slowly descends to sit in a chair and moves from a standing to a sitting position, the quadriceps muscles must eccentrically contract to control the rate of descent or the person would suddenly fall into the chair.

Important Concepts

In an eccentric contraction, tension is produced; however, lengthening of the muscle occurs.

ISOMETRIC

In an isometric contraction, tension is produced, but no joint movement or action occurs (Fig. 5-4, *C*). Isometric exercise involves a muscle contraction against a force with no significant movement occurring. Examples include pushing or pulling against an immovable object or holding a weight in a particular position. Isometric exercises are used when joint movement is restricted or impossible. A form of isometric exercise is a muscle-setting exercise. Setting exercises are muscle contractions performed without movement or resistance. An example is a quadriceps set. (The word "set" is used to describe an isometric contraction.) If the quadriceps contracts as the knee is

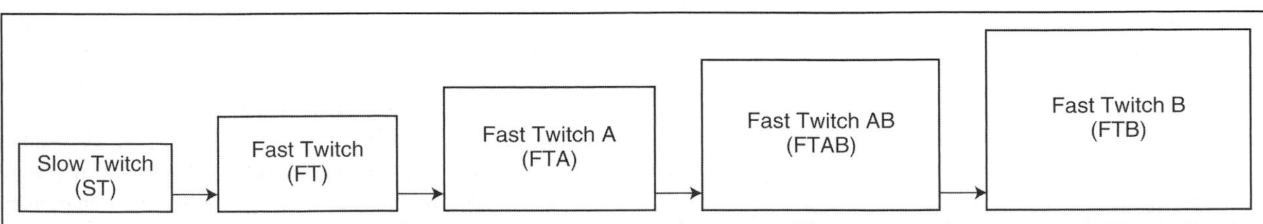

FIG 5-3 Progressive orderly recruitment of muscle fibers during contraction.

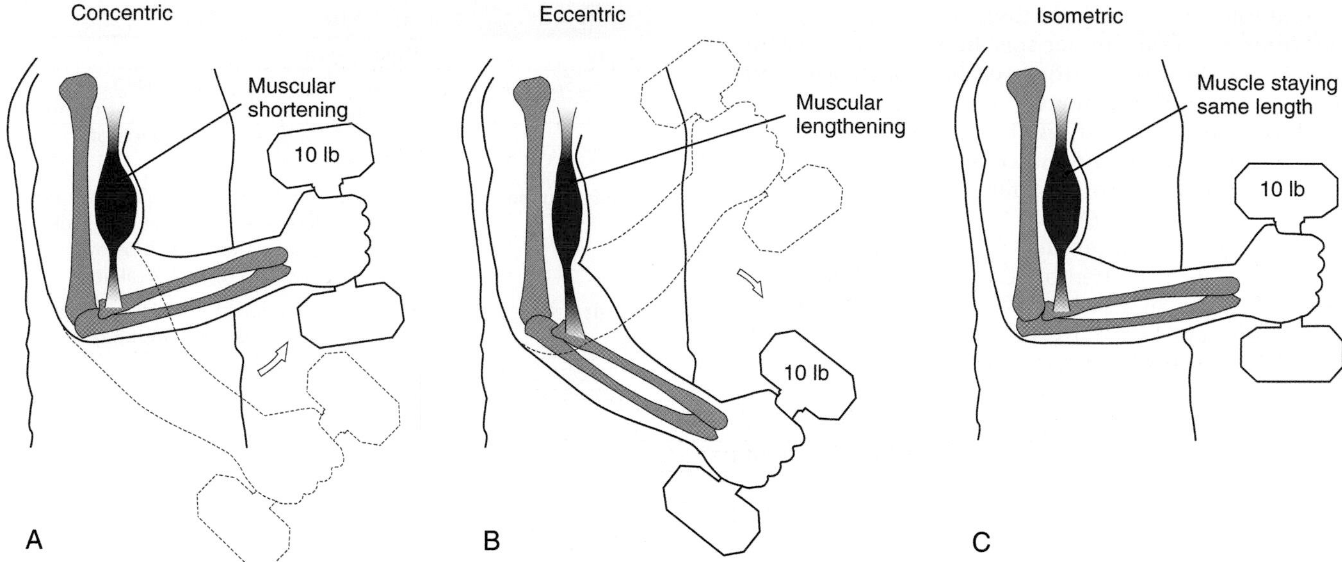

FIG 5-4 The three types of muscular activation: concentric (**A**), eccentric (**B**), and isometric (**C**). *(From Mansfield PJ, Neumann DA:* Essentials of kinesiology for the physical therapist assistant, *St Louis, 2009, Mosby.)*

held straight, tension is produced within the muscle, but no change in joint angle occurs. Clinically, setting exercises are used to decrease pain, facilitate muscle contraction, increase circulation, and retard muscle **atrophy.**

> **Important Concepts**
>
> In an isometric contraction, tension is produced, but no joint movement or action occurs.

ISOTONIC

Isotonic muscle contraction is not an accurate name for what happens physiologically. The name implies that the resistance, force, load, or tension remains constant, but actually the tension or force created in a muscle during this type of action must change as the joint angle changes. For example, when one lifts a barbell (constant resistance), the amount of force generated by the contracting muscle varies at different angles during the movement, even though the weight itself remains constant. This variation occurs because changes in the muscle length and the muscle tendon angle of pull alter the mechanical advantage of the muscle throughout the movement, resulting in variations of force-developing capacity. A more precise and descriptive term, *isoinertial,*[56] can be used in place of isotonic. The term *isotonic* is used in this book to describe the action of variable velocities of movement with a constant load. Examples of isotonic resistance equipment are barbells, dumbbells, and ankle weights, which are collectively referred to as *free weights.*

> **Important Concepts**
>
> In an isotonic contraction, the resistance, force, load, or tension remains constant, whereas the tension created changes as the joint angle changes.

ISOKINETIC

In an isokinetic contraction, the speed or velocity of movement is held constant regardless of the magnitude of force applied to the resistance. Any force applied results in an equal reaction force supplied by the machine throughout a given range of motion (ROM); this is accomplished by a rate-limiting computerized dynamometer. Examples of isokinetic equipment are Cybex, Biodex, Lido, and Kin-Com. Isokinetic exercise is called *accommodating resistance.* The theoretical construct is that if a patient provides maximal effort during a repetition, the machine will provide variable resistance, stressing the muscle maximally throughout the full ROM, in contrast to the resistance provided with isotonic exercise. This equipment also provides an object force measurement throughout the ROM of a joint and can be a valuable tool for strength assessment.

> **Important Concepts**
>
> In an isokinetic contraction, the speed or velocity of movement is held constant regardless of the magnitude of force applied to the resistance.

DEFINITIONS OF STRENGTH AND POWER

Strength is a broad term. Generally, strength is the ability of a muscle to generate force, or more specifically the maximum force generated by a single muscle or related muscle group.[51] Other definitions of strength include "[t]he ability to exert force under a given set of conditions defined by body position, the body movement by which force is applied, movement type, and movement speed"[36] and "[t]he maximal force a muscle or muscle group can generate at a specified velocity."[46] The American Physical Therapy Association defines muscle strength as "the muscle force exerted by a muscle or group of muscles to overcome resistance under specific set of circumstances," muscle performance as "the capacity of a muscle or group of muscles to generate forces," muscle power as "the work produced per unit time or the product of strength and speed," and muscle endurance as "the ability to sustain forces repeatedly or to generate forces over a period of time."[5] Functional strength has been described as the ability of the neuromuscular system to produce, reduce, or control forces, contemplated or imposed, during functional activities in a smooth, coordinated manner.[42]

To help clarify strength clinically, it may be most useful to consider strength in terms that describe performance, as follows:

- **Work** is used to describe the result or product of a force exerted on an object and the distance the object moves.[36]
  - This term is expressed as work = force × distance.
- Force can be described as either linear or rotary.[67]
  - Linear force is described as force = mass × acceleration.
  - Rotary force is expressed as force = mass × angular acceleration.
- Torque is the ability to cause rotational movement.
  - Torque is expressed as torque = force × perpendicular distance from the axis of rotation.
- **Power** is defined as the time rate of doing work, which can be expressed in several ways.[56]
  - Power = work/time = force × [distance/time]
  - Power = force × [distance/time]
  - Power = force × velocity
- Velocity is defined as a vector that describes displacement.

Overall, these terms help describe resultant muscular performance as it relates to the development of strength.

MEASURING STRENGTH

Strength can be measured by the following six methods:

1. Manual muscle testing (MMT)
2. Cable tensiometry
3. Dynamometry
4. Isotonic 1 repetition maximum (RM) lift
5. Isokinetics
6. Functional strength assessment

MMT is an isometric method of muscle testing that is designed to measure muscle strength requiring no equipment other than the examiner's hands. This technique was introduced in the early 1900s, and its use is widely accepted in the health care professions.[62] It is used to obtain a general grade of isometric contraction capacity of a muscle at a specific joint angle against a manually applied force or gravity. Performing MMT requires extensive time, effort, and attention to detail while performing the correct technique to ensure that the results obtained are as accurate as possible.[62] The tester must have a comprehensive and detailed understanding of kinesiology to reproduce accurately and consistently manual grading of muscle strength (performance). The grading scale for this test is clinically easy to use and is outlined in Table 5-1. The disadvantage of isometric strength testing is that because muscle length is held constant, isometric strength testing provides muscle strength data at only one point in the range.[60] MMT is valid from grades 0 to 5; however, when MMT scores exceed grade 4, MMT loses its ability to discriminate between gradations of strength. In cases in which measurement and documentation of strength level are critical above MMT grade 4, an alternative form of measuring strength should be used.[60]

TABLE 5-1 Manual Muscle Test Scale

Score	Description
Grade 5/normal	Patient can hold position against maximum resistance and has complete ROM. There is a wide range of normal.
Grade 4/good	Patient can hold position against strong to moderate resistance and has full ROM. Grade 4/good and below represents true clinical weakness.
Grade 3+/fair +	Patient can complete full ROM against gravity and hold end position against mild resistance.
Grade 3/fair	Patient can tolerate no resistance but can perform movement through full ROM.
Grade 2+/poor +	Patient has full ROM in gravity-eliminated position and can take some resistance.
Grade 2/poor	Patient has full ROM in gravity-eliminated position.
Grade 2–/poor –	Patient can complete partial ROM in gravity-eliminated position.
Grade 1/trace	Examiner can detect visually or by palpation some contractile activity.
Grade 0/zero	Muscle is completely quiescent on palpation or visual inspection.

ROM, range of motion.
From Hislop HJ, Montgomery J: *Daniels and Worthingham's muscle testing: techniques of manual examination,* ed 7, St Louis, 2002, Saunders.

Important Concepts

Performing MMT requires extensive time, effort, and attention to detail while performing the correct technique to ensure that the results obtained are as accurate as possible.[62] The tester must have a comprehensive and detailed understanding of kinesiology to reproduce accurately and consistently manual grading of muscle strength (performance).

Cable tensiometry is used for isometric measurement of a muscle's strength (Fig. 5-5). This tool is essentially a mechanical form of MMT. The tensiometer provides the advantage of versatility for recording force measurements at virtually all angles of a joint's ROM and may be more sensitive for grading muscle strength above grade 4. This method is used primarily to measure strength in normal subjects in research projects. Many tests were developed in the 1950s to describe static force or isometric strength by use of the cable tension method.[15,16]

Dynamometry is used extensively in physical therapy. Hand-held dynamometers (Fig. 5-6) are used to quantify grip strength, and the standing-back dynamometer is used to evaluate back extension strength. In this latter example, many factors contribute to the subject's ability to generate tension or force during the back pull, including the subject's motivation, degree of pain (if any), arm length, leg length, height, weight, and the obvious contribution from other muscle groups. These variables make dynamometry an unreliable, nonspecific testing tool.

An isotonic 1 RM lift is used to test strength using commercially available exercise equipment or barbells and dumbbells. In this method, the patient performs a single, full ROM lift, such as a bench press (Fig. 5-7), shoulder press, or arm curl, for a particular muscle group. Applying this method is difficult because the tester and patient must first establish a reasonable starting weight through trial and error, fatigue becomes a factor if many trials are needed, and precise performance or execution of the proper lift is determined subjectively by the tester. This method is best used for normal subjects, in a sports medicine environment, or with uninvolved body parts not necessary for stabilization of a disabled joint.

Perhaps the most widely used and clinically relevant method of objective, reproducible strength testing is through isokinetics. The data collected with isokinetic

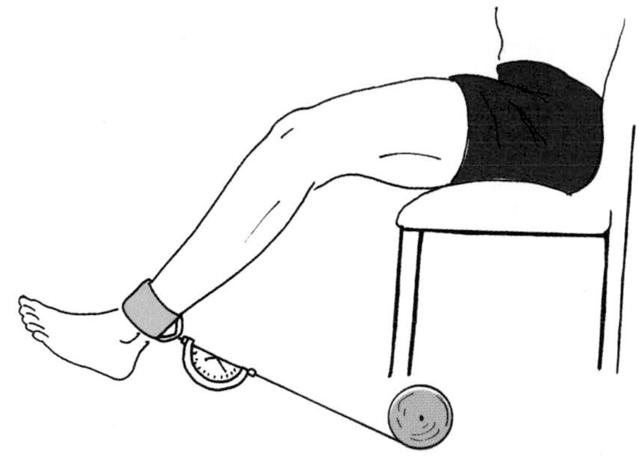

FIG 5-5 Seated cable tensiometer for quantifying isometric quadriceps strength.

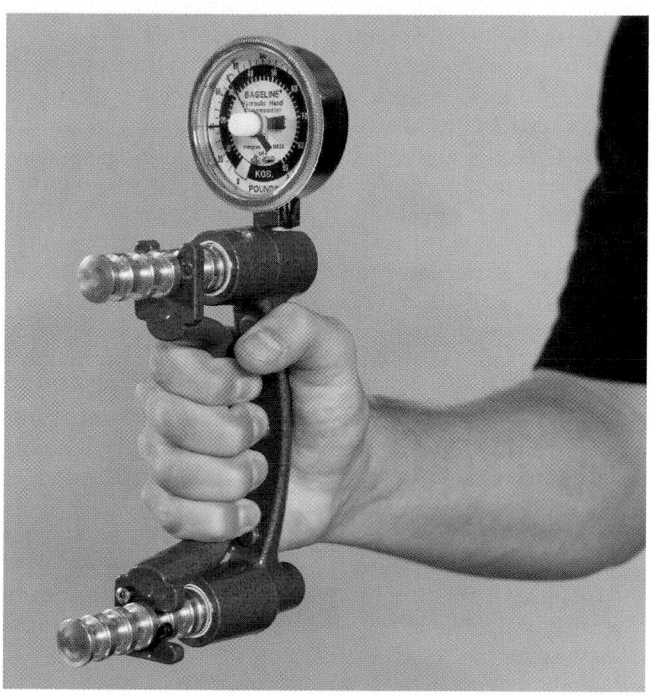

FIG 5-6 Hand-held grip dynamometer for measuring grip strength. *(From Evans RC:* Illustrated orthopedic physical assessment, *ed 3, St Louis, 2009, Mosby.)*

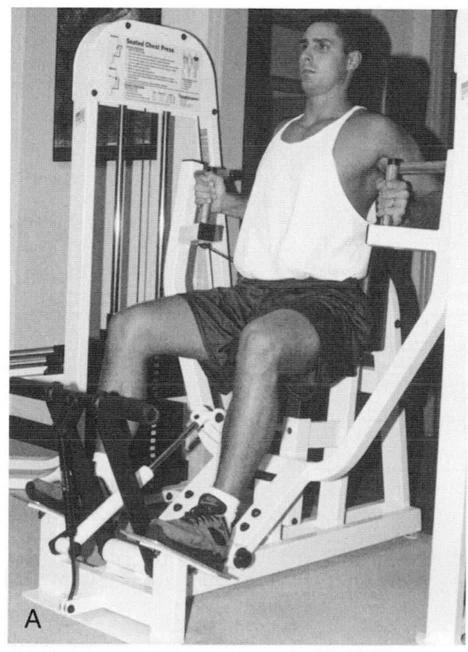

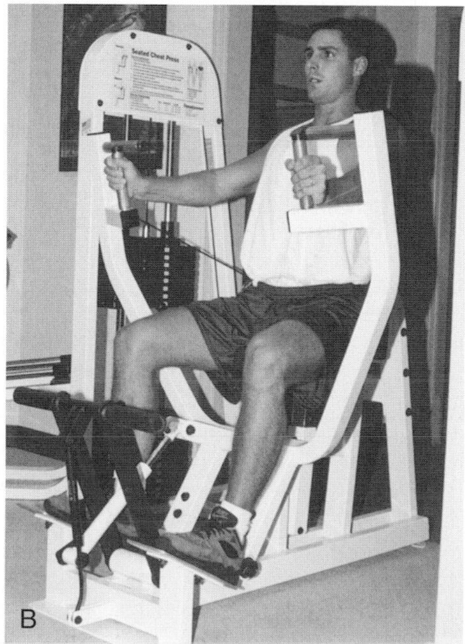

FIG 5-7 Concentric and eccentric 1 RM lift test. This is a generalized nonspecific method to determine strength with commercial isotonic equipment. **A,** Starting position. **B,** End position.

testing document strength (force production), torque, power, and work.[61] As stated, isokinetics employs a fixed speed, or velocity, of movement that allows for maximum loading throughout the full ROM. If a patient experiences pain during any part of the test or does not apply a maximum force throughout the entire ROM, the velocity remains constant with a variable resistance that is totally accommodating to the individual.[19] To test for strength, slow speeds (30°/sec to 60°/sec) are generally used.[49] Because isokinetic equipment can be interfaced with computers, a hard-copy graph of the data can be used for evaluation and exercise prescription. In addition to being a valid and reliable tool for strength testing, isokinetics can evaluate neuromuscular endurance, speed of muscle contraction, and muscular power.[41]

The determination of an individual's readiness to return to normal levels of activity is a common issue in rehabilitation. To resolve this issue, clinicians have incorporated functional testing after rehabilitation. Functional testing involves the evaluation of broad skills necessary to perform complex movements versus traditional methods that focus on isolated joint testing. This testing is particularly important when dealing with athletes who may be returned to activity too soon after rehabilitation because of inaccuracies in the assessment of their functional ability resulting from more traditional assessment methods.[18]

Examples include the following:

- One-leg hop for distance: The patient performs a single-leg hop for distance with each lower extremity.
- Single-leg triple hop for distance: The patient performs a single-leg triple hop for distance with each lower extremity.
- Timed single-leg hop (minitrampoline): The patient hops on the trampoline a maximum number of times in 30 seconds.
- Vertical jump: The patient performs a double-leg vertical jump for height.

> **Important Concepts**
>
> Functional testing involves the evaluation of broad skills necessary to perform complex movements versus traditional methods that focus on isolated joint testing. This testing is particularly important when dealing with athletes who may be returned to activity too soon after rehabilitation because of inaccuracies in the assessment of their functional ability resulting from more traditional assessment methods.

COMPARISON OF MUSCLE CONTRACTION TYPES

Generally, muscle contractions are characterized by the amount of tension the contraction produces and the amount of energy liberated (ATP use) by the contraction. The most common clinically applicable way to strengthen muscle is with concentric and eccentric contractions using isotonic (isoinertial)[56] **progressive resistive exercise (PRE).** Ankle or cuff weights, hand-held weights (dumbbells), and weight machines are examples of isotonic equipment used in physical therapy practice.* Elftman[23] demonstrated that the production of maximal force of contraction by various methods occurs in a predictable fashion, as shown in Fig. 5-8.

The force of contraction is expressed as the amount of tension developed per unit of contractile tissue. In terms of energy liberated (ATP use), eccentric muscle contractions use the least ATP, and concentric contractions use the most (Fig. 5-9).[3]

*Companies that produce lines of exercise equipment for strength training used in fitness and physical therapy facilities include Cybex, Nautilus, Rehab Systems, Body Masters, Universal, and Paramount. This equipment is typically available in single-station and multistation units.

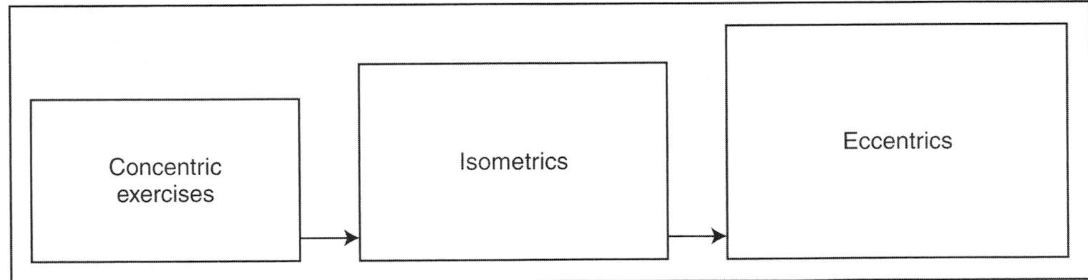

FIG 5-8 Progression of maximal force production from least to most.

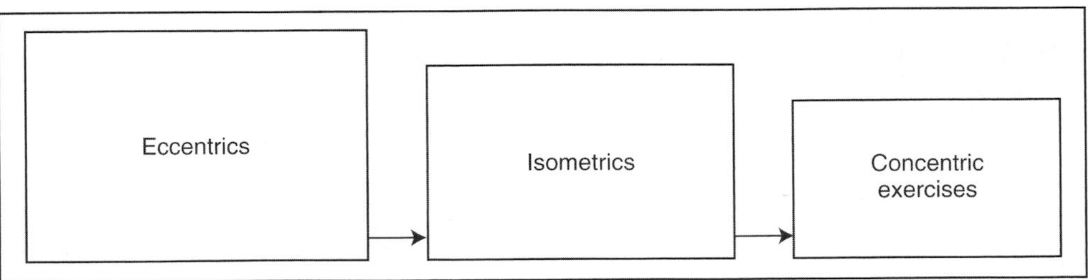

FIG 5-9 Relative amounts of ATP used in muscle contraction.

Based on this information, it appears that eccentric muscle contractions are more energy efficient and produce greater tension per contractile unit than concentric and isometric contractions. However, Davies[19] pointed out that much of the tension produced by eccentric muscle contraction results from stress imposed on the noncontractile serial elastic components (perimysium, epimysium, and endomysium) of the muscle. Eccentric muscle contractions stimulate both contractile and noncontractile elements, whereas concentric contractions and isometrics focus on the contractile elements.[61]

The PTA must consider the context in which each muscle contraction type is used clinically. Fundamentally implementing multiple muscle contraction types during all phases of rehabilitation is well supported.[8,35,70] In comparing muscle contraction types, it is best to view the decision concerning which type to use, when to use it, and in what pathologic conditions it should be used as a progression or continuum rather than a choice of one type over another. Davies[19] described a classic model of exercise progression (Box 5-1) that can be used as a general guide. Certain criteria must be established for the progression from one type of contraction to another.

First, exercise variables and parameters must be understood so that necessary adjustments can be made in a patient's exercise prescription (Box 5-2).The criteria established for progressing from one exercise mode to another are based on many factors and are patient specific. In general, pain usually dictates the time frame for progression, although swelling also does to a lesser degree. The sequence proceeds from the least intense to more challenging exercises with increased joint forces and metabolic demands. Some of the advantages and disadvantages of concentric and eccentric isotonic exercise and isokinetic exercise equipment are outlined for general comparison in Table 5-2.

BOX 5-1 Davies Model of Exercise Progression (1985)

- Isometric/eccentric contractions, multiple angle
- Isometrics (submaximal effort)
- Multiple-angle isometrics (maximal effort)
- Short arc concentric isokinetics (submaximal effort)
- Short arc isotonics—concentric/eccentric
- Short arc concentric isokinetics (maximal effort)
- Full ROM concentric isokinetics (submaximal effort)
- Full ROM isotonics—concentric/eccentric
- Full ROM concentric isokinetics (maximal effort)
- Full ROM eccentric isokinetics (submaximal effort)
- Full ROM eccentric isokinetics (maximal effort)

From Davies G: *A compendium of isokinetics in clinical usage and rehabilitation techniques,* ed 3, Onalaska, WI, 1987, S & S Publishers.
ROM, range of motion.

MUSCLE RESPONSE TO EXERCISE

Strength training must be individually tailored to meet the goals of recovery. As stated by DeLee,[21] "Function increases with use; functions we do not use, we lose. The intensity, duration, and frequency of activity are all related to the functional capacity that is developed."

Muscle tissue morphology is mutable; that is, it has the ability to change. Muscle mutability has two distinct categories: **hypertrophy** and atrophy.

BOX 5-2 Therapeutic Exercise Parameters

Frequency	Daily, 3 days a week, 2 days a week (once daily, twice daily)
Intensity	Amount of resistance, full ROM, short arc of motion, velocity of contraction (slow, moderate, fast)
Duration	6 weeks, 8 weeks, 10 weeks
Type of resistance	Isotonic, isokinetic
Muscle contraction type	Concentric, eccentric, isometric
Degree of resistance	Total amount of weight or force applied
Number of repetitions	1 to 15
Number of sets	1 to 5
Length of rest between sets	Short rest for aerobic-metabolic pathway, long rest (2 to 3 minutes) for anaerobic pathways
Order of exercise	Exercise large muscle groups first, progress to smaller muscle groups
Degrees of effort	Low intensity (submaximal effort), high intensity (maximal effort)

ROM, range of motion.

TABLE 5-2 Comparison of Isotonics versus Isokinetics

Commercially Available Machines and Free Weights	Isokinetics
ADVANTAGES	
• Low cost (relative) • Has concentric and eccentric components • Easy to instruct patients • Objective increase in muscle performance by increasing weight • Can perform static or isometric contractions	• Can exercise over a wide velocity (0° to ≥300°) • Accommodates to pain and fatigue • Low compressive forces at high speeds • Provides objective permanent record of data • Valid and reliable
DISADVANTAGES	
• Momentum is involved • Not safe if patient has pain during the motion of lifting	• Very expensive • Some models do not provide eccentrics • Takes time to switch machine for other body parts (time-consuming)

The stimuli for adaptive changes in skeletal muscle are described as frequency, intensity, and duration.[12] Human skeletal muscle responds and adapts to these stimuli and is characterized by the nature, rate, magnitude, and duration of the stimulus.[8] In a clinical situation, the stimulus provided to human muscle is the conditioning or training program. These programs are based on certain principles that lead to the necessary adaptive changes, which affect function.

Important Concepts

The stimuli for adaptive changes in skeletal muscle are described as frequency, intensity, and duration.[12]

The principles of overload, specificity, and reversibility[25] and progression and transfer of training[6] provide the foundation for the strength training programs used in physical therapy and are as follows:

The overload principle[6] is the guiding principle of exercise prescription. If muscle performance is to improve, a load that exceeds the metabolic capacity of the muscle must be applied. A muscle must be challenged to perform at a level greater than that to which it is accustomed.

The **specific adaptations to imposed demands (SAID) principle**[25] in part defines specific adaptations and alterations in response to highly specific demands. After injury, muscle reeducation helps the patient adapt and prepare for return to function.

Specificity[6] is the training of a patient in a specific manner to produce a specific adaptation or training outcome.

The progression principle[6] dictates that the intensity of program must become progressively greater to continue to make gains.

The transfer of training[6] principle describes the carryover of training effects from one variation of exercise or task to another.

The reversibility principle[25] indicates that changes in a body's systems are transient unless training-induced improvements are regularly used for functional activities or a person participates in a maintenance program. This can begin within 1 to 2 weeks after cessation of exercises.

Important Concepts

The overload principle[6] is the guiding principle of exercise prescription. If muscle performance is to improve, a load that exceeds the metabolic capacity of the muscle must be applied. A muscle must be challenged to perform at a level greater than that to which it is accustomed.

In general, type I muscle fibers (red [high myoglobin content] and oxidative) respond more favorably to low-intensity (low tension), high-volume (sets and repetitions) exercise than type II (white [low myoglobin content] and glycolytic) muscle fibers. High-volume, low-intensity exercise is repetitive, and gross muscle movements occur (e.g., bicycling, running, swimming, rowing). In this type of training, oxidative capabilities increase and relative percent of oxygen increases in type I muscle fibers in the specific muscle or muscle groups used.

In strength training programs, a desirable and predictable morphologic adaptive change is hypertrophy, which is the compensatory increase in individual muscle fiber size as a result of increases in and synthesis of the contractile proteins actin and myosin.[32] Type II muscle fibers increase more than type I fibers; this can be observed in comparing the body types of long-distance runners with the larger, more muscular physiques of sprinters. The physiques of long-distance runners and most aerobic athletes are thinner, possess less body fat, and have smaller muscles that are more adapted to endurance activities. Highly specific, or absolute strength, programs use a high-tension (heavy loads) and low-volume protocol. This type of training program requires relatively short bouts of progressive overload to stimulate the type II muscle fibers.

Biochemical adaptations of muscle occur in specifically applied strength training programs. After intense strength training, significant increases appear in glycogen, ATP, and creatine phosphate; increased activity and quantity of enzymes involved with anaerobic glycolysis, creatine kinase, and myokinase also are seen.[17]

Hyperplasia (the development of new muscle fibers) or longitudinal fiber splitting may occur in response to high-intensity strength training programs. Gonyea and colleagues[33] reported in animal studies that an increase of 19% of the total number of muscle fibers occurred in cat forelimb muscles after weight lifting. This phenomenon has not been proven in humans. The predominant change in response to high-intensity strength training programs is hypertrophy of existing skeletal muscle fibers. The relative contribution (if any) of hyperplasia or muscle fiber splitting has not been determined.[12] Induced hypertrophy in injured or postoperative muscle tissue is important because hypertrophy relates to a potential to generate greater tension.

Passive stretching of innervated muscle tissue creates tension and results in fiber hypertrophy. The change in fiber size associated with this stretch-induced hypertrophy results from increased protein turnover.[12] This feature has clinical relevance in muscle recovery during immobilization.

DELAYED ONSET MUSCLE SORENESS

The clinical features of exercise-induced muscle soreness are diffuse and general, occurring in the absence of specific, intense injury.[58] Acute muscle strain can be differentiated from exercise-induced soreness primarily by the history leading to the injury. With an acute strain, the patient is able to relate a specific event or episode that caused the injury.[58]

Based on this distinction, the PTA can identify complaints of diffuse muscle soreness resulting from new or unaccustomed exercise.[58] However, if the patient can describe a history of local, intense pain after a specific episode, an acute muscle strain must be considered.[58]

Although the PTA does not interpret and define complaints of pain without consulting with the physical therapist (PT), the assistant must be able to identify and describe accurately the nature and disposition of any pain, based on the patient's complaints and relevant history, and be able to communicate this information to the PT.

After a specific exercise program, muscle soreness is an anticipated by-product of intense eccentric exercise.[29,30,41,53,66,69] The degree and presence of after-exercise muscle soreness appear to be greater with these eccentric programs than with concentric exercise programs.[11,41,53,55,66,73]

Symptoms of **delayed onset muscle soreness (DOMS)** include pain, swelling, tenderness, reduced ROM, and stiffness.[3,41,53,66] Albert[3] reported five general theories concerning the process of DOMS:

1. Lactic acid theory
2. Torn tissue theory
3. Tonic muscle spasms theory
4. Connective tissue damage theory
5. Tissue fluid theory

Important Concepts

Symptoms of DOMS include pain, swelling, tenderness, reduced ROM, and stiffness.[3,41,53,66]

The lactic acid and tonic muscle spasms theories do not appear to be related to DOMS.[1,2,63,76] Studies[50,52] showed evidence that the primary cause of muscle soreness after exercise is skeletal muscle damage. Greater tensions produced by eccentric exercise contribute to the initial muscle damage, although isometric and concentric contractions are not absolved of producing latent muscle soreness. Isometric exercise and concentric exercise can produce DOMS even in well-trained athletes.

Conventional methods of treating DOMS are listed in Table 5-3. Treatment of DOMS remains controversial. One study[65] found ice, a traditional treatment method, to be ineffectual, whereas other studies[7,26] found vibration and compression, nontraditional treatment methods, to be effective.

A review[68] of the current strategies for treating DOMS revealed the following:

- Pharmacologic aids, nonsteroidal antiinflammatory drugs (NSAIDs): Although there is some inconsistency in findings, NSAIDs such as ibuprofen have the potential to alleviate some symptoms of DOMS.
- Therapeutic treatments using physical modalities: Treatment using conventional therapies, such as icing, massage, or stretching, also proved inconsistent. Nonconventional treatments such as acupuncture, herbal remedies, and hyperbaric oxygen therapy were found to have limited use. However, the review did indicate that of all the therapies examined, icing the affected area appeared to be the most effective.
- Dietary methods using nutritional supplements: Additional supplementation with antioxidants (vitamins C and E) and supplements such as arnica, coenzyme Q and L-carnitine appears to be of little use.

The authors concluded that "It would appear that we are still no closer to establishing a conclusive approach to the treatment of the symptoms of DOMS. In the interim, several possible treatments, such as the use of NSAIDs and cryotherapy (icing), have the potential to help alleviate the pain associated with DOMS."

The most prudent approach appears to be to ease into any unfamiliar exercises (especially eccentrics). If patients experience DOMS, they should be educated that with appropriate rest and recovery, DOMS should run its course in 2 to 3 days, and they will be able to get back to their training relatively pain-free.

TABLE 5-3 Suggested Treatment Techniques for Delayed Onset Muscle Soreness

Type	Efficacy
Rest	None
Nonsteroidal antiinflammatory drugs	Highly successful
Steroidal antiinflammatory drugs	Moderately successful
Electrical stimulation	Proposed only
Exercise	Highly successful
Transcutaneous electrical nerve stimulation	Highly successful
Stretching	Mixed success
Iontophoresis	Not successful
Cryotherapy	Not successful
Calcium antagonists	Proposed only

From Albert M: *Eccentric muscle training in sports and orthopaedics,* New York, 1991, Churchill Livingstone.

VELOCITY OF MUSCLE CONTRACTIONS

Muscle contraction velocity and speed of limb movement are not the same. If two arms are bending at the same speed but one arm is holding a weight, the muscle bending the arm with more weight must produce a greater speed of contraction to overcome the resistance. More tension is developed in the muscle lifting the heavier arm, even though the speed of limb movement is the same.

Slower speeds of muscle contraction can produce greater force and tension than the same muscle moving at a higher rate of speed. A slower contracting muscle moving a heavy resistance can produce greater tension than a faster contracting muscle lifting a lighter resistance.[55] When slow speeds of full arc resistance exercise are used to generate greater tension and strength, joint compression forces and torque are increased as well. To minimize the negative or unwanted effects of joint compression (Fig. 5-10), a program of isometric exercise may be more appropriate in some instances.

Strength programs initially focus on using slow-speed tension to produce isometric contractions and spare the negative effects of excessive joint motion, torque, and compressive forces found in full ROM slow-speed isotonic (concentric and eccentric) exercises. Fast and slow contraction speeds can be distinguished with isokinetic exercise. By controlling the speed of limb movement with an isokinetic apparatus, better control of joint compression forces can be achieved. (Speed is defined isokinetically as control of limb movement, not the actual speed of muscle contraction.) A slow speed of limb movement using an isokinetic apparatus may be 60°/sec, and a fast speed may be 300°/sec.

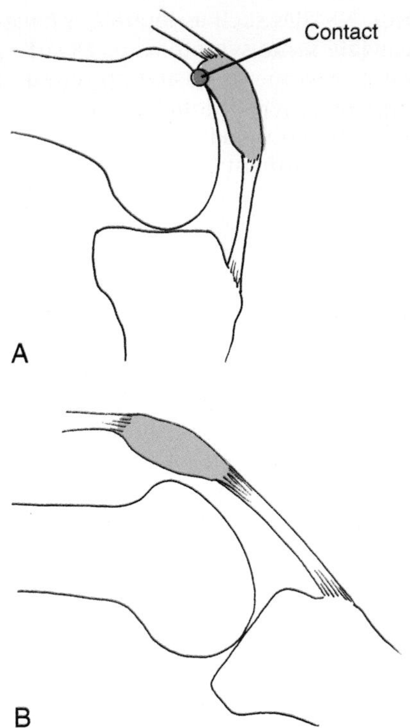

FIG 5-10 **A,** With the knee flexed to 90°, there are resultant increases in patellofemoral compression with excursion of the knee (leg) into extension. **B,** With the knee in extension, there is less patellofemoral compression.

Higher speeds of limb movement require the resistance to be lighter than in a slower moving limb with greater resistance. Isokinetic testing and exercise use the concept of velocity spectrum training, which is the ability to control limb speeds within a range of slow to fast speeds. Higher speeds of limb movement produce less joint compression and lower forces relative to slow-speed, high-resistance training.

Functionally, human limbs move at various speeds and with various degrees of motion. Velocity spectrum training allows a patient to train at speeds of motion that more closely approximate normal human limb speeds.[10,59,78] For example, a training program using the velocity spectrum concept may include submaximal contractions at slow speeds (60°/sec to 90°/sec) for two sets of 8 to 12 repetitions, then contractions at incrementally increasing speeds up to 24°/sec or higher for two or three sets of 15 repetitions. This program may not be appropriate for athletes because the functional speeds of movements in athletics far exceed the capability of the isokinetic dynamometer.

In a comparison of isokinetic and isotonic exercise, most isotonic exercise is performed at approximately 60°/sec,[19] whereas isokinetic exercise can be adjusted specifically to train the affected area at speeds more closely duplicating normal functional speeds of movement. The higher velocity contractions used with isokinetic exercise allow for the following:

- Improved functional speeds of contraction
- Reduced joint compression forces
- Accommodation of patient's pain (the patient will not undergo more force than he or she can safely produce)

Using velocity spectrum training with isokinetics allows the progression from multiple-angle isometrics (0°/sec) to slow speeds (60°/sec) for greater tension and torque and to higher speeds (240°/sec and faster) for functional activities and lower compressive forces.

CLINICALLY RELEVANT EXERCISE PROGRAMS

Although there are many strength training protocols, three broad fundamental strength protocols are used extensively in physical therapy. The DeLorme[22] **progressive resistance exercise (PRE)** protocol is still used widely for strength training programs after injury to the musculoskeletal system. This program uses the classic and well-recognized exercise of three sets of 10 repetitions of resistance. Its protocol states that the patient must establish a maximum weight that can be lifted for 10 repetitions; this is termed the 10 RM. To initiate the program, the patient performs 10 repetitions at half (50%) of the predetermined 10 RM. The next set of exercise is performed at three fourths (75%) of the 10 RM. Finally, the third set is performed for 10 repetitions at the established 10 RM (100%).

The DeLorme protocol calls for an arbitrary increase in resistance each week. It allows for a systematic and gradual progression during each exercise session by providing a warmup period using submaximal contractions before the 10 RM.

An example of a DeLorme protocol that provides progressive loading with a warmup built in follows:

- Set 1 = 10 repetitions at 50% of 10 RM
- Set 2 = 10 repetitions at 75% of 10 RM
- Set 3 = 10 repetitions at 100% of 10 RM

Performing three sets of 10 repetitions at the same resistance is a common clinical practice. However, it is not the DeLorme protocol and is less efficient because it does not overload the muscle in the same manner, and it does not involve a built-in warmup.

The Oxford program[79] is the opposite of the DeLorme protocol. Although it begins by establishing the individual's 10 RM, the second set is performed at three fourths (75%) of the 10 RM, and the following set is performed at half (50%) of the established 10 RM. Each set involves 10 repetitions. The method reportedly takes advantage of the muscle's fatigue during exercise.

There are fundamental differences in philosophy between the DeLorme PRE protocol and the Oxford technique. The DeLorme program calls for a progressive overload during each session by adding resistance while the muscle fatigues. The Oxford technique calls for reducing resistance as the muscle fatigues. Both programs were developed in the 1950s, and since then many variations and combinations have been used to discover the most effective and efficient means to regain strength after an injury.

The Oxford regimen provides regressive loading and takes into consideration muscle fatigue:

- Set 1 = 10 repetitions at 100% of 10 RM
- Set 2 = 10 repetitions at 75% of 10 RM
- Set 3 = 10 repetitions at 50% of 10 RM

To control objectively the progression or resistance with exercise programs, Knight[45] established the daily adjustable progressive resistance exercise (DAPRE) technique. Instead of using three sets of 10 repetitions as DeLorme and Oxford did, Knight's program calls for four sets with variable repetitions. The protocol calls for establishing the patient's 6 RM instead of 10 RM, with the number 6 based on research by Berger[9] as the optimum number of repetitions for developing strength.

The first set is performed at half (50%) of the established working weight for 10 repetitions. The second set is performed at three fourths (75%) of the 6 RM for six repetitions. The third set is performed at the full previously established maximum weight, but the patient is asked to perform as many repetitions as possible with this weight. The number of repetitions performed in this set is used to determine the weight used in the fourth set. The goal of this technique is to establish a maximum resistance that can be performed for six repetitions.

As the individual's strength increases, the number of repetitions in the third set increases, which increases the weight in the fourth set. The hallmark of this program is understanding the guidelines used to adjust the working weight of the third and fourth sets.[21] The DAPRE adjusted working weight guide is as follows:

Set 1	10 repetitions	50% of 6 RM
Set 2	6 repetitions	75% of 6 RM
Set 3	Maximum repetitions	100% of 6 RM
Set 4	Maximum repetitions	Adjust weight based on number of repetitions performed in set 3

Third Set Number of Repetitions	Fourth Set Change
0 to 2	Reduce weight 5 to 10 pounds
3 to 4	Reduce weight 5 to 10 pounds
5 to 7	Keep weight the same
8 to 12	Increase weight 5 to 10 pounds
13 or more	Increase weight 10 to 15 pounds

The rationale for the weight adjustments described in the preceding list is to modify resistance during the fourth set to maintain the goal of keeping repetitions between five and seven, whereas encouraging maximum resistance to influence strength increases and morphologic changes, such as hypertrophy.

In this protocol, the exact weight used by the patient is highly specific and tailored to the individual and goals of recovery. Adjustments in weight are made to accommodate the specific healing constraints of the injury and the individual tolerance level of the patient. Extremely close communication and supervision of the patient are necessary. With the DeLorme PRE program and Oxford program, the patient works with a percentage of an established weight each session and advances in resistance once each week. The DAPRE protocol requires daily adjustments; it takes advantage of the fact that submaximal work does not provide the necessary stimulus for maximal gains in strength. By reducing the volume of repetitions to six and adjusting the weight so that a maximal load is used for six repetitions, the intensity of work is increased.

The National Strength and Conditioning Association[6] makes the following recommendations:

Training Goal	Load (%1 RM)	Goal Repetitions	Goal Sets
Strength	≥85	≤6	2-6
Power	80-90	1-2	3-5
Hypertrophy	67-85	6-12	3-6
Muscle endurance	≤67	≥12	2-3

Other protocols have suggested[71] that by initially focusing on muscular hypertrophy, a greater potential for strength would exist. Because the cross-sectional area of muscle would be increased by a program of higher volume, the potential to develop greater amounts of tension is increased by reducing the volume of exercise and increasing the loads used.

The rule of tens is followed in isometric exercise protocols that are commonly used in rehabilitation.[61] This rule states that the patient must perform 10-second contractions for 10 repetitions with a 10-second rest between each repetition.[19] The patient is taught to perform isometric contractions by gradually developing tension for 2 seconds, maintaining a maximal contraction for 6 seconds, then gradually decreasing tension for 2 seconds (Fig. 5-11).

While one is performing isometric exercise, an overflow of strength occurs approximately 10° above and below the angle (Fig. 5-12) at which the exercise is occurring.[44] Multiple-angle isometrics are taught at 10° increments to achieve strength gains throughout a described ROM.

A circuit training program is a predetermined, organized sequence of exercise. Traditionally, this type of program is used for general body conditioning and total fitness. A general circuit program calls for the performance of one or two exercises for each body part in sequence (Table 5-4). Usually a rest period of 30 seconds to 1 minute is allowed between sets. If resistance exercise equipment is used, circuit weight-training programs also tax the aerobic metabolic pathway to a degree. The movement from one station to another does not allow for maximum recovery and high-intensity loads, but it does provide an adequate stimulus for aerobic and anaerobic work.

The clinical delivery of specific exercise protocols depends on many factors. The patient's pathologic

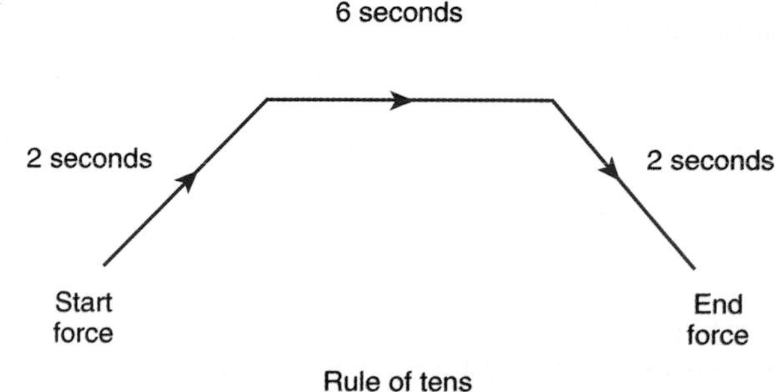

FIG 5-11 Isometric contractions by rule of tens. *(From Davies G: A compendium of isokinetics in clinical usage and rehabilitation techniques, ed 3, Onalaska, WI, 1987, S & S Publishers.)*

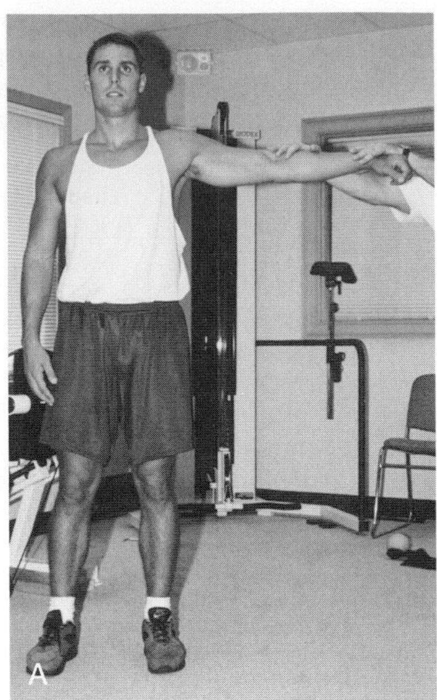

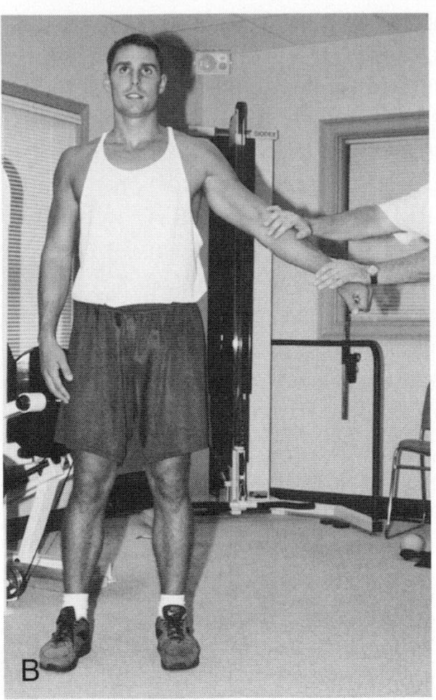

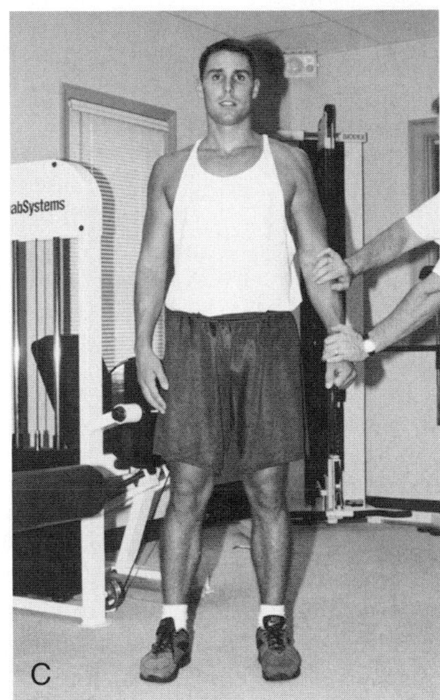

FIG 5-12 Multiple-angle isometric shoulder abduction. **A,** Isometric hold in approximately 90° of abduction. **B,** Midrange isometric shoulder abduction. **C,** Isometric set in 0° of abduction.

TABLE 5-4 Sample Circuit Weight Training Program

Exercise	Repetitions	Sets	Rest
Leg press	10	2	30 sec between each set
Leg extension	10	2	30 sec between each set
Leg curl	10	2	30 sec between each set
Bench press	10	2	30 sec between each set
Supine fly	10	2	30 sec between each set
Shoulder press	10	2	30 sec between each set
Lateral pull-down	10	2	30 sec between each set
Bent over row	10	2	30 sec between each set
Bicep curl	10	2	30 sec between each set
Triceps press-down	10	2	30 sec between each set

condition; time constraints for healing of specific tissues; and degree of swelling, pain, function, and motivation all play a role in determining the most appropriate program to use and when to use it. In making an organized, systematic progression from one program to another, following specific guidelines is a responsible and appropriate plan for strength training programs for a wide variety of musculoskeletal system injuries.

PLYOMETRICS

Plyometric exercises are intense power-generating exercises that are traditionally confined to sport-specific functional training near the end of a rehabilitation program. *Plyo* comes from the Greek word *plythein,* meaning to increase, and *metric* refers to measure. **Plyometrics** is a system of exercising that uses the stretch reflex to develop muscle contraction speed.[77]

Important Concepts

Plyometric exercises are intense power-generating exercises that are traditionally confined to sport-specific functional training near the end of a rehabilitation program. *Plyo* comes from the Greek word *plythein,* meaning to increase, and *metric* refers to measure.

Plyometric exercises are also highly adaptable for use with the general orthopedic patient population. However, the inherent nature of plyometrics requires the patient to be prepared for high-intensity, task-specific, dynamic exercise.

The principles behind plyometrics are based on the neurophysiologic responses from the Golgi tendon organs and muscle spindles.[77] The most rudimentary example of plyometrics is the depth jump (Fig. 5-13). As the patient's foot contacts the ground (amortization phase), the muscle

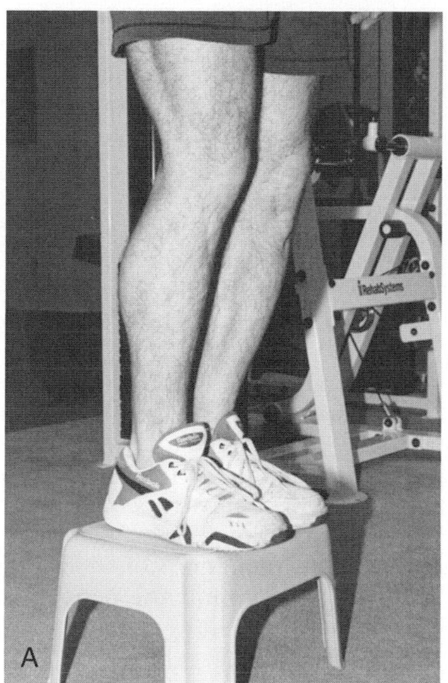

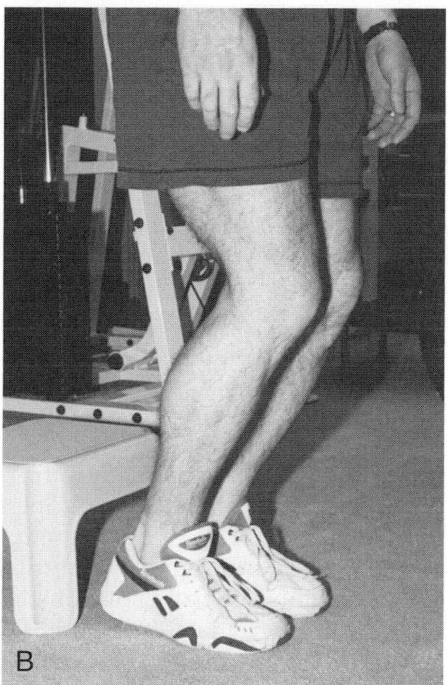

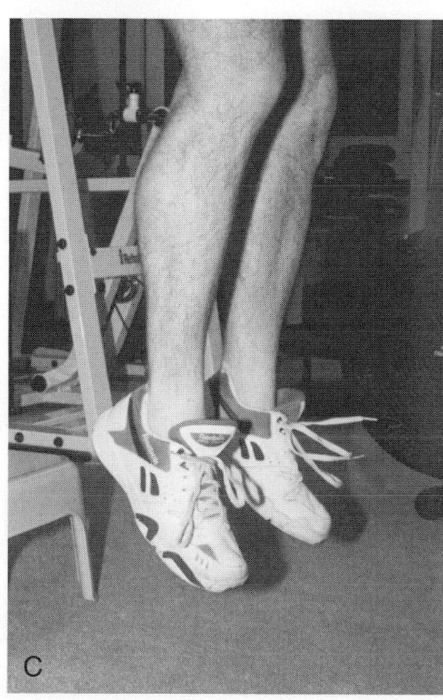

FIG 5-13 Plyometric depth jump. **A,** Starting position on a short stool. **B,** Without jumping up, the patient steps off the stool down to the ground with both feet simultaneously. The time spent on the ground is called the amortization phase. **C,** Rapid concentric contraction follows the amortization phase, which results in a powerful leap.

spindles respond by causing a reflex muscular contraction. Albert[3] stated, "The greater and more quickly a load is applied to a muscle, the greater the firing frequency of the muscle spindle with a corresponding stronger muscle contraction." The fundamental goal of plyometric exercise is to minimize the amortization phase of the exercise, which, in this example, is contact with the ground.

All forms of jumping, skipping, and hopping can be used in a plyometric exercise program.[77] Upper body exercises, such as throwing and catching a weighted object, are examples of plyometrics. An isotonic supine leg press hop is an example of plyometrics used to develop rapid, eccentric loading with a corresponding rapid, concentric contraction.

Plyometrics must be used judiciously and principally as an end component in a phase progression program. The fundamental concept of plyometrics involves ballistic, high-velocity movement patterns, which cannot be used during early rehabilitation when tissues are still healing. Plyometrics can be added to increase function as the patient progresses from one program or phase to another.

Many isotonic strength training programs involve lifting a load from a seated, supine, or standing position. These exercises are meant to isolate and strengthen specific muscle groups throughout a single plane of motion. Plyometrics focus on weight-bearing functional activities that duplicate high-velocity, multiplane, normal human movement.[77] The PTA must recognize that the value of plyometrics is primarily to prepare the patient to return to function. Not all patients recovering from an orthopedic injury require an intense plyometric exercise program. However, if the patient desires to return to dynamic sporting activities, or his or her job requires dynamic or ballistic physical labor, plyometrics are appropriate conditioning to enable one to withstand high levels of eccentric and concentric loads.

CLOSED KINETIC CHAIN EXERCISE

During any exercise, if the distal portion of the exercising segment is weight bearing or fixed, it is a **closed kinetic chain (CKC) exercise.** An **open kinetic chain (OKC) exercise** involves the distal segment moving freely in space, such as a seated knee extension. A CKC is best described as a system of interdependent articulated links. For example, in a weight-bearing leg (Fig. 5-14), as the knee is flexed, the entire chain or link system joining the ankle to the knee and to the hip is affected. In an OKC system, such as the arm (Fig. 5-15), the shoulder and elbow are fixed, whereas the distal wrist segment moves freely in space. Davies[20] stated, "In a closed kinetic chain, motion at one joint will produce motion at all of the other joints in the system in a predictable manner."

Important Concepts

During any exercise, if the distal portion of the exercising segment is weight bearing or fixed, it is a CKC exercise. An OKC exercise involves the distal segment moving freely in space, such as a seated knee extension.

The human body functions as a combination of open and closed chain activities such as walking and stair climbing. The primary advantage of CKC exercises is the highly functional nature of the exercises, which use concentric and eccentric muscle contractions synchronously to produce functional movement. In a strength training program, combinations of OKC and CKC exercises should be used to condition the patient to perform purposeful, functional activities.

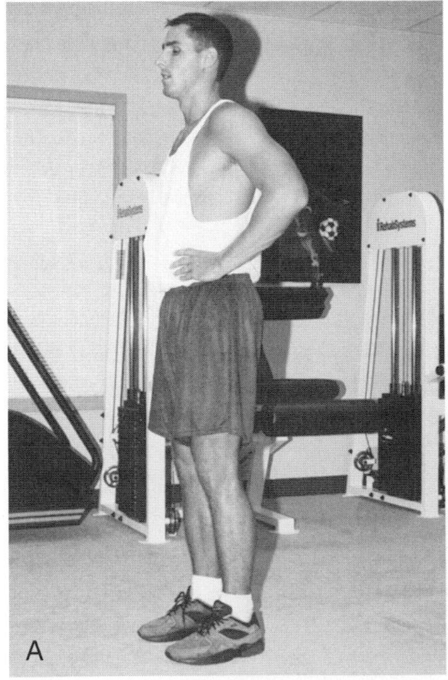

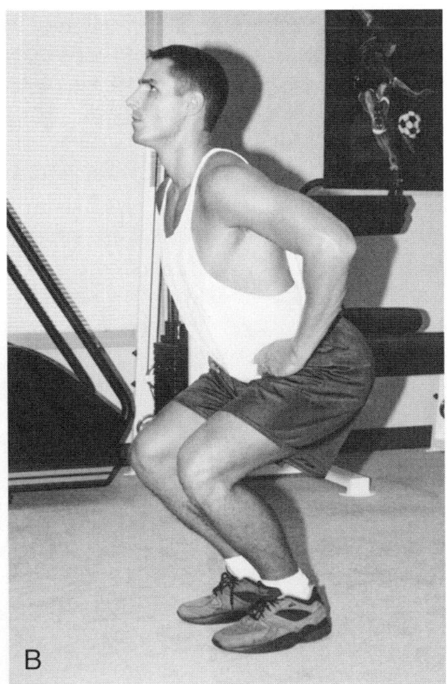

FIG 5-14 A closed kinetic chain. **A,** Starting position of a standing squat or leg bend maneuver. **B,** Motion of the knee produces predictable motion in all joints within the kinetic chain. With knee flexion, the resultant change in joint position of the ankle, hip, and spine is noticeable.

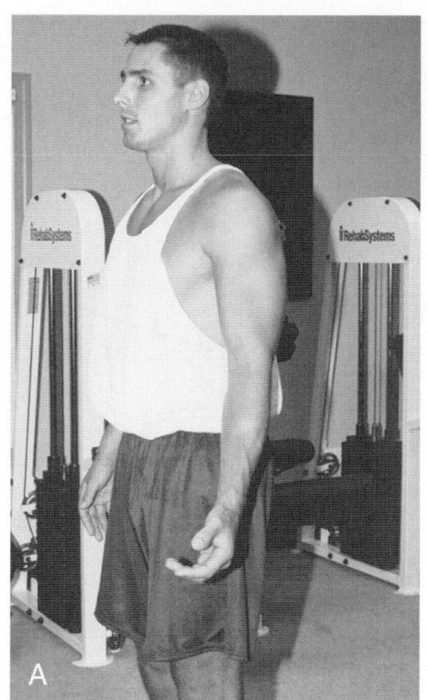

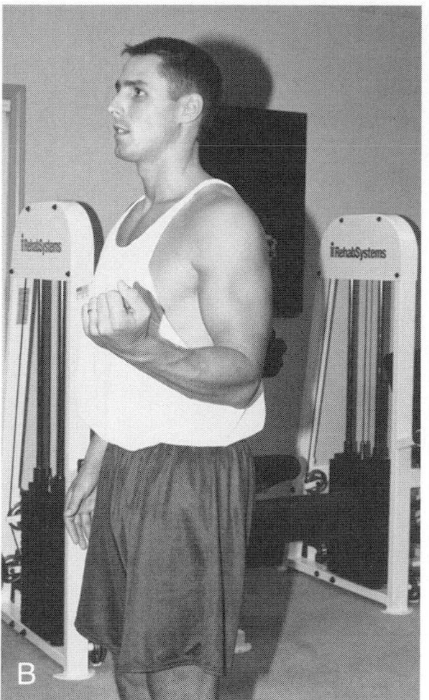

FIG 5-15 An open kinetic chain. **A,** Beginning position of elbow flexion. **B,** The distal arm and wrist segments move freely in space.

In knee rehabilitation programs,[14,57] quadriceps strengthening can be achieved through knee extension exercises (which are open chain) or leg press exercises or squats (which are closed chain). In many cases, patients are introduced to therapeutic exercises by way of submaximal isometric muscle contractions. More intense and demanding exercises are added as pain, strength, and function allow. OKC resistance exercises can be employed to stimulate growth in strength further. In some cases, the PT institutes CKC exercises early in the recovery phase of rehabilitation. For example, CKC exercises are frequently used within the first few weeks after anterior cruciate ligament reconstructive surgery. In addition, selected open chain exercises (exercises that do not place unwanted forces on the newly repaired tissues) are used. CKC exercises may not be appropriate for some patients with osteoarthritis or other conditions where vertical, compressive loads would exacerbate the condition.

The general rationales for using CKC exercises in rehabilitation programs are as follows:

- In theory, CKC exercises are more functional than OKC exercises (this can be refuted).
- Loading of the affected joint produces an increase in kinesthetic awareness.
- Improved neuromuscular coordination is achieved.
- CKC exercises are nonisolation exercises that produce muscular cocontractions.

Caution must be used when prescribing CKC activities during rehabilitation when pain, swelling, dysfunction, or muscle weakness is present.[20] Because an articulated joint system is being exercised under these conditions (e.g., limited ROM, pain, swelling), unpredictable compensation may occur in the joints superior and inferior to the affected joint.[20] OKC exercises must be used to isolate and strengthen the weakened area before progressing to CKC exercises.

PERIODIZATION OF STRENGTH TRAINING PROGRAMS

Periodization involves a predictable pattern of exercise volume, intensity, and rest periods that enhance strength-developing capabilities.[72] Its main components are cycles, or periods, of strength training. Many fundamental strength programs call for a PRE system without consideration for variations in frequency, intensity, duration, and recovery. The periodization model takes into consideration progressive cycles of various training loads and degrees of intensity during strength programs.[72]

Important Concepts

Periodization involves a predictable pattern of exercise volume, intensity, and rest periods that enhance strength-developing capabilities.[72] Its main components are cycles, or periods, of strength training.

Periodization can involve any of three cycles: microcycle, mesocycle, or macrocycle. The microcycle is the smallest unit of time (usually weeks), and accumulated microcycles form a mesocycle. The mesocycle is traditionally a few months long and consists of multiple microcycles that vary in volume, frequency, and intensity. The macrocycle is the largest segment of time (it can be 1 year) and involves a collection of mesocycles.

Periodization of strength training programs in the clinical rehabilitation setting was originally designed for and used extensively in athletes and is justified by following a series of defined protocols directed specifically at developing strength while minimizing fatigue and overtraining of a patient recovering from an orthopedic condition. The fundamental goals and objectives of a classic periodization program are outlined in Fig. 5-16. This is only a basic example, which must be modified to meet the specific

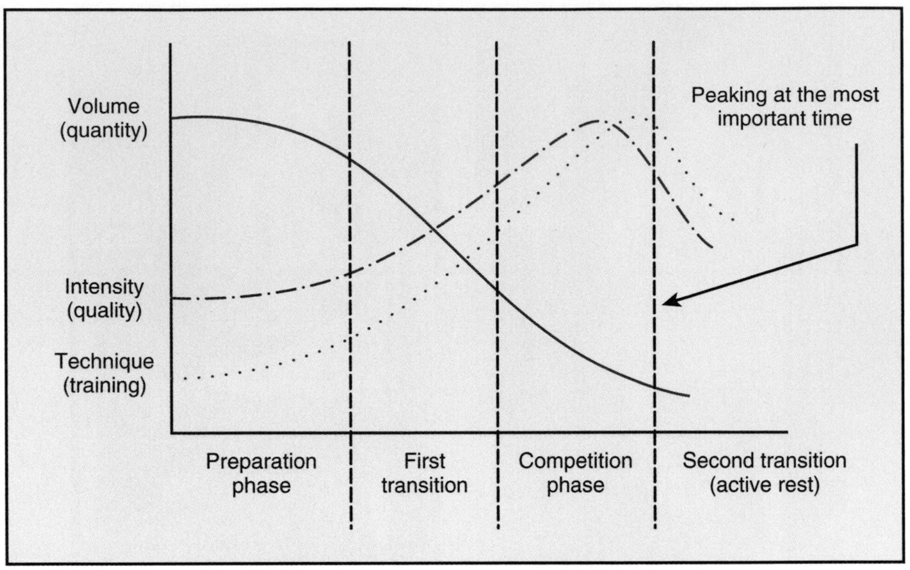

FIG 5-16 Classic periodization model. *(From Stone MH, O'Bryant H, Garhammer J, et al.: A theoretical model of strength training,* NSCA Journal, *4(4):36-39, August 1982.)*

rehabilitation goals for recovering patients. It can be adapted for many patients who require strength as part of their rehabilitation program.

In a periodization program, instead of constantly striving to increase resistance during each treatment or each week by use of the same system of sets and repetitions for a recovering patient, an attempt should be made to cycle the program into specific phases. In general, the first phase (microcycle) strives to develop basic strength and muscular hypertrophy. There are small alterations in sets (between three and six sets) and repetitions (between 8 and 12 repetitions) in each week of rehabilitation, and a high volume of exercise is used, dictating a lower intensity level (approximately 65% to 70% of 1 RM). This phase can be called the *preparatory phase* or *initial rehabilitation protocol.* The second phase (mesocycle) is designed to enhance strength by increasing the loads used (85% of 1 RM) and decreasing the volume of exercise to three to five sets of four to six repetitions. This phase as well as the first phase may last 2 or 3 months. During each mesocycle, there are numerous microcycles (weeks) in which various changes are made to reduce chronic overwork. The second phase of this basic example is called the *first transition phase* or *active rehabilitation phase.*

The traditional athletic model for this modified periodization program is described in Fig. 5-17. The strength protocol should be modified to fit the specific needs of each individual.

Preparation → Transition 1 → Competition → Transition 2 (active rest)

Phase	Hypertrophy	Basic strength	Strength & power	Peaking or maintaining
Sets	3 - 10	3 - 5	3 - 5	1 - 3
Reps	8 - 12	4 - 6	2 - 3	1 - 3
Days/wk	3 - 4	3 - 5	3 - 5	1 - 5
Times/day	1 - 3	1 - 3	1 - 2	1
Intensity cycle (weeks)	2 - 3/1	2 - 4/1	2 - 3/1	—
Intensity	low	high	high	very high to low
Volume	high	moderate to high	low	very low

FIG 5-17 Traditional athletic model of a modified periodization program. *(From Stone MH, O'Bryant H, Garhammer J, et al.: A theoretical model of strength training,* NSCA Journal, *4(4):36-39, August 1982.)*

Strength Training for Older Populations

Strength training programs for elderly adults include special considerations. Declines in muscle performance, force-generating capabilities, and concomitant muscle mass are well documented in elderly adults.[40,48] Strength training programs for elderly adults are focused on delaying muscle atrophy, improving function, and increasing force-generating capabilities by stimulating muscle hypertrophy. Resistance exercise programs for healthy older adults show significant improvements in muscle strength, muscle volume (hypertrophy), and other parameters of muscle structure and function.[75] According to Thompson,[75] studies show that "Given an adequate training stimulus, older men and women show similar gains compared to young individuals after resistive training." In addition, McCartney and colleagues[52] reported that "Long term resistance training in older people is feasible and results in increases in dynamic muscle strength, muscle size, and functional capacity."

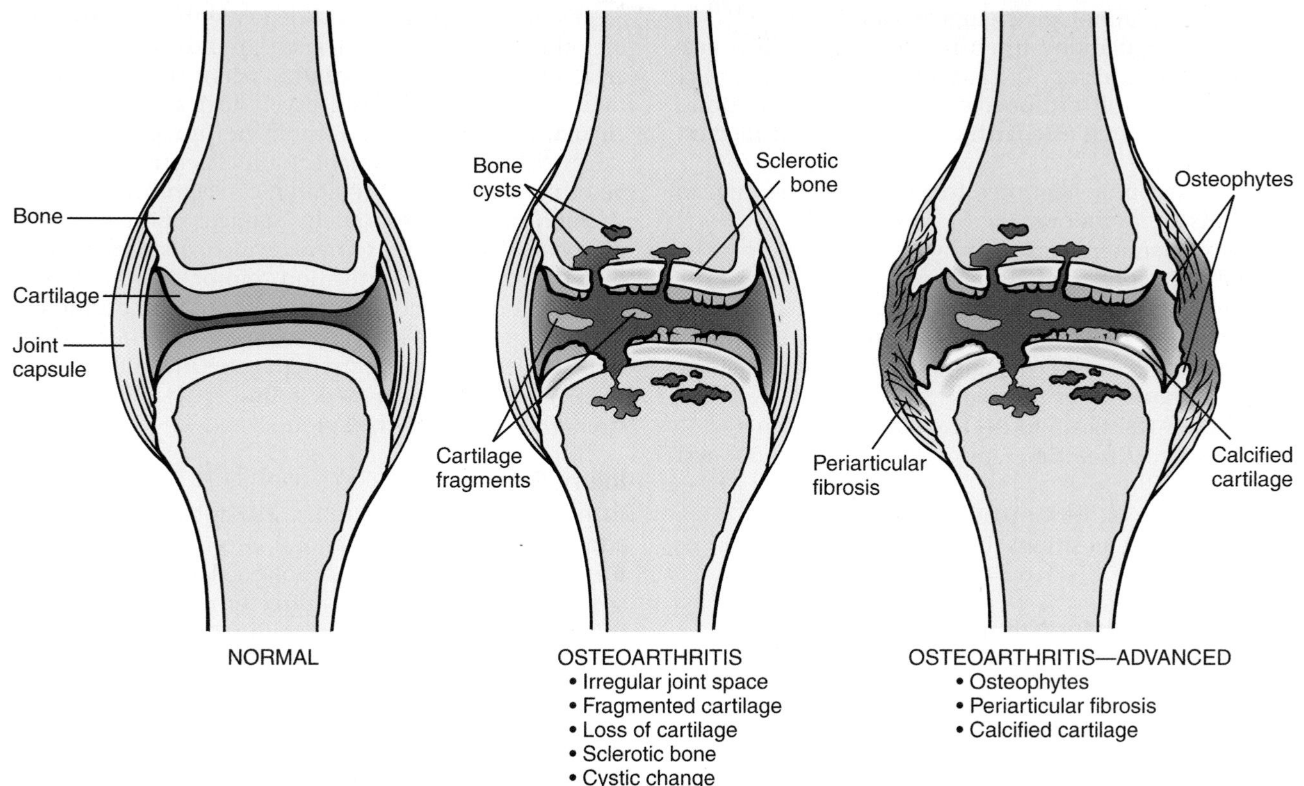

FIG 5-18 Schematic presentation of the pathologic changes in osteoarthritis. Fragmentation and loss of cartilage denude the subchondral bone, which undergoes sclerosis and cystic change. Osteophytes form on the lateral sides and protrude into the adjacent soft tissues, causing irritation, inflammation, and fibrosis. *(From Damjanov I:* Pathology for the health professions, *ed 3, St Louis, 2006, Saunders.)*

A study by Evans[24] concluded that "exercise may minimize or reverse the syndrome of physical frailty, which is so prevalent among the most elderly. Because of their low functional status and high incidence of chronic disease, there is no segment of the population that can benefit more from exercise than the elderly."

Another study by Henwood and Taaffe[38] found that cessation of training resulted in only a modest loss of muscle power and strength, which was recouped with retraining. This finding is important, considering that elderly adults tend to take extended vacations and have family commitments that require breaks from training.

One must consider multiple morbidities and degenerative joint disease when developing strength training programs for elderly adults. Unstable, chronic, and complex medical problems may preclude certain types of strength training programs. For example, in cardiovascular disease, chronic obstructive pulmonary disease, and other conditions, a protocol of general, very low-intensity gross body movement may be more beneficial and safer than isometric or isotonic resistance exercise. In advanced cases of osteoarthritis of the knee and hip, it is prudent to avoid vertical compression loads and full ROM heavy isotonic exercise. Pain and swelling from osteoarthritic lesions, bone spurs, and osteophytes (Fig. 5-18) can be exacerbated by the tibiofemoral vertical compressive loads involved in leg press or squatting exercises.

In general, studies have found that high-intensity resistance training promotes force-generating capabilities in aged muscle[43] and that resistance training enhances muscle hypertrophy in elderly people.[13,31] One study[27] comprising a very small population of very old (89- to 90-year-old) men and women showed the beneficial effects of isotonic resistance exercise for this age group. When the study subjects trained for 8 weeks, three times per week, the force-generating capacity of the trained muscles increased 174% ± 31%. The muscle mass of this group increased 9% ± 4.5%. In addition, two subjects improved in ambulation, no longer requiring the use of a cane. A hypothesis drawn from these findings suggests that increased force-generating capacity can be correlated with increased function.[39]

The previously outlined PRE protocols (DeLorme, Oxford, and Knight DAPRE protocols) may be inappropriate for disabled elderly persons. However, modifications of these programs have provided some guidance in developing strength programs for elderly adults.[39] Frontera and colleagues[31] stated, "The isotonic resistance protocol that produced the greatest increases in force-generation capacity and attenuated atrophy to the greatest extent in older human muscle was three sets of eight repetitions of exercise performed at an intensity of 80% of a muscle's 1 RM, 3 days a week for 12 weeks." Studies also supported the need to monitor heart rate, blood pressure, respirations, and subtle signs of distress closely during any exercise program for elderly persons.[39]

As with any resistance program to elicit strength, intensity of effort is the key element in the magnitude of functional or morphologic change in muscle tissue.[13,31] In the elderly population, intensity of effort must take into account age, history of cardiovascular or pulmonary disease, history of orthopedic pathologic conditions, present disease states, osteoarthritis, and multiple medical comorbidities.

General recommendations for strength training in older adults are as follows[4,51]:

- Get physician approval
- Initially, supervise closely
- Monitor vital signs
- Start with low resistance and low number of repetitions
- Progress by increasing repetitions, then by increasing small amounts of resistance
- Avoid high resistance to decrease stress on joints
- Train two to three times per week with 48-hour rest intervals
- Use a balance of flexion and extension exercises
- Use supported positions if a decrease in balance is noted

Strength Training for Younger Populations

A clear definition of the age range of this special population must be established at the outset to clarify and define the application of resistance exercise and the physiologic adaptation to the precise mode of training. *Prepubescent* and *child* are synonymous terms used to describe boys and girls before the onset of secondary sex characteristics.[34] The general range of prepubescence is 11 years for girls and 13 years for boys.[34] The terms *pubescent* and *adolescent* are synonymous descriptive terms for girls 12 to 18 years old and for boys 14 to 18 years old.[34]

In general, these definitions correspond to the classic Tanner stage classification system. Tanner stage I represents preadolescence or ages before the onset of secondary sex characteristics. Tanner stages II through IV describe various levels of development of secondary sex characteristics within adolescence. Tanner stage V is defined as adulthood.[34] Other definitions that must be clarified are strength, weight training, resistance training, and weightlifting. The terms *strength training, weight training,* and *resistance training* are used to describe submaximal PRE to improve strength, whereas weightlifting describes an attempt to lift maximum weight for a single repetition as a competitive sporting event. Examples are Olympic weightlifting (e.g., clean and jerk, snatch lift) and powerlifting (e.g., bench press, squat, dead lift). The appropriate terminology must be specific to denote the precise intent of the mode of exercise. The terms *PRE, weight training, resistance training,* and *strength training* are appropriate and practical in the context of orthopedic rehabilitation.

Physiologic Adaptations

Preadolescent children (Tanner stage I) do not possess circulating androgenic-anabolic hormones (testosterone) that act to stimulate hypertrophy, muscular strength, and secondary sex characteristics. Historically, this single irrefutable fact has led many researchers to state, "prepubertal boys do not significantly improve strength or increase muscle mass in a weight training program because of insufficient circulating androgens."[34] However, strength acquisition is complex and dependent on many factors, including hypertrophy, increases in muscle cross-sectional area, motor activation, central nervous system stimulation, genetic control, and psychological drive as well as circulation levels of endogenous hormones.[34]

Several leading researchers and scientists have identified that preadolescent children can significantly increase strength with appropriately applied resistance exercise protocols.[34] However, current evidence strongly suggests that neuromuscular activation, motor coordination, and intrinsic muscular adaptations contribute to preadolescent strength gains.[34] When investigating the effectiveness of nine studies supporting strength gains in children younger than 13 years, researchers found a 71.6% increase in strength versus a control group.[35]

Injury Risk

In nonpathologic conditions, PRE for preadolescent and adolescent children is safe and effective, provided that a few conditions are strictly followed. Also, the nature of the specific type of training is directly related to the risk of injury. Unsupervised weight training poses no greater risk for injury compared with other sports or recreational activities common to this age group.[34]

Injuries specific to this age group include disruption of the primary growth centers of ossification, the physeal plates. The secondary growth centers, the apophyses, are at risk of injury from traumatic and chronic traction at these sites.

Specific sites of injury occurring from nonsupervised weightlifting include the wrist, shoulder, elbows, lumbar spine, and knee. It is estimated that more than 17,000 injuries occur annually to adolescents participating in nonsupervised weightlifting or powerlifting.[34] Other researchers found no evidence of subclinical or clinical manifestations of musculoskeletal injury in prepubertal boys participating in 20 weeks of resistance training on the basis of bone scans and serum extraction of creatine phosphokinase (a marker of muscle damage).[34]

Well-supervised, submaximal resistance exercise with use of nonballistic, slow, controlled motions is effective and safe for preadolescent and adolescent children. The mechanism of physiologic adaptations of resistance exercise for this population is primarily a result of motor unit recruitment, motor control, and neuromuscular activation. Morphologic changes via hypertrophy do not play a role in strength development in preadolescent children.[34]

Relevant Clinical Applications

The specific therapeutic intervention of strength development in children follows a parallel progression of bone and soft tissue healing. Each contraction type (isometric, concentric, eccentric) is appropriately used during the defined stages of tissue healing (acute inflammatory, stage I; fibroplasia, stage II; and maturation, stage III), depending on radiographic confirmation of osseous union and stability as well as soft tissue healing constraints. In concert with specifically applied flexibility techniques (autogenic and reciprocal inhibition; see Chapter 4), strength acquisition in children using the foundation of

BOX 5-3 American Academy of Pediatrics Recommendations for Strength Training

- A medical evaluation by a pediatrician is needed before starting a strength training program.
- Children should be able to complete 8 to 15 repetitions in a set. The greatest benefits and smallest risks occur when 8 to 15 repetitions can be performed with a given weight before adding weight in small increments.
- The goal is not lifting as much as the child can. Instead, children can slowly begin adding weight in small increments as they are able to finish their sets easily.
- Be sure to include a warmup and cooldown with all workouts.
- Aerobic conditioning and all major muscle groups should be included in the strength training program.
- Workouts should last about 20 to 30 minutes and be done two to four times a week.
- Ensure that children are well supervised as they start lifting weights, especially if they are lifting at home and are not supervised by a trainer at school or a gym.

Adapted from the American Academy of Pediatrics. Strength training by children and adolescents. *Pediatrics.* 2008;121:835-840.

therapeutic exercise parameters—frequency, intensity, duration, muscle contraction type, degree of resistance, number of repetitions, number of sets, length of rest between sets, speed of contraction, and order of exercise—and a clearly defined model of exercise progression (see Davies model of exercise progression), preadolescent children can be expected to develop strength primarily by neurogenic activation.

Although the American Academy of Pediatrics does not approve weightlifting, powerlifting, and bodybuilding, it does approve of strength training programs for children and teens. Training may use free weights, the individual's own body weight, machines, or other resistance devices to attain this goal (Box 5-3).

THERAPEUTIC EXERCISE EQUIPMENT USED IN STRENGTH TRAINING

The most commonly used strength training tools are ankle or cuff weights. These extremely versatile pieces of equipment are easily adapted to many programs, body parts, and age groups. TheraBand, surgical tubing, or latex rubber bands are popular, inexpensive, highly adaptable, very portable (for home use), and effective tools. They allow for diagonal patterns of resistance and patterns involving a single plane. Some manufacturers have added handles to ends of thick rubber cords to enhance the versatility of this equipment.

Dumbbells also are used extensively in physical therapy. Inexpensive, portable, and versatile, dumbbells also can be used to develop excellent ROM and unilateral or bilateral motions. Barbells also can be used but are cumbersome. Barbells are effective in sports medicine practices where young athletes should develop overall strength and fitness, but they are not generally used in acute rehabilitation environments or hospital physical therapy departments.

Wall pulleys or cable column systems are used in most rehabilitation departments. The amount of resistance used with pulleys can vary from a few pounds to more than 100 pounds. Cable columns are extremely useful for upper extremity and lower extremity strength training and can be used for many age groups and conditions. They also allow for use of diagonal movements such as those used in proprioceptive neuromuscular facilitation.

There are many commercially available isotonic exercise systems.* Generally, isotonic exercise machines are fairly adaptable, provide a wide range of resistance (5 to 500 pounds for some leg machines), and are mechanically adjustable to accommodate different body types. Individual pieces can be expensive (≥$3000 for a single leg press machine), and a full system may cost $30,000 or more. Various types of muscle contractions can be used with isotonic exercise machines, including concentric and eccentric contractions, isometric static holds, and unilateral or bilateral movements; these exercises can be done using a wide degree of contraction velocities. As discussed, 1 RM testing can be performed on isotonic systems.

Space availability also is a consideration when one acquires exercise equipment. Although the footprint of many of these machines is small, a space of several hundred square feet to a few thousand feet may be needed for complete systems. Most of these systems use weight stacks, cables, straps, cams, and chains, but some use pneumatic (air), hydraulic, or electromagnetic resistance.

Isokinetic exercise systems are used extensively in physical therapy practices for testing, documentation, medicolegal presentations, rehabilitation, and velocity spectrum training. These systems generally are very expensive, with a single multijoint system costing $40,000 or more.†

These systems are extremely adaptable to most major body parts (knee, ankle, hip, wrist, elbow, shoulder, and back attachments are available with most systems), and therapeutically these systems are perhaps the most versatile of all strength training tools. Protocols and training modes that are generally available with most isokinetic systems are as follows:

- Passive
  - Continuous passive motion
  - Active assistive ROM
- Isometric
  - Multiple-angle isometrics
- Isotonic: Types of contraction modes
  - Concentric/eccentric
  - Concentric/concentric
  - Eccentric/concentric
  - Eccentric/eccentric
- Isokinetic: Types of contraction modes
  - Concentric/eccentric
  - Concentric/concentric
  - Eccentric/concentric
  - Eccentric/eccentric

*Popular systems include the Universal, Paramount, Nautilus, Body Masters, and Cybex systems.

†Popular multijoint systems are the Cybex, Lido, Kin-Com, Biodex, Isotechnologies, and Ariel systems.

BOX 5-4 Example of Knee Rehabilitation: Protocol Versatility Using Isokinetic Technology

To Gain Knee Motion
- Continuous passive motion

To Initiate Muscle Contractions
- Use isometric mode; progress to multiple-angle isometric, from 0° to 120° of knee motion at 20° increments

To Progress Strength
- Use isotonic modes—for example, knee extension (concentric)
- Quadriceps followed by knee flexion (eccentric)
- Quadriceps from 60°/sec to 180°/sec (five sets: 60°, 90°, 120°, 150°, and 180°)

Progress to Isokinetics
- Knee extension (concentric)
- Quadriceps followed by concentric hamstrings velocity spectrum training (eight sets: 30°, 60°, 90°, 120°, 150°, 180°, 210°, and 240°)

BOX 5-5 Application for Inertial Training

Conditions	Indications
Submaximal plyometrics	Painful arc remediation
Neuromuscular training	Mechanical, reproducible joint pain
Training of tendon tissue	Capsular afferents and coordination
Alteration of electromechanical delay	Proposed prevention of bone loss
Physiologic crossover effects	

From Albert M: *Eccentric muscle training in sports and orthopaedics,* New York, 1991, Churchill Livingstone.

Isokinetic systems typically function from 0°/sec to 350°/sec to 400°/sec. These systems are designed to isolate, test, and rehabilitate single joints. It is very time-consuming to change from one leg to another or from one joint (knee) to another (ankle). The versatility of these systems is demonstrated in Box 5-4.

The impulse inertial exercise apparatus is a system used for submaximal plyometric training. The impulse system provides limited ROM (by design), high-velocity, low-intensity, concentric, and eccentric loading. The application of inertial exercise involves rapid, coordinated, cyclic, and dynamic motions with reduced loads or resistance. The impulse system can be used for upper and lower extremity exercise. Extremely adaptive components with various handles allow for the duplication of sports such as tennis, racquetball, and golf. Clinically, this system is used mainly for neuromuscular coordination and strength in limited degrees of motion. The clinical delivery of inertial exercise is demonstrated in Box 5-5.[3]

GLOSSARY

Actin: A thin protein that, with myosin, is actively involved with the mechanics of muscular contraction.

Atrophy: Shrinking or wasting of muscle fiber size as a result of lack of use or disease.

Closed kinetic chain (CKC) exercise: Exercise performed while the distal portion of the exercising segment is weight bearing or fixed.

Concentric: A type of contraction in which tension is produced and shortening of the muscle takes place.

Delayed onset muscle soreness (DOMS): Muscle soreness that is secondary to exercise, characterized by increasing pain or discomfort during the subsequent 24 to 72 hours that subsides within a few days.

Eccentric: A type of contraction in which tension is produced and lengthening of the muscle takes place.

Endomysium: A noncontractile connective tissue that surrounds each individual muscle fiber.

Epimysium: Noncontractile connective tissue that surrounds the body of an individual muscle.

Fasciculi: Bundles of fibers within the muscle that are surrounded by perimysium.

Fast-twitch (FT) (type II, white glycolytic) muscle fibers: Anaerobic muscle fibers that contract at a higher speed than type I fibers and with more force; mainly used in activities that require speed, strength, and power.

Hypertrophy: The compensatory increase in individual muscle fiber size as a result of increases in and synthesis of the contractile proteins actin and myosin.

Isometric: A type of contraction in which tension is produced, but no joint movement or action takes place.

Myofibrils: Threadlike fibrils within muscle fibers that are composed of myofilaments.

Myosin: A thick protein that, with actin, is actively involved with the mechanics of muscular contraction.

Open kinetic chain (OKC) exercise: Exercise performed while the distal segment moves freely in space.

Perimysium: A noncontractile connective tissue that surrounds the fasciculi.

Plyometrics: A system of exercising that uses the stretch reflex to develop muscle contraction speed.

Power: The time rate of doing work: Power = Work/Time.

Progressive resistance exercise (PRE): The practical application of the overload principle to improve muscular strength and size; resistance is gradually and continually increased to keep pace with strength gains as training progresses.

Specific adaptations to imposed demands (SAID) principle: A principle that in part defines specific adaptations and alterations in response to highly specific demands.

Slow-twitch (ST) (type I, red oxidative) muscle fibers: Aerobic muscle fibers that have relatively low myosin-ATPase and glycolytic activity and slower calcium handling ability and shortening speed; specialized for muscular endurance activities.

Strength: The ability of a muscle to generate force; the maximum force generated by a single muscle or related muscle group.

Tension: The condition of a muscle being stretched or strained.

Work: The result or product of a force exerted on an object and the distance the object moves: Work = Force × Distance.

REFERENCES

1. Abraham WM: Factors in delayed muscle soreness. *Med Sci Sports Exer* 9:11, 1977.
2. Abraham WM: Exercise induced muscle soreness. *Phys Sports Med* 7:57, 1979.
3. Albert M: *Eccentric muscle training in sports and orthopaedics*, New York, 1991, Churchill Livingstone.
4. American College of Sports Medicine: *ACSM's guidelines for exercise testing and prescription*, ed 8, Baltimore, 2009, Lippincott Williams & Wilkins.
5. American Physical Therapy Association: *Guide to physical therapy practice*, ed 2, Alexandria, VA, 2003, American Physical Therapy Association.
6. Baechle TR, Earle RW: *Essentials of strength training and conditioning*, ed 2, Champaign, IL, 2000, Human Kinetics.
7. Bakhtiary AH, Safavi-Farokhi Z, Aminian-Far A: Influence of vibration on delayed onset of muscle soreness following eccentric exercise. *Br J Sports Med* 41:145, 2007.
8. Belka D: Comparison of dynamic, static, and combination training on dominant wrist flexor muscles. *Res Q* 39:244, 1968.
9. Berger RA: Optimum repetitions for the development of strength. *Res Q Exerc Sport* 33:334–338, 1962.
10. Brinkman JR, et al: Rate and range of knee motion in ambulation. *Phys Ther* 62:632, 1982.
11. Byrnes WC, et al: Delayed onset muscle soreness following repeated bouts of downhill running. *J Appl Physiol* 59:7109, 1985.
12. Caplan A, et al: Skeletal muscle. In Woo SL-Y, Buckwalter J, editors: *Injury and repair of the musculoskeletal soft tissues*, Rosemont, IL, 1988, American Academy of Orthopaedic Surgeons.
13. Charette SL, et al: Muscle hypertrophy response to resistance training in older women. *J Appl Physiol* 70:1912–1916, 1991.
14. Chu DA: Rehabilitation of the lower extremity. *Clin Sports Med* 14:205–222, 1995.
15. Clarke HH: Improvements of objective strength tests of muscle groups by cable tension methods. *Res Q* 21:399, 1950.
16. Clarke HH, et al: New objective strength tests of muscle groups by cable tension methods. *Res Q* 23:136, 1952.
17. Conroy BP, Earle RW: Bone, muscle and connective tissue adaptations to physical activity. In Baechle TR, editor: *Essentials of strength training and conditioning*, Champaign, IL, 1994, Human Kinetics.
18. Cordova M, Armstrong C: Reliability of ground reaction forces during a vertical jump: implications for functional strength assessment. *J Athl Train* 31:342–345, 1996.
19. Davies GJ: *A compendium of isokinetics in clinical usage and rehabilitation techniques*, ed 3, Onalaska, WI, 1987, S & S Publishers.
20. Davies GJ: *Course notes. Open and closed kinetic chain exercises and their application to testing and rehabilitation: advances on the knee and shoulder*, Cincinnati, 1993, Cincinnati Sports Medicine and Orthopaedic Center.
21. DeLee J: Therapeutic exercise modalities. In DeLee JC, Drez D, Jr, Miller MD, editors: *Orthopaedic sports medicine*, Philadelphia, 1989, Mosby.
22. DeLorme TL, Watkins A: *Progressive resistance exercise*, New York, 1951, Appleton-Century.
23. Elftman H: Biomechanics of muscle. *J Bone Joint Surg* 48:363, 1966.
24. Evans WJ: Exercise training guidelines for the elderly. *Med Sci Sports Exerc* 31:12–17, 1999.
25. Faulkner JA: New perspectives in training for maximum performance. *JAMA* 205:741–746, 1986.
26. Fedorko BF: *The effects of continuous compression as a therapeutic intervention on delayed onset muscle soreness following eccentric exercise*, University of Pittsburgh, 2007. PhD (dissertation).
27. Fiatarone MA, et al: High intensity strength training in nonagenarians: effects on skeletal muscle. *JAMA* 263:3029–3034, 1990.
28. Fraleigh J: Strength training: not just for the young. *Montvale* 71:41, 2008.
29. Francis KT: Delayed muscle soreness: a review. *J Orthop Sports Phys Ther* 5:10, 1983.
30. Friden J, Sjostrom M, Ekblom B: Myofibrillar damage following intensive eccentric exercise in man. *Int J Sport Med* 4:170–176, 1983.
31. Frontera WR, et al: Strength conditioning in older men: skeletal muscle hypertrophy and improved function. *J Appl Physiol* 64:1038–1044, 1988.
32. Gollnick PD: Fiber number and size in overloaded chicken anterior latissimus dorsi muscle. *J Appl Physiol* 54:1292, 1983.
33. Gonyea W, Ericson GC, Bonde-Peterson F: Skeletal muscle fiber splitting induced by weight-lifting exercise in cats. *Acta Physiol Scand* 99:105–109, 1977.
34. Guy JA, Michel LJ: Strength training for children and adolescents. *J Am Acad Orthop Surg* 9:26–31, 2001.
35. Hakkinen K, Komi PV: Effect of different combined concentric and eccentric muscle work regimes on maximal strength development. *J Hum Mov Stud* 7:33, 1981.
36. Harman E: Strength and power: a definition of terms. *J Strength Cond Res* 15:18–20, 1993.
37. Henneman E, Somjen G, Carpenter DO: Excitability and inhibitability of motoneurons of different sizes. *J Neurophysiol* 28:599–620, 1965.
38. Henwood TR, Taaffe DR: Detraining and retraining on older adults following long-term muscle power or muscle strength specific training. *J Gerontol A Biol Sci Med* 63:751–758, 2008.
39. Hopp JF: Effects of age and resistance training on skeletal muscle: a review. *Phys Ther* 73:361–373, 1993.
40. Jzankoff SP, Norris AH: Effect of muscle mass decreases on age-related BMR changes. *J Appl Physiol* 43:1001–1006, 1977.
41. Kellis E, Baltzopoulos V: Isokinetic eccentric exercise. *Sports Med* 19:202–222, 1995.
42. Kisner C, Colby LA: *Therapeutic exercise: foundations and techniques*, ed 5, Philadelphia, 2002, Davis.
43. Klitgaard H, et al: Function, morphology and protein expression of aging skeletal muscle: a cross-sectional study of elderly men with different training backgrounds. *Acta Physiol Scand Suppl* 140:41–54, 1990.
44. Knapik JJ, et al: Angular specificity and test mode specificity of isometric and isokinetic strength training. *J Orthop Sports Phys Ther* 5:58–65, 1983.
45. Knight KL: Quadriceps strengthening with the DAPRE technique: case studies with neurological implications. *Med Sci Sport Exerc* 17:646–650, 1985.
46. Knuttgen H, Kramer W: Terminology and measurement in exercise performance. *J Appl Sports Sci Res* 1:1–10, 1987.
47. Kruger J, Carlson S, Kohl H, III: Trends in strength training: United States, 1998-2004. *Morb Mortal Wkly Rep* 55:769–772, 2006.
48. Kuta I, Parizkova J, Dycka J: Muscle strength and lean body mass in old men of different physical activity. *J Appl Physiol* 29:168–171, 1970.
49. Mangine R, Heckman TP, Eldridge VL: Improving strength, endurance and power. In Scully RM, Barnes MR, editors: *Physical therapy*, Philadelphia, 1989, Lippincott.
50. McAllister RM, Amann JF, Laughlin MH: Skeletal muscle fiber types and their vascular support. *J Reconstr Microsurg* 9:313–317, 1993.
51. McArdle WD, Katch VL: *Exercise physiology: energy, nutrition, and human performance*, ed 5, Baltimore, 2002, Lippincott Williams & Wilkins.
52. McCartney N, et al: Long-term resistance training in the elderly: effects on dynamic strength, exercise capacity, muscle, and bone. *J Gerontol Appl Biol Sci Med Sci* 50:97–104, 1995.
53. Miles MP, Clarkson PM: Exercise-induced muscle pain, soreness, and cramps. *J Sports Med Phys Fitness* 34:203–216, 1994.
54. Newham DJ, et al: Pain and fatigue after concentric and eccentric muscle contractions. *Clin Sci* 64:55, 1983.
55. Newham DJ, et al: Ultrastructural changes after concentric and eccentric contractions of human muscle. *J Neurol Sci* 61:109–122, 1983.
56. Norkin CC, Levangie PK: *Joint structure and function: a comprehensive analysis*, ed 2, Philadelphia, 1992, Davis.

57. Nyland J, et al: Review of the afferent neural system of the knee and its contribution to motor learning. *J Orthop Sports Phys Ther* 19:2–11, 1994.
58. Page P: Pathophysiology of acute exercise induced muscular injury: clinical implications. *J Athl Train* 30:29–34, 1995.
59. Palmieri G: Weight training and repetition speed. *J Appl Sport Sci Res* 1:36–38, 1987.
60. Reese NB: *Muscle and Sensory Testing*, ed 2, St Louis, 2005, Saunders.
61. Rothstein JM, Lamb RL, Mayhew TP: Clinical uses of isokinetic measurements: critical issues. *Phys Ther* 67:1840, 1988.
62. Schmitt WH, Cuthbert SC: Common errors and clinical guidelines for manual muscle testing: "the arm test" and other inaccurate procedures. *Chiropr Osteopat* 16:1746, 2008.
63. Schwane J, et al: Blood markers of delayed onset muscle soreness with downhill treadmill running. *Med Sci Sports Exerc* 13:80, 1981.
64. Seguin R, Nelson ME: The benefits of strength training for older adults. *Am J Prev Med* 25(Suppl 2):141–149, 2003.
65. Sellwood KL, Brukner P, Williams D, et al: Ice-water immersion and delayed-onset muscle soreness: a randomised controlled trial. *Br J Sports Med* 41:392, 2007.
66. Smith LL, et al: Impact of a repeated bout of eccentric exercise on muscular strength, muscle soreness and creatine kinase. *Br J Sports Med* 28:267–271, 1994.
67. Soderberg G: *Kinesiology: Application to Pathological Motion*, Baltimore, 1986, Williams & Wilkins.
68. Sports Injury Bulletin: DOMS treatment: a review of the current strategies for treating DOMS (website). http://www.sportsinjurybulletin.com/archive/doms-treatment.html#.
69. Stauber WT: Eccentric action of muscles: physiology, injury and adaptation. *Exerc Sport Sci Rev* 19:157, 1989.
70. Steadman JR: Rehabilitation of athletic injury. *Am J Sports Med* 7:147, 1979.
71. Stone M: Literature review: explosive exercise and training. *J Strength Cond Res* 15:6–19, 1993.
72. Stone MH, et al: Periodization. *NSCA J Part I reprinted* 15(1):29, 1993.
73. Talag TS: Residual muscular soreness as influenced by concentric, eccentric and static contractions. *Res Q Exerc Sport* 44:458, 1973.
74. Talmadge RJ, Roy RR, Edgerton VR: Muscle fiber types and function. *Curr Opin Rheumatol* 5:695–705, 1993.
75. Thompson LV: Aging muscle: characteristics and strength training. *Issues Aging* 18:25–30, 1995.
76. Waltrous B, Armstrong R, Schwane J: The role of lactic acid in delayed onset muscular distress. *Med Sci Sports Exerc* 13:80, 1981.
77. Wilk KE, et al: Stretch-shortening drills for the upper extremities: theory and clinical application. *J Orthop Sports Phys Ther* 17:225–239, 1993.
78. Wyatt MP, Edwards AM: Comparison of quadriceps and hamstring torque values during isokinetic exercise. *J Orthop Sports Phys Ther* 3:48–56, 1981.
79. Zinowieff AN: Heavy resistance exercise: the Oxford technique. *Br J Phys Med* 14:129, 1951.

REVIEW QUESTIONS

Multiple Choice

1. Which muscle fiber type is highly oxidative and is fatigue resistant?
   a. Type I
   b. Type II
   c. Type IIA
   d. Type IIB
2. The body of an individual muscle is surrounded by which connective tissue?
   a. Perimysium
   b. Epimysium
   c. Fasciculi
   d. Endomysium
3. Muscle fasciculi are surrounded by which connective tissue?
   a. Perimysium
   b. Epimysium
   c. Endomysium
   d. Exomysium
4. In which muscle contraction type does the muscle shorten while tension is being produced?
   a. Concentric
   b. Isometric
   c. Eccentric
   d. None of the above
5. Which of the following is a way in which muscle strength can be measured?
   a. MMT
   b. Cable tensiometry
   c. Dynamometry
   d. All of the above
6. In which grade of MMT can the patient complete a full ROM against gravity and hold end position against mild resistance?
   a. 5
   b. 4
   c. 3
   d. 2
7. In which grade of MMT does the patient have full ROM in the gravity-eliminated position only?
   a. 5
   b. 4
   c. 3
   d. 2
8. Which form of muscle contraction is the most energy efficient and produces the greatest amount of tension per contractile unit?
   a. Concentric
   b. Isometric
   c. Eccentric
   d. Isokinetic
9. A training goal to increase muscle strength would require the use of which load as a percentage of a patient's 1 RM?
   a. 85
   b. 80 to 90
   c. 67 to 85
   d. 67
10. A training goal to increase muscle endurance would require the use of which load as a percentage of a patient's 1 RM?
    a. 85
    b. 80 to 90
    c. 67 to 85
    d. 67
11. Which exercise program calls for an arbitrary increase in resistance each week allowing for a gradual progression during each exercise session?
    a. Oxford
    b. DeLorme
    c. DAPRE
    d. None of the above

12. In which system of kinetic chain linkage does the entire system produce predictable patterns of movement in all other joints?
    a. Open kinetic chain
    b. Closed kinetic chain
13. Which of the following statements regarding resistance training for older adults is true?
    a. There is a minimal need for supervision.
    b. Physician approval is needed.
    c. Start with high resistance and high repetitions for best results.
    d. Progress by increasing resistance first and then repetitions.
14. Which of the following are considered contractile tissues?
    a. Epimysium
    b. Perimysium
    c. Actin and myosin
    d. Endomysium
15. Which of the following is not a symptom of DOMS?
    a. Pain
    b. Swelling
    c. Ecchymosis
    d. Tenderness

Short Answer

16. Organize the following five muscle fiber types into a numeric sequence of recruitment, proceeding from the lowest force requirements (1) to the greatest (5):
    ____ Fast-twitch (type II)
    ____ Fast-twitch (type IIAB)
    ____ Slow-twitch (type I)
    ____ Fast-twitch (type IIA)
    ____ Fast-twitch (type IIB)
17. Organize the following muscle contraction types in orderly sequence from greatest (3) to least (1) use of ATP:
    ____ Eccentrics
    ____ Concentrics
    ____ Isometrics
18. Organize the following muscle contraction types in orderly sequence from greatest (3) to least (1) force production:
    ____ Concentrics
    ____ Isometrics
    ____ Eccentrics
19. List the five ways muscular strength is measured.
20. A patient returns to the outpatient physical therapy department and reports localized, specific muscle pain and describes an isolated event of lifting a box, which immediately increased pain. Describe the appropriate course of action the PTA will take to manage this patient's complaints of increased pain.

Fill in the Blank

21. Aerobic exercises require muscle fibers that are primarily ________.
22. Exercise-induced muscle soreness is also known as ________.
23. Higher speeds of limb movement during resistance training require the resistance to be ________ than in a slower moving limb with greater resistance.
24. ________ is the ability of a muscle to generate maximum force.
25. An ________ contraction occurs when tension is produced in a muscle but no joint movement or action takes place.

True/False

26. The terms *isokinetic* and *isotonic* do not describe muscle contractions but rather are terms used to define and describe events using true muscle contractions.
27. Clinically it is important to choose one contraction type throughout the course of recovery from injury.
28. In terms of muscle hypertrophy, type I fibers hypertrophy more than type II fibers.
29. Stretching an innervated muscle creates tension, which results in muscle hypertrophy.
30. High-intensity strength training for elderly adults is not safe or effective and does not lead to improved function.

Chapter 6

Endurance

Jason Brumitt

CHAPTER OUTLINE

LEARNING OBJECTIVES

1. Recognize the differences between muscular and cardiovascular endurance.
2. Define activities and exercises that are aerobic or anaerobic.
3. Describe benefits associated with cardiovascular fitness training.
4. Compare moderate-intensity and vigorous-intensity exercises.
5. Describe methods to measure exercise intensity.
6. Describe the role of aerobic exercise for patients with an orthopedic injury.
7. Define the training parameters to improve muscular endurance.

KEY TERMS

Borg Rating of Perceived Exertion Scale
Cardiovascular endurance
Catabolism
Karvonen method
Maximal heart rate (MHR)
Maximal oxygen uptake ($\dot{V}O_2max$)
Muscular endurance
Oxidative system
Target heart rate (THR)

The ability to perform repetitive activities, participate in recreational pursuits, or compete in sports requires adequate endurance capacity. The performance of an endurance activity (or exercise) may require involvement from a person's muscular system, cardiovascular system, or both. **Muscular endurance** describes the ability of a muscle or muscles to perform at a particular level for a prolonged period of time. **Cardiovascular endurance** describes the ability of one's cardiovascular system to allow the performance of prolonged aerobic activities. Both the muscular and the cardiovascular systems require training to maintain or improve endurance capacity. In addition, training both systems helps to improve one's fitness level, reduces the risk of developing certain acute or chronic conditions, and helps restore function after injury. This chapter defines muscular and cardiovascular conditioning, reviews the metabolic pathways associated with each form of endurance training, discusses the physical and physiologic changes that occur when performing an endurance fitness program, presents the recommended minimum training requirements, and addresses the functional role of endurance training for the rehabilitation client.

CARDIOVASCULAR TRAINING

ENERGY METABOLISM FOR AEROBIC TRAINING

The **catabolism** of macronutrients (carbohydrates, proteins, and fats) creates energy for the human body. These fuel sources are ultimately converted into adenosine triphosphate (ATP), the main energy source for muscular function. Three metabolic pathways (Box 6-1) in the human body are responsible for the production of ATP. Energy metabolism may occur either with (aerobic metabolism) or without (anaerobic metabolism) the presence of oxygen.

Important Concepts

ATP is the main energy source for muscular function.

When an endurance-based activity is initiated, the initial production of ATP is supplied by the ATP–creatine phosphate (ATP-CP) and glycolysis systems. The ATP-CP system can provide enough ATP for only approximately 10 seconds of activity, and the glycolysis system can supply only up to an additional 2 minutes worth of ATP.

Continuation of an endurance-based activity requires the constant supply of oxygen for the body to continue to produce ATP.[2,11,25] The **oxidative system** produces approximately 19 times the ATP (38 to 39 ATP, depending on the fuel substrate) as produced by the phosphagen energy system (2 ATP).[11,25]

BENEFITS OF CARDIOVASCULAR FITNESS TRAINING

More than 60% of adults in the United States are considered overweight or obese.[17,21] Obesity is a leading risk factor for developing heart disease, diabetes, hypertension, and some cancers. Obesity may also contribute to the development of certain musculoskeletal injuries.[15] An individual with a chronic disease who initiates an aerobic exercise program may experience a decrease in the severity of symptoms associated with the disease. Likewise, participating in a regular aerobic fitness program may help to reduce the risk of developing a chronic disease.

Important Concepts

Participation in a regular exercise program has physical and physiologic benefits for clients. Initiation of an aerobic exercise program may help to decrease musculoskeletal pain, improve cardiorespiratory health, and reduce the risk of developing a chronic disease.

There are many positive physical and physiologic changes that occur when one participates in a cardiovascular fitness program. Individuals who participate in a cardiovascular fitness program have a lower risk of developing many chronic diseases, including cardiovascular disease, type 2 diabetes, and some cancers.[3,5,12,16,18,19,26,29,32,33]

BOX 6-1 Metabolic Pathways in the Human Body Responsible for the Production of Adenosine Triphosphate

- ATP-CP system
- Glycolysis
- Oxidative system

ATP-CP, adenosine triphosphate–creatine phosphate.

Additional training benefits associated with regular participation in an aerobic exercise program include reduction and control of one's weight, an increase in muscular strength, a reduction in the risk of falls, and a reduced mortality.[9,13]

The most notable physical and physiologic changes associated with regular participation in an aerobic exercise training program are the following[4,23,25]:

- Increased size and number of mitochondria
- Increased myoglobin content
- Increased heart weight and size
- Increased cardiac output and stroke volume
- Improved mobilization and use of fat and carbohydrates
- Selective hypertrophy of type I slow twitch oxidative muscle fibers
- Decreased resting heart rate and submaximal heart rate
- Decrease in adipose tissue
- Increased blood volume and hemoglobin
- Reduced systolic and diastolic blood pressure
- Significantly improved oxygen extraction rates from the blood

MINIMUM AEROBIC EXERCISE GUIDELINES FOR AMERICANS

The U.S. Centers for Disease Control and Prevention (CDC) has provided physical activity guidelines for children, adults, healthy pregnant or postpartum women, and older adults.[1,9] Table 6-1 presents the minimum aerobic exercise guidelines suggested to improve aerobic fitness.[1,9]

EXERCISE GUIDELINES FOR ADULTS

The minimum exercise guidelines for adults, older adults, and healthy pregnant or postpartum women are based on the volume of moderate-intensity or vigorous-intensity aerobic activity one performs.[9] The CDC has provided relative and absolute guidelines to help one appreciate the intensity of an exercise session.[9] The talk test may be used to determine the relative intensity of an exercise session.[9] If one is able to talk during exercise, the exercise is of moderate intensity. If one is unable to speak more than a few words before needing to pause for a breath, one is likely performing a vigorous-intensity exercise. The

TABLE 6-1 Minimum Weekly Aerobic Exercise Guidelines for Adults

Intensity Level	Adults	Older Adults (≥65 years old)	Healthy Pregnant or Postpartum Women
Moderate-intensity aerobic activity	2 hours and 30 minutes weekly	2 hours and 30 minutes weekly	2 hours and 30 minutes weekly
Vigorous-intensity aerobic activity	1 hour and 15 minutes weekly	1 hour and 15 minutes weekly	May continue vigorous-intensity activities, such as running, if these exercises were being performed before pregnancy.
Combination	Equal amount of moderate- and vigorous-intensity aerobic activity	Equal amount of moderate- and vigorous-intensity aerobic activity	NA

NA, not applicable.
From Centers for Disease Control and Prevention: *Physical activity for everyone* (website). www.cdc.gov/physicalactivity/everyone/guidelines/index.html. Accessed March 15, 2013.

absolute intensity guidelines are based on the amount of energy one typically uses during 1 minute of exercise.[9] Examples of moderate-intensity exercises include walking briskly, water aerobics, doubles tennis, and cycling at a pace less than 10 miles per hour.[9] Running, swimming laps, singles tennis, cycling faster than 10 miles per hour, and hiking are examples of vigorous-intensity exercises.[9]

Important Concepts

The talk test is an effective method to assess clinically the relative intensity of an exercise. The ability to talk during exercise suggests that the exercise is of moderate intensity, whereas the inability to talk without having to pause for breath suggests that the exercise is of vigorous intensity.

The CDC recommends that as an adult's fitness level improves, the adult should increase the level of moderate-intensity aerobic activity to 5 hours a week, or the level of vigorous-intensity aerobic activity to 2½ hours a week, or an equal mix of both types.[9]

Important Concepts

The CDC recommends adults should perform, at a minimum, 2½ hours of moderate-intensity exercise each week.

EXERCISE GUIDELINES FOR CHILDREN

The number of children and adolescents who are considered overweight or obese has at least doubled during the past 20 years.[21] More recent studies have demonstrated that an obese child has a greater likelihood of being an obese adult.[31] To combat pediatric obesity, children and adolescents need to participate in daily physical activity. A lack of physical education in many school districts limits the opportunities during the day for a child to exercise.[20]

The CDC recommends that children perform at least 60 minutes of moderate-intensity exercises each day.[9,30] In addition, children should perform vigorous-intensity exercises at least three times a week.[9] The physical therapy team may play a crucial role in educating a family about the importance of daily physical activity for a child as well as developing and implementing a fitness program for the child.[8]

Important Concepts

There has been an increase in childhood obesity. The CDC recommends children should perform at least 60 minutes of moderate-intensity exercise each day. This can be achieved via play, after-school programs, or supervised sports.

ADDITIONAL METHODS TO MEASURE EXERCISE INTENSITY

In a clinical exercise physiology setting, the efficiency of one's aerobic fitness may be determined by measuring the maximum volume of oxygen consumed during exercise. This measurement has been termed the **maximal oxygen uptake (Vo_2max)**.[2,11,25] Using this number, a clinician can prescribe a particular exercise intensity based on a percentage of the client's Vo_2max.

Most physical therapy clinics do not possess the equipment necessary to record a patient's Vo_2max. Several methods have been developed that allow clinicians to measure and prescribe a particular exercise intensity without needing "high-tech" equipment.

The talk test, described in the previous section, is one way to determine a client's aerobic exercise intensity. Two other methods used to measure aerobic intensity are the **target heart rate (THR)** and estimated **maximum heart rate (MHR)** method and the perceived exertion method.[9]

TARGET HEART RATE AND ESTIMATED MAXIMUM HEART RATE

The CDC recommends that an individual who is performing moderate-intensity exercise should do so at a THR range of 50% to 70% of one's maximum heart rate (beats per minute [bpm]).[9] When an individual performs vigorous-intensity exercise, the individual's THR should be 70% to 85% of the MHR.[9] How is the MHR measured? To calculate a client's MHR, his or her age is subtracted from 220 (e.g., 220 − 30). To establish the THR, the MHR is multiplied by the desired intensities. These two calculations (Table 6-2) provide the lower and upper limit THRs for someone who is performing moderate-intensity or vigorous-intensity exercises.[9]

Important Concepts

Aerobic intensity can be assessed by measuring heart rate in beats per minute. Moderate-intensity exercise is performed at 50% to 70% of one's MHR, and vigorous-intensity exercise is performed at 70% to 85% of one's MHR.

The **Karvonen method** has been suggested as an alternative method of calculating THR.[25] The Karvonen method differs from the aforementioned technique in that it accounts for one's resting heart rate. In the previous example (see Table 6-2), the THR for a 30-year-old individual performing moderate-intensity exercise is 95 to 113 bpm. If this individual has a resting heart rate of 70 bpm, the THR range would be 130 to 154 bpm (Table 6-3).

TABLE 6-2 Target Heart Rate Calculations for a 30-Year-Old Adult

	Moderate-Intensity Exercise	Vigorous-Intensity Exercise
Formula	MHR × (0.50) or (0.70)	MHR × (0.70) or (0.85)
Lower limit	(220 − 30) × 0.50 = 95 bpm	(220 − 30) × 0.70 = 113 bpm
Upper limit	(220 − 30) × 0.70 = 113 bpm	(220 − 30) × 0.85 = 162 bpm

MHR = 220 − age.
bpm, beats per minute; *MHR,* maximum heart rate.

TABLE 6-3 Target Heart Rate Calculations Using the Karvonen Method

	Moderate-Intensity Exercise
Formula	MHR (or HR_{max}) = 220 − 30 = 190
50% MHR	[(190 − 70) × 0.50] + 70 = 130
70% MHR	[(190 − 70) × 0.70] + 70 = 154

THR = [(HR_{max} − HR_{rest}) × % Intensity] + HR_{rest}.
HR_{rest}, resting heart rate; *HR_{max},* maximum heart rate; *MHR,* maximum heart rate; *THR,* target heart rate.

BORG RATING OF PERCEIVED EXERTION

The **Borg Rating of Perceived Exertion Scale** may be used to assess exercise intensity based on an individual's perception of exertion. While the client is exercising, the clinician asks him or her to rate how hard he or she is exercising based on the Borg scale. The Borg scale ranges from 6 to 20 points, with a 6 corresponding to "no exertion at all" and a 20 corresponding to "maximal exertion."[7] The client should be asked to view the scale each time when measuring perceived exertion. The Borg scale has also been found to correlate with heart rate.[6,7] This is a helpful feature allowing the clinician to monitor exercise intensity level based on an estimate of heart rate. To determine heart rate from the Borg scale, multiply the perceived rating (e.g., 13) by a factor of 10 (e.g., 130 bpm).

METHODS OF AEROBIC TRAINING

Aerobic conditioning programs are either continuous or discontinuous. Continuous aerobic activities provide no rest interval during the entire bout of exercise. Examples of continuous activities are jogging, walking, running, cycling, and stair climbing.

Important Concepts

Continuous aerobic activities are commonly prescribed in outpatient orthopedic physical therapy settings. The upper body ergometer (UBE) is used in rehabilitation of patients with upper extremity injuries. The stationary cycle, the recumbent bicycle, the elliptical machine, and the stair-climber are used to rehabilitate patients with lower extremity injuries.

Discontinuous aerobic activities are also known as *interval training activities.* A discontinuous aerobic exercise routine may include similar exercises used during continuous aerobic programs; however, during interval training, repeated exercise bouts are interspersed with rest intervals. Discontinuous training routines may be beneficial for patients who have limited exercise tolerance.

AEROBIC EXERCISE FOR PATIENTS WITH AN ORTHOPEDIC INJURY

Patients with an orthopedic injury will benefit from the inclusion of aerobic exercise as part of their rehabilitation program. The physical therapy team must consider tissue healing parameters when implementing an exercise. An acute injury or surgery may require a period of rest (or activity avoidance) to avoid additional injury or protect the surgical repair.

Evidence suggests that aerobic fitness activities should be included in a rehabilitation program for a patient recovering from a back injury.[27] Riding a stationary bicycle or walking on a treadmill (Fig. 6-1, *A, B*) may help to facilitate initial aerobic training. However, sitting on the saddle seat of a stationary ergometer may be uncomfortable or provoke symptoms for some patients with back pathology. A recumbent cycle, with its large bucket seat (Fig. 6-1, *C*) to provide lumbar support, may be preferred by many clients. Some postsurgical patients (e.g., a patient after total knee replacement) may also prefer to use a recumbent cycle because of the relative ease of getting on and off compared with an upright stationary cycle. Patients who are unable to tolerate land-based aerobic exercises may benefit from walking on an underwater treadmill. Immersion in the water can provide enough buoyancy during walking, unloading the spine, to allow the patient to exercise without exacerbating symptoms (Fig. 6-1, *D*).

Important Concepts

Patients with chronic low back pain may benefit from regular participation in an aerobic exercise program. The severity of a patient's symptoms guides the aerobic exercise prescription. For example, patients who experience pain when walking on land may benefit from participating in an aquatic exercise program.

Patients who have sustained a lower extremity injury or are recovering after surgery involving a lower extremity can maintain or improve cardiorespiratory fitness using the UBE (Fig. 6-2, *A*). The UBE is ideal for individuals for whom bearing weight or performing range of motion activities with their involved lower extremity is contraindicated. The single-leg stationary bicycle ergometer exercise (Fig. 6-2, *B*) may also be safely initiated by a patient before beginning double-leg cycling.

Important Concepts

The UBE is frequently prescribed to help rehabilitate patients with upper extremity injuries; however, patients with lower extremity injuries can also benefit from starting their aerobic training program with this machine. For example, physical therapists may initiate training on the UBE for a patient 1-week status post anterior cruciate ligament surgery. The patient likely would be unable to perform a full revolution on the stationary cycle with the postsurgical lower extremity but would be able to perform bilateral upper extremity revolutions with the UBE.

Older patients with hip, knee, or ankle osteoarthritis (degenerative joint disease) may also benefit from a training program using the UBE. The vertical compressive loads experienced during treadmill walking, stair climbing, or stationary cycling may cause or increase symptoms in these patients.

Patients with upper extremity conditions can use a stationary cycle or treadmill for endurance training. Patients also can be instructed to perform one-arm cycling

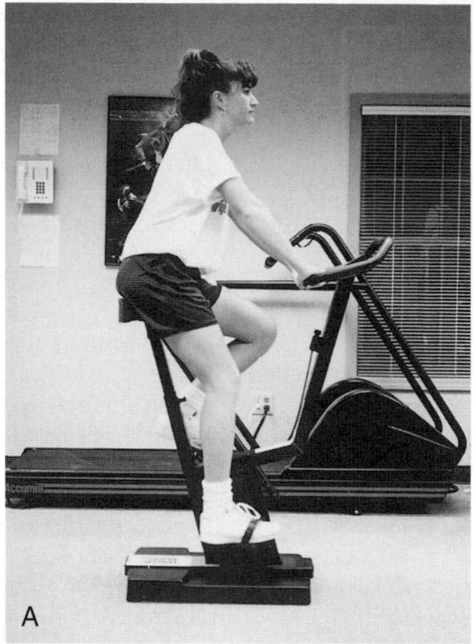

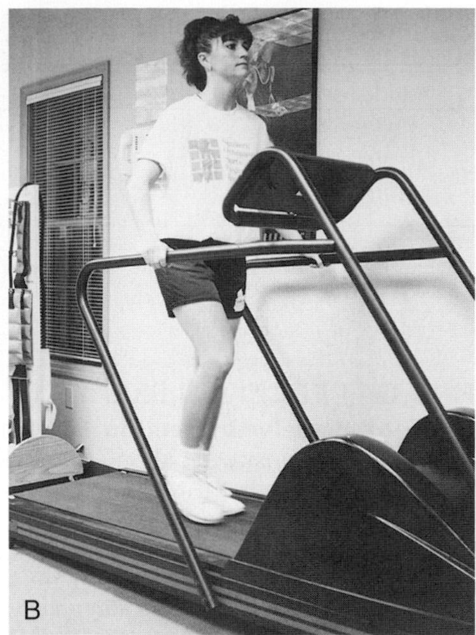

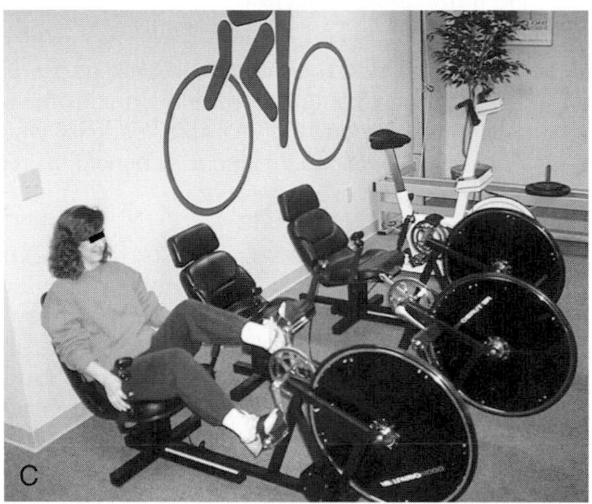

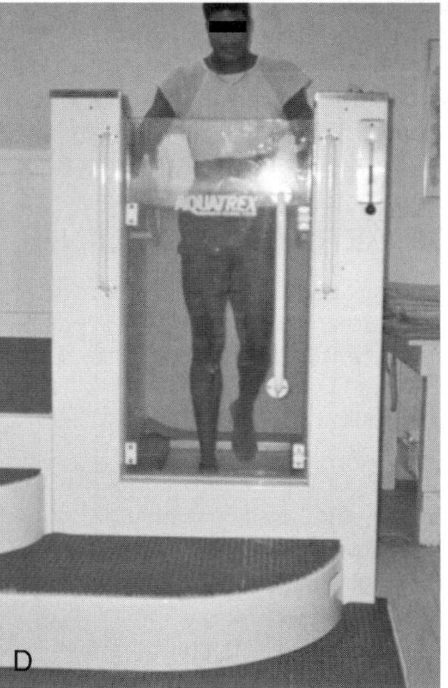

FIG 6-1 **A,** Seated stationary bicycle ergometer. **B,** Standard treadmill. **C,** Recumbent bicycle ergometer. The large bucket seat used in a recumbent position may allow some patients to tolerate seated aerobic activities. **D,** Underwater treadmill. The buoyancy of the water may allow early vertical loading and the initiation of normalized gait mechanics.

on the UBE (Fig. 6-3) to maintain aerobic fitness and develop upper extremity strength.

Modifications can be made on stationary cycles to allow for continued aerobic conditioning after an ankle injury or surgery. Typically, the seat height should allow for slight knee flexion (~10°) at the end of the pedal stroke. With the seat in normal position, the foot generally plantar flexes toward the end of the pedal stroke, causing strain to the anterior talofibular ligament. The seat height is lowered for a patient with a severe ankle sprain to allow for a complete pedal stroke and to keep the ankle joint in neutral (Fig. 6-4).

Stair climbing, seated rowing, and cross-country ski machines are popular aerobic tools but must be used judiciously. Stair climbers require the patient to be correctly positioned vertically and to maintain balance (holding the hand rails) to perform the exercise correctly. Stair climbers are inappropriate or unsafe for many patients during the acute stage of recovery or the period immediately after orthopedic surgery. Rowing machines require both a pulling motion with the arms and hip and knee flexion and extension. These simultaneous motions make modifications for use with specific orthopedic problems quite difficult. Cross-country ski machines require bilateral,

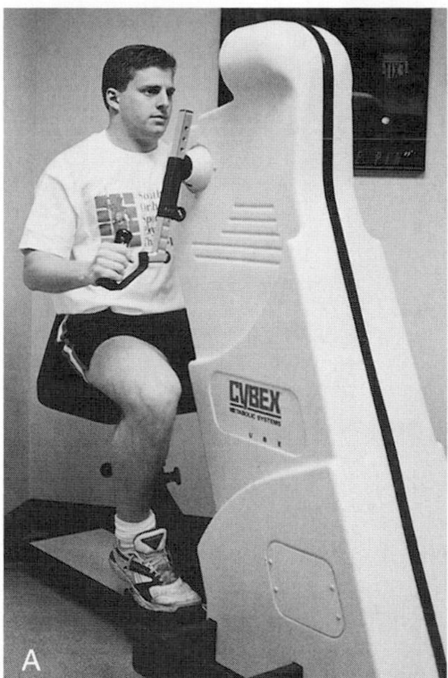

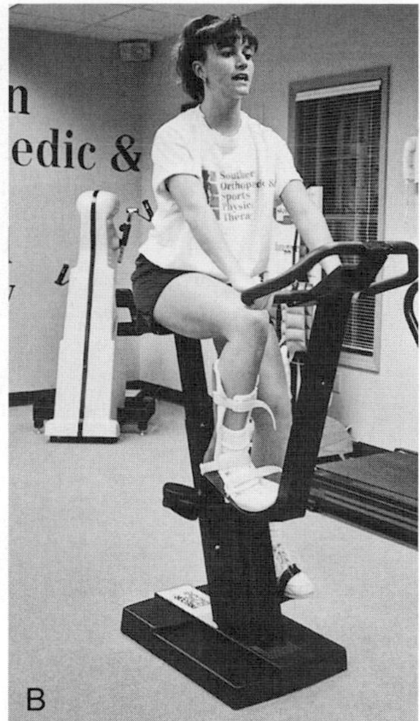

FIG 6-2 **A,** For patients with lower extremity injuries, an upper body ergometer allows continued aerobic activities during periods of immobilization. **B,** In some cases, a single-leg stationary cycle ergometer can be used for cardiovascular fitness during periods of immobilization.

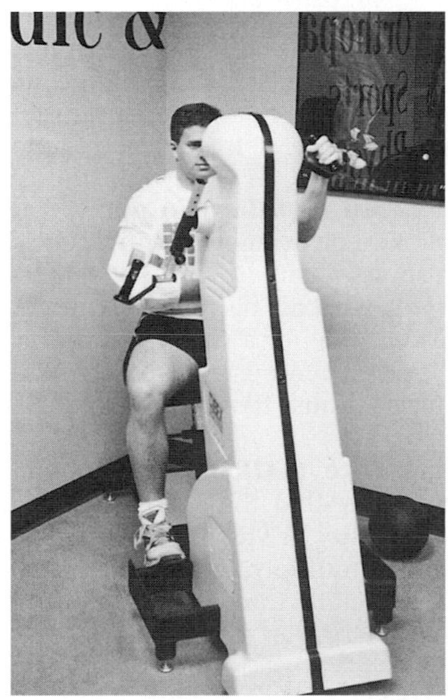

FIG 6-3 A one-arm, upper body cycling activity with an upper body ergometer is also an effective aerobic exercise activity.

reciprocal leg and arm motions and are difficult to modify for patients with acute orthopedic disorders. However, stair climbers, rowing machines, and cross-country ski machines can be effective tools in aerobic conditioning programs after the acute phase of recovery from injury or surgery.

MUSCULAR ENDURANCE TRAINING

Even though they share the term *endurance,* muscular endurance and cardiovascular endurance are not the same thing. One can demonstrate functional muscular endurance but not possess functional cardiovascular endurance. What is the difference? As mentioned earlier in the chapter, cardiovascular endurance involves the ability of one's cardiovascular system to perform an aerobic activity. For an activity to be considered aerobic, the oxidative energy system is used. Muscular endurance exercises typically use only the ATP-CP and glycolysis energy systems.

TABLE 6-4 Training Variables Associated with Training Goals

Training Goal	Repetitions Goal	Load (% of 1 RM)	Rest Interval between Sets (min)
Power	1-2	80-90	2-3
Strength	≤6	≥85	2-3
Hypertrophy	6-12	67-85	2-3
Endurance	≥15	≤67	1-2

RM, repetition maximum.

The key variables that define how a muscle is being trained are the number of repetitions performed during a set, the amount of weight lifted during the set, and the period of rest between sets. To increase muscular endurance, sets of high repetitions should be performed. At least 15 repetitions should be performed per set.[2,10] Each repetition should be performed at or below 67% of one's 1 RM (repetition maximum). A period of 1 to 2 minutes should be allowed for rest in between each set. Table 6-4 compares variables associated with the four main types of muscular training: power, strength, hypertrophy, and endurance.

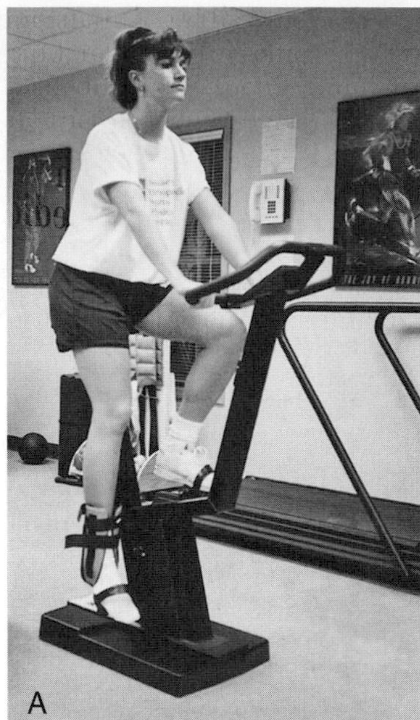

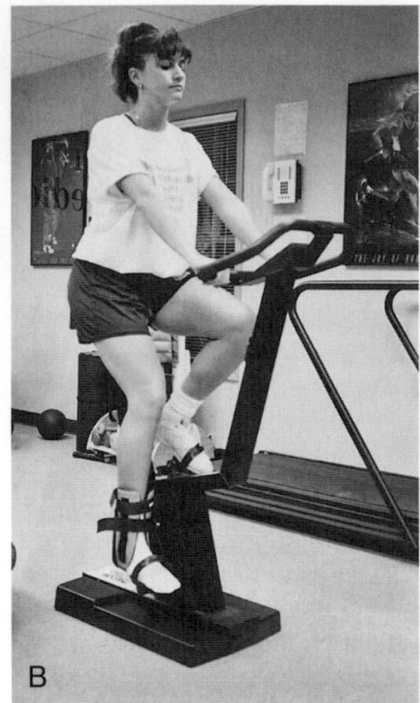

FIG 6-4 **A,** Normal seat elevation of a seated bicycle ergometer allows for greater plantar flexion motion. Plantar flexion may be contraindicated with acute and subacute sprains of the lateral ligament complex of the ankle. **B,** With the saddle seat lowered, the affected ankle can be maintained in a more appropriate neutral position during periods of aerobic activity on the cycle ergometer.

Important Concepts

To increase muscular endurance capacity, a patient should perform a minimum of 15 repetitions per set at 67% of one's 1 RM. Often it is not feasible or safe to assess the 1 RM of a rehabilitation patient. Physical therapists may initiate a patient's training program using low loads (e.g., 1 to 2 pounds) as long as the patient is able to perform repetitions without reproduction of symptoms. As a patient is able to perform the desired number of repetitions and sets successfully, weight is gradually progressed by 1 to 2 pounds.

Muscular endurance training plays a key role when rehabilitating patients with an orthopedic injury.[14,22,24,27,28] Using the muscular endurance training principles allows the physical therapy team to prescribe strengthening exercises during the subacute phase of healing (see Chapter 13), while reducing the risk of overstressing the healing tissue.

GLOSSARY

Borg Rating of Perceived Exertion Scale: A scale used to assess exercise intensity based on an individual's perception of exertion.

Cardiovascular endurance: The ability of one's cardiovascular system to allow the performance of prolonged aerobic activities.

Catabolism: A metabolic process that breaks down compounds, such as degradation of glucose to CO_2 and H_2O, causing the release of energy.

Karvonen method: An alternative (to the Borg scale) method of calculating target heart rate.

Maximal heart rate (MHR): The maximum number of beats per minute that the heart is able to pump. MHR is measured by subtracting the patient's age from 220.

Maximal oxygen uptake ($\dot{V}O_2max$): The maximum volume of oxygen consumed during exercise. This measurement shows a patient's level of aerobic fitness.

Muscular endurance: The ability of muscles to perform at a particular level for a prolonged period of time.

Oxidative system: An energy system known as the *aerobic system* because its operation requires a constant supply of O_2.

Target heart rate (THR): The optimum number of beats per minute that the heart should pump during moderate-intensity or vigorous-intensity exercise. THR is calculated by multiplying the patient's MHR by either 0.70 (for moderate intensity) or 0.85 (for vigorous intensity).

REFERENCES

1. American College of Sports Medicine Position Stand: The recommended quantity and quality of exercise for developing and maintaining cardiorespiratory and muscular fitness, and flexibility in healthy adults. *Med Sci Sports Exerc* 30(6):975–991, 1998.
2. Baechle TR, Earle RW, Wathen D: Resistance training. In Baechle TR, Earle RW, editors: *Essentials of strength training and conditioning*, ed 3, Champaign, IL, 2008, Human Kinetics.
3. Ballard-Barbash R, Hunsberger S, Alciati MH, et al: Physical activity, weight control, and breast cancer risk and survival: clinical trial rationale and design considerations. *J Natl Cancer Inst* 101(9):630–643, 2009.
4. Barnard RJ, Edgerton VR, Peter JB: Effects of exercise of skeletal muscle. I. Biochemical and histochemical properties. *J Appl Physiol* 28(6):762–766, 1970.
5. Blair SN, Morris JN: Healthy hearts—and the universal benefits of being physically active: physical activity and health. *Ann Epidemiol* 19(4):253–256, 2009.

6. Borg G: Psychophysical bases of perceived exertion. *Med Sci Sports Exerc* 14(5):377–381, 1982.
7. Borg G: *Borg's perceived exertion and pain scales*, Champaign, IL, 1998, Human Kinetics.
8. Brumitt J: The role of the certified strength and conditioning specialist in preventing childhood obesity. *Strength Cond J* 28(4):54–56, 2006.
9. Centers for Disease Control and Prevention: *Physical activity for everyone* (website). www.cdc.gov/physicalactivity/everyone/guidelines/index.html. Accessed March 15, 2013.
10. Cooper LW, Powell AP, Rasch J: Master's swimming: an example of successful aging in competitive sport. *Curr Sports Med Rep* 6(6):392–396, 2007.
11. Cramer JT: Bioenergetics of exercise and training. In Baechle TR, Earl RW, editors: *Essentials of strength training and conditioning*, ed 3, Champaign, IL, 2008, Human Kinetics.
12. Dalleck LC, Allen BA, Hanson BA, et al: Dose-response relationship between moderate-intensity exercise duration and coronary heart disease risk factors in postmenopausal women. *J Womens Health (Larchmt)* 18(1):105–113, 2009.
13. Donnelly JE, Blair SN, Jakicic JM, et al: American College of Sports Medicine position stand. Appropriate physical activity intervention strategies for weight loss and prevention of weight regain for adults. *Med Sci Sports Exerc* 41(2):459–471, 2009.
14. Durall CJ, Udermann BE, Johansen DR, et al: The effects of preseason trunk muscle training on low-back pain occurrence in women collegiate gymnasts. *J Strength Cond Res* 23(1):86–92, 2009.
15. Durstine JL, Moore GE: *ACSM's exercise management for persons with chronic diseases and disabilities*, ed 2, Champaign, IL, 2003, Human Kinetics.
16. Firestone B, Mold JW: Type 2 diabetes: which interventions best reduce absolute risks of adverse events? *J Fam Pract* 58(6):E1, 2009.
17. Flegal KM, Carroll MD, Ogden CL, et al: Prevalence and trends in obesity among US adults, 1999-2000. *JAMA* 288(14):1723–1727, 2002.
18. Giada F, Biffi A, Agostoni P, et al: Exercise prescription for the prevention and treatment of cardiovascular diseases: part II. *J Cardiovasc Med (Hagerstown)* 9(6):641–652, 2008.
19. Giada F, Biffi A, Agostoni P, et al: Joint Italian Societies' Task Force on Sports Cardiology. Exercise prescription for the prevention and treatment of cardiovascular diseases: part I. *J Cardiovasc Med (Hagerstown)* 9(5):529–544, 2008.
20. Grunbaum JA, Kann L, Kinchen S, et al: Youth risk behavior surveillance—United States, 2003. *Morb Mortal Wkly Rep* 53(SS–2):1–95, 2004.
21. Hedley AA, Ogden CL, Johnson CL, et al: Prevalence of overweight and obesity among U.S. children, adolescents, and adults. *JAMA* 291(23):2847–2850, 2004.
22. Kell RT, Asmundson GJ: A comparison of two forms of periodized exercise rehabilitation programs in the management of chronic nonspecific low-back pain. *J Strength Cond Res* 23(2):513–523, 2009.
23. Kiessling K: Effects of physical training on ultrastructural features in human skeletal muscle. In Pernow B, Saltin B, editors: *Muscle metabolism during exercise*, New York, 1971, Plenum Press.
24. Lorig KR, Sobel DS, Stewart AL, et al: Evidence suggesting that a chronic disease self-management program can improve health status while reducing hospitalization: a randomized trial. *Med Care* 37(1):5–14, 1999.
25. McArdle WD, Katch FI, Katch VL: *Exercise physiology. energy, nutrition, and human performance*, ed 4, Baltimore, 1996, Williams & Wilkins.
26. McGavock JM, Eves ND, Mandic S, et al: The role of exercise in the treatment of cardiovascular disease associated with type II diabetes mellitus. *Sports Med* 34(1):27–48, 2004.
27. McGill SM: *Low back disorders. Evidence-based prevention and rehabilitation*, ed 2, Champaign, IL, 2007, Human Kinetics.
28. Nikander R, Mälkiä E, Parkkari J, et al: Dose-response relationship of specific training to reduce chronic neck pain and disability. *Med Sci Sports Exerc* 38(12):2068–2074, 2006.
29. Sandrock M, Schulze C, Schmitz D, et al: Physical activity throughout life reduces the atherosclerotic wall process in the carotid artery. *Br J Sports Med* 42(10):539–544, 2008.
30. Strong WB, Malina RM, Blimkie JR, et al: Physical activity recommendations for school-age youth. *J Pediatr* 146:732–737, 2005.
31. Styne DM: Childhood and adolescent obesity. *Pediatr Clin North Am* 48:823–854, 2001.
32. Taylor RS, Brown A, Ebrahim S, et al: Exercise-based rehabilitation for patients with coronary heart disease: systematic review and meta-analysis of randomized controlled trials. *Am J Med* 116(10):682–692, 2004.
33. Thompson PD, Buchner D, Piña IL, et al: Exercise and physical activity in the prevention and treatment of atherosclerotic cardiovascular disease: a statement from the Council on Clinical Cardiology (Subcommittee on Exercise, Rehabilitation, and Prevention) and the Council on Nutrition, Physical Activity, and Metabolism (Subcommittee on Physical Activity). *Arterioscler Thromb Vasc Biol* 23:e42–e49, 2003.

REVIEW QUESTIONS

Multiple Choice

1. The ATP-CP system is capable of supplying enough ATP to last for approximately how many seconds of activity?
   a. 10
   b. 20
   c. 40
   d. 60
2. How many ATP are produced (per fuel substrate) by the oxidative system?
   a. 25
   b. 38
   c. 49
   d. 70
3. Obesity is a risk for all of the following medical conditions except:
   a. Musculoskeletal injuries.
   b. Heart disease.
   c. Hypertension.
   d. Influenza.
4. The CDC recommends that adults should perform a minimum of ___________ moderate-intensity aerobic activity *or* a minimum of ____________ vigorous-intensity aerobic activity per week.
   a. 2 hours, 1 hour
   b. 2 hours and 30 minutes, 1 hour
   c. 2 hours and 30 minutes, 1 hour and 15 minutes
   d. 3 hours, 2 hours
5. If one is able to talk during exercise, that exercise is considered to be of _________ intensity.
   a. Easy
   b. Moderate
   c. Vigorous
   d. Severe
6. All of the following are examples of moderate-intensity exercise except:
   a. Running.
   b. Water aerobics.
   c. Cycling.
   d. Doubles tennis.
7. The CDC recommends that children should perform how many minutes of moderate-intensity exercise at a minimum each day?
   a. 15
   b. 30

c. 45
d. 60

8. The THR when performing a vigorous-intensity exercise should be what percentage of one's MHR?
   a. 10% to 20%
   b. 50% to 70%
   c. 60% to 80%
   d. 70% to 85%
9. The ______ Rating of Perceived Exertion scale is used to assess exercise intensity based on one's perception of exertion.
   a. Karvonen
   b. Borg
   c. Davies
   d. Rauh
10. A 70-year-old patient with a recent total knee replacement (status post 3 weeks) has been referred to physical therapy to improve range of motion, increase strength, and improve cardiovascular fitness. Which of the following exercise machines would the physical therapist most likely have the patient start on to facilitate cardiovascular fitness training?
    a. Treadmill
    b. Elliptical
    c. Recumbent cycle
    d. Stairmaster
11. In general, the seat height on a stationary cycle should allow for approximately how many degrees of knee flexion at the end of the pedal stroke?
    a. 10
    b. 40
    c. 75
    d. 90
12. When developing a training program to facilitate muscular endurance capacity, a minimum of how many repetitions should be performed per set?
    a. 8
    b. 10
    c. 12
    d. 15
13. Which of the following exercises would not be performed for high repetitions?
    a. Side-lying external rotation for the shoulder
    b. Side plank
    c. Olympic lifts
    d. Crunches
14. During which stage of the healing process would high-repetition, low-load exercises first be prescribed?
    a. Acute
    b. Subacute
    c. Maturation
    d. Chronic
15. As a guide, when performing exercises to promote muscular endurance, each repetition should be performed at ____% of one's 1 RM.
    a. 50
    b. 67
    c. 80
    d. 85

Short Answer

16. According to the CDC, what is the minimum number of hours a week that an adult should perform moderate-intensity aerobic exercises?
17. Moderate-intensity exercise should be performed at what percentage (range) of one's MHR?
18. Calculate the MHR for a 40-year-old man.
19. A 25-year-old football player has fractured his right fibula. The orthopedic surgeon believes that he can return to competition in 3 to 4 weeks. At this moment, the football player is not allowed to bear weight on his right lower extremity. Which exercises would be most appropriate for him to maintain cardiovascular fitness?
20. How does the Karvonen method differ from the standard method of calculating target heart rate?

Fill in the Blank

21. The Borg scale has a range of numbers starting at _______ and ending at _______.
22. Discontinuous aerobic activities are also known as _______ activities.
23. To increase muscular endurance, sets of at least _______ repetitions should be performed at or below _______ percent of one's 1 repetition maximum.
24. The _______ is ideal for individuals who are contraindicated from either bearing weight or performing range of motion activities with their involved lower extremity.
25. Cardiovascular endurance describes the ability of one's cardiovascular system to allow the performance of prolonged _______.

True/False

26. Cardiovascular endurance and muscular endurance are the same thing.
27. A distance runner primarily uses the glycolytic pathway to produce ATP.
28. Vigorous-intensity exercise should be performed at 70% to 85% of one's MHR.
29. The UBE should be prescribed only to patients with upper extremity injuries.
30. An inability to talk during exercise suggests that the exercise is of moderate intensity.

Chapter 7

Balance and Coordination

Bryan Riemann

CHAPTER OUTLINE

LEARNING OBJECTIVES

1. Define and contrast balance and coordination.
2. Discuss the mechanoreceptor system and define four mechanoreceptors.
3. List static and dynamic balance and coordination tests and activities.
4. Define proprioception and kinesthetic awareness.
5. Discuss several factors that contribute to balance dysfunction.
6. Identify functional closed kinetic chain proprioceptive exercises.
7. Discuss the rationale for proprioceptive training for the upper extremity.

KEY TERMS

Balance
Base of support
Coordination
Golgi tendon organs
Mechanoreceptors
Muscle spindles
Neuromuscular control
Postural equilibrium
Proprioception

EXERCISE IN ORTHOPEDIC DISORDERS

Rehabilitation after an acute injury, surgery, immobilization, or chronic orthopedic condition must address all the components of normal function. Regaining lost strength, reducing pain and swelling, improving flexibility, enhancing local muscular endurance, and building cardiovascular fitness are vital areas requiring specific therapeutic interventions. Sometimes less apparent, but equally important, is the need to address the motor control and neuromuscular elements to promote synchronous, fluid, and stable motor function of the injured part within the context of the distal and proximal body parts. Secondary to the interdependence of coordination, posture, and balance in gait and functional movements, attention must also be directed to these elements for complete recovery from injury. Long-term convalescence reduces strength, flexibility, and cardiorespiratory fitness as well as the use of vestibular and afferent neural input needed for balance and coordination.

Important Concepts

Motor control and neuromuscular elements, both distally and proximal to the injured part, need to be addressed to promote synchronous, fluid, and stable motor function of the injured segment.

DEFINITIONS OF BALANCE, PROPRIOCEPTION, NEUROMUSCULAR CONTROL, AND COORDINATION

Balance is often defined as the ability to maintain the center of mass over the **base of support**.[11] However, this definition is appropriate only when the base of support is fixed, such as standing in a constant location on two feet. The base of support is defined as the area contained within the parts of the body making physical contact with the external environment (Fig. 7-1).[7] During dynamic situations, such as gait and functional activity, the base of support does not remain fixed to a constant location. Rather, as part of locomotion, the base of support moves, increasing the challenge to the elements responsible for maintaining balance. For this reason, the concept of balance also needs to include consideration of these circumstances.

Important Concepts

Destabilizing forces arising from gravity, perturbations, and voluntary movements all challenge the maintenance of the center of mass within the limits of stability.

Postural equilibrium is a broader term that refers to balancing all forces acting on the body's center of mass to maintain the center of mass within the limits of stability with optimal joint segment alignment.[9] Forces that

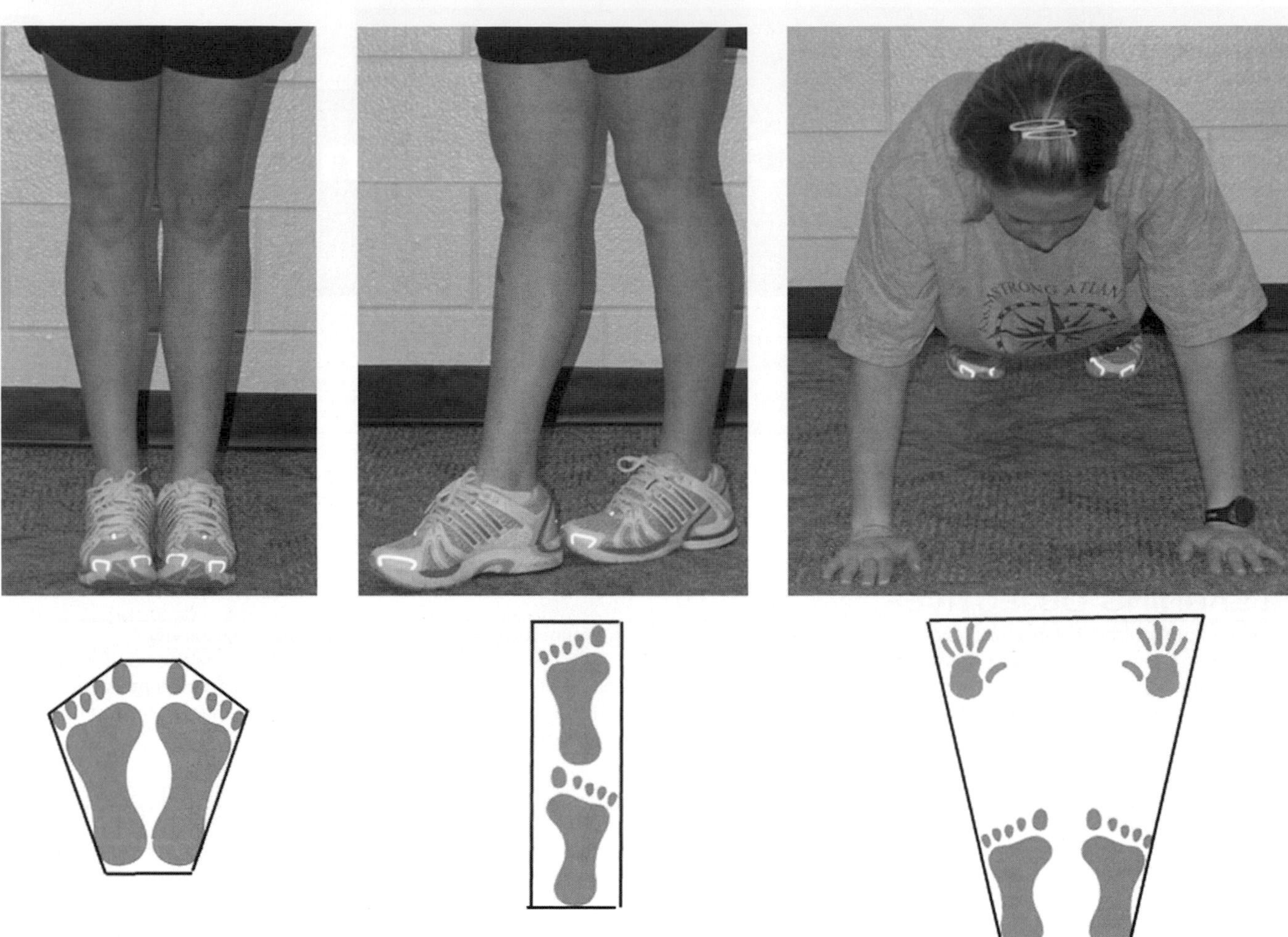

FIG 7-1 The base of support encompasses the perimeter around the feet, hands, or hands and feet making contact with the external environment.

challenge postural equilibrium arise from gravity, unexpected perturbations (i.e., stumbling over an unforeseen obstacle), or performance of voluntary motor activities (i.e., picking up a bag of groceries). Maintaining postural equilibrium is accomplished by the postural control system, the collection of sensory sources (somatosensory, vision, and vestibular), the central nervous system, and the musculoskeletal system. The somatosensory sources relevant to postural equilibrium are the mechanoreceptor populations located on the plantar surface of the foot and those residing in joint, muscle, connective, and ligamentous tissues. Because these tissues are often damaged during orthopedic injury, postural equilibrium may be disturbed after injury because of sensory disruptions, musculoskeletal disruptions, or both.[7] Performing motor tasks effectively and efficiently requires not only postural equilibrium, but also effective coordination of the many muscles serving to move and stabilize the joints on which they cross.

Important Concepts

Performing motor tasks effectively requires not only postural equilibrium but also effective coordination of the many muscles serving to move and stabilize the joints on which they cross.

Coordination has been defined as the ability to produce patterns of body and limb motions in the context of environmental objects and events.[14] For example, picking up an object from a table requires coordinating the shoulder, elbow, and wrist joints through all of the muscles acting on these joints to put the hand and fingers into position so that the object can be grasped. Essential to coordinating joint positions is sufficient sensory (afferent) information regarding joint position, movement (kinesthesia), and movement resistance/tension. The afferent information contributing to these three elements, joint position, movement (kinesthesia), and movement resistance/tension, is referred to as **proprioception**.[11] When the proprioception elements are consciously perceived, they are referred to as the conscious perceptions of proprioception.[11] Proprioception is vital for neuromuscular control. From a joint stability perspective, **neuromuscular control** refers to the subconscious activation of muscles occurring in preparation for and in response to joint motion and loading.[11]

MECHANORECEPTORS

Mechanoreceptors are the sensory receptors that are responsible for converting mechanical events (e.g., movement, tension) into neural signals that can be conveyed to the central nervous system.[5] As mentioned previously, mechanoreceptors are located in muscle, tendon, ligament, joint capsules, and skin and connective (fascial) tissues. Each mechanoreceptor has specific stimuli (e.g., light touch versus tissue lengthening) and thresholds (e.g., magnitude of stimuli required) to which it will respond.[4] Mechanoreceptors most susceptible to disruption during orthopedic injury include the receptors located in the musculotendinous tissues, ligaments, and joint capsules. Mechanoreceptors located in the musculotendinous tissues include the muscle spindles and Golgi tendon organs. **Muscle spindles** are responsible for conveying information regarding muscle length and rate of length change. Unique to muscle spindles is their adjustable sensitivity via the gamma motor neurons. **Golgi tendon organs**, located across a musculotendinous junction, are responsible for conveying information regarding muscle tension. Located in the ligaments and joint capsules are Ruffini receptors, pacinian corpuscles, Golgi tendon–like endings, and free nerve endings. Collectively, based on their threshold and adaptation characteristics, these four mechanoreceptors provide the central nervous system with information regarding speed of joint position and movement and host tissue load levels.

Important Concepts

During orthopedic injury, the musculoskeletal tissues and the populations of mechanoreceptors residing in the tissues may be disrupted. The ability to maintain postural equilibrium may be disrupted because of sensory disruptions, musculoskeletal disruptions, or both.

BALANCE AND COORDINATION TESTS

To prescribe appropriate balance and coordination exercises, it is essential to have data related to present balance and coordination status. Most often, coordination is evaluated by using simple tests such as those outlined in Box 7-1. Although quantifying a patient's coordination abilities can be easily accomplished by counting the number of repetitions completed in a given time frame or the number or percentage of successes per number of attempts, qualitatively examining and describing the patient's abilities and difficulties (e.g., steadiness, control, speed) can also be useful. Although many tests can be used to conduct bilateral comparisons (e.g., affected limb compared with unaffected limb), the clinician must keep in mind that better coordination should be expected in the dominant limb, particularly in the upper extremity. Because coordination involves multiple elements, including sensory organs, muscle function, and central nervous system centers, deficits in coordination revealed by these assessments often require follow-up assessments to determine the source or sources of coordination deficiency.

Functionally, periods of single-leg stance are often interspersed in many activities of daily living, such as walking, turning, climbing stairs, and putting on a pair of pants. During activities of daily living, one does not usually concentrate solely on maintaining balance but rather on the details of the task (e.g., reaching up to

Important Concepts

Deficits identified during balance and coordination assessments may require more specific follow-up testing to identify the source or sources of the deficits.

Balance tests and specific balance treatment activities are rarely separated, and the same movements are used for fundamental balance exercises and clinically relevant balance tests. Three sensory sources—somatosensory, visual, and vestibular—contribute afferent information to the central nervous system so that appropriate muscle actions can be selected. By manipulating the conditions in which balance tasks are conducted, different aspects of the postural control system may be more selectively challenged.[7] For example, having a patient stand with eyes closed heightens the patient's reliance on somatosensory and vestibular information. In addition, manipulating the base of support and support surface characteristics can change the challenge imposed on the postural control system. For example, compared with double-leg stance, single-leg stance requires that the postural control system reorganize itself over a narrow and short base of support, with the additional advantage that bilateral comparisons can be made.

Important Concepts

By manipulating the sensory, task, and environmental conditions in which balance tasks are performed, different aspects of the postural control system may be more selectively challenged.

BOX 7-1 Coordination Tests

Rapid alternating movement: An alternating movement test in which the patient places the hands on the thighs (palms down) and then turns the hands over (palms up) and lifts them off the thighs as quickly as possible. The patient then rapidly returns to the starting position to complete 10 repetitions.

Finger to nose: A reciprocal motion test in which the patient touches the tip of the index finger to the tip of the nose.

Finger opposition: A reciprocal motion test in which the patient alternately touches the tip of each finger with the tip of the thumb.

Fixation-position hold: A static position test in which the arms are held horizontally or the knees are extended.

Heel on shin: A reciprocal motion and accuracy test in which the patient is supine and is asked to slide the heel of one leg from the ankle to the knee of the opposite leg.

Pronation-supination: A reciprocal motion test in which the palms are rotated up and down.

Tapping foot or hand: A reciprocal motion test in which the patient is asked to tap the ball of one foot repeatedly while keeping the heel in contact with the floor. With the hand, the patient is asked to tap the hand on the knee.

Throwing and catching a ball: A reciprocal motion test in which the patient is asked to receive and deliver a ball.

remove the correct book from a shelf). Additionally, during activities of daily living, situations arise where unexpected challenges (perturbations) to postural equilibrium occur. Comprehensive balance assessment and training frequently requires a progressive battery of specific tasks of incremental difficulty and should include not only static stances with varying bases of support and support surface characteristics but also tasks that involve voluntary movement and task completion and unexpected perturbations.[7]

Important Concepts

Comprehensive balance assessment and training often requires a progressive battery of specific tasks of incremental difficulty including various stances, support surfaces, unexpected perturbations, and voluntary movements.

Evidence directly supports the notion that a battery of tests be used to determine overall postural control performance because the performance of static balance tasks is mildly to moderately related but unrelated to functional reaching or hopping movements.[12] Close observation of the patient's protective reactions during loss of balance is a critical component of all balance tests and training activities. Immediate corrective action by the patient to maintain balance is necessary to move the patient from low-level balance activities to more challenging, complex maneuvers.

Box 7-2 summarizes common progressions used with respect to stances, support surfaces, and vision. For example, the static double-leg stance test with the eyes open is often the first test performed. This simple test is made more challenging by having the patient maintain balance on both legs with his or her eyes closed. Next, the patient can stand on a high-density foam surface with eyes open and closed, followed by standing on low-density foam with eyes open and closed. After that, the patient can stand on inclined or declined surfaces and unstable surfaces such as minitrampolines, rocker boards, and wobble boards, again using the eyes open to eyes closed progression. Similar eyes open to eyes closed and support surface progressions can be used with the patient using single-leg and tandem stances.

After a patient has mastered static stances under various visual and support surface conditions, balance tasks can be progressed to include concurrent voluntary movements and tasks. Reaching tasks are a practical and functional test that determine a patient's ability to perform simple daily tasks. Tests can be performed with the patient seated or standing using the upper or lower extremity (Fig. 7-2). Patients are offered a target that is slightly out of reach to test their ability to shift their center of mass to their limits of stability. Automatic activities, such as catching a ball, can also be performed in sequence from a seated to a standing position. The velocity, angle, and direction of throwing the ball to the patient challenge the patient's ability to move arms and trunk rapidly out of the static balance state and back to equilibrium.

More dynamic balance tests requiring the patient to maintain a base of support, negotiate a single-plane or multidirectional movement, and keep the body in motion are also useful. Walking in a straight line for a prescribed functional distance (e.g., from a chair to the bathroom) is a simple test to administer. Adding directional changes, such as turning a corner or negotiating a random series of obstacles, provides information concerning the patient's dynamic balance. Additional challenges can be assessed by asking the patient to tandem walk (heel-to-toe walking), walk on their toes only, and walk on their heels only. Similar to the coordination tests, deficits uncovered during these balance assessments may require more specific follow-up testing to identify the source or sources of the deficits.

Quantifying performance during many of the previously mentioned tasks can be done using noninstrumented or instrumented measures. Noninstrumented measures include variables such as length of time in equilibrium,[3,7] error scoring systems,[8,10] and distances reached with arms or legs.[1,6] During the dynamic tests, such as tandem walking (straight line, heel-to-toe sequencing), the distance traveled during a specified time period can be recorded. Instrumented measures often involve technology that records the forces exerted on a support surface (force platforms) (Fig. 7-3) or sensors that detect movement and position of the support surface (Fig. 7-4). In addition to providing objective measures of balance performance, some instrumented measures provide real-time biofeedback (Fig. 7-5) to facilitate weight transfer within base of support boundaries, with some commercial devices providing interactive applications that require the patient to transfer his or her weight to complete various games.

Important Concepts

Quantifying balance performance can be done using similar tasks as used during training exercises employing noninstrumented or instrumented measures.

BOX 7-2 Progressive Balancing Exercises

Seated: Eyes open, eyes closed, manually applied postural stress. Throwing and catching a ball.
Seated: Uneven surface, less stable surface (Swiss ball). Eyes open, eyes closed.
Standing: Double-leg standing—eyes open, eyes closed, manually applied postural stress, weight shifting
Single-leg standing—eyes open, eyes closed, postural stress
Surface changes: All standing drills can be advanced by changing the inclination and type of surface:
- Concrete
- Carpet (short, dense, thick)
- Asphalt
- Tile (slick), linoleum
- Grass, loose gravel, dirt

Minitrampoline: Double-leg standing—eyes open, eyes closed, hopping
Single-leg standing—eyes open, eyes closed, hopping
Foam padding: Double-leg and single-leg standing, ambulation, eyes open, eyes closed
Balancing devices: rocker boards, BAPS Biomechanical Ankle Platform System, Biodex Balance SD, seated position, standing position, double-leg and single-leg standing, eyes open, eyes closed

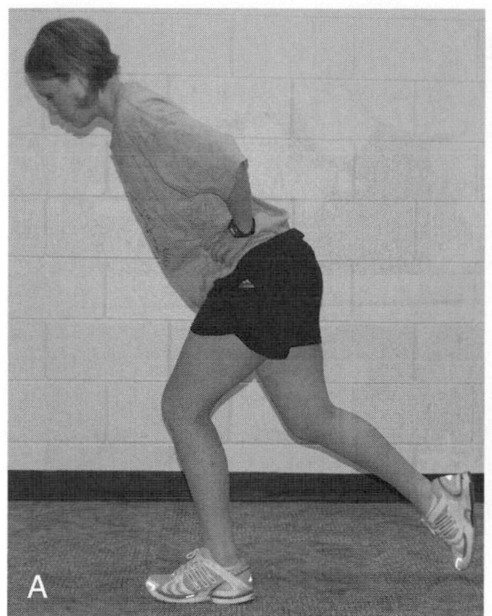

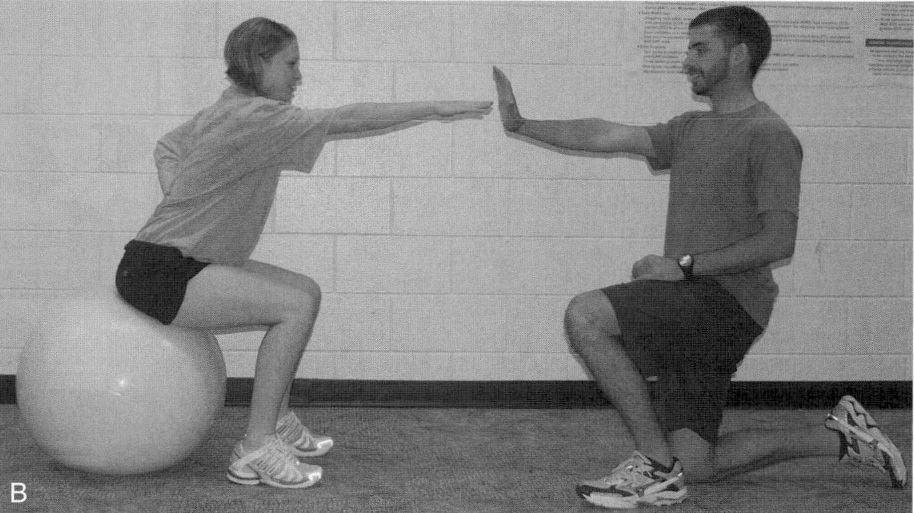

FIG 7-2 Reaching tasks can be completed with the upper or lower extremity in standing and seated positions. For a patient who has mastered reaching tasks from a stable sitting base, sitting on a physioball increases the challenge.

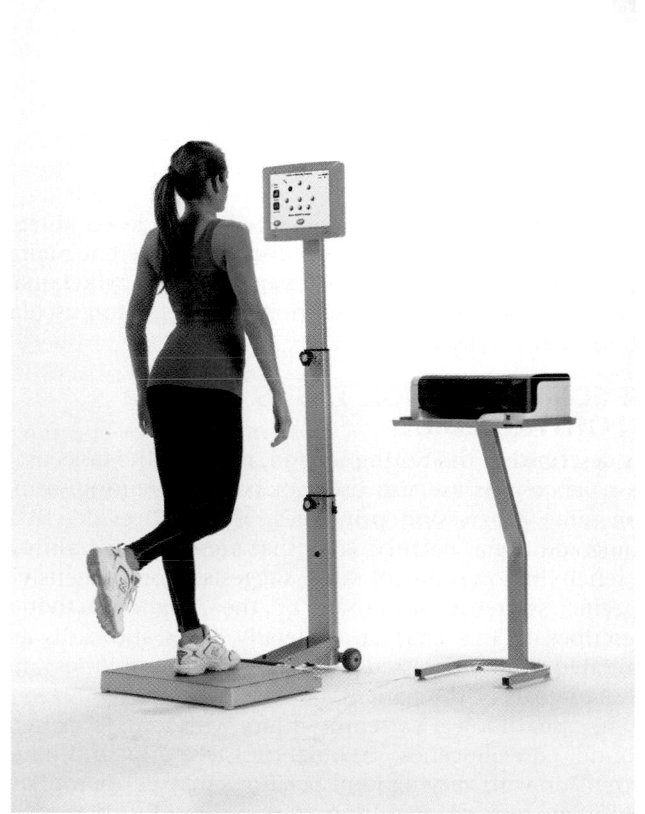

FIG 7-3 Biodex Biosway balance system. *(Courtesy Biodex Medical Systems, Inc., Shirley, NY.)*

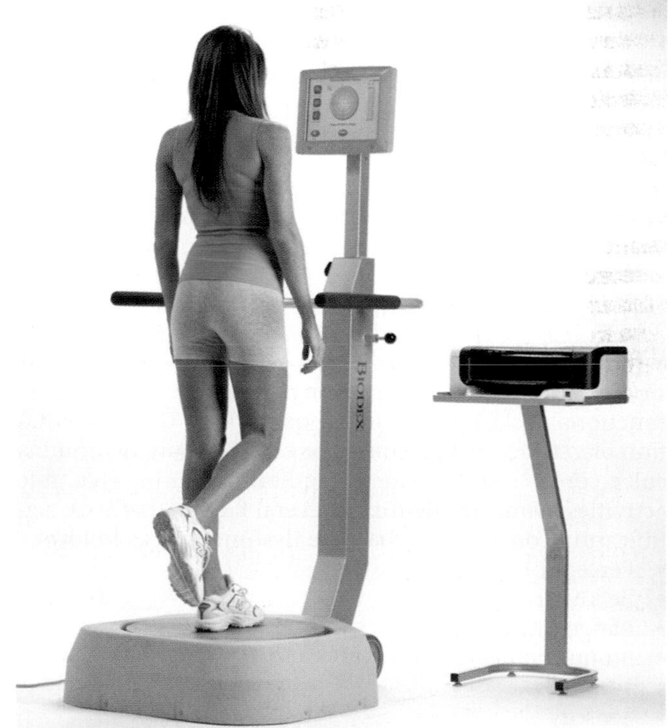

FIG 7-4 Biodex Balance System SD. *(Courtesy Biodex Medical Systems, Inc., Shirley, NY.)*

Shumway-Cook and Horak[13] designed a method of assessing the influence of various sensory sources on balance in standing subjects. This method requires the patient to maintain standing balance under different intersensory conditions that eliminate, isolate, or alter visual and surface orientation inputs. The original protocol consists of six different conditions through the use of two different surfaces (firm, foam) and three different visual conditions (eyes open, eyes closed, conflict dome); however, in many clinical settings, the protocol is shortened to include only two of the visual conditions (eyes open, eyes closed). By observing changes in the amount of sway or using a forceplate to quantify sway, the clinician can determine which of the three sensory sources (vision, somatosensory, vestibular) a patient relies on for balance as well as the degree to which the patient can

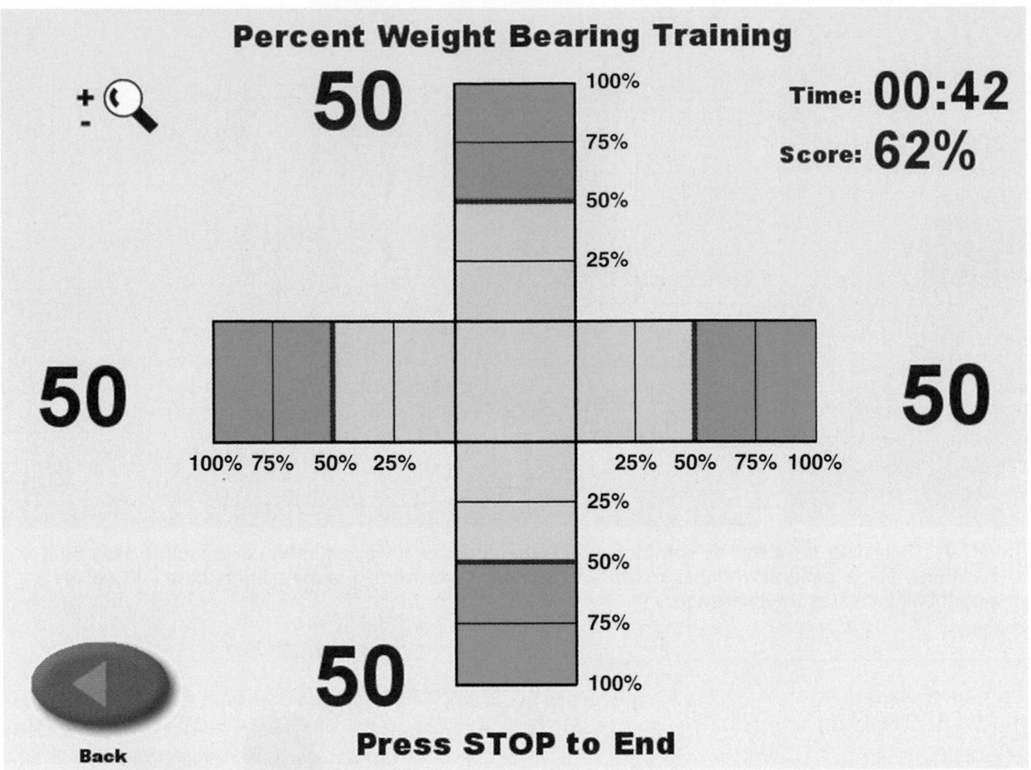

FIG 7-5 Example of an interactive real-time interface to facilitate weight transfer within the base of support boundaries. *(Courtesy Biodex Medical Systems, Inc., Shirley, NY.)*

adapt reliance on the remaining senses during situations of intersensory conflict.

BALANCE TRAINING IN ORTHOPEDICS

In concert with regaining strength and motion, specific functional tasks must be incorporated into the rehabilitation plan to accentuate muscular coordination, neuromuscular control, and postural equilibrium during dynamic activities. Duncan[2] identified several factors that may significantly contribute to balance dysfunction, as follows:

- Perception
- Behavior
- Range of motion
- Biomechanical alignment
- Weakness
- Sensory
- Synergistic organization strategy
- Coordination
- Adaptability

Many studies have demonstrated how injury, surgery, immobilization, and rehabilitation programs without specific balance and proprioceptive training can have a profound negative effect on balance and neuromuscular control. It can be concluded from these studies that the physical therapist assistant must clearly recognize that injury, surgery, and non–weight-bearing immobilization negatively affect the proprioceptive pathways and use of proprioceptive information by the central nervous system for neuromuscular control and balance. Functional balance and coordination training combined with closed kinetic chain (CKC) resistive exercises allows for afferent neural input from peripheral joint mechanoreceptors, which may promote restoration of proprioception, neuromuscular control, and balance.

SPECIFIC BALANCE TASKS IN ORTHOPEDICS

As described in the testing section, many of the tasks used as balance tests are also used for balance training, using the same progression principles. This section describes some additional balance tasks that are used for training. A rehabilitation protocol rarely suggests a comprehensive, specific sequence using all of the balance activities described in this chapter. Generally, tasks and drills are initiated and progressed according to the abilities and desired goals of the patient.

In cases of lower extremity injury with long-term, bed-bound convalescence, manual resistive hip and knee extension with varying joint positions may be appropriate to initiate restoration of normal proprioceptive pathways. When a patient may assume an upright position, progressive balance training may begin in a seated position. Similar progressive sequencing as with the standing tasks can be used, with the patient first attempting to maintain balance with the eyes open and then with the eyes closed. Progressions can include movements such as reaching tasks and the lifting of objects. Manually applied external forces (perturbations) can be applied while the patient's eyes are closed to initiate reflexive balance training. Comparable to using foam and unstable surfaces for standing

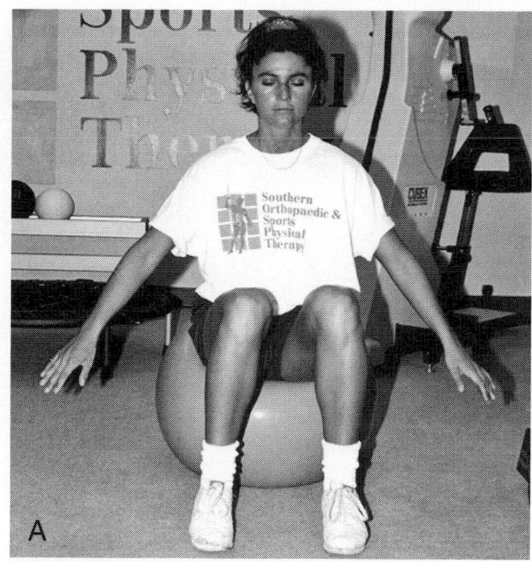

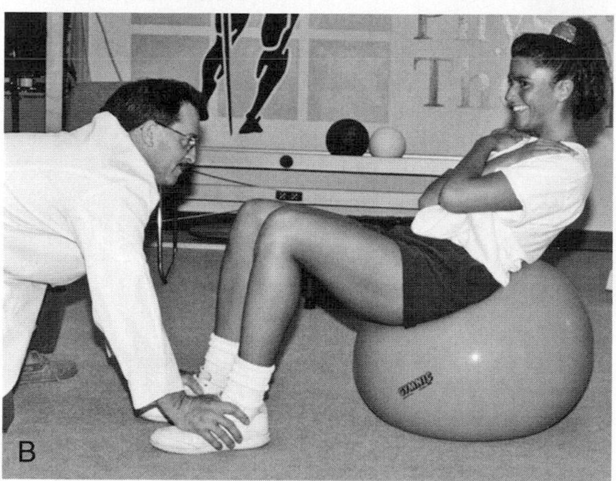

FIG 7-6 **A,** Sitting trunk balance can be progressed using a physioball to challenge and test a patient's ability to demonstrate protective reactions and appropriate muscular corrective action while seated. **B,** Supported partial direct sit-ups for improving trunk balance and strength on a large-diameter physioball.

progressions, a large physioball or Swiss ball can be used as part of a seated static and dynamic balancing program to increase the challenge to the postural control system (Fig. 7-6, *A*). The physioball, which is a demanding exercise apparatus, has many creative uses in balancing and strengthening programs for patients with various orthopedic conditions. One very challenging exercise is the performance of support sit-ups on the physioball (Fig. 7-6, *B*). This particular exercise is for an active population and not for all patients.

When a patient is weight bearing, progressive balance training can begin with vertical weight bearing (double-leg standing). For proper gait mechanics, weight shifting (changing base of support from one leg to another) is critical. After the patient masters double-leg standing static balance, the physical therapist assistant should begin training the patient to shift balance from one leg to the other. The next progressions can include the aforementioned visual, support surface, and base of support progressions. For teaching and safety purposes, all single-leg balance drills should be initiated on the uninvolved limb. As confidence and motor learning progress, the patient performs the balance activity on the involved limb. In all cases of balance training, manual support and spotting are provided as required. As a means to document progress, the length of time the patient can maintain equilibrium can be recorded.

Other functional CKC exercises that replicate the specific demands of daily activities or athletic skills serve to restore coordination and balance as well as the factors contributing to balance dysfunction listed in the previous section. Progressively demanding tasks are sometimes omitted from rehabilitation programs, with reliance put on increased clinical strength tests, greater range of motion grades, and reduced pain and swelling as objective data leading to discharge from formal therapy. Examples of functional CKC exercises include double-leg and single-leg squats on stable and unstable surfaces, forward and backward gait, sidestepping (lateral steps), heel-to-toe walking, and braiding steps (carioca). Progressively challenging tasks that stimulate the patient's ability to negotiate obstacles and make multidirectional changes while in motion safely and accurately are important.

Important Concepts

Progressively demanding coordination and balance tasks that aim to replicate the demands of daily activities are needed at all stages of rehabilitation.

It is important that advanced functional balance drills, such as hopping, be included in the programs of patients returning to high levels of physical activity. Hopping drills can range from simple vertical leaps to challenging combinations of vertical and horizontal patterns. Hopping is useful with an athletic population and can be done on a flat, hard surface or on a minitrampoline (Fig. 7-7, *A*). The forgiving, uneven rebound surface of the minitrampoline adds an appropriate challenge for progressive balance training. Additionally, a wobble board (Fig. 7-7, *B*) or other commercially available balance training system that provides an adjustable unstable surface (see Fig. 7-3) can be used to challenge single-leg or double-leg proprioception. Using the minitrampoline after hip, knee, or ankle injury for static standing balance and for single-leg or double-leg hopping is unique and challenging for many patients. As with other balance drills, single-leg or double-leg standing or hopping can progress from eyes open to eyes closed.

Important Concepts

Upper extremity coordination and balance training is an important component to upper extremity rehabilitation, particularly for patients returning to vigorous upper extremity activities.

Inclusion of tasks in which sudden perturbations challenge balance is also an important component of a

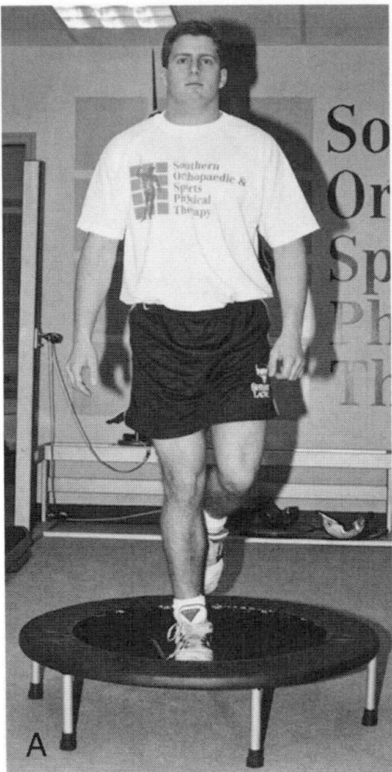
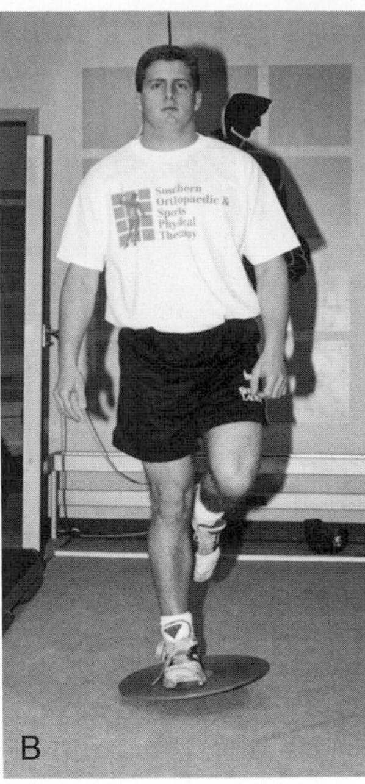

FIG 7-7 **A,** A minitrampoline provides a unique, challenging, and forgiving surface to encourage balance and proprioception while hopping or standing. **B,** A wobble board can be used to challenge single-leg or double-leg proprioception and balance.

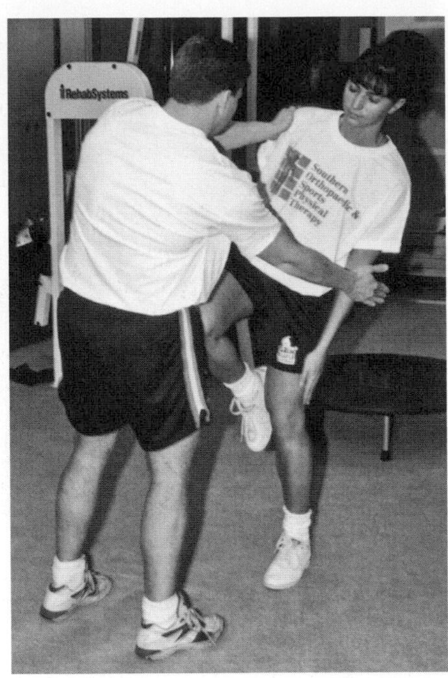

FIG 7-8 To test and challenge a patient's protective reactions, the clinician can apply a sudden external force while the patient's eyes are closed. Close protection and support must be provided by the clinician during this activity.

balance training program. For example, the clinician can apply sudden force to the patient while the patient is standing on one leg with the eyes closed (Fig. 7-8). Applying manual postural stresses in different directions and with varying degrees of force can further challenge the ability to "right" or correct balance. Another method of perturbing balance is to use elastic tubing secured to a patient. The clinician begins the task by applying tension through the tubing. By suddenly releasing the tubing, the patient is presented with an immediate challenge to postural equilibrium.

Many commercial training devices have been developed to assist with balance training. Wobble and balance boards can be used for both lower and upper extremity conditions (Fig. 7-9). This device is very adaptable, portable, and affordable for many physical therapy environments. Initially, double-leg support progresses to single-leg standing. One of the most challenging balance drills is performing single-leg standing on a balance board with the eyes closed.

BALANCE AND PROPRIOCEPTIVE TRAINING FOR THE UPPER EXTREMITY

Many household chores involve the repetitive use of the arms and shoulders to lift, pull, and carry. Industrial workers, manual laborers, and assembly line workers all use their arms and shoulders in vigorous weight-bearing positions (weight bearing in these instances refers to overhead lifting, pulling, and climbing maneuvers). Athletes in particular use their arms and shoulders to perform sports skills. Gymnasts require extraordinary flexibility, strength, and glenohumeral stability during demanding upper body, weight-bearing activities. With the upper extremity in contact with a secure surface, it is incorporated into defining the base of support.

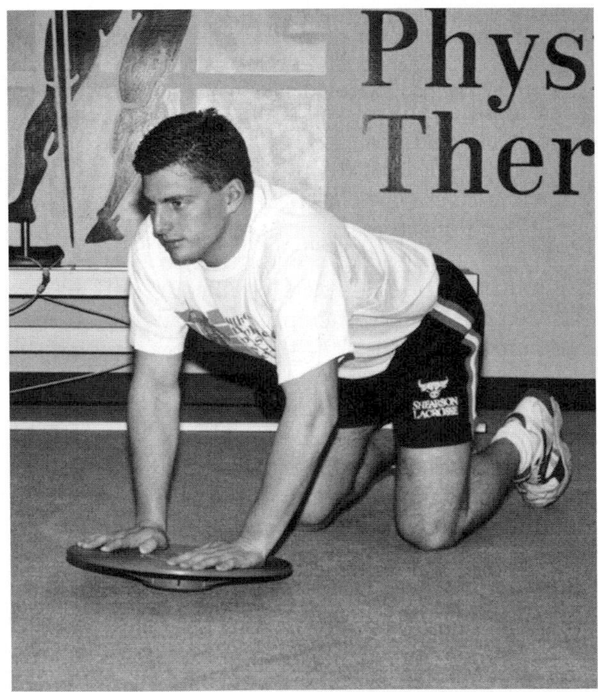

FIG 7-9 For upper extremity proprioception and balance training, a wobble board can be used; initially, both arms are involved. As the patient gains strength, balance, and confidence, one arm can be used.

As mentioned, injury, surgery, and immobilization lead to significant alterations in proprioception. Specific

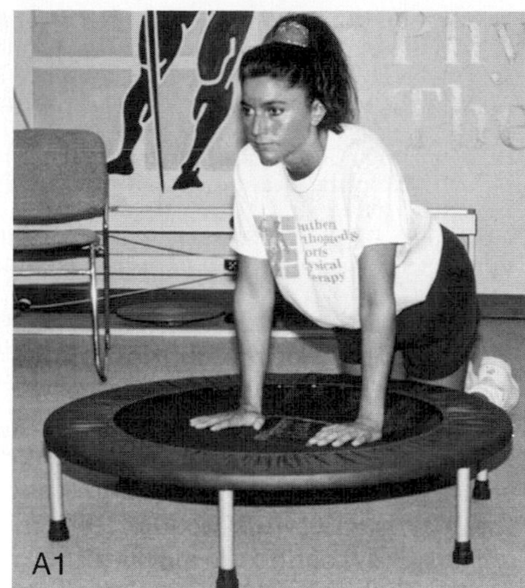

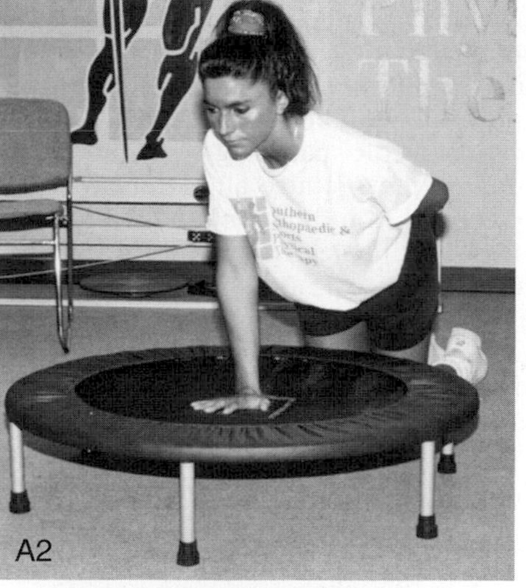

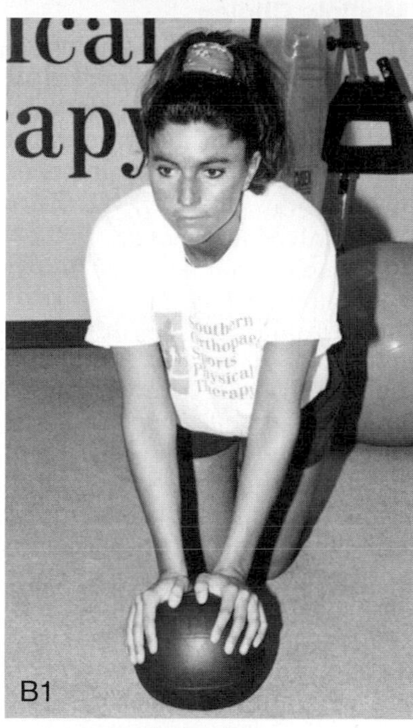

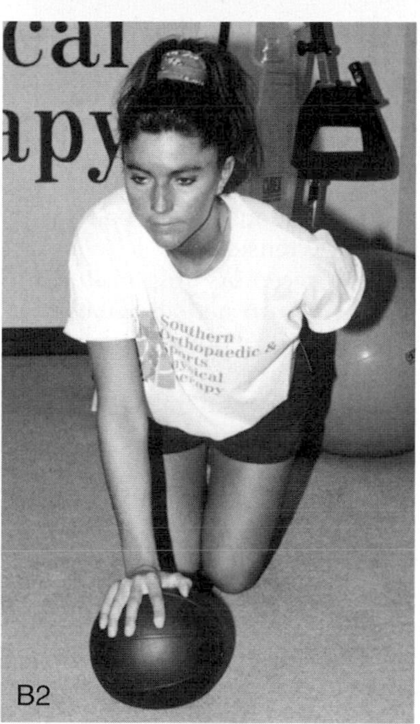

FIG 7-10 **A1,** The minitrampoline can be used to encourage closed chain proprioception for the upper extremities. **A2,** Progressing this activity will have the patient perform one-arm balancing, push-ups, and hopping maneuvers on the forgiving surface of the minitrampoline. **B1,** A small physioball (Plyoball) can be used to encourage dynamic closed chain proprioception for the upper extremities. **B2,** Closed chain, weight-bearing activities can be progressed by having the patient balance and support on one arm on a Plyoball.

proprioceptive exercises have been proposed that, when used in conjunction with proprioceptive neuromuscular facilitation exercises, rhythmic stabilization strengthening exercises, and general range of motion, may contribute to improved proprioception in the upper extremity.

The upper extremities can be progressed in much the same way as the lower extremities. Although many of these exercises are often considered to be specific for an athletic population, they can be adapted to general orthopedic patients who must rely on dynamic vigorous weight-bearing shoulder and arm activities to accomplish tasks of daily living. With both arms in contact with the ground, weight shifting between the arms can be conducted on firm and unstable surfaces. In addition, while in a similar position, eyes open and eyes closed, balancing can be conducted on the same support surfaces used for standing balance (Figs. 7-9 and 7-10, *A1, A2*). Beginning with two arms, this exercise can be intensified by having the patient use one arm with the eyes open and closed. Global stability of the glenohumeral joint can be enhanced effectively with the use of medicine balls and physioballs (Fig. 7-10, *B1, B2*). The patient begins the progression of this exercise by kneeling in front of the ball and placing both hands on the ball. As the exercise progresses, extraordinary joint stability, strength, and balance are required to maintain equilibrium.

SUMMARY

Underlying all motor activities are specific processes to ensure that postural equilibrium is maintained. Disruptions to balance, postural equilibrium, and coordination often accompany orthopedic pathology. Additionally, orthopedic conditions often produce alterations in proprioception, motor control, coordination, and neuromuscular control, requiring specific elements to be incorporated into rehabilitation programs to promote their restoration. Often the same tasks used for balance assessments can be used for training. Progressions can be made by changing stances, support surfaces, visual conditions, and tasks. Similar progressions can be incorporated into upper extremity rehabilitation programs.

GLOSSARY

Balance: The ability to maintain the center of mass over the base of support.[12]

Base of support: The area contained within the parts of the body making physical contact with the external environment.[9]

Coordination: The ability to produce patterns of body and limb motions in the context of environmental objects and events.[13]

Golgi tendon organs: Fibers responsible for conveying information regarding muscle tension.

Mechanoreceptors: Sensory receptors responsible for converting mechanical events into neural signals that can be conveyed to the central nervous system.[7]

Muscle spindles: Fibers responsible for conveying information regarding muscle length and rate of length change.

Neuromuscular control: Subconscious activation of muscles occurring in preparation for and in response to joint motion and loading.[12]

Postural equilibrium: The balance of all forces acting on the body's center of mass to maintain it within the limits of stability with optimal joint segment alignment.[1]

Proprioception: The afferent information contributing to joint position, joint movement (kinesthesia), and movement resistance/tension.

REFERENCES

1. Bellew J, Fenter P: Control of balance differs after knee or ankle fatigue in older women. *Arch Phys Med Rehabil* 87:1486–1489, 2006.
2. Duncan P: *Balance dysfunction: implications for geriatric and neurological rehabilitation. Course Notes*, 1994, Advanced Educational Seminars, Inc.
3. Ekdahl C, Jarnlo G, Andersson S: Standing balance in healthy subjects. *Scand J Rehabil Med* 21:187–195, 1989.
4. Erikson R: Stimulus coding in topographic and nontopographic afferent modalities: on the significance of the activity of individual sensory neurons. *Psychol Rev* 75:447–465, 1968.
5. Grigg P: Peripheral neural mechanisms in proprioception. *J Sport Rehabil* 3:2–17, 1994.
6. Hertel J, Braham R, Hale S, Olmstead-Kramer L: Simplifying the star excursion balance test: analyses of subjects with and without chronic ankle instability. *J Orthop Sports Phys Ther* 36(3):131–137, 2006.
7. Riemann B: Is there a link between chronic ankle instability and postural instability? *J Athl Train* 37(4):386–393, 2002.
8. Riemann B, Caggiano N, Lephart S: Examination of a clinical method of assessing postural control during a functional performance task. *J Sport Rehabil* 8:171–183, 1999.
9. Riemann B, Guskiewicz K: Contribution of peripheral somatosensory system to balance and postural equilibrium. In Lephart S, Fu F, editors: *The Role of Proprioception and Neuromuscular Control in the Management and Rehabilitation of Joint Pathology*, Champaign, IL., 2000, Human Kinetics, pp 37–51.
10. Riemann B, Guskiewicz K, Shields E: Relationship between clinical and forceplate measures of postural stability. *J Sport Rehabil* 8: 71–82, 1999.
11. Riemann B, Lephart S: The sensorimotor system, part I: The physiologic basis of functional joint stability. *J Athl Train* 37(1):71–79, 2002.
12. Riemann B, Schmitz R: The relationship between various modes of single leg postural control assessment. *Int J Sports Phys Ther* 7(3):257–266, 2012.
13. Shumway-Cook A, Horak F: Assessing the influence of sensory interaction on balance. *Phys Ther* 66:1548–1550, 1986.
14. Turvey M: Coordination. *Am Psychol* 45(8):938–953, 1990.

REVIEW QUESTIONS

Multiple Choice

1. Proprioception and the mechanoreceptor system provide information concerning which of the following?
   a. Joint displacement
   b. Joint position, direction, and speed
   c. Pressure and stretch
   d. Pain
   e. All of the above
2. Muscle spindles are responsible for which of the following?
   a. Pain
   b. Muscle tension
   c. Pressure
   d. Muscle length change
   e. All of the above
3. Free nerve endings are type IV mechanoreceptors and are involved with which of the following?
   a. Pain and inflammation
   b. Posture
   c. Muscle stretch
   d. Ligament tension
   e. None of the above
4. Which of the following are measures that can be used to document balance performance objectively?
   a. Record length of time in equilibrium
   b. Count the number of compensatory errors
   c. Record distance the upper or lower extremity can reach from a standing position
   d. All of the above
   e. None of the above
5. A critical safety component to all balance and proprioception activities is the patient's ability to demonstrate which of the following?
   a. Increased range of motion
   b. Improved strength
   c. Protective reactions
   d. Faster gait
   e. All of the above
6. A challenging functional balance test and activity requires the patient to do which of the following?
   a. Maintain balance with eyes closed while standing
   b. Ambulate and negotiate obstacles

c. Maintain balance while seated, performing trunk rotation
d. Maintain balance while seated, performing marching

7. Which of the following factors contributes to balance dysfunction?
   a. Perception
   b. Weakness
   c. Range of motion
   d. Coordination
   e. All of the above
8. Which of the following tasks should be incorporated into a comprehensive balance training program?
   a. Quiet stances
   b. Quiet stances while performing other tasks
   c. Ambulatory and location tasks
   d. Perturbations
   e. All of the above
9. Which of the following stances has the smallest base of support?
   a. Double-leg stance
   b. Push-up position
   c. Single-leg stance
   d. Tandem stance
10. Having a patient stand on a foam surface affects which of the following sensory sources?
   a. Visual
   b. Vestibular
   c. Somatosensory
11. Which of the following describes a progress of balance training tasks going from easiest to more complex?
   1. Double-leg stance on foam surface with eyes open
   2. Double-leg stance on firm surface with eyes closed
   3. Double-leg stance on firm surface reaching for object
   4. Tandem (heel-to-toe) walking
      A. 2 → 1 → 3 → 4
      B. 1 → 2 → 3 → 4
      C. 2 → 3 → 1 → 4
      D. 3 → 2 → 1 → 4
12. Perturbation balance training helps the patient develop:
   a. Static stance balance.
   b. An ability to correct sudden disruptions or challenges to balance.
   c. Balance during voluntary movements.
13. Kinesthesia refers to sensory information regarding:
   a. Joint position.
   b. Joint movement.
   c. Movement resistance/tension.
   d. Joint orientation with respect to gravity.
14. A comprehensive balance testing and training battery includes which of the following?
   a. Different stances—double, single, tandem
   b. Different support surfaces—firm, foam, biomechanical ankle platform system
   c. Different tasks—static stance, reaching, catching a ball
   d. Functional tasks—walking, squatting, turning
   e. All of the above
15. Which of the following exercises can be used for closed chain proprioception activities after upper extremity injuries? (Choose all that apply.)
   a. Push-ups
   b. Minitrampoline
   c. Physioball or Plyoball
   d. Biceps curls
   e. Pendulum exercise

Short Answer

16. Define and contrast balance, postural equilibrium, and coordination.
17. Discuss the functions and locations of mechanoreceptors.
18. List static and dynamic balance and coordination tests and activities in a progressive order of challenge.
19. Discuss several factors that contribute to balance dysfunction.
20. Discuss the rationale for proprioceptive training for the upper extremity.

Fill in the Blank

21. The reach test shows the patient's ability to reach and challenge the limits or borders of the ______________.
22. ____________________ refers to the sensory sources that report joint position and movement to the central nervous system.
23. Destabilizing forces arising from gravity, ____________, and voluntary movements all challenge the maintenance of the center of mass within the limits of stability.
24. In a progressive balance testing or training battery, the _________-leg stance is often the first one used.
25. Similar to the lower extremity, upper extremity balance tasks should begin with _______ _________ and progress to ______ ________.

True/False

26. Single-leg and double-leg stances are examples of balance tests and are never used as treatment activities.
27. A higher degree of balance is necessary to maintain equilibrium while standing and walking on low-density foam compared with high-density foam.
28. Injury, surgery, immobilization, and non–weight-bearing convalescence have a profoundly negative effect on the afferent neural input system.
29. Rehabilitation programs that do not address balance, coordination, and proprioception can result in poor restoration of function and increase the risk of reinjury.
30. Proprioception and balance exercises are not required in patients after shoulder surgery because the shoulder is a non–weight-bearing structure.

Part II

Review of Tissue Healing

The physical therapist assistant (PTA) must understand the general healing mechanisms of specific tissues to make sound clinical recommendations, develop a progression of rehabilitation exercises, and identify promptly problems associated with injury, immobilization, or the postoperative period. Trauma, surgery, and prolonged immobilization profoundly affect bone and soft tissues. Different tissues (ligament, tendon, bone, muscle, cartilage) heal or remodel at different rates.[2] To understand the events and factors that negatively influence tissue healing, the PTA must be aware of the response of tissues to trauma, surgery, and immobilization.

When beginning therapeutic exercises after an acute traumatic injury, surgery, cast removal, or immobilization, initial clinical information must include which specific tissues are involved; the length of time of immobilization; weight-bearing status during immobilization; and which surgical procedure, if any, was performed. These points help the clinician recognize healing constraints of specific tissues as well as indications and contraindications for modifying therapeutic interventions and functional activities. This part provides information concerning the composition of connective tissue and the effects of immobilization, physical stress, exercise, joint protection, inflammation, repair, and remodeling on these tissues. Part II provides excellent clinical foundations for specific exercises and progressions that are discussed in later chapters describing management of patients with orthopedic conditions by region (Chapters 17-23) and condition (Chapters 24-27).

Three overlapping, interrelated series of events initiate healing: phase I, inflammatory response; phase II, proliferation; and phase III, remodeling and tissue maturation (Fig. II-1).[3]

The five cardinal signs of an acute inflammatory reaction are redness, swelling, pain, heat, and loss of function. The acute phase of inflammation lasts 24 to 48 hours, and the entire inflammatory response is generally complete after 2 weeks.[3]

Immediately after injury, vasoconstriction, stimulated by serotonin,[1,5] limits blood and fluid loss for a few minutes. A platelet plug occludes small vessels surrounding the injury site, blocking the flow of blood and fluids away from the site. Other strong chemical mediators responsible for vascular constriction and later tissue permeability are histamine (permeability), serotonin (vasoconstriction), bradykinin (permeability), and prostaglandins (inflammatory regulation, permeability, and pain) (Fig. II-2).[2]

A principal feature of the inflammatory response to injury is the process of ridding the injured area of tissue debris (autolytic wound débridement). This process occurs via neutrophils that migrate to the injury site.[3] Other phagocytic cells, macrophages, and lymphocytes help produce enzymes that foster this process.[4]

The proliferation phase is characterized by fibroplasia, myofibroblast activity, and organization and production of collagen (Fig. II-3).[3] Collagen formation begins about 5 days after injury.[3] Type III immature collagen predominates, providing very limited structural strength to the injury site. The synthesis, orientation, and deposition of new collagen are random, which reduces strength of scar formation.

Phase III, the remodeling phase, begins about 2 weeks after injury and can last a few months to 1 year or more.[1] In remodeling, as the name implies, new collagen and connective tissue gradually reorient along the lines of physical stress imposed on the injured site.[1] If tissues are immobilized for prolonged periods, new collagen is laid down in a highly disorganized and random manner. Active stress or muscular contractions with progressive joint motion promotes longitudinally organized, stronger, more functional collagen arrangements.[1]

Box II-1 outlines basic healing mechanisms.

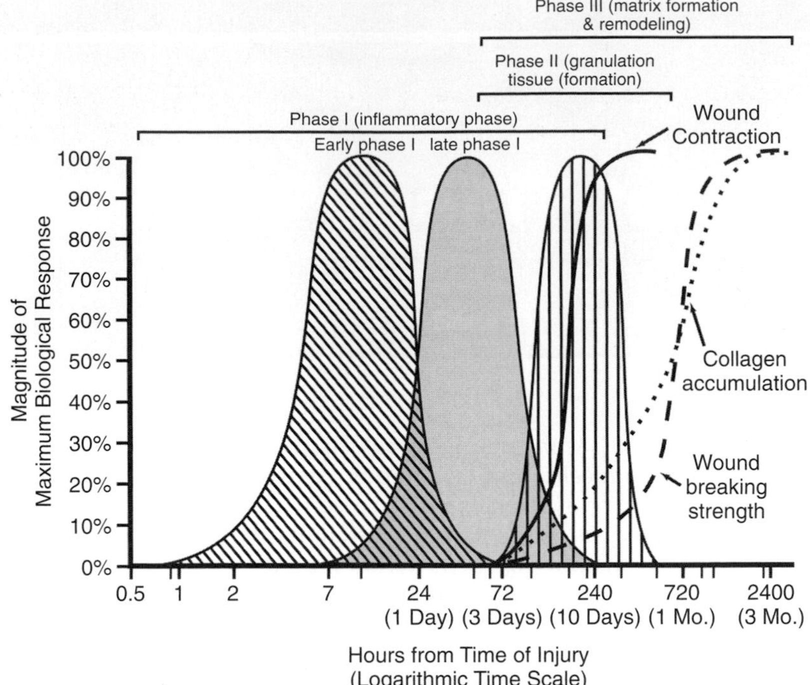

FIG II-1 The three overlapping phases of wound repair. *(From Kloth LC, McCulloch JM, Feedar JA:* Wound healing: alternatives in management, *Philadelphia, 1990, FA Davis.)*

BOX II-1 Review of Basic Healing Mechanisms

Days 2–4

Scar tissue composition: A clot forms in the wound. Connective tissue cells infiltrate the area, with macrophages attracting fibroblasts. In this initial stage of scarring, the tissue is very fragile and easily disrupted because of the predominance of weak and unstable type III collagen. Adhesion is by cellular attachments, and stretching of the scar causes tearing of the cells.

Days 5–21

Fibroplasia and contraction: This stage is very cellular. The scar increases in bulk because of fibroplasia, with an increase in the quantity of collagen fibers. This is a highly active stage of collagen synthesis and degradation. Treatment to increase range of motion and function of a joint can be very effective during this stage because of the collagen remodeling process.

Days 21–60

Consolidation: The scar contains well-organized collagen. The tissue gradually changes from predominantly cellular to fibrous, with a large amount of collagen fibers. There is a gradual increase in strength of the scar because of an increased stable covalent bonding. During this time, there is a continuous decrease in the ability of the scar to respond to treatment.

Days 60–360

Maturation: Type I collagen fibers are compact and large. The fully mature scar is only 3% cellular and almost totally collagenous. Response to treatment is poor, and hypertrophic and keloid scar tissue increases when stretched in multiple directions.

From Currier D, Nelson R: Mechanisms of connective tissue, In Currier D, Nelson R, editors: *Dynamics of human biologic tissues,* Philadelphia, 1992, FA Davis.

WOUNDS

REACTION: INFLAMMATION

Definition: Inflammation is part of the reaction phase and consists of a cellular and vascular response. Normally, this phase lasts 2–5 days.

The inflammatory process

After bleeding is stopped, cellular and vascular responses to the injury are initiated. This is the body's natural damage-control mechanism: it protects the body from foreign objects at the wound site, cleans the site, and brings cells necessary for directing healing in the next stage to the site.

Collagen's work

Collagen's role during the reaction phase is to help mediate some of the activities of the inflammation process.

Attracts plasma components, absorbs fluids and stops bleeding.

Cleans the wound, removes bacteria and debris by absorption.

Attracts white cells. Provides environment for macrophages.

How the body reacts to injury

Three steps are characteristic of the inflammation phase:

Step 1

Vasodilation

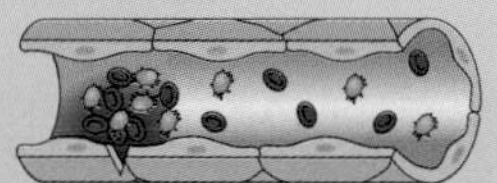

Swollen vessel brings more blood and plasma components to the wound site.

Step 2

Increased permeability

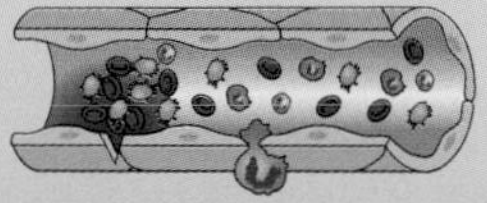

Allows more white cells to travel through the vessel wall to combat foreign bodies.

Step 3

Cellular response

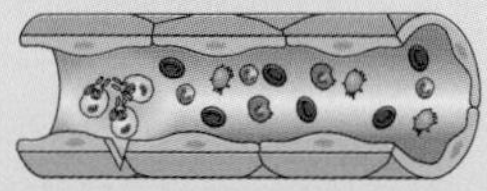

White cells ingest bacteria, debris, and dead cells. Exhausted white cells build up in plasma, forming pus.

Evolution of cellular response

PMNs are the first cells to the injury site but must be replaced by larger cells and macrophages for wound healing to progress normally.

PMN

Polymorphonuclear leukocytes (PMNs) are white cells responsible for cleaning the wound site. They provide resistance to microorganisms and are scavengers of tissue debris and foreign materials.

Monocytes

These intermediary white cells replace PMNs and eventually become macrophages. Monocytes function similarly to PMNs.

Macrophage

Toward the end of the reaction phase, the macrophage is the most common white cell present in the tissue and is the major mediator of inflammation and repair in wound healing.

Signs of inflammation

The four classic clinical signs of inflammation are: rubor (redness), tumor (swelling), calor (heat or warmth), and dolor (pain).

Rubor

The injury turns red because more blood is present in the area (a result of vasodilation).

Tumor

Swelling is caused by increased fluid mobility and accumulation of body fluids in the tissue.

Calor

The wounded area is heated by warm blood flowing into the region.

Dolor

Pain is caused by the pressure from the swelling of nearby tissue and the accumulation of white cell by-products.

FIG II-2 The inflammatory process and cellular response to injury. *(Adapted from BioCore, Inc., Topeka, KS.)*

WOUNDS

REGENERATION & REMODELING

Definition: During the regeneration phase damaged tissue is replaced by new tissue which is, in turn, strengthened during the remodeling phase.

Recreating tissue

Macrophages from the inflammation phase cause fibroblasts to migrate into the wound bed. These cells divide and deposit collagen and become the basis of new tissue called the granulation bed. This tissue eventually is covered by epithelial cells and becomes a scar.

How the body repairs itself

Tissue is regenerated from the bottom up in the following sequence:

Step 1

Granulation

Cells migrate into the wound area and deposit a matrix, which fills the tissue void. This tissue is usually red.

Step 2

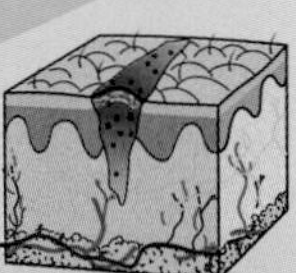

Epithelialization

After a healthy granulation bed is formed, a two- to three-cell layer epidermis forms over the surface.

Step 3

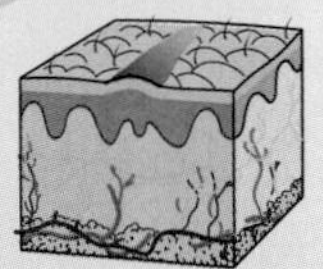

Contracture

About 20 days after injury, the wound can withstand normal stresses. This scar tissue is usually pink.

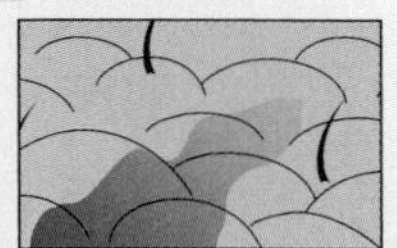

Remodeling

The final stage of wound healing yields tissue, which has regained most of the original tissue strength.

Collagen's work

Collagen is the matrix which the new tissue is built upon.

- Attracts cells to the wound site. Provides optimal environment for cellular growth and vascularization. Promotes formation of granulation tissue.
- Provides a bridge for epithelial cells to cross the wound site. Integral factor in angiogenisis.
- Reconstruction of tissues accelerated by collagen. Reduces contracture and scarring.
- Consolidation of collagen fibers strengthens the scar.

Key cell: fibroblast

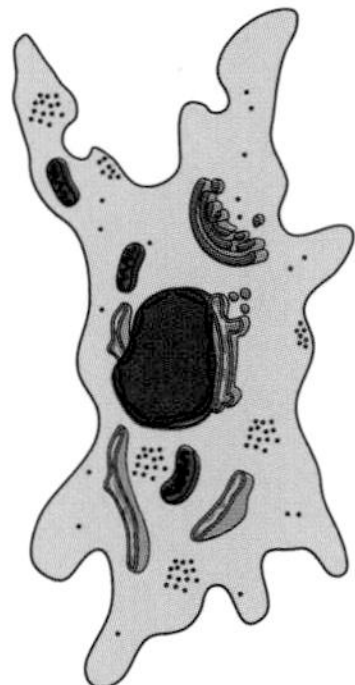

The fibroblast

A generic term for cells which establish, maintain, and repair tissues. Fibroblasts are usually present in all tissues.

Fibroblastic activity

The functions of the fibroblast include deposition, maintenance, degradation, and rearrangement of tissue structures. The fibroblast plays a crucial role in producing new granulation tissue by releasing collagen into the wound bed.

It is also responsible for wound contracture. It does this by pulling on the collagen fibers.

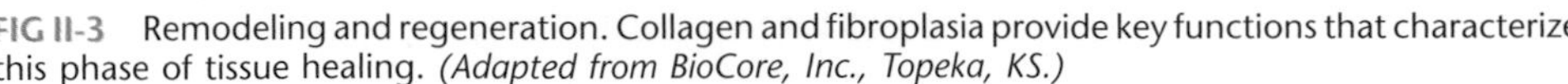

FIG II-3 Remodeling and regeneration. Collagen and fibroplasia provide key functions that characterize this phase of tissue healing. *(Adapted from BioCore, Inc., Topeka, KS.)*

REFERENCES

1. Bushbacher R: Tissue injury and healing. In *Practical guide to musculoskeletal disorders: diagnosis and rehabilitation*, Boston, 1994, Andover Medical Publishers.
2. Cummings GS, Tillman LJ: Remodelling of dense connective tissue in normal adult tissues. In Currier DP, Nelson RM, editors: *Dynamics of human biologic tissues*, Philadelphia, 1992, FA Davis.
3. Kloth LC, Miller KH: The inflammatory response to wound healing. In Kloth LC, McCulloch JM, Feedar JA, editors: *Wound healing: alternatives in management, contemporary perspectives in rehabilitation*, Philadelphia, 1990, FA Davis.
4. Laub R, Huybrechts-Godin G, Peeters-Joris C, et al: Degradation of collagen and proteoglycan by macrophages and fibroblasts. *Biochim Biophys Acta* 721:425–433, 1982.
5. Vander AJ, Sherman JH, Luciano DS: *Human physiology: the mechanisms of body function*, ed 3, Minneapolis, 1980, McGraw-Hill.

Chapter 8

Composition and Function of Connective Tissue

Erik P. Meira

CHAPTER OUTLINE

LEARNING OBJECTIVES

1. Outline components of connective tissue.
2. Discuss the sequence of overlapping events of inflammation.
3. Define fibroplasia.
4. Identify the sources of coagulation.
5. Describe and discuss the various cells of inflammation and their function.
6. Discuss the molecular cascade of arachidonic acid metabolic pathways of lipoxygenase and cyclooxygenase.
7. Define cytokines and growth factors, and discuss their various functions.

KEY TERMS

Apoptosis
Cellular necrosis
Glycosaminoglycans (GAGs)
Ground substance
Maturation
Regeneration
Remodeling
Repair

CONNECTIVE TISSUE PROPERTIES

The functions of various connective tissues are to bind cells together to form and organize tissues, organs, and systems and to provide a mechanical link between musculoskeletal junctions and the articulations of joints. Generally, connective tissues are composed of cells and the extracellular matrix that they produce. Extracellular matrix is defined as the noncellular components of connective tissue.[4]

Two classic functions of connective tissues are mechanical support for bone and soft tissues and intercellular exchange of oxygen, blood, water, gases, cells, and wastes. Basic mechanical support functions of connective tissues, such as bone, ligament, tendon, muscle, and cartilage,[1,3] are to provide stability and shock absorption in joints,[2] provide a mechanical link system between bones, and transmit muscle forces.[4]

Intracellular exchange relies on the circulation of blood to supply tissues with nutrients and oxygen and to provide removal of extracellular waste and gases. The basic aggregate components of the extracellular matrix of connective tissues are (1) elastin; (2) collagen; (3) ground substance; (4) proteoglycans and **glycosaminoglycans (GAGs)**; and (5) lipids, phospholipids, proteins, and glycoproteins.

Important Concepts

The basic aggregate components of the extracellular matrix of connective tissues are (1) elastin; (2) collagen; (3) ground substance; (4) proteoglycans and GAGs; and (5) lipids, phospholipids, proteins, and glycoproteins.

Elastin is a noncollagenous glycoprotein in which molecules are arranged randomly as a constituent of extracellular connective tissue matrix. Elastin is found in varying amounts in tissues requiring high levels of physiologic motion (elasticity). Two special amino acids, desmosine and isodesmosine, are found in elastin. They are directly responsible for the cross-linking arrangement of elastin fiber and its unique ability to deform under stress and then return to its original orientation and shape. Elastin fibers primarily contain the amino acids glycine, proline, alanine, and valine. Characteristically, elastin fibers can elongate about 70% without undergoing fiber disruption.[4]

In contrast to elastin, collagen is the most abundant component of the connective tissue matrix, and 12 to 19 distinct types of collagen exist.[4] Types of collagen are classified according to their structure and tissue distribution. Biochemical properties of connective tissues such as ligament, cartilage, tendon, bone, and muscle depend on the specific predominant types of collagen found in the extracellular matrix. The characteristic extensive network of cross-links in collagen significantly contributes to the stability and strength of the extracellular matrix. The basic histochemical profile of collagen includes the amino acids glycine, hydroxyproline, proline, and hydroxylysine. Of these amino acids, proline generally is responsible for resisting tensile forces in collagen.[4] Fibroblasts stimulate collagen synthesis through assembly of polypeptide chains of proline and lysine, which aggregate into a triple helix monomer.[4] **Ground substance** is an amorphous nonfibrous aqueous-gel component of the connective tissue matrix. Generally, this substance is responsible for facilitating intercellular exchange of water, oxygen, cells, and gases as well as providing mechanical support between various tissues.

Proteoglycans are protein and mucopolysaccharide macromolecules subclassified as GAGs. Generally, GAGs are responsible for the compressive strength of the cartilage matrix. Proteoglycans are extremely hydrophilic, so they attract and bind water. The major and distinct types of GAGs found in cartilage are chondroitin sulfate, keratan sulfate, and dermatan sulfate; chondroitin sulfate represents almost 90% of all GAGs in cartilage. These large proteoglycans, specifically chondroitin and keratan, bind together to form a distinct type of GAG referred to as *aggrecan*. Various types of connective tissues, such as ligament, cartilage, tendon, and muscle, contain varying amounts of these large proteoglycans that relate directly to the specific biomechanical and biochemical nature of all connective tissues. The networking capacity of proteoglycans and collagen within all forms and types of connective tissue contributes to the classically distinct nature of strength, stiffness, rigidity, and flexibility of connective tissues.[4]

Noncollagenous proteins and glycoproteins are minor constituents in terms of volume in the extracellular matrix of connective tissues. Generally, these molecules function in matrix organization and cell matrix interactions. They also help with orientation and maintenance of matrix structure. Two important glycoproteins found in the extracellular matrix are fibronectin and laminin. Fibronectin regulates the spread of cells and has strong chemotactic properties that attract and bind various connective tissue cells. Fibronectin is synthesized by many connective tissue cells, including osteoblasts, and may play a role in cell matrix interactions during osteoblast **maturation.** Laminin is a multifunctional glycoprotein found in the extracellular matrix that is important in establishing epithelial tissue and basement membranes during wound healing.

Lipids represent less than 1% of human articular cartilage matrix. The specific function of lipids and phospholipids is not clearly known. However, the presence of lipids in extracellular connective tissue matrix varies with the onset of osteoarthritis.[4]

Specific connective tissue organization of muscle fibers is systematically arranged by endomysium connective tissue. Muscle fibers collectively are bound together to form fascicles. These fascicles are supported by perimysium connective tissue. The connective tissue membrane surrounding the entire muscle is called *epimysium*. Muscle tissue is unique in that it consists of contractile elements that respond to stimuli and passive or elastic elements that resist stretching. Muscle tissue and noncontractile connective tissues such as endomysium, perimysium, and epimysium demonstrate characteristic load deformation viscoelastic properties in response to specific stimuli. Human skeletal muscle exhibits the same viscoelastic properties as other dense connective tissues. In fetal development, these noncontractile connective tissues act as tissue scaffolds to hold, support, and provide continuity of gross form and structure of the muscle belly. In addition, loose connective tissue of the perimysium serves as a channel for nutrient arteries and vessels as well as nerves that supply the muscle fibers.[4]

REVIEW OF TISSUE HEALING

Healing of biologic tissue is characterized by predictable, orderly, and sequential phases of **repair**. In essence, healing can be broadly classified as a series of three overlapping events: (1) inflammatory response, (2) proliferation, and (3) **remodeling** and tissue maturation. All musculoskeletal tissue proceeds to heal and repair by these individually unique processes.

INFLAMMATORY RESPONSE

Directly after trauma, platelets migrate to the injury site and release specific growth factors and chemical mediators, which stimulate homeostasis and initiate the repair process. A fibrin scaffold structure is formed within the trauma bed, creating a matrix that allows for platelet aggregation and adherence to the injury site. This process of platelet activation stimulates synthesis of thrombin and fibrin and the random organization of clot formation. Platelet plug formation is essentially a four-step process: (1) adhesion, (2) aggregation, (3) secretion, and (4) procoagulant activity (Fig. 8-1).

Important Concepts

Acute inflammation is a transient initial phase of injury repair that lasts approximately 5 to 7 days.

Adhesion of platelets is the deposition of these cells on the subendothelial matrix. Platelets have a surface receptor glycoprotein that binds to a sticky protein substance referred to as *von Willebrand factor* found in the subendothelial matrix. Endothelial cells synthesize von Willebrand factor, which is released into the circulating plasma and deposited in the subendothelial matrix in response to exposure from injury.[1,3] Aggregation is simply platelet-to-platelet

WOUNDS

REACTION: HEMOSTASIS

Definition: The first stage in wound healing is hemostasis (hemo, *blood*; stasis, *standing*). It leads to clot formation and arrest of blood loss from severed blood vessels.

How bleeding is stopped

When a blood vessel is damaged, a series of reactions are initiated to arrest bleeding. The hemostatic process involves at least four interelated steps: adhesion, accumulation and cohesion, platelet surface clotting, and consolidation.

Collagen's work

To facilitate platelet activation and serve as a cofactor in blood coagulation.

Activation

The collagen surface activates platelets causing them to change shape, become sticky and release chemicals.

Accumulation/adhesion

In response to collagen, platelets stick to the vessel wall and themselves creating an initial plug.

Cofactor for blood coagulation

Collagen is a catalyst for the body's natural clotting mechanism.

Formation of a hemostatic plug

Platelets form a net that is a foundation for the clotting mechanism to build upon.

Step 1

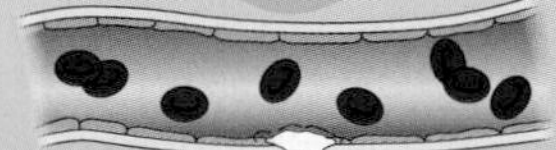

Immediately after vessel rupture, platelets are activated in response to contact with collagen.

Step 2

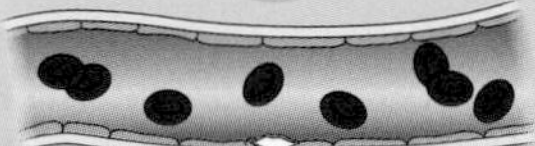

Platelets become sticky and adhere to the collagen as well as themselves and form a barrier to restrict blood loss.

Step 3

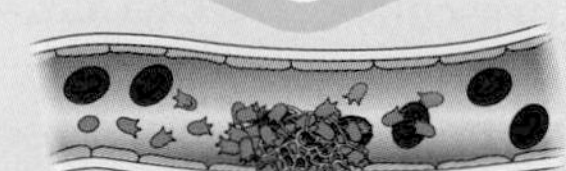

The second phase of the clotting mechanism kicks in to reinforce the platelets barrier and forms a solid clot.

Step 4

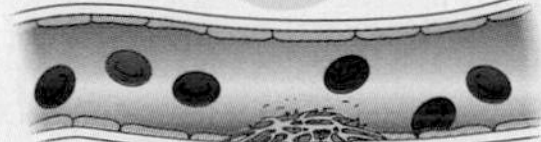

Finally, the scab contracts and becomes stable, preparing the wound for the next phase of healing.

Key cell: Platelet

The blood cell responsible for initial response to the rupture of a blood vessel.

Platelets initiate hemostasis by sticking together and forming a net.

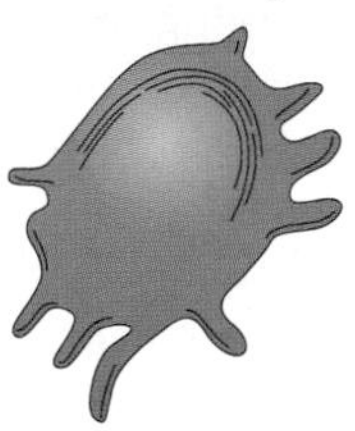

Function

The platelet's sole responsibility is to form a plug to limit blood loss when a vessel is ruptured.

Structure

A platelet is a disk-shaped, nonnucleated blood cell. It has a cytoplasm and is highly granulated. It also contains many tube-like structures.

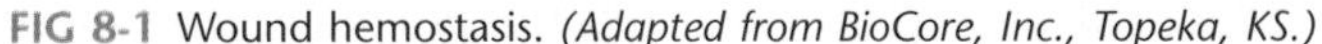

FIG 8-1 Wound hemostasis. *(Adapted from BioCore, Inc., Topeka, KS.)*

cohesion via the surface fibrinogen receptor complex of the platelets. Secretion is the release of numerous platelet-derived growth factors (PDGFs) by stimulated platelets. The aggregating stimulators of serotonin, thrombospondin, and thromboxane also are secreted. Procoagulant activity refers to the process of thrombin formation and ensures that coagulation occurs at the site of the platelet plug.

INFLAMMATION

Initially triggered by the release of histamine from mast cells in the surrounding tissue, the inflammatory response is amplified by cytokines (signaling molecules) such as interleukin (IL)-1 and tumor necrosis factors (TNFs) that are activated by leukocytes (white blood cells). These leukocytes are involved with phagocytosis, or the engulfment of cellular debris. Cytokines stimulate vascular permeability allowing mononuclear cells to mobilize, proliferate, and differentiate into monocytes at the injury site. Other cytokines such as PDGF, insulinlike growth factor (IGF), and transforming growth factor (TGF)-β help organize the specific sequence of migration of neutrophils, macrophages, and then fibroblasts to the injury site.

Important Concepts

The inflammatory process is triggered by the release of histamine from mast cells in the tissue surrounding the injury site.

FIBROPLASIA

Several days (5 to 7) after the injury, the relative population of fibroblasts increases, whereas inflammatory cells and proinflammatory factors decrease. At this stage, there is a proliferation of reparative cells. Fibroblasts stimulate PDGF and TGF-β, among others, to synthesize and deposit extracellular matrix constituents of fibronectin, laminin, collagen, and GAGs.[1,3,4]

This phase also includes angiogenesis, the neovascular budding that helps reestablish oxygen-rich and growth factor–rich blood to new, fragile healing tissue. Angiogenic growth factors involved with the stimulation of this neovascularization are fibroblast growth factor (FGF), TNF-β, and wound angiogenesis factor. Endothelial cells from intact vascular membranes are mobilized to form new tissue from the secretion of specific enzymes and collagens. The end stages of angiogenesis signal vascular capillary and network tube formation, creating new vascular basement membranes that directly communicate with the injury site.[1,3,4]

REMODELING AND TISSUE MATURATION

The remodeling phase of injury repair is essentially a balance between the deposition, organization, modification, and maturation of necessary collagen and the enzymatic (proteolytic) degradation of excess collagen. There is a systematic regression of inflammatory cells during this phase as well (Fig. 8-2).

Collagenases are enzymes of the metalloproteinase family that act to fragment collagen. The regulation of the rate of collagen synthesis and degradation (turnover) is mediated by specific growth factors such as PDGF, ILs, TGF-β, and TNF-β.[4]

Important Concepts

Remodeling is a balance between the deposition, organization, modification, and maturation of necessary collagen and the degradation of excess collagen.

Cummings and Reynolds[2] described remodeling as "the process by which the architecture of connective tissue alters in response to stress." Collagen fibers align parallel to the direction of applied stress, which increases the strength of the scar tissue union. Remodeling also includes absorption of collagen fibers that lie in opposing directions. If controlled properly, the effect of the remodeling phase is that the fibrous union becomes stronger and more supple with fewer adhesions.

Because of the vascularity, the dense cell population of myofibroblasts, and the nature of its small fragile collagen fibers, new scar tissue is able to remodel quickly. Collagen fibers are initially small and disorganized, and they form a spongy, randomly oriented tissue. As remodeling continues, larger, more parallel fibers replace the smaller fibers and orient across the wound, which forms a stronger yet supple repair (Fig. 8-3).[2]

GENERAL CELL TYPES INVOLVED IN INJURY REPAIR

Various cells with complex interactions are involved with tissue homeostasis, injury, and repair processes. Generally, cell membranes are plasma-based with a relatively selective permeable barrier, which promotes bidirectional flow of molecules. The major components of cellular plasma membranes are proteins and lipids. The major relevant class of cell membrane lipids is phospholipids.

CELLULAR STRUCTURE

Organelles define various component structures within cells. Smooth endoplasmic reticulum as a cell organ is involved with the synthesis of steroid hormones, particularly cholesterol. Rough endoplasmic reticulum organelles are actively involved with protein synthesis and secretion. Within cells, the Golgi apparatus functions primarily as a storage and modification organ for various proteins that have been synthesized in the rough endoplasmic reticulum. Lysosomes and peroxisomes are cellular compartment structures that are involved with enzymatic degradation and oxidation of protein and fatty acids. Mitochondria, the powerhouses of the cell, are actively involved with adenosine triphosphate production and protein synthesis.[1,3]

PROTEOGLYCANS AND GLYCOPROTEINS

Proteoglycans are macromolecules consisting of a protein core and bound polysaccharide units referred to as GAGs. GAGs are major components of ground substance within the extracellular matrix of various connective tissues, such as ligament, capsule, muscle, tendon, cartilage, nerve, vessel, and bone. GAGs are synthesized within the

WOUNDS

HEALING PROCESS

Definition: A *wound* is created when the anatomic integrity of the tissue is disrupted. Healing is the process whereby the integrity of the tissue is restored.

How the body heals

Regardless of the nature, type or size of a wound, the healing process is universal. A simple shaving cut and a third-degree burn follow the same specific steps in the course of healing. Collagen is a key element of each wound healing step for every wound.

Healing is a continuous process with distinct phases that overlap. Healing is divided into three phases to describe dominant activity at any given time.

Collagen's work

Collagen provides a favorable environment for the wound healing process in several ways:

- Helps in the formation of a plug to stop bleeding.
- Cleans the wound, removes bacteria and debris by absorbtion. Provides environment for macrophages.
- Provides optimal environment for cells. Integral factor in angiogenisis. Provides optimal environment for vascularization. Promotes formation of granulation tissue.
- Reconstruction of tissues accelerated by collagen. Reduces contracture and scarring.

Injury

Hemostasis

Sticky blood platelets adhere to exposed collagen to form a plug for broken blood vessels. As more platelets collect they adhere not only to the vessel wall, but to one another, forming a plug.

Step 1

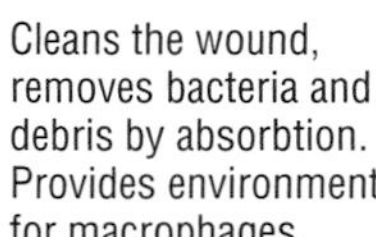

Reaction

Vascular and cellular response to injury give rise to inflammation, the hallmark of this phase. Blood flow is decreased by vasodilation and white cells are brought in to combat infection.

Step 2

Regeneration

The body begins repairing itself by generating red, vascular (granulation) tissue to replace the scab and debris in the wound. This is followed by restoration of the epidermis and subsequent wound closure.

Step 3

Remodeling

Collagen content of the wound continues to increase with a corresponding increase in wound strength. The end result is a relatively weak and brittle tissue called a scar.

Step 4

Healed wound

Obstacles

Wound healing is disturbed by deficiencies, drugs and disease.

Infection

Challenge by bacteria, fungus, or virus to the wound may slow or interrupt healing. In order to resume the normal healing process, contamination or infection must be controlled.

Necrosis

Tissues that lack blood flow may become necrotic and die. This arrests the healing process. The tissue must be removed for the healing process to resume.

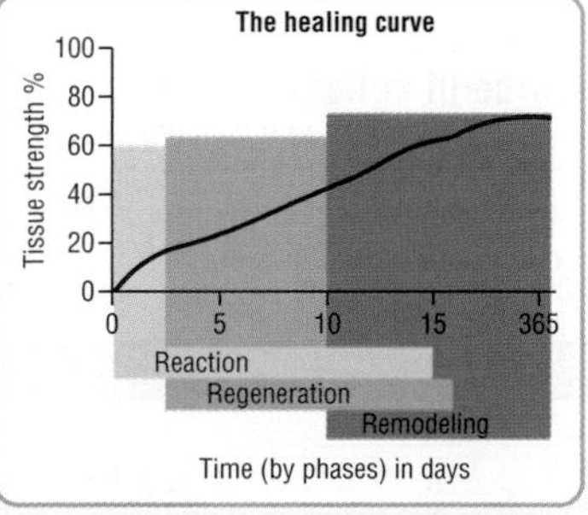

FIG 8-2 Remodeling and tissue maturation. *(Adapted from BioCore, Inc., Topeka, KS.)*

COLLAGEN

Overview

Definition: Collagen is the most abundant protein found in the body. It is safe enough to be used as a food product and versatile enough to handle problems ranging from fluid absorption to regeneration of tissue.

Collagen and the body

Collagen fibers give strength and structure to tissues in the body. Fibroblast cells produce collagen which forms tissue structures. Tissues contain collagen fibers arranged in three dimensions. Collagen fibers contain smaller units called fibrils. Fibrils are organized collagen molecules. Each molecule is a rope-like structure with three strands. Each strand has a specific sequence determining collagen type and function.

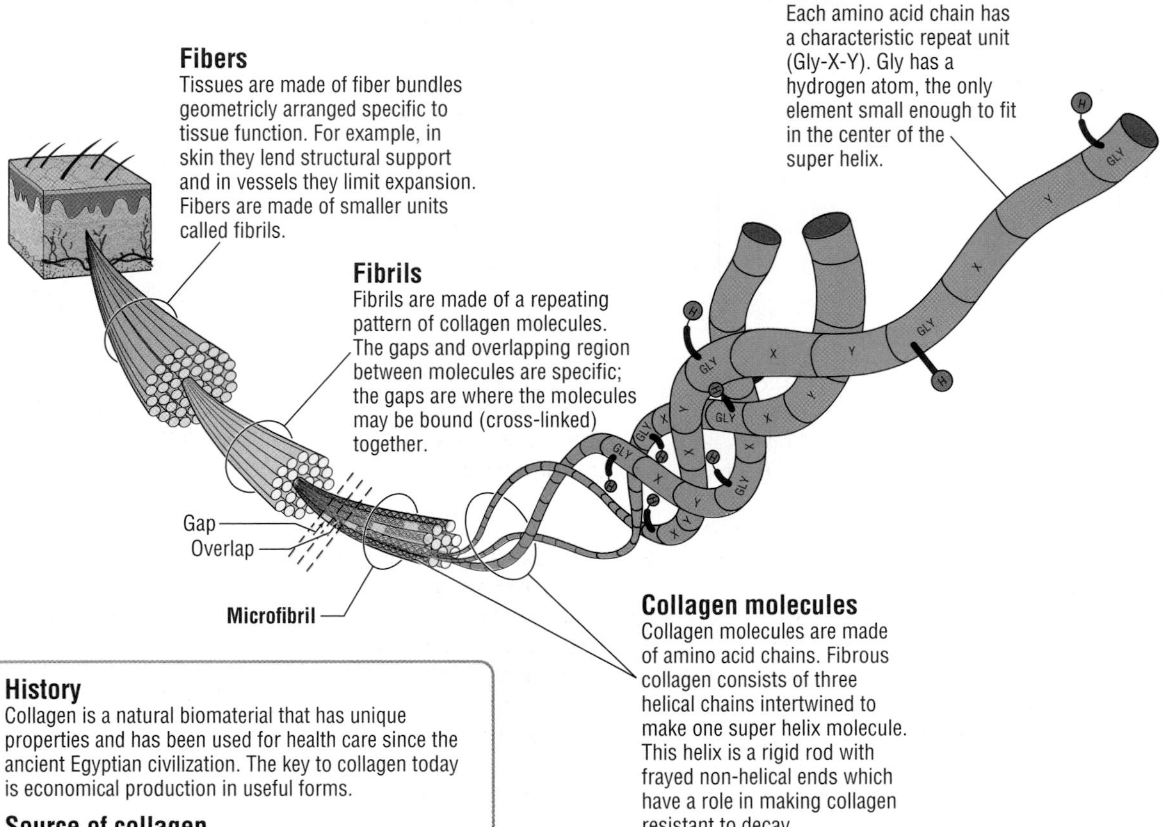

History

Collagen is a natural biomaterial that has unique properties and has been used for health care since the ancient Egyptian civilization. The key to collagen today is economical production in useful forms.

Source of collagen

The most abundant and well characterized collagen is type I extracted from bovine (cow) hide. However, collagen can be obtained from many sources including porcine (pig) skin, chicken tendon, bovine tendon, etc.

Tracing collagen through the body

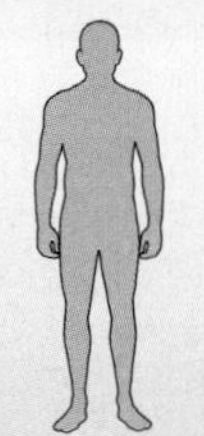

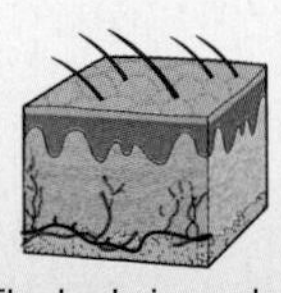

The body is made of **tissues**

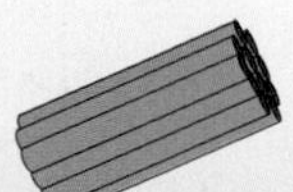

Tissues are made of bundles of fibers; fibers are made of **fibrils**

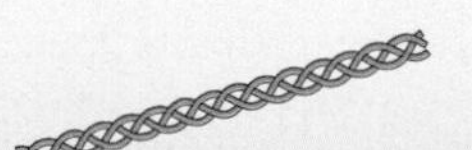

Fibrils are made of **collagen molecules**

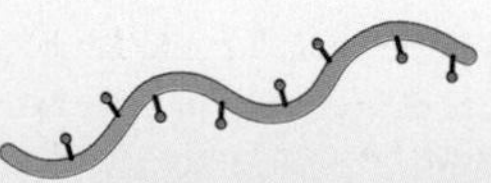

Collagen molecules are made of **chains of amino acids**

FIG 8-3 Collagen overview. *(Adapted from BioCore, Inc., Topeka, KS.)*

endoplasmic reticulum and Golgi apparatus of the fibroblast cells in connective tissues. Several GAGs are identified in musculoskeletal tissues that significantly contribute to structure, composition, and function of the extracellular matrix of tissues, as follows: (1) chondroitin sulfate, (2) dermatan sulfate, (3) keratan sulfate, (4) hyaluronate, (5) aggrecan, (6) decorin, and (7) biglycan.[1,3]

Generally, GAGs carry a high negative charge that renders them hydrophilic. Within articular cartilage, GAGs are continuously synthesized, assembled, degraded, and secreted by the extracellular matrix to establish a relative homeostatic environment. Enzymatic degradation of GAGs occurs within lysosome organelles of the chondrocytes.[1,3,4]

Glycoproteins are molecules that organize and maintain the structure of the extracellular matrix. In articular cartilage, these are fibronectin, laminin, anchorin, and tenascin.

CELLS OF INFLAMMATION AND REPAIR

The complex cascade of molecular events during the inflammatory phase are mediated by cytokines acting through endocrine (distant cells), paracrine (adjacent cells), or autocrine (same cells) stimulation.

POLYMORPHONUCLEAR LEUKOCYTES

Granulocytes, or polymorphonuclear leukocytes, differentiate into neutrophils, basophils, and eosinophils when stimulated by cytokine growth factors and colony-stimulating factors. Neutrophils, the most abundant granulocytes, are leukocytes that migrate to damaged tissue after mediation and activation of cytokines, platelet factor 4, and TGF-β that are released by platelets. A primary function of neutrophils is initial phagocytosis of foreign matter, bacteria, and cellular debris from the damaged tissue site. Neutrophils also contribute to the immune system inflammation process by stimulation, vasodilation, and vascular permeability assisting with transportation and migration of molecules and cytokine growth factor–PDGF propagating events to minimize intense inflammatory reactions further.

MONONUCLEAR LEUKOCYTES

Mononuclear leukocytes are single-nucleus cells that are derived from pluripotent hematopoietic stem cells, which differentiate into monocytes and lymphocytes. Circulating monocytes are mobilized to damaged tissue, where they are activated and become macrophages. Noted as *scavenger cells,* macrophages are leukocytes that display three essential functions during the inflammatory process: (1) phagocytosis, (2) antigen presentation, and (3) production of cytokine growth factors.[1,3,4]

Macrophages synthesize and secrete numerous cytokines, such as TGF-β, PDGF, TGF-α, and IL-1. The release of these cytokines stimulates proliferation of fibroblasts and collagen deposition and degradation of collagen by secreting enzymes (collagenases) also, which denatures collagen during the inflammatory and remodeling phases.[1,3,4]

FIBROBLASTS

Fibroblasts, important and highly specialized cells, are actively involved with collagen production of various stages of injury repair. Fibroblastic cell proliferation is activated by cytokines released by platelets and leukocytes. PDGF is responsible for the stimulation of fibroblast proliferation. Fibroblasts serve a critical function in wound healing mechanics. Fibronectin is a glycoprotein produced by fibroblasts that acts to bind collagen within the extracellular matrix of healing tissue. Myofibroblasts are specialized contractile cell types that are important during the later stages of wound repair, contracting the edges of the wound.

Important Concepts

Fibroblasts, important and highly specialized cells, are actively involved with collagen production of various stages of injury repair.

PROSTAGLANDINS, THROMBOXANES, AND LEUKOTRIENES

Prostaglandins and thromboxanes are lipid-derived powerful and important mediators of inflammatory reactions (Fig. 8-4) that are metabolized from arachidonic acids within the cells. Arachidonic acid metabolism is initiated by the degradation of cell membrane phospholipids by phospholipase enzymes. This cell membrane degradation releases arachidonic acid–synthesized cyclooxygenase enzymes, such as COX-1 and COX-2, which results in metabolic conversion to prostaglandins and thromboxanes.

Prostaglandins are generally of three forms[1,3]: (1) prostaglandin E_2, which stimulates smooth muscle relaxation and vasodilation; (2) prostaglandin I_2, which is synthesized in endothelial cells and incites vascular dilation and inhibition of platelet adhesion; and (3) prostaglandin F_2, which is a potent vasoconstrictor and stimulates smooth muscle contractions. These molecules are capable of producing pain and stimulating synthesis of pain-producing chemicals.[1,3] Thromboxanes are synthesized by platelets and are products of the cyclooxygenase pathway along with prostaglandins. These cell-signaling molecules are potent vasoconstrictors and smooth muscle contractors. Leukotrienes are products of an alternative arachidonic acid metabolic pathway. In this pathway, lipoxygenase is converted to leukotrienes, which act as smooth muscle contractors; lipoxygenase also stimulates bronchoconstriction and is a strong mediator of various other inflammatory chemicals (chemotactic).[1,3]

Various pharmacologic agents involved with antiinflammatory action—corticosteroids and nonsteroidal antiinflammatory drugs (NSAIDs)—target arachidonic acid for the inhibition of prostaglandins, thromboxanes, and leukotrienes. Specifically, corticosteroids inhibit production of arachidonic acid metabolites (cyclooxygenase and lipoxygenase) by inhibiting the conversion of cell membrane phospholipids to arachidonic acid. Conversely, NSAIDs are post–arachidonic acid inhibitors of the specific cyclooxygenase (COX-1, COX-2) metabolic pathway.

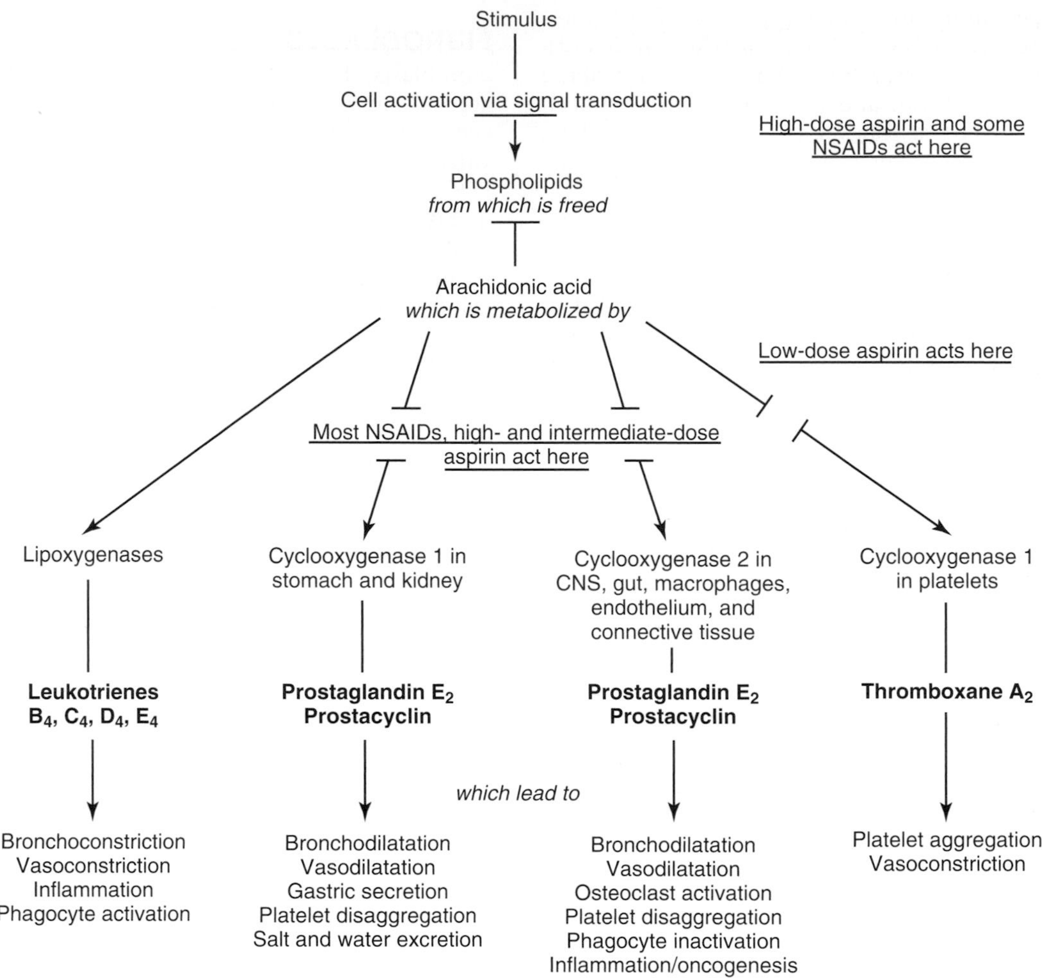

FIG 8-4 The inflammatory cascade. *CNS,* central nervous system; *NSAIDs,* nonsteroidal antiinflammatory drugs. *(From Goldman L, Bennett JC:* Cecil textbook of medicine, *ed 21, Philadelphia, 2000, Saunders, p. 115.)*

Important Concepts

Various pharmacologic agents involved with antiinflammatory action—corticosteroids and NSAIDs—target arachidonic acid for the inhibition of prostaglandins, thromboxanes, and leukotrienes.

CYTOKINES

Cytokines, including many growth factors, are a large and complex group (>100 identified) of protein-soluble peptide signaling molecules that are synthesized and secreted by all musculoskeletal tissues. They are used for cellular communication and stimulate cell proliferation, differentiation, and regulation of normal growth, homeostasis, injury, disease, and repair (Table 8-1). Generally referred to as *mitogenic,* cytokines are powerful and important immunologic mediators that coordinate and amplify various repair processes of injured musculoskeletal tissues.[1,3]

Cytokines are named for either the biologic actions they perform or the tissue on which they exert action. TNF-α is a proinflammatory cytokine synthesized and secreted by macrophages, lymphocytes, and monocytes. The biologic effects and anatomic target tissues are varied and diverse. General target tissues include stimulation of leukocytes, mononuclear phagocytes, vascular endothelial cells, fibroblasts, chondrocytes, and synovial macrophages. TNF-α activates granulocytes and stimulates other proinflammatory cytokines, which are also important regulators of bone resorption. IL-1 is also a proinflammatory cytokine that is synthesized by various cells. Tissue targets include monocytes, synovial macrophages, fibroblasts, chondrocytes, and endothelial cells. Biologically mediated effects include inhibition of extracellular matrix synthesis within chondrocytes, stimulation of fibroblast proliferation, proliferation of T cells, and stimulation of other proinflammatory cytokine synthesis. IL-7 is also a proinflammatory growth factor responsible for additional cytokine secretion and stimulation of prostaglandins in epithelial, endothelial, and fibroblastic cells.

TGF-β is a potent immunosuppressive cytokine with strong anabolic activity in cartilage. TGF-β reduces enzymatic degradation activity specifically within cartilage. In addition, TGF-β promotes wound healing, bone formation, and neovascular activity.[1,3,4]

TABLE 8-1 Types and Functions of Cytokines

Type	Primary Functions
Interleukins	
IL-1	Augments immune response; inflammatory mediator; promotes maturation and clonal expansion of B cells; enhances activity of NK cells; activates T cells and macrophages
IL-2	Induces proliferation and differentiation of T cells; activation of T cells, NK cells, and macrophages; stimulates release of other cytokines (IFN-α, TNF, IL-1, IL-6)
IL-3 (multicolony colony-stimulating factor)	Hematopoietic growth factor for hematopoietic precursor cells
IL-4	B-cell growth factor; stimulates proliferation and differentiation of B cells; induces differentiation into T_H2 cells; stimulates growth of mast cells
IL-5	B-cell growth and differentiation; promotes growth and differentiation of eosinophils
IL-6	T- and B-cell growth factor; enhances inflammatory response; promotes differentiation of B cells into plasma cells; stimulates antibody secretion; induces fever; synergistic effects with IL-1 and TNF
IL-7	Promotes growth of T and B cells
IL-8	Chemotaxis of neutrophils and T cells; stimulates superoxide and granule release
IL-9	Enhances T-cell survival; mast cell activation
IL-10	Inhibits cytokine production by T and NK cells; promotes B-cell proliferation and antibody responses; potent suppressor of macrophage function
IL-11	Synergistic action with IL-3 and IL-4 in hematopoiesis; multifunctional regulator of hematopoiesis and lymphopoiesis; osteoclast formation; elevates platelet count; inhibits proinflammatory cytokine production
IL-12	Promotes IFN-α production; induction of T helper cells; activates NK cells; stimulates proliferation of activated T and NK cells
IL-13	B-cell growth and differentiation; inhibits proinflammatory cytokine production
IL-14	Stimulates proliferation of activated B cells
IL-15	Mimics IL-2 effects; stimulates proliferation of T and NK cells
IL-16	Proinflammatory cytokine; chemoattractant of T cells, eosinophils, and monocytes
IL-17	Promotes release of IL-6, IL-8, and G-CSF; enhances expression of adhesion molecules
IL-18	Induces IFN-α, IL-2, and GM-CSF production; important role in development of T helper cells; enhances NK activity; inhibits production of IL-10
IL-19	Similar to IL-10
IL-20	Similar to IL-10
IL-21	Similar to IL-2, IL-4, and IL-5
IL-22	Similar to IL-10
IL-23	Similar to IL-12; promotes memory T-cell proliferation
IL-24	Similar to IL-10
IL-25	Promotes T_H2 cytokine production
IL-26	Similar to IL-10
IL-27	Similar to IL-12
Interferons	
IFN-α	Inhibit viral replication; activate NK cells and macrophages; antiproliferative effects on tumor cells
IFN-β	Is produced by fibroblasts and epithelial cells and is involved in humoral immune responses against viruses
IFN-γ	Activates macrophages, neutrophils, and NK cells; promotes B-cell differentiation; inhibits viral replication
TNF	Activates macrophages and granulocytes; promotes immune and inflammatory responses; kills tumor cells; is responsible for extensive weight loss associated with chronic inflammation and cancer
Colony-stimulating factors	
G-CSF	Stimulates proliferation and differentiation of neutrophils; enhances functional activity of mature PMNs
GM-CSF	Stimulates proliferation and differentiation of PMNs and monocytes
M-CSF	Promotes proliferation, differentiation, and activation of monocytes and macrophages
Erythropoietin	Stimulates erythroid progenitor cells in bone marrow to produce red blood cells

G-CSF, granulocyte colony-stimulating factor; *GM-CSF,* granulocyte-macrophage colony-stimulating factor; *IFN,* interferon; *IL,* interleukin; *M-CSF,* macrophage colony-stimulating factor; *NK,* natural killer; *PMNs,* polymorphonuclear neutrophils; T_H2, helper T2; *TNF,* tumor necrosis factor.
Adapted from Lewis SM. *Medical-surgical nursing: assessment and management of clinical problems,* ed 7, St Louis, 2008, Mosby.

IGF regulates many musculoskeletal functions. Generally, IGF stimulates proteoglycan synthesis, chondrocyte proliferation, and osteoblast matrix synthesis. Target cells for neovascularization include platelets and endothelial cells.

PDGF contributes significant stimulation toward the repair process of musculoskeletal and vascular tissue. Cell types activated by PDGF include platelets, neutrophils, macrophages, fibroblasts, and endothelial cells. Biologic activity activated by PDGF includes homeostasis, initiation of wound repair cascade phagocytic activity, synthesis, and deposition of extracellular matrix constituents and angiogenesis activity.

Vascular endothelial growth factor (VEGF) is an important angiogenic cytokine that stimulates endothelial cell proliferation. VEGF significantly contributes to

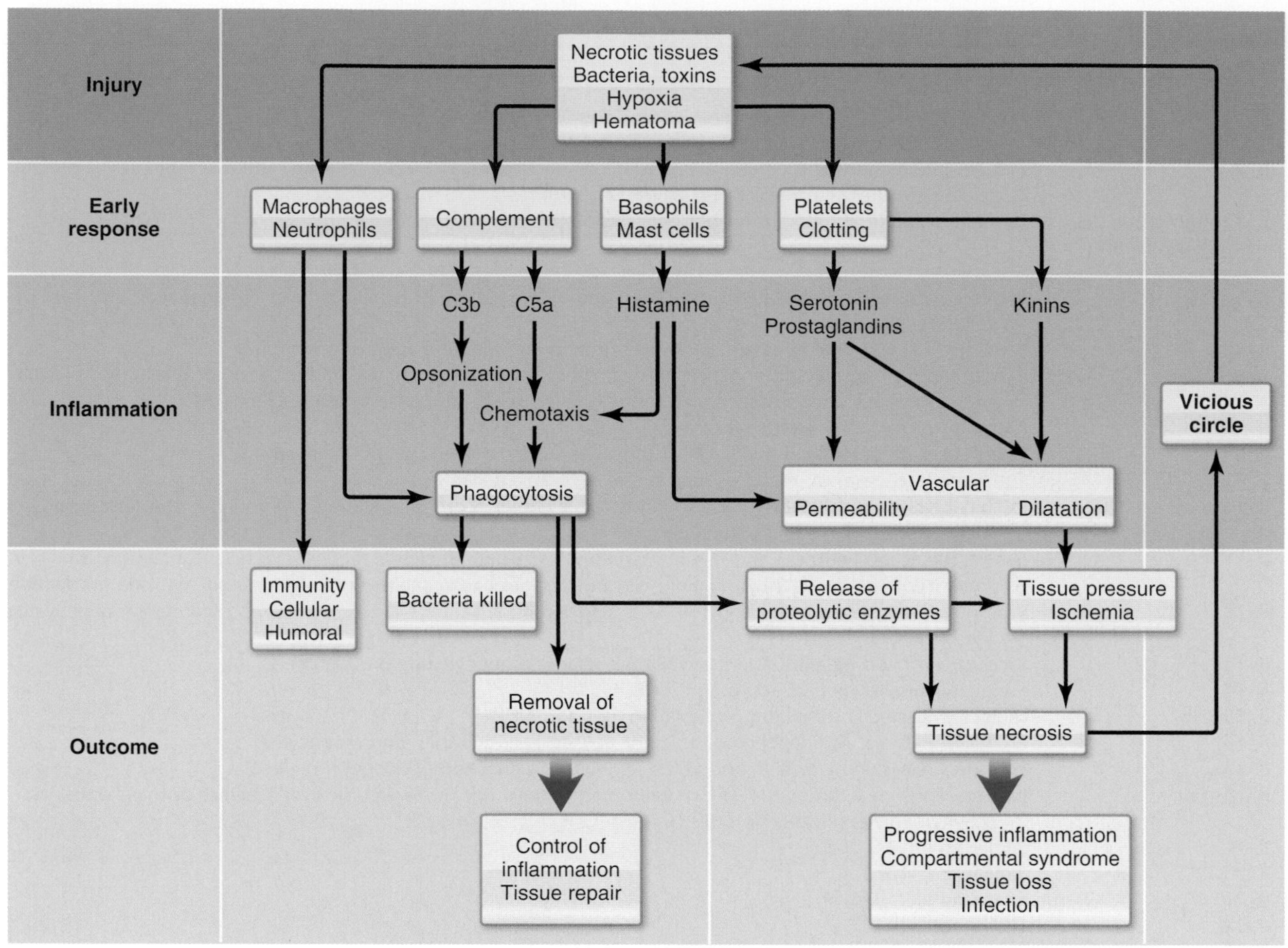

FIG 8-5 Results of the necrotic process: cellular, hematologic, and immunologic responses to injury lead to repair or further destruction. *(Modified from Browner BD, Levine A, Jupiter J, et al:* Skeletal trauma, *ed 4, Philadelphia, 2009, Saunders.)*

neovascularization. In addition, VEGF has been identified in the hypertrophic zone of calcified cartilage in the epiphyseal plate. VEGF stimulates endothelial cell ingrowth in this area, possibly enhancing cartilage conversion to bone. VEGF also is responsible for the release of degradative enzymes in the extracellular matrix.

FGF stimulates cell proliferation of cartilage matrix and bone tissue. FGF is also an effective angiogenic stimulant for revascularization after injury and promotes epithelial cell activity during remodeling and neovascular growth.

Important Concepts

FGF is an effective angiogenic stimulant for revascularization after injury and promotes epithelial cell activity during remodeling and neovascular growth.

Overall, tissue disruption and subsequent repair processes initiate and propagate complex cellular events mediated by cytokines. Cytokines regulate, stimulate, and express other growth factors to synthesize, proliferate, excrete, and mobilize numerous molecules involved with extracellular matrix deposition, cartilage synthesis, vascular growth, enzymatic degradation, and modulation of inflammatory immune reactions during injury and repair of musculoskeletal and neurovascular repair (Fig. 8-5).[1,3]

GENERAL CELL INJURY AND REPAIR

Cellular hypertrophy is an adaptive response to a specific applied stimulus when cells and tissues are able to cope physiologically with unusual or stressful demands that do not rupture the cell's phospholipid membrane or damage the mitochondria. This situation is essentially a reversible cell injury.[1,3]

Cells also can become irreversibly damaged. Hypoxia, caused by ischemia, is the most common cause of irreversible cell injury. Tissue or **cellular necrosis** refers to the aggregate morphologic changes after irreversible cell injury. When cells are damaged, specific organelles (lysosomes) are involved with autolysis, or self-killing, leading to tissue necrosis. Cells of the immune system are involved with the process of heterolysis through phagocytosis and degranulation from active circulating T cells. **Apoptosis** refers to programmed cellular, organelle, and nuclear disassembly and death. In contrast to necrosis, in which organelles rupture, cell phospholipid membranes tear from intracellular swelling, and inflammatory reactions occur from cell debris. Apoptosis is more organized and systematic without inducing an inflammatory response. Apoptosis is an efficient, controlled process of orderly cellular, organelle, and nuclear shrinkage and disassembly of intracellular structures.[1,3]

GENERAL REPAIR AND REGENERATION PROCESS

The term ***regeneration*** specifically refers to injured tissue being replaced with identical or similar tissue. The process occurs from the activation of various cytokine growth factors that stimulate the synthesis, differentiation, and proliferation of specialized cells that regenerate the damaged tissue. Repair processes involve adaptive scar tissue replacement within the damaged musculoskeletal tissue rather than regenerative similar tissue. Fibroplasia, extracellular matrix synthesis, deposition, and collagen formation serve as the foundation for intrinsically repaired tissue.

Specific cells are subclassified according to identified healing characteristics. Labile cells are cells that are proliferative and capable of regeneration after injury. For example, epithelial cells are labile, requiring continued proliferation and regeneration throughout life. Stable cells typically are not continuously regenerating. However, they are capable of regeneration after injury with appropriate stimulation from various cytokines. Permanent cells are cells that cannot regenerate after surgery. Permanent cells require fibroplasia, matrix synthesis, and collagen formation with adaptive scar tissue.

GLOSSARY

Apoptosis: Programmed cell death; no inflammation reaction; cell shrinkage with maintenance of organelles.

Cellular necrosis: Swelling of cells, loss of organelle structure, rupture of cell membrane, breakdown of cell nucleus, and inflammation.

Glycosaminoglycans (GAGs): The most common GAGs are hyaluronic acid, chondroitin sulfate, heparan sulfate, dermatan sulfate, and keratan sulfate.

Ground substance: The space between cells and collagen fibers composed of water, salts, and proteoglycans.

Maturation: The process of maturing of granulation tissue to relative avascular fibrous tissue.

Regeneration: Traumatized tissue is replaced by biochemically similar tissues resulting from stimulation and proliferation of local specialized cells.

Remodeling: Collagen and fibrous tissue organization and orientation to a stable scar.

Repair: Traumatized tissue is replaced with scar.

REFERENCES

1. Cell biology. In *United States medical licensing examination, step I. The Princeton review*, ed 3, New York, 2000, Random House.
2. Cummings GS, Reynolds CA: Principles of soft tissue extensibility of joint contracture management. In Wadsworth C, editor: *Strength conditioning. Applications in orthopaedics*, LaCrosse, WI, 1998, APTA, Inc.
3. Kent TH, Hart MN: Injury, inflammation, and repair. In *Introduction to human disease*, ed 3, Norwalk, CT, 1993, Appleton & Lange.
4. Mankin HJ, Mow VC, Buckwalter JA, et al: Articular cartilage structure, composition, and function. In Buckwalter JA, Einhorn TA, Simon SR, editors: *Orthopedic basic science, biology, and biomechanics of the musculoskeletal system*, ed 2, Rosemont, IL, 2000, American Academy of Orthopedic Surgeons.

REVIEW QUESTIONS

Multiple Choice

1. Which two amino acids are directly responsible for the cross-linking of elastin fiber and its unique ability to deform under stress and then return to its original orientation and shape?
   a. Glycine and proline
   b. Desmosine and isodesmosine
   c. Alanine and valine
   d. Hydroxyproline and hydroxylysine
2. What is a noncollagenous glycoprotein in which molecules are arranged randomly as a constituent of extracellular connective tissue matrix?
   a. Elastin
   b. Collagen
   c. Ground substance
   d. GAGs
3. What is the most abundant component of the connective tissue matrix?
   a. Lipids
   b. Collagen
   c. Proteoglycans
   d. Elastin
4. Which amino acid is generally responsible for resisting tensile forces in collagen?
   a. Glycine
   b. Hydroxyproline
   c. Lysine
   d. Proline
5. ________________ is an amorphous nonfibrous aqueous-gel component of the connective tissue matrix.
   a. Elastin
   b. Collagen
   c. Ground substance
   d. GAGs
6. What regulates the spread of cells and has strong chemotactic properties that attract and bind various connective tissue cells?
   a. Fibronectin
   b. Laminin
   c. Anchorin
   d. Tenascin
7. What is a multifunctional glycoprotein found in the extracellular matrix that is important in establishing epithelial tissue and basement membranes during wound healing?
   a. Decorin
   b. Aggrecan
   c. Laminin
   d. Biglycan
8. Approximately how long does the acute inflammation phase of injury repair last?
   a. 5 to 7 days
   b. 7 to 14 days
   c. 30 days
   d. 3 months

9. ________________ migrate(s) to the injury site directly after trauma and release(s) specific growth factors and chemical mediators, which stimulate homeostasis and initiate the repair process.
   a. Mast cells
   b. Histamine
   c. Cytokines
   d. Platelets
10. What are (is) initially released from mast cells in the surrounding tissue that initially trigger(s) the inflammatory response after injury?
    a. Cytokines
    b. Histamine
    c. Leukocytes
    d. IGF
11. What is the neovascular budding that helps reestablish oxygen-rich and growth factor–rich blood to new, fragile healing tissue?
    a. Aggregation
    b. Collagenase
    c. Remodeling
    d. Angiogenesis
12. What is the process by which the architecture of connective tissue alters in response to stress?
    a. Remodeling
    b. Angiogenesis
    c. Collagenase
    d. Aggregation
13. What is a glycoprotein produced by fibroblasts that acts to bind collagen within the extracellular matrix of healing tissue?
    a. Biglycan
    b. Fibronectin
    c. Laminin
    d. Decorin
14. What growth factor stimulates cell proliferation of cartilage matrix and bone tissue?
    a. IGF
    b. TGF-β
    c. PDGF
    d. FGF
15. ________________ is an efficient, controlled process of orderly cellular, organelle, and nuclear shrinkage and disassembly of intracellular structures.
    a. Apoptosis
    b. Angiogenesis
    c. Cellular necrosis
    d. Collagenases

Short Answer

16. Name the five basic aggregate components of the extracellular matrix of connective tissues.
17. How is muscle tissue unique?
18. What are the four steps of platelet plug formation?
19. What is balanced during the remodeling phase of injury repair?
20. How do corticosteroids limit inflammation?

Fill in the Blank

21. Healing of biologic tissue is characterized by predictable, orderly, and sequential phases of repair. These phases are broadly classified into a series of three overlapping events: inflammatory response, ________________, and remodeling and tissue maturation.
22. These large proteoglycans, specifically chondroitin and keratan, bind together to form a distinct type of GAG referred to as ________________.
23. Carrying a high negative charge renders GAGs ________________.
24. Angiogenic growth factors involved with the stimulation of neovascularization are ________________, ________________, and ________________.
25. The connective tissue membrane surrounding the entire muscle is called ________________.

True/False

26. Elastin is a collagenous proteoglycan.
27. There are essentially three types of collagen found in musculoskeletal tissue.
28. GAGs are responsible for the tensile strength of cartilage matrix.
29. Chondroitin sulfate represents approximately 90% of all GAGs in cartilage.
30. NSAIDs are used to affect the cyclooxygenase pathway of arachidonic acid.

Chapter 9

Ligament Healing

Robert C. Manske, John DeWitt

CHAPTER OUTLINE

LEARNING OBJECTIVES

1. Define and discuss the inflammatory response to injury.
2. Describe the phases of healing and sequence of events characteristic of each phase.
3. Identify the five cardinal signs of inflammation.
4. Describe the effects of immobilization on ligaments.
5. Discuss the effects of stress and exercise on ligaments.
6. Identify and discuss practical clinical applications of stress deprivation and protected motion during phases of ligament healing.

KEY TERMS

Collagen
Continuous passive motion (CPM)
Immobilization
Inflammatory reaction
Ligament
Sprain

LIGAMENT ANATOMY

A skeletal **ligament** is uniformly classified as a band of grossly parallel, fibrous, dense connective tissue that "ties" or "binds" bones together at or near the margins of bony articulations.[45] Macroscopic gross examination reveals ligaments to be opaque, white band or cordlike tissue. Ligaments are composed of up to six genetically distinct types of **collagen**, although type I collagen represents the major fibrillar component (approximately 85%). Ligaments also contain fibroblasts, extracellular matrix, and varying amounts of elastin.[30] Type I collagen, the predominant structural collagen in the body, is structurally very strong in mature scars. Conversely, type III collagen is assembled in thin filaments and is more elastic in nature. This type of collagen is usually seen in immature scars and is more prevalent in newborns and young children. Proteoglycans are also found in ligamentous tissue. Proteoglycans are protein-sugar conjugates that have major water-binding properties and appear to be responsible for controlling water composition and distribution in ligaments.[22]

Important Concepts

Skeletal ligaments are uniformly classified as bands of grossly parallel, fibrous, dense connective tissue that "tie" or "bind" bones together at or near the margins of bony articulations.[45]

Certain ligaments (e.g., ligamentum nuchae) contain greater amounts of elastin, which contributes to different mechanical properties compared with ligaments with less elastin. Most ligaments are composed of less than 2% of elastin; however, this component may be an important contributor to low load recovery of ligaments.[21] Although considered hypovascular, ligaments demonstrate relative uniform microvascularity that originates from their origin and insertion sites.[45] Estimates are that only 1.5% of the extracellular matrix of the rabbit medial collateral ligament (MCL) is occupied by blood vessels.[36] Ligaments have a more ligament-specific blood supply that may be more functional and aids in promoting healing.[21] For example the popliteal artery gives rise to numerous branches that supply the knee joint. Although major branches of the middle and inferior genicular arteries supply the anterior cruciate ligament (ACL), it appears that even smaller branches supply synovium that covers the ACL. The MCL is supplied by the superior and inferior genicular arteries and is more highly vascularized in its superficial portion, whereas deeper portions are comparably less vascularized.[7]

Ligaments have a rich sensory innervation of specialized mechanoreceptors and free nerve endings that contribute to proprioception and pain, respectively. Ligament attachment to bone is by direct or indirect transition. Direct ligament insertion into bone represents a gradual change from specific ligament fiber to fibrocartilage to calcified fibrocartilage to bone. With indirect insertion, the superficial layers of ligament fibers attach directly in the periosteum, whereas the deep fibers transition to bone by way of Sharpey's perforating fibers.[45]

MECHANICAL PROPERTIES

Characteristic behavior of ligament substance (e.g., stress-strain, tensile loading) is directly influenced by collagen composition, proteoglycans, glycosaminoglycans (GAGs), orientation of fibers, and actions between extracellular matrix and ground substance. Anatomic location of various ligaments (extraarticular versus intraarticular) and cellular, histologic, ultrastructural, and biochemical differences strongly influence ligament mechanical and viscoelastic behavior. These unique differences between various ligaments influence intrinsic healing abilities, physical therapy procedures, and surgical intervention.

INJURY AND REPAIR

Similar to other vascular tissues, extraarticular ligaments heal in a highly structured, organized, and predictable fashion. Generally, the sequential cascade of events overlaps four stages of repair: phase I, homeostasis and degeneration; phase II, inflammation; phase III, proliferation and migration; and phase IV, remodeling and degeneration.[20]

> **Important Concepts**
>
> Four phases of repair include homeostasis and degeneration, inflammation, proliferation and migration, and remodeling and degeneration.

In contrast, intraarticular ligaments, although they demonstrate an intense vascular response to injury, do not heal spontaneously. The environment of intraarticular synovial fluid tends to dilute hematoma formation between the ends of the injured ligaments, while preventing fibrin clot organization and ultimately limiting the intrinsic healing mechanism.[45]

> **Important Concepts**
>
> The environment of intraarticular synovial fluid tends to dilute hematoma formation between the ends of the injured ligaments, while preventing fibrin clot organization and ultimately limiting the intrinsic healing mechanism.[45]

The **inflammatory reaction** to trauma represents phase I of the injury and repair cascade. Initially, the injured ends of the ligament retract and usually demonstrate a highly disorganized appearance. As the ligamentous microvascularity is disrupted, a hematoma forms between the damaged ends of tissue.

Phase II is marked by a release of extremely potent chemical mediators of vasodilation, cell wall permeability, and pain in response to fibrin clot formation. Prostaglandins, histamine, bradykinins, and serotonin are mobilized to the trauma site to increase capillary permeability and profuse dilation of blood vessels. This action allows migration of specific inflammatory polymorphonuclear cells and lymphocytes to the injured tissue to initiate the action of ingestion (phagocytosis) to remove bacteria and dead tissue. The predominant cell types present during the acute inflammatory phase are neutrophils and lymphocytes. Monocytes are referred to as *macrophages* as they become phagocytes.[45]

The production of type III collagen, extracellular matrix, and, within 2 days, proteoglycans by fibroblasts initiates the beginning of phase III matrix and cellular proliferation. Fibroblasts rapidly synthesize new extracellular matrix containing high concentrations of water; GAGs; and relatively weak, fragile, and immature type III collagen. Neovascularization (angiogenesis) begins as granulation tissue tenuously attaches to the damaged gap. The concentration of water, GAGs, and type III collagen gradually decreases over several weeks. Inflammatory cytokines are slowly removed from the injured site. Fibroblastic activity synthesizes type I collagen during this highly cellular phase of repair. There is a marked decrease in vascularity within the repair tissue as the collagen concentration increases. Matrix organization continues as the fibrils of type I collagen slowly arrange and align in response to appropriately applied stress. As the density of collagen, elastin, and proteoglycans increases, the tensile properties of repaired tissue also increase.[44]

Remodeling and maturation of intrinsically repaired ligament tissue is a slow process that characteristically lasts 1 year or more. This phase IV tissue repair process is an overlapping transition from the matrix and cellular proliferation phase of tissue healing. During this final phase, active matrix synthesis decreases, and type III collagen transitions to type I, improving stiffness. The hallmark of phase IV remodeling is collagen organization and increases in tensile strength of the repair tissue.

Intrinsically repaired extraarticular ligament does not return to normal, biochemically or biomechanically. Even after considerable time and remodeling of dense connective tissue, ultimate tensile strength may approach only 50% to 70% of normal ligaments 1 year after injury.[32,45]

> **Important Concepts**
>
> Healing of intrinsically repaired extraarticular ligament results in ultimate tensile strength that approaches 50% to 70% of normal ligaments even after 1 year.

The most common injury of joints is ligament **sprain.** The knee and ankle joints are common areas of sprains, with knee ligament sprains, particularly of the MCL, occurring in 25% to 40% of all knee injuries.[13,37]

> **Important Concepts**
>
> An injury to a skeletal ligament is termed a *sprain.*

Not all ligaments heal at the same rate or to the same degree.[6] For example, the ACL does not appear to heal as well as the MCL of the knee.[46] Factors affecting ligament healing include blood supply and function.[23,46]

Three key conditions must be present for ligaments to remodel or heal properly:[6]

1. Torn ligament ends must be in contact with each other.
2. Progressive, controlled stress must be applied to the healing tissues to orient scar tissue formation.
3. The ligament must be protected against excessive forces during the remodeling process.

The continuum of the healing process outlined here is ligament specific. Healing is related to blood supply, degree of injury, and mechanical stresses applied to the ligament.[6]

NONSURGICAL REPAIR VERSUS SURGICAL REPAIR

Ligaments can be repaired surgically or allowed to heal conservatively without surgery, depending on the degree of injury and involvement of supporting tissues. Investigators have shown that untreated ligaments heal by way of scar tissue proliferation rather than true ligament regeneration.[16] Untreated ligament tears are biochemically inferior, possessing a large portion of type III immature collagen, and generally are not healed at 40 weeks after injury.[16]

The following is a list of grades of injury occurring to ligament tissue. They are graded by severity:

Grade I: Microscopic tearing of the ligament without producing joint laxity
Grade II: Tearing of some ligament fibers with moderate laxity
Grade III: Complete rupture of the ligament with profound instability and laxity

Grade I and II ligament sprains are most common, with only 15% of all knee sprains classified as grade III.[8] Generally, grade I and II ligament sprains can be treated with protective bracing and comprehensive and progressive rehabilitation with appropriate strengthening to provide dynamic muscular support. With grade I and II ligament sprains of the knee (ACL, MCL, posterior cruciate ligament, and lateral collateral ligament), good to excellent results can be anticipated in 90% of cases treated nonsurgically.[6] Surgical repair of a grade III sprain frequently involves repair of associated tissues. Cartilage (menisci) injury and injury related to the MCL, lateral collateral ligament, or posterior cruciate ligament often are seen with primary ACL grade III injury.

Important Concepts

Following is a list of grades of injury occurring to ligament tissue, graded by severity:

Grade I: Microscopic tearing of the ligament without producing joint laxity
Grade II: Tearing of some ligament fibers with moderate laxity
Grade III: Complete rupture of the ligament with profound instability and laxity

REPAIR VERSUS NONREPAIR

The decision to repair a torn ligament surgically is based on several intrinsic and extrinsic factors. The most clinically relevant example is to contrast the differences between tears of extraarticular MCLs with intraarticular ACL. In addition to the severity of injury (grade), the anatomic location (biomechanical influences) and vascular supply must be considered.

By virtue of its extracapsular anatomy, the MCL provides for a greater periarticular vascular response and the ability to protect the ligament from unwanted forces (e.g., varus, valgus, and internal and external rotation) and allows for an appropriate environment to stimulate healing and propagation of motion, collagen synthesis organization and orientation, proteoglycan concentration, and joint function. All three distinct grades (grades I, II, and III) of isolated MCL tears appear to heal uneventfully without surgical repair. Although a fibrous repair gap may exist between torn ends of the ligament, resulting in inferior mechanical resistance to tensile loads, the greater cross-sectional area of the healed ligament provides for biochemical properties (e.g., ultimate tensile load to failure) that more closely resemble an uninjured ligament.[45]

Conversely, the relatively pristine environment of the ACL is not conducive to intrinsic repair. When healing of extraarticular ligaments such as the MCL was compared with healing of the ACL, it was found that the mechanical stabilization between the ACL and the environment surrounding it is different. Although the cells of the ACL and its vascularity are capable of healing, there was no structural place to rejoin the two ends of the ligament for cells to remodel.[29,42] The lack of a tissue scaffold between the two torn ends of the ACL is the key mechanism behind failed healing. In addition, the difficulty of protecting the injured ACL from unwanted deforming forces by using commercial or custom braces contributes to and maintains a high-stress force environment of the ACL that limits healing.

Important Concepts

The lack of tissue scaffold between the two torn ends of the ACL is the key mechanism behind failed healing.

It was reported in the early 1980s that patellar tendon ACL grafts undergo a functional adaptation and remodeling termed *ligamentization*.[5] In this process, the continuous postoperative remodeling process takes the graft from a tendon toward a tissue that closely resembles that of the structural properties of a ligament. This process of ligamentization follows several distinct phases, as follows: necrosis, in which the vascular supply is diminished after initial replacement, native cells diminish, and hypocellularity occurs; revascularization, which begins during the first 6 to 8 weeks at which time the acute inflammatory response should be under control; cellular proliferation, which occurs as the tissue begins to become more vascularized and fibroblastic activity creates collagen and elastin; and finally, collagen formation and maturation, which occur as a long-term process in which the tissue gradually assumes a normal ligament appearence.[9,39] Early studies on ligamentization were done using a patellar tendon graft source. However, more recent evidence substantiates that a similar staged healing process occurs for hamstring graft ligamentization.[35]

Important Concepts

Ligamentization is the continuous process by which postoperative remodeling takes an ACL graft from a tendon toward a tissue that more closely resembles the structural properties of a ligament.

EFFECTS OF IMMOBILIZATION

Although it is unclear why, ligamentous complexes are sensitive to load and load history. **Immobilization**, surgery, injury, and rehabilitation of ligaments must take into consideration not only the healing response of the ligament itself but also that of the ligament-bone interface. Stress deprivation of the ligament and ligament-bone complexes resulting from prolonged immobilization after injury or surgery can have significant and profound negative effects. Joint stiffness after immobilization is related to adhesion formation, active shortening of dense connective tissue (ligament), and decreases in water content.[6] Studies show a gradual deterioration in ligament strength and stiffness,[2-4] loss of bone, weakening of cartilage and tendons, significant muscle atrophy, and negative effects on joint mechanics after periods of immobilization (Box 9-1).[1] Immobilization also affects ligament-bone complexes. Studies report that loss of bone directly beneath the junction of ligament and bone reduces the strength of the insertion site and the entire ligament-bone complex.[31]

Important Concepts

Stress deprivation of the ligament and ligament-bone complexes resulting from prolonged immobilization after injury or surgery can have significant and profound negative effects.

BOX 9-1 Effects of Immobilization on Ligament Tissue and Associated Structures

- Reduced physiologic motion
- Decreased afferent neural input
- Muscular atrophy
- Ligament shortening
- Reduction of water content, proteoglycans, and glycosaminoglycans
- Bone loss, periosteal bone reabsorption
- Articular (hyaline cartilage) erosion
- Reduced ligament weight
- Reduced ligament size
- Reduced ligament strength
- Adhesion formation
- Increased ligament laxity
- Joint stiffness related to synovial membrane adherence

From Kloth LC, McCulloch JM, Feedar JA: *Wound healing: alternatives in management,* Philadelphia, 1990, FA Davis.

Rigid immobilization of joints produces chemical and morphologic changes in ligaments 2 and 4 weeks after injury, respectively.[17] After 8 weeks of immobilization, ligaments lose 20% of their weight; significant atrophy results, and marked infiltration of periarticular connective tissue is observed surrounding the ligament.[17] Although immobilization may be needed to promote healing of damaged tissues, the extended use of rigid immobilization should be limited. As an alternative, limited range of motion braces (Fig. 9-1) can be used to protect healing structures, decrease unwanted external forces, and allow for progressive motion of involved joints to minimize the negative effects of immobilization.

The biochemical, histochemical, and morphologic changes that occur in ligament and dense connective tissue in response to immobilization are related to the length of time tissues are immobilized. In addition, structure and mechanical function of ligament substance and ligament-bone insertion complexes (direct insertion and indirect periosteal insertion with Sharpey's perforating fibers) are significantly affected in response to the quality and duration of immobilization.

The effects of immobilization on dense connective tissue have been described by Cummings and Reynolds.[11]: After only 2 weeks of immobilization, animal studies revealed increased GAG synthesis and concentration, decreased water content, thickening of the joint capsule and ligaments, adaptive muscle shortening, and adhesion formation of unopposed articular surfaces. After 4 weeks of immobilization, the biochemical and morphologic changes become more pronounced, with a reduction of GAGs, fissures in articular cartilage, increased ligament stiffness, and decreased capsular remodeling. After 6 weeks of immobilization, joint mobility becomes significantly

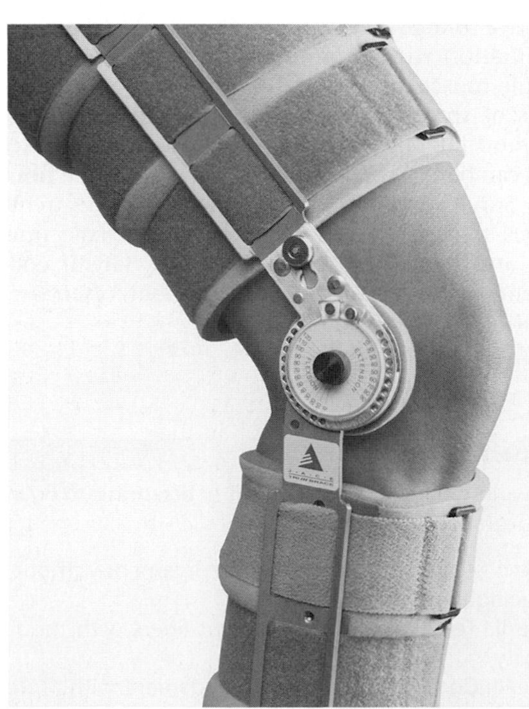

FIG 9-1 Limited range of motion long leg brace.

limited, with thickening noted in the joint capsule, ligaments, and cartilage and decreased ligamentous compliance. Joint immobilization causes a progression of dense connective tissue remodeling, resulting in joint stiffness.

During the first 2 weeks, adaptive muscle shortening appears to be the primary limiting factor in joint mobility. As immobilization extends to 4 weeks, changes in GAG synthesis and water concentration become more pronounced, resulting in a loss of normal fiber lubrication, spacing, and connective tissue disorganization. As the immobilization period approaches 6 weeks, morphologic and biochemical changes become more evident as the dense connective tissue remodels in a shortened position.[45]

Specifically, immobilization causes more pronounced mechanical and biochemical changes in ligament-bone complex insertion sites compared with ligament substance alone. Generally, the area of bone directly beneath the ligament-bone insertion site becomes osteoporotic with osteoclastic activity, resulting in pronounced bone resorption, loss of cortex, and reduced strength of the entire ligament-bone insertion complex.[45]

EXERCISE

As stated, stress deprivation of ligaments secondary to immobilization results in atrophy.[16,17,32,34,46] Conversely, motion, stress, and general physical activity prescribed for healing ligaments produce hypertrophy and increased tensile strength.[6,17] Research shows that ligament and ligament-bone complex strength is related to the mode and duration of exercise used during rehabilitation.[6] Tipton and colleagues[44] showed that endurance types of exercise are more effective in producing larger diameter collagen than nonendurance types of exercise. In addition, the long-term detrimental effects of prolonged immobilization on ligament-bone insertion sites are reversible.[6] The effects of mobilization and exercise are seen 4 months to 1 year after immobilization.[6]

Important Concepts

Research shows that ligament and ligament-bone complex strength is related to the mode and duration of exercise used during rehabilitation.[6]

EFFECTS OF REMOBILIZATION AND EXERCISE

The negative biomechanical, biochemical, and morphologic changes incurred with immobilization generally are reversible. However, there are therapeutically relevant differences between ligament substance and ligament-bone insertion complexes after immobilization.

As stated, ligament substance once injured may regain only 50% to 70% of normal tensile strength after 1 year or more of remodeling.[45] Ligament-bone insertion complexes tend to remodel and regain tensile strength more slowly than ligament tissue after immobilization and therapeutically directed reconditioning. The clinical significance of delayed ligament-bone insertion healing compared with midsubstance tissue repairs is manifested by the relative increase in avulsion injury during this protracted healing interval.[45]

Generally, ligament substance and ligament-bone complexes are sensitive to exercise. These tissues become stronger depending on the type and duration of exercise prescribed. The orientation, composition, synthesis, and concentration of type I collagen and ultimate load to failure, increase in tensile strength, and stiffness of ligament and ligament-bone complexes are observed with appropriately directed exercise.[45]

Dense fibrous tissue (e.g., tendon or ligament) responds not only to frequency, intensity, and duration of exercise but also to the specific type of load applied to the tissue. The structural and biochemical adaptation of dense fibrous tissue varies according to compressive or tensile loads. Tissues subjected to repeated compressions respond by synthesizing larger and greater amounts of proteoglycans than tissues exposed to tension loads. Generally, after injury to ligaments, appropriate controlled motion and exercise stimulate ligament repair by improving matrix organization and composition, increasing the weight of injured ligaments, and promoting normalized collagen synthesis and strength.[45]

Important Concepts

Generally, after injury to ligaments, appropriate controlled motion and exercise stimulate ligament repair by improving matrix organization and composition, increasing the weight of injured ligaments, and promoting normalized collagen synthesis and strength.[45]

CONTINUOUS PASSIVE MOTION

Motion, exercise, and protected progressive stress can influence and determine the degree and type of healing that occur after trauma and subsequent immobilization.[33] Studies have demonstrated that healing is dramatically different in immobilized joints compared with joints moved passively through limited motion.[18] Gelberman and colleagues[18] showed that joints moved passively have well-organized, longitudinally oriented collagen fibers in which no adhesions are present. Conversely, joints that were immobilized demonstrated scar tissue and adhesions.

The concept of early protected motion applied to healing soft tissues has resulted in the development of **continuous passive motion (CPM)** (Fig. 9-2). CPM is a technique used in the treatment of knee joint contractures; postoperative ACL reconstructions; joint effusions; knee, elbow, and ankle fractures (after immobilization); joint arthrosis; and total knee arthroplasty.[28] Early motion after surgery or immobilization acts to enhance and facilitate connective tissue strength, size, and shape; evacuate joint hemarthrosis (bloody effusion within the joint space); improve joint nutrition; inhibit adhesions; initiate normal joint kinematics; reduce articular surface changes; and minimize other deleterious effects of prolonged immobilization.[28] With postoperative ACL reconstruction, no stretching out of the graft occurs when CPM is used.[10,12,33,38] CPM can be used postoperatively; can be applied in the operating room; or can be used a few days after surgery, immediately on cast removal, or during the early phases of rehabilitation.

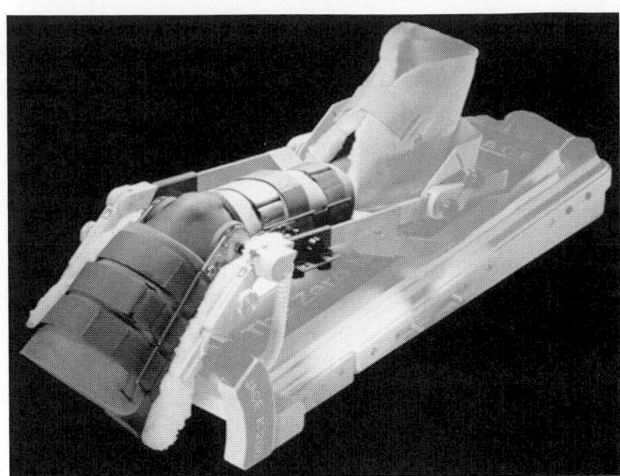

FIG 9-2 Continuous passive motion machine.

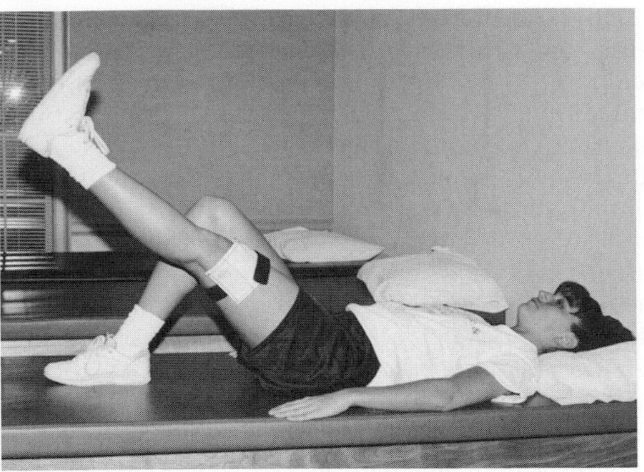

FIG 9-3 Supine straight leg raises with the resistance placed proximal to the knee joint to reduce anterior translatory forces after anterior cruciate ligament reconstructive surgery.

CPM devices have been designed for use on many body parts.[28] The knee is the most common; the ankle, shoulder, elbow, wrist, hand, and hip joints also benefit from CPM. The CPM machine is calibrated in cycles per minute and degrees of motion. Progressive increases in the cycle mode and degrees of motion are made gradually so as not to initiate pain or increase the time necessary for healing.

CPM usually is used in conjunction with other agents to reduce swelling and pain. Among these are ice packs, oral or intravenous analgesics, antiinflammatory medications, transcutaneous electrical nerve stimulation, and joint compression bandages.

Although CPM may be helpful to decrease postoperative pain after ACL reconstruction, systematic reviews suggest that there is no substantial advantage to using CPM and no difference in long-term outcomes. It is recommended as an adjunct rather than a replacement for a postoperative exercise program.[40,49]

Important Concepts

Although CPM may be helpful to decrease postoperative pain after ACL reconstruction, systematic reviews suggest that there is no substantial advantage to using CPM and no difference in long-term outcomes.

PRACTICAL CONSIDERATIONS

The time constraints and healing mechanics of ligaments are well documented.[6,8,16,26,31,32,43,46,50] Careful consideration must be given to the progression of therapeutic exercises and functional activities for patients with ligament injuries. Usually the absence of pain and swelling is an exceedingly poor indicator of healing tissue. With an ACL reconstruction, pain and swelling normally subside within a few weeks, but return of functional joint motion requires a couple of months. Strength values gradually increase, with muscle hypertrophy following slowly.

As the outward clinical signs point to healing, the ligament, being a dynamic tissue, continues to remodel and mature for up to 1 year. Protection of the joint is critical during healing. Functional knee braces with range-limiting devices can have a protective effect for MCL injuries; however, no evidence exists that supports the routine use of functional bracing after ACL reconstruction.[48,49] Initiating progressive resistance exercises after knee ligament injury or surgery, while maintaining joint protection, can be challenging. Placing the resistance (weight) above the joint line during straight leg raises (Fig. 9-3) after ACL surgery can be the first phase of progressive resistance while protecting the healing ligament and retraining quadriceps activation.

To strengthen hip adduction with MCL sprain, resistance initially is applied above the knee joint line so as not to overstress the healing MCL (Fig. 9-4). As the time constraints of healing allow, progressive strengthening of the adductors can involve loading the joint more distally, if joint protection is applied. Awareness of the time necessary for healing and duration of immobilization after trauma, weight-bearing status, and degree of injury guide the physical therapist assistant (PTA) in making clinical recommendations about the progression of exercise and the placement of force during rehabilitation.

Developing a progressive therapeutic exercise and functional activities program with ankle sprains is similarly challenging. Generally, a grade II anterior talofibular ligament sprain does not produce significant pain or functional limitations after a few weeks of conservative treatment involving splinting, crutch walking (non–weight bearing progressing to full weight bearing), ice, compression, and elevation. The PTA should protect the ligament for many weeks after injury because ligament healing is a slow process (Fig. 9-5).

Encouraging weight bearing as soon as tolerated, while protecting the joint, helps to establish normal joint kinematics and gait. Protecting the ligaments from further stress not only involves external bracing but, more importantly, includes avoidance of motions that place unwanted force on the healing ligaments. For example, the anterior talofibular ligament of the ankle is stressed with plantar flexion and inversion. To protect the ligaments, these two motions should be avoided during the early (postacute) and middle phases of rehabilitation.

Early protected motion is encouraged after ligament injury, repair, or immobilization, but caution should be

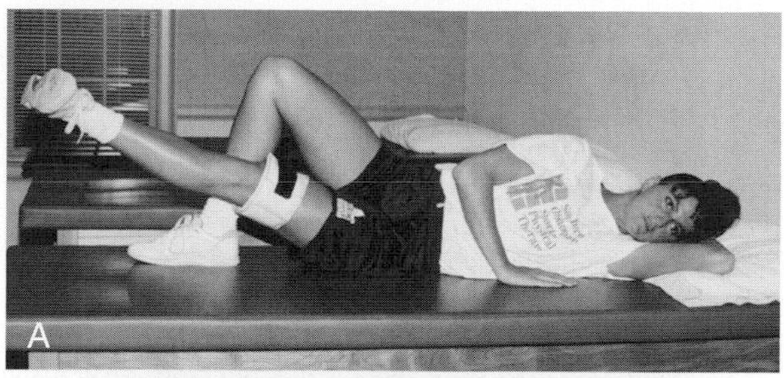

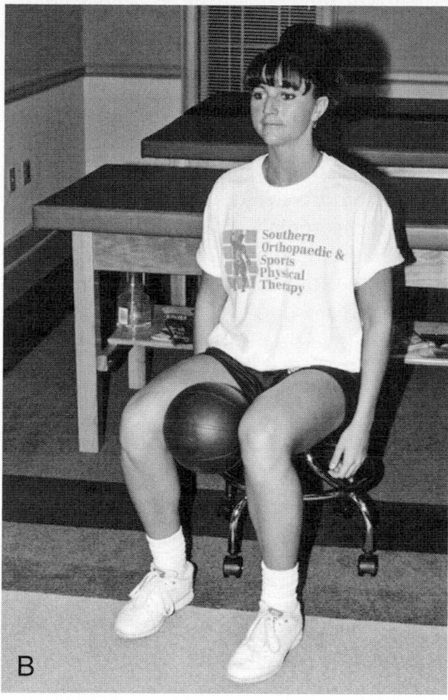

FIG 9-4 **A,** Side-lying hip adduction exercise with the resistance placed proximal to the knee joint to protect the healing medial collateral ligament. **B,** Isometric hip adduction with the use of a ball placed proximal to the joint line.

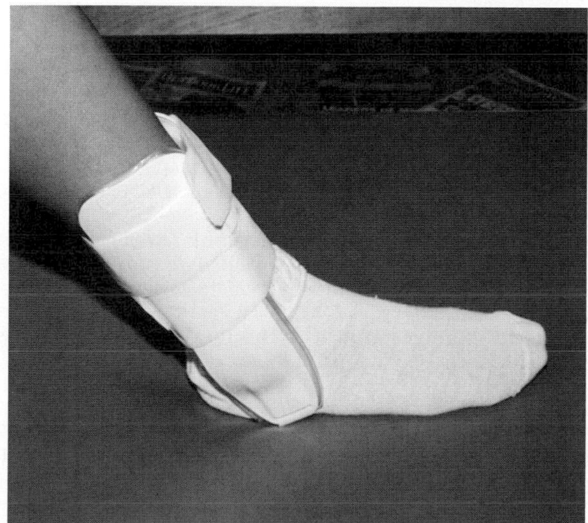

FIG 9-5 Joint protection from unwanted forces is essential for many weeks after ligament injuries. Shown here is an air-stirrup brace for a lateral ligament complex sprain of the ankle.

used to avoid overstressing the ligament or duplicating motions that place unwanted strain too soon after injury. The acute and postacute phases of rehabilitation after ligament injury or repair usually involve pain management techniques, swelling reduction, muscle reeducation (isometric muscle contraction and functional muscle stimulation), CPM, active range of motion, ligament protection devices via range-adjustable bracing, and weight-bearing gait maneuvers with crutches as needed. During this early phase of recovery, it is particularly important to avoid excessive motions that may disrupt the intentional scar formation needed for joint stability. The degree of motion, direction of forces, and velocity of joint movement applied during this early postacute phase must be joint specific, functional, and protected. For example, with a cruciate ligament sprain, movements that are allowed include knee flexion and extension but no rotary or torque-producing motions. After an MCL sprain, knee flexion and extension motion can be initiated in the postacute phase (within limits); however, no valgus stress should be applied. As stated, the reason for ligament protection, maintenance of joint stability, and improved motion is that collagen fiber growth and parallel alignment are stimulated by early tensile loading within the normal physiologic range of the healing ligament.

Table 9-1 outlines the stages of ligament healing and subsequent therapeutic interventions that enhance the healing of ligament tissues.

EFFECTS OF SMOKING ON LIGAMENT HEALING

Smoking and tobacco use are leading causes of preventable morbidity and mortality in the United States. Nicotine has been implicated in the pathogenesis of various diseases by increasing platelet aggregation; reducing microvascular prostacyclin levels; and after surgery, inhibiting fibroblasts, red blood cells, and macrophages.[24,51] Assessment of literature related to ligament healing and smoking revealed that two basic science studies examined the effect of smoking on the healing of surgically induced ruptures of the MCL of mice. Exposure to smoke in mice with surgically ruptured MCL resulted in significant decreases in cellular density and decreases in type I collagen gene expression, strength, and stiffness compared with control mice.[19,47] Studies examining the effects of smoking on ACL injuries and postoperative rehabilitation after reconstruction showed that smoking status had impact and was a significant factor in (1) permanent disability discharge from the U.S. Army, (2) decreases in subjective International Knee Documentation Committee scores, (3) decreases in mean overall International Knee Documentation

Important Concepts

Nicotine has been implicated in the pathogenesis of various diseases by increasing platelet aggregation; reducing microvascular prostacyclin levels; and, after surgery, inhibiting fibroblasts, red blood cells, and macrophages.[24,51]

TABLE 9-1 Therapeutic Considerations during Stages of Ligament Healing

Timeline	Immediate	Day 3-14	Day 14-60	Day 60-360
Description	Hemostasis and degeneration; weak, fragile tissue[20,43]	Inflammation; vasodilation and scar formation; break down and remove dead cells; unstable type III collagen[20]	Proliferation and migration; angiogenesis; very gradual changes in collagen strength; tissue changes from cellular to fibrous[20,43]	Remodeling and maturation
Treatment	RICE, pain management techniques (TENS, oral IV analgesics); Non–weight bearing or weight bearing as tolerated; can initiate CPM (within limited range of motion); protection of ligaments from unwanted stress—usually adjustable range braces or hinged casts; strict, rigid, long-term cast immobilization should be minimized; isometric muscle contractions; contralateral limb exercise as tolerated	Continue RICE; active progressive motion; continued ligament protection; progressive weight bearing; protected, controlled, active resisted exercise; cycling (for motion); isometric exercise progression; electrical muscle stimulation; initiate gentle multiangle static holds (isometrics); avoid excessive motion	Continue RICE as needed; begin low-load static stretch if needed, preheating tissues if needed; full weight bearing; isokinetic exercise with continued ligament protection with bracing; eccentric isotonic exercise; progressive concentric isotonic exercise; hydrotherapy—swimming; progressive cycling; initiate CKC exercise	Prolonged low-load static stretching; progressive advanced isokinetic and isotonic exercise; cycling—stair climbs; proprioception-balance-coordination exercise; advanced CKC exercise, progressing to plyometric exercise; jogging, running, jumping; maintain joint protection with functional bracing as needed

CKC, closed kinetic chain; *CPM,* continuous passive motion; *IV,* intravenous; *RICE,* rest, ice, compression, elevation; *TENS,* transcutaneous electrical nerve stimulation.

Committee scores, (4) decreased rate of return to sport, (5) increased objective ligament laxity, (6) decreased activity levels based on validated activity scales, and (7) decreased quality of life.[14,15,25,27,41]

GLOSSARY

Collagen: The primary protein of connective tissue in the human body; there are 25 different forms and types.

Continuous passive motion (CPM): A form of rehabilitation that is typically instituted immediately after surgery when there is anticipation that a joint restriction may occur. This form of treatment uses a device known as a *continuous passive motion machine,* which gently moves the joint through a controlled range of motion decided on by the physician in charge of the patient's care.

Immobilization: An attempt to render a joint in a fixed position. Immobilization is used in rehabilitation to decrease stressful activity to a joint that is inherently unstable. Typically immobilization is prescribed for as short a duration as possible because complications can result from extended immobility.

Inflammatory reaction: A physiologic reaction to injury and tissue damage; its main functions are to defend the body against harmful destruction, dispose of dead tissues, and promote healing of injured tissue.

Ligament: Dense connective tissue.

Sprain: An injury to a ligament or capsular structure. Sprains are graded by their severity. A grade I sprain indicates minimal damage to tissue, whereas a grade III sprain indicates complete rupture of the ligament or capsule.

REFERENCES

1. Akeson WH: An experimental study of joint stiffness. *J Bone Joint Surg Am* 43:1022–1034, 1961.
2. Akeson WH, Amiel D, Abel MF, et al: Effects of immobilization on joints. *Clin Orthop Relat Res* 219:28–37, 1987.
3. Akeson WH, Woo SL-Y, Amiel D, et al: The chemical basis of tissue repair: the biology of ligaments. In Hunter LY, Funk FJ, editors: *Rehabilitation of the injured knee*, St Louis, 1984, Mosby.
4. Amiel D, Akeson WH, Harwood FL, et al: Stress deprivation effect on metabolic turnover of the medial collateral ligament collagen: a comparison between 9- and 12-week immobilization. *Clin Orthop Relat Res* 172:265–270, 1983.
5. Amiel D, Kleiner JB, Rouz RD, Harwood FL, Akeson WH: The phenomenon of "ligamentization": anterior cruciate ligament reconstruction with autogenous patellar tendon. *J Orthop Res* 4:162–172, 1986.
6. Andriacchi TP, DeHaven KE, Dahners LE, et al: Ligament: injury and repair. In Woo SL-Y, Buckwalter J, editors: *Injury and repair of the musculoskeletal soft tissues*, Rosemont, IL, 1988, American Academy of Orthopaedic Surgeons.
7. Bray RC: Blood supply of ligaments: a brief overview. *Orthopaedics* 172:69–79, 1995.
8. Buschbacher R: Tissue injury and healing. In *Musculoskeletal disorders: a practical guide for diagnosis and rehabilitation*, Boston, 1994, Andover Medical Publishers.
9. Claes S, Verdonk P, Forsyth R, Bellemans J: The "ligamentization" process in anterior cruciate ligament reconstruction: what happens to the human graft? A systematic review of the literature. *Am J Sports Med* 39:2476–2483, 2011.
10. Coutts RD, Toth C, Kaita JH: The role of continuous passive motion in the rehabilitation of the total knee patient. In Hungerford DS, Krackow KA, Kenna RV, editors: *Total knee arthroplasty: a comprehensive approach*, Baltimore, 1984, Williams & Wilkins.
11. Cummings GS, Reynolds CA: Principles of soft tissue extensibility and joint contracture management. In Wadsworth C, editor: *Strength and conditioning applications in orthopedics*, LaCrosse, WI, 1998, Orthopedic section, APTA.
12. Davis D: Continuous passive motion for total knee arthroplasty. *Phys Ther* 64:709, 1984.
13. DeHaven KE, Lintner DM: Athletic injuries: comparison by age, sport and gender. *Am J Sports Med* 14:218–224, 1986.

14. Dunn WR, Lincoln AE, Hinton RY, Smith GS, Amoroso PJ: Occupational disability after hospitalization for the treatment of an injury of the anterior cruciate ligament. *J Bone Joint Surg Am* 85:1656–1666, 2003.
15. Dunn WR, Spindler KP: Predictors of activity level 2 years after anterior cruciate ligament reconstruction (ACLR): a Multicenter Orthopaedic Outcomes Network (MOON) ACLR cohort study. *Am J Sports Med* 38:2040–2050, 2010.
16. Frank C, Woo SL, Amiel D, et al: Medial collateral ligament healing: a multidisciplinary assessment in rabbits. *Am J Sports Med* 11:379–389, 1983.
17. Gamble JG, Edwards CC, Max SR: Enzymatic adaptation in ligaments during immobilization. *Am J Sports Med* 12:221–228, 1984.
18. Gelberman RH, Van de Berg JS, Lundborg GN, et al: Flexor tendon healing and restoration of the gliding surface: an ultrastructural study in dogs. *J Bone Joint Surg Am* 65:70–80, 1983.
19. Gill CS, Sandell LH, El-Zawawy HB, Wright RW: Effects of cigarette smoking on early medial collateral ligament healing in a mouse model. *J Orthop Res* 24:2141–2149, 2006.
20. Goodman CC, Tepper SH, McKeough DM: Injury, inflammation, and healing. In Goodman CC, Fuller KS, editors: *Pathology: implications for the physical therapist*, St Louis, 2009, Saunders.
21. Hildebrand KA, Hart DA, Rattner JB, Marchuk LL, Frank CB: Ligament injuries: pathophysiology, healing, and treatment considerations. In Magee DJ, Zachazewski JE, Quillen WS, editors: *Scientific foundations and principles of practice in musculoskeletal rehabilitation*, St Louis, 2007, Saunders.
22. Ilic MZ, Carter P, Tyndall A, et al: Proteoglycans and catabolic products of proteoglycans present in ligament. *Biochem J* 385:381–388, 2005.
23. Inoue M, McGurk-Burleson E, Hollis JM, et al: Treatment of the medial collateral ligament I: the importance of anterior cruciate ligament on the varus-valgus knee laxity. *Am J Sports Med* 15:15–21, 1987.
24. Jorgensen LN, Kallehave F, Christensen E, Siana JE, Gottrup F: Less collagen production in smokes. *Surgery* 123:450–455, 1998.
25. Karim A, Pandit H, Murray J, Wandless F, Thomas NP: Smoking and reconstruction of the anterior cruciate ligament. *J Bone Joint Surg Br* 88:1027–1031, 2006.
26. Kloth LC, Miller KH: The inflammatory response to wound healing. In Kloth LC, McCulloch JM, Feedar JA, editors: *Wound healing: alternatives in management, contemporary perspectives in rehabilitation*, Philadelphia, 1990, FA Davis.
27. Kowalchuk DA, Harner CD, Fu FH, Irrgang JJ: Prediction of patient-reported outcome after single-bundle anterior cruciate ligament reconstruction. *Arthroscopy* 25:457–463, 2009.
28. McCarthy MR, O'Donoghue PC, Yates CK, et al: The clinical use of continuous passive motion in physical therapy. *J Orthop Sports Phys Ther* 15:132–140, 1992.
29. Murray MM, Spector M: The migration of cells from the ruptured human anterior cruciate ligament into collagen-glycosaminoglycan regeneration templates in vitro. *Biomaterials* 22:2393–2402, 2001.
30. Niyibizi C, Visconoti CS, Kavalkovich K, Woo SL: Collagens in an adult bovine medial collateral ligament: immunofluorescence localization by confocal microscopy reveals that type XIV collagen predominates at the ligament-bone junction. *Matrix Biol* 14:743–751, 1995.
31. Noyes FR, DeLucas JL, Torvik PJ: Biomechanics of anterior cruciate ligament failure: an analysis of strain-rate sensitivity and mechanisms of failure in primates. *J Bone Joint Surg Am* 56:236–253, 1974.
32. Noyes FR, Keller CS, Grood ES, et al: Advances in the understanding of knee ligament injury, repair and rehabilitation. *Med Sci Sports Exerc* 16:427–443, 1984.
33. Noyes FR, Mangine RE: Early motion after open arthroscopic anterior cruciate ligament reconstruction. *Am J Sports Med* 1:149–160, 1987.
34. O'Donoghue DH, Frank GR, Jeter WJ: Repair and reconstruction of the anterior cruciate ligament in dogs: factors influencing long-term results. *J Bone Joint Surg Am* 53:710–718, 1971.
35. Pauzenberger L, Syré S, Schurz M: "Ligamentization" in hamstring tendon grafts after anterior cruciate ligament reconstruction: a systematic review of the literature and a glimpse into the future. *Arthroscopy* 29:1712–1721, 2013.
36. Petersen W, Tillmann B: Structure and vascularization of the cruciate ligaments of the human knee joint. *Anat Embryol (Berl)* 200:325–334, 1999.
37. Powell J: 636,000 injuries annually in high school football. *Athl Train* 22:19–22, 1987.
38. Salter RB, Simmonds DF, Malcolm HW: The effects of continuous passive motion on the healing of articular cartilage defects: an experimental investigation in rabbits. *J Bone Joint Surg Am* 57:570–571, 1975.
39. Scheffler SU, Unterhauser FN, Weiler A: Graft remodeling and ligamentization after cruciate ligament reconstruction. *Knee Surg Sports Traumatol Arthrosc* 16:834–842, 2008.
40. Smith TO, Davies L: The efficacy of continuous passive motion after anterior cruciate ligament reconstruction: a systematic review. *Phys Ther Sport* 8:141–152, 2007.
41. Spindler KP, Huston LH, Wright RW, et al: The prognosis and predictors of sports function and activity at minimum 6 years after anterior cruciate ligament reconstruction: a population cohort study. *Am J Sports Med* 39:348–359, 2011.
42. Spindler KP, Murray MM, Devin C, et al: The central ACL defect as a model for failure of intra-articular healing. *J Orthop Res* 24:401–406, 2006.
43. Tillman LJ, Cummings GS: Biologic mechanisms of connective tissue mutability. In Currier DP, Nelson RM, editors: *Dynamics of human biologic tissues*, Philadelphia, 1992, FA Davis.
44. Tipton CM, James SL, Mergner W, et al: Influence of exercise on strength of medial collateral knee ligaments of dogs. *Am J Physiol* 218:894–902, 1970.
45. Woo SL, An K-N, Frank CB: Anatomy, biology, and biomechanics of tendon and ligament. In Buckwalter JA, Einhorn TA, Simon SR, editors: *Orthopedic basic science, biology, and biomechanics of the musculoskeletal system*, ed 2, Rosemont, IL, 2000, American Academy of Orthopaedic Surgeons.
46. Woo SL, Gomez MA, Inoue M, et al: New experimental procedures to evaluate the biomechanical properties of healing canine medial collateral ligaments. *J Orthop Res* 5:425–432, 1987.
47. Wright R, Mackey RB, Silva M, Steger-May K: Smoking and mouse MCL healing. *J Knee Surg* 23:193–199, 2010.
48. Wright RW, Fetzer GB: Bracing after ACL reconstruction: a systematic review. *Clin Orthop Relat Res* 455:162–168, 2007.
49. Wright RW, Preston E, Fleming BC, et al: A systematic review of anterior cruciate ligament reconstruction rehabilitation: part I: continuous passive motion, early weight bearing, postoperative bracing, and home-based rehabilitation. *J Knee Surg* 21:217–224, 2001.
50. Zarro V: Mechanisms of inflammation and repair. In Michlovitz S, editor: *Thermal agents in rehabilitation*, Philadelphia, 1986, FA Davis.
51. Zelvin S, Gourlay SG, Benowitz NL: Clinical pharmacology of nicotine. *Clin Dermatol* 16:557–564, 1998.

REVIEW QUESTIONS

Multiple Choice

1. Which of the following statements is true?
   a. Ligaments contain primarily type II collagen.
   b. Collagen is a yellow-colored tissue.
   c. Ligaments contain proteoglycan.
   d. Ligaments contain large amounts of elastin.
2. Proteoglycans are:
   a. Fats.
   b. Hydrophobic.
   c. Carbohydrates.
   d. Proteins.
3. Which phase of ligament repair occurs as the ligament retracts and looks highly disorganized?
   a. Phase I
   b. Phase II
   c. Phase III
   d. Phase IV

4. What is the ultimate tensile strength of a normal repaired ligament after 1 year?
   a. 20% to 30%
   b. 30% to 50%
   c. 50% to 70%
   d. 70% to 90%
5. What is the grade of ligament tear that occurs when there is only microscopic injury to the ligament and there is not any actual laxity of the ligament?
   a. Grade I
   b. Grade II
   c. Grade III
   d. None of the above
6. Which degree of ligament injury occurs when there is moderate tearing and moderate instability exists?
   a. Grade I
   b. Grade II
   c. Grade III
   d. None of the above
7. Which degree of ligament injury occurs when there is a complete rupture of the entire ligament with profound instability?
   a. Grade I
   b. Grade II
   c. Grade III
   d. None of the above
8. What is ligamentization?
   a. Tendon healing
   b. Ligament healing
   c. Tendon remodeling to ligamentlike tissue
   d. Ligament healing to tendonlike tissue
9. Which of the following statements regarding effects of immobilization on ligaments is true?
   a. Immobilization produces no morphologic changes.
   b. Ligaments lose up to 20% of their weight after 8 weeks of immobilization.
   c. Extended use of immobilization should be condoned.
   d. Immobilization does not cause loss of ligament strength.
10. Which of the following are effects of prolonged immobilization during ligament healing?
    a. Muscular atrophy
    b. Ligament shortening
    c. Articular erosion
    d. Adhesion formation
    e. All of the above
11. Dense fibrous tissues such as ligaments respond to:
    a. Frequency of stress.
    b. Intensity of stress.
    c. Duration of exercise.
    d. All of the above
12. Which of the following statements is true?
    a. The ACL heals well conservatively.
    b. Ligament ends do not need contact to heal.
    c. Progressive stress must be applied to ligament.
    d. Excessive stress is important for healing.
13. CPM devices have been used on which types of ligaments?
    a. Knee
    b. Hip
    c. Shoulder
    d. All of the above
14. During the immediate stage of ligament healing, which of the following are true?
    a. Soft tissue is weak and fragile.
    b. Vasodilation and scar formation occur.
    c. Proliferation and angiogenesis occur.
    d. Remodeling and maturation occur.
15. The predominant cell types present during the acute inflammatory phase are:
    a. Neutrophils and lymphocytes.
    b. Polymorphonuclear cells and lymphocytes.
    c. Monocytes and phagocytes.
    d. Phagocytes and polymorphonuclear cells.

Short Answer

16. Name the four phases of tissue healing.
17. Name the five cardinal signs of inflammation.
18. Organization and production of collagen occur during which phase of healing?
19. Discuss the rationale for continuing or discontinuing external support as it relates to the healing constraints of ligament tissue after 2 weeks of progressive rehabilitation for a ligament sprain of the ankle.
20. What does the term *ligamentization* mean?

Fill in the Blank

21. For torn ligaments to heal properly, the torn ends must be in ________________ to one another.
22. To orient collagen fibers and promote a functional scar, ________________ must be applied.
23. After injury or surgery to a ligament, protection against ________________ must be strictly enforced.
24. Systematic reviews indicated that after ACL reconstruction, the use of ____________ does not provide a substantial advantage.
25. ____________ has been shown to decrease cellular density and decrease collagen expression, strength, and stiffness in healing ligaments.

True/False

26. Ligaments heal through a process of tissue regeneration.
27. Strict, long-term, rigid cast immobilization is necessary to allow for proper ligament healing.
28. The specific type and duration of exercise used during rehabilitation is not related to ligament and ligament–bone complex strength.
29. The long-term detrimental effects of immobilization on ligament and ligament-bone complex are not reversible.
30. Pain is an excellent guide to judge the degree of healing a ligament has achieved.

Chapter 10

Bone Healing

Robert C. Manske, B. J. Lehecka

CHAPTER OUTLINE

LEARNING OBJECTIVES

1. Identify and describe the phases of bone healing.
2. Discuss the objectives that serve as the foundation of fracture management and bone healing.
3. Define osteoblasts, osteoclasts, and osteocytes.
4. Define and discuss Wolff's law.
5. Discuss stress deprivation, immobilization, and normal physiologic stress as they apply to fracture healing.
6. Identify three complications of bone healing.
7. Outline and describe six areas of descriptive organization of classifying fractures.
8. Describe the five types of pediatric fractures defined by Salter and Harris.
9. Define pathologic fractures and list four types.
10. Discuss how osteoporosis affects fractures.
11. Define osteomalacia.
12. List common methods of fracture fixation, fixation devices, and fracture classifications.
13. Discuss clinical applications of rehabilitation techniques used during bone healing.

KEY TERMS

Bone matrix
Bone types
Cancellous bone
Cortical bone
Osteoblasts
Osteoclasts
Osteocytes
Piezoelectric effect
Remodeling
Repair

Orthopedic conditions involving bone tissue are extremely common ailments treated in physical therapy. The physical therapist assistant (PTA) must appreciate the organized, dynamic nature of bone healing and must recognize the various methods of treating injuries to bone. Bone tissue is not a static structure, but a living, dynamic tissue that can actively adapt to its changing needs.

STRUCTURE AND FUNCTION

Bone is an intense metabolically active tissue. Bone has unique mechanical characteristics that are determined primarily by the structural components of bone tissue. Chemically complex, bone tissue is approximately 65% mineral and 35% organic matrix including lipids, collagen, and noncollagenous protein (Fig. 10-1). The major organic constituent of bone is type I collagen, representing about 90% of the dry weight of bone.[41] The remaining 10% is composed of noncollagenous matrix proteins, lipids, phospholipids, proteoglycans, and phosphoproteins. The principal inorganic component of bone is a crystalline calcium phosphate hydroxyapatite.[41] This compound is generally brittle, tolerating only small amounts of deformation before fracture. The remaining tissue volume includes fluid-filled vascular channels and cellular spaces.[16]

Important Concepts

Bone tissue is living tissue that is constantly adapting with high metabolic activity.

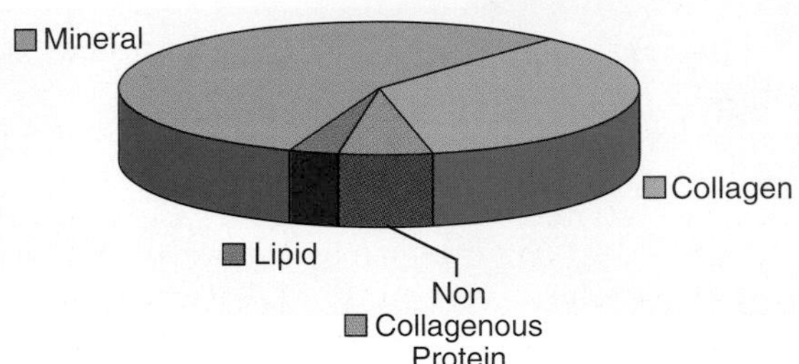

FIG 10-1 The solid matter of bone is distributed as shown in this pie chart. *(From Bullough PG:* Orthopedic pathology, *ed 5, St Louis, 2010, Mosby.)*

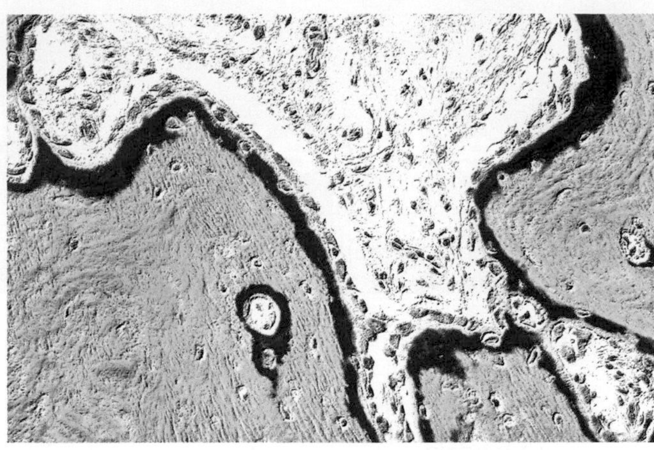

FIG 10-3 Photomicrograph of an undecalcified specimen showing a layer of active, plump osteoblasts at a bone surface. The layer of red-stained tissue beneath the osteoblastic layer represents unmineralized matrix or osteoid. The green-staining material represents calcified bone matrix. *(From Bullough PG:* Orthopedic pathology, *ed 5, St Louis, 2010, Mosby.)*

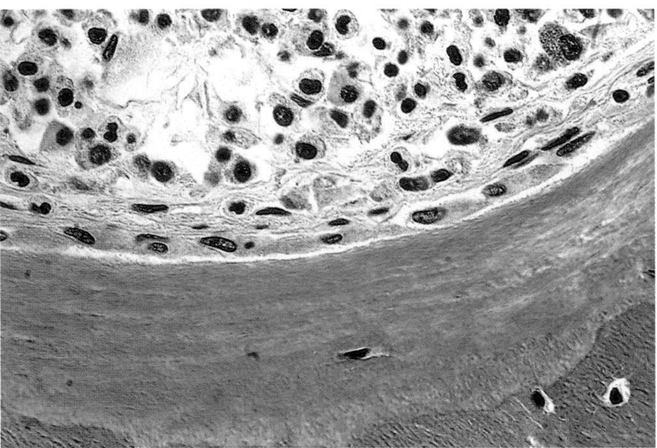

FIG 10-2 Photomicrograph of an actively forming bone surface. A layer of flat active osteoblasts with abundant basophilic cytoplasm lines the smooth formative surface. *(From Bullough PG:* Orthopedic pathology, *ed 5, St Louis, 2010, Mosby.)*

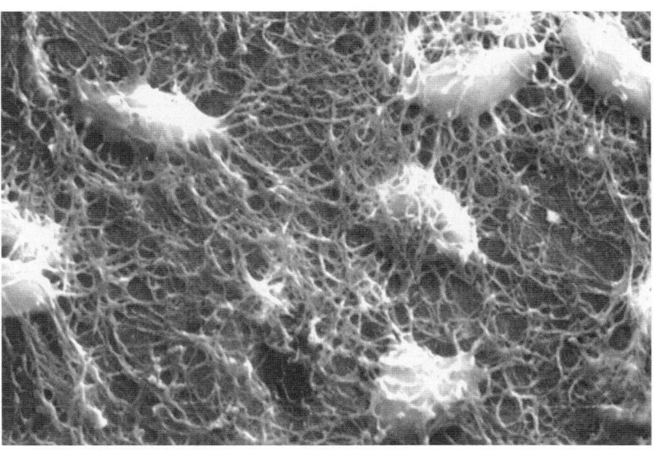

FIG 10-4 Scanning electron photomicrograph demonstrating the osteocytes and their connecting canaliculi. *(From Bullough PG:* Orthopedic pathology, *ed 5, St Louis, 2010, Mosby.)*

BONE CELLS

There are three types of bone cells. **Osteoblasts** are functionally distinct cells that form **bone matrix** (osteoid) and synthesize type I collagen[41] and are commonly found on a bony surface. These cells are unique in that they have a large volume of endoplasmic reticulum, Golgi apparatus, and mitochondria to synthesize collagen and secrete matrix proteins.[41]

Osteoblasts and **osteocytes** are distinguished more by their location than by their structure and function.[20] Osteoblasts are responsible for synthesis, deposition, and mineralization of bone. They are derived from bone marrow and secrete procollagen on all active bone surfaces. When the osteoblast is done forming bone, it can become an osteocyte. Osteoblasts synthesize bone matrix by forming a layer on the bone surface (Figs. 10-2 and 10-3). Osteoblasts become surrounded by mineralized matrix and are buried into the substance of bone tissues, becoming osteocytes.

Osteocytes actually are osteoblasts that are embedded within newly formed mineralized bone matrix.[41] Chemically, osteocytes differ from osteoblasts in that they demonstrate fewer organelles and a greater nucleus-to-cytoplasmic ratio.[41] These cells represent approximately 90% of mature skeletal tissue and function metabolically to control extracellular concentrations of calcium and phosphorus.[41] Osteoid, osteocyte, and osteocytic osteoblasts are cells that are in an intermediate changeover from osteoblast to osteocyte; the pure distinction between cells may be related more to developmental stage than differing cell types.[45]

Osteoclasts are giant cell multinucleated bone resorption cells. Osteoclasts synthesize a specific acid phosphatase enzyme and produce hydrogen ions, which lower the pH environment.[41] The reduced pH increases the solubility of the crystalline phosphate-hydroxyapatite that functions to remove the organic matrix crystals via acid proteolytic degradation.[41] These enzymes remove a thick layer of osteoid covering, allowing osteoclasts to bind to bone and begin resorption if needed (Fig. 10-4).[6]

Important Concepts

Osteoblasts are responsible for synthesis deposition and mineralization of bone. Osteoclasts are cells that are responsible for resorption of bone cells.

TYPES OF BONE

The microscopic organization and classification of bone tissue involves two distinct forms that change or adapt as we age: (1) normal, mature lamellar bone and (2) weak, fragile, immature woven bone (Fig. 10-5). Woven bone is structurally immature, embryologically (primary) fragile, and weak with a random disorganized collagen arrangement.[4] This random arrangement of collagen fibers allows strength in all directions, while preferring strength in no specific direction. This form of bone is not nearly as strong as mature bone. This specific type of bone is more commonly seen in embryos and newborns but can also be seen in adults in fracture **repair** callus, bone tumors, and various bone pathologies.[41]

A unique feature of woven bone is that it can be deposited without any previous part of a cartilaginous model existing.[29] The primary function of woven bone is to provide temporary, quick-acting mechanical support for injured skeletal tissue.

Early after birth (approximately 2 months to 4 years), woven bone slowly remodels into organized, structurally mature lamellar bone. A clinically relevant feature of woven bone is that its specific mechanical behavior is termed *isotropic;* that is, woven bone does not conform to Wolff's law, so its biomechanical reaction to applied forces and stress is similar in all planes.[4] The disorganized arrangement of collagen fibers in woven bone strongly contributes to this unique characteristic (Fig. 10-6).[4]

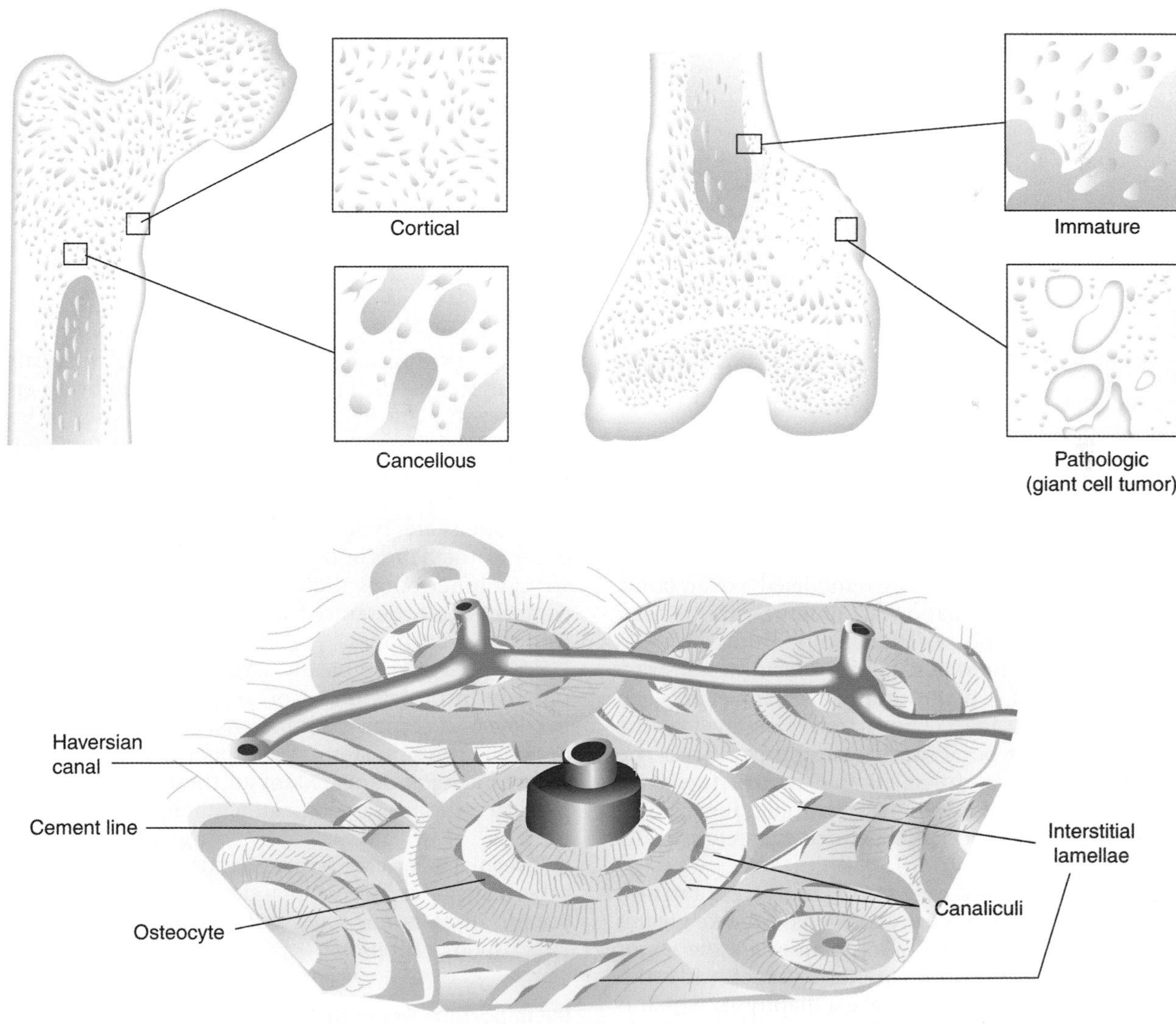

FIG 10-5 Types of bone. Cortical bone consists of tightly packed osteons. Cancellous bone consists of a meshwork of trabeculae. In immature bone, there is unmineralized osteoid lining the immature trabeculae. Atypical osteoblasts and architectural disorganization are seen in pathologic bone. *(From Brinker MR, Miller MD:* Fundamentals of orthopaedics, *Philadelphia, 1999, Saunders.)*

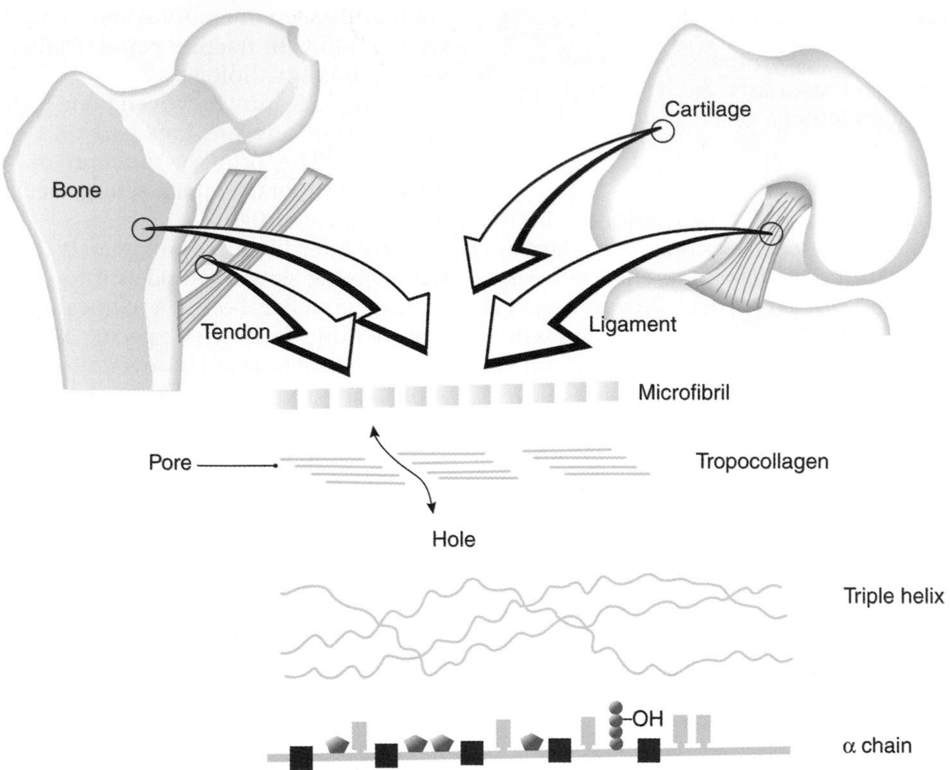

FIG 10-6 Microstructure of collagen. Collagen is composed of microfibrils that are packed in a quarter-standard fashion to form tropocollagen. Note hole and pore regions for mineral deposition (for calcification). Tropocollagen is made up of a triple helix of chains of polypeptides. *(From Brinker MR, Miller MD:* Fundamentals of orthopaedics, *Philadelphia, 1999, Saunders.)*

Important Concepts

Woven bone is structurally immature, fragile, and weak compared with lamellar bone with its stronger, more mature bone. Woven bone is found in infants and newly formed fracture callus.

Lamellar bone refers to mature remodeled woven bone. Mature bone begins formation at about 1 month after birth[15] and comprises most of the skeleton by age 4 years.[3] The collagen arrangement in lamellar bone is highly structured and organized. These bundles lie parallel to each other, although they may change from one layer to the next, giving lamellar bone much strength similar to the various layers of plywood (Fig. 10-7). This structure gives normal mature lamellar bone anisotropic mechanical properties that are stress oriented, which characteristically respond to Wolff's law.[4]

Bones are classified not only into various types but also by their shape. Long bones are considered to have greater length than width. Examples of long bones are the femur and the humerus. These bones are tube shaped with widening at each end. Long bones have a diaphysis, which is the tubular-shaped midportion that houses **cancellous bone** and the intermedullary canal where blood cells are formed (Fig. 10-8). The proximal and distal ends of the long bone widen to form a metaphysis, which continues to widen even more into the epiphysis or the end of the bone. In growing children, before skeletal maturity, the metaphysis and the epiphysis are separated by an epiphyseal growth plate. This can be a common area of fracture before skeletal maturity, at which time the two ends fuse and demarcation is not detectable.

Short bones are described as such because their main dimensions are typically of equal length. These bones occur in the hands and feet. Short bones are composed of spongy inner bones that are enclosed by a thick layer of compact bone. Sesamoid and accessory bones are other forms of short bones.

Flat bones are typically larger and appear to serve a purpose in protection of organs. These bones consist of two layers of compact bone with a portion of spongy bone between. The ribs, sternum, scapula, and skull bones constitute most flat bones. Many of these flat bones are actually curved and serve as attachment sites for multiple muscles.

Irregular bones are bones that do not seem to fit in the other categories. These include skull, vertebrae, and hip bones. These bones have a thin cortical exterior with a larger spongy interior.

Important Concepts

Bones come in many sizes and shapes to allow them to be useful in a variety of purposes. Some are flat and thin, and others are thicker. Some bones are smooth, whereas others have areas that protrude and areas that are rough.

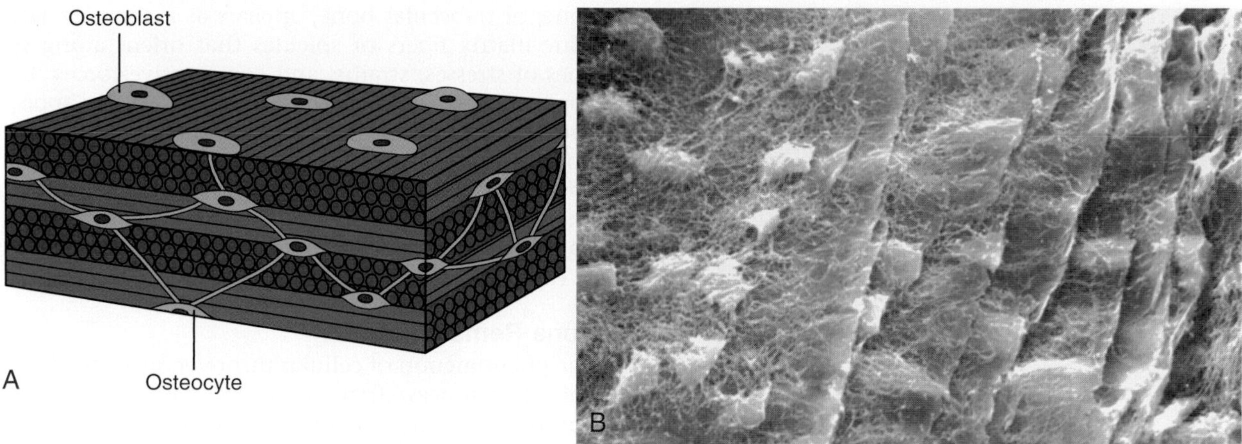

FIG 10-7 **A,** Diagrammatic representation of the layered (lamellar) appearance of bone shows how the alternating dark and light layers are explained by change in direction of the collagen fibers in each layer. **B,** Scanning electron photomicrograph demonstrating collagenous lamellae (layers) of the bone with the osteocytes between the lamellae. *(From Bullough PG:* Orthopedic pathology, *ed 5, St Louis, 2010, Mosby.)*

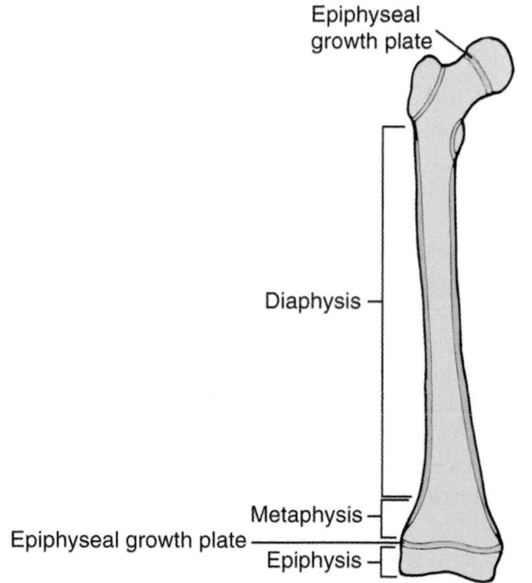

FIG 10-8 Long bone components. *(From Cameron MH, Monroe L:* Physical rehabilitation for the physical therapist assistant, *St Louis, 2011, Saunders.)*

MACROSCOPIC STRUCTURE OF BONE

All bone tissue has a limiting surface shell or cortex. Enclosed by this cortical shell are planes and rows of osseous tissue that is structurally organized as either cancellous bone (trabecular bone) or **cortical bone** (compact bone). Cancellous bone is located at the metaphysis of long bones, the vertebrae, and other cuboid bones.[4]

Cortical bone, also known as *compact bone,* is located in the diaphyseal portion of long bones. Compact bone is very dense and hard on all surfaces, allowing it to function structurally and for protection. Approximately 80% to 90% of the volume of cortical bone is calcium.[22] The thickness of cortical bone varies considerably within a single bone and between bones. In a long bone such as the femur, the cortex in the mid-diaphysis may reach more than a quarter of in inch, whereas the ends may be much thinner (Fig. 10-9). The major structural subunit of cortical bone (compact bone) is the osteon. As described by Bostrom and colleagues,[4] the osteon is a central component of the haversian system.

Haversian bone is the most complex type of cortical bone. It comprises vascular channels circumferentially surrounded by lamellar bone. This complex arrangement of bone around the vascular channel is called the *osteon.* The osteon is an irregular, branching, and anastomosing cylinder composed of a more or less centrally placed neurovascular canal surrounded by cell permeated layers of bone matrix.[4] Primary osteons are osteons that develop into mature bone, whereas as new haversian canals are constantly formed, secondary osteons form on top of the old.

Conversely, trabecular or cancellous bone is uniformly less dense with a large surface area and is significantly metabolically more "active" than cortical bone.[4] Although cortical bone (compact bone) has four times the mass of trabecular bone, the metabolic activity of trabecular bone is eight times greater than that of cortical bone.[4] This makes sense because cancellous bone is concentrated more where compressive forces predominate, such as in vertebral bodies and ends of long bones (Fig. 10-10). Because bone turnover is a surface-oriented event, the profound surface area of trabecular bone explains the greater cellular exchange of cancellous bone.[4]

Periosteum is a thin fibrous covering to all bone except at the musculotendinous insertion and at the articular ends. It attaches to bone cortex by collagen fibers known as Sharpey's fibers. In adults, this periosteum is firmly attached, whereas it is loosely adherent in children (Fig. 10-11).

Bone Architecture

Characteristic differences between cortical bone and trabecular bone are best distinguished by the density and porosity of these two **bone types**. Visually, cancellous

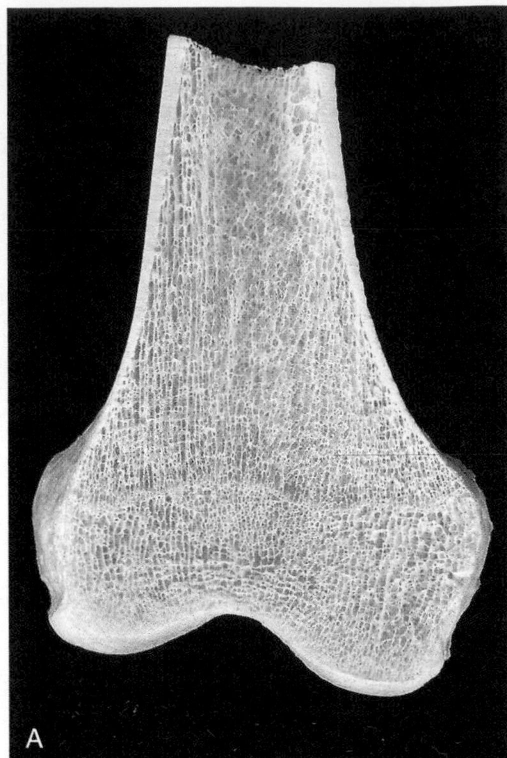

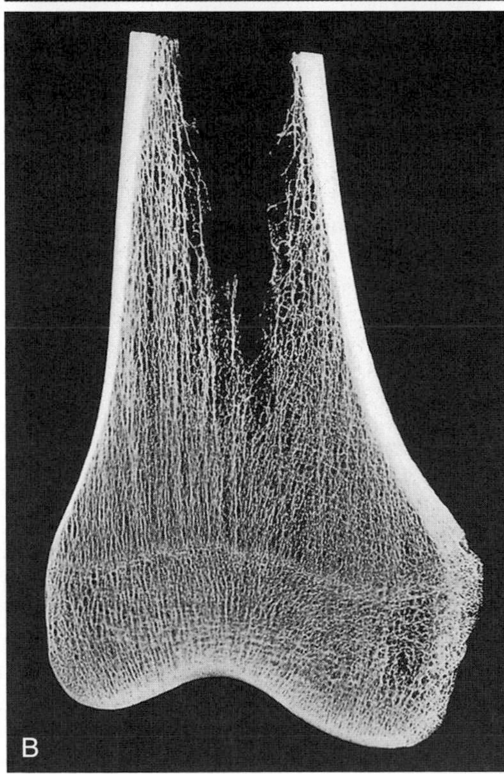

FIG 10-9 **A,** Cleaned and macerated specimen of a lower femur demonstrates the decrease in cancellous bone and the thickening of the cortex as one approaches the diaphysis. **B,** Radiograph of the same specimen. Note the arrangement of the trabecular bone and the horizontal plate of bone that marks the site of the cartilage growth plate—the "epiphyseal scar." *(From Bullough PG:* Orthopedic pathology, *ed 5, St Louis, 2010, Mosby.)*

bone, or trabecular bone, appears as a complex lattice of bone matrix fibers or spicules that orient along specific lines of stresses, strains, and compressive forces. Cortical bone, also known as compact bone, is dense in appearance and is subject to bending, torsion, and compressive forces. Cortical bone also is defined as bone with less than 30% porosity. Trabecular bone is generally 50% to 90% porous. The structure and material characteristics of cortical and trabecular bone are distinguished by the relative density of each.

Bone Remodeling

The phenomenon of cellular turnover, or **remodeling**, of bone is a process that occurs on the surface of various portions of bone (periosteal, endosteal, trabecular, and haversian canal).[41] Generally, bone remodeling is a lifelong activity that responds to mechanical stress (torsion bending, compression, tension) according to Wolff's law.[4] In simplified terms, Wolff's law states that intermittent physiologic loads applied to bone stimulate adaptive responses. Removal of mechanical forces on the bone has the opposite effect. That is, when bone does not receive appropriate physiologic stress, osteoclastic activity overwhelms osteoblast production, which reduces bone mass (Fig. 10-12). The Hueter-Volkmann law is the reverse of Wolff's law and is more specifically applied to compression and tensile forces acting on physeal growth plates. Simply stated, the Hueter-Volkmann law suggests that compression forces limit bone growth, whereas tensile stress stimulates growth.[4]

Osseous tissue also is responsive to piezoelectric charges. In conjunction with mechanical forces strengthening compression and tensile stress, compression produces an electronegative charge that acts to stimulate osteoblast activity. Tensile stress produces an electropositive charge that stimulates osteoclastic activity. Mechanical laws of stress (Wolff's law) produce electromechanical changes that act to maintain equilibrium between bone formation and bone resorption.

Important Concepts

Osseous tissue also is responsive to piezoelectric charges. In conjunction with mechanical forces strengthening compression and tensile stress, compression produces an electronegative charge that acts to stimulate osteoblast activity. Tensile stress produces an electropositive charge that stimulates osteoclastic activity.

VASCULAR SUPPLY TO BONE

The adult skeletal system receives 5% to 10% of the body's total cardiac output.[41] Bone receives blood supply from three distinct but interconnected systems: (1) the nutrient artery, (2) metaphyseal-epiphyseal system, and (3) periosteal systems (Fig. 10-13).

The arterial vascular system provides the origin of the nutrient system via a nutrient foramen in the diaphysis of long bones. The total number of nutrient vessels and

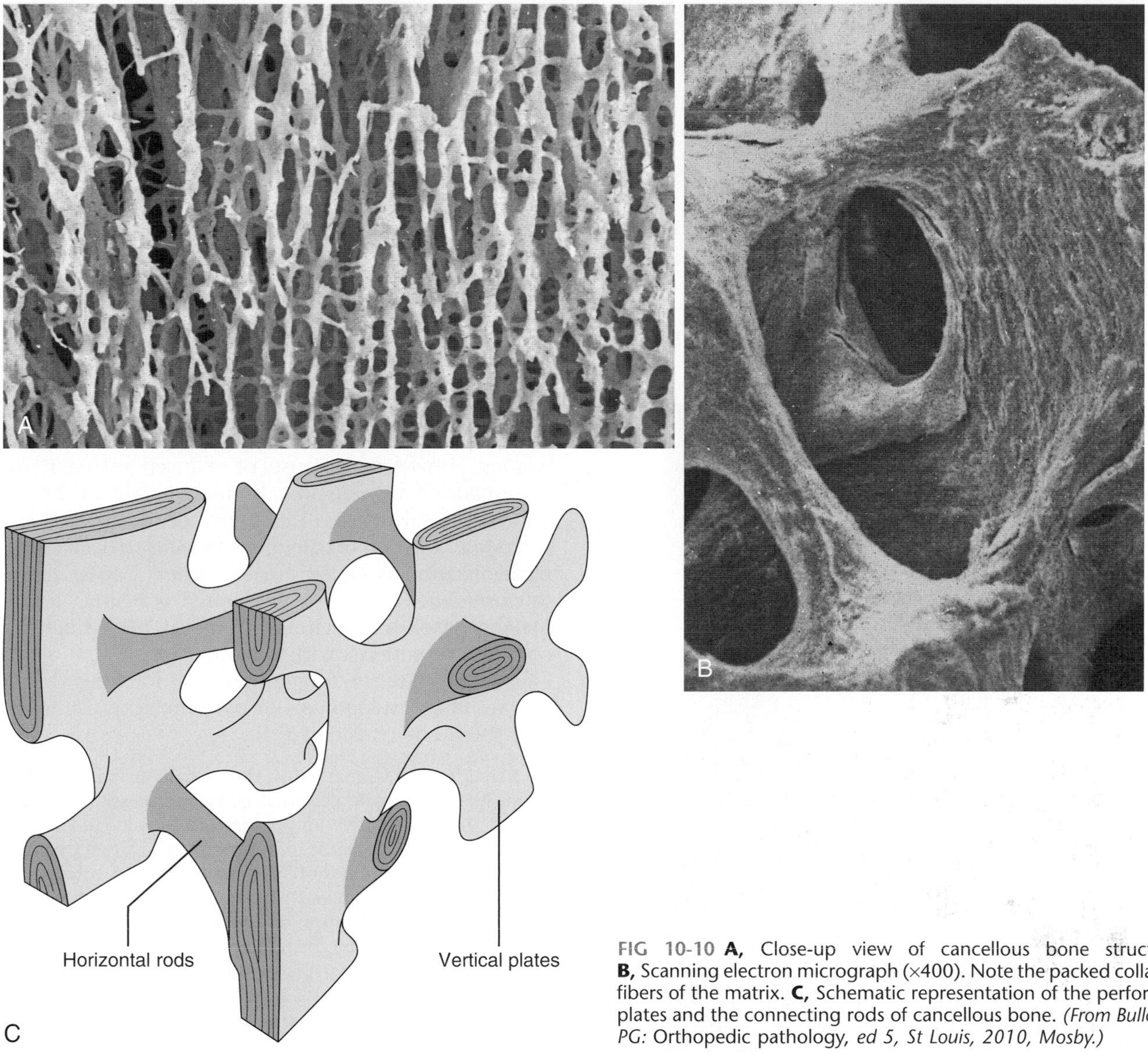

FIG 10-10 **A,** Close-up view of cancellous bone structure. **B,** Scanning electron micrograph (×400). Note the packed collagen fibers of the matrix. **C,** Schematic representation of the perforated plates and the connecting rods of cancellous bone. *(From Bullough PG:* Orthopedic pathology, *ed 5, St Louis, 2010, Mosby.)*

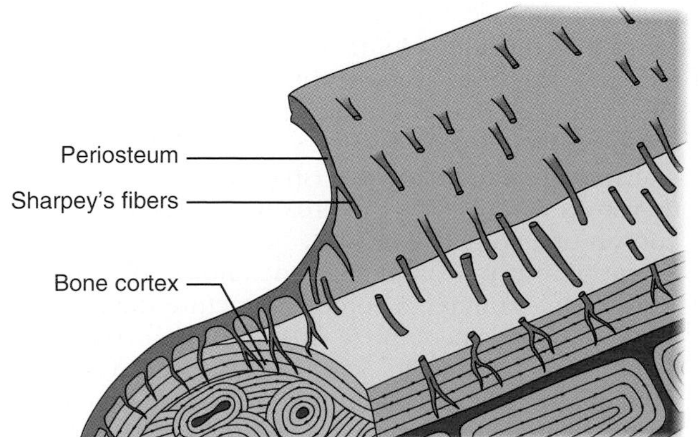

FIG 10-11 Sharpey's fibers are direct continuations of the periosteal collagen fibers around which the circumferential lamellae of the cortical bone have grown, firmly anchoring the periosteum. *(From Bullough PG:* Orthopedic pathology, *ed 5, St Louis, 2010, Mosby.)*

foramen varies with each bone.[4] The nutrient arteries enter the medullary space and then ascend and descend into the arterioles within the endosteal surface supplying the diaphyseal area of long bones.[4] The metaphyseal-epiphyseal system is supplied by a periarticular complex system of the genicular arteries that penetrates the thin cortices of the metaphysis of long bones.[4] Muscular attachment to the periosteal cortical sites of bone provides nutrition through the periosteal capillary system.[4]

Fractures, internal fixation devices, external fixation, and prosthetic joint implants devitalize the microcirculation of the cortical-periosteal and endosteal portion of the bone. The resultant ischemia of bone can lead to nonunion and bone infections.[4] These important clinical ramifications of disruption of bone circulation are evident when initiating therapeutic interventions of early weight bearing and closed kinetic chain resistance exercise after fractures or joint replacement.

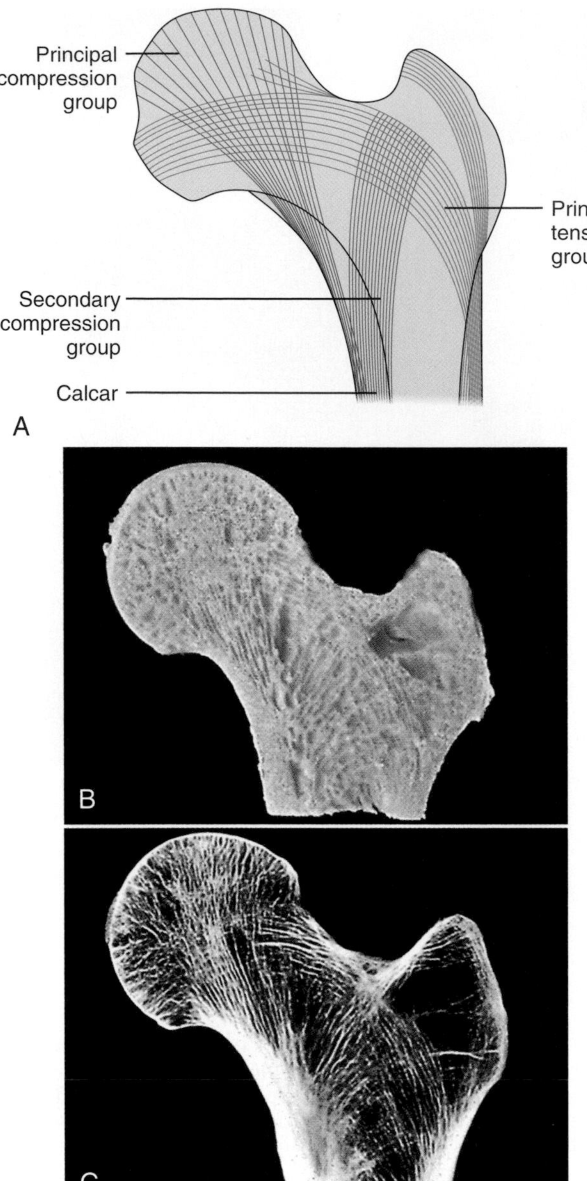

FIG 10-12 **A,** Wolff's law is well demonstrated in the head and neck of the femur, in which the bone trabeculae radiate from the articular surface down onto the medial cortex of the femoral neck (the calcar), which is much thicker than the cortex on the lateral side of the femoral neck. **B,** In this slice through the upper end of the femur, the marrow fat has been washed out of the specimen to demonstrate the distribution of the cancellous bone. **C,** Perhaps the best way to demonstrate clearly the arrangement of the bone trabeculae is by radiography of the specimen. *(From Bullough PG:* Orthopedic pathology, *ed 5, St Louis, 2010, Mosby.)*

Important Concepts

Surgical devices can sometimes disrupt the natural healing process by devitalizing the circulation of cortical-periosteal and endosteal portions of bone. Delayed healing or non-union of fractures can result. These concepts are important when beginning weight bearing or instituting closed kinetic chain exercises.

OSTEOPOROSIS

Osteoporosis is an age-related heterogeneous bone disease characterized by decreased bone tissue. Osteoporosis occurs when osteoblast (bone formation) activity is surpassed by osteoclast (bone resorption) activity (Fig. 10-14).[27] This situation creates weaker bones that are subjected to greater rates of fracture. More than 1 million fractures a year can be attributed to osteoporosis[33]; vertebral body compression fractures are the most common.

Causes of osteoporosis may be multifactorial, including hormonal alterations after menopause, prolonged immobilization, diseases, and prolonged steroid administration. Women are at greater risk for developing osteoporosis for several reasons. Age-related cortical bone loss generally begins at about age 40 years,[27] with the rate thereafter being approximately 0.5% annually for both men and women. However, because of reduced estrogen during menopause,[27] women lose bone at a rate of 2% to 8% annually, resulting in a much greater total loss.

Poor absorption of calcium that leads to decreased bone mineralization is called *osteomalacia*.[33] Causes include a calcium-deficient diet, accelerated calcium loss, and malabsorption of calcium.[27] Femoral neck fractures are common in patients with osteomalacia.[33]

To appreciate the fragile nature of fractures that occur as a result of osteoporosis or osteomalacia, the following case should be considered:

> A frail, elderly woman with osteoporosis sustains resultant multilevel thoracic vertebral body compression fractures. Bed rest with relative immobilization is ordered. She experiences further decrease in bone strength caused by immobilization. Rehabilitation is complicated by osteoporosis and fractures. Combined with the general overall negative effects of immobilization on the body's systems, the effects of immobilization on the remaining skeletal tissue interfere with exercise, sitting, progressive ambulation, and functional activities, forming a vicious cycle that will need to be broken for a functional recovery to occur.

CLASSIFICATIONS OF FRACTURES

By definition, a fracture is any abnormal disruption in the normal anatomic continuity of a bone, an epiphyseal plate, or a cartilaginous joint surface.[39] The classification of fractures takes into account the following criteria[38,39]:

- Site of injury—the area of insult on the bone itself. An epiphyseal fracture describes the site, as does an intraarticular fracture or diaphyseal (shaft) fracture. Generally, the site is described as the proximal, middle, or distal portion of a bone (Fig. 10-15).
- Extent of injury—complete or incomplete (Fig. 10-16). As the name implies, a complete fracture traverses the bone entirely. Incomplete fractures are commonly described as hairline cracks or greenstick fractures.
- Configuration or direction of abnormality—the direction of the fracture. In a transverse fracture, the fracture line goes straight across (horizontally) through the bone; an oblique fracture crosses the bone diagonally. A spiral fracture describes a torsion or rotational injury where the fracture line literally spirals through the

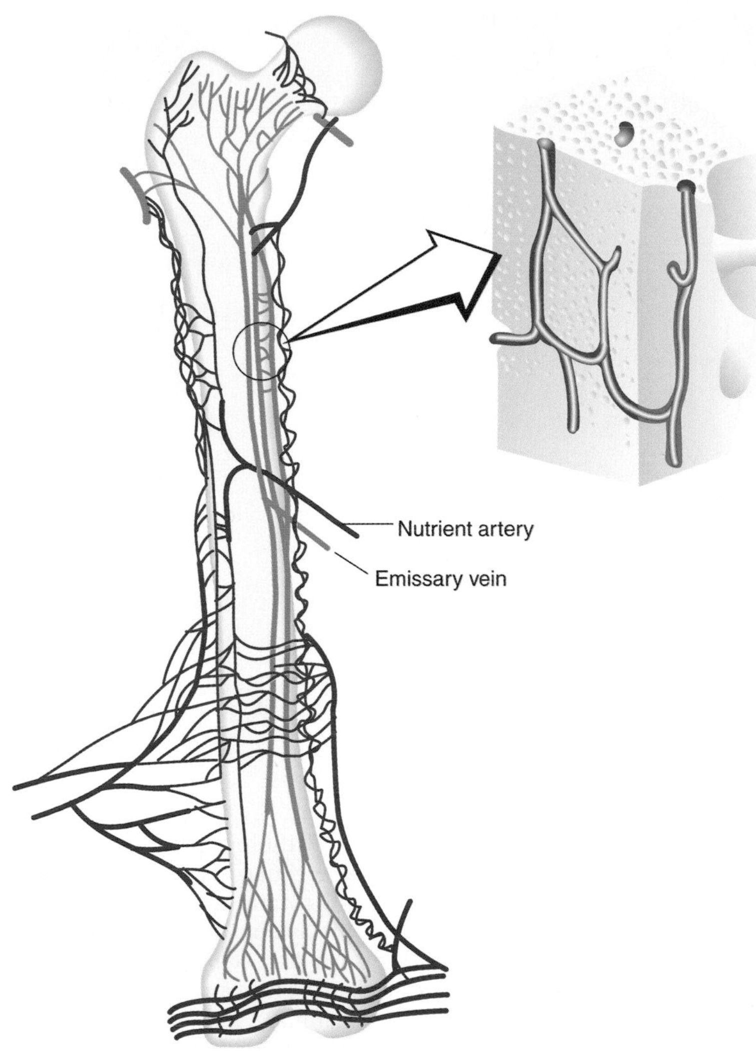

FIG 10-13 Blood supply to the bone. *(From Brinker MR, Miller MD:* Fundamentals of orthopaedics, *Philadelphia, 1999, Saunders.)*

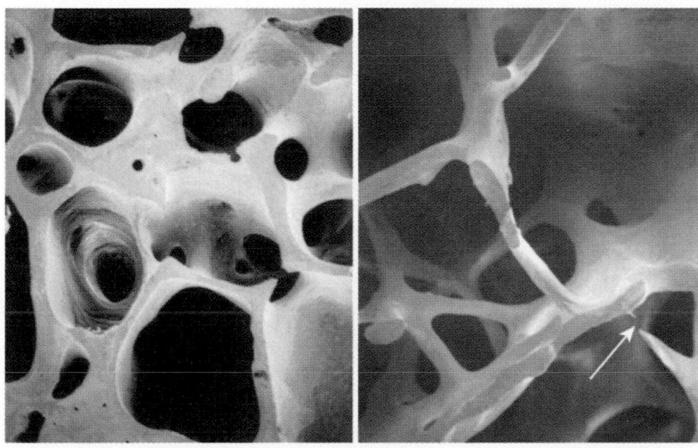

FIG 10-14 Normal and osteoporotic bone. *Arrow* on osteoporotic bones shows trabecular microfracture. *(From Patton KT, Thibodeau GA:* Anatomy and physiology, *ed 7, St Louis, 2010, Mosby.)*

bone. An impacted fracture is a long-axis compression injury where the fracture fragments are forced together. The fracture is classified as comminuted when more than two fragments are present.

- Relationship of fracture fragments to each other—can be displaced, nondisplaced, angulated, twisted, rotated, or overriding. An example is an avulsion fracture where a portion of bone is pulled away as part of a musculotendinous attachment or ligament-bone attachment.
- Relationship of fracture fragments to the environment—whether the injury is open (compound fracture) or closed (simple).
- Complications—resulting in delayed union, nonunion, or malunion of the fracture fragments. An uncomplicated course of healing is called *uneventful*.

Pediatric fractures have a special classification of injuries involving the epiphysis. Depending on the type of epiphyseal fracture, the eventual growth of the bone can be profoundly affected.

The fracture classification of Salter and Harris is outlined in Figure 10-17. Type I Salter-Harris fractures,

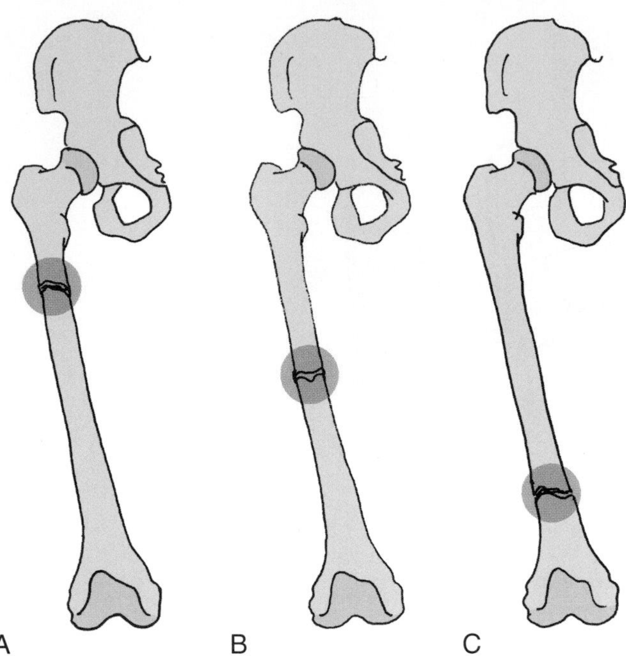

FIG 10-15 Fracture classification, site of injury. **A,** Proximal fracture of the femur. **B,** Middle fracture of the femur. **C,** Distal fracture of the femur.

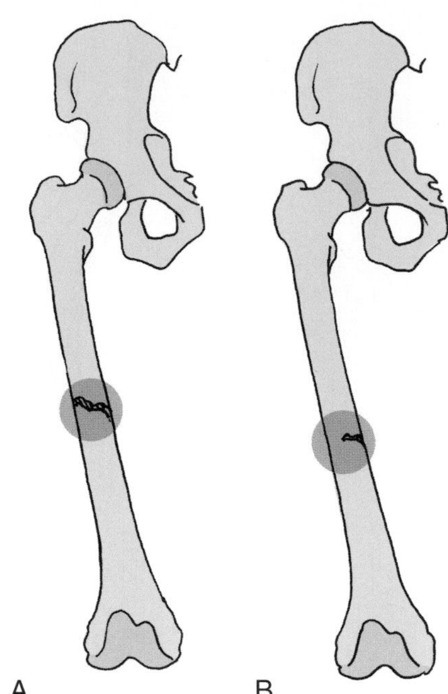

FIG 10-16 Fracture classification, extent of injury. **A,** Complete fracture of the femur. **B,** Incomplete fracture of the femur.

modified by Rang,[33,37-39] are transverse fractures through the physis. Type II fractures are the same as type I but also have a metaphyseal fragment. Type III fractures involve the physis and the epiphysis. Typically, these are intraarticular fractures. Type IV fractures are the same as type III but include the metaphysis. These are significant injuries that can lead to a reduction in bone growth. Type V fractures are severe injuries classified as crush injuries to the physis. This type of fracture also can lead to growth arrest. The PTA should also be aware of the Arbeitsgemeinschaft für Osteosynthesefragen (AO) classification system, which is universally applied to fracture patterns and the devices used for internal fixation. This classification system is discussed later in this chapter.[32]

Important Concepts

The Salter-Harris fracture classification is one of the most common systems of identification and is based on the fracture and its location to the physis.

Other fractures that are commonly seen in children are incomplete fractures. Incomplete fractures typically occur because the bones of a child are more flexible than the bones of an adult. A buckle fracture is one in which a deformation or "bending" of the cortex occurs on one side of the bone. A greenstick fracture is one that involves a linear fracture through one cortical surface and a flexing deformation of the opposite surface. A bowing fracture is one that may be caused by multiple microfractures along the length of a long bone so that the entire bone is bent or curved.

Pathologic fractures are caused by tumors[33] (malignant or primary bone disease), osteoporosis (most common), microtrauma from repetitive overload (stress fractures), or metastatic bone disease (second most common). These usually occur in an elderly person secondary to osteoporosis and can happen spontaneously or with very minor trauma.[33]

COMPONENTS OF BONE HEALING

Most of the adult skeleton (80%) is composed of compact, cortical bone. Approximately 20% of the skeleton is cancellous or spongy bone. Compact bone is extremely dense and unyielding to bending, whereas cancellous bone is more elastic and less dense than cortical bone.[33]

Three types of cells take part in the highly dynamic, reparative process in bone. Osteoblasts help form and synthesize bone. Osteocytes are mature bone cells that account for approximately 90% of all bone tissue. Osteoclasts are active in bone resorption.

The normal dynamic process of bone synthesis and resorption is termed *remodeling*. Remodeling and stress occur together, which profoundly influences bone shape, density, internal architecture, and external configuration.[1,24,28,33] With normal bone remodeling, weight-bearing forces and muscular contractions provide the stress needed for bone formation and adaptation. The absence of physiologic loading, or stress, is detrimental to bone, ligament, cartilage, muscle, and tendons as well as the cardiorespiratory system. Wolff's law[1] states that intermittently applied stress, as well as changes in function of bone, causes definite changes.[5,28] After a fracture, treatment may involve rigid cast immobilization and non–weight bearing over a

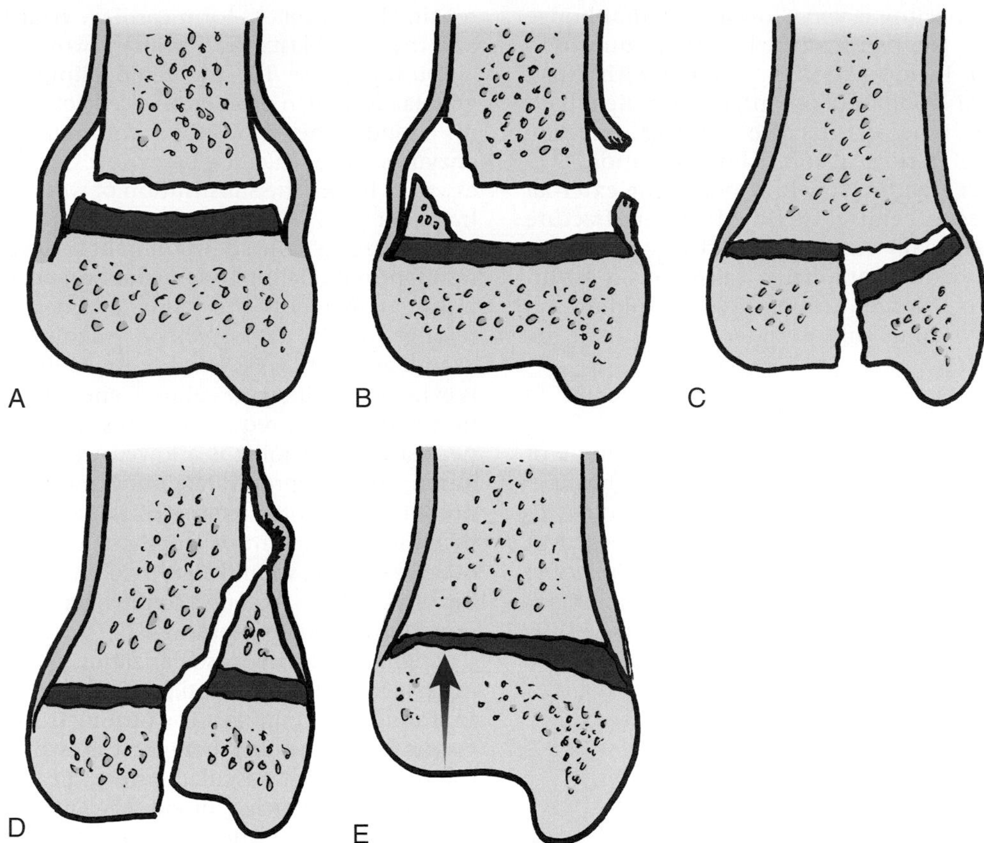

FIG 10-17 Salter-Harris fracture classification. **A,** Type I is a transverse fracture through the physis. **B,** Type II is the same as type I but also has a metaphyseal fragment. **C,** Type III is an intraarticular fracture that involves the physis and the epiphysis. **D,** Type IV is the same as type III but also involves the metaphysis. **E,** Type V is a crush injury to the physis.

period of weeks. This decreased stress on the bone causes rapid osteoclast activity (bone resorption) and decreased osteoblast activity.[34] Although the removal of stress is paramount for healing, the decrease in external force also causes significant bone loss.[33] Bone loss caused by immobilization is reversible after progressive weight bearing, active motion, resistive exercise, and vertical loading (closed kinetic chain exercise).[33] It is recommended that strict, long-term, rigid cast immobilization be minimized whenever possible.

Although normal stresses promote bone development, excessive stress also can lead to gradual bone resorption.[28] Stress that is unrelenting and does not allow for osteoblastic repair of bone can lead to pathologic accelerated bone resorption and eventual stress fracture.[1,24,28]

Bone remodeling is also influenced by electrical charges when forces are applied to bone. The **piezoelectric effect** describes a negative electrical charge toward the concave, or compression, side of a force applied to a bone. An electropositive charge is seen on the tension, or convex, side of the bone. The negative-charge side responds by stimulating osteoblasts, whereas the positive-charge side (tension side) responds by increasing osteoclast activity.[33]

BONE INJURY AND REPAIR

Injury repair and eventual regeneration of osseous tissue is a complex process that involves the bone marrow, bone cortex, periosteum, and external soft tissues. Trauma to the bone disrupts the biologic, mechanical, structural, architectural, and histochemical environment of bone. Classic descriptions of fracture healing are divided into primary (direct) cortical healing and secondary (indirect) fracture healing. The spontaneous natural course of fracture repair can be described as interfragmentary stabilization by periosteal and endosteal callus formation and by interfragmentary fibrocartilage differentiation, restoration of continuity and bone union by intramembranous and endochondral ossification, substitution of avascular and necrotic areas by haversian remodeling, modeling of the fracture site, and functional adaptation.[1,4,5,11,14,26]

Fracture healing responses differ according to the nature of stabilization provided (direct, internal, compression-appositional, alignment fixation versus cast immobilization). That is, rigid internal fixation results in primary-direct cortical healing, which is an attempt by the cortex of bone to reestablish mechanical and anatomic continuity. In primary fracture healing, the new bone grows directly across the bone ends to unite the fracture site.

This form of bone healing is very slow and cannot bridge a fracture gap, and the two fractured ends are unable to appose each other. Rigid fixation is required with direct contact of cortical bone and an intact intramedullary vasculature. This type of fracture healing response usually is devoid of periosteal soft callus formation. Secondary or indirect fracture repair is noted for external periosteal soft tissue callus bridging between fracture fragments. In secondary healing, a cartilage matrix is initially formed, which gradually takes on a callus appearance. This method of healing involves adding stability by creating a callus that is larger (wider) than the two opposing bones.

PHASES OF FRACTURE REPAIR

In general, most fractures heal with a combination of primary cortical healing and secondary-indirect healing. The phases of fracture repair are divided into six sequences of events that ultimately lead to functional remodeling of the injured bone.[26] Phase I is inflammation and hematoma formation, phase II is chondrocyte formation and angiogenesis, phase III is cartilage and calcification, phase IV is cartilage removal, phase V is bone formation, and phase VI is bone remodeling.[26]

Important Concepts

Fracture healing occurs through six different phases. Phase I is inflammation and hematoma formation, phase II is chondrocyte formation and angiogenesis, phase III is cartilage and calcification, phase IV is cartilage removal, phase V is bone formation, and phase VI is bone remodeling.

Phase I, inflammation and hematoma formation, is characterized by fibrin clot formation. This occurs because small blood vessels near the site of injury are torn and result in internal bleeding. The fracture site creates formation of the inflammatory response. Because of increased vascularity from the injury, a hematoma forms and begins the process of clot formation. The extent of bleeding and hematoma that is formed depends on the degree of injury and amount of fracture displacement. The presence of the fibrin clot between fracture fragments acts as a rich source of activating inflammatory molecules essential to the complex cascade of intense cellular activity required for fracture repair. Many cellular processes are involved during this phase that are responsible for attracting, regulating, and differentiating cells that serve to propagate the development of cartilage and revascularization of bone. Animal models demonstrate intramembranous and endochondral bone formation during the first 2 weeks after fracture.[26] This early mass of tissue formed during bone healing is termed a *callus*. The callus is an early precursor to mature calcified bone.

The presence of cartilage within the fracture repair matrix at this point is the hallmark of phase II, the reparative phase. Chondrocytes form a V-shaped wedge of tissue between the ends of fractured bone. The matrix formed is type I and II cartilage. Calcification of chondrocytes (cartilage) requires specific enzyme release for phosphate and calcium interactions. In the initial process of phase II repair, chondroblasts form cartilage near the fracture site, and the osteoblasts form primary woven bone.

During phase III, the remodeling phase, there is a gradual decline in proliferative cell activity and an increase in chondrocyte deposition and release of proteolytic enzymes. The calcification process of fibrocartilage is essential before the substitution of woven bone within the fragment gap. When fibrocartilage is calcified, the ultimate integrity and development of woven bone with resultant remodeling to lamellar bone depends on revitalization (vascularity) of injured bone. Eventually, bone reforms into its natural shape. At this time, radiographic examination shows a fracture line still present, but there is evidence of the bone callus. Generally, rigid immobilization is no longer required at this time. Movement of the nearest affected joint is allowed with caution. If healing has occurred appropriately, movement at the site should not elicit pain or a feeling of bone fragment movement by either the patient or the therapist. Pain or a sensation of bone shifting should alert the PTA to contact the attending physical therapist (PT) or the referring physician before more movement is performed.

Angiogenesis (neovascularization) is critical for delivering oxygen, nutrients, inflammatory cells, and fibroblasts to stimulate and support the healing fracture. The vascular response to a healing fracture varies over time. Initially, the three distinct vascular systems of bone are disrupted significantly, reducing blood flow. Over the next several days after fracture, the circulation increases and peaks at approximately 2 weeks.[26] Although there is a relative increase in vascular budding, the dramatic volume of cellular activity creates a state of hypoxia at the fracture that is highly conducive for cartilage formation.[26]

PROCESS OF BONE HEALING

Bone healing can be characterized by the following sequence of events:

- Fracture occurs.
- Bleeding occurs, and a hematoma results.
- Granulation tissue is formed by the hematoma (soft callus formation).
- Osteoblasts produce new bone, and a bony or hard callus is formed.
- The callus is gradually reabsorbed, and the anatomic contour of the bone is regained.

As with soft tissue, the immediate inflammatory response lasts 24 to 48 hours and is characterized by the development of granulation tissue, blood clotting, and fibroblast and osteoblast proliferation.[5,33] The repair phase of bone healing signals the development of bone scarring, or callus formation, which is usually detected within the first 2 weeks after injury. The degree of callus formation depends on anatomic alignment of the fragments and the degree and quality of immobilization. If motion occurs through the fracture site during this phase, a soft bone callus (primarily of cartilage) bridges the fragments.[5,33] This type of callus also forms if the union between the fragments is poor, even when immobilization prevents motion.

Primary cortical healing (hard callus) forms with anatomic alignment and fragment apposition, immobilization, negligible gap size, and appropriately applied progressive stress.[13] The remodeling phase of bone healing can take several years to complete and is strongly influenced by Wolff's law.[1]

As with ligament healing, protection of the injury site is vital to a successful outcome. There is an exceedingly narrow line to follow with respect to motion after bone injury. In many cases, a reducing plan of immobilization is used to secure the bone fragments, protect the fracture, and provide needed motion for healing. For example, a rigid cast can be applied for 2 to 4 weeks, and then a limited range hinge brace can be used to protect the healing structures and initiate physiologic motion within set limits. Depending on the severity of the insult, some fractures may require secure immobilization for extended periods to allow for proper healing.

Overall, healing times vary with the age and health of the patient and with the location and type of fracture incurred. In general, without complications, children heal within 4 to 6 weeks, adolescents heal within 6 to 8 weeks, and adults heal within 10 to 18 weeks.

Important Concepts

Overall, fracture healing times vary with the age and health of the patient and with the location and type of fracture incurred. In general, without complications, children heal within 4 to 6 weeks; adolescents, within 6 to 8 weeks; and adults, within 10 to 18 weeks.

EFFECTS OF IMMOBILIZATION ON BONE TISSUE

A major goal for bone healing to occur is to immobilize the fracture site. However, when bone tissue does not receive physiologic loads (ambulation, vertical loads, and muscle contractions), the normal remodeling processes are negatively affected. The rate of normal bone remodeling changes when immobilization lasts slightly longer than 1 week.[14] The "turnover" or remodeling of bone during immobilization is characterized by a loss of calcium, resulting in localized bone loss. Immobilization leads to a reduction in the hardness of bone related to the duration of immobilization.[14] By 3 months, bone strength is only 55% to 60% of normal.[44] The relationship between soft tissue structures and bone during periods of immobilization reflects the interdependence of muscular contractions, forces acting on joints, compressive loads, circulation (blood flow affecting nutrition), and motion in maintaining bone remodeling equilibrium.

A definite contrast is seen in the care of healing bone tissue. It is necessary to immobilize the fracture fragments so that healing can occur, yet minimize the negative effects of immobilization through the judicious application of progressive motion, exercise, and weight bearing. The length of time needed to regain bone strength after immobilization is considerably longer than the duration of immobilization. The length of the immobilization is an important component in the overall process of healing bone tissue.

COMPLICATIONS

Occasionally the process of bone healing leads to three distinct complications:

1. Delayed union
2. Nonunion
3. Malunion

In delayed union, the dynamic biologic repair processes of bone healing occur at a slower rate than anticipated. Brashear and Raney[5] described delayed union as clinically detectable when firm callus is not present at 20 weeks (for fractures of the tibia and femur) and at 10 weeks (for fractures of the humerus). An important cause of delayed union is "inadequate or interrupted immobilization."[5] Rehabilitation can significantly affect the healing process either positively or negatively. If therapeutic interventions are begun too soon or too vigorously, delayed union may occur because of excessive motion occurring at the fracture site. The tradeoff when caring for patients with delayed bone union is the need to provide extended periods of immobilization for healing. However, cast braces and walking casts can be used to provide the weight bearing (Wolff's law) necessary to enhance healing. In nonunion, the healing processes have stopped. Nonunion occurs when there is significant and severe associated soft tissue trauma, poor blood supply, and infections.

In malunion, healing results in a nonanatomic position (Fig. 10-18). Malunion is caused by ineffective immobilization and failure to maintain immobilization for an adequate period of time. For appropriate bone healing to occur, anatomic alignment (apposition) of fragments, adequate fixation (external or internal), and length of time of immobilization must occur in concert. If these factors are not balanced, the chance of complications is increased. Regardless of the type of complication, fracture healing fails or is delayed 5% to 10% of the time.[8,12]

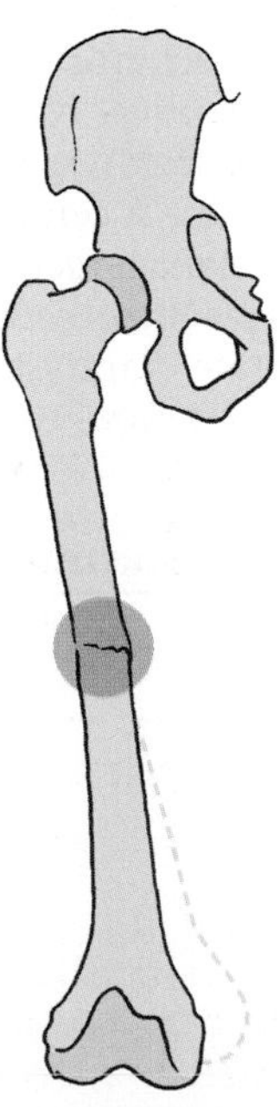

FIG 10-18 Malunion of the femur. *Dotted line* indicates normal anatomic alignment.

Important Concepts

Complications of fracture healing include delayed union, nonunion, and malunion.

FRACTURE FIXATION: BIOLOGY AND BIOMECHANICS

Rigid anatomic fixation of bone results in primary repair or direct cortical reconstruction. This process generally inhibits periosteal soft tissue bridging callus. The repair process of rigid internal fixation is characterized by haversian remodeling and osteon formation. *Creeping substitution* is a term used to describe osteoclastic cutting cones traversing the cortical fracture fragments, followed by osteoblast formation and revascularization of bone.

The precise application of various internal fixation devices (intermedullary rods, bone plates, and compression screws) to stimulate primary cortical healing is not without inherent risks. The surgical placement of bone plates requires "stripping" the periosteum where the screws and plates are to be fixed. This process devascularizes the periosteal blood supply. In addition, the areas beneath the plate increase the porosity of bone and weaken the mechanical and structural behavior and the architecture of the injured bone. With intramedullary rod application, the medullary canal must be "reamed" to allow for proper anatomic placement of the rod. The nutrient arterial system, metaphyseal-diaphyseal system, and medullary circulation are disrupted. During the surgical placement of screws and plates, the surgeon attempts to apply these devices by hand-held screw devices and manual torque wrenches instead of using high-speed drills that might create thermal necrosis of bone and soft tissue, which could contribute to increased bone devitalization.[40,44]

Conversely, nonoperative fracture management involves a complex series of interactions, which stimulate the thermal, chemical, mechanical, and electrical environment of periosteal and cortical bone (Table 10-1).[11,26]

Secondary fracture healing results in a series of sequential states that overlap to a certain extent. In cases of nonoperative fracture management, the type of repair is referred to as *secondary-periosteal callus.* The natural healing sequence of nonoperative diaphyseal fractures includes a period of instability (phase I), in which essentially no true biologic support is provided to the fracture site. The fracture stimulates an autoactivated response to repair the site naturally. Blood emanates from the ruptured vessels and fills the gap site. The fracture hematoma and proliferative cellular activation provide no mechanical protection of the fragments. Macrophages remove necrotic tissue and generate granulation tissue for undifferentiated mesenchymal cells originating an initial stabilizing callus.

The second phase is the development of the soft callus. Phase II is characterized by the soft tissue compliance provided by the peripheral structures surrounding the fracture fragments. The formation, organization, and gradual maturation of cellular activity in and around the injury site provides for greater stability.[26] As stated by Latta and colleagues,[26] "peripheral structures supply early vascularization and soft tissue repair. Peripheral soft tissues provide a compliant strength which leads to reduction of acute symptoms long before there is radiographic evidence of healing." Phase III demonstrates a radiographic confirmation of thin "hard callus" (bony ridge).

Generally, hematoma and cartilage are prevalent along with a gradual revascularization of the interfragmentary gap of soft and hard callus formation. Radiographic confirmation of the disappearance of the fracture line is characteristic of phase IV, the fracture line consolidation phase.

During this stage of nonoperative diaphyseal fracture management, there is a subtle, gradual shrinkage of the central soft callus bone with remodeling, consolidation of the fracture line, and maturation of hard bony callus. This process is termed *endochondral ossification,* and the cellular dynamics of the process are similar to the cellular dynamics that occur in a normal growth plate.

Finally, in phase V structural remodeling, there is gradual contraction and shrinkage of callus with resultant reorganization and configuration of normal bone anatomy and topography. This is a gradual process in which controlled mechanical stresses can result in gradual maturation and strengthening of the fractured region.

External Fixation and Fracture Repair

External fixators are used in a wide variety of clinical situations and allow for modification of stiffness and rigidity of fixation during fracture healing.[5,36] The geometric composite construct of these elaborate frame configurations usually can be altered by several orders of magnitude.

TABLE 10-1 Type of Fracture Healing Based on Type of Stabilization

Type of Immobilization	Predominant Type of Healing	Comments
Cast (closed treatments)	Periosteal bridging callus	Endochondral ossification
Compression plate	Primary cortical healing (remodeling)	Cutting cone-type remodeling
Intramedullary nail	Early—periosteal bridging callus Late—medullary callus	Endochondral ossification
External fixator	Dependent on extent of rigidity Less rigid—periosteal bridging callus More rigid—primary cortical healing	
Inadequate	Hypertrophic nonunion	Failed endochondral ossification Type II collagen predominates

From Brinker MR, Miller MD: *Fundamentals of orthopaedics,* Philadelphia, 1999, Saunders.

Several factors significantly contribute to the stability, rigidity, stiffness, and compression of the fracture site and the mechanical properties of the frame.[36] The number of pins used; the length, diameter, and type of pin material; the number of side bars set in the spacing between pins; the spacing between side bars and bone surface; pin-bone contact; and proximal-distal pin spacing all contribute to the material characteristics of stability, stiffness, and compression of the fracture site.[11,36]

Fracture healing characteristics using external fixators depend on the rigidity obtained by the device. Overall, the more rigid the fixation, the earlier the radiographic confirmation of bone union. Less rigid fixators create greater periosteal callus formation, whereas rigid fixators characteristically stimulate direct primary cortical fracture healing.[11,36]

As stated, a unique advantage of external fixation is the ability to alter or modify rigidity during various stages of fracture healing. Several models demonstrate the effect of dynamization (mechanisms used to decrease stiffness of the fixation or mechanisms that allow for controlled micromotion between fracture fragments) on blood flow and bone callus formation.[11,26,31,36,41] A 25% increase in fracture site micromotion resulted in a 400% increase in regional blood flow and substantially more callus formation with animals receiving semirigid external fixators compared with rigid external fixation.[36]

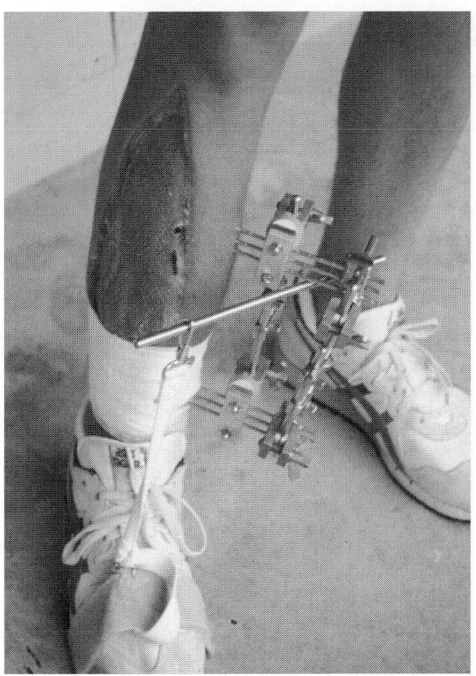

FIG 10-19 External fixation device (external fixator).

> **BOX 10-1 AO Classification System**
>
> The AO classification system was designed by the Association for the Study of Internal Fixation (ASIF) or Arbeitsgemeinschaft für Osteosynthesefragen [AO]) as a method of grading, identifying, and classifying fixation devices as well as fractures themselves. The ASIF was founded in 1956 to develop instrumentation screws, plates, and other devices related to internal fixation, and since that time the AO classification system has come to be widely accepted and universally applied.[8] In clinical practice, the PTA may frequently see the AO classification used to describe certain devices used for internal fixation, such as the ones discussed in this chapter.

Bone Fixation Devices

When caring for patients who have sustained fractures, the PTA must be aware of various methods used to immobilize or stabilize the fracture so that a clear understanding of the extent of trauma can be appreciated. This knowledge also allows the PTA to understand the degree of tissue healing necessary before vigorous rehabilitation exercises can be undertaken.

The remarkable sensitivity of bone to normal biologic stress is well known.[1,28,33,39] After fracture, an attempt is made to stabilize the fracture, bring the fragments together by apposition (approximation) and alignment, and remove or minimize forces that may slow the normal healing process. Two general methods of immobilization are used in the treatment of fractures. In one method, the area is immobilized by external fixation devices. This method involves the use of casts, traction, splints, and braces as well as the external fixation devices employed with significant open (compound comminuted) fractures where the risk of infection is present (Fig. 10-19). These ominous-looking devices help fix the fracture site, while allowing care of the open wounds with skin grafts, tissue flaps, or débridement. These are classified as external fixation devices because the pins used to immobilize the fracture do not contact the fragments directly but are used to hold the bone segments in rigid alignment and anatomic apposition. With closed (simple) fractures, various rigid lightweight fiberglass casts, plaster casts, hinged-plaster casts, and adjustable-range hinged braces are used for immobilization.

The second method of immobilization uses internal fixation devices and is best for displaced fractures where external fixation does not provide the degree of immobilization necessary to effect healing. (See Box 10-1 for the background on the AO classification system, designed by the Association for the Study of Internal Fixation [ASIF] or Arbeitsgemeinschaft für Osteosynthesefragen [AO].) Internal fixation is called *open reduction with internal fixation (ORIF)* and involves surgically exposing the fracture site to reduce, approximate, and align the bone fragments. The materials used for ORIF procedures include metals (stainless steel and metal alloys of cobalt-chromium-molybdenum and titanium) and nonmetals (high-density polyethylene, polymethyl methacrylate, silicones, and ceramics). Metal internal fixation devices frequently are combinations of screws, staples, pins, nails, tension-band wires, and various plates. The placement of these materials can affect the delivery of certain therapeutic agents, such as ultrasound. Also, a hole or tunnel defect in a bone, with or without a screw in it, effectively reduces the overall strength of the bone up to 50%.[33] Even after screw removal, the bone does not regain normal strength for up to 1 year.[33]

TABLE 10-2 Internal Fixation Devices

Type	Use
Compression plate	Diaphyseal fractures
Intramedullary rod	Lower extremity diaphyseal fractures (femur, tibia); removed at 1 or 2 years
Reconstruction plate	Used in pelvic and distal humerus fractures
Tension wires	Patella fractures and olecranon fractures
Sliding hip screws	Intertrochanteric hip fractures
Condylar screws	Distal femur fractures
Cannulated screws	Femoral neck fractures

From Miller M: *Review of orthopaedics,* Philadelphia, 1992, Saunders.

Metal internal fixation devices occasionally loosen and can "back out," as is the case with screws. If the PTA notes signs of hardware loosening (pain, swelling, or crepitus), he or she must immediately consult with the supervising PT and physician. Many metal fixation devices are designed to be left in place, as with most plates, but these devices should be removed if metal allergic reactions occur. Table 10-2 lists the various internal fixation devices.

Important Concepts

ORIF involves surgically exposing the fracture site to reduce, approximate, and align the bone fragments.

FACTORS INFLUENCING BONE HEALING

Several key factors are implicated in delayed biologic fracture repair. Tobacco smoke, malnutrition, inadequate reduction of the fragments, excessive motion from inadequate immobilization, poor vascular supply, soft tissue interposition between fracture fragments, and infection significantly limit spontaneous fracture repair.[4,11]

Cigarette smoke is a vasoconstrictor that may reduce blood supply to the injury site. In addition, smoking directly interferes with osteoblast formation.[44] Protein, malnutrition, and calorie deprivation reduce skeletal muscle mass and may contribute to reduced periosteal and cortical bone formation.[11] Poor reduction of the fracture fragments and inadequate immobilization create excessive motion and reduced vascular supply to the bone (Box 10-2).[44] Occasionally, a sleeve of soft tissue becomes interposed within the fracture site, significantly reducing primary cortical and secondary periosteal bridging callus and rendering the fragments devitalized.

Infectious organisms have many deleterious effects on implants and the host bone environment. Orthopedic implant loosening, bone resorption, bone destruction, and reactive periosteal elevation can occur in the presence of infection.[11] The risk for orthopedic infection is extremely low (<1% to 2%). On implantation of a prosthetic device, there is an immediate race for the surface—a contest between tissue cell integration and bacterial adhesion to the same surface. If bacteria win, they can live in an enclosed colony called a *biofilm.* Because bacteria in this state are slow-growing, they are not easily eradicated with antibiotics. About 25% of these cases occur within 4 weeks of surgery; 25% of subacute infections occur within 1 year. Late infections (50%) develop after 2 years of pain-free use.[7] The only consistent finding with these infections is pain at the site of the implant; the PTA should be aware that pain can occur in acute, subacute, and late phases.

STIMULATION OF FRACTURE REPAIR

Several methods are available to augment, stimulate, or enhance fracture repair. Bone grafts are used to fill osseous defects and stabilize fractures. Bone autografts are taken from the same individual. Allograft bone tissue is tissue from the same species. An example of a fresh autograft is harvesting bone from the iliac crest to transpose (heterotopic transportation) to the lumbar spine for fusion.

Cadaveric bone allografts must be sterilized chemically. This process renders all cells nonviable. In both autografts and allografts, the implanted graft acts as a scaffold to support the growth of host bone tissue. This process is known as *passive osteoconduction.*[11] The implant bone tissue gradually becomes revascularized with stimulation and transportation of osteoblasts into the new graft. This process is referred to as *osteoinduction.*[11] Although the sequence of events is similar (passive osteoconduction, gradual revascularization, and osteoinduction) with both graft materials, allogeneic bone requires a longer time for creeping substitution to take place. Additional materials used for osteoconduction that support vascular ingrowth, growth, attachment, division, and remodeling of bone include ceramics, bioactive glass, and synthetic polymers.[11]

Ceramic bone graft substitutes include hydroxyapatite and tricalcium phosphate. Some of these graft substitutes are formed from marine coral and crystalline hydroxyapatite. These bone substitutes generally have been shown to be as effective as autograft bone.[11]

Two clinically relevant methods of fracture healing augmentation are electromagnetic field application and low-intensity ultrasound. The use of exogenously applied pulsed electromagnetic fields over nonunion fractures is based on the piezoelectric effect in response to load deformation of crystalline-collagen components of Wolff's law.[11] The use of specific electrical stimulation waveforms to induce bone formations is supported by scientific investigation and clinical observation that electrical stimulation affects endochondral bone formation and connective tissue repair. Pulsed electromagnetic field therapy has been advocated because it is a noninvasive means of fracture management in delayed healing or nonunion fractures.[2,10,42]

Basic science research suggests that the use of nonthermal, low-intensity ultrasound (30 mW/cm^2) has very strong biological value to bone healing owing to signal transduction and gene expression; stimulation of chondroblasts and osteoblasts and increasing blood flow; and enhancement of greater mechanical and histologic influence on endochondral and periosteal bone healing.[23,43,46] Various studies have demonstrated that use of brief low-intensity ultrasound on the order of 20 minutes per day can reduce the time to fracture union.[11,19,21,25,30,35]

BOX 10-2 Biologic and Mechanical Factors Influencing Fracture Healing

Biologic Factors	Mechanical Factors
Patient age	Soft tissue attachments to bone
Comorbid medical conditions	Stability (extent of immobilization)
Functional level	Anatomic location
Nutritional status	Level of energy imparted
Nerve function	Extent of bone loss
Vascular injury	
Hormones	
Growth factors	
Health of soft tissue envelope	
Sterility (in open fractures)	
Cigarette smoke	
Local pathologic conditions	
Level of energy imparted	
Type of bone affected	
Extent of bone loss	

From Brinker MR, Miller MD: *Fundamentals of orthopaedics,* Philadelphia, 1999, Saunders.

A systematic review[9] of the use of low-intensity pulsed ultrasound for fractures that assessed randomized controlled trials determined that many of the studies had only moderate-quality to low-quality evidence for its use. Studies rarely included functional endpoints, and two of the highest quality studies showed no difference in functional outcome with the use of ultrasound. A more recent Cochrane review[17] stated that although a potential benefit of ultrasound for the treatment of acute fractures in adults cannot be ruled out, the currently available evidence from a set of clinically heterogeneous trials is insufficient to support the routine use of this intervention in clinical practice.

CLINICAL APPLICATION OF REHABILITATION TECHNIQUES DURING BONE HEALING

Immobilization after bone injury may not be total and depends on fracture type. Stable fracture patterns (transverse, short oblique, and minimally displaced) can generally be treated with aggressive mobilization of adjacent joints and partial weight bearing with physician approval. Full weight bearing is allowed when fracture healing is demonstrated on follow-up radiography. Unstable fracture patterns (comminuted, long oblique, and most spiral fractures) are generally treated surgically followed by protected weight bearing with mobilization of adjacent joints. Weight bearing is restricted until fracture healing is documented via radiograph. The nonimmobilized structures should be exercised throughout the period of immobilization. For example, a program of lower extremity strengthening and endurance activities (stationary cycle, treadmill, and leg extension) should be instituted for patients with upper extremity fractures. The same principle applies for patients with lower extremity fractures. Endurance activities can be either single-leg stationary cycling or upper body ergometer exercises in these cases.

Specific exercises for the injured area frequently involve isometric muscle contractions. Therapeutic exercise programs during bone healing are designed to minimize muscle atrophy while maintaining or improving muscular strength. Muscle contractions provide forces acting to approximate fragments, improve circulation, promote motion to nonimmobilized body parts, and stimulate the piezoelectric effect.

The cast or brace serves as resistance in the initial phases of active range of motion exercises involving the affected limb. Ankle weights can be applied to the cast or brace for added resistance in later stages. It is best to apply the external resistance superior to the injury site at first, such as in ligament injuries. A more distal application of external force may produce excessive, unwanted shearing or torque through the fracture site.

Occasionally, electrical muscle stimulation is used during cast immobilization to help retard atrophy and maintain strength. A small "window" is cut in the cast to allow the application of the electrodes. The patient is instructed to isometrically contract simultaneously with the electrically evoked muscle contraction. The benefits of electrical stimulation on muscle tissue during immobilization are controversial. The piezoelectric effect is enhanced by applying a negatively charged electrode to stimulate osteoblast activity, which is called *direct current* (any current in which electrons flow in one direction). An externally applied electrode with an external power source is called *inductive coupling.*[33]

Continuous passive motion devices are used in some cases of intraarticular or extraarticular fractures of the tibia and femur.[18] Although this appears to conflict with the notion of secure immobilization leading to bone healing, Salter and colleagues[40] found positive effects of continuous passive motion on the development of chondrocytes and the reduction of intraarticular synovial adhesions when judiciously applied to healing intraarticular fractures.

The goals of rehabilitation programs during immobilization of healing fractures are as follows:

- Improve the overall fitness of the patient
- Promote motion of unaffected, nonimmobilized joints
- Minimize muscle atrophy (isometrics and muscle stimulators)
- Maintain or improve muscular strength
- Protect the healing structures; avoid unwanted, premature, or excessive motion
- Teach safe and effective transfers and gait activities (with cumbersome long-leg plaster casts or external fixators)

After immobilization, progressive exercise must be directed cautiously. Motion and circulation can be promoted by using various thermal agents. Strengthening exercises should systematically progress through isometrics, concentric and eccentric resistance, isokinetics, and closed kinetic chain resistance exercises. Balance, coordination, and proprioceptive exercises are also included during the postimmobilization phases of rehabilitation. Stationary cycle ergometers, upper body ergometers, stair climbers, and treadmills are tools that can enhance cardiorespiratory fitness during and after immobilization.

Communication of the PTA with the PT and the referring physician forms the foundation of the development of an appropriate rehabilitation plan. This requires a dialogue between the PTA, PT, and physician concerning the patient's adherence to postfracture guidelines. It is extremely helpful to avoid confusing the patient by having all health care providers on the same page regarding immobilization time frames and weight-bearing status.

GLOSSARY

Bone matrix: Organic components—40% dry weight of bone, collagen, proteoglycans, glycoproteins, and phospholipids.

Bone types: Normal bone is lamellar. Immature or pathologic bone is woven, not stress oriented. Mature lamellar bone is cortical or cancellous.

Cancellous bone: Spongy or trabecular. Fractures generally progress at 6 weeks. Examples are calcaneus, vertebral body, radius, pelvis, and tibia.

Cortical bone: Constitutes 80% of adult skeleton.

Osteoblasts: Form bone; have increased endoplasmic reticulum, increased Golgi apparatus, and increased mitochondria.

Osteoclasts: Resorb bone. Bone resorption generally is more rapid than bone formation.

Osteocytes: Constitute 90% of mature skeleton; former osteoblasts that serve to maintain bone.

Piezoelectric effect: Compression side of bone is electronegative and stimulates osteoblasts. Tension side of bone is electropositive and stimulates osteoclasts.

Remodeling: Occurs long after fracture has healed clinically. Woven bone formed during the repair phase is replaced with lamellar bone. Bone remodeling is affected by mechanical function according to Wolff's law. Removal of external stress can lead to significant bone loss. Bone remodels in response to stress and responds to piezoelectric charges.

Repair: Primary callus forms in about 2 weeks. Soft callus involving endochondral ossification occurs if fracture is not in continuity. Amount of callus is indirectly proportional to degree of immobilization. Primary cortical healing occurs with immobilization and near-anatomic reduction.

REFERENCES

1. Bassett C: Effect of force on skeletal tissue. In Downey JA, Darling RC, editors: *Physiological basis of rehabilitation medicine*, Philadelphia, 1971, Saunders.
2. Bassett CA, Pilla AA, Pawluk RH: A non-operative salvage of surgically-resistant pseudarthroses and non-unions by pulsing electromagnetic fields, a preliminary report. *Clin Orthop Relat Res* 124:128–143, 1977.
3. Bennell K, Dannus P: Bone. In Kolt GS, Snyder-Mackler L, editors: *Physical therapies in sports and exercise*, London, 2003, Churchill Livingstone.
4. Bostrom MPG, Boskey A, Kaufman JK, et al: Form and function of bone. In Buckwalter JA, Einhorn TA, Simon SR, editors: *Orthopaedic basic science: biology and biomechanics of the musculoskeletal system*, Rosemont, IL, 2000, American Academy of Orthopaedic Surgeons.
5. Brashear HR, Raney RB: *Fracture principles, fracture healing. Handbook of orthopaedic surgery*, St Louis, 1986, Mosby.
6. Buckwalter JA, Glimcher MJ, Cooper RR, et al: Bone biology. *J Bone Joint Surg Am* 77:1256–1277, 1995.
7. Bullough PG: Tissue response to and complications of orthopaedic implants. In *Orthopedic pathology*, 5th ed, St Louis, 2010, Mosby.
8. Busse JW, Bhandari M, Kulkarni AV, et al: The effect of low-intensity pulsed ultrasound therapy on time to fracture healing: a meta-analysis. *Can Med Assoc J* 166:437–441, 2002.
9. Busse JW, Kaur J, Mollon B, et al: Low intensity pulsed ultrasonography for fractures: systematic review of randomised controlled trials. *BMJ* 338:b351, 2009.
10. Chao EY, Inoue N: Biophysical stimulation of bone fracture repair, regeneration and remodeling. *Eur Cell Mater* 6:72–84, 2003.
11. Day SM, Ostrum RE, Chao EYS, et al: Bone injury regeneration and repair. In Buckwalter JA, Einhorn TA, Simon SR, editors: *Orthopaedic basic science: biology and biomechanics of the musculoskeletal system*, Rosemont, IL, 2000, American Academy of Orthopaedic Surgeons.
12. Einhorn TA: Enhancement of fracture-healing. *J Bone Joint Surg Am* 77:940–956, 1995.
13. Einhorn TA: The cell and molecular biology of fracture healing. *Clin Orthop Relat Res* 355:S7–S21, 1998.
14. Engles M: Tissue response. In Donatelli R, Wooden MJ, editors: *Orthopedic physical therapy*, New York, 1989, Churchill Livingstone.
15. Frankel VH, Nordin M: Biomechanics of bone. In Nordin M, Frankel VH, editors: *Basic biomechanics of the musculoskeletal system*, ed 3, Philadelphia, 2001, Lippincott Williams & Wilkins.
16. Frost HM: Mechanical determinants of skeletal architecture. In Albright JA, Brand RA, editors: *The scientific basis of orthopaedics*, ed 2, Norwalk, CT, 1987, Appleton-Lange.
17. Griffin XL, Costa ML, Parsons N, Smith N: Ultrasound and shockwave therapy for acute fractures in adults. *Cochrane Database Syst Rev* (2):CD008579, 2012.
18. Hamilton HW: Five years' experience with continuous passive motion. *J Bone Joint Surg Br* 64:259, 1982.
19. Heckman JD, Ryaby JP, McCabe J, et al: Acceleration of tibial fracture healing by non-invasive, low-intensity pulsed ultrasound. *J Bone Joint Surg Am* 76:26–34, 1994.
20. Holtrop ME: Hall BK. In: *Bone, light and electron microscopic structure of bone-forming cells*, vol 1, Boca Raton, FL, 1992, CRC Press.
21. Huber M, Prantl L, Gehmert S: Successful treatment of nonunion in severe finger injury with low-intensity pulsed ultrasound (LIPUS): a case report. *J Med Case Rep* 6:209, 2012.
22. Khan K, McKay H, Kannus P, et al: *Physical activity and bone health*, Champaign IL, 2001, Human Kinetics.
23. Khan Y, Laurencin CT: Fracture repair with ultrasound: clinical and cell-based evaluation. *J Bone Joint Surg Am* 90:138–144, 2008.
24. Kisner C, Colby LA: *Therapeutic exercise: foundations and techniques*, Philadelphia, 1990, FA Davis.
25. Kristiansen TK, Ryaby JP, McCabe J, et al: Accelerated healing of distal radius fractures with the use of specific, low-intensity ultrasound. A multi-center, prospective, randomized, double-blind, placebo-controlled study. *J Bone Joint Surg Am* 79:961–973, 1997.
26. Latta LL, Sarmiento A, Zych GA: Principles of nonoperative fractures. In Brown BD, Jupiter JB, Trafton PG, editors: *Skeletal trauma: fractures, dislocations, ligamentous injuries*, ed 2, Philadelphia, 1998, Saunders.
27. Lewis CB, Bottomley JM: *Geriatric physical therapy: a clinical approach*, New York, 1994, Appleton & Lange.
28. Li GP, Zhang SD, Chen G, et al: Radiographic and histologic analyses of stress fracture in rabbit tibias. *Am J Sports Med* 13:285–294, 1985.
29. Martin RB, Burr DB: *Structure, function, and adaptation of compact bone*, New York, 1989, Raven Press.
30. Mayr E, Rudzki MM, Rudzki M, et al: Acceleration by pulsed, low-intensity ultrasound of scaphoid fracture healing. *Handchir Mikrochir Plast Chir* 32:115–122, 2000.
31. Mazzocca AD, Caputo AE, Brown BD, et al: Principles of internal fixation. In Brown BD, Jupiter JB, Levine AM, et al, editors: *Skeletal trauma: fractures, dislocations, and ligamentous injuries*, Philadelphia, 1998, Saunders.
32. McRae R: *Practical fracture treatment*, New York, 1994, Churchill Livingstone.

33. Miller MD: *Review of orthopaedics*, Philadelphia, 1992, Saunders.
34. Morris JM: Fatigue fractures. *Calif Med* 108:268–274, 1968.
35. Nolte PA, van der Krans A, Patka P, et al: Low-intensity pulsed ultrasound in the treatment of nonunions. *J Trauma* 51:693–703, 2001.
36. Pollak AN, Ziran BH: Principles of external fixation. In Brown BD, Jupiter JB, Levine AM, et al, editors: *Skeletal trauma: fractures, dislocations, ligamentous bone injuries*, ed 2, Philadelphia, 1998, Saunders.
37. Rang M: *Children's fractures*, Philadelphia, 1974, JB Lippincott.
38. Rothstein JM, Roy SH, Wolf SL: *The rehabilitation specialists' handbook*, Philadelphia, 1991, FA Davis.
39. Salter RB: *Textbook of disorders and injuries of the musculoskeletal system*, ed 2, Baltimore, 1983, Williams & Wilkins.
40. Salter RB, Hamilton HW, Wedge JH, et al: Clinical applications of basic research on continuous passive motion for disorders and injuries of synovial joints. A preliminary report of a feasibility study. *J Orthop Res* 1:325–342, 1983.
41. Shenk RK: Biology of fracture repair. In Brown BD, Jupiter JB, Levine AM, et al, editors: *Skeletal trauma: fractures, dislocations, ligamentous bone injuries*, ed 2, Philadelphia, 1998, Saunders.
42. Shi HF, Cheung WH, Qin L, Leung AH, Leung KS: Low-magnitude high-frequency vibration treatment augments fracture healing in ovariectomy-induced osteoporotic bone. *Bone* 46:1299–1305, 2010.
43. Sisda PA, Gruen GS, Pape HC: External adjuncts to enhance fracture healing: what is the role of ultrasound. *Injury* 39:1095–1105, 2008.
44. Steinburg FU: *The immobilized patient: functional pathology and management*, New York, 1980, Plenum.
45. Vernon-Roberts B: Morphological and functional interrelationships of bone cells and matrix. *Aust N Z J Med* 9:1–8, 1979.
46. Watanabe Y, Matsusita T, Bhandari M, Zdero R, Schemitsch EH: Ultrasound for fracture healing: current evidence. *J Orthop Traumatol* 24:S56–S61, 2010.

REVIEW QUESTIONS

Multiple Choice

1. Which of the following is a true statement about bone tissue?
   a. It is metabolically inactive.
   b. A major component is noncollagenous matrix.
   c. It is very brittle and can tolerate small deformation.
   d. It is composed of 50% collagen.
2. Which form of bone tissue is found surrounded by mineralized matrix because it is buried within mineralized bone matrix?
   a. Osteoblast
   b. Osteocyte
   c. Osteoclast
   d. Osteoid
3. Which form of cell is a giant cell multinucleated bone resorption cell?
   a. Osteoblast
   b. Osteocyte
   c. Osteoclast
   d. Osteoid
4. Woven bone is more commonly found in:
   a. Embryos.
   b. Newborns.
   c. Tibia fracture.
   d. All of the above
5. Which form of bone is equal in length and main dimensions and is usually found in the hands and feet?
   a. Short bones
   b. Flat bones
   c. Irregular bones
   d. Long bones
6. Which of the following bones are composed of two layers of compact bone and have the main purpose of protection of underlying structures?
   a. Short bones
   b. Flat bones
   c. Irregular bones
   d. Long bones
7. Which of the following statements about cellular responses to osseous tissue is true?
   a. Remodeling to bone occurs for up to 3 months after injury only.
   b. Removal of mechanical forces creates increased osteoblastic activity.
   c. Intermittent physiologic loads create osteoblastic activity.
   d. Compressive forces stimulate bone growth.
8. Which law states that compression forces limit bone growth, whereas tensile stress stimulates growth?
   a. Shankman's
   b. Wolff's
   c. Hueter-Volkman
   d. Volkman's
9. Which law states that intermittent physiologic loads applied to bone stimulate adaptive responses?
   a. Shankman's
   b. Wolff's
   c. Hueter-Volkman
   d. Volkman's
10. Which of the following statements about osteoporosis is true?
    a. Age is not a factor.
    b. Medial tibial stress fractures are most common.
    c. Osteoblastic activity is surpassed by osteoclast activity.
    d. Osteoporosis is most commonly caused by lack of dietary dairy products.
11. Which fracture type traverses the entire bone?
    a. Spiral
    b. Transverse
    c. Complete
    d. Incomplete
12. Which fracture type is caused by a torsion or rotational injury?
    a. Transverse
    b. Spiral
    c. Impact
    d. Comminuted
13. Which Salter-Harris fracture is transverse through the physis and has a metaphyseal fragment?
    a. Type I
    b. Type II
    c. Type III
    d. Type IV
14. Which form of fracture usually is due to repetitive microtrauma?
    a. Tumor
    b. Osteoporosis
    c. Stress
    d. Metastatic disease

15. Which phase of fracture repair occurs as inflammation and hematoma formation?
    a. Phase I
    b. Phase II
    c. Phase III
    d. Phase IV

Short Answer

16. Name and describe the two general methods used to immobilize fractures, and give clinical examples of instances in which each of these methods would be used.
17. When treating a patient with an ORIF procedure in which a screw was used to stabilize a fracture, the PTA must be cautious of hardware loosening and "backing out." List three clinical signs of hardware loosening.
18. Describe the three different types of bone cells and contrast their significance in bone adaptation.
19. Compare and contrast woven versus lamellar bone.
20. Describe Wolff's law of bone remodeling.

Fill in the Blank

21. Mature bone begins formation at about age _________ and comprises most of the skeleton by age _________.
22. The _________ describes a negative electrical charge toward the concave, or compression, side of a force applied to a bone.
23. _________ is a term used to describe osteoclastic cutting cones traversing the cortical fracture fragments, followed by osteoblast formation and revascularization of bone.
24. The three distinct complications of bone healing are _________, _________, and _________.
25. Women lose bone at a rate of _________% to _________% annually

True/False

21. Compact bone heals faster than cancellous bone.
22. A reduced rate of bone healing (delayed union) can occur when physical therapy interventions are applied too soon or too vigorously.
23. When treating patients recovering from fractures, active exercise of all nonimmobilized joints is necessary.
24. Collagen constitutes about 50% of the dry weight of bone, whereas lipids and proteins constitute the remaining 50%.
25. Pulsed electromagnetic field therapy has been advocated because it is a noninvasive means of fracture management in delayed healing or nonunion fractures.

Chapter 11

Cartilage Healing

Erik P. Meira

CHAPTER OUTLINE

LEARNING OBJECTIVES

1. Discuss the composition and function of articular cartilage.
2. Identify common causes of injury to articular cartilage.
3. Describe the sequence of healing and the extent of intrinsic repair of articular cartilage.
4. Define invasive and noninvasive techniques of stimulating articular cartilage repair.
5. Define and describe the composition and function of fibrocartilage.
6. Identify and discuss common mechanisms of injury to fibrocartilage.
7. Describe the mechanisms of intrinsic healing of the meniscus.

KEY TERMS

Angiogenesis
Articular cartilage
Chondrogenesis
Chondromalacia
Deep zone
Hyaline cartilage
Hydrophilic
Menisci (singular, meniscus)

Understanding the mechanisms involved in the healing of articular (hyaline) cartilage and fibrocartilage guides the appropriate application of rehabilitation techniques. Proper rehabilitation techniques are based on the foundation of intrinsic cartilage repair (**chondrogenesis**), time necessary for healing, and extrinsic reparative interventions. Osteoarthritis, **chondromalacia** (softening of **hyaline cartilage**), meniscal lesions, labral tears, and many other cartilage pathologies are common problems the physical therapist assistant (PTA) sees clinically. Understanding the function, injury, and repair of articular cartilage and fibrocartilage helps the PTA execute appropriate rehabilitation techniques.

ARTICULAR CARTILAGE

COMPOSITION

Articular cartilage (or hyaline cartilage) covers the ends of bones of synovial joints. It is composed primarily of water (approximately 65% to 80%),[11,13] which provides for load deformation of the cartilage surface.[16] The tensile strength of articular cartilage depends on type II collagen, which is approximately 20% of the total composition of articular cartilage.[19] Proteoglycans contribute 10% to 15% of the structure of articular cartilage. These proteoglycans are composed of glycosaminoglycans (GAGs), which are partly responsible for bearing the compressive strength of articular cartilage. Finally, chondrocytes (mature cartilage cells) make up 2% to 5% of the articular cartilage.[1,16,19]

Important Concepts

The tensile strength of articular cartilage depends on type II collagen, which is approximately 20% of the total composition of articular cartilage.

Articular Cartilage Zones

Articular cartilage is not homogeneous. The composition of articular cartilage varies considerably among four distinct zones: superficial zone, middle or transitional zone, deep zone, and zone of calcified cartilage. The superficial zone of articular cartilage is composed of water and parallel, highly organized collagen fibrils with very limited concentration of proteoglycans.[14] The middle or transitional zone of articular cartilage demonstrates randomly arranged, large-diameter collagen and rounded chondrocytes.[14] The **deep zone** is rich in proteoglycans and lowest in water concentration. In this zone, collagen is large with a more organized structure that is arranged vertically.[14]

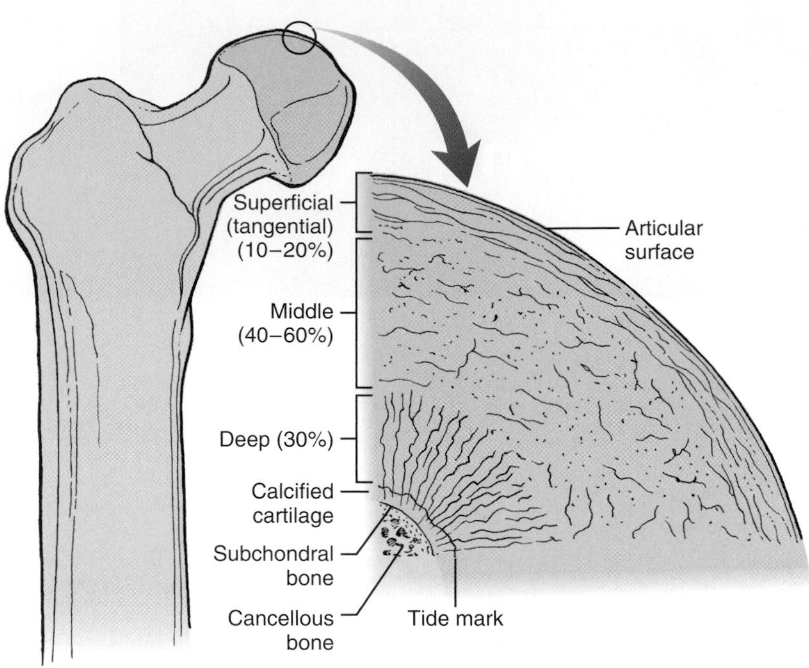

FIG 11-1 Articular cartilage layers. *(Modified from Brinker MR, Miller MD, editors:* Fundamentals of orthopaedics, *Philadelphia, 1999, Saunders.)*

TABLE 11-1 Articular Cartilage Layers

Layer	Width (μm)	Characteristic	Orientation	Function
Gliding zone (superficial)	40	↓ Metabolic activity	Tangential	vs. Shear
Transitional zone (middle)	500	↑ Metabolic activity	Oblique	vs. Compression
Radial zone (deep)	1000	↑ Collagen size	Vertical	vs. Compression
Tidemark	5	Undulation barrier	Tangential	vs. Shear
Calcified zone	300	Hydroxyapatite crystals		Anchor

↑, increased; ↓, decreased.
From Brinker MR, Miller MD: *Fundamentals of orthopaedics,* Philadelphia, 1999, Saunders.

The zone of calcified cartilage is the deepest zone that separates cartilage tissue from subchondral bone. This small distinct layer is composed mainly of cells, cartilage, matrix, and inorganic salts (Fig. 11-1 and Table 11-1).

Collagen in Articular Cartilage

Articular cartilage is an extremely unique biologic tissue with durable and permeable characteristics. Collagen represents more than 50% of the entire dry weight of articular cartilage.[14] Most collagen in articular cartilage is type II; however, the extracellular matrix also contains types V, VI, IX, X, XI, and XIV.[1]

Clinicians must recognize the composition of various collagen types to appreciate fully the remarkable resilience of articular cartilage tissue. Collagen in general contains various amounts of proline, hydroxyproline, and hydroxylysine. The proline content of collagen provides a structure that is highly resistant to tensile forces. Conversely, hydroxyproline composition of collagen provides for the compressive stability of articular cartilage. Articular cartilage is composed of collagen types that are distinct in organization, structure, and fiber arrangement. These characteristics are consistent with the zones of cartilage and their unique physiologic requirements of compression, tension, stiffness, strength, and durability (Table 11-2).[14]

Vascular Supply of Articular Cartilage

Vascularized tissues heal in an organized, predictable fashion. Trauma to vascular tissue incites an intense cascade of events characterized by hemorrhage, inflammation, and fibrin clot formation. **Angiogenesis**, or neovascularization, is the hallmark of intrinsic repair through mobilization of repair molecules and undifferentiated cells capable of synthesizing matrix and new tissue.[14]

Important Concepts

Articular cartilage is a nonhomogeneous and avascular structure that lacks the ability to stimulate, regulate, or organize intrinsic repair.

Conversely, articular cartilage is a nonhomogeneous and avascular structure that lacks the ability to stimulate, regulate, or organize intrinsic repair.[1] Without an intense

TABLE 11-2 Overview of Collagen Types

Type	Location
I	Bone Tendon Meniscus Anulus of intervertebral disk Skin
II	Articular cartilage Nucleus pulposus of intervertebral disk
III	Skin Blood vessels
IV	Basement membrane
V	Articular cartilage (in small amounts)
VI	Articular cartilage (in small amounts)
VII	Basement membrane
VIII	Basement membrane
IX	Articular cartilage (in small amounts)
X	Hypertrophic cartilage Associated with calcification of cartilage (matrix mineralization)
XI	Articular cartilage (in small amounts)
XII	Tendon
XIII	Endothelial cells

From Brinker MR, Miller MD: *Fundamentals of orthopaedics,* Philadelphia, 1999, Saunders.

vascular response to injury, articular cartilage cannot form a fibrin scaffold or mobilize cells to repair the defect. Chondrocytes are essentially trapped within the dense extracellular matrix and are incapable of traveling to the damaged site via a vascular access channel.[14]

This makes spontaneous healing of superficial wounds to articular cartilage limited. Because chondrocytes do not fill the defect, weak, fragile proteoglycans surround the injury. Deep injuries that communicate below the deep, calcified zone into subchondral bone produce a vascular inflammatory response to a limited extent. As expected, a fibrin clot forms a repairlike tissue but ultimately demonstrates a biochemically and mechanically weak scar of fibrocartilage.[1]

FUNCTION

The viscoelastic structure of articular cartilage, by virtue of its component parts of collagen, water, and proteoglycans, makes articular cartilage incredibly durable.[16,19] Generally, articular cartilage is only 2 to 4 mm thick, yet it is capable of bearing compressive loads many times greater than body weight.[24] Articular cartilage is resistant to wear; has an extremely low coefficient of friction; and is responsible for influencing and dissipating compression, shear, and tension forces within synovial joints.[1,16,19,24]

IMMOBILIZATION AND RESPONSE TO HEALING

Articular cartilage requires physiologic stress (e.g., cyclical compression) to maintain its unique environment as a strong, tough, fatigue-resistant, permeable, and low-friction tissue.[14,15] The biochemical components of proteoglycans or GAGs, chondrocytes, matrix-molecules, and collagen significantly contribute to its structure, composition, and mechanical properties.[14,15]

Important Concepts

The viscoelastic structure of articular cartilage, by virtue of its component parts of collagen, water, and proteoglycans, makes articular cartilage incredibly durable.

Articular cartilage is also permeable. The chondrocytes within the cartilage must receive nutrition to remain viable. The synovial fluid surrounding the articular cartilage provides the necessary nutrients through diffusion, convection, or both.[19] Diffusion and convection are achieved through joint motion and normal physiologic weight bearing. Normal joint motion is needed to maintain the cartilage integrity, fluid movement (lubrication between articulating surfaces), and nutrition of hyaline cartilage.[19]

Just as collagen is varied and distinct among the zones of articular cartilage, so are proteoglycans distributed in different concentrations between zones. Because these proteoglycan molecules—including chondroitin sulfate, keratan sulfate, and dermatan sulfate—bind and attract water (**hydrophilic**), their concentration and distribution among zones influence the various mechanical wear characteristics of articular cartilage.[14,15] The removal of normal physiologic loading, unloading, and joint motion has profoundly negative effects on the biochemical and mechanical characteristics of articular cartilage.[14,15]

Important Concepts

Immobilization, or the removal of normal physiologic loading, unloading, and joint motion, has profoundly negative effects on the biochemical and mechanical characteristics of articular cartilage.

The significance of articular cartilage atrophy and degeneration is related to the magnitude and duration of immobilization. Joint contact surfaces experience greater degenerative changes than noncontact areas of articular cartilage (Table 11-3).[14,15]

Chondrocyte necrosis and subchondral bone degenerative lesions occur with prolonged rigid immobilization. Generally, immobilization and lack of physiologic stress cause a reduction in the synthesis and concentration of proteoglycans, which ultimately leads to surface fibrillation, fissures, and ulceration of the various zones of articular cartilage.[14,15]

INJURY

Articular cartilage can be damaged in many ways.[1,19,24] Erosion and degeneration of the articular surface can be seen clinically in patients ranging from young athletes to elderly individuals. Causes of degenerative joint disease include related joint instability, blunt trauma, repetitive overloading, and immobilization.[24] Articular cartilage degeneration is generally characterized by three progressively

TABLE 11-3 Biochemical Changes of Articular Cartilage

Biochemical Structure	Aging	Osteoarthritis
Water content (hydration; permeability)	↓	↑
Collagen	Content remains relatively unchanged	Becomes disorderly (breakdown of matrix framework) Content ↓ in severe osteoarthritis Relative concentration ↑ (because of loss of proteoglycans)
Proteoglycan content (concentration)	↓ (length of the protein core and GAG chains also decreases)	↓
Proteoglycan synthesis	↓	↑
Proteoglycan degradation	↓	↑
Chondroitin sulfate concentration (includes chondroitin 4-sulfate and chondroitin 6-sulfate)	↓	↑
Chondroitin 4-sulfate concentration	↓	↑
Keratin sulfate concentration	↑	↓
Chondrocyte size	↑	
Chondrocyte number	↓	
Modulus of elasticity	↑	↓

GAG, glycosaminoglycan; ↑, increased; ↓, decreased.
From Brinker MR, Miller MD: *Fundamentals of orthopaedics,* Philadelphia, 1999, Saunders.

overlapping events (Fig. 11-2).[24] Initially, the hyaline cartilage begins to fray or fibrillate. Progressive destruction leads to blistering of the articular surface. Further joint deterioration leads to splitting or clefting (fissuring) of the surface; this affects the deeper layers of cartilage and eventually progresses to denuded bone.[24]

Although blunt trauma, progressive friction abrasion, and a focal concentration of weight-bearing forces mechanically erode articular cartilage, joint immobilization does not cause these mechanical changes. However, joint immobilization may lead to loss of the load-bearing structural compression-resistant component GAGs.[19] Such loss is related to decreased normal joint loading and motion, which is needed for cartilage nutrition.

Articular cartilage erosion can occur after trauma, penetrating injury, infection, excessive shearing loads, joint immobilization, or reduction of normal joint mechanics. The therapeutic application of exercise and functional activities must be adjusted and modified to minimize the progressive destruction of tissue in patients who have a range of osteoarthritic changes to articular cartilage.

HEALING AND REPAIR

Articular cartilage defects heal differently, depending on the extent or depth of the injury.[1,16,19,24] Less serious, more superficial lesions of articular cartilage do not spontaneously remodel or heal as well as deeper or full-thickness injuries because of the lack of vascularization. Healing of these superficial layers occurs through proteoglycans and limited chondrocyte proliferation, but the strength, composition, and durability of this healing tissue are inferior compared with normal articular cartilage.[19]

Superficial articular cartilage defects do not heal as well as deeper injuries because these injuries do not stimulate an inflammatory reaction.[19] The thickness of the articular cartilage (2 to 4 mm) forms a barrier between the superficial layers of the cartilage and subchondral blood vessels, effectively eliminating any contact among fibrin, fibroblasts, and inflammatory response cells (neutrophils, macrophages). In effect, the chondrocytes do not adhere to the defect and do not fill the injury site with new tissue.

Deeper wounds or full-thickness injuries expose subchondral bone blood vessels to the defect site, which stimulates the acute inflammatory response. Full-thickness cartilage injuries heal spontaneously with large amounts of type I collagen. Approximately 20% of the repaired defect remains type I collagen 1 year after injury.[19] Although full-thickness injuries heal considerably better than superficial wounds, the quality of the scar formed within the defect remains inferior to normal articular cartilage because of the lack of type II collagen. The healed scar does not maintain its integrity over time.[19] In animal model studies, various types and depths of articular cartilage defects are created to evaluate these repair processes (Fig. 11-3).

Important Concepts

Although full-thickness injuries heal considerably better than superficial wounds, the quality of the scar formed within the defect remains inferior to normal articular cartilage because of the lack of type II collagen.

Overview of Nonoperative Management for Articular Cartilage Pathology

When treating patients recovering from injury, immobilization, or other damage to articular cartilage, appropriate physical therapy measures are measures that stimulate cartilage repair. Noninvasive therapeutic measures can be beneficial in the treatment of articular cartilage injury. Limited weight-bearing activities can arrest symptoms of pain and swelling in some cases. Reducing compressive

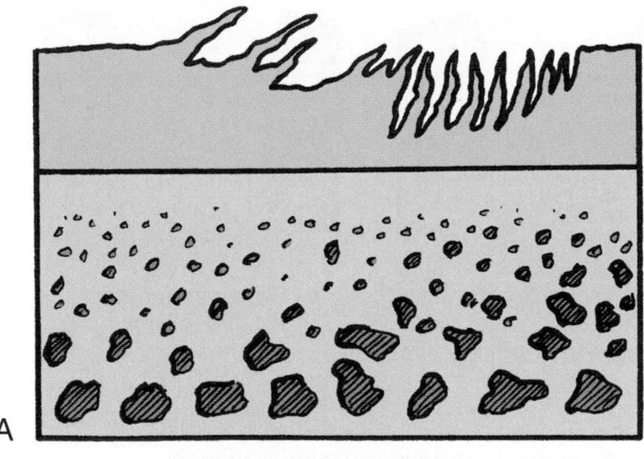

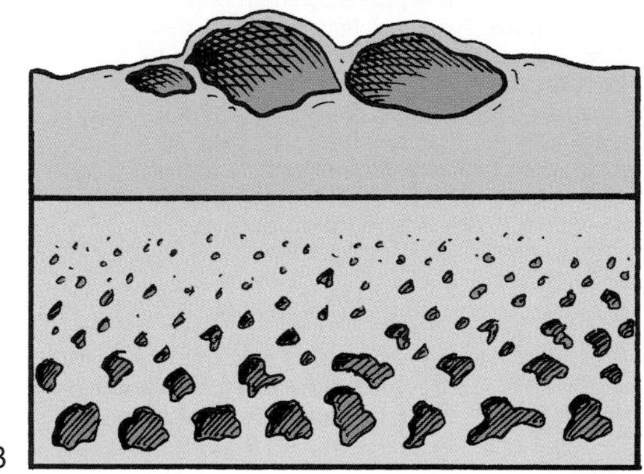

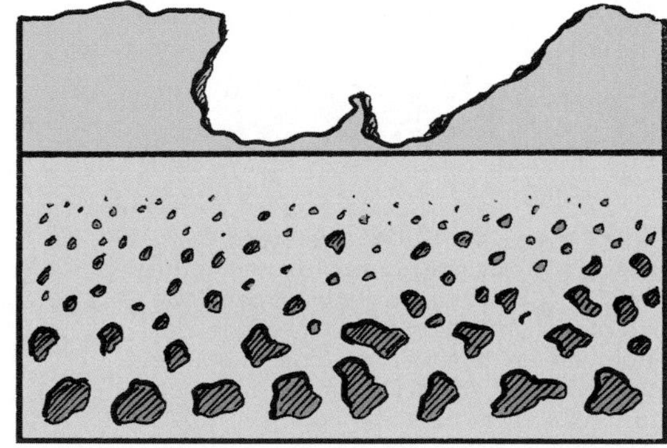

FIG 11-2 Articular cartilage degeneration generally is characterized by three progressive overlapping stages. **A,** Fibrillation or fraying of articular cartilage. **B,** Blistering of articular surface. **C,** Splitting, clefting, or fissuring of articular surface.

loads is a critical first step in the care of articular cartilage defects. Patients can maintain strength with isometric exercise or limited open kinetic chain progressive-resistive exercise.

Continuous passive motion (CPM) is sometimes used in the care of patients with articular cartilage injury. The benefits from the use of CPM appear to be limited to full-thickness hyaline cartilage defects.[21,22] Salter and colleagues[21,22] demonstrated that CPM used on full-thickness cartilage injury in rabbits showed healing of the defect with tissue resembling hyaline cartilage. Salter and colleagues,[20-22] who believe that CPM can help stimulate chondrocyte formation, also found that using CPM with full-thickness hyaline cartilage injuries improves articular cartilage nutrition by enhancing fluid mechanics, inhibiting adhesions, and clearing the joint of noxious material.

Maintaining near-normal joint motion through modified exercise regimens and weight-bearing activities (depending on the location and severity of the articular defect) is necessary for healing of cartilage injuries and maintenance of hyaline cartilage nutrition.

Viscosupplementation through Intraarticular Hyaluronic Acid Injection. Hyaluronic acid is a proteoglycan constituent of articular cartilage matrix and synovial fluid. Fibroblasts and synoviocytes synthesize hyaluronic acid into the joint space of the knee.[26]

The normal, nonpathologic human adult knee contains approximately 2 mL of synovial fluid with a hyaluronic acid concentration of 2.5 to 4.0 mg/mL.[26] Osteoarthritis creates a deficit in volume and molecular mass of hyaluronic acid.[26] This reduction in hyaluronic acid causes lower viscosity, high stress concentration, and lowered elastic properties of the synovium and articular cartilage matrix.[26]

Injecting hyaluronic acid is thought to benefit the osteoarthritic knee by reducing pain and inflammation, replenishing decreased volume of hyaluronic acid, and stimulating intrinsic synovial synthesis of hyaluronic acid.[26] Hyaluronic acid injections are shown to reduce inflammation by limiting prostaglandins, reducing circulating proinflammatory cytokine, and decreasing the release of arachidonic acid from synovial fibroblasts.[26]

Typically, commercially available hyaluronic acid preparations are injected into the affected knee joint once a week for 3 weeks. At the present time, there is no consensus about the clinical efficacy of hyaluronic acid intraarticular injections. Several clinical trials have demonstrated no increased joint function or pain relief compared with traditional nonsteroidal antiinflammatory agents or intraarticular steroidal preparations. However, clinical trials of hyaluronic acid injections versus placebo favor its use. The rate of side effects is approximately 1% per injection. Local site reactions of pain, warmth, and swelling are most common and last 1 to 2 days.[26]

Overview of Operative Management for Articular Cartilage Pathology

Various surgical interventions that are designed to stimulate an intense inflammatory response are at the disposal of the surgeon.

Microfracture. Articular cartilage repair is promoted when the injury site can go through the inflammatory process and when factors lead to chondrocyte proliferation. With some cartilage defects, surgically abrading or fracturing multiple small holes through the cartilage layers down to bone stimulates bleeding and initiates the healing process (Fig. 11-4).[2]

Initially, the bleeding response produces a "superclot" over the chondral defect. The desired outcome of this penetrating technique is the development of fibrocartilage consisting of type I collagen, which attempts to fill the

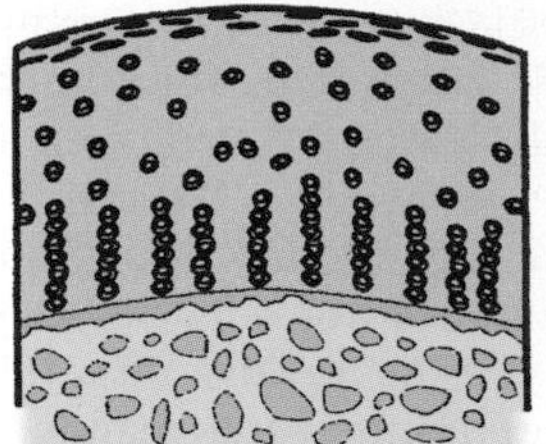

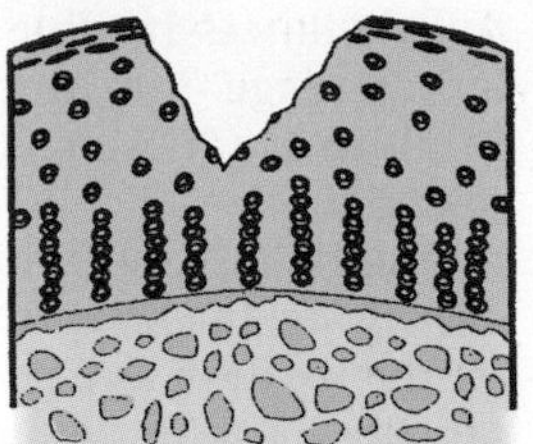

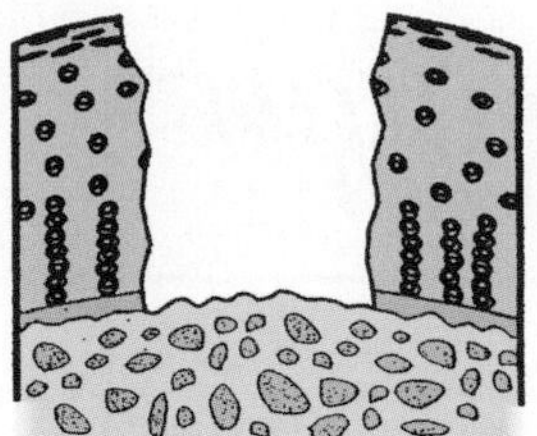

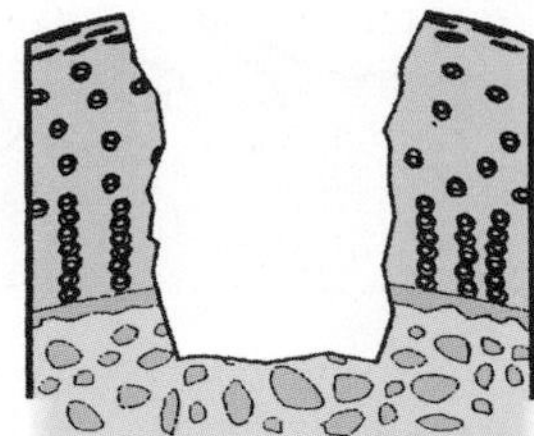

FIG 11-3 Various types and depths of articular cartilage defects or lesions that can be created in animal models to evaluate repair processes in articular cartilage. **A,** Normal articular cartilage is typically organized histologically into zones. **B,** A partial-thickness (superficial or shallow) defect penetrating to the middle zone is isolated from the blood supply and marrow space. Such a defect typically does not elicit or demonstrate a repair response. **C,** A lesion that penetrates to the subchondral bone but does not penetrate into the marrow space, if truly isolated from the marrow, will not repair. However, even a very small communication of the lesion with the marrow blood supply will elicit a repair response. Full-thickness lesions usually are in this category. **D,** A defect that penetrates through all zones of the articular cartilage and penetrates into the marrow space typically demonstrates a repair response that results in fibrocartilaginous tissue. *(Modified from Jackson DW, Scheer MJ, Simon TM: Cartilage substitutes: overview of basic science and treatment options,* J Am Acad Orthop Surg *9:42, 2001.)*

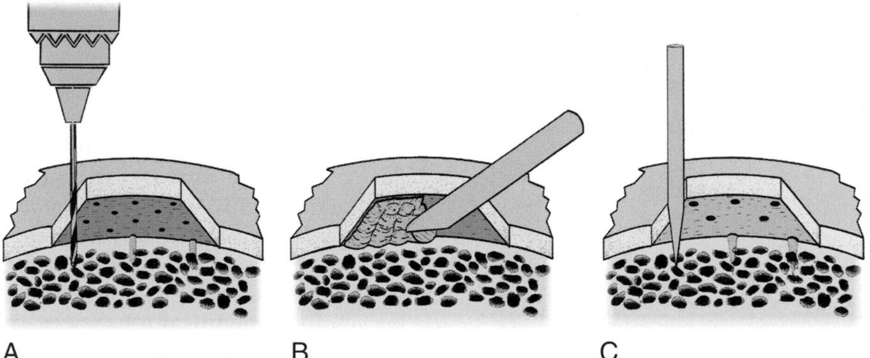

FIG 11-4 Various methodologies currently used to elicit repair tissue in articular cartilage defects. **A,** Current methods involve penetrating the underlying bone end plate by drilling, as proposed in the Pridie procedure. Variations include abrasion **(B)** and microfracture **(C)**. All these techniques penetrate the subchondral bone to open communication with a zone of vascularization to initiate fibrin clot formation and obtain the potential benefit of vascular ingrowth or migration of more primitive mesenchymal cells from the bone marrow. These communications open the defect to the migration of many types of cells, including fibroblasts and inflammatory cells. These cells may compete with a limited number of the primitive mesenchymal cells to occupy the fibrin matrix, contributing to various repair scenarios. These methods penetrate the subchondral bone plate and tidemark, but the intent is not to disrupt the integrity of the subchondral bone. Large disruption or removal of the subchondral bone end plate may result in detrimental mechanical, structural, and biologic changes. *(Modified from Jackson DW, Scheer MJ, Simon TM: Cartilage substitutes: overview of basic science and treatment options,* J Am Acad Orthop Surg *9:45, 2001.)*

defect. Being different from the type II collagen of normal articular cartilage, the repair tissue that forms from microfracture is histochemically and biochemically fragile and weak compared with structurally intact articular cartilage. The repair also lacks the anatomically distinct layers of differing collagen types characteristic of normal articular cartilage, which provide additional protection from compression, shear, and tensile loads.[2]

Microfracture has been shown to provide short-term functional improvement, but long-term efficacy is still unknown.[17] Outcomes are highest when performed on younger patients with cartilage defects that are surrounded by normal articular cartilage.[2]

Osteochondral Autografts. Full-thickness articular lesions (osteochondral) can be surgically filled with transplanted plugs of intact bone and articular cartilage using the technique of mosaicplasty or osteochondral autograft transplantation system (Fig. 11-5). The surgeon prepares the lesion by removing all nonviable surrounding tissue from the crater, creating precise borders of the lesion. Multiple full-thickness bone plugs are surgically harvested from a relatively non–load-bearing surface of the femur, usually the superior lateral femoral condyle or, less often, the inferior condylar notch. Harvest site morbidity is a concern because full-knee range of motion provides significant contact pressure of the mentioned harvest sites.[10] These cylindrical osteochondral plugs become revascularized (incorporated) into the lesion. These "press-fit" plugs contain viable hyaline cartilage, which tends to survive over time and remains structurally stable.[2,10]

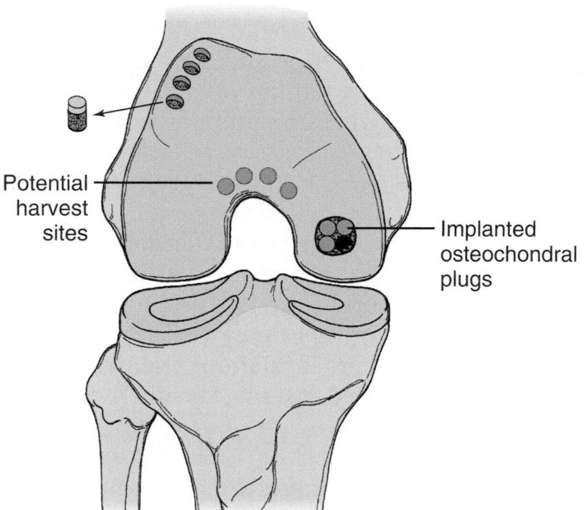

FIG 11-5 Osteochondral plug transplantation technique. The lesion site is prepared by débriding any loose articular cartilage, and the number and size of the plugs to be used for repair are determined. The holes to receive the plugs are drilled in the floor of the lesion. With use of specialized harvesting instrumentation, the osteochondral plugs are procured from suitable sites so as to approximate the surface geometry of the lesion site. The plugs are implanted to the appropriate depth into the holes placed in the lesion base. *(Modified from Jackson DW, Scheer MJ, Simon TM: Cartilage substitutes: overview of basic science and treatment options,* J Am Acad Orthop Surg *9:48, 2001.)*

Several key factors may compromise the outcome of the osteochondral autograft transplantation system technique. The convex geometry of the femoral condyles contributes to a relative joint incongruence because the shape of the plugs may not match the surrounding surface with anatomic precision. In addition, the depth placement of the chondral plugs is critical because the donor plugs may collapse or settle over time or may be inserted with too much "pride" (the surface of the plugs may sit too high above the horizon of the chondral plate).[10]

Autologous Chondrocyte Implantation. Because of substantial variations in collagen types, orientation, proteoglycan content, extracellular matrix composition, and avascularity of the four anatomically distinct zones of articular cartilage, a tissue implantation procedure is available to generate a biologic substitute tissue.[2,10] The autologous chondrocyte implantation procedure calls for two separate surgical interventions. First, the surgeon harvests articular cartilage from the superomedial edge of the trochlea or the lateral edge of the intercondylar notch. This harvested tissue is sent to a specific laboratory, where the chondrocytes are enzymatically separated from the extracellular matrix, cultured, and multiplied. The second procedure typically occurs 6 to 18 weeks after harvesting. At this time, a periosteal patch may be harvested from the proximal medial tibia.[2] However, concern regarding hypertrophy of the periosteum has led to the development of second-generation patches such as porcine-derived collagen.[5,8] This patch is secured with fibrin glue and sutures over the defect. The cultured chondrocytes are injected under the patch to fill the defect with biologically active viable chondrocytes (Fig. 11-6).

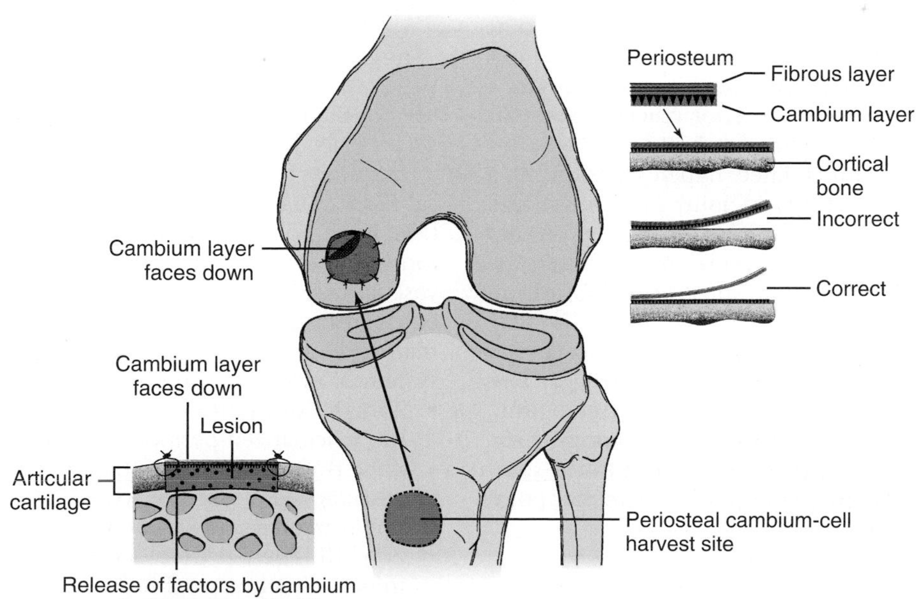

FIG 11-6 Autologous chondrocyte implantation technique. Articular cartilage is procured, and its chondrocytes are enzymatically released and expanded in cell culture. When a sufficient number of cells are obtained, a second operation is performed for implantation of the cultured cells. A periosteal flap with matching geometry is harvested and sutured in place with the cambium cell layer facing the defect (down). Care must be taken to ensure that the cambium cells remain attached to the periosteal fibrous layer (*insets*). *(Modified from Jackson DW, Scheer MJ, Simon TM: Cartilage substitutes: overview of basic science and treatment options,* J Am Acad Orthop Surg *9:46, 2001.)*

FIBROCARTILAGE

Understanding fibrocartilage injury and repair is a necessary foundation for the appropriate delivery of rehabilitation programs. The PTA also must be aware of the differences in healing between articular cartilage and fibrocartilage.

COMPOSITION

Fibrocartilage is found within many synovial joints, with its presence in the hip, knee, and shoulder being the most commonly clinically relevant. A large percentage of fibrocartilage is water.[12] The collagen in fibrocartilage is almost entirely type I collagen. Proteoglycans and elastin (0.6%) complete the components of fibrocartilage.[3]

> **Important Concepts**
>
> The collagen in fibrocartilage is almost entirely type I collagen.

FUNCTION

The **menisci** of the knee are semilunar (C-shaped) fibrocartilage tissues that have several functions. Generally, the meniscus dissipates extreme compressive (vertical) loads. By virtue of its anatomic position within the knee and its collagen makeup, the meniscus acts as a mechanical buffer between the load-bearing surfaces of the tibia and the femur. The meniscus of the knee also functions as a shock absorber.[3] Studies have shown that a knee without a meniscus has 20% less shock-absorbing capacity than normal knees.[25]

The meniscus may also function as a secondary restraint in joint stability. Several factors influence its effect, including ligament stability, joint surface congruency, and joint compression loads.[3] Significant joint instability does not occur with an isolated, total meniscectomy. However, a meniscectomy combined with anterior cruciate ligament injuries produces profound joint instability.[23]

The meniscus also limits knee hyperextension as a passive restraint and functions in joint lubrication and nutrition.[12] Normal physiologic joint motion promotes the lubricating effects of a thin layer of fluid between the joint surfaces. The meniscus may spread this lubrication medium during motion.[18]

The glenoid labrum of the shoulder and the acetabular labrum of the hip are also made up of fibrocartilage. This fibrocartilage surrounds the glenoid and acetabulum, respectively, providing increased joint surface congruency. The role of the labrum is to provide stability to the joint through this increased congruency and as an anchor point for other structures.

INJURY

Injuries to the meniscus can be traumatic or degenerative. Traumatic intraarticular fibrocartilage tears usually occur in a younger population (<40 years old) and generally result from a combination of compression, torque, acceleration, or deceleration. These events usually occur during running, jumping, twisting, and dynamic change-of-direction activities.

Degenerative meniscal tears typically occur in an older population (>40 years old). Patients with these injuries do not present with a history of sudden trauma, but rather with a minor event that precipitates complaints of pain and dysfunction.[3]

Injuries to the glenoid labrum often occur through direct trauma or repetitive stress. Detachment of the anterior-inferior labrum (Bankart lesion) is a common injury produced by anterior shoulder dislocation. The long head of the biceps tendon attaches to the superior labrum. Tears of the superior labrum anterior to posterior lesions are sometimes caused by trauma but are often caused by repetitive stress from the biceps tendon during throwing activities.

The most common injury to the acetabular labrum is through repeated bony contact seen in femoroacetabular impingement. The labrum can become torn or detached over time as the femur repeatedly makes contact during deep hip flexion or internal rotation. Traumatic tears also occur, typically in hip extension.

HEALING

The vascular anatomy of fibrocartilage profoundly influences the type of healing that occurs and the degree of remodeling, such as with articular cartilage. The peripheral borders of the medial and lateral meniscus of the knee are vascularized 10% to 30% of the width of the tissue.[3] If an injury occurs within a nonvascular region of the meniscus, spontaneous, intrinsic repair is impossible because no vascular supply communicates with the injury site. However, if the injury extends to the periphery where the cartilage is vascularized, healing is possible through the inflammatory-response mechanism.

> **Important Concepts**
>
> The vascular anatomy of fibrocartilage profoundly influences the type of healing that occurs and the degree of remodeling.

Decisions regarding surgical repair or excision of meniscal tissue are based on the extent of the injury and location. If the tear is within the vascularized peripheral border (only 15% to 20% of all meniscal injuries occur within the vascularized bed of the meniscus), arthroscopic repair can be done by placing sutures in the meniscus to approximate the torn tissue.[3] Surgeons refer to the following zone system of evaluating meniscal injuries[9]:

- Zone I: Both portions of the meniscus are torn within the vascularized periphery—"red-on-red"
- Zone II: One portion of the meniscus is torn within the vascularized periphery, whereas the other portion is in the avascular region—"red-on-white"
- Zone III: There is no blood supply on either side of the injury—"white-on-white"

Both red-on-red and red-on-white zones are considered reparable. When injuries occur in an avascular portion of the meniscus, the surgeon must perform either a partial or a total meniscectomy. However, in animal studies,[4] when an injury was present within the white-on-white nonvascularized zone III area of the meniscus, researchers surgically created a "vascular access channel" to connect the blood supply of the periphery to the area of injury without circulation.[3,4] These changes allowed blood vessels to migrate to the injury site and provided an avenue for repair.

In labral injuries of the hip and shoulder, torn or frayed fibrocartilage is similar to the white-on-white lesions in the meniscus. Because of a lack of blood supply, these are simply débrided. Labral detachments are more similar to the red-on-white lesions in the meniscus and usually respond well to surgical repair. Before reattachment, a bleeding bone bed is exposed to promote healing down of the labrum.

GLOSSARY

Angiogenesis: The physiologic process during healing of bodily tissues in which new capillary blood vessels are formed from preexisting vasculature.

Articular cartilage: Concentration of collagen, proteoglycans, and water influences tensile forces, compression, shear, and permeability.

Chondrogenesis: Intrinsic cartilage repair.

Chondromalacia: Softening of hyaline cartilage.

Deep zone: Largest part of the articular cartilage. Contains the largest collagen fibrils and has the highest proteoglycan content and lowest water content.

Hyaline cartilage: A synonym for articular cartilage.

Hydrophilic: A quality of a molecule that causes it to bind to and attract water.

Menisci (*singular,* meniscus): Semilunar (C-shaped) fibrocartilage tissues in the knee that act as a mechanical buffer between the load-bearing surfaces of the tibia and the femur.

REFERENCES

1. Alford JW, Cole BJ: Cartilage restoration, part 1: basic science, historical perspective, patient evaluation, and treatment options. *Am J Sports Med* 33(2):295–306, 2005.
2. Alford JW, Cole BJ: Cartilage restoration, part 2: techniques, outcomes, and future directions. *Am J Sports Med* 33(2):443–460, 2005.
3. Arnoczky SP, Adams M, DeHaven K, et al: Meniscus. In Buschbacher JA, Woo SL-Y, editors: *Injury and repair of the musculoskeletal soft tissues*, Rosemont, IL, 1988, American Academy of Orthopaedic Surgeons.
4. Arnoczky SP, Warren RF: The microvasculature of the meniscus and its response to injury. An experimental study in the dog. *Am J Sports Med* 11:131–141, 1983.
5. Bartlett W, Skinner JA, Gooding CR, et al: Autologous chondrocyte implantation versus matrix-induced autologous chondrocyte implantation for osteochondral defects of the knee. *J Bone Joint Surg Br* 87:640–645, 2005.
6. Brief AA, Maurer SG, Di Cesare PE: Use of glucosamine and chondroitin sulfate in the management of osteoarthritis. *J Am Acad Orthop Surg* 9:71–78, 2001.
7. Clegg DO, Reda DJ, Harris CL, et al: Glucosamine, chondroitin sulfate, and the two in combination for painful knee osteoarthritis. *N Engl J Med* 354:795–808, 2006.
8. Haddo O, Mahroof S, Higgs D, et al: The use of chondrogide membrane in autologous chondrocyte implantation. *Knee* 11:51–55, 2004.
9. Hammesfahr JR: Surgery of the knee. In Donatelli R, Wooden MJ, editors: *Orthopaedic physical therapy*, New York, 1989, Churchill Livingstone.
10. Jackson DW, Scheer MJ, Simon TM: Cartilage substitutes: overview of basic science and treatment options. *J Am Acad Orthop Surg* 9:37–52, 2001.
11. Jaffe FF, Mankin HJ, Weiss H, et al: Water binding in the articular cartilage of rabbits. *J Bone Joint Surg Am* 56:1031–1039, 1974.
12. MacConaill MA: The function of intraarticular fibrocartilages, with special reference to the knee and inferior radio-ulnar joints. *J Anat* 66:210–227, 1932.
13. Mankin HJ: The water of articular cartilage. In Simon WH, editor: *The human joint in health and disease*, Philadelphia, 1978, University of Pennsylvania Press.
14. Mankin HJ, Mow VC, Buckwalter JA, et al: Articular cartilage structure, composition, and function. In Buckwalter JA, Einhorn TA, Simon SR, editors: *Orthopaedic basic science, biology, and biomechanics*, ed 2, Rosemont, IL, 2000, American Academy of Orthopaedic Surgeons.
15. Mankin JH, Mow VC, Buckwalter JA, et al: Articular cartilage repair and osteoarthritis. In Buckwalter JA, Einhorn TA, Simon SR, editors: *Orthopaedic basic science, biology, and biomechanics*, ed 2, Rosemont, IL, 2000, American Academy of Orthopaedic Surgeons.
16. Miller MD: *Review of orthopaedics*, Philadelphia, 1992, Saunders.
17. Mithoefer K, McAdams T, Williams RJ, et al: Clinical efficacy of the microfracture technique for articular cartilage repair in the knee: an evidence-based systematic analysis. *Am J Sports Med* 10(10):1–11, 2009.
18. Radin EL, Bryan RS: The effect of weight bearing on regrowth of the medial meniscus after meniscectomy. *J Trauma* 12:169, 1970.
19. Rosenberg L: Articular cartilage. In Woo SL-Y, Buckwalter JA, editors: *Injury and repair of the musculoskeletal soft tissues*, Rosemont, IL, 1988, American Academy of Orthopaedic Surgeons.
20. Salter RB, Hamilton HW, Wedge JH, et al: Clinical application of basic research on continuous passive motion for disorders and injuries of synovial joints: a preliminary report of a feasibility study. *J Orthop Res* 1:325–342, 1984.
21. Salter RB, Mister RR, Bell RS, et al: Continuous passive motion and the repair of full-thickness articular cartilage defects: a one year follow-up. *Trans Orthop Res Soc* 7:167, 1982.
22. Salter RB, Simmonds DF, Malcolm BW, et al: The biological effect of continuous passive motion on healing of full-thickness defects in articular cartilage. An experimental investigation in the rabbit. *J Bone Joint Surg Am* 62:1232–1251, 1980.
23. Shoemaker SC, Markolf KL: The role of the meniscus in the anterior-posterior stability of the loaded anterior cruciate-deficient knee. Effects of partial versus total excision. *J Bone Joint Surg Am* 68:71–79, 1986.
24. Threlkeld JA: Electrical stimulation of articular cartilage. In Currier DP, Nelson RM, editors: *Dynamics of human biologic tissues*, Philadelphia, 1992, FA Davis.
25. Voloshin AS, Wosk J: Shock absorption of meniscectomized and painful knees: a comparative in vivo study. *J Biomed Eng* 5:157–161, 1983.
26. Watterson JR, Esdaile JM: Viscosupplementation: therapeutic mechanisms and clinical potential in osteoarthritis in the knee. *J Am Acad Orthop Surg* 8:277–284, 2000.

REVIEW QUESTIONS

Multiple Choice

1. What provides for load deformation of the surface of articular cartilage?
   a. Collagen
   b. Lipids
   c. Water
   d. Chondrocytes
2. On what collagen type does the tensile strength of articular cartilage depend?
   a. Type I
   b. Type II
   c. Type V
   d. Type IX

3. Chondrocytes (mature cartilage cells) make up what percentage of the articular cartilage?
   a. 2% to 5%
   b. 27% to 33%
   c. 50% to 65%
   d. 78%
4. Which zone of articular cartilage is rich in proteoglycans and lowest in water concentration?
   a. Superficial
   b. Middle or transitional
   c. Deep
   d. Zone of calcified cartilage
5. Collagen represents what percentage of the entire dry weight of articular cartilage?
   a. Less than 10%
   b. 15% to 20%
   c. 35% to 40%
   d. More than 50%
6. What component of collagen provides a structure that is highly resistant to tensile forces?
   a. Proline
   b. Hydroxyproline
   c. Lysine
   d. Hydroxylysine
7. What component of collagen provides for the compressive stability of articular cartilage?
   a. Proline
   b. Hydroxyproline
   c. Lysine
   d. Hydroxylysine
8. Deep injuries that communicate below the deep, calcified zone into subchondral bone fill in with what type of tissue?
   a. Articular cartilage
   b. Fibrocartilage
   c. Hyaline cartilage
   d. Type II collagen
9. In general, how thick is articular cartilage?
   a. 0.5 to 1 mm
   b. 1 to 2 mm
   c. 2 to 4 mm
   d. 4 to 6 mm
10. What is needed to maintain the cartilage integrity, fluid movement (lubrication between articulating surfaces), and nutrition of hyaline cartilage?
    a. Immobilization
    b. Normal joint motion
    c. High shear loads
    d. Adequate rest periods
11. Which area of the joint experiences greater degenerative changes of articular cartilage from immobilization?
    a. Noncontact areas
    b. Lateral
    c. Medial
    d. Joint contact surfaces
12. What collagen type is lacking after full-thickness injuries to articular cartilage have healed?
    a. Type I
    b. Type II
    c. Type V
    d. Type IX
13. A reduction in which of the following causes lower viscosity, high stress concentration, and lowered elastic properties of the synovium and articular cartilage matrix?
    a. Hyaluronic acid
    b. Lipids
    c. Chondrocytes
    d. Chondroitin sulfate
14. The repair tissue that forms from what operative intervention is histochemically and biochemically fragile and weak compared with structurally intact articular cartilage?
    a. Autologous chondrocyte implantation
    b. Osteochondral autograft
    c. Microfracture
    d. Osteotomy
15. What collagen type makes up almost the entirety of fibrocartilage?
    a. Type I
    b. Type II
    c. Type V
    d. Type IX

Short Answer

16. Explain how chondrocytes receive nutrients to remain viable.
17. How do proteoglycan molecules—including chondroitin sulfate, keratan sulfate, and dermatan sulfate—influence the various mechanical wear characteristics of articular cartilage?
18. Describe in general how immobilization and lack of physiologic stress cause cartilage degeneration.
19. Name the three progressively overlapping events that characterize articular cartilage degeneration.
20. Name four functions of the menisci of the knee.

Fill in the Blank

21. The _________ zone of articular cartilage is composed of water and parallel, highly organized collagen fibrils with very limited concentration of proteoglycans.
22. Articular cartilage is an extremely unique biologic tissue with both _________ and _________ characteristics.
23. The _________ structure of articular cartilage, by virtue of its component parts of collagen, water, and proteoglycans, makes articular cartilage incredibly durable.
24. Articular cartilage requires _________ to maintain its unique environment as a strong, tough, fatigue-resistant, permeable, and low-friction tissue.
25. The removal of normal physiologic _________, _________, and _________ has profoundly negative effects on the biochemical and mechanical characteristics of articular cartilage.

True/False

26. Articular cartilage is a nonhomogeneous and avascular structure that lacks the ability to stimulate, regulate, or organize intrinsic repair.
27. Less serious, more superficial lesions of articular cartilage spontaneously remodel or heal as well as deeper

or full-thickness injuries owing to the lack of vascularization.

28. Joint immobilization may lead to loss of the load-bearing structural compression-resistant component GAGs.
29. Hyaluronic acid is a proteoglycan constituent of articular cartilage matrix and synovial fluid.
30. If an injury were to occur to the central nonvascular portion of the meniscus, spontaneous intrinsic repair is possible.

Chapter 12

Muscle and Tendon Healing

Jason Brumitt

CHAPTER OUTLINE

LEARNING OBJECTIVES

1. Recognize the macrostructure and microstructure of muscle and tendon.
2. Describe the two main types of muscle fibers.
3. Describe the three mechanisms for a muscle injury.
4. Describe the associated tendon pathology of the injury mechanism.
5. Name the functional unit of a tendon and its structural significance.
6. Describe the difference between a supraphysiologic and a subfailure load and how each type may contribute to an injury.
7. Define how a muscle strain differs from a ligament sprain.
8. Describe the differences between a tendinitis and a tendinosis.
9. Describe the effects of aging on tendons.
10. Name and describe the three phases of connective tissue healing.
11. Describe the effects of immobilization on connective tissue.
12. Discuss clinical applications of therapeutic interventions based on the stages of connective tissue healing.

KEY TERMS

Endomysium
Epimysium
Muscle sprain
Muscle strain
Perimysium

Skeletal muscles, and by extension their tendons, are responsible for human movement. Injury to a muscle or a tendon may have a significant impact on one's functional ability. A muscle or tendon injury may range in severity from minor pain with minimal functional loss to severe pain with prolonged or permanent functional loss. A person who has sustained a muscle or tendon injury may benefit from a supervised clinical rehabilitation program.

For many patients who have sustained a muscle or tendon injury, a conservative physical therapy treatment program may help reduce pain, increase range of motion (ROM) and strength, and restore functional abilities. To maximize a patient's recovery, communication between the physical therapist (PT) and the physical therapist assistant (PTA) is crucial. The PTA should be told how and when the patient was injured and be able to integrate that knowledge to appreciate the patient's current stage of healing. Using this information is crucial to understanding why one patient is progressing and tolerating treatment, whereas a different patient's progress is plateauing or regressing.

The purpose of this chapter is to review the functional anatomy of the muscle and tendon, present the pathomechanics associated with common muscle and tendon injuries, identify the various types of muscle and tendon injuries, present an overview of the body's response to injury and the healing process, and present evidence-based and evidence-supported treatments to facilitate muscle and tendon healing.

MUSCLE AND TENDON FUNCTIONAL ANATOMY

MACROSTRUCTURE OF MUSCLES AND TENDONS

Functional movement of the human body is performed by the interaction of more than 600 skeletal muscles and their respective tendons. Skeletal muscles are complex tissues consisting of muscle fibers, connective tissue, blood supply, and innervating nerves. Tendons, fibrous connective tissue consisting of collagen fibers, extend from the skeletal muscle to provide an attachment to bone. The contraction of a muscle creates movement about a joint through the tension applied to the tendon.

The transition zone between the muscle and the tendon is known as the *musculotendinous junction*. The anatomic arrangement at the musculotendinous junction allows for the transmission of force from the muscle to the tendon. The attachment between a tendon and a bone is known as the *tendo-osseous junction*.

MICROSTRUCTURE OF MUSCLES

A muscle consists of muscle fibers and connective tissue (Fig. 12-1). There are three layers of connective tissue: the **epimysium**, the **perimysium**, and the **endomysium**. The epimysium surrounds the muscle and (along with the perimysium and the endomysium) is continuous with the muscle's tendons. Within the muscle, groups of muscle fibers (known as a *fasciculus*) are surrounded by the perimysium. Within each fasciculus, each individual muscle fiber is surrounded by the endomysium.

A muscle fiber (muscle cell) is divided further into myofibrils and myofilaments (see Fig. 12-1). Each muscle fiber is surrounded by a sarcolemma, the cellular membrane of the muscle fiber. Within the muscle fiber, the myofibrils are contained within the sarcoplasm. The myofibrils are bundles of the contractile proteins myosin and actin grouped together as a sarcomere (the basic functional unit of the myofibril). The interaction between the myosin and actin during contraction of the muscle contributes to functional movement. The structural relationship between the contractile and noncontractile components allows skeletal muscles to perform concentric (shortening) and eccentric (lengthening) muscle contractions as well as return to a resting position.[18]

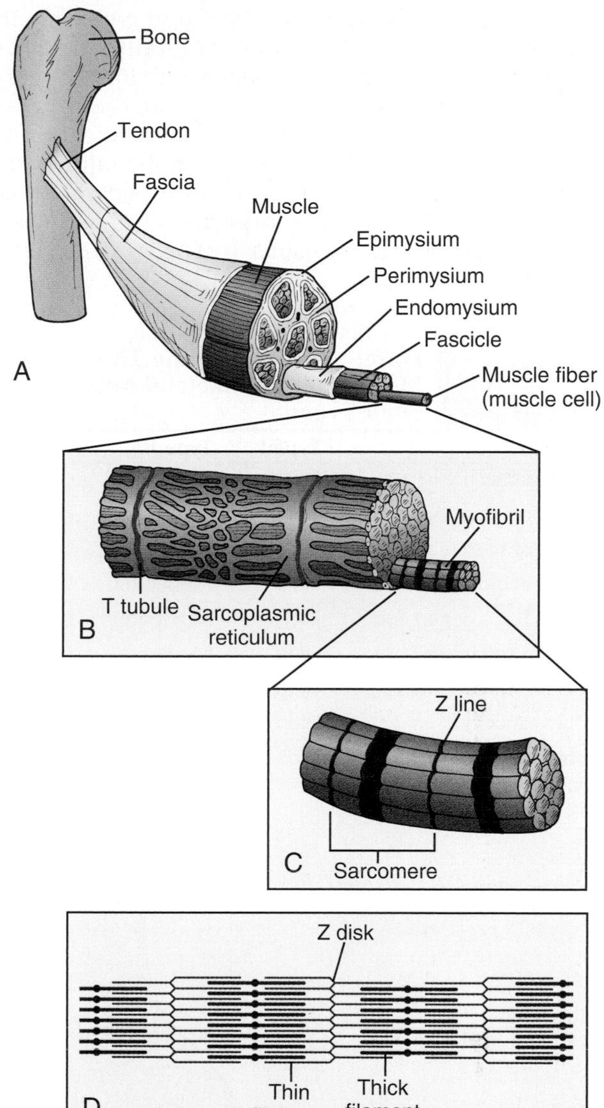

FIG 12-1 Macrostructure and microstructure of human skeletal muscle. **A,** Skeletal muscle organ composed of bundles of contractile muscle fibers held together by connective tissue. **B,** Greater magnification of a single fiber showing small fibers, myofibrils, in the sarcoplasm. **C,** Myofibril magnified further to show sarcomere between successive Z lines. Cross striae are visible. **D,** Molecular structure of a myofibril showing thick and thin myofilaments. *(From Cameron MH, Monroe LG:* Physical rehabilitation: evidence-based examination, evaluation, and intervention, *St Louis, 2007, Saunders.)*

Muscle Fiber Types

Several types of muscle fibers have been identified in skeletal muscle. The differences between muscle fibers are based on the shape of the fiber and its function. There are two general categories of muscle fiber types: fast twitch (FT) and slow twitch (ST). The term *twitch* relates to the time it takes the muscle fiber (and its associated nerve) to contract and relax.

ST muscle fibers are also known as *type I muscle fibers*. The type I fibers appear red because of the presence of myoglobin, an oxygen-binding protein. This is an important feature of the type I muscle fiber because it is specifically adapted for continuous aerobic activity; the type I muscle fibers are generally fatigue resistant. Examples of muscle groups consisting of a high number of type I fibers are the soleus and the erector spinae, postural muscles that either must contract repetitively or require being held for long durations.

ST muscle fibers possess a high endurance capacity, whereas FT muscle fibers, also known as *type II muscle fibers*, are specialized for more anaerobic activities. There are several types of FT fibers that are differentiated by their resistance to fatigue, their functional use, and the type of myosin heavy chain protein complex present (Table 12-1).[27]

The literature describes at least eight types of named muscle fibers: I, IC, IIA, IIB, IIC, IID, IIX (IIB), and IIAX.[7,9,12,15,27,30,31,35] However, this does not mean that there are eight distinct fiber types. Rather, there appears to be an inconsistency in the literature as to how the fibers are named.[7,9,12,15,27,30,31,35] Although the PTA can appreciate that there is variability among sources about the actual number of different fiber types, it is more important to appreciate the two broad categories of muscle fibers: type I and type

II. Type I are the slow, oxidative fibers, and type II are the fast, glycolytic fibers. There are significant differences between the two main types that have functional implications. The exercise prescription strategy used during different phases of the healing process should take into account the primary fiber composition of the injured skeletal muscle. The characteristics of the three most common fiber types in human skeletal muscle—types I, IIA, and IIB—are compared in this chapter (see Table 12-1).[7,31,35]

TABLE 12-1 Physical and Physiologic Differences among the Three Most Common Skeletal Muscle Fiber Types

Parameter	Type I	Type IIA	Type IIB
Cell body size	Small	Medium	Large
Conduction velocity	Slow	Fast	Fast
Number of muscle fibers	Few	More	Most
Rate of force development	Slow	Moderate	Fast
Absolute force generation	Low	Moderate	High
Resistance to fatigue	High	Moderate	Low
Mitochondrial density	High	High	Low
Aerobic capacity	High	Moderate	Low
Myoglobin content	High	Low	Low

MICROSTRUCTURE OF TENDONS

Tendons serve two functions: (1) to facilitate movement or joint stability by transmitting forces between muscle and bone and (2) to store energy for later movement. An example of the latter function is the energy created during plyometric exercises. The series elastic component stores elastic energy created during plyometric exercises in response to an eccentric stretch of the muscle. Tendons have the ability to withstand significant physiologic loads; however, they may be at risk of injury by trauma, degeneration, or overuse. A tendon's structure is divided into three locations: muscle-tendon junction, midsubstance, and bone-tendon junction.

Tendons are dense connective tissue consisting of fibroblasts (cells) and an extracellular matrix composed of collagen fibers, elastin, and ground substance (Fig. 12-2). The fibroblasts are responsible for synthesizing components of the extracellular matrix.[28] The ground substance provides support to collagen fibers.[28] The collagen fibers, which are oriented in a parallel arrangement, provide strength to resist tensile forces.

The structural hierarchy of tendons is similar to skeletal muscle. Collagen fibrils are grouped together into the tendon's basic functional unit, the collagen fiber. Groups of collagen fibers (primary fiber bundle) form a subfascicle.[16] Several subfascicles grouped together form a fascicle

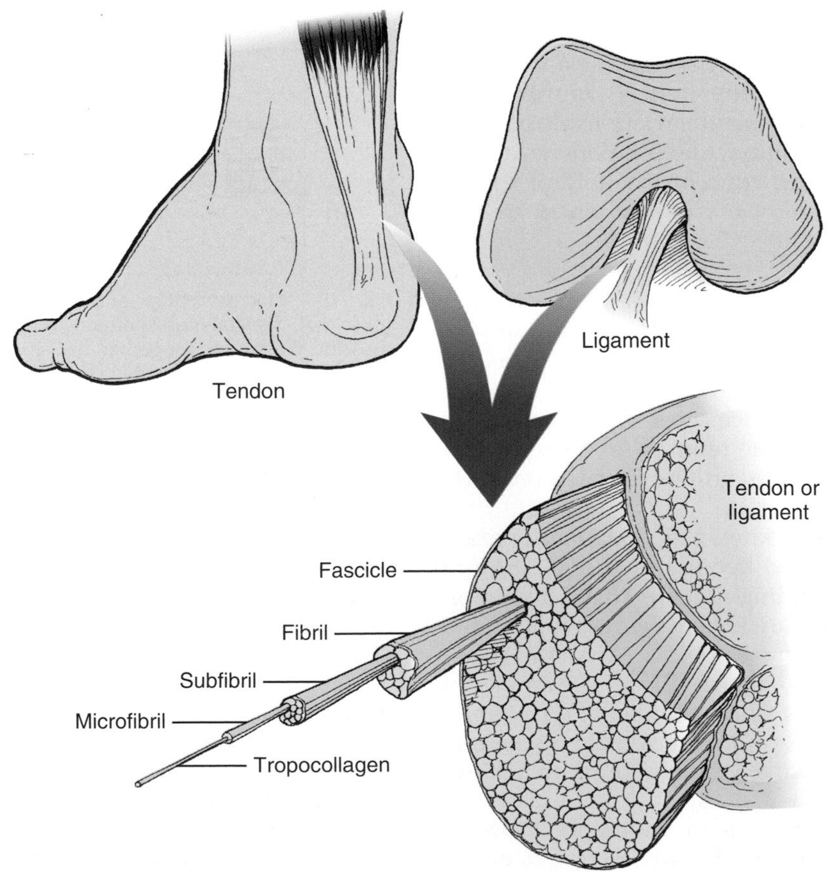

FIG 12-2 Macrostructure and microstructure of tendon. *(Modified from Brinker MR, Miller DS:* Fundamentals of orthopaedics, *Philadelphia, 1999, Saunders.)*

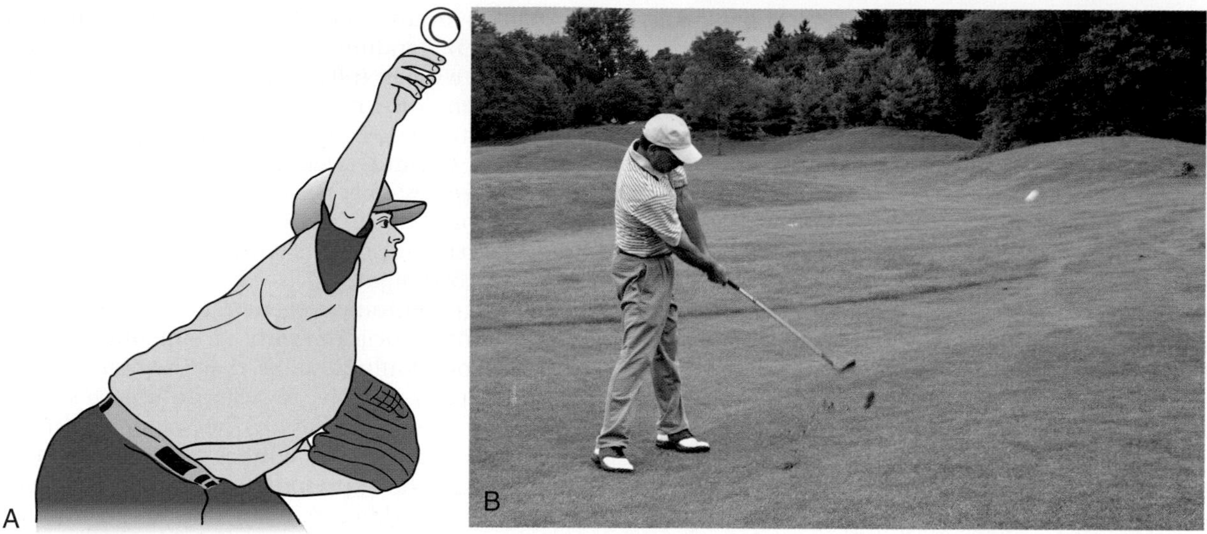

FIG 12-3 **A,** Deceleration phase of the pitching motion. **B,** Follow-through phase of the golf swing. (**A,** *Modified from Ellenbecker T:* Clinical examination of the shoulder, *St Louis, 2005, Saunders.* **B,** Photo courtesy iStock.com.)

(secondary fiber bundle).[16] Several fascicles grouped together form a tertiary bundle.[16] These three groups (bundles) are surrounded by a connective tissue called the *endotenon*.[16] The epitenon surrounds the entire tendon as a fine, loose connective tissue sheath.[16,28] Blood vessels and nerves are also contained within the epitenon.[28] The paratenon is a loose areolar connective tissue attaching to the outer portion of the epitenon.[16,28] The function of the paratenon is to allow gliding over adjacent structures.[16]

The transition from the tendon into its osseous attachment site includes several connective tissue changes.[16] The first change is from the primary tendon structure into fibrocartilage. Next, the fibrocartilage converts into a mineralized fibrocartilage. The mineralized fibrocartilage secures the attachment of the tendon to the bone. In addition to this arrangement, collagen fibers from the tendon pass through these transition zones and attach to the bone. These fibers are known as *Sharpey's fibers*.

MUSCLE AND TENDON INJURIES

The human body experiences a range of physical loads and stresses during activities, work, and sports. These forces on the body, whether they are a one-time supraphysiologic load that is greater than a tissue's tolerance or a subfailure load that is experienced for a prolonged period of time, may contribute to a musculoskeletal injury.

Examples from sports are presented to help illustrate the significant loads and stresses that may be experienced by some athletes. During the deceleration phase of pitching a baseball, the pitcher's shoulder rotates up to 7000° per second with 400 newtons (N) of posterior shear forces, 300 N of inferior shear forces, and 1000 N of compressive forces experienced at the glenohumeral joint (Fig. 12-3, *A*).[20] Over time, these shear and compressive forces may increase the baseball pitcher's risk of sustaining a shoulder injury.[20,21,34] During the golf swing, a golfer may experience compressive loads in the lumbar spine that are eight times his or her body weight (Fig. 12-3, *B*).[11] To provide some perspective, a distance runner experiences compressive loads that are equal to three times his or her body weight during the run. To reduce the risk of injury, muscles and tendons must possess the ability to stretch or deform in response to the applied load. When an applied load supersedes the ability of the muscle or tendon to resist tensile forces, the muscle or tendon is at a higher risk of injury.

MUSCLE AND TENDON INJURY MECHANISMS

A patient's rehabilitation program is developed by the PT based on the patient's medical history, the patient's subjective report, and the PT's physical evaluation of the patient. When guiding a patient through his or her treatment program, the PTA should be familiar with the patient's diagnosis and mechanism of the injury. Possessing this knowledge helps the PTA advance the rehabilitation program per the PT's plan and alerts the PTA to cease treatment and consult with the PT when the patient demonstrates a negative response to treatment.

A muscle injury may be caused by disease, a direct (external) mechanism, or an indirect (internal) mechanism. Some diseases may have profound effects on the muscular system and contribute to significant disability. Examples of diseases that weaken muscles include muscular dystrophy, multiple sclerosis, Parkinson's disease, and Huntington's disease. Patients who have a neuromuscular disease may benefit from treatment by the physical therapy team. However, for purposes of this chapter, the pathomechanics and only the rehabilitation strategies for direct and indirect muscle injuries are addressed.

A direct muscle injury occurs when an external force applied to the body results in a trauma. Examples of direct muscle injuries include a contusion caused by a blunt trauma or a deep laceration caused by a sharp implement. In each of these examples, the applied supraphysiologic load was greater than the muscle's maximum tissue tolerance. An indirect muscle injury occurs independent of an applied external force. Indirect muscle injuries are the result of either a supraphysiologic load (e.g., a violent or excessive muscular stretch or excessive muscular stretch combined with an eccentric muscular contraction) or repeated insults (e.g., overuse injury) to the tissue without proper time for recovery.[8,18] Indirect muscle injuries primarily occur at the musculotendinous junction; however, they may also occur in the muscle belly itself.[18]

A **muscle strain,** frequently referred to as a muscle tear, is an indirect injury (Box 12-1). A pulled hamstring (sometimes referred to as a *hammy*) is an example of a common muscle strain experienced in sports.[5,6,26] Muscle strains can cause significant pain and greatly reduce function.[5,6,26] Hamstring injuries can result in a lengthy rehabilitation period and a slow return to sport for an athlete.[25] Muscles that cross two joints, such as the hamstrings, are frequently strained.[8,25] Sports medicine specialists believe that these muscles may become injured in response to an intense eccentric load.[8] Many of the most frequently strained muscles are composed of type II muscle fibers, the fibers that are least resistant to fatigue.[8]

Muscle strains are frequently described by the degree of damage to the muscle. Table 12-2 presents the characteristics associated with a first-degree, second-degree, or third-degree muscle strain.

Important Concepts

The severity of a muscle injury influences how quickly a patient is progressed through a rehabilitation program.

Because muscle attaches to bone via tendon, the two structures are interrelated and are frequently injured together (e.g., musculotendinous junction muscle strains). However, many injuries seen clinically are specific to the tendon itself (e.g., tendinitis or Achilles tendon ruptures).

BOX 12-1 Sprain versus Strain

The terms *strain* and *sprain* do not mean the same thing. A strain is a muscle or tendon injury. A strain to the muscle, tendon, or musculotendinous unit may be caused by one of several mechanisms, including direct impact, violent stretch or eccentric overload, or overuse. A sprain is an injury to a ligament. Ligament sprains occur in response to a violent stretching mechanism above physiologic capacity. A muscle and a ligament may be injured during the same mechanism; however they are two distinct injuries.

Tendon injuries range from tendinitis to tendinosis (Table 12-3). Tendinitis is an acute injury of the tendon associated with an inflammatory response. A patient with a "true" tendinitis may present to physical therapy with pain, functional loss, and signs associated with inflammation (pain, warmth, swelling, redness). A patient with tendinitis often describes performing an unfamiliar, repetitive activity from 1 day to a week before seeking medical attention. If a patient presents with a tendon injury that lacks inflammatory signs, it is likely that the patient has tendinosis—a chronic, degenerative change of the tendon that is not associated with an inflammatory process. Patients commonly describe that they have experienced pain for many months to years before seeking medical attention. Common locations where one might develop a tendinosis include the Achilles tendon, the quadriceps tendon, and the supraspinatus tendon. The manner in which each condition is treated differs greatly. A tendon may also rupture, requiring surgical repair.

Important Concepts

A tendinitis is marked by classic inflammatory signs and symptoms—pain, inflammation, redness, and warmth. Tendon injuries not associated with inflammatory signs and symptoms may be the result of degeneration.

Microtrauma results when a tendon experiences strain levels that overload the tissue's tensile capabilities. A frequent, repeated strain to the tendon continues the microtrauma (damage) to the microstructure of the tendon. An injury occurs when the rate of damage surpasses the ability of the tendon to repair itself. Over time, if the tendon fails to heal, a tendinosis region develops.

TABLE 12-3 Tendon Injury Classifications

Injury	Classification
Tendinitis	Acute injury to tendon with associated inflammatory response
Tendinosis	Degeneration to tendon, not associated with inflammatory process, secondary to one or more factors (e.g., microtrauma, age-related changes)
Peritenonitis	Inflammation of peritenon only
Tenosynovitis	Inflammation of tendon synovial membrane
Tenovaginitis	Inflamed, thickened tendon sheath

TABLE 12-2 Characteristics of First-Degree, Second-Degree, and Third-Degree Muscle Strains

Parameter	First Degree	Second Degree	Third Degree
Extent of damage to muscle	Tear of a few muscle fibers	Tear of approximately half of muscle fibers	Tear (rupture) of entire muscle
Muscle weakness	Minor	Moderate (significant)	Major
Loss of function	None to minor	Moderate	Major
Pain	Minor	Moderate to major	None (lack of pain is associated with third-degree strain because the nerve is often significantly damaged during the injury)
Swelling	Minimal to none	Noticeable degree of swelling	Significant degree of swelling

Some tendons may also be at risk for significant tearing or rupturing. With tendon rupture, surgical intervention is necessary to restore function. Orthopedic surgeons frequently perform repairs to the tendons of the supraspinatus (in addition to the other rotator cuff muscles), extensor carpi radialis brevis, quadriceps tendon, and Achilles tendon.

AGE EFFECTS ON TENDONS

Over time, the aging tendon has an increased risk of sustaining an injury.[33] PTAs frequently provide treatment for patients who are 40 years old and older who have experienced a tendon injury. In some cases, patients receive conservative physical therapy treatment, whereas in other cases, patients may require invasive procedures such as injections or surgical repair.

Pathomechanics Associated with the Aging Tendon

As one ages, the stresses that would have been tolerated in youth can contribute to an overuse injury or a tendon rupture. The aging tendon is usually smaller in size (compared with its size during youth or young adulthood) with a decrease in total number of collagen fibers. In addition, the ability of the aging tendon to turn over collagen fibers decreases.[28,33] The inability to add new collagen fibers at the same rate, or at all, limits the body's effectiveness in repairing microtrauma. Over time, repeated subfailure loads to a tendon result in a tendon rupture. In addition, because of the smaller overall size, the tendon has a lower capacity to resist certain tensile loads.

INJURY AND HEALING

As an immediate response to a muscle or tendon injury, the human body initiates the healing process. For a patient to experience optimal recovery from a muscle or tendon injury, his or her body must successfully complete the three stages of healing: acute, subacute, and chronic.[1,23,28] The events that occur during each of the three stages are fairly consistent among connective tissues. Table 12-4 provides a timeline overview of events that occur during the healing process. A chronic pain syndrome may develop if the body fails to progress appropriately through these three stages.

Important Concepts

There are three stages of healing after a muscle or tendon injury—acute, subacute, and chronic. Physical therapy interventions should take into account the unique features associated with each stage of healing.

TABLE 12-4 Timeline of Cellular Events Occurring during the Healing Process

Time Frame (Postinjury)	Events
Immediate to 48 hours	Rupture of blood and lymphatic vessels with initial vasoconstriction—coagulation Clot formation Vasodilation occurs shortly after initial injury Immediate swelling—cellular (exudate) components from vessels fill wound site Patient experiences hallmark signs and symptoms of inflammation (redness, warmth, pain, and swelling) Phagocytosis (process of removing injured and dead cellular material) Chemical mediators attracted to the area to control inflammatory process
Day 2-4	Decrease in inflammation Decrease in clot size (reabsorption) Increase in granulation tissue (fibroblasts, myofibroblasts, and capillaries) Repair process initiated Angiogenesis—process of developing a new blood supply to injured region
Day 4-21	Initiation of fibroplasia (scar formation) Fibroblastic activity (produces collagen, elastin, and ground substance) Growth of scar ceases at the end of the phase
Day 21-60	Remodeling of scar Collagen thickens and strengthens

ACUTE STAGE (INFLAMMATORY PHASE)

The onset of the acute stage begins immediately in response to injury. Trauma incites a complex series of chemical events that mobilize cells and chemotactic agents to the injury site to stimulate coagulation (clot formation), control hemorrhage (bleeding), and synthesize new collagen.

The inflammatory response, a hallmark sign associated with the acute stage, is the immediate physiologic response designed to protect the injured area, stop the progression of cellular damage, and stimulate the body's repair process. The signs and symptoms associated with an inflammatory response are redness (rubor), swelling (tumor), heat or warmth (calor), and pain (dolor). The redness and warmth of the injured site are due to the damage to blood and lymphatic vessels, dilation of the blood vessels, and increased permeability allowing exudate to fill the area. Swelling in the injured area is due to exudate. Exudate consists of plasma and serum proteins that have leaked out of the vessels and into the surrounding tissue. Their function is to repair the injured site, but excessive exudate can cause significant swelling. Swelling increases the pressure within the injured area and applies a mechanical stress to free nerve endings, causing pain.

It may take up to 6 days for the body to complete the cellular and vascular activity associated with the acute stage. However, the acute phase may continue for an additional period of time if the injured area is continually stressed (e.g., a football athlete who keeps playing despite pain).

SUBACUTE PHASE (REPAIR AND HEALING)

Repair of the injured tissue (starting the third day after the injury) is initiated and proceeds for up to 3 weeks. Growth of capillaries into the injured region and fibroblastic activity are initiated early in this phase. Fibroblasts are cells that synthesize new collagen. This new collagen, which replaces the clot material, is formed and oriented in haphazard fashion as it is first laid down. Although new, this collagen is structurally immature (thin and weak). If this area is overstressed with activity or aggressive therapy, it may be injured.

Angiogenesis begins during the subacute phase. Angiogenesis is the process of new growth of blood vessels to supply the injured area. This neovascularization is necessary for continued soft tissue injury healing. The new blood supply carries oxygen and nutrients to the region.

Important Concepts

Newly formed collagen during the subacute phase of healing is weak and thin. This newly formed collagen may be damaged if the patient performs exercises that reproduce symptoms or pain.

CHRONIC STAGE (MATURATION AND REMODELING)

The scar tissue that was initially formed after the injury has stopped growing by the end of the third week. The body is now ready to enter the chronic phase of healing, which is highlighted by tissue remodeling and strengthening. During this phase, the collagen is remodeled along the line of forces that it experiences. Applying the appropriate volume of stress to the healing tissue helps to facilitate the functional growth of the collagen and the improvement in its tensile strength capability. This process may occur for 12 to 18 months after the date of the original injury.

EFFECTS OF IMMOBILIZATION

Patients who have been immobilized for any period of time after an injury experience significant changes to the muscle and tendon. Perhaps the most profound change in human skeletal muscle during immobilization is atrophy. The degree of atrophy depends on the duration of immobilization and the position or stretch imposed on the muscle. If a muscle in a joint is immobilized in a shortened position, the muscle fiber decreases in length, and there is an associated decrease in the number of sarcomeres. This muscle may atrophy more than a muscle that has been casted in a lengthened position. Muscles that are immobilized in a shortened position are also less extensible after cast removal than muscles that have been immobilized in a lengthened position.

Muscle fiber types are also affected by position during immobilization. When muscles are immobilized in a shortened position, type I muscle fibers atrophy (decrease in number of fibers and fiber diameter) far more than type II fibers. When a large percentage of type I muscle fibers atrophy during periods of immobilization, the relative number of type II fibers increases.

BOX 12-2 Effects of Immobilization of Skeletal Muscle Tissue (Shortened)

- Muscle atrophy (type I)
- Decreased sarcomeres
- Increased protein breakdown
- Decreased muscle extensibility after immobilization
- Decreased muscle weight
- Decreased force-generating capacity
- Increase in connective tissue
- Decreased anaerobic glycolytic enzymes
- Decreased aerobic oxidative enzymes

Muscle atrophy also results in a decrease in muscle weight. Muscle that has atrophied and lost weight also loses its ability to generate force and tension. The greatest amount of atrophy occurs within the first week of immobilization, and muscle fiber size decreases by approximately 17% within 3 days of immobilization. Box 12-2 depicts the various physiologic changes that occur in skeletal muscle when immobilized in a shortened position.

If a tendon has to be immobilized because of injury or surgery, the collagen that is formed by the fibroblasts is oriented in a haphazard fashion. During immobilization, the tissue lacks the stimulus to orient the new collagen fibers in a functional parallel orientation. There is also an increased risk of development of adhesion between the disorganized collagen fibers. After immobilization, the tendon is at risk for reinjury for a period of time because of the limited tensile capacity of the repaired tissue. Failure to continue with a home exercise program after formal discharge from physical therapy can limit a patient's full return to function. Inactivity after an injury (or in general) can result in a decrease in quantity and size of collagen fibers.

MUSCLE REPAIR AND HETEROTOPIC BONE FORMATION

Can muscle cells be repaired after an injury? There is some debate within the scientific community; however, the current state of thought is that a special cell known as a *satellite cell* can increase in number and convert into muscle cells. Further research is necessary at this time to explain or refute this notion.

Occasionally, injury to a muscle (e.g., severe blunt injury, deep contusion, surgical exposures, certain fractures) may result in heterotopic bone formation (ectopic bone formation). Heterotopic bone formation after blunt trauma to muscle is known as *myositis ossificans*.[22] Generally, if the contusion is severe (deep versus superficial), there may be a periosteal reaction that stimulates undifferentiated mesenchymal cells to proliferate during the first 3 to 4 days after the trauma. During the next 5 to 8 days, cartilage develops with gradual calcification and neovascularization with subsequent bone deposition.

EVIDENCE-BASED THERAPEUTIC INTERVENTIONS FOR INJURED MUSCLES AND TENDONS

No two muscle or tendon injuries should be rehabilitated the same way. There is no "cookbook" or "one size fits all" approach to physical therapy. Instead, the PT must develop the patient's rehabilitation program based on several factors, including the tissue (or tissues) injured, the severity of the injury, the current stage of healing, the findings from the patient's musculoskeletal examination, and the patient's short-term and long-term goals. This section presents evidence-based therapeutic interventions for muscle and tendon injuries based on the stages of tissue repair. Evidence-based and evidence-supported rationales are used when available.

ACUTE STAGE: IMMEDIATE RESPONSE FOR A MUSCLE OR TENDON INJURY

When an athlete is injured, a sports medicine team consisting of the PT, the PTA, or the PTA with a dual credential as a certified athletic trainer provides the first line of treatment. Many sports certified PTs who are dual-credentialed as certified athletic trainers or who are sports certified specialists (board-certified sports physical therapist by the American Physical Therapy Association) provide game coverage within their community. The immediate treatment provided by the sports medicine team for an athlete who has been sidelined because of a sport-related injury includes protection, rest, ice, compression, and elevation (PRICE).

If an athlete sustains an injury that impairs function or if continued sports participation might worsen the injury, the athlete should be removed from competition and allowed to rest the injured area. If possible, the injured region should be elevated. Elevation of the joint or extremity should be above the level of the heart (e.g., an athlete who has injured his or her leg should have the lower extremity elevated and supported while the athlete lies on his or her back). Elevating the extremity reduces the swelling that occurs immediately after injury. Ice should be immediately applied to the injured area to reduce further inflammatory damage and control pain. Compression should be applied in conjunction with the ice for up to 20 minutes, every 30 minutes to 1 hour. Finally, the injured region should be protected from further injury. For example, an athlete who has sprained an ankle might benefit from the use of bilateral crutches and decreased weight-bearing stress. Depending on the severity of the injury, the athlete should be referred to the emergency department to rule out a fracture (if necessary) or to the appropriate sports medicine or orthopedic physician the following day.

ACUTE STAGE: TREATMENT IN THE PHYSICAL THERAPY CLINIC

The clinical goals associated with the acute stage are to facilitate healing to the injured tissue, control or reduce the effects of the inflammation, decrease pain, initiate controlled movement to restore ROM, and reduce the loss of muscular strength. Physical agents are frequently used during the acute stage of healing to decrease pain, reduce inflammation, facilitate healing, and restore muscular function. In addition, passive range of motion (PROM) and active assisted range of motion (AAROM) exercises are initiated to maintain or restore movement around the joint. Manual therapy techniques are performed to reduce pain and improve soft tissue and joint mobility. Isometric strengthening may also be performed during this phase to retard strength loss. Table 12-5 lists evidence-supported treatments for patients in the acute stage of healing.

Patients should be provided with a home exercise program to perform between sessions. The effectiveness of each technique should be assessed during and between treatment sessions. Treatments that fail to have an impact on the patient's recovery should be terminated. In addition, treatments that worsen the patient's state should be stopped immediately. Failure to remove stress to the injured tissue during the acute phase may increase swelling, pain, and the length of this phase.

TABLE 12-5 Evidence-Supported Treatments for Patients in Acute Stage of Healing

Goal	Treatment	Relevant Study
Facilitate healing of injured tissue	Ultrasound	Noonan,[24] Reilly[29]
	Cryotherapy	Jarvinen,[13] Noonan,[24] Reilly,[29] Thompson[32]
Control or reduce effects of inflammation	Ultrasound	Noonan,[24] Reilly[29]
	Cryotherapy	Jarvinen,[13] Noonan,[24] Reilly,[29] Thompson[32]
	Massage	Brumitt,[2] Reilly[29]
Decrease pain	Ultrasound	Noonan[24]
	Cryotherapy	Jarvinen,[13] Noonan,[24] Reilly,[29] Thompson[32]
	Massage	Brumitt,[2] Reilly[29]
	Joint mobilization	Brumitt[3,4]
Restore ROM	PROM (manual or self techniques	Brumitt,[4] Meier,[19] Noonan[24]
	AAROM (self techniques)	Brumitt,[4] Meier[19]
	Massage	Brumitt,[2] Reilly[29]
	Joint mobilization	Brumitt[3,4]
Restore muscular strength	Isometric exercises	Brumitt,[3,4] Frohm,[10] Jarvinen,[13] Meier,[19] Noonan[24]

AAROM, active assisted range of motion; *PROM,* passive range of motion; *ROM,* range of motion.

Important Concepts

The primary treatments performed during the acute phase of healing are directed toward reducing pain and modulating the inflammatory response. In addition, PROM and AAROM are prescribed to initiate restoration of motion. Isometric exercises may be appropriate for some patients; however, strengthening exercises should not be performed if they reproduce pain.

SUBACUTE STAGE: TREATMENT IN THE PHYSICAL THERAPY CLINIC

The clinical goals during the subacute phase are to restore full active range of motion (AROM) and PROM, initiate muscular strengthening, continue to address residual swelling, reduce pain, and initiate functional movement tasks. During the subacute phase of healing, the body deposits immature collagen fibers in the injured region. Prescribing therapeutic exercises that appropriately stress the injured region helps to promote the normal healing process and the development of a mobile scar. However, overstressing the area may injure the new collagen fibers. Pain during exercise should be avoided. It must be made clear to patients that they should stop performing an exercise if it reproduces their pain.

A primary goal of this phase is to progress and restore ROM. During the acute phase, PROM and AAROM exercises are prescribed. As tolerated, the patient should be progressed to AROM techniques and static stretching exercises. Typically, multiple sets and repetitions of AROM exercises are prescribed. Manual therapy techniques (e.g., joint mobilization, massage) may continue to be necessary to restore joint and soft tissue mobility. Static stretching exercises should initially be performed gently, holding each stretch for 30 seconds.[13,24,37]

The prescription of resisted exercises assists the collagen orientation and improves tensile capabilities. Initially, exercises should be performed with high repetitions and low weights. Performing a muscular endurance program allows the patient to gain strength gradually while reducing the risk of damaging the new collagen fibers. Patients can be instructed to perform 15 to 25 repetitions of one to two sets per exercise. The initial number of exercises prescribed by the PT depends on the patient's presentation. The inclusion of neuromuscular electrical stimulation may further assist the restoration of muscular strength.[19]

Important Concepts

Patients should perform a higher volume of repetitions initially during the subacute stage of healing. Performing high-repetition, low-load exercises allows the patient to develop muscular endurance capacity without overloading the newly formed collagen.

CHRONIC STAGE: TREATMENT IN THE PHYSICAL THERAPY CLINIC

During the chronic stage of healing, collagen aligns to the stresses applied, and the tissue is maturing and remodeling. Physical therapy interventions should facilitate this process through the continued prescription of therapeutic exercises.

Increasing the endurance capacity of the muscle may be continued as necessary, but now the therapy team should be able to progress strengthening as tolerated. Exercise prescription should be functional in nature and should account for muscle fiber structure within muscle groups. For example, muscles of the core (type I muscle fibers) should continue to be trained using endurance training strategies. Strength training variables may be applied to muscle groups containing higher percentages of type II muscle fibers. When the patient is pain-free, plyometrics or power training may be initiated if functionally necessary (e.g., athletes, industrial workers).[4]

SPECIAL CONSIDERATIONS: TENDON REPAIRS AND TENDINOSIS

A patient who has been referred to physical therapy with a postoperative tendon repair requires special consideration. Failing to follow the physician's postoperative protocol may put the repaired tendon at risk for injury or rerupturing.

Patients who have been referred with a tendinosis diagnosis benefit from performance of eccentric exercises. A growing body of evidence suggests that the inclusion of eccentric exercises helps to reduce pain and restore function in individuals with a tendinosis at the Achilles tendon or patella tendon.[10,14,17,36]

Important Concepts

Evidence suggests that prescription of eccentric exercises is preferred for patients with a diagnosis of tendinosis. A typical training program consists of performing three sets of 15 repetitions per eccentric exercise, performed one to two times a day for up to 12 weeks. Eccentric exercise training programs allow for patients to experience pain during performance.

SUMMARY

Successful rehabilitation after a muscle or tendon injury occurs when members of the rehabilitation team effectively communicate with one another regarding the patient's diagnosis and progression. When possible, the therapy team should use evidence-based rehabilitation interventions. If evidence-based rehabilitation programs are not available in the literature, the rehabilitation professional should select interventions that are appropriate for the patient's current stage of healing.

GLOSSARY

Endomysium: An internal connective sheath that covers the muscle fibers; one of three layers of connective tissue that surrounds the muscle and is continuous with the muscle's tendons.

Epimysium: The outermost layer of tissue covering that becomes continuous with tendons; one of three layers of connective tissue that surrounds the muscle and is continuous with the muscle's tendons.

Perimysium: Covers groups of individual muscle fibers into bundles; one of three layers of connective tissue that surrounds the muscle and is continuous with the muscle's tendons.

Muscle sprain: An injury to a ligament.

Muscle strain: An injury to a muscle or tendon.

REFERENCES

1. Alaseirlis DA, Li Y, Cilli F, et al: Decreasing inflammatory response of injured patellar tendons results in increased collagen fibril diameters. *Connect Tissue Res* 46:3–8, 2005.

2. Brumitt J: The role of massage in sports performance and rehabilitation: current evidence and future direction. *N Am J Sports Phys Ther* 3(1):7–21, 2008.
3. Brumitt J, McIntosh L, Rutt R: Comprehensive sports medicine treatment of an athlete who runs cross-country and is iron deficient. *N Am J Sports Phys Ther* 4(1):13–20, 2009.
4. Brumitt J, Sproul A, Lentz P, et al: In-season rehabilitation of a division III female wrestler after a glenohumeral dislocation. *Phys Ther Sport* 10(3):112–117, 2009.
5. Cohen S, Bradley J: Acute proximal hamstring rupture. *J Am Acad Orthop Surg* 15(6):350–355, 2007.
6. Croisier JL: Factors associated with recurrent hamstring injuries. *Sports Med* 34(10):681–695, 2004.
7. den Hoed MD, Hesselink MKC, Westerterp KR: Skeletal muscle fiber-type and habitual physical activity in daily life. *Scand J Med Sci Sports* 19:373–380, 2009.
8. Dugan SA, Frontera WR: Muscle fatigue and muscle injury. *Phys Med Rehabil Clin N Am* 11(2):385–403, 2000.
9. Eriksson A, Kadi F, Malm C, et al: Skeletal muscle morphology in power-lifters with and without anabolic steroids. *Histochem Cell Biol* 124:167–175, 2005.
10. Frohm A, Saartok T, Halvorsen K, et al: Eccentric treatment for patellar tendinopathy: a prospective short-term pilot study of two rehabilitation protocols. *Br J Sports Med* 41(7):7, 2007.
11. Hosea TM, Gatt CJ, Jr: Back pain in golf. *Clin Sports Med* 15(1):37–53, 1996.
12. Hostler D, Schwirian CI, Campos G, et al: Skeletal muscle adaptations in elastic resistance-trained young men and women. *Eur J Appl Physiol* 86:112–118, 2001.
13. Jarvinen TA, Kaariainen M, Jarvinen M, et al: Muscle strain injuries. *Curr Opin Rheumatol* 12(2):155–161, 2000.
14. Jonsson P, Alfredson H: Superior results with eccentric compared to concentric quadriceps training in patients with jumper's knee: a prospective randomized study. *Br J Sports Med* 39(11):847–850, 2005.
15. Kadi F: Adaptation of human skeletal muscle to training and anabolic steroids. *Acta Physiol Scand Suppl* 646:1–52, 2000.
16. Kannus P: Structure of the tendon connective tissue. *Scand J Med Sci Sports* 10:312–320, 2000.
17. Magnussen RA, Dunn WR, Thomson AB: Nonoperative treatment of midportion Achilles tendinopathy: a systematic review. *Clin J Sports Med* 19(1):54–64, 2009.
18. Matzkin E, Zachazewski JE, Garrett WE, et al: Skeletal muscle: deformation, injury, repair, and treatment considerations. In Magee DJ, Zachazewski JE, Quillen WS, editors: *Scientific foundations and principles of practice in musculoskeletal rehabilitation*, St Louis, 2007, Saunders.
19. Meier W, Mizner RL, Marcus RL, et al: Total knee arthroplasty: muscle impairments, functional limitations, and recommended rehabilitation approaches. *J Orthop Sports Phys Ther* 38(5):246–256, 2008.
20. Meister K: Injuries to the shoulder in the throwing athlete. Part one: biomechanics/pathophysiology/classification of injury. *Am J Sports Med* 28(2):265–275, 2000.
21. Meister K: Injuries to the shoulder in the throwing athlete. Part two: evaluation/treatment. *Am J Sports Med* 28(4):587–601, 2000.
22. Miller AE, Davis BA, Beckley OA: Bilateral and recurrent myositis ossificans in an athlete: a case report and review of treatment options. *Arch Phys Med Rehabil* 87(2):286–290, 2006.
23. Molloy T, Wang Y, Murrell G: The roles of growth factors in tendon and ligament healing. *Sports Med* 33(5):381–394, 2003.
24. Noonan TJ, Garrett WE, Jr: Muscle strain injury: diagnosis and treatment. *J Am Acad Orthop Surg* 7(4):262–269, 1999.
25. Orchard J, Best TM, Verrall GM: Return to play following muscle strains. *Clin J Sport Med* 15(6):436–441, 2005.
26. Petersen J: Holmich P: Evidence based prevention of hamstring injuries in sport. *Br J Sports Med* 39(6):319–323, 2005.
27. Pette D, Staron RS: Transitions of muscle fiber phenotypic profiles. *Histochem Cell Biol* 115:359–372, 2001.
28. Platt MA: Tendon repair and healing. *Clin Podiatr Med Surg* 22:553–560, 2005.
29. Reilly T, Ekblom B: The use of recovery methods post-exercise. *J Sports Sci* 23(6):619–627, 2005.
30. Rodriguez LP, Lopez-Rego J, Calbet JAL, et al: Effects of training status on fibers of the musculus vastus lateralis in professional road cyclists. *Am J Phys Med Rehabil* 81:651–660, 2002.
31. Sciote JJ, Horton MJ, Rowlerson AM, et al: Specialized cranial muscles: how different are they from limb and abdominal muscles? *Cells Tissues Organs* 174:73–86, 2003.
32. Thompson C, Kelsberg G, St Anna L, et al: Clinical inquiries. Heat or ice for acute ankle sprain? *J Fam Pract* 52(8):642–643, 2003.
33. Thompson LV: Effects of age and training on skeletal muscle physiology and performance. *Phys Ther* 74:71–81, 1994.
34. Wang Q: Baseball and softball injuries. *Curr Sports Med Rep* 5(3):115–119, 2006.
35. Wang YX, Zhang CL, Yu RT, et al: Regulation of muscle fiber type and running endurance by PPARdelta. *PLoS Biol* 2(10):e294, 2004.
36. Woodley BL, Newsham-West RJ, Baxter GD: Chronic tendinopathy: effectiveness of eccentric exercise. *Br J Sports Med* 41(4):188–198, 2007.
37. Woods K, Bishop P, Jones E: Warm-up and stretching in the prevention of muscular injury. *Sports Med* 37(12):1089–1099, 2007.

REVIEW QUESTIONS

Multiple Choice

1. The transition zone between the muscle and the tendon is known as the:
   a. Musculotendinous junction.
   b. Myotendinous junction.
   c. Tendon-osseous junction.
   d. Musculotendinous articulation.
2. There are three layers of connective tissue associated with muscle fibers. The layer that surrounds the muscle and that is continuous with the muscle's tendon is the:
   a. Ectomysium.
   b. Endomysium.
   c. Perimysium.
   d. Epimysium.
3. The contractile proteins located in the muscle's sarcomere are known as:
   a. Myofibril and sarcolemma
   b. Myosin and actin
   c. Myofibril and actin
   d. Myosin and sarcolemma
4. Which type of muscle fiber is generally fatigue resistant?
   a. Type I
   b. Type II
   c. Type IIa
   d. Type IIb
5. Muscles, such as the ________________, contain a higher percentage of type I muscle fibers, allowing for a high level of ___________________.
   a. rectus femoris; explosive power
   b. soleus; explosive strength
   c. erector spinae; muscular endurance capacity
   d. biceps brachii; muscular endurance capacity
6. Muscle injuries may be the result of a disease, a direct mechanism, or an indirect mechanism. Which of the following would be considered a direct mechanism?
   a. Parkinson's disease
   b. Violent stretch to the hamstring muscle during sprinting
   c. Multiple sclerosis
   d. Injury resulting from football tackle

7. Which of the following signs or symptoms would not be associated with a tendinosis?
   a. Swelling
   b. Pain
   c. Muscular weakness
   d. Reported history of functional limitation or pain for many years
8. All of the following tendons are common locations that might develop a tendinosis except which one?
   a. Achilles tendon
   b. Quadriceps tendon
   c. Short head biceps tendon
   d. Supraspinatus tendon
9. Which stage of healing is marked by an inflammatory response?
   a. Acute stage
   b. Subacute stage
   c. Chronic stage
   d. Maturation stage
10. It may take up to ______ days to complete the cellular and vascular activity associated with the acute stage.
    a. 1
    b. 3
    c. 6
    d. 10
11. All of the following are features of the subacute phase of healing except which one?
    a. Fibroblasts synthesize new collagen
    b. Collagen is organized along functional lines of stress
    c. New collagen is thin and weak
    d. Capillaries grow into the injured region
12. Angiogenesis is _______________, and it is initiated during _______________.
    a. the creation of new peptides; subacute phase of healing
    b. new growth of blood vessels; subacute phase of healing
    c. new growth of blood vessels; chronic phase of healing
    d. creation of new peptides; chronic phase of healing
13. Maturation and remodeling of tissue after an injury may take _____________ months.
    a. 1 to 3
    b. 2 to 6
    c. 5 to 10
    d. 12 to 18
14. Heterotopic bone formation after blunt trauma is known as :
    a. Myositis ossificans.
    b. Mesenchymal cells.
    c. Bony proliferation.
    d. Osteogenesis imperfecta.
15. Which of the following treatments would most likely not be performed during the acute stage of healing?
    a. PRICE
    b. PROM exercises
    c. Isometric exercises
    d. Eccentric exercises

Short Answer

16. Name the three degrees of a muscle strain and provide characteristics for each type.
17. Describe the changes that occur in the aging tendon, and explain how these factors affect the ability of the body to repair itself.
18. Name the four cardinal signs of inflammation.
19. A patient has been referred to an outpatient physical therapy clinic with a diagnosis of right shoulder rotator cuff strain. She strained her shoulder 8 days ago. Her orthopedic physician prescribed her an anti-inflammatory medication, which she started taking 3 days ago. She has also been icing her shoulder two to three times a day for 30 minutes per session. Based on the aforementioned information, identify the patient's current stage of healing and describe typical interventions (and the clinical rationale) performed during this stage of healing.
20. Discuss the reasons why an aging tendon becomes injured or fails to heal.

Fill in the Blank

21. The process of new growth of blood vessels to an injured area is called _______________.
22. The three stages of healing are _____________, _____________, and _____________.
23. The "R" in PRICE stands for _____________________.
24. Current evidence suggests that _____________ ________ should be included in a rehabilitation program for patients with a diagnosis of tendinosis.
25. The _____________ are bundles of the contractile proteins myosin and actin grouped together as a sarcomere.

True/False

26. A tendon injury results in a permanent functional loss.
27. The subfascicle is the basic functional unit of a tendon.
28. During the subacute stage of healing, it is appropriate in all cases to prescribe strengthening exercises that cause pain.
29. The greatest amount of muscle atrophy occurs the third week after an injury.
30. Isotonic exercises during the subacute phase of healing initially should be in the range of 15 to 25 repetitions per set.

Chapter 13

Neurovascular Healing and Thromboembolic Disease

Barbara Smith

CHAPTER OUTLINE

LEARNING OBJECTIVES

1. Identify neural anatomy.
2. Discuss the vascular supply to nerve tissue.
3. Understand the mechanical behavior of nerve tissue.
4. Identify the causes and classification of nerve injury.
5. Discuss intrinsic nerve healing.
6. Describe methods of surgical repair of nerve injury.
7. Identify structure and composition of vascular tissue.
8. Discuss the vascular response to injury.
9. Explain the various signs and symptoms of vascular injury.
10. Discuss the pathophysiology of thromboembolic disease.
11. Recognize risk factors of deep vein thrombosis and pulmonary emboli.

KEY TERMS

Anoxia
Axonotmesis
Compression neuropathy
Creep
Deep vein thrombosis (DVT)
Double crush syndrome
Dyspnea
Endoneurium
Epineurium
"Hard" signs
Intermittent pneumatic compression
Intimal hyperplasia
Ischemia
Low-molecular-weight heparin (LMWH)
Neurapraxia
Neurorrhaphy
Neurotmesis
Perineurium
Pleuritic pain
Pulmonary embolism (PE)
"Soft" signs
Tachypnea
Thromboembolic disease
Traction neuropathy
Tunica adventitia
Tunica intima
Tunica media
Virchow's triad
Warfarin (Coumadin)

PERIPHERAL NERVE INJURY

In general, peripheral nerves sustain mechanical, thermal, chemical, and ischemic injuries. As an organ system, the peripheral nervous system (PNS) is highly vascularized. A mechanical insult to nerve (e.g., compression, stretch, or severance) stimulates an intense inflammatory reaction.

VASCULAR SUPPLY

Peripheral nerve has a complex and extensive blood supply. The PNS requires an ongoing nutritive energy supply for maintenance of nerve conduction. Longitudinal extrinsic vessels connect with regional feeding vessels forming a vascular plexus within the **epineurium, perineurium,** and **endoneurium** connective tissue network within the nerve fiber (Figs. 13-1 and 13-2).[2,10]

> **Important Concepts**
>
> The blood supply to peripheral nerves is a complex arrangement of superficial longitudinal and segmental longitudinal arterial systems.

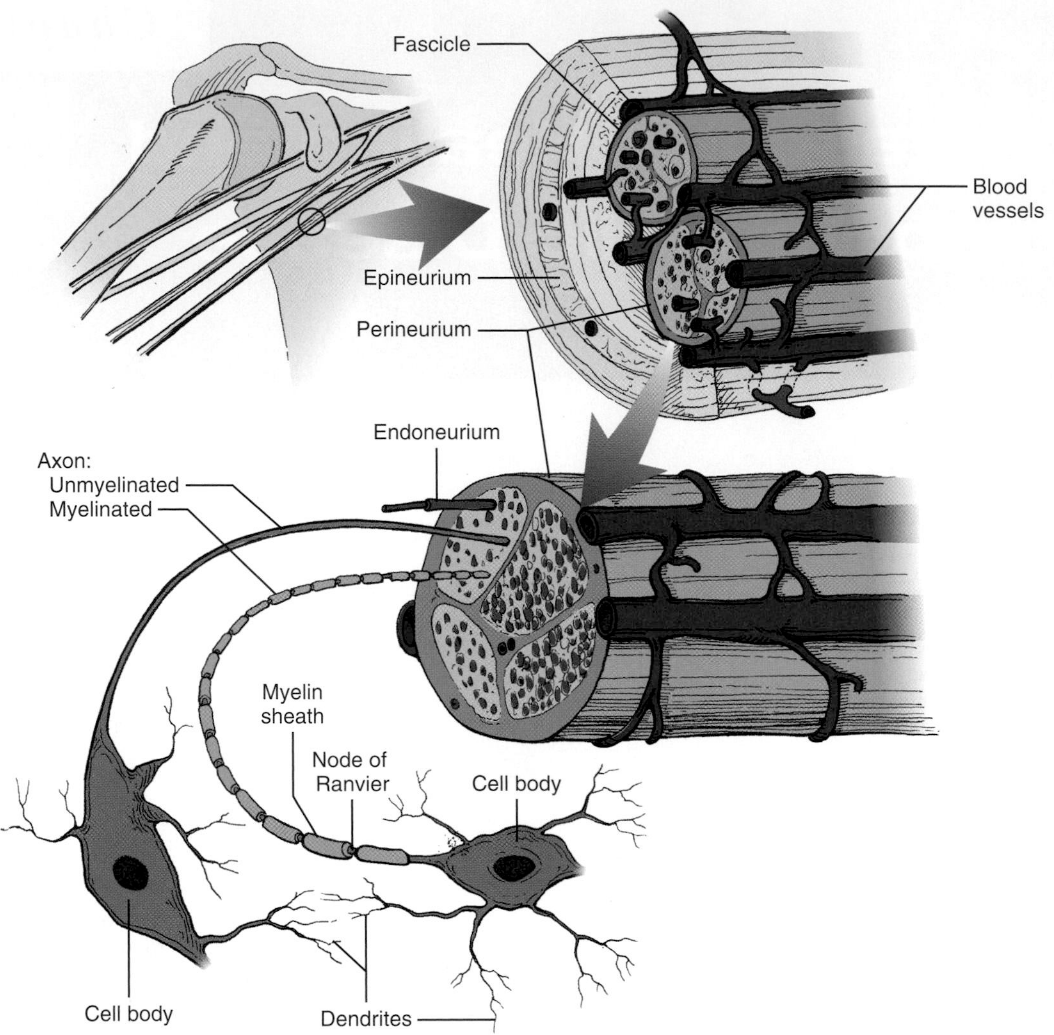

FIG 13-1 Nerve architecture. *(From Brinker MR, Miller MD:* Fundamentals of orthopaedics, *Philadelphia, 1999, Saunders.)*

The initial response to nerve trauma is a predictable response similar to that seen after vascular tissue trauma. After a brief period of vasoconstriction, vascular permeability increases because of the release of potent chemical mediators such as serotonin and histamine.[10] The result is edema within the connective tissue barriers (epineurium, perineurium, endoneurium) of the nerve fiber. The dramatic change in fluid pressure and tissue edema adversely affect oxygen transport, nutrition, ion content of nerve cells, and conductivity of the traumatized nerve fiber.[10]

Important Concepts

Connective tissue components of peripheral nerve are epineurium, perineurium, and endoneurium.

MECHANICAL BEHAVIOR OF NERVE

Nerve tissue is highly deformable, expressing viscoelastic mechanical behavior similar to other soft tissue. Essentially, two load deformation terms are used to quantify a tissue's ability to adapt structurally and mechanically to time-dependent forces. ***Creep*** is a term used to describe the tissue's ability to change or "creep" to a new length in response to a constant, applied load. The greater the load (stress), the faster the tissue deforms or creeps. *Stress relaxation* is similar to creep, in that it is a time-dependent phenomenon. It occurs when a material is elongated (strained) to a given dimension and then maintained at that length. In this situation, there is a reduction in the amount of stress required to maintain the fixed length. Peripheral nerve tissue responds with this viscoelastic behavior by showing ultimate load-to-failure values of 20% to 60%. Although peripheral nerve tissue may tear when the nerve is elongated to approximately 20% more than its resting length, ischemic changes, which profoundly affect nerve function, may occur when a nerve is stretched less than or equal to 15% of its resting length.[1,17]

CAUSES AND CLASSIFICATION OF NERVE INJURY

Trauma to peripheral nerve is due to mechanical, thermal, chemical, and vascular injury. Mechanical sources cause contusion, concussion, stretch, compression, laceration, and transection.[8,11] Classification of nerve injury provides

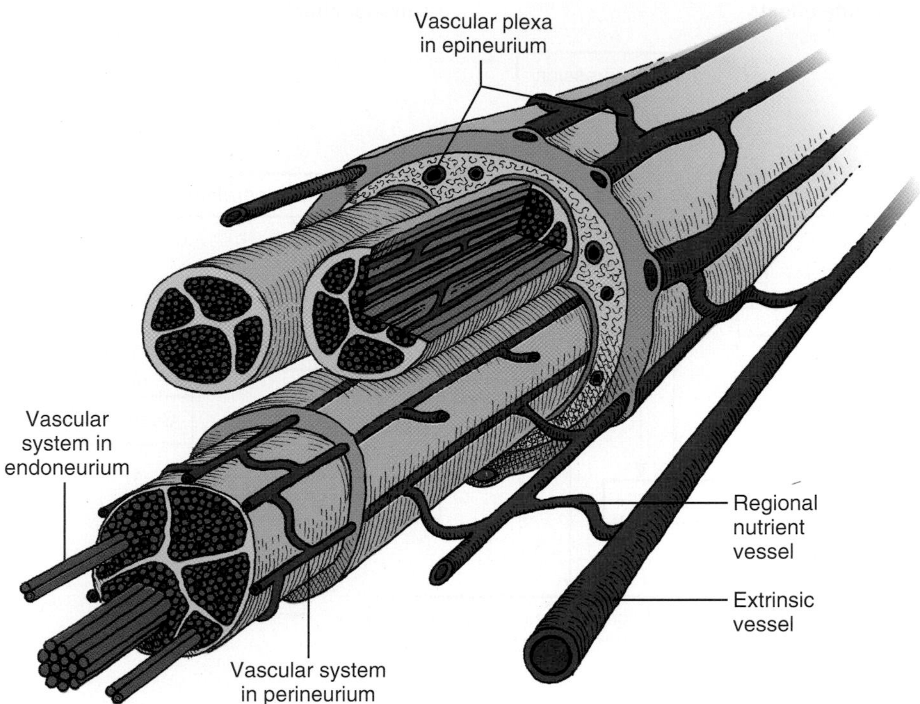

FIG 13-2 Blood supply of a peripheral nerve. *(Adapted from Lundborg G:* Nerve injury and repair, *New York, 1988, Churchill Livingstone.)*

concise and anatomic descriptions. However, the clinical reliability of this system is debatable. Many injuries cannot be classified into a single grade. The three most common categories of nerve injury are **neurapraxia, axonotmesis,** and **neurotmesis.**[8]

Neurapraxia is the reduction in nerve conduction at the site of injury, usually secondary to compression. The lesion is local, the continuity of the axon is maintained, and all pathologic changes associated with neurapraxia generally are reversible if the cause is removed. Functional recovery occurs within weeks or months.[8,11]

In axonotmesis, the epineurium remains intact, whereas damage to the perineurium and endoneurium occurs to varying degrees. Because the epineurium is undamaged, functional recovery without surgery may occur. However, as greater amounts of perineurium and endoneurium are involved, surgery is required to achieve the most functional recovery.[11]

Neurotmesis is diagnosed when the entire nerve trunk is transected or ruptured. The total loss of nerve continuity requires surgical adaptation and coaptation. The prognosis depends on the nature of the injury and local and general factors, such as patient age and timing of the repair.[8,10]

In a very broad sense, a pure motor nerve is a greater risk for injury than a pure sensory nerve. A gross prediction is that peripheral nerves usually fail to conduct impulses related to motion (first), proprioception, touch, temperature, and pain (last). Recovery of these abilities occurs in the reverse order.[11]

COMPRESSION AND TRACTION NEUROPATHY

Nerve compression injuries are acute or chronic in origin. In both cases, the physiologic consequence of compression or traction on peripheral nerve tissue is mechanical disruption of the nerve fiber and **ischemia.**[11] Anatomically, certain peripheral nerves have a greater risk of compression because of the surrounding arrangement of soft tissue and bone, which limits the nerve's three-dimensional motion. Specifically at risk in the lower extremity are the common peroneal nerve behind the fibular head and the lateral femoral cutaneous nerve within the inguinal ligament (meralgia paresthetica).[1] In the upper extremity, nerves most susceptible to mechanical disruption are the radial nerve within the spiral groove of the humerus and the median nerve within the soft tissue confines of the carpal tunnel arch. Spinal nerve roots are more susceptible to compression injury than peripheral nerves because spinal nerve roots have no epineurium.[3,12]

The biologic responses of the PNS to acute and chronic compression include obstruction of intraneural blood vessels, tissue **anoxia,** local ischemia, nerve fiber deformation, increased vascular permeability, intraneural edema, and fibroblastic proliferation with resultant decreased nerve gliding.[3,12]

Traction neuropathy, or stretch neuropathy, is classified as acute or chronic with the magnitude of injury classified as neurapraxia, axonotmesis, and neurotmesis as described. A practical and common description of acute

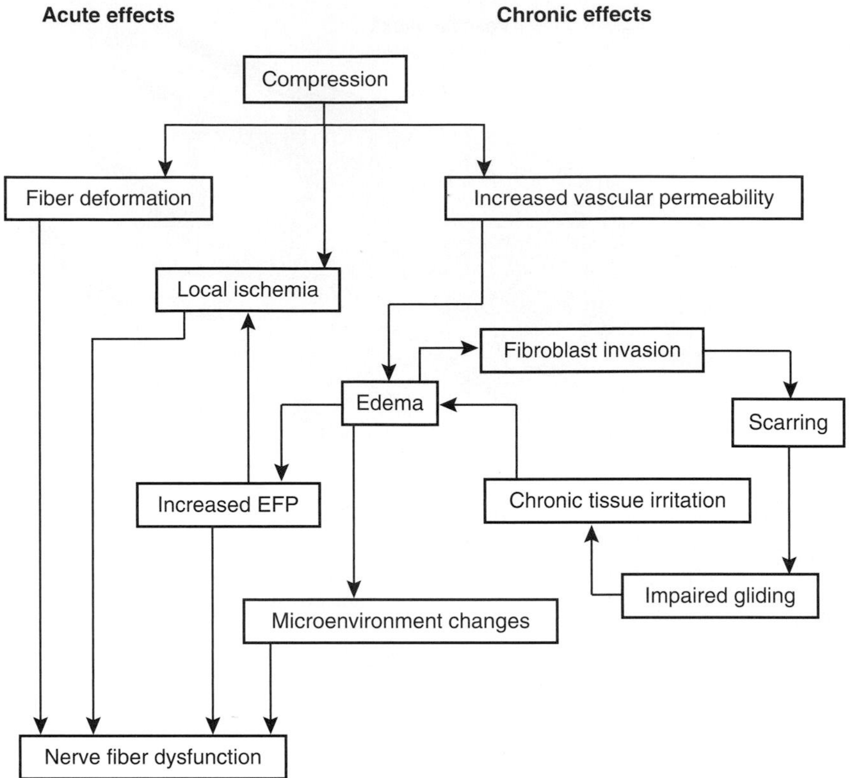

FIG 13-3 Effects of compression on intraneural tissue. *EFP*, effective filtration pressure. *(From Lundborg G:* Nerve injury and repair, *ed 2, New York, 2004, Churchill Livingstone.)*

traction neurapraxia is the "burner" or "stinger" experienced by athletes, in which the plexus is compressed between the shoulder pad and the superior medial scapula when the pad is compressed into Erb's point.[14]

Occasionally with lengthy surgical procedures, prolonged wide surgical field exposure leads to inadvertent stretch of surrounding peripheral nerve tissue. Surgical procedures may also require prolonged tourniquet application, with cuff pressures occluding neural blood supply.[10,11]

Physical therapy (e.g., range of motion [ROM] exercise) after prolonged joint immobilization may cause traction neurapraxia secondary to premature and intensive stretch. During the protection phase of postoperative care or during prolonged immobilization, slow, controlled stretch, devoid of high velocity or force, protects nerve from unwanted injury.[11,17]

Some patients may experience signs and symptoms of peripheral nerve compression or entrapment at more than one level of the same nerve. The term ***double crush syndrome*** is used to describe these signs and symptoms. The most common examples are carpal tunnel median nerve **compression neuropathy** and cervical nerve root injury. Another example is nerve entrapment neuropathy at the elbow along with a cervicothoracic root lesion. To explain this syndrome, it is hypothesized that a compression lesion at one level of the nerve makes the same nerve more susceptible to injury at another site.[1,3] It is suggested that compression reduces nerve conduction, blood supply, and the amount of plasma membrane proteins. These reductions adversely influence other segments, making them more sensitive to mechanical or compressive forces.[3,10]

METHODS OF PERIPHERAL NERVE REPAIR

The term ***neurorrhaphy*** is synonymous with direct coaptation or surgical apposition of corresponding nerve stumps or fascicles.[8,10,11] This specific intervention is reserved for neurotmesis with complete disruption of nerve continuity. The basic objectives for surgical repair (neurorrhaphy) are to maximize the number of axons that regenerate across the lesion and to reinnervate distal sites accurately (e.g., proximal motor axons reach distal motor axons) (Figs. 13-3 and 13-4).[1,8,10,11]

Important Concepts

The term for direct surgical repair is *neurorrhaphy*. For this primary repair, skeletal stability is essential. Too much tension or too little tension on the repair decreases functional recovery. Moderate tension improves outcomes.

Skeletal stability and a well-vascularized tissue bed are essential for effective, direct coaptation. The procedure requires that appropriate tension be applied at the injury site.[8,10,11] Animal studies show that repairs subject to minimal tension produce better results than tension-free repairs.[10,11] Overall, four steps are prerequisites for direct coaptation: (1) clean preparation of traumatized nerve stumps; (2) manual approximation of tissue stumps with correct tension; (3) direct connection between nerve fascicles at both nerve endings or interposing nerve graft; and

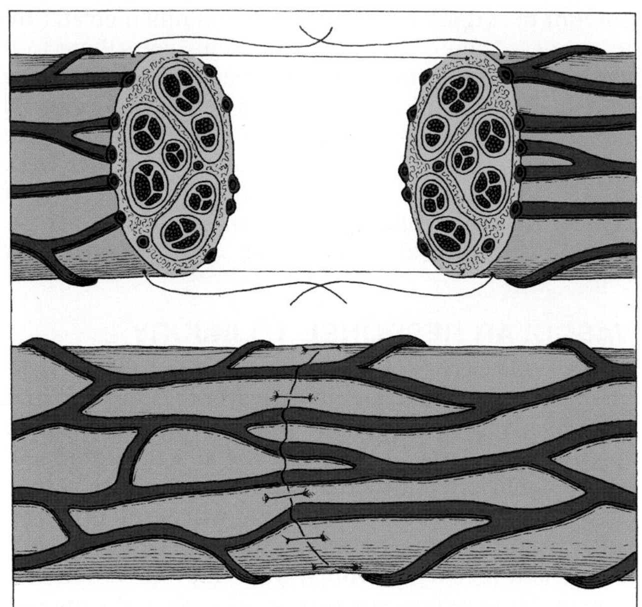

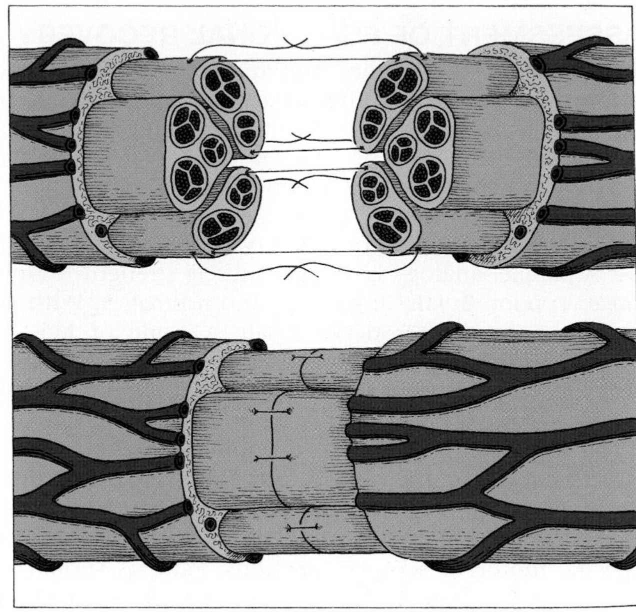

FIG 13-4 **A,** Epineurial neurorrhaphy. **B,** Group fascicular neurorrhaphy. *(From Lundborg G:* Nerve injury and repair, *ed 2, New York, 2004, Churchill Livingstone.)*

(4) maintenance of coaptation with sutures, fibrin glue, or interstitial clot.[8,10,11]

When primary repair cannot be achieved without undue tension on nerve endings, autografts may be used for indirect coaptation. The most common autograft source for peripheral nerve repair is the sural nerve.[8,11] Other sources are the anterior branch of the medial antebrachial cutaneous nerve, the lateral femoral cutaneous nerve, and the superficial radial nerve. The use of autografts must be carefully considered because their use sacrifices healthy nerves and puts the donor site at risk for morbidity and local disturbances of sensory function.[8]

Without repair, denervated tissues undergo many changes. Denervated bone becomes osteoporotic, joint capsule and periarticular soft tissues become fibrotic, and muscle atrophies leading to decreased muscle volume. During the first month after unrepaired nerve injury, muscle loses up to 30% of its weight, and approximately 60% is lost by the end of the second month of denervation.[11]

Good to excellent results can be expected in approximately 50% of surgically repaired peripheral nerves. A few generalizations can be made concerning reconstruction. Better results occur in younger patients and patients with prompt repairs, more distal repairs, and shorter grafts.[8,11]

RECOVERY AFTER PERIPHERAL NERVE INJURY

Repair site protection is the most important factor after peripheral nerve coaptation or autograft. Overzealous ROM exercise during early recovery can easily disrupt fragile healing of fascicle sutures and axonal regeneration. Typically, postoperative splinting is used to maintain appropriate tension and mechanical properties of the repaired nerve.[17] Compressive dressings help to decrease venous congestion and edema. Cautious use of ROM exercises encourages venous return, muscle activation, and lymphatic flow and reduces the potential for muscle and connective tissue adhesions.[11,17] Vascular supply to the healing and repaired nerve tissue must be continuously enhanced to influence axonal regeneration. Superficial heat application may encourage peripheral vascular blood flow to the healing tissues. Electrical stimulation may be beneficial to initiate muscle contraction, increase blood flow, and stimulate removal of cellular debris.[12] Neuromuscular and sensory reeducation exercises are initiated early and progressed continuously during all phases of peripheral nerve recovery after injury with or without surgical repair. Continuous stimulation of distal target sites of reinnervation is essential to redirect axonal regeneration and to facilitate reeducation. Various sensory stimulation tactics are used to decrease hypersensitivity. Reintroduction of light touch, pressure, vibration, thermal stimuli, and texture and stimulation of the mechanoreceptor system (proprioception and kinesthesia) are critical components of functional recovery of nerve injury or repair.[11]

Not only do changes occur at the site of injury and distal to it, but also central changes occur. The somatosensory cortex, even in adults, is rapidly altered after injury. The correct amount of sensory input from the affected area is necessary to reexpand cortical representation from the injured extremity. Animal studies show that the injured part may need repeated and substantial practice of functional movements to induce expansion of the contralateral cortical area that controls movement of the affected extremity.[12]

Important Concepts

Rehabilitation after peripheral nerve injury includes splinting for protection of healing tissue, warmth to propagate blood flow, ROM to prevent adhesion, and motor and sensory stimulation to facilitate reeducation.

ASSESSMENT OF FUNCTIONAL RECOVERY

To document the quality and quantity of motor and sensory nerve recovery after injury or surgical repair, an objective grading system is used to determine the level of functional recovery. The Mechanical Research Council Grading System is used for continued assessment of motor and sensory recovery.[11,12] Motor recovery is graded M0 through M5, and sensory recovery is graded S0 through S4. A parallel analogy is manual muscle strength testing: trace, 1; poor, 2; fair, 3; good, 4; and normal, 5. With an excellent result after nerve repair, a grade of M5, S4 describes full motor reinnervation and complete sensory recovery. A good result is described as M3, S3; a fair result is M2, S2; and a poor result is M0 to M1, S0 to S1.

By establishing objective documentation relating to functional motor and sensory nerve recovery after injury or surgical repair, appropriate physical therapy interventions can be explored to stimulate, regulate, or enhance specific motor or sensory functions. Patients should be encouraged to identify daily stresses that fall under a continuum of low to extreme stress on the injured or repaired extremity. Through activity modification, education, and physical therapy intervention, the patient may be able to achieve a better balance of stresses and improve functional recovery or prevent further injury or reinjury.[17]

VASCULAR INJURY

The peripheral vascular system frequently is damaged by trauma, surgery, or disease. The importance of bone and soft tissue vascularization after injury is well documented and firmly established. Without a continuous supply of oxygen, red blood cells, and proliferative cells, bone and soft tissues become anoxic and necrotic and eventually cease to function. The complex relationship between the causes of vascular tissue injury and the vascular response to injury is important for the patient's functional recovery.

STRUCTURE AND COMPOSITION

Grossly, vessels consist of three basic components: endothelial cells, smooth muscles, and connective tissue. Arteries and veins consist of three identifiable concentric layers (lamina) that form lumen or "walls." The innermost layer is the **tunica intima** (interna), consisting of connective tissue, endothelial cells, and a basement membrane. The middle layer is the **tunica media,** composed of smooth muscle cells and connective tissue. The outermost layer is the **tunica adventitia** (externa), made up of fibrous connective tissue that blends with loose surrounding connective tissue. Between the tunica media and externa is an external elastic membrane (elastica externa). The internal elastic lamina (elastica interna) lies between the internal and intermediate tunicae. The outermost walls of large vessels contain their own microvascular system. Nerves of the sympathetic nervous system innervate the arterial tunicae.[16]

Although veins contain the same three layers of tunicae, the relative percentage of smooth muscle and elastic components is less than that of arteries. In addition, the amount of connective tissue in veins is much greater than in arteries. These anatomic distinctions contribute to the vasomechanical differences between the highly elastic muscular arteries and the relatively less elastic veins. The biochemical composition within the vascular system varies greatly depending on regional requirements. Generally, the peripheral vascular system is composed of extracellular matrix, collagens, elastin, proteoglycans, and squamous epithelial (endothelial) and smooth muscle cells.[16]

VASCULAR RESPONSE TO INJURY

As with other types of soft tissue, injuries to vessels incite an organized, predictable inflammatory response with distinct overlapping sequential events: coagulation, inflammation, fibroplasia, and remodeling and maturation. The most significant histochemical event in the vascular response is **intimal hyperplasia,** where smooth muscle cells proliferate after arterial injury. Depending on the nature and severity of injury, the cell proliferation of the damaged lumen may thicken vessel walls, reducing blood flow.[5]

MECHANISMS OF INJURY

Vascular injury from traction, avulsion, compression, or penetration can occur during orthopedic surgery (Table 13-1). Total knee arthroplasty (TKA) poses a risk to the popliteal artery as well. Total hip arthroplasty may put the common or external iliac artery at risk for injury. Identifiable arterial injury can occur because of shoulder dislocation and humeral neck fractures, resulting in axillary artery injury. Supracondylar humeral fractures and elbow dislocation can lead to brachial artery injury. Posterior knee dislocation and supracondylar femoral fracture can result in popliteal artery injury (Table 13-2).[7]

SIGNS AND SYMPTOMS OF VASCULAR INJURY

General signs and symptoms of peripheral artery injury are classified as either "hard" or "soft." **"Hard" signs** and symptoms include the traditional indications of pulselessness, pallor, paresthesias, pain, and paralysis. Overt signs of bleeding and a rapidly spreading hematoma are additional signs that warrant immediate surgical repair.[7]

"Soft" signs include a possible history of arterial bleeding, hematoma over a peripheral artery, and a neurologic deficit originating in a nerve adjacent to the injured artery. After specific fractures, dislocation, and selected surgical procedures (e.g., glenohumeral or posterior knee dislocation, TKA), continuous reassessment of peripheral pulses (radial or dorsalis pedis) is essential to identify potential vascular injury. Also routinely assessed are skin color, temperature, presence of edema, and digital capillary refill.[5]

DIAGNOSTIC STUDIES

Doppler flow detection and duplex ultrasonography are used for noninvasive diagnosis of arterial occlusion. Duplex ultrasonography is a combination of ultrasound imaging and pulsed Doppler flow detection. With Doppler flow, a comparison is made with the noninvolved

TABLE 13-1 Arterial Injuries Associated with Orthopedic Operative Procedures

	Orthopedic Procedure	Artery Injured
Upper extremity	Clavicular compression plate/screw	Subclavian artery
	Anterior approach to the shoulder	Axillary artery
	Closed reduction humeral fracture	Brachial artery
Lower extremity	Total hip arthroplasty	Common or external iliac artery
	Nail or nail-plate fixation of intertrochanteric or subtrochanteric hip fracture	Profunda femoris artery
	Subtrochanteric osteotomy	Profunda femoris artery
	TKA	Popliteal artery
	Anterior or posterior cruciate reconstruction	Popliteal artery
	External fixator pin	Superficial femoral, profunda femoris, popliteal, or tibial arteries
Spine	Anterior spinal fusion	Abdominal aorta
	Lumbar spine fixation device	Abdominal aorta
	Resection of nucleus pulposus	Right common iliac artery and vein, inferior vena cava

TKA, total knee arthroplasty.
From Browner BD, Levine AM, Jupiter JB, et al: *Skeletal trauma,* ed 4, Philadelphia, 2009, Saunders.

TABLE 13-2 Arterial Injuries Associated with Fractures and Dislocations

	Fracture or Dislocation	Artery Injured
Upper extremity	Fracture of clavicle or first rib	Subclavian artery
	Anterior dislocation of shoulder	Axillary artery
	Fracture of neck of humerus	Axillary artery
	Fracture of shaft or supracondylar area of humerus	Brachial artery
	Dislocation of elbow	Brachial artery
Lower extremity	Fracture of shaft of femur	Superficial femoral artery
	Fracture of supracondylar area of femur	Popliteal artery
	Posterior dislocation of the knee	Popliteal artery
	Fracture of proximal tibia or fibula	Popliteal artery, tibioperoneal trunk, tibial artery, or peroneal artery
	Fracture of distal tibia or fibula	Tibial or peroneal artery

From Browner BD, Levine AM, Jupiter JB, et al: *Skeletal trauma,* ed 4. Philadelphia, 2009, Saunders.

extremity. In this way, an arterial pressure index (API) is calculated by dividing the Doppler systolic pressure of the involved extremity by that of the noninvolved extremity. Arterial injury can be predicted with 97% accuracy when the API is less than 0.90.[4,7] Percutaneous arteriography is the gold standard and most commonly used invasive technique for diagnosis of suspected arterial injury. This technique requires injection of dye proximal (antegrade) or distal (retrograde) to the suspected injury, then multiple sequential plain film radiographs are taken of the area.[7]

METHODS OF VASCULAR REPAIR

An analogy of repair techniques can be drawn from peripheral nerve repair. Generally, direct vascular repair, including arteriorrhaphy/venorrhaphy or anastomosis, involves direct suturing of the traumatized vessel. Interpositional grafting uses an autograph or synthetic graft material (polytetrafluoroethylene or polyethylene terephthalate [Dacron]).[5,7]

THROMBOEMBOLIC DISEASE

Thromboembolic disease, caused by a **deep vein thrombosis (DVT)** that may progress to **pulmonary embolism (PE)**, is one of the most common causes of mortality and morbidity in hospitalized patients. Total hip arthroplasty and TKA place patients at increased risk of developing thromboembolic disease.[6]

RISK FACTORS

Several intrinsic and extrinsic conditions are identified as additive risk factors in the potential development of thromboembolic disease. Surgery, trauma, obesity, pregnancy, age older than 40 years, use of oral contraceptives, and immobility are well-known causative factors. In addition, history of DVT and varicose veins, smoking, family history, and congestive heart failure contribute as risk factors. The type of surgery has little effect on the incidence of DVT. Rather, other factors (e.g., heart disease, length of immobilization) determine the incidence.[6,15]

Important Concepts

Risk factors for DVT include age greater than 40 years, prior history of DVT, malignancy, trauma, immobility, lower extremity surgical procedures, cardiovascular disease, varicosity, and obesity.

PATHOPHYSIOLOGY OF THROMBOEMBOLISM

Most thrombi start in the valve cusps of the deep lower leg veins. Critical components of the coagulation cascade are prothrombin, thrombin, fibronectin, and fibrin. The result of this cascade is stimulation of platelet adherence to vessel walls. Eventually, this buildup of blood cells creates a thrombus. A dislodged clot from the thrombus is referred to as an embolus. PE is a life-threatening consequence; the lower lobes of the lungs are involved four times more often than the upper lobes.[15]

VIRCHOW'S TRIAD

Three factors generally lead to development of DVT. Categorically referred to as **Virchow's triad,** these factors are hypercoagulability; venous stasis (e.g., caused by immobilization, obesity, heart disease); and venous injury, especially with endothelial damage (e.g., caused by surgery, trauma, previous DVTs). Damage exposes the vessel walls to collagen, basement membrane, and von Willebrand's factor increasing platelet activity and number. The initial trauma shifts the balance more toward coagulation than fibrinolysis and ultimately DVT formation.[15]

Important Concepts

Virchow's triad includes hypercoagulability, venous stasis, and vessel wall damage.

Vessel wall injury and stasis are directly related to orthopedic surgical procedures, such as total joint arthroplasty (TJA) and repair of pelvic and femoral fractures. Once a DVT has formed, without treatment, one of three processes occurs. The thrombus undergoes partial or complete lysis with complete or near-complete recanalization of the thrombosed blood vessel. The thrombus becomes more organized, resulting in further proximal vessel occlusion. The thrombus dislodges, completely or partially escaping to a proximal site in the vascular system as an embolus.[15]

SIGNS AND SYMPTOMS OF DEEP VEIN THROMBOSIS

Very high levels of suspicion must accompany all complaints of proximal thigh, inguinal, and lower leg pain after TJA, pelvic or femoral fractures, spinal surgery, and general trauma. Most signs and symptoms are nonspecific, such as diffuse complaints of leg pain and tenderness, edema, palpable warmth, skin discoloration, and dilated superficial veins. The most important signs and symptoms of DVT are tenderness and swelling. Calf asymmetry of more than 3 cm (when measured 10 cm below the tibial tuberosity) is also abnormal and, if new, indicates the presence of DVT until proved otherwise.[13] Both extremities require assessment because studies show that thrombosis is generally present bilaterally even when injury is limited to one lower extremity.[15]

DIAGNOSTIC STUDIES

Duplex ultrasonography is a common noninvasive diagnostic technique for suspected DVT. This test combines venous system Doppler flow detection and ultrasound imaging with manual compression of the suspected vein. Veins that do not easily compress with normal pressure on the transducer are considered positive for DVT. Generally, thrombi in the inguinal area, deep proximal thigh, and popliteal area are considered more dangerous than deep calf vein thrombi because distal clots are smaller and less frequently associated with major complications.[15]

Important Concepts

Signs and symptoms of DVT include peripheral edema, warmth, skin discoloration, prominent superficial veins, leg pain, and tenderness.

PULMONARY EMBOLI

Pulmonary emboli are a result and complication of DVT. A dislocated deep vein thrombus may travel to the pulmonary artery or obstruct pulmonary blood supply. The result is hypoxia from constriction of the bronchioles, mediated by vasoactive substances such as serotonin, histamine, and prostaglandins. The effect is pulmonary infarction, shock, right heart failure, and occasionally death.[9,15]

Signs and Symptoms

Generally, **tachypnea** (>18 breaths per minute) is the most common sign of PE. **Dyspnea** is the most frequent symptom. The patient may also complain of **pleuritic pain,** develop a cough or hemoptysis, or report feeling apprehensive. These signs and symptoms are usually related to the size of the embolus and the patient's cardiopulmonary status.[9,15]

Important Concepts

Clinical probability estimate of suspected pulmonary emboli is defined as a high probability that PE exists with dyspnea, tachypnea, or pleuritic pain in a patient with recent lower extremity injury or surgery.

TREATMENT OF THROMBOEMBOLIC DISEASE

Selective use of prophylactic anticoagulants decreases the incidence of DVT in patients undergoing elective surgery without altering the operative plan. Patients undergoing TJA are treated with heparin or **low-molecular-weight heparin (LMWH)**. The judicious use of LMWH has proven to be safe and effective in DVT prevention and treatment. The patient's response to LMWH is more predictable than the response to heparin, and the rate of bleeding complications is less than with heparin.[6,15]

If prophylactic anticoagulants are not administered preoperatively, administration of anticoagulation medication begins 12 to 24 hours postoperatively. **Warfarin (Coumadin)**, an oral anticoagulant, is used simultaneously with heparin or during the transition from intravenous or subcutaneous anticoagulation. Warfarin is indicated for prophylaxis and treatment of DVT or PE. The duration of therapy may be 3 to 6 months postoperatively, depending on the patient's risk factors and possibility of recurrence.[6,15]

Nonpharmacologic treatment of DVT includes early mobilization and judicious exercise after surgery and use of antiembolism stockings or **intermittent pneumatic compression.** Contraindications for use of antiembolism stockings are arterial compromise or peripheral neuropathy. Use of pneumatic compression devices is not advised in the presence of local ulceration, cellulitis, and arterial insufficiency. Bent knee and semisitting positions increase the incidence of postoperative thromboembolic complications. Patients should be as mobile as possible as early as possible after surgery.[9]

GLOSSARY

Anoxia: The absence or deficiency of oxygen reaching the tissues.

Axonotmesis: Loss of continuity of axons, with varying degrees of injury to the perineurium and endoneurium.

Compression neuropathy: Signs and symptoms resulting from pressure on the nerve because of the surrounding arrangement of soft tissue and bone.

Creep: Ability of tissue to change or "creep" to a new length in response to a constant, applied load.

Deep vein thrombosis (DVT): Local coagulation or clotting in vein lying deep below the skin.

Double crush syndrome: A term used to describe signs and symptoms of peripheral nerve compression or entrapment at more than one level of the same nerve.

Dyspnea: Shortness of breath; the most frequent symptom of pulmonary embolism.

Endoneurium: The dense connective tissue sheath that surrounds a nerve trunk.

Epineurium: The loose delicate connective tissue between individual nerve fibers.

"Hard" signs: Symptoms of peripheral artery injury that include the traditional indications of pulselessness, pallor, paresthesias, pain, and paralysis.

Intermittent pneumatic compression: A medical form of therapy in which air is pumped into an inflatable sleeve surrounding a limb in an effort to improve venous circulation and decrease edema.

Intimal hyperplasia: The most significant histochemical event in the vascular response, where smooth muscle cells proliferate after arterial injury.

Ischemia: Inadequate blood supply to an organ or part of the body.

Low-molecular-weight heparin (LMWH): A class of anticoagulant medications.

Neurapraxia: Axon maintains continuity, no distal degeneration, usually secondary to compression.

Neurorrhaphy: Surgical apposition of corresponding nerve stumps or fascicles.

Neurotmesis: Complete physiologic disruption of a nerve.

Perineurium: The connective tissue sheath that surrounds bundles of nerve fibers.

Pleuritic pain: A type of chest pain that is sharp or stabbing in nature; usually made worse when one breathes in or coughs.

Pulmonary embolism (PE): Blockage of an artery in the lung by fat, air, blood clot, or tumor cells.

"Soft" signs: Symptoms of peripheral artery injury that include a possible history of arterial bleeding, hematoma over a peripheral artery, and a neurologic deficit originating in a nerve adjacent to the injured artery.

Tachypnea: Condition of breathing less than 18 breaths per minute; the most common sign of pulmonary embolism.

Thromboembolic disease: A condition caused by formation in a blood vessel of thrombus that breaks loose and is carried by the bloodstream to plug another vessel.

Traction neuropathy: Signs and symptoms owing to stretch on a nerve from various causes.

Tunica adventitia: The outermost layer of the lumen, composed of fibrous connective tissue that blends with loose surrounding connective tissue.

Tunica intima: The innermost layer of the lumen, consisting of connective tissue, endothelial cells, and a basement membrane.

Tunica media: The middle layer of the lumen, composed of smooth muscle cells and connective tissue.

Virchow's triad: The three factors that lead to deep venous thrombosis development.

Warfarin (Coumadin): An oral anticoagulant that is used simultaneously with heparin or during the transition from intravenous or subcutaneous anticoagulation.

REFERENCES

1. Bodine SC, Lieber RL: Peripheral nerve physiology, anatomy, and pathology. In Buckwalter JA, Einhorn TA, Simon SR, editors: *Orthopaedic basic science, biology, and biomechanics of the musculoskeletal system*, ed 2, Rosemont, IL, 2000, American Academy of Orthopaedic Surgeons.
2. Brinker MR, O'Connor DP: basic Sciences. In Miller MD, Thompson SR, Hart JA, editors: *Review of orthopaedics*, ed 6, Philadelphia, 2012, Saunders.
3. Brunton LM, Chhabra AB: Hand, upper extremity and microvascular surgery. In Miller MD, Thompson SR, Hart JA, editors: *Review of orthopaedics*, ed 6, Philadelphia, 2012, Saunders.
4. Cole P, Levy B, Watson JT, et al: Tibial plateau fracture. In Browner BD, Levine AM, Jupiter JB, et al, editors: *Skeletal trauma: basic science, management, and reconstruction*, ed 4, Philadelphia, 2009, Saunders.
5. Davies MG: Intimal hyperplasia. In Cronenwett JL, Johnston KW, editors: *Rutherford's vascular surgery*, ed 7, Philadelphia, 2010, Saunders.
6. Falck-Ytter Y, Francis CW, Johanson NA, et al: Prevention of VTE in orthopedic surgery patients. *Chest* 141:278S–325S, 2012.
7. Feliciano DV: Evaluation and treatment of vascular injuries. In Browner BD, Levine AM, Jupiter JB, et al, editors: *Skeletal trauma: basic science, management, and reconstruction*, ed 4, Philadelphia, 2009, Saunders.
8. Hébert-Blouin M-N, Spinner RJ: Cameron JL, Cameron AM, editors: *Current surgical therapy*, ed 10, St Louis, 2011, Mosby.
9. Ikeda B, Goodman CG: The respiratory system. In Goodman CG, Fuller KS, editors: *Pathology: implications for the physical therapist*, ed 3, Philadelphia, 2009, Saunders.
10. Jabaley ME: Primary nerve repair. In Slutsky DJ, Hentz VR, editors: *Peripheral nerve surgery*, Philadelphia, 2006, Churchill Livingstone.
11. Lee SK, Wolfe SW: Peripheral nerve injury and repair. *J Am Acad Orthop Surg* 8(4):243–252, 2000.
12. Lundborg G: *Nerve injury and repair: regeneration, reconstruction, and cortical remodeling*, ed 2, Philadelphia, 2004, Churchill Livingstone.
13. Mangione S: The extremities and peripheral vascular system. In Mangione S, editor: *Physical diagnosis secrets*, ed 2, St Louis, 2008, Mosby.

14. Milweski MD, Hart JA, Miller MD: Sports medicine. In Miller MD, Thompson SR, Hart JA, editors: *Review of orthopaedics*, ed 6, Philadelphia, 2012, Saunders.
15. Roberts CS, Gleis GE, Seligson D: Diagnosis and treatment of complications. In Browner BD, Levine AM, Jupiter JB, et al, editors: *Skeletal trauma: basic science, management, and reconstruction*, ed 4, Philadelphia, 2009, Saunders.
16. Sumpio B, Huang C: Arterial wall biology. In Cronenwett JL, Johnston KW, editors: *Rutherford's vascular surgery*, ed 7, Philadelphia, 2010, Saunders.
17. Topp KS, Boyd BS: Structure and biomechanics of peripheral nerves: nerve responses to physical stresses and implications for physical therapist practice. *Phys Ther* 86:92–109, 2006.

REVIEW QUESTIONS

Multiple Choice

1. Connective tissue barriers of peripheral nerve tissue include which of the following? (Circle all that apply.)
   a. Endoneurium
   b. Myosin
   c. Perineurium
   d. Epineurium
2. As an organ system, how can the peripheral nervous system be described?
   a. Moderately vascularized
   b. Minimally vascularized
   c. Highly vascularized
   d. Avascular
3. What is the common load-to-failure value for peripheral nerve tissue?
   a. 10% to 30%
   b. 20% to 60%
   c. 25% to 45%
   d. 70% to 90%
4. What is the term for a local peripheral nerve lesion, with anatomic continuity of the axon maintained and all pathologic changes generally reversible?
   a. Axonotmesis
   b. Neurapraxia
   c. Neurotmesis
   d. Neuralgia
5. What is the biologic response of the peripheral nervous system to acute or chronic compression or traction? (Circle all that apply.)
   a. Epineurial deformation
   b. Anoxia
   c. Decreased vascular permeability
   d. Intraneural edema
6. "Burner" or "stinger" is a term used to describe which classification of nerve pathology?
   a. Axonotmesis
   b. Neurapraxia
   c. Neurotmesis
   d. Neuropathy
7. What is the innermost lamina of blood vessels?
   a. Tunica media
   b. Tunica adventitia
   c. Tunica intima
   d. Elastica interna
8. What are the gross anatomic components of blood vessels? (Circle all that apply.)
   a. Skeletal muscle
   b. Endothelial cells
   c. Macrophages
   d. Connective tissue
9. What is intimal hyperplasia?
   a. Decreased perfusion
   b. Connective tissue proliferation
   c. Smooth muscle cell proliferation
   d. Reduced epithelial cells
10. What vascular injury may result from supracondylar humerus fracture or elbow dislocation?
    a. Ulnar artery
    b. Axillary artery
    c. Brachial artery
    d. Subclavian artery
11. Which of the following are "hard" signs of vascular injury? (Circle all that apply.)
    a. Pain
    b. Pallor
    c. Pulselessness
    d. All of the above
12. What are risk factors for developing thromboembolic disease?
    a. Total hip replacement
    b. TKA
    c. Immobility
    d. All of the above
13. What are parts of Virchow's triad? (Circle all that apply.)
    a. Venous stasis
    b. Hypertension
    c. Endothelial cell wall injury
    d. Hypercoagulability
14. What are signs of DVT? (Circle all that apply.)
    a. Dilated superficial veins
    b. Cool skin
    c. Edema
    d. Skin discoloration
15. Which nerve injury occurs when the entire nerve is transected?
    a. Neuropraxia
    b. Axonotmesis
    c. Neurotmesis
    d. None of the above

Short Answer

16. What are other terms for acute traction neurapraxia?
17. Name the syndrome that describes a compressive nerve lesion at the proximal location that may involve the distal segment of the same nerve.
18. Name the three layers of blood vessels from deep to superficial.
19. Total hip or knee arthroplasty poses a risk to which arteries?
20. Describe "hard" signs of vascular injury.

Fill in the Blank

21. __________ is a term used to describe the tissue's ability to change to a new length in response to a constant, applied load.
22. Ischemic changes may occur when a nerve is stretched less than or equal to _________% of its resting length.

23. A pure motor nerve is at greater risk for injury than a pure _________ nerve.
24. _________ describes the signs and symptoms of peripheral nerve compression or entrapment at more than one level of the same nerve.
25. Arterial injury can be predicted with 97% accuracy when the API is less than _________.

True/False

26. Axonotmesis results in disruption of the epineurium, perineurium, and endoneurium.
27. Meralgia paresthetica is compression of L4-L5 nerve roots.
28. Neurotmesis results in total loss of nerve trunk continuity.
29. Proximal nerve compression reduces conductivity, blood supply, and the number of plasma membrane proteins that decrease the quality of the distal nerve segments, making the nerve less sensitive to mechanical or compressive deforming forces.
30. Animal studies demonstrate that tension-free surgical repairs are essential for complete healing.

Part III

Basis for Movement

In this section, the physical therapist assistant (PTA) is introduced to rudimentary concepts and compulsory scientific principles related to biomechanics and kinesiology, gait, and peripheral joint mobilization techniques. The study of biomechanics supports the application of principles of kinesiology when providing therapeutic interventions. The utility of biomechanics in all clinical settings is demonstrated in the daily provision of gait analysis, manual muscle testing, goniometric assessments, therapeutic exercise modifications, facilitated balance and coordination activities, posture assessment, application and adjustment of prosthetic devices, recognition of abnormal movement patterns, and use of rehabilitation strategies to correct aberrant mechanics.

A basic, yet essential, component of orthopedic physical therapy management is the instruction and application of proper gait techniques after injury or disease of the musculoskeletal system. To instruct patients safely and properly in the use of assistive devices and apply fundamental gait techniques effectively, the PTA must understand the components of the gait cycle, both normal and pathologic, and be able to instruct patients in appropriate gait patterns and identify deviations. This section clarifies and describes the gait cycle and introduces basic terms, definitions, and concepts. In addition, the PTA is introduced to proper gait pattern instruction, weight-bearing status, and the identification of gait abnormalities.

The delegation of selected mobilization techniques is entirely at the discretion of the physical therapist, and the application of peripheral joint mobilization is not universally accepted as a routine domain of clinical practice for the PTA. The information concerning peripheral joint mobilization is provided as a means of making the PTA aware of the rationale for improving arthrokinematic motion and for the reduction of pain as identified and prescribed by the physical therapist.

The presentation of introductory mechanics in this section precedes orthopedic pathologies and therapeutic interventions by pulling together essential basics of anatomy, physiology, tissue healing, kinesiology, and principles of therapeutic exercise, providing the student PTA and practicing clinician a sound practical and scientifically based understanding of the essentials of human movement on which sound treatment approaches can be developed by the chapters that follow in the sections on management of orthopedic patients.

Chapter **14**

Fundamentals of Normal and Abnormal Gait

Thomas W. Kernozek, John D. Willson

CHAPTER OUTLINE

LEARNING OBJECTIVES

1. Define and describe basic components of the gait cycle.
2. Discuss the two phases of gait.
3. Identify and describe each component of the two phases of gait.
4. Define and describe common gait deviations.
5. Identify appropriate gait patterns.
6. Outline and describe terms used to define weight-bearing status during gait.
7. Identify and discuss the appropriate use of assistive devices.

KEY TERMS

Antalgic gait
Stance phase
Step
Stride
Swing phase
Trendelenburg gait
Trendelenburg sign
Vaulting

Rehabilitation professionals should understand the terminology and the requirements of what is described as normal locomotion or gait. Gait is often evaluated in a clinical setting as an important activity of daily living skill that links musculoskeletal or neurologic impairment with a functional movement performance. Gait is a repetitive and cyclic movement pattern. The joints that make up the lower extremities and pelvis work together as a series of linked segments or kinetic chain. As with any linked system, the motion at one segment can greatly influence the motion of another. For example, a lack of knee extensor strength may lead to performance change during gait such as an avoidance of knee flexion that could be perceptible to the observer. Rehabilitation professionals who are aware of what constitutes a normal gait pattern can recognize this gait deviation and plan effective interventions.

GAIT CYCLE TERMINOLOGY AND PHASES OF GAIT

The definition of the gait cycle is based on a reference extremity (e.g., the right foot) from a defined event such as heel contact until the next occurrence of that event (contact with the heel of that same foot). The gait cycle is often based on 100% and can be broken down further into the **stance phase** and the **swing phase** (Fig. 14-1). The stance phase is defined as the portion of the gait cycle when the foot is in contact with the ground, and the swing phase is the portion of the gait cycle when the foot is off the ground. A **step** is defined as contact on one foot until contact with the other (right to left or left to right). A **stride** is defined as contact with one foot until contact with the same foot (right to right or left to left). The stance phase of the gait cycle is typically about 60% of the gait

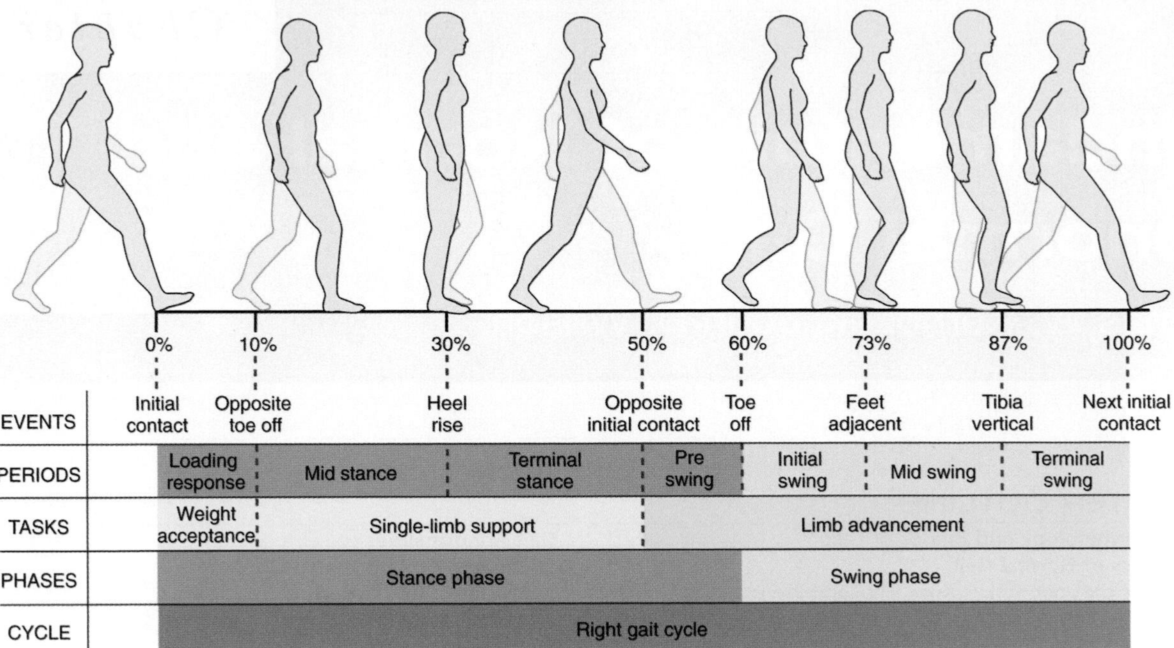

FIG 14-1 Terminology to describe the events of the gait cycle. Initial contact corresponds to the beginning of stance when the foot first contacts the ground at 0% of gait cycle. Opposite toe off occurs when the contralateral foot leaves the ground at 10% of gait cycle. Heel rise corresponds to the heel lifting from the ground and occurs at approximately 30% of gait cycle. Opposite initial contact corresponds to the foot contact of the opposite limb, typically at 50% of gait cycle. Toe off occurs when the foot leaves the ground at 60% of gait cycle. Feet adjacent takes place when the foot of the swing leg is next to the foot of the stance leg at 73% of gait cycle. Tibia vertical corresponds to the tibia of the swing leg being oriented in the vertical direction at 87% of gait cycle. The final event is initial contact again, which is the start of the next gait cycle. These eight events divide the gait cycle into seven periods. Loading response, between initial contact and opposite toe off, corresponds to the time when the weight is accepted by the lower extremity, initiating contact with the ground. Midstance is from opposite toe off to heel rise (10% to 30% of gait cycle). Terminal stance begins when the heel rises and ends when the contralateral lower extremity touches the ground, from 30% to 50% of gait cycle. Preswing takes place from foot contact of the contralateral limb to toe off of the ipsilateral foot, which is the time corresponding to the second double-limb support period of the gait cycle (50% to 60% of gait cycle). Initial swing is from toe off to feet adjacent, when the foot of the swing leg is next to the foot of the stance leg (60% to 73% of gait cycle). Midswing is from feet adjacent to when the tibia of the swing leg is vertical (73% to 87% of gait cycle). Terminal swing is from a vertical position of the tibia to immediately before heel contact (87% to 100% of the gait cycle). The first 10% of the gait cycle corresponds to a task of weight acceptance—when body mass is transferred from one lower extremity to the other. Single-limb support, from 10% to 50% of the gait cycle, serves to support the weight of the body as the opposite limb swings forward. The last 10% of stance phase and the entire swing phase serve to advance the limb forward to a new location. *(From Neumann DA:* Kinesiology of the musculoskeletal system: foundations for physical rehabilitation, *ed 2, St Louis, 2010, Mosby.)*

cycle, whereas the swing phase is about 40% (see Fig. 14-1). The reason why the stance and swing phases are not 50% is due to the relatively short period of double support (10%) within the gait cycle. This small portion of support phase is the period where the weight is transferred from one limb to the other.

The stance phase has been described as having two basic functions: weight acceptance and single-limb support. The swing phase has one primary function: limb advancement.[16] Figure 14-1 depicts the phases within the stance and swing phases of the gait cycle. Contact with the floor is often made with the heel (often called *heel contact* or *initial contact*). Perry[16] described the first 15% of the gait cycle portion as when the foot functions as a heel rocker or first rocker. This phase is also described as the *loading response*. During this part of the gait cycle, impact forces tend to be large at 1 to 1.5 times body weight, depending on the speed of locomotion. With the use of a force platform, researchers have quantified the magnitude of these impact forces during walking by measuring ground reaction forces. Figure 14-2 depicts the ground reaction forces in walking at 1.5 m/sec. When the foot becomes flat on the ground, the tibia advances forward over the stance foot. Perry[16] described this as the ankle rocker or second rocker. This phase of the gait cycle is also called *midstance phase*. The *terminal stance phase* begins when the heel is raised off the ground (about 40% of the stance phase) until the opposite foot makes ground contact. The final phase of stance phase of the gait cycle is the *preswing phase,* which begins with heel strike of the contralateral limb and ends with toe off. When the heel is lifted from the floor (heel off), this can also be described as the toe rocker or third rocker.

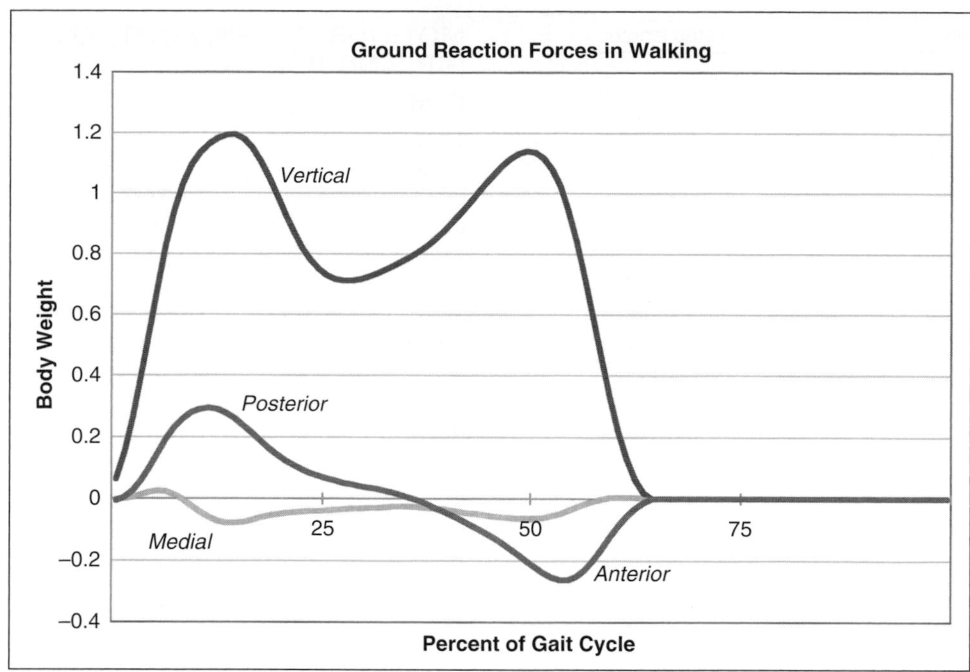

FIG 14-2 The ground reaction forces of a single foot contact are depicted during typical walking over the gait cycle. The vertical ground reaction force is associated with the loading into the floor, which is transmitted back to the person. These vertical loads are typically highest (one times body weight) and vary in magnitude with walking speed. The first impact peak is associated with the loading response, and the second is associated with terminal stance. The lowering of the vertical ground reaction force during midstance is largely due to the reaction forces being attenuated by dorsiflexing the ankle and flexing the knee during stance. Medial-lateral forces in typical walking are the smallest. The medially directed ground reaction force accelerates a person's center of mass toward the contralateral leg for the subsequent foot strike. The positive portion of the anterior-posterior ground reaction force describes the amount of braking where the person's center of mass is behind the extended foot during the loading response. During midstance, these forces get smaller and then change direction as the person pushes into the ground to propel himself or herself forward. This negative portion of the anterior-posterior curve is associated with propulsion when the person's center of mass is in front of the stance foot. From examining these curves, one can determine that the stance phase is approximately 60% of the gait cycle and that the extremity is not in contact with the ground during the remainder of the cycle making these forces zero. These data were processed with The MotionMonitor software (Innovative Sports Training, Chicago, IL) on 25 healthy, college-age participants walking at a self-selected gait speed at the University of Wisconsin La Crosse Strzelczyk Clinical Biomechanics Laboratory. Data were collected from an eight-camera three-dimensional motion analysis system, electromyography measurements, and integrated force platforms.

The swing phase of the gait cycle has three portions: preswing, midswing, and terminal swing phases. The preswing phase begins with double-limb support and ends with toe off. This phase primarily comprises the foot moving off the ground and is critical for limb advancement. This phase takes place as the gait cycle is 60% and 75% complete. Midswing phase is 75% to 85% of the gait cycle, when the swing limb advances in front of the stance limb. The terminal swing phase completes the remainder of the swing phase until a second heel contact with the same extremity.

CHARACTERISTICS OF NORMAL GAIT

Many factors can influence gait, such as age, pain, strength, range of motion (ROM), walking speed, and fitness level. The extent of the influence of such factors can be quantified by taking simple measurements to characterize and assess a person's walking performance with the use of a tape measure, goniometer, and stopwatch. The measures are stride or step length, step width (walking base), foot progression angle, walking speed, and cadence. Typical stride length reported from the literature is 1.33 to 1.63 m in healthy individuals.[4,5,7,9-12,15,18] Men generally have a greater step length than women. Step width, or the horizontal distance between feet while walking, is 0.61 to 9.0 cm.[11,12,17,20] Foot progression angle or angle of toe out has been reported to be 5.1° to 6.8°. Various definitions for foot placement are shown in Figure 14-3. The average typical walking speed is 1.49 m/sec for men and 1.40 m/sec for women, between 3 and 4 miles per hour for both genders.[2-4,14,18,21] Average walking speed can be measured over a specific distance with a stopwatch. Speed can be calculated by taking the distance over the elapsed time taken to walk the prescribed distance. Walking speed is based on cadence (number of steps per minute) and step length. Average cadence is 107 to 125 steps per minute.[2-4,14,18,21] To increase walking speed, one can increase

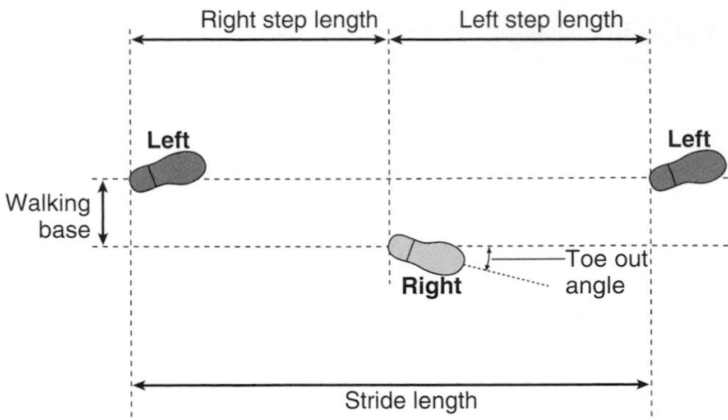

FIG 14-3 Terms used to describe foot placement on the ground. *(From Whittle MW:* Gait analysis: an introduction, *ed 4, St Louis, 2008, Butterworth-Heinemann.)*

cadence or step length. Self-selected walking speed is typically slower in women than in men. With the slower gait speed, there appears to be a shorter step length and faster cadence for women than men. All measurements of gait are largely dependent on walking speed.

As walking speed increases, stance time generally decreases compared with swing time. Most of the reduction in stance time comes from a reduction in double support time (owing to the reduction in stance time on both limbs). Overall, these simple measures of gait can give the clinician a clinical impression of the overall quality of the gait pattern. These measures are often called the *temporal spatial measures of gait.*

Normal gait is not symmetric.[18] Small asymmetries in gait are often considered typical. With slower walking speeds, greater amounts of asymmetry have been observed in healthy individuals with normal gait. One must be able to identify if these subtleties in normal gait have clinical relevance.

Important Concepts

Asymmetry exists in normal gait. It is up to the clinician to evaluate the clinical relevance of asymmetries with respect to a patient's goals.

Movement patterns of the joints can provide additional insight to an individual's gait. Researchers in motion analysis laboratories have provided detailed three-dimensional data on the range of joint motion during walking. Sagittal plane motion patterns are the largest motions and represent the most studied parameters; frontal plane and transverse plane motion patterns are smaller motions that have been less studied. Estimations of these motions can be visually observed by the health care professional at a distance from the side for sagittal motions or from the front or behind for frontal plane motions as the patient is walking. Pure transverse plane rotation is difficult to observe in a clinical setting because an aerial perspective is required. One likely has to combine side and front views to estimate transverse plane motion.

MOTIONS OF THE FOOT, ANKLE, KNEE, HIP, AND PELVIS

Foot

There are several joints within the foot with some motion occurring at each of the joints during gait. However, most of the required motion at the foot is from the first metatarsophalangeal joint. At the instant of heel off during the terminal stance phase of gait, the first metatarsophalangeal joint typically hyperextends 45° to 55° as the ankle actively plantar flexes. The first metatarsophalangeal joint returns to nearly 0° during the remainder of the gait cycle. A limitation in this passive hyperextension may cause compensations in other joints in the chain.[19]

Rearfoot motion is movement based on the motion of the posterior aspect of the heel relative to the posterior aspect of the lower leg in the frontal plane. This motion has been used as an estimation of the triplanar motion of pronation that occurs during the stance phase of gait when the foot everts, abducts, and dorsiflexes. When the posterior aspect of the heel is more everted relative to the lower leg, the foot is considered to be in a more pronated position. With foot contact, the rearfoot is slightly inverted and immediately begins to evert or pronate until the midstance phase. At the instant of heel off during the beginning of terminal stance phase, the rearfoot is nearly neutral and then begins to invert until toe off. This inversion of the rearfoot is thought to describe the triplanar motion of supination during terminal stance when the foot inverts, adducts, and plantar flexes.

Ankle

At ground contact, the ankle is primarily in a neutral position (0°, at a right angle to the tibia, neither plantar flexed nor dorsiflexed). Figure 14-4 depicts the typical ankle, knee, and hip motion during the gait cycle. After contact, the ankle plantar flexes about 5° so that the foot becomes flat on the ground.[16] This motion is controlled eccentrically by the ankle dorsiflexor muscles. Next, the tibia rotates over the stance foot resulting in maximum ankle dorsiflexion. This motion is generally controlled eccentrically by the ankle plantar flexor muscles. During the preswing phase of gait, the ankle plantar flexes to propel the person forward. An inadequate amount of plantar flexion may be due to a lack of ankle power, resulting in a reduction in step length during gait. During swing, the ankle must dorsiflex to allow for foot clearance as that leg steps forward for ground contact.

Knee

The knee is close to full extension at ground contact. The knee flexes 10° to 15° as the foot becomes flat on the ground during the initial 15% of the gait cycle. Knee flexion facilitates the absorption of forces during impact as the quadriceps muscles function eccentrically. After foot flat, the knee extends until about 40% of the gait cycle. As the ankle plantar flexes during terminal stance phase, the knee flexes to about 35° at toe off. Knee flexion during this phase reduces the overall length of the limb allowing for adequate foot ground clearance. The knee continues to flex to its maximum at about 60° during

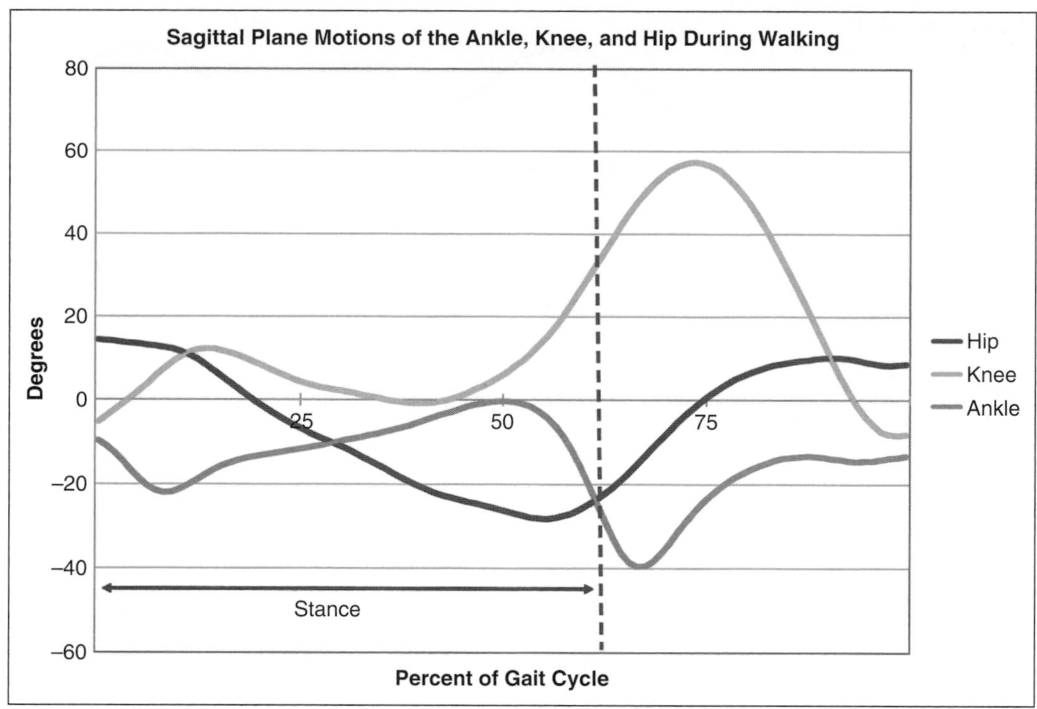

FIG 14-4 The sagittal plane motions of the ankle, knee, and hip are depicted during the gait cycle. The *dashed vertical line* depicts the beginning of the swing phase. Angles near zero depict that the joints are in a more neutral (anatomic) position. The hip begins in flexion and then extends until nearly the end of stance. The knee is flexed during the loading response and extends before flexing to its maximal amount during preswing. The ankle is near neutral at initial contact and plantar flexes as the foot becomes flat on the floor. As the tibia moves forward over the fixed foot, the ankle dorsiflexes and then rapidly plantar flexes as the heel first and then the remainder of the foot leaves the ground. The ankle reaches maximum plantar flexion during preswing and then dorsiflexes again for foot clearance. These data were generated from a motion study of 25 healthy, college-age participants walking at a self-selected gait speed at the University of Wisconsin La Crosse Strzelczyk Clinical Biomechanics Laboratory (see Fig. 14-2).

midswing. Later in midswing and terminal swing, the knee extends to nearly full extension in preparation for ground contact.[16] The knee motion reported during gait in the frontal plane is minimal (within 10° of abduction and adduction during the entire gait cycle) and appears to be quite variable.[1,3,8] A small amount of medial rotation of the knee that occurs during early stance and appears to be linked with foot pronation has been reported.[8] During midstance and throughout the swing phase, the knee appears to rotate laterally back to neutral. Rearfoot pronation is accompanied by tibial medial rotation with knee flexion; this is thought to be important for shock absorption occurring with foot impact with the ground. Tibial lateral rotation occurs later in stance with foot supination and is accompanied by knee extension.

Hip

The hip is flexed to about 20° to 30° at ground contact. This is typically the maximum amount of hip flexion observed during normal gait. After this, the hip extends to a hyperextension angle of about 10° to 25° at about 50% of the gait cycle. Hip flexion is started at preswing and continues until nearly ground contact.[16]

Pelvis

There is a small amount of pelvic motion apparent during the gait cycle in which the pelvis goes through a symmetric pattern of excursion twice. In general, the pelvis tilts anteriorly, and on the swing leg the pelvis rotates forward whenever either hip extends. The pelvis also has a considerable amount of oscillating motion in the frontal and transverse planes (up to 10° of total motion). During the first 10% to 15% of the gait cycle, the pelvis rotates and laterally tilts toward the swing leg contributing to hip adduction on the stance leg. From about 20% to 60% of the gait cycle, the pelvis rotates and tilts away from the swing leg contributing to hip abduction.[16]

JOINT MOTION AND ENERGY EXPENDITURE

Coordinated lower extremity movement patterns are thought to minimize the vertical oscillation of the body center of mass (COM). The body COM is nearly at the height of a person's navel and is in the center of the body anterior to the sacrum. Movement of the COM oscillates up and down and from side to side during normal gait (Fig. 14-5). Vertical oscillation of the COM has been related to energy expenditure. Greater energy expenditure is

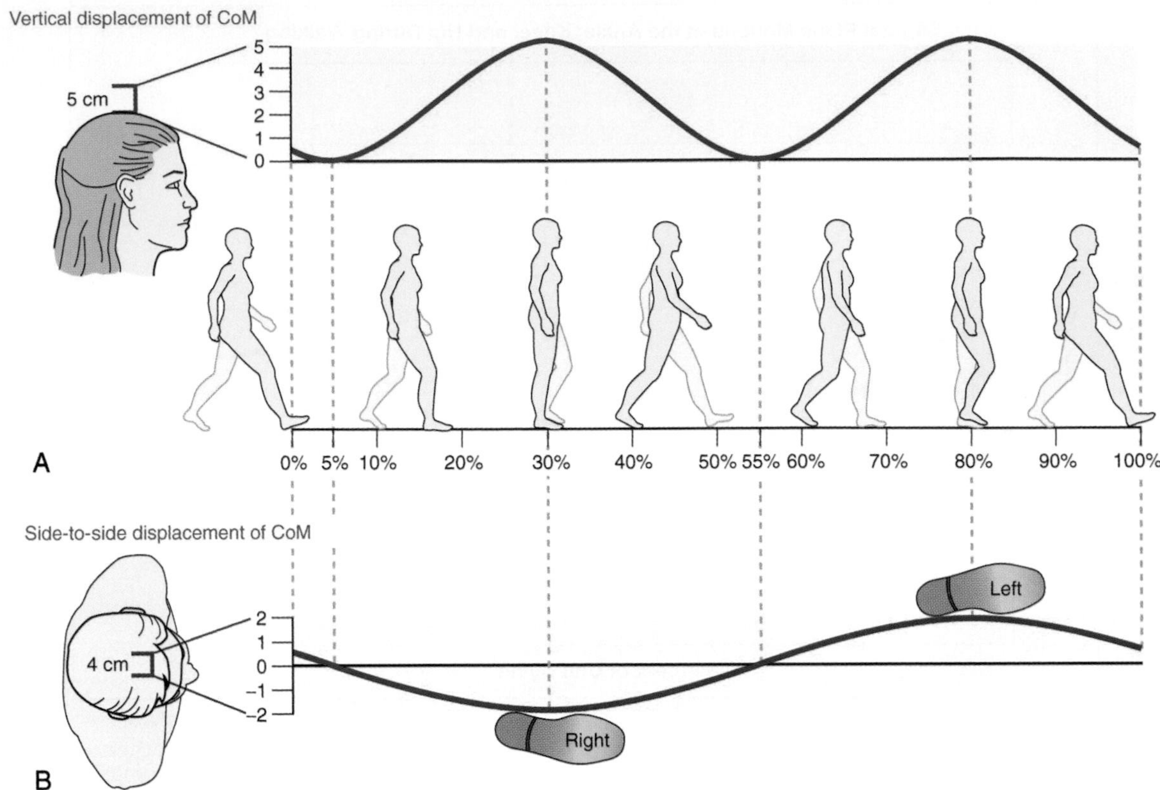

FIG 14-5 Center of mass (COM) displacement during gait. **A** and **B,** The vertical and the medial-lateral displacements of the COM are illustrated. The COM is at its lowest and most central position, in the medial-lateral direction, in the middle of double-limb support (5% and 55% of the gait cycle)—a position of relative stability with both feet on the ground. Conversely, the COM is at its highest and most lateral position at midstance (30% and 80% of the gait cycle)—a position of relative instability. During single-limb support, the trajectory of the COM is never directly over the base of support. This factor is illustrated in **B,** with the vertical projection of the COM always medial to the footprints. *(From Neumann DA:* Kinesiology of the musculoskeletal system: foundations for physical rehabilitation, *ed 2, St Louis, 2010, Mosby.)*

thought to be related to greater oscillation of the body COM. In general, the COM oscillates nearly 5 cm in the vertical direction and horizontally toward the stance limb.[6] The COM is typically highest during midstance and lowest during double support phases of gait. Lower extremity gait deviations may result in excessive COM motion, resulting in greater fatigue because of the higher metabolic cost.

Important Concepts

Large variations in COM position increase the metabolic cost of gait and limit gait efficiency.

MUSCLE ACTIVATION

Timing of muscle activation appears to be critical generally occurring in short bursts during gait (Fig. 14-6). Much of the muscle action within the gait cycle is eccentric. Eccentric forces by the muscles are used to control the rate of joint motion.

Foot and Ankle

The tibialis anterior is active eccentrically at heel contact to control the rate of ankle plantar flexion until the foot is flat on the ground (Fig. 14-7). A second period of activity by the tibialis anterior is during early swing phase when it dorsiflexes the ankle to allow for foot clearance. The extensor digitorum and extensor hallucis longus have a similar role in helping control the rate of plantar flexion during the loading response. They may also be activated during late midswing and terminal swing for propulsion in combination with the ankle plantar flexors. The ankle plantar flexors (gastrocnemius and soleus) are active during most of the stance phase; they are active eccentrically during the first 10% to 40%, when they control the rate for tibial advancement over the foot, to a high burst of concentric activity at preswing (at heel off) until inactivity at toe off.[13] The tibialis posterior is primarily active during 5% to 35% of the gait cycle and is thought to limit excessive foot pronation. Later in stance, the tibialis anterior and posterior function concentrically to help supinate the foot to create a rigid lever for effective push off by the ankle plantar flexors.[19]

Knee

During terminal swing, the quadriceps muscle group begins to become activated in preparation for weight acceptance during stance. At the instant of heel contact,

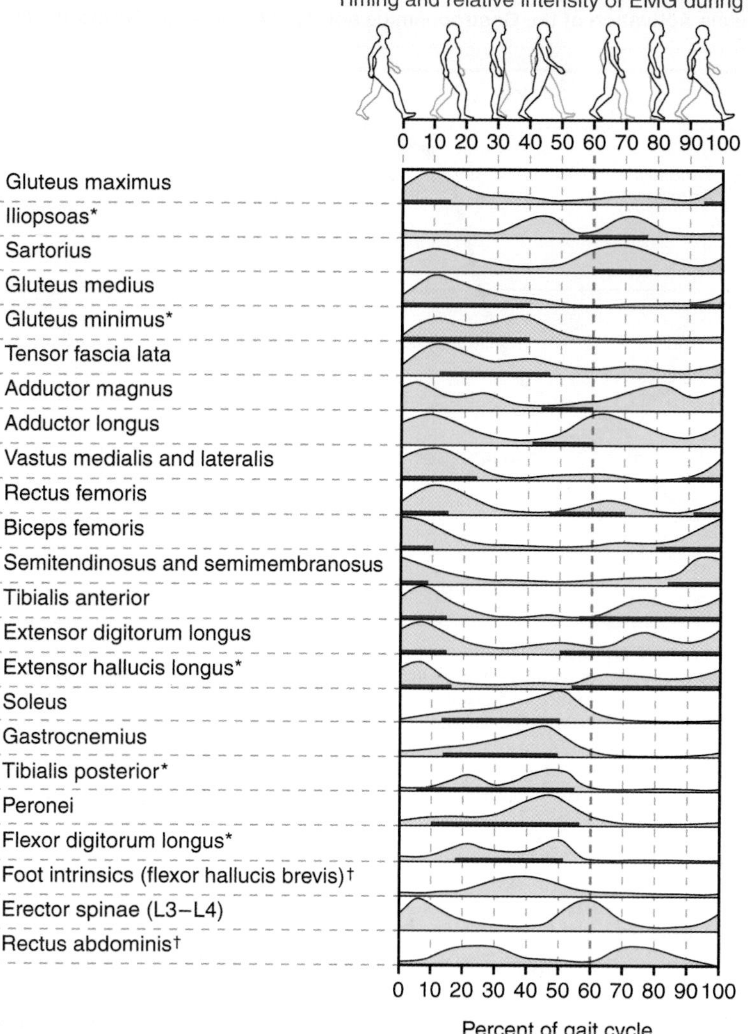

FIG 14-6 Timing *(dark red bars)* and relative intensity of muscle activation *(light red shading)* during gait. *(Muscle timing data from Knutson LM, Soderberg GL: EMG: use and interpretation in gait. In Craik RL, Oatis CA, editors:* Gait analysis: theory and application, *St Louis, 1995, Mosby. Relative intensity of muscle activation data from Winter DA:* The biomechanics and motor control of human gait: normal, elderly and pathological, *ed 2, Waterloo, Canada, 1991, University of Waterloo Press. *Bechtol CO: Normal human gait. In Bowker JH, Hall CB, editors:* Atlas of orthotics: American Academy of Orthopaedic Surgeons, *St Louis, 1975, Mosby. †Carlsöö S:* How man moves: kinesiological methods and studies, *New York, 1972, Crane, Russak & Company. Figure from Neumann DA:* Kinesiology of the musculoskeletal system: foundations for physical rehabilitation, *ed 2, St Louis, 2010, Mosby.)*

the quadriceps is highly active eccentrically to control the rate of knee flexion and absorb impact forces during the loading response phase. Later during midstance while in single-limb support, the quadriceps acts concentrically to extend the knee. During preswing, there may be some quadriceps activity to help flex the hip. The hamstrings are most active near the instant of heel contact and through approximately the first 10% of the stance phase. Before heel contact, the hamstrings slow the rate of knee extension, and early in stance assist with hip extension and enhance knee stability with coactivation with the quadriceps. Minimal activation of the hamstrings is necessary during preswing and swing.[13,16,19]

Hip

The gluteus maximus is active during terminal swing to slow the rate of hip flexion and to prepare for weight acceptance during stance. This muscle becomes most active at the instant of heel contact for hip extension with assistance from the hamstrings and to prevent trunk flexion. The gluteus maximus remains active during the first 30% of the gait cycle.[16] The iliacus and psoas muscles are active eccentrically during toe off to slow down the rate of hip extension and are concentrically active to flex the hip during preswing. These hip flexors are active only during the first 50% of swing and are partially assisted by the quadriceps for limb advancement and foot clearance.

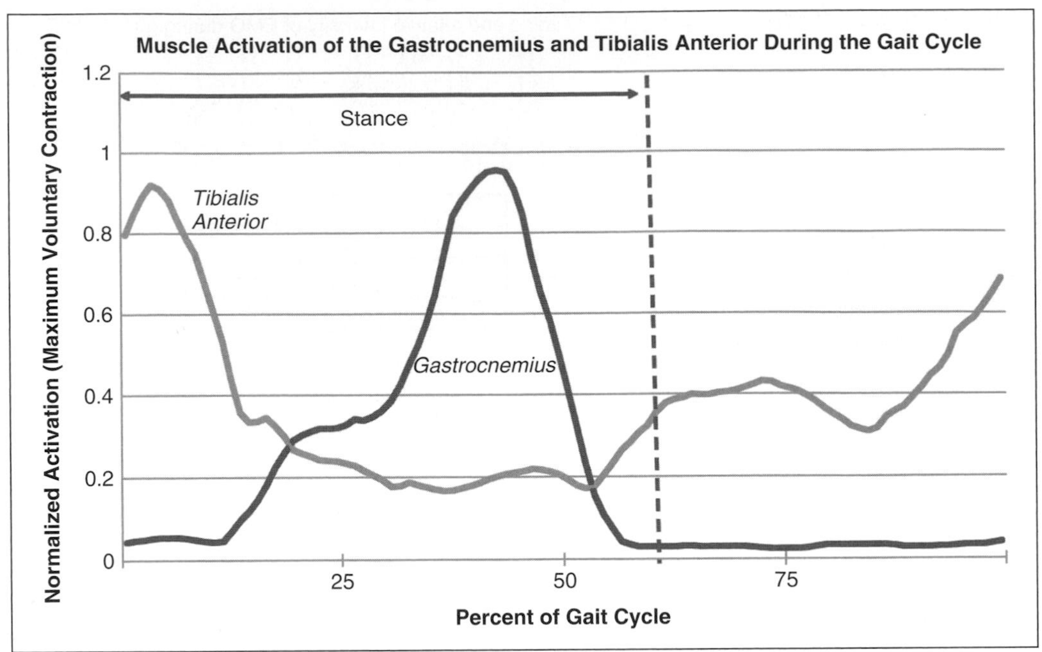

FIG 14-7 Muscle activation patterns of the gastrocnemius and tibialis anterior are depicted during the gait cycle for walking. The activation of the tibialis anterior occurs during the loading response to control the rate of plantar flexion and again late in terminal stance and preswing for foot clearance with the ground. The gastrocnemius is active eccentrically during midstance and again with a higher magnitude concentrically as the foot plantar flexes during preswing. These data were generated from a motion study of 25 healthy, college-age participants walking at a self-selected gait speed at the University of Wisconsin La Crosse Strzelczyk Clinical Biomechanics Laboratory (see Fig. 14-2).

The hip abductors (gluteus medius, gluteus minimis, and tensor fascia lata) help control pelvis motion in the frontal plane during single-leg stance.[19] The gluteus medius is also active in terminal swing in preparation for heel contact. It is assisted by the gluteus minimus during the first 40% of the gait cycle to control pelvis tilt toward the swing limb during stance and may control the alignment of the femur in the frontal plane. The hip adductors and rotators are also active during stance. The role of the hip rotators during gait may be important to enable control of the motion between the pelvis and the femur during stance.[13]

GAIT ABNORMALITIES

The ability to move our bodies from one location to another is an important aspect of functional independence. The normal gait pattern described so far in this chapter is the method many consider to be the most economical method to achieve this end. However, pain during gait and various permanent or temporary neurologic or musculoskeletal impairments affect normal gait. The consequences of nearly every deviation from normal gait include increased energy consumption to move a given distance, decreased gait speed, abnormal joint loading, and, in some cases, decreased safety. For some people, the additional energy required for ambulation may be so great that frequent rests are necessary over relatively short distances. The health care professional must be able to identify and describe gait abnormalities to make appropriate recommendations to the patient or other health care professionals to minimize the impact of the gait abnormality on functional independence.

Important Concepts

Pain or limitation in any linked segment of the lower extremity may elicit gait abnormalities.

Just as normal gait is a complex interaction of musculoskeletal and neuromuscular systems, adaptations or compensations in response to pain or limitations in either system are frequently equally complex. There may be many ways for a person to compensate for or adapt to a given impairment. As a consequence, the same impairment may not result in the same gait abnormality among different people. The way that a person compensates for a musculoskeletal or neuromuscular limitation may change, leading to different gait abnormalities over time for one person with the same limitation.

Important Concepts

The same pain or limitation may result in very different gait abnormalities in different people.

The clinical presentation and potential causes of several common gait abnormalities are briefly discussed in the remainder of this chapter. As previously noted, the joints that make up the lower extremities work together as a series of linked segments or kinetic chain. As with any linked system, motion at one segment can greatly influence the motion of another. Observed gait abnormalities may be due to pain or a limitation in any portion of the kinetic chain.

ANTALGIC GAIT

Antalgic gait is a general term used to describe a gait pattern accompanied by pain. It can assume many forms, but generally there is an observable reduction in motion at the painful joint and asymmetry in temporal-spatial gait parameters, with a reduction in stance time on the involved limb and a rapid swing phase of the uninvolved limb being most common. Patients who experience pain during walking as a consequence of weight bearing frequently find it more comfortable to walk if they reduce the magnitude of the loads delivered to the painful leg during the stance phase of gait. This reduction is typically accomplished by leaning the trunk toward (hip pain) or away (knee or ankle pain) from the side of the painful lower extremity joint during the stance phase.

LATERAL TRUNK BENDING

As described, lateral trunk bending may be observed among patients attempting to minimize joint compression loads and pain during ambulation. Lateral trunk bending may also be observed as a compensation for weakness of the hip abductors. During the stance phase of walking, patients with marked hip abductor weakness may lean toward the stance leg of the weak abductors to minimize the force required of these muscles to prevent downward movement of the pelvis on the side of the swing leg (contralateral pelvis drop). This lateral trunk bending is a compensation for ipsilateral hip abductor weakness and is most commonly referred to as ***Trendelenburg gait***. The clinician may observe lateral trunk bending toward each side during the single-leg stance phase of each leg among people who have bilateral hip abductor weakness, a presentation most commonly referred to as *waddling*. People who walk with a wide step width (walking base) or have unequal leg length may also demonstrate increased lateral trunk bending.

CONTRALATERAL PELVIS DROP

Excessive downward movement of the pelvis for the swing leg may also occur during walking. This movement is most frequently observed as a consequence of a musculoskeletal impairment, such as hip abductor weakness, or a neuromuscular disease affecting gluteus medius recruitment. Specifically, this movement occurs when the hip abductors do not produce enough force to resist the torque created by the weight of the trunk acting medially to the hip joint during the single-leg stance phases of the gait cycle. This gait deviation is known as *increased contralateral pelvic drop* or the ***Trendelenburg sign***.

POSTERIOR TRUNK LEAN

Patients may demonstrate a posterior trunk lean during either the early stance or the early swing phase of the gait cycle. During early stance, a patient may lean posteriorly to move the line of gravity of the trunk behind the hip joint. This tends to reduce the demands placed on the gluteal muscles to resist hip flexion during the loading phase and, as such, is a gait deviation frequently employed by individuals with weak hip extensors. Conversely, individuals may lean posteriorly during early swing in an effort to pull the femur anteriorly and advance the swing leg as a compensation for hip flexor insufficiency or hip extensor spasticity.

ANTERIOR TRUNK LEAN

Anterior trunk lean is most commonly observed during the stance phase of gait. However, timing of the anterior trunk lean may vary according to the impairment causing this gait abnormality. Anterior trunk lean during early stance is often a compensation for quadriceps weakness. Shortly after heel strike, the magnitude and direction of the reaction force from the ground are posterior to the knee joint, which tends to produce knee flexion under the eccentric control of the knee extensors. If the knee extensors cannot generate enough force to resist knee flexion, a person may lean forward to move the ground reaction force anterior to the knee joint (Fig. 14-8). Moving the ground reaction force anterior to the knee joint changes the effect of the ground reaction force to one that tends to cause knee extension rather than knee flexion, diminishing the need for knee extension strength to resist knee flexion. Quadriceps weakness is a common consequence of poliomyelitis. This compensation is a common gait deviation among individuals who have had poliomyelitis.

Anterior trunk lean during midstance or terminal stance is often a compensation for decreased ankle dorsiflexion ROM. To continue to ambulate forward, the ankle typically dorsiflexes before initial contact of the contralateral leg to allow the person's COM to pass anterior to the stance leg base of support. Among individuals with ankle plantar flexor spasticity, plantar flexor contracture, or pes equinus deformity, the ankle may not permit sufficient dorsiflexion at this stage of the gait cycle, and the person may need to lean the trunk forward to move his or her COM anterior to the foot (Fig. 14-9).

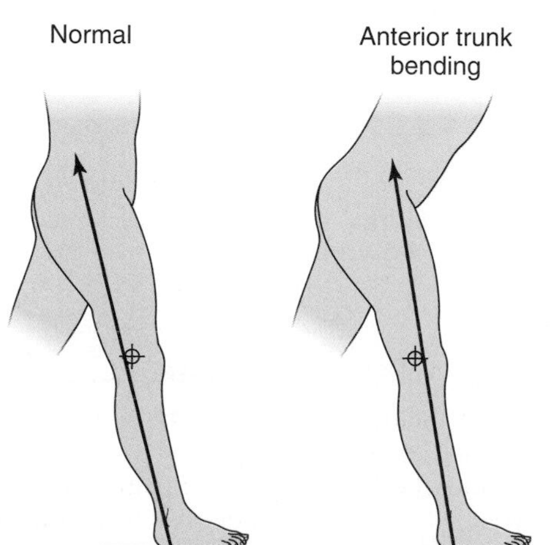

FIG 14-8 Anterior trunk bending. In normal walking, the line of force early in the stance phase passes behind the knee; anterior trunk bending brings the line of force in front of the knee, to compensate for weak knee extensors. *(Modified from Whittle MW:* Gait analysis: an introduction, *ed 4, St Louis, 2008, Butterworth-Heinemann.)*

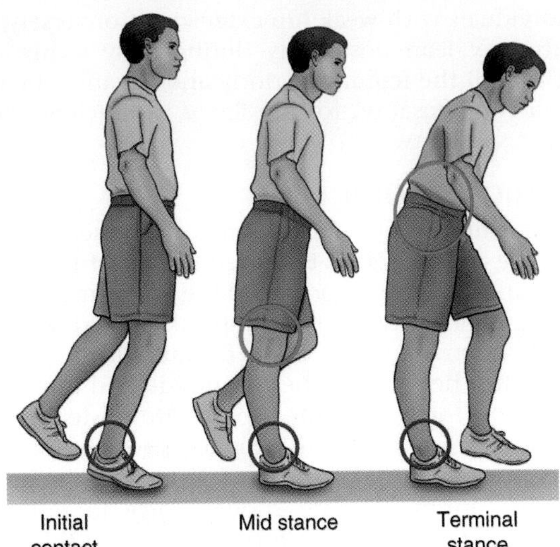

FIG 14-9 Individuals with an ankle plantar flexion contracture make initial contact with the ground with the forefoot region. At midstance, bringing the heel to the ground results in knee hyperextension. Forward lean of the trunk occurs in terminal stance as a strategy to maintain forward progression of the center of mass. *(From Neumann DA:* Kinesiology of the musculoskeletal system: foundations for physical rehabilitation, *ed 2, St Louis, 2010, Mosby.)*

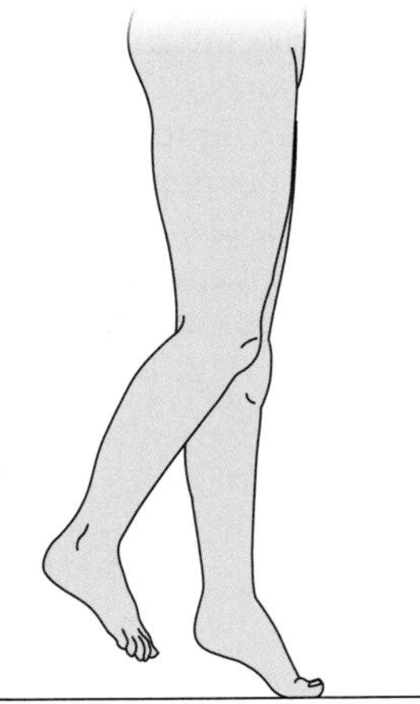

FIG 14-10 Vaulting. The subject goes up on the toes of the stance phase leg to increase ground clearance for the swing phase leg. *(Modified from Whittle MW:* Gait analysis: an introduction, *ed 4, St Louis, 2008, Butterworth-Heinemann.)*

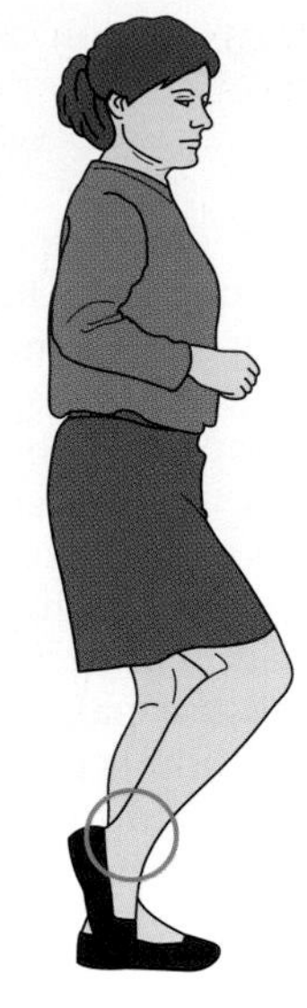

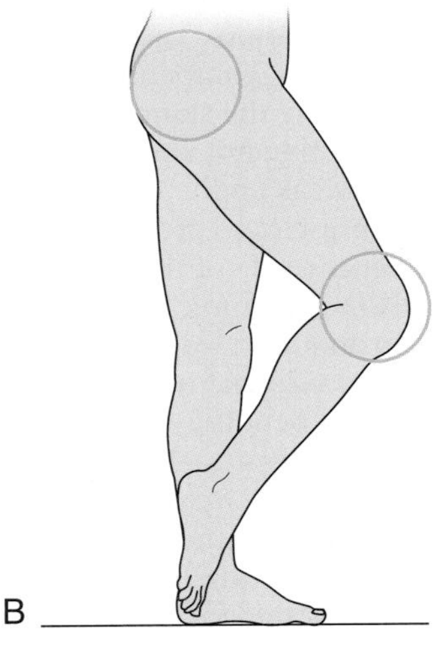

FIG 14-11 **A,** Weak ankle dorsiflexors may result in a foot drop during swing phase, requiring excessive hip and knee flexion for the toes to clear the ground as the limb is advanced forward during swing. **B,** Steppage. Increased hip and knee flexion improve ground clearance for the swing phase leg, in this case, necessitated by a foot drop. *(**A,** Modified from Neumann DA:* Kinesiology of the musculoskeletal system: foundations for physical rehabilitation, *ed 2, St Louis, 2010, Mosby;* ***B,*** *modified from Whittle MW:* Gait analysis: an introduction, *ed 4, St Louis, 2008, Butterworth-Heinemann.)*

EXCESSIVE ANKLE PLANTAR FLEXION

Increased ankle plantar flexion is frequently observed in both the stance and the swing phase of the gait cycle. Increased ankle plantar flexion during and after midstance of the stance leg is commonly referred to as **vaulting** (Fig. 14-10). This is frequently a compensatory mechanism intended to increase ground clearance for the swing leg and is common among individuals with an impairment that prevents shortening of the swing leg during the swing phase, such as an ankle plantar flexion contracture, ankle dorsiflexor weakness, knee or hip extensor spasticity, or hip flexor weakness. Ankle plantar flexion of the stance leg may also be an indication of decreased ankle dorsiflexion ROM, particularly if the person demonstrates heel rise very shortly after contralateral toe off (early in midstance). In either case, the effect is a characteristic bouncing appearance, indicative of large vertical oscillations of the person's COM.

Increased ankle plantar flexion may also be observed in the swing phase of the gait cycle. This gait deviation is frequently the result of injury to the common fibular nerve, weakness of the ankle dorsiflexors, or spasticity or contracture of the ankle plantar flexors (Fig. 14-11, *A*).

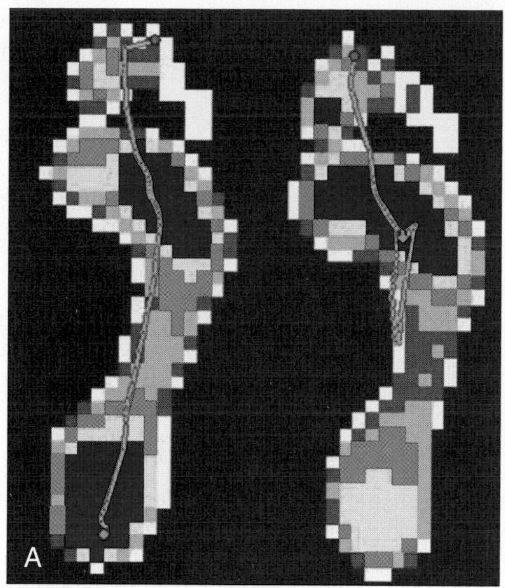

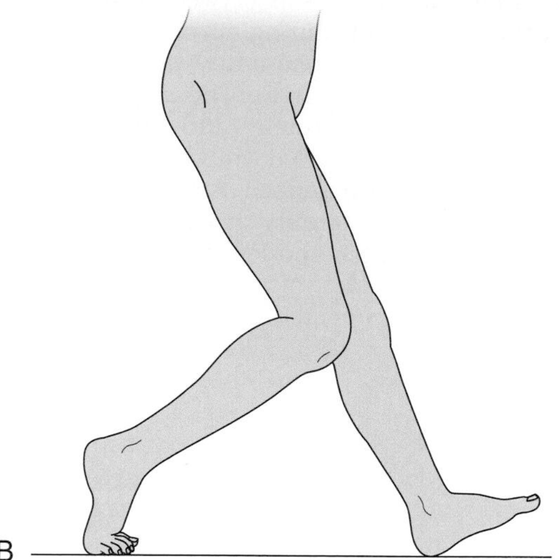

FIG 14-12 **A,** The typical progression of the center of pressure is from the heel (starting at the *dark red dots*) to the forefoot and toes (at the *light red dots*) as on the left figure. This was obtained with a pressure platform while walking barefoot. Ground contact with the forefoot as on the left figure shifts the center of pressure largely anterior, where it travels posterior toward the heel before moving anterior again toward the forefoot and toes. **B,** Excessive knee flexion. In late stance phase, there is increased knee flexion, caused by a flexion contracture of the hip. *(**B,** Modified from Whittle MW:* Gait analysis: an introduction, *ed 4. St Louis, 2008, Butterworth-Heinemann.)*

Compensations for increased swing phase ankle plantar flexion are typically necessary to avoid tripping secondary to toe drag during contralateral leg stance phase. These compensations often include vaulting on the stance leg, increased hip or knee flexion of the swing leg (steppage gait) (Fig. 14-11, *B*), or hip circumduction of the swing leg (described later). A combination of these compensations may also be used to increase ground clearance during the swing phase.

HIP CIRCUMDUCTION

Individuals who advance the swing leg in a lateral semicircular pattern rather than in a straight plane from posterior to anterior are said to be circumducting the hip. Ground clearance of the swing leg is increased using this swing pattern. Hip circumduction is a common compensation used to advance the swing leg if a person lacks hip flexion, knee flexion, or ankle dorsiflexion ROM. Individuals may also circumduct the hip if they lack hip flexion strength to swing the leg forward. In this case, the swing leg may be advanced by first externally rotating the hip and using the hip adductors rather than the hip flexors to pull the femur forward.

INCREASED KNEE FLEXION

Excessive knee flexion is most noticeable during either the loading response or the terminal stance phase of the gait cycle, when the knee would normally be nearly fully extended. Increased knee flexion at initial contact would almost certainly be accompanied by initial contact with the midfoot or forefoot rather than the heel. As the remainder of the foot comes in contact with the ground, the center of pressure first moves posteriorly and then anteriorly during stance rather than the typical posterior to anterior progression (Fig. 14-12, *A*). One consequence of this progression is that much of the forward momentum of the COM may be lost during early stance, minimizing the gait economy normally preserved by the foot and ankle rockers. Increased knee flexion during stance phase may be the consequence of numerous impairments, including a knee flexion contracture, knee pain or knee joint effusion, or a hip flexion contracture (Fig. 14-12, *B*).

Increased knee flexion and hip flexion during gait is referred to as *crouch gait* and is commonly observed in individuals with spastic diplegia as a consequence of cerebral palsy (Fig. 14-13). Increased knee flexion in such individuals may be due to spasticity of the hamstrings, hip flexors, or both. Careful gait and clinical analysis is required to develop the best course of surgical or conservative treatment for these patients.

GAIT PATTERN INSTRUCTION

Instructing patients in the proper use of assistive devices and identifying appropriate gait patterns are relevant clinical tasks for the physical therapist assistant (PTA). Several patterns are outlined here.

A four-point gait pattern is described as advancing the crutch opposite the uninvolved limb first, followed by the involved limb, then advancing the crutch toward the uninvolved limb, then finally advancing the uninvolved limb (Fig. 14-14). If the injured limb is the left leg, the four-point gait pattern looks like this:

Right crutch × left foot × left crutch × right foot

The four-point gait pattern attempts to duplicate the normal reciprocal motion that occurs between the upper extremities and the lower limbs during normal gait.

A three-point gait pattern is commonly taught using bilateral axillary crutches (Fig. 14-15). The sequence of events begins by advancing both crutches and the involved limb first followed by the uninvolved limb.

A two-point gait pattern is described as advancing the left crutch and right lower extremity at the same time, then advancing the right crutch and left lower extremity together. This gait pattern is similar to the four-point gait pattern in which normal reciprocal motion and walking rhythm is encouraged.

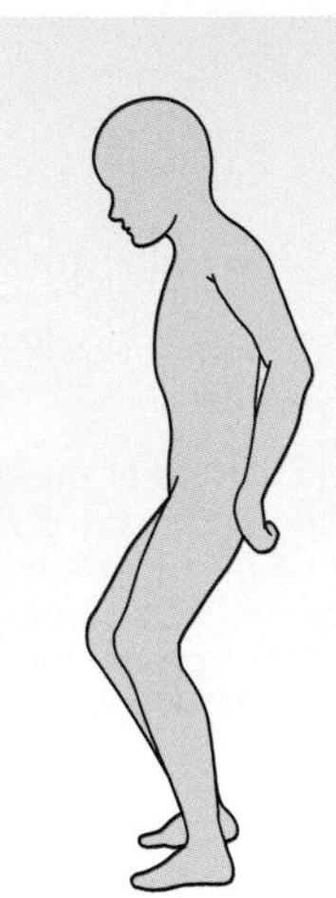

FIG 14-13 Position of body at midstance in a 12-year-old child with crouch gait, following Achilles tendon lengthening for spastic diplegia. *(Adapted from Sutherland DH, Cooper L: The pathomechanics of progressive crouch gait in spastic diplegia,* Orthop Clin North Am *9:143-154, 1978. In Whittle MW:* Gait analysis: an introduction, *ed 4, St Louis, 2008, Butterworth-Heinemann.)*

A tripod gait pattern is used for bilateral nonfunctioning limbs. Crutches are advanced, then the entire lower body is advanced. With a tripod gait, the body can be lifted and advanced to the crutch or swung through and beyond the contact point of the crutches.

WEIGHT-BEARING STATUS

Depending on the healing constraints of injured tissues (bone, ligament, tendon, cartilage, and muscle), certain weight-bearing restrictions are imposed to protect the injured tissues from excessive stresses and loads and to promote normal physiologic healing. If an injured limb is unable to support any weight, non–weight bearing (NWB) status is assigned until sufficient healing has taken place to allow the limit to accept some amount of weight safely. Partial weight bearing (PWB) is frequently graded in a percentage of the patient's weight (e.g., 20%, 40%, 50%) or in pounds of load applied to the floor from the involved limb. When teaching PWB with orders to apply a certain amount of weight (e.g., 20 pounds, 50 pounds), a bathroom scale can acquaint the patient with exactly how much weight is necessary to bear on the injured limb. The terms *touch down weight bearing* (TDWB) and *toe touch weight bearing* can be used synonymously to describe minimal contact of the involved limb with the ground. Generally, TDWB is used for balance purposes initially. As healing and pain allow, progressive weight bearing can be instituted. Weight bearing as tolerated (WBAT) is assigned to patients in whom pain tolerance is the predominant limiting factor. The patient is allowed to bear as much

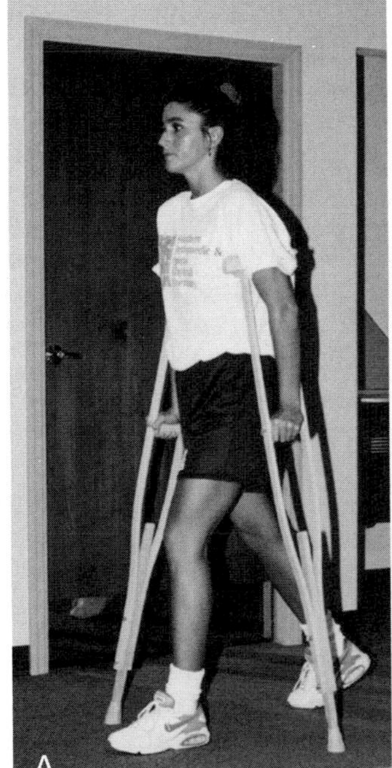

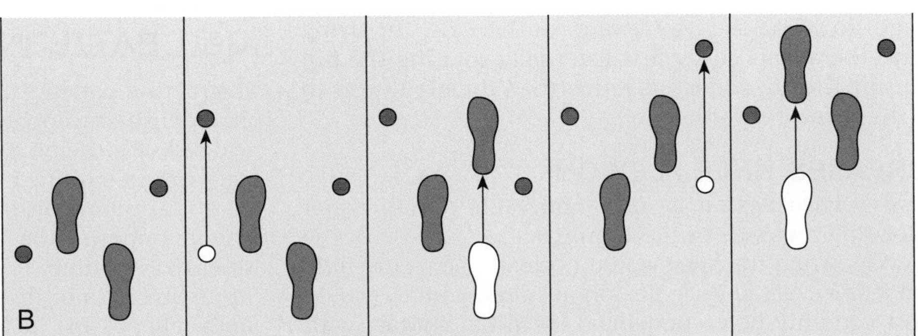

FIG 14-14 Four-point gait. One crutch or leg is moved at a time in the following pattern: left crutch–right leg–right crutch–left leg. *(**B,** From Whittle MW:* Gait analysis: an introduction, *ed 4, St Louis, 2008, Butterworth-Heinemann.)*

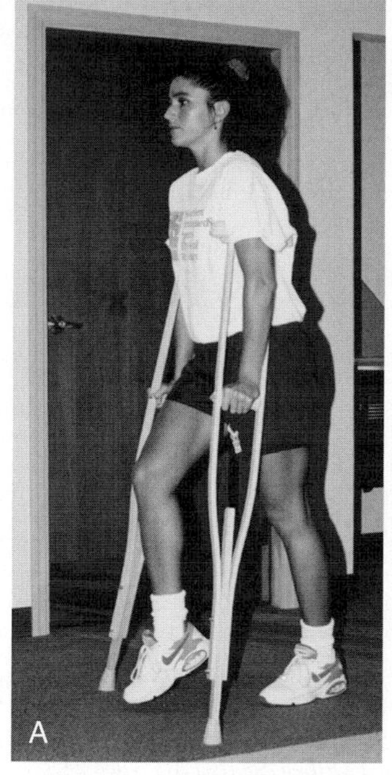

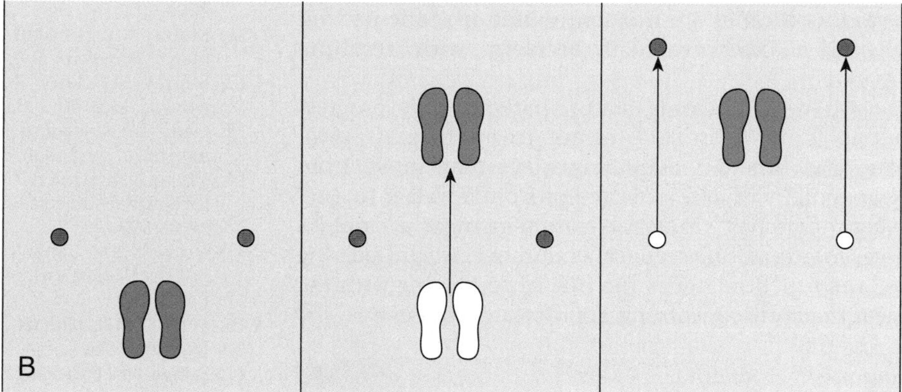

FIG 14-15 Three-point gait. **A,** Three-point step-through gait in someone taking weight on both crutches. **B,** The legs are advanced together (weight bearing on uninvolved limb), in front of the line of the crutches, then the crutches are advanced together, in front of the line of the legs. *(**B,** From Whittle MW:* Gait analysis: an introduction, *ed 4, St Louis, 2008, Butterworth-Heinemann.)*

weight on the injured limb as is comfortable. When a patient no longer requires an assistive device to accommodate pain or healing of injured tissues, full weight bearing (FWB) status is generally allowed.

Weight-bearing status is a progressive process that involves constant assessment and reassessment of pain, joint stability, tissue healing constraints, and function. A patient with severe injuries progresses through each designation of weight bearing as follows:

NWB × TDWB × PWB × WBAT × FWB

Less severe injuries may begin anywhere along the continuum and progress from there.

NEGOTIATING STAIRS WITH ASSISTIVE DEVICES

Ascending and descending stairs, steps, or curbs requires prudent instruction and careful supervision with necessary tactile and verbal cueing. The safety of the patient is the principal concern. Perhaps no other gait training technique elicits as much anxiety as negotiating stairs. The PTA must clearly articulate the fundamentals of ascending and descending the stairs, while both validating the patient's fears and providing confidence, encouragement, and a safe environment for instruction.

When instructing patients to ascend stairs using bilateral axillary crutches, the first step is to encourage the use of a handrail, if one is available. As the patient uses the handrail, both crutches are placed in the hand opposite the handrail. The patient should be instructed to use the handrail on the side of the injured limb if possible because this may provide an added sense of stability and support. Ascending a step requires the uninvolved leg to step up first, then the involved limb and crutches are advanced up to the same step.

When descending steps, the same instructions about the use of the handrail next to the injured limb should be repeated. The first step when descending stairs is to advance the crutches or cane to the step. The injured limb is then advanced down to the step, followed by the uninjured limb. It may help patients to remember, "up with the good, down with the bad," when cueing them as to which limb to advance up or down the stairs. When providing support for the patient during stair climbing, the PTA should stand behind the patient while giving appropriate verbal cues and physical support at the waist. As a safety precaution, an interlocking gait belt should be applied and used during all phases of gait training. When instructing patients during stair descent, it is best to stand in front of the patient. However, enough space must be allowed between the therapist and patient to permit a technically correct and safe descent. When no handrail is available, the patient should follow the same steps except that both crutches are used as with normal walking with crutches.

SELECTION OF ASSISTIVE DEVICES

The initial selection of assistive gait devices depends largely on the age and activity level of the patient, the severity of the injury, and the weight-bearing status. Walkers can be prescribed for an elderly person because a walker is inherently more stable and easy to use. Children may find a pediatric walker easier and safer to use than axillary crutches.

Axillary crutches provide less stability than a walker but allow greater mobility. Canes provide the least stability of all assistive devices. However, some types of canes provide more stability than others. For example, a wide-based quadripod cane (four points) allows more stability than a narrow-based quadripod cane or a single-point cane. A hemi-walker provides a wider, more stable base of support than a wide-based quadripod cane. Hemi-walkers and quadripod canes are frequently used by patients who have had a cerebrovascular accident with resulting hemiparesis.

As with weight-bearing status, patients may progress from one form of assistive device to another. As pain, healing, and function allow, a patient may move from using an axillary crutch to a cane or from a walker to a set of axillary crutches. Constant reassessment of a patient's balance, coordination, strength, endurance, weight-bearing status, and function guides the PTA in consulting with the physical therapist concerning appropriate gait devices.

Important Concepts

Consideration of pain, balance, coordination, strength, weight-bearing status, and environmental factors guides the selection of an assistive device suitable for each patient.

GLOSSARY

Antalgic gait: A general term used to describe a gait pattern accompanied by pain.

Stance phase: The portion of the gait cycle during which the foot is in contact with the ground.

Step: Contact with one foot until contact with the other (right to left or left to right).

Stride: Contact with one foot until contact with the same foot (right to right or left to left).

Swing phase: The portion of the gait cycle during which the foot is off the ground.

Trendelenburg gait: Lateral trunk bending as a compensation for ipsilateral hip abductor weakness.

Trendelenburg sign: A term used to refer to contralateral pelvic drop.

Vaulting: Increased ankle plantar flexion during and after midstance of the stance leg.

REFERENCES

1. Apkarian J, Naumann S, Cairns B: A three dimensional kinematic and dynamic model of the lower limb. *J Biomech* 22:143–155, 1989.
2. Auvinet B, Berrut G, Touzard C, et al: Reference data for normal subjects obtained with an accelometric device. *Gait Posture* 16:124–134, 2003.
3. Chao EY, Laughman RK, Schneider E, et al: Normative data of knee joint motion and ground reaction forces in adult level walking. *J Biomech* 16:219–233, 1983.
4. Cho SH, Park JM, Kwon OY: Gender differences in three dimensional gain analysis in 98 healthy Korean adults. *Clin Biomech (Bristol, Avon)* 19:145–152, 2004.
5. Hageman PA, Blanke DJ: Comparison of gait of young women and elderly women. *Phys Ther* 66:1382–1386, 1986.
6. Inman VT, Ralston HJ, Todd F: *Human walking*, Baltimore, 1989, Williams & Wilkins.
7. Kadaba MP, Ramakrishman HK, Wooten ME, et al: Repeatability of kinematic, kinetic and electromyographic data in normal adult gait. *J Orthop Res* 7:849–860, 1989.
8. Lafortune MR, Cavanaugh PR, Sommer HJ, et al: Three dimensional kinematics of the human knee during walking. *J Biomech* 25:347–357, 1992.
9. Larsson LE, Odenrick P, Sandlund B, et al: The phases of the stride and their interaction in human gait. *Scand J Rehabil Med* 12:107–112, 1980.
10. Menz HB, Latt MD, Tiedemann A, et al: Reliability of the Gaitrite walkway system for the quantification of temporal-spatial parameters of gait in young and older people. *Gait Posture* 20(1):20–25, 2004.
11. Murray MP, Drought AB, Kory RC: Walking patterns of normal men. *J Bone Joint Surg Am* 46:335–360, 1964.
12. Murray MP, Kory RC, Sepic SB: Walking patterns of normal women. *Arch Phys Med* 51:637–650, 1979.
13. Oatis CA: *Kinesiology: the mechanics and pathomechanics of human movement*, ed 2, Baltimore, 2009, Lippincott Williams & Wilkins.
14. Oberg T, Karszina A, Oberg K: Basic gait parameters: reference data for normal subjects, 10–79 years of age. *J Rehabil Res Dev* 30:210–223, 1993.
15. Ostrosky KM, VanSwearingen JM, Burdett RG, et al: A comparison of gait characteristics in young and old subjects. *Phys Ther* 74:637–646, 1994.
16. Perry J: *Gait analysis: normal and pathological function*, Thorofare, NJ, 1992, Slack.
17. Sekiya N, Nagasaki H, Ito H, et al: Optimal walking in terms of variability of step length. *J Orthop Sports Phys Ther* 26:266–272, 1997.
18. Senden R, Grimm B, Heylingers IC, et al: Acceleration-based gait test for healthy subjects: reliability and reference data. *Gait Posture* 30:192–196, 2009.
19. Simoneau G: Kinesiology of walking. In Neumann DA, editor: *Kinesiology of the musculoskeletal system: foundations for physical rehabilitation*, St Louis, 2002, Mosby.
20. Stolze H, Kuhtz-Buschbeck JP, Mondwurf C, et al: Retest reliability of spatiotemporal gait parameters in children and young adults. *Gait Posture* 7:125–130, 1998.
21. Winter DA, Patla AE, Frank JS, et al: Biomechanical walking changes in the fit and healthy elderly. *Phys Ther* 70:340–347, 1990.

REVIEW QUESTIONS

Multiple Choice

1. Movement of the tibia over the foot during early stance phase has been described as the:
   a. Heel rocker.
   b. Ankle rocker.
   c. Toe rocker.
   d. Knee rocker.
2. Which of the following events marks the end of one gait cycle for the right leg?
   a. Heel strike of the left leg
   b. Toe off of the right leg
   c. Heel strike of the right leg
   d. Toe off of the left leg
3. Which of the following is not typically associated with greater gait velocity?
   a. Faster cadence
   b. Longer step length
   c. Decreased double support time
   d. Increased stance time
4. During normal gait, the greatest motion occurs at the hip, knee, and ankle in which plane?
   a. Sagittal
   b. Frontal
   c. Transverse
   d. Movement is equal in all planes

5. Rearfoot motion during normal gait can be best characterized as:
   a. Initially everted, followed by inversion until midstance, then eversion until toe off.
   b. Initially everted, followed by eversion until midstance, then inversion until toe off.
   c. Initially inverted, followed by eversion until midstance, then inversion until toe off.
   d. Initially inverted, followed by inversion until midstance, then eversion until toe off.
6. Which of the following events occur after initial contact during normal gait?
   a. Knee flexion and concentric quadriceps activity
   b. Knee flexion and eccentric quadriceps activity
   c. Knee extension and concentric quadriceps activity
   d. Knee extension and eccentric quadriceps activity
7. At what point in the normal gait cycle is the body COM highest?
   a. Initial contact
   b. Midstance
   c. Double support phase
   d. Toe off
8. Decreased stance time and a rapid swing phase of the contralateral limb are common gait deviations observed among people with:
   a. Pain on the weight-bearing side.
   b. Decreased knee extension strength.
   c. Decreased first metatarsophalangeal joint ROM.
   d. Decreased knee flexion strength.
9. A commonly observed compensation for insufficient hip abductor force during gait is:
   a. Contralateral pelvic drop.
   b. Lateral trunk lean toward the stance leg.
   c. Increased gait speed.
   d. Longer step length.
10. Quadriceps weakness is often associated with which gait abnormality?
    a. Hip circumduction
    b. Anterior trunk lean
    c. Crouch gait
    d. Vaulting
11. Which of the following gait deviations is associated with the Trendelenburg sign?
    a. Increased trunk lean toward the stance leg
    b. Increased knee flexion and ankle dorsiflexion during stance phase
    c. Increased pelvic drop on the swing leg side
    d. Increased posterior trunk lean
12. Which of the following gait deviations is not typically employed to increase ground clearance for the swing leg?
    a. Hip circumduction of the swing leg
    b. Vaulting on the stance leg
    c. Steppage gait
    d. All of these may increase ground clearance for the swing leg
13. What is the order of events for a person ascending stairs with axillary crutches?
    a. Uninvolved limb first, then crutches, then involved limb
    b. Crutches first, then involved limb, then uninvolved limb
    c. Involved leg first, then crutches, then uninvolved limb
    d. Crutches first, then uninvolved limb, then involved limb
14. When a patient using axillary crutches is ascending stairs with a hand rail on either side, the patient should be advised to:
    a. Avoid using the hand rail in favor of the crutches.
    b. Carry the crutches and use the hand rail on the uninvolved side.
    c. Put the crutches together under the uninvolved side and use the hand rail on the involved side.
    d. Put the crutches together under the involved side and use the hand rail on the uninvolved side.
15. Which of the following assistive devices provides the most stability but the least mobility?
    a. Standard walker
    b. Two axillary crutches
    c. One axillary crutch
    d. Cane

Short Answer

16. What is the term used to describe linear distance between right and left feet during gait?
17. Name the components of the stance phase of gait.
18. Name the components of the swing phase of gait.
19. Name a primary action of the foot-flat period of the stance phase of gait.
20. On which side of the injured limb should a single crutch or cane be used?

Fill in the Blank

21. The double support phase typically represents only ________________ of the gait cycle.
22. Patients demonstrating a posterior trunk lean during early stance phase may be suspected to have weakness of the ________________.
23. Increased knee flexion and hip flexion during gait is referred to as ________________.
24. The sequence of events that begins by advancing both crutches and the involved limb first followed by the uninvolved limb is described as a ________________.
25. ________________ describes the weight-bearing status that permits minimal contact of the involved limb with the ground.

True/False

26. During gait, an individual's center of gravity displaces vertically and horizontally.
27. Non–weight-bearing status allows the patient to place minimal weight on the involved limb.
28. Partial weight-bearing status allows the patient to place a prescribed amount of resistance on the involved limb. The amount of weight is determined by the physician and is carried out in physical therapy through grading the resistance by a percentage of the patient's weight (e.g., 20%, 30%, 50%).
29. Knee flexion during the swing phase of gait is the result of strong hamstring contraction that begins during preswing.
30. The hip is flexed to about 25-30° at ground contact.

Chapter 15

Concepts of Joint and Soft Tissue Mobilization

Robert C. Manske, Justin Rohrberg, B. J. Lehecka

CHAPTER OUTLINE

LEARNING OBJECTIVES

1. Discuss the general and applied concepts of peripheral joint mobilization.
2. Define terms and principles of peripheral joint mobilization.
3. Define and describe the convex–concave rule.
4. Define the five grades of mobilization.
5. Identify and describe terms of joint end-feel.
6. Define and describe capsular and noncapsular patterns.
7. Identify common indications and contraindications for mobilization.
8. Discuss the clinical basics and applications of peripheral joint mobilization.
9. Identify and discuss the role of the physical therapist assistant in assisting the physical therapist with the delivery of peripheral joint mobilization.

KEY TERMS

Arthrokinematics
Capsular pattern
Compression
Manipulation
Mobilization
Tension

To provide comprehensive musculoskeletal rehabilitation, the physical therapist assistant (PTA) needs to understand the basic concepts related to joint **mobilization**. The PTA must be able to apply accurately and skillfully the mobilization techniques as delegated by the physical therapist (PT). This chapter focuses primarily on concepts, definitions, and general rationales for peripheral joint mobilization, including mobilization theory and compulsory scientific principles.

FUNDAMENTAL PRINCIPLES OF MOBILIZATION

A healthy joint is one that moves without limitation. In synovial joints, movement stimulates biologic activity by moving synovial fluid to areas of avascular articular cartilage. Additionally, strength and resiliency of capsular tissue and periarticular tissue are maintained via joint movement. Immobilization causes a host of negative consequences, such as fatty infiltration, articular adhesions, and physiologic changes to the strength and tolerance of ligaments, tendons, and capsular tissue. The term *mobilization* refers to an attempt to restore joint motion or mobility or decrease pain associated with joint structures using manual, passive accessory joint movement.[4,22]

Joint mobilizations are passive, skilled manual therapy techniques applied to joints and related soft tissues at varying speeds and amplitudes using physiologic or accessory motions for therapeutic purposes.[1] Range of motion (ROM) involves physiologic movements that are active or passive motions at a given joint through one of the traditional cardinal planes of flexion, extension, abduction, adduction, or internal and external rotation.

Important Concepts

Joint mobilizations are passive, skilled manual therapy techniques applied to joints and related soft tissues at varying speeds and amplitudes using physiologic or accessory motions for therapeutic purposes.[1]

Physiologic movements are sometimes called *osteokinematic,* classic, or traditional movements because they are movements of the actual bones of a given joint system. These motions can be visualized by the naked eye and are commonly measured by goniometric assessment. Osteokinematic motions occur in the cardinal planes of movement such as frontal, sagittal, and transverse. Hip, knee, and shoulder flexion movements are examples of osteokinematic movements. All of these movements can occur under volitional control. Arthrokinematic movements are movements that occur at the bone ends, without regard to the larger physiologic movement. These movements are not under volitional control. These types of movements are accessory movements involving motions specific to articulating joint surfaces.[4,22] These accessory joint motions are referred to as *glide or slide, spin,* and *roll.*[4,14] Because these are passive movements at the actual joint level, they are sometimes referred to as *arthrokinematic motions*. Accessory and physiologic joint motions occur together during active ROM. If full accessory motion does not occur, there is a limitation in normal physiologic cardinal plane movements. However, accessory joint motion cannot be selectively recruited, meaning a patient cannot selectively perform joint roll, glide, or spin movements independently.[4] The application of accessory joint motion is defined as "joint play" or "motion that occurs within the joint as a response to an outside force but not as a result of voluntary movement."[4]

Important Concepts

Accessory joint motions are referred to as *glide* or *slide, spin,* and *roll.*[4,14]

An arthrokinematic glide movement and an arthrokinematic slide movement are essentially the same. Gliding and sliding occurs as a specific point on one portion of the articular surface comes into contact with a series of locations on the corresponding joint surface. An analogy would be a car wheel sliding on ice when brakes are applied. One part of the tire glides or slides across a series of locations of the ice surface. When the elbow is flexed doing a biceps curl, the convex olecranon rolls anteriorly and glides or slides posteriorly on the relatively fixed concave trochlea of the distal humerus.

The arthrokinematic movement termed *spin* occurs when a portion of one joint spins or rotates, clockwise or counterclockwise, around a stationary longitudinal axis. An example is when a forearm goes through the motion of supination and pronation. At the radiohumeral joint, the radial head spins on the capitellum of the distal humerus.

Rolling occurs when multiple points of contact on one joint surface come into contact with multiple points of contact on the corresponding joint surface. An analogy for this movement would be a car tire driving normally where the tire surface makes contact with different portions of the road. In human joints, this occurs as the convex distal femur rolls forward and glides posteriorly on the concave tibia as a person moves from a seated to standing position.

JOINT CONGRUENCY AND POSITION

The concept of joint congruency and the terms *close-packed* and *loose-packed* joint positions are pertinent to the discussion of various grades of mobilization. Congruence refers to articular position with regard to concave and convex joint surfaces. A joint is congruent when both articulating surfaces are in contact throughout the total surface area of the joint.[4,14] However, the study of **arthrokinematics** (joint movement) states that joints are rarely in total congruence. As joints move, the accessory motions of glide or slide, spin, and roll alter total joint congruence.

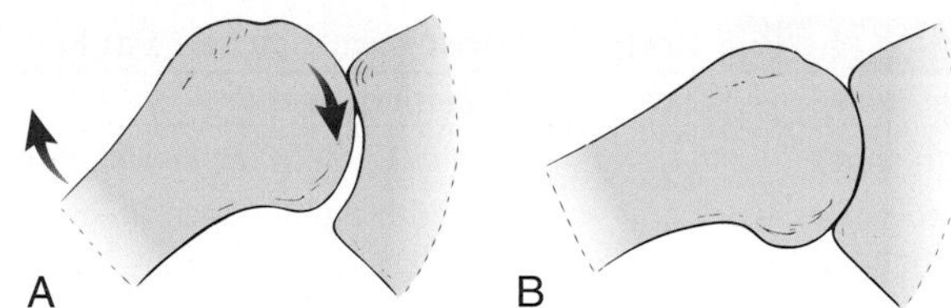

FIG 15-1 The congruence of articular surfaces. **A,** Loose-packed position. **B,** Close-packed position. *(Modified from Gould JA: Orthopaedic and sports physical therapy, ed 2, St Louis, 1990, Mosby.)*

MacConaill and Basmajian[14] described close-packed positions as the most congruent positions of a joint, where the joint articular surfaces are aligned, the capsule and ligaments are taut, and joint volume is minimal (Fig. 15-1). Generally, a close-packed position is used for testing the integrity and stability of ligaments and capsular structures. However, the close-packed position described by MacConaill and Basmajian[14] is not used for mobilization techniques. The close-packed position is one of stability. When the elbow and knee are fully extended, the ligaments and joint capsule are taut, allowing no freedom of movement. The knee and elbow in extension serve as two excellent examples of joints in their close-packed position.

Important Concepts

MacConaill and Basmajian[14] described close-packed positions as the most congruent positions of a joint, where the joint articular surfaces are aligned, the capsule and ligaments are taut, and joint volume is minimal.

Any joint position other than the close-packed position is a loose-packed position. The position in which the joint capsule and ligaments are most relaxed and loose and allow the maximum amount of joint play is referred to as the joint's *resting position.*[4] When the knee joint is flexed to 30°, the intracapsular space is increased, and supporting ligaments become more relaxed. The loose-packed position is ideal for applying joint mobilization techniques, but painful, stiff, and dysfunctional joints are rarely in ideal resting positions for the application of joint mobilization. Table 15-1 lists resting and close-packed positions of major joints in the human body.[16] If a joint has a limitation of arthrokinematic movement in which the close-packed position cannot be achieved, ground reaction forces and gravitational forces are not distributed through the joint optimally, and additional stress and work must be taken by the periarticular muscles. If this dysfunctional movement pattern continues, a condition of muscle overuse can ensue.

CONVEX–CONCAVE RULE

Anatomically, all articular surfaces are either convex or concave,[4,22] although the surfaces of some joints are not overtly of either shape. In these cases, fibrocartilage

TABLE 15-1 Resting (Loose) and Closed-Packed Position of Joints

Joint	Resting Position	Closed-Packed Position
Facet (spine)	Midway between flexion and extension	Extension
Temporomandibular	Mouth slightly open (freeway space)	Clenched teeth
Glenohumeral	55° abduction, 30° horizontal adduction	Abduction and lateral rotation
Acromioclavicular	Arm resting by side in normal physiologic position	Arm abducted to 90°
Sternoclavicular	Arm resting by side in normal physiologic position	Maximum shoulder elevation
Ulnohumeral (elbow)	70° flexion, 10° supination	Extension
Radiohumeral	Full extension, full supination	Elbow flexed 90°, forearm supinated 5°
Proximal radioulnar	70° flexion, 35° supination	5° supination
Distal radioulnar	10° supination	5° supination
Radiocarpal (wrist)	Neutral with slight ulnar deviation	Extension with radial deviation
Carpometacarpal	Midway between abduction-adduction and flexion-extension	
Metacarpophalangeal (all)	Slight flexion	
Metacarpophalangeal (fingers)		Full flexion
Metacarpophalangeal (thumb)		Full opposition
Interphalangeal	Slight flexion	Full extension
Hip	30° flexion, 30° abduction, slight lateral rotation	Full extension, medial rotation
Knee	25° flexion	Full extension, lateral rotation of tibia
Talocrural (ankle)	10° plantar flexion, midway between maximum inversion and eversion	Maximum dorsiflexion
Subtalar	Midway between extremes of ROM	Supination
Midtarsal	Midway between extremes of ROM	Supination
Tarsometatarsal	Midway between extremes of ROM	Supination
Metatarsophalangeal	Neutral	Full extension
Interphalangeal	Slight flexion	Full extension

ROM, range of motion.
From Magee DJ: *Orthopedic physical assessment,* ed 5, St Louis, 2008, Saunders.

enhances and modifies the contour of the joint surfaces. On the convex joint surface, more cartilage is found at the center of the surface. Alternatively, on a concave joint surface, more cartilage is found at the periphery.[4]

The convex–concave rule specifically states, "When the concave surface is stationary and the convex surface is moving, the gliding movement in the joint occurs in a direction opposite to the bone movement."[4] Conversely, if the convex surface is fixed while the concave surface is mobile, the gliding motion occurs in the same direction as the bone movement.[4] This occurs because the convex bone surface maintains an axis of rotation during joint motion (Fig. 15-2). The concept of accessory joint motions (glide or slide, spin, and roll) as they apply to joint congruency and the convex–concave rule is illustrated by MacConaill's classification of accessory movements (Fig. 15-3).

Important Concepts

The convex–concave rule specifically states, "When the concave surface is stationary and the convex surface is moving, the gliding movement in the joint occurs in a direction opposite to the bone movement."[4] Conversely, if the convex surface is fixed while the concave surface is mobile, the gliding motion occurs in the same direction as the bone movement.[4]

MOBILIZATION GRADES

Maitland[17] described five grades of physiologic and accessory joint motions used in mobilization (Fig. 15-4). The terms *velocity, oscillation,* and *amplitude* of movement are used to describe the degree of force and rate of motion applied during the different grades of mobilization, as follows:

- Grade I mobilization: A small oscillation or small amplitude joint motion that occurs only at the beginning of the available ROM.
- Grade II mobilization: A larger amplitude motion occurring from the beginning of the ROM to near midrange.
- Grade III mobilization: A large amplitude motion that occurs from midrange of motion to the end of the available range.
- Grade IV mobilization: A small oscillation or amplitude of motion that occurs at the very end range of the available joint motion.
- Grade V mobilization: "A high velocity thrust of small amplitude at the end of the available ROM."[4] This grade is not applied to mobilization techniques used by PTAs and is not addressed in this text.

In general terms, a grade I or II amplitude oscillation is used to treat pain or when joint motion produces pain.[4,22] Alternatively, grade III and IV mobilizations are used to treat joint restrictions.[4,22]

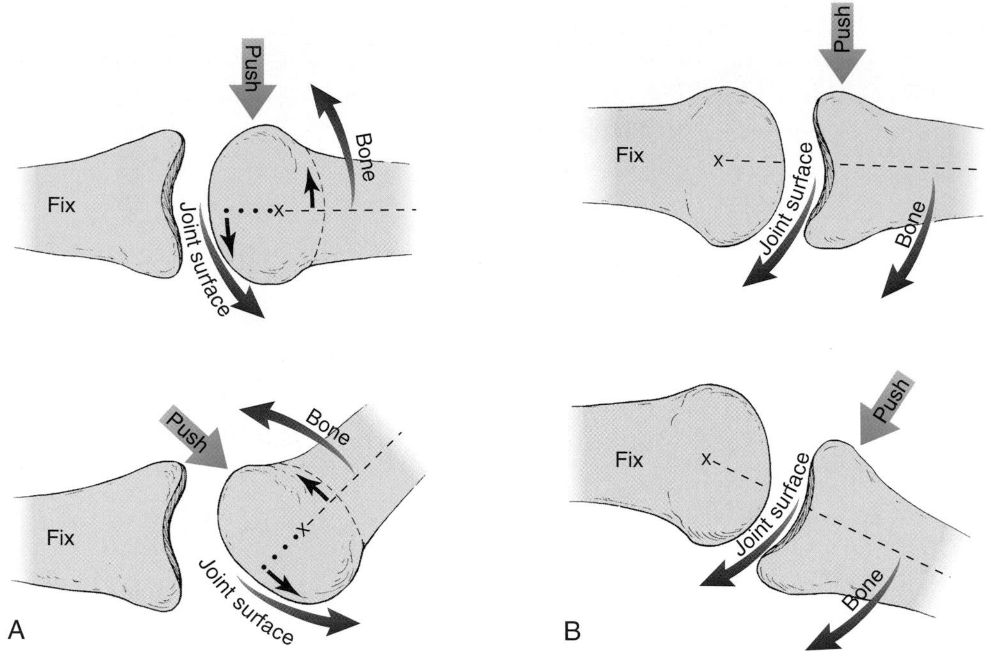

FIG 15-2 **A,** Convex surface moving on concave surface. **B,** Concave surface moving on convex surface with a combination of roll, spin, and glide occurring in both simultaneously. *(Modified from Gould JA:* Orthopaedic and sports physical therapy, *ed 2, St Louis, 1990, Mosby.)*

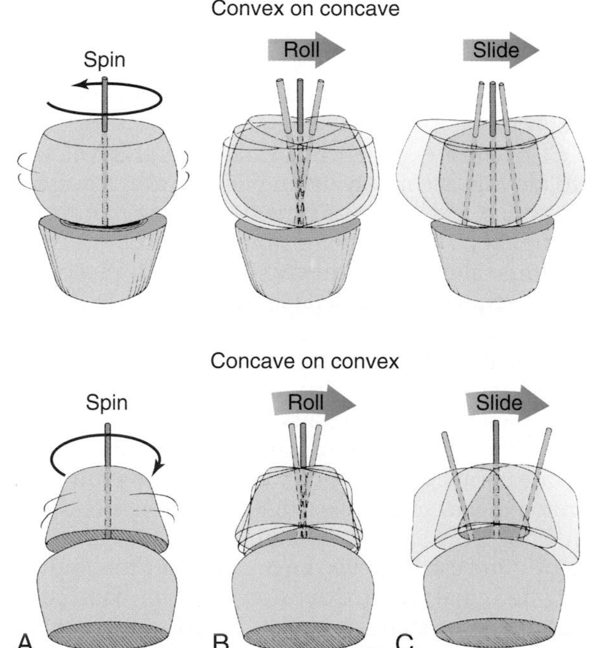

FIG 15-3 MacConaill's classification of accessory movements. **A,** Spin. **B,** Roll. **C,** Glide. *(Modified from Gould JA:* Orthopaedic and sports physical therapy, *ed 2, St Louis, 1990, Mosby.)*

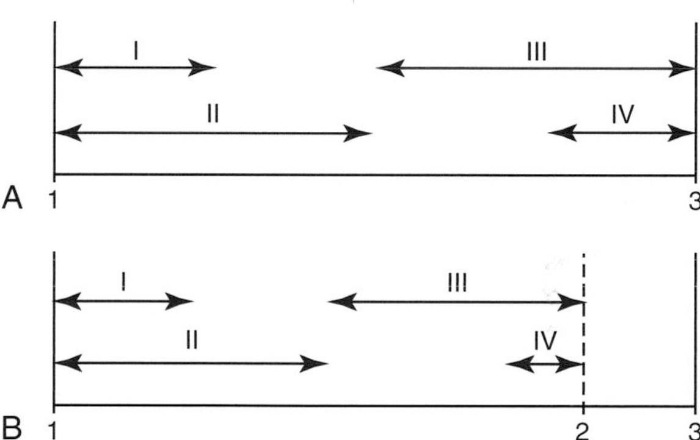

FIG 15-4 **A,** Grades of oscillations used in manual therapy. **B,** Grades of oscillations used in manual therapy in relation to a joint with limited motion. *1,* starting position of movement; *2,* point of limitation of movement; *3,* anatomic limit of movement. *(From Gould JA:* Orthopaedic and sports physical therapy, *ed 2, St Louis, 1990, Mosby.)*

Important Concepts

In general terms, a grade I or II amplitude oscillation is used to treat pain or when joint motion produces pain.[4,22] Alternatively, grade III and IV mobilizations are used to treat joint restrictions.[4,22]

Translational movements during joint mobilization techniques can be performed in one of two planes. Joint mobilizations can be performed perpendicular or parallel to the treatment plane. The treatment plane is described as a line running perpendicular to, or at a right angle to, a line running from the axis of joint rotation in the convex surface to the center of the concave articular surface.[12] A translational joint mobilization technique (glide) is one in which the articulating surface glides along a line parallel to the treatment plane.

Traction is also used as a manual therapy technique either by itself or along with various mobilization techniques (Fig. 15-5). A traction technique is a joint mobilization technique that translates one articular surface in a

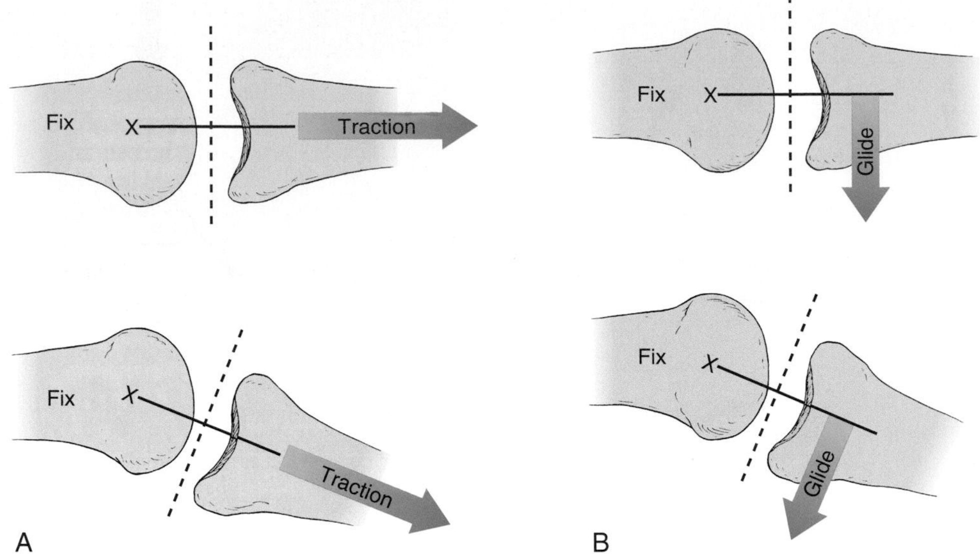

FIG 15-5 **A,** Traction. **B,** Glide. *(From Gould JA:* Orthopaedic and sports physical therapy, *ed 2, St Louis, 1990, Mosby.)*

perpendicular direction away from the treatment plane. Traction can be classified in grades or stages.[12,17] Generally, grade I or stage I traction is used to relieve pain and to minimize compressive joint forces during mobilization. The term *piccolo traction* describes a stage I traction technique. The force used to deliver grade I traction is not enough to separate the joint surfaces, but rather neutralizes joint pressure.[4]

As a general rule, distraction techniques cannot stretch or increase length of any specific portion of a joint cavity; rather, they are for general overall mobility. Translational glide techniques are used specifically to treat a single portion of a restricted joint capsule or tight structure. The term *slack* refers to the amount of normal looseness found in nonpathologic joint capsules and describes various degrees of joint tightness with stage II and III traction. Stage II traction is defined as being able to "take up the slack" in the capsule of the joint being stretched; it is commonly used to treat pain. Stage III traction is more substantial and involves stretching of the soft tissues. These techniques are performed to stretch out joint tightness.

JOINT END-FEEL

There are various qualities of joint tightness or "play" during the application of passive joint movements. Three types of end-feel have been defined in normal, nonpathologic joints.[7,16] Bone-to-bone end-feel refers to a sudden, hard, nonyielding sensation felt at the end ROM. Generally, end-feel is not painful. Terminal elbow extension in which the olecranon process contacts the olecranon fossa is an example of a sudden bone-to-bone end-feel.

Another normal end-feel is soft tissue approximation. This type of joint end-feel is characterized by a "yielding **compression**" as is typically encountered with knee or elbow flexion.[16] The end-feel that occurs with soft tissue approximation results from muscular tissue compression during joint flexion. The hamstring and calf muscles buttress and compress against each other during knee flexion, delivering a soft tissue approximation end-feel.

The third normal joint end-feel is described as a hard or springy tissue stretch. The characteristic feature of this end-feel is "elastic resistance" or "rising **tension**."[16] This type of end-feel is the most common normal feel at the end range of joints. Terminal knee extension and wrist flexion provide a springy stretch that defines tissue stretch.

The PTA must experience normal joint end-feel and be able to identify accurately distinguishing characteristics of bone-to-bone end-feel, soft tissue approximation, and tissue stretch.[7] The PTA performing mobilization is likely to encounter abnormal joint end-feel also. Its precise identification requires considerable didactic and hands-on experience.[7]

Multiple types of abnormal end-feel exist. The first type is termed *muscle spasm*. The major component is pain accompanied by a sudden halt of movement that prevents full ROM.[4,7,16] Another abnormal end-feel is called a *springy block,* or internal derangement, during which full motion is limited by a soft or springy sensation occasionally accompanied by pain. If a meniscus is torn in a knee, frequently the cartilage becomes caught in the joint, preventing terminal knee extension and its characteristic normal tissue stretch and feel. In an empty end-feel, motion is very limited by significant pain without muscle spasm. Clinically, this end-feel is not characterized by any mechanical block or restriction. A fourth abnormal end-feel is termed a *loose end-feel.*[4] Its primary feature is joint hypermobility, with minimal resistance felt at the end ROM signifying extraordinary joint looseness. Lastly, a capsular end-feel[16] is analogous to a normal tissue stretch, but the elastic resistance is encountered before the normal ROM. This end-feel is related to a capsular restriction.[16] Table 15-2 lists normal and pathologic end-feels and examples of each.[2]

TABLE 15-2 Normal and Pathologic End-Feels

End-Feel	Description and Example
Normal	
Capsular	Firm, forcing the shoulder into full external rotation
Bony	Abrupt, moving the elbow into full extension
Soft tissue approximation	Soft; flexing the normal knee or elbow
Muscular	Rubbery; tension of tight hamstrings
Pathologic	
Adhesions and scarring	Sudden; sharp arrest in one direction
Muscle spasm	Rebound; usually accompanies pain felt at the end of restriction
Loose	Ligamentous laxity; a hypermobile joint
Boggy	Soft, mushy; joint effusion
Internal derangement	Springy; mechanical block such as a torn meniscus
Empty	No resistance to motion

From Andrews J, Harrelson G, Wilk K: *Physical rehabilitation of the injured athlete,* ed 3, St Louis, 2004, Saunders; source material from Cyriax JH: *Textbook of orthopedic medicine,* vol 1, ed 6, Baltimore, 1975, Williams & Wilkins.

CAPSULAR AND NONCAPSULAR PATTERNS

The PTA must be aware that certain limitations of motion can be caused by lesions specific to the capsule or synovial tissues of a joint. All joints controlled by muscle activity possess a characteristic "**capsular pattern** of proportional limitation."[16] Each joint has its own capsular pattern. For example, in the shoulder joint, the capsular pattern "involves external rotation as the most limited movement, abduction as less limited, internal rotation still less limited, and flexion as the least limited movement."[4,7] Any "characteristic pattern of limitation" is called a *capsular pattern.*

If a lesion causes a restriction of movement that does not correspond to a characteristic, predetermined capsular pattern, it is called a *noncapsular pattern.*[4,16] Cyriax[7] identified three possible causes of noncapsular pattern restrictions:

1. Ligamentous adhesions: These frequently cause pain and limitation of motion. A noncapsular pattern exists when injury to the capsule or accessory ligaments causes a restriction in one direction while other motions remain unaffected and pain-free.
2. Internal derangements: These include displaced or loose cartilaginous or bony fragments within the joint. The limitation of movement depends on the size and location of the fragment. For example, if the medial meniscus becomes wedged in the joint, knee extension is affected, although flexion remains normal.
3. Extraarticular lesions: These adhesions result from injury outside the joint. Muscular adhesions or acutely inflamed structures are examples. Causes include bursitis, muscle strains, and neural tissue irritation.

TABLE 15-3 Joint Restrictions from Noncapsular Pattern

Type	Description
Ligament adhesions	These occur when adhesions form around a ligament after an injury and may cause pain or a restriction of mobility. Some movements are painful, some are slightly limited, and some are pain-free
Internal derangement	Restriction in joint mobility is the result of a loose fragment within the joint. The onset is sudden; pain is localized; and movements that engage against the block are limited, whereas all others are free
Extraarticular limitation	Loss in joint mobility results from adhesions in structures outside the joint. Movements that stress the adhesions are limited and painful

From Andrews J, Harrelson G, Wilk K: *Physical rehabilitation of the injured athlete,* ed 3, St Louis, 2004, Saunders.

Table 15-3 lists joint restrictions from noncapsular patterns.[2]

INDICATIONS AND CONTRAINDICATIONS FOR MOBILIZATION

Patient safety should always be considered when applying joint mobilization or **manipulation** techniques. Cautions or contraindications for joint mobilization and manipulation are listed in Table 15-4 and Box 15-1.[15] Extreme caution must be employed before applying mobilization techniques in the early stages after trauma such as surgery or during times of immobilization. Although pain is an indication for the use of mobilization, care must be taken to avoid retarding or impairing the sequence of tissue healing during the acute inflammatory phase.

Pain and joint restrictions are rarely independent impairments. However, in many instances of severe joint limitations, there may be only mild complaints of pain. There may also be little or no joint restriction but significant pain. Naturally, varying degrees of pain and joint limitations occur as either major or minor components; pain is a relative indication for joint mobilization, depending on which stage of tissue healing is present. If an injury is acute or a patient is recovering immediately after a surgical procedure, mobilization may not be indicated because it is best not to disturb an immature scar. Healing that proceeds in an organized fashion encourages mature collagen formation. When injured tissues have progressed from the acute, intense, inflammatory phase to fibroplasia and scar maturation, mobilization is warranted to stress and remodel the scar.[22]

There are a few relative and absolute contraindications to the application of joint mobilization. Extreme caution is needed when considering mobilization in cases of osteoporosis, rheumatoid arthritis, joint hypermobility, and the presence of neurologic symptoms; all are considered

TABLE 15-4 Factors Involving Patient Anatomy or Physiology to Consider as a Caution or Contraindication for Mobilization or Manipulation

Type of Element	Description
Bony elements	Fractures (presently healing) Dislocations (presently healing) Past or present cancers that metastasize to bone (e.g., breast, bronchus, prostate, thyroid, kidney, bowel, lymphoma) Active bone infection (cautionary with past bone infections, e.g., osteomyelitis, tuberculosis, congenital anomalies) Gross foraminal or spinal canal encroachment on radiograph or other imaging examination
Vascular elements	Vertebral artery insufficiency Vascular disease (e.g., aneurysm, atherosclerosis) Signs of vascular insufficiency in that region Bleeding disorders Aortic graft
Neurologic elements	CNS disease or signs and symptoms of CNS injury Spinal cord disease or signs and symptoms of spinal cord injury Cauda equina disease or signs and symptoms of cauda equina injury Multiple/bilateral level nerve root involvement
Soft tissue elements	Collagen disease (e.g., Ehlers-Danlos syndrome) Connective tissue instability Acute posttraumatic stage of healing
Metabolic disease	Bone disease (e.g., osteoporosis)
Systemic disease/condition	Asthma, hemophilia, pregnancy
Inflammatory diseases	Acute active inflammation (e.g., rheumatoid arthritis, inactive inflammatory disease)
Medications patient may be taking	Anticoagulants (e.g., heparin/caution with aspirin) Any medication that affects collagen (e.g., corticosteroids or tamoxifen or any medication that is linked to osteoporosis) Antidepressants

CNS, central nervous system.
From Maffey LL: Arthrokinematics and mobilization of musculoskeletal tissue: the principles. In Magee DJ, Zachazewski JE, Quillen WS, editors: *Scientific foundations and principles of practice in musculoskeletal rehabilitation,* St Louis, 2007, Saunders.

Important Concepts

Extreme caution is needed when considering mobilization in cases of osteoporosis, rheumatoid arthritis, joint hypermobility, and the presence of neurologic symptoms; all are considered relative contraindications.[4,22]

relative contraindications.[4,22] Pregnancy and spondylolisthesis are also relative contraindications. Absolute contraindications include bone diseases of the area treated, malignancy of the area treated, acute inflammatory and infectious arthritis, central nervous system disorders, and vascular disorders of the vertebral artery.[4,22]

CLINICAL APPLICATION OF JOINT MOBILIZATION

Safe and effective joint mobilization requires the patient to be placed in a comfortable position. It also requires the joint to be mobilized to be placed in its maximal resting or loose-packed position.[14] Before mobilization, patient compliance and relaxation can be facilitated by the judicious use of moist heat, ultrasound, transcutaneous electrical nerve stimulation, electrical muscle stimulation, ice, exercise, and the timely use of any physician-prescribed analgesics or muscle relaxant medications. If pain is the predominant feature of the joint to be mobilized, grade I and II mobilizations can be employed safely.

Oscillations help modulate or minimize pain when using grade I and II mobilizations. Manually applied joint oscillations occur at a rate of 1 to 3 per second, or 60 to 180 per minute.[4,17] Typically, a mobilization grade technique is applied for 20 to 60 seconds only four or five times. This approach is recommended for the treatment of painful conditions on a daily basis or until pain is reduced. These smaller amplitude mobilization techniques are used to stimulate mechanoreceptors within the joint that can limit pain perception transmission at the spinal cord or brainstem level through a hypoalgesic response mediated by the noradrenergic descending pain pathways from the periaqueductal gray area.[23]

It is common to perform grade I and II mobilizations to a joint to decrease pain before more aggressive mobilization techniques. Some irritable conditions require a short bout of smaller oscillation techniques before techniques designed to gain mobility.

A program of mobilization is carried out two to three times per week for the treatment of joint restrictions.[4] Piccolo or stage I traction can be used simultaneously with grade I or II mobilization or by itself to reduce pain and neutralize joint pressure. When the limitation of joint motion is greater than the complaints of pain, grade III

BOX 15-1 Factors Involving the Clinician and Patient Relationship to Consider as a Contraindication for Mobilization or Manipulation

- Insufficient subjective assessment of the patient—inadequate information about coexisting conditions, disease, or medication, or in general the patient has an inability to communicate or is an unreliable historian
- Poor appraisal of the patient as a reliable historian
- Patient is intoxicated or heavily medicated
- Patient age—children (skeletal maturity, consent issues) or elderly (tissue health/integrity issues)
- Failure to discuss assessment findings and treatment options with patient
- Failure to receive or to agree with patient consent
- Insufficient scanning examination or detailed biomechanical examination
- Inappropriate findings, end-feel, or patient response with the following:
  - Scanning examination
  - Biomechanical testing
  - Stress testing (positive for level desire to treat or cautionary if above or below joint/level treating)
  - Dizziness reproduction testing
- Clinician's insufficient awareness of contraindications and conditions requiring extra care and gentleness
- Clinician's physical limitations for the technique (e.g., size, strength, speed, fatigue)
- Lack of clinician's confidence for the technique
- Lack of proper equipment for the technique (e.g., not using a high/low plinth)
- Pain in the position of the technique
- Patient's joint placed in a fully close-packed position

From Maffey LL: Arthrokinematics and mobilization of musculoskeletal tissue: the principles. In Magee DJ, Zachazewski JE, Quillen WS, editors: *Scientific foundations and principles of practice in musculoskeletal rehabilitation,* St Louis, 2007, Saunders.

and IV mobilizations can be used to help stretch the capsule and soft tissues around the joint.

The pathologic condition of the joint to be mobilized must be thoroughly understood before applying any mobilization technique. For example, it is critical to avoid stressing the anterior capsule of the shoulder after an anterior dislocation, although mobilization to improve shoulder abduction may be warranted.[22]

In every case of joint mobilization, the PTA must constantly observe and document the patient's tolerance, pain response, and swelling to determine whether to halt the procedure, reduce the grade of motion, or consult with the PT about advancing the grade of mobilization.

Important Concepts

In every case of joint mobilization, the PTA must constantly observe and document the patient's tolerance, pain response, and swelling to determine whether to halt the procedure, reduce the grade of motion, or consult with the PT about advancing the grade of mobilization.

As stated at the beginning of this discussion, the PT is responsible for delegating selected peripheral joint mobilization techniques to the PTA. Although peripheral joint mobilization beyond active and passive ROM is an area of treatment not usually delegated to the PTA, understanding peripheral joint mobilization techniques and having an awareness of rudimentary concepts and principles of mobilization provide the PTA with a broad understanding of the rationale for the application of certain techniques.

MOBILIZATION EVIDENCE

The medical literature contains limited high-level evidence via randomized controlled clinical trials (RCTs) assessing the effectiveness of joint mobilization techniques. The following studies describe evidence for or about mobilization at various joints.

There are mixed reviews in the ankle. Lin and colleagues[13] reported that the incorporation of large amplitude grade III anterior-posterior glides to the talus for 4 weeks did not enhance their outcomes at 24 weeks after ankle fractures. This study is in direct contradiction to Green and coworkers,[8] who used an experimental group given anterior-posterior joint mobilizations to the talus after an acute ankle sprain compared with a control group that was treated with rest, ice, compression, and elevation (RICE). After the intervention period, the experimental group required fewer treatments, had greater improvements in ROM at the ankle, and experienced greater increases in stride speed, indicating the addition of joint mobilizations had a positive impact on outcomes.

In the hip, Hoeksma and associates[10] showed in a single-blind RCT of 109 patients with osteoarthritic hips that manual therapy resulted in 81% success rates for the experimental group compared with only 50% for the control group. The experimental group demonstrated better outcomes in regard to pain, stiffness, hip function, and ROM after 5 weeks (nine sessions) of manual therapy treatments of hip joint distraction followed by a hip traction manipulation. These beneficial changes remained after 29 weeks. Similar benefits of mobilization have been seen in patients with knee osteoarthritis who demonstrated immediate pain relief and increased ROM after treatment.[21]

In the shoulder, Senbursa and colleagues[19] performed a RCT to compare the effectiveness of two treatments for shoulder impingement—soft tissue and joint mobilization or an independent exercise program. There were 30 patients with impingement who were randomly assigned to one of the treatment approaches and followed for 3 months. The manual therapy group received a prescription of 12 sessions of joint mobilization and demonstrated significant decreases in pain and increases in ROM. Conroy and Hayes[6] examined the usefulness of joint mobilizations on 14 patients with impingement syndrome. Subjects were randomly assigned to an exercise program alone or an exercise program with joint mobilizations. The results were mixed, with the mobilization group demonstrating less 24-hour pain and less pain with a subacromial compression test but no differences in ROM and function.

Bang and Deyle[3] compared supervised exercise versus supervised exercise combined with manual therapy to the upper quarter in patients with impingement syndrome. The manual therapy approach consisted mainly of grade

I to V oscillatory caudal glides of the glenohumeral joint in varying degrees of flexion and abduction. Significant improvements were found in pain reduction, function, and strength in patients who received manual therapy in addition to supervised exercises. Manske and colleagues[18] performed a RCT of stretching versus stretching plus posterior shoulder capsular mobilizations to assess for efficacy in treating a tight posterior shoulder. The main outcome measure was internal rotation motion loss. Using 39 randomly assigned subjects with at least a 10° loss of internal rotation, it was found that the addition of posterior shoulder joint mobilization to a stretching program resulted in trends toward increased motion.

A Cochrane review performed by Gross and colleagues[9] assessed mobilization and manipulation in patients with mechanical neck disorders. Outcomes were based on pain relief, functional improvement, or overall disability improvement. Studies included single session and multiple session manipulative therapy. Mobilization alone was found to have little to no effect on outcomes based on four RCTs in which mobilization was tested against cold pack, transcutaneous electrical nerve stimulation, and ultrasound, among others. Also, little evidence was found to support the use of mobilization and manipulation for pain relief and improvement in function. Mobilization and manipulation with the addition of exercise was found to have positive results for pain relief, functional improvement, or overall disability improvement. Although this finding is encouraging for patients experiencing acute to chronic pain in the cervical spine, the authors also noted studies that compared manipulation plus exercise with exercise alone with little difference between these groups.

A review of the literature by Hurwitz and associates[11] looked at studies examining the use of mobilization and manipulation in the management of neck pain and headaches. Neck pain was categorized into acute, subacute, or chronic neck pain. In the studies reviewed, the authors found that mobilization provided some statistically significant decreases in pain compared with other treatment options. Manipulation of the cervical spine in patients experiencing subacute and chronic neck pain and tension-induced headaches showed subjective improvements compared with other therapies; however, the authors noted risks involved with cervical manipulation. These risks included paralysis and death, with rates of injury occurring in 5 to 10 per 10 million manipulations.

In a study investigating the safety of mobilization to the thoracic spine, Sran and colleagues[20] used 12 cadavers to determine the in vitro effects of spinal mobilization to the sixth thoracic vertebra. Loading of the spinous process of T6 was performed using mechanical compression to the point of failure. The average amount of force to failure in the cadaver models was 479 ± 162 Newtons (N). These results varied significantly compared with the in vivo effects of mobilization, where two physiotherapists applied an average load of 145 ± 38 N. The amount of force applied in this study showed that posterior-to-anterior mobilization when applied with care has a fairly significant margin of error before fracture occurs.

Management of low-back pain is difficult and a common problem in patients encountered by the PT and PTA. The use of manipulation or mobilization to address the dysfunction associated with the low back is becoming increasingly popular. A systematic review of the literature by Bronfort and colleagues[5] showed there was some evidence to support use of manipulation and mobilization of the spine in the management of acute and chronic low-back pain. In acute episodes, the authors concluded that manipulation was better suited to relieve pain than other treatment techniques, including mobilization and diathermy. For chronic low-back pain, the authors concluded that manipulation with the addition of strengthening exercises had evidence to support its use in the reduction of pain and disability.

GLOSSARY

Arthrokinematics: Study of motion within joints. Description of joint typography.

Capsular pattern: Limitation of movement or a pattern of pain at a joint that occurs in a predictable pattern.

Compression: Occurs when two forces or loads are applied toward each other.

Manipulation: Passive intervention motion of high velocity at end ranges of available joint motion.

Mobilization: Passive intervention motion within and at end range of joint motion with varying degrees of speed and amplitude.

Tension: Occurs when two forces are applied in opposite directions.

REFERENCES

1. American Physical Therapy Association: Guide to physical therapist practice. Second edition. American Physical Therapy Association. *Phys Ther* 81:9–746, 2001.
2. Andrews J, Harrelson G, Wilk K: *Physical rehabilitation of the injured athlete*, ed 3, St Louis, 2004, Saunders.
3. Bang MD, Deyle GD: Comparison of supervised exercise with and without manual physical therapy for patients with shoulder impingement syndrome. *J Orthop Sports Phys Ther* 30:126–137, 2000.
4. Barak T, Rosen ER, Sofer R: Basic concepts of orthopaedic manual therapy. In Gould JA, editor: *Orthopaedic and sports physical therapy*, ed 2, St Louis, 1990, Mosby.
5. Bronfort G, Haas M, Evans RL, et al: Efficacy of spinal manipulation and mobilization for low back pain and neck pain: a systematic review and best evidence synthesis. *Spine* 4:335–356, 2004.
6. Conroy DE, Hayes KW: The effect of joint mobilization as a component of compressive treatment for primary shoulder impingement syndrome. *J Orthop Sports Phys Ther* 28:3–14, 1998.
7. Cyriax J: *Textbook of orthopaedic medicine*, vol 1, *Diagnosis of soft tissue lesions*, ed 8, London, 1982, Baillière Tindall.
8. Green T, Refshauge K, Crosbie J, et al: A randomized controlled trial of passive accessory joint mobilization on acute ankle inversion sprains. *Phys Ther* 81:984–994, 2001.
9. Gross AR, Hoving JL, Haines TA, et al: A Cochrane review of manipulation and mobilization for mechanical neck disorders. *Spine* 29:1541–1548, 2004.
10. Hoeksma HL, Dekker J, Ronday HK, et al: Comparison of manual therapy and exercise therapy in osteoarthritis of the hip: a randomized clinical trial. *Arthritis Care Res* 51:722–729, 2004.
11. Hurwitz EL, Aker PD, Adams AH, et al: Manipulation and mobilization of the cervical spine: a systematic review of the literature. *Spine* 21:1746–1759, 1996.
12. Kaltenborn F: *Mobilization of extremity joints: examination and basic treatment techniques*, Oslo, 1980, Olaf Norlis Bokhandel.
13. Lin CWC, Moseley AM, Haas M, et al: Manual therapy in addition to physiotherapy does not improve clinical or economic outcomes after ankle fracture. *J Rehabil Med* 40:433–439, 2008.

14. MacConaill MA, Basmajian JV: *Muscles and movements: a basis for human kinesiology*, Baltimore, 1969, Williams & Wilkins.
15. Maffey LL: Arthrokinematics and mobilization of musculoskeletal tissue: the principles. In Magee DJ, Zachazewski JE, Quillen WS, editors: *Scientific foundations and principles of practice in musculoskeletal rehabilitation*, St Louis, 2007, Saunders.
16. Magee DJ: *Orthopedic physical assessment*, ed 5, St Louis, 2008, Saunders.
17. Maitland G: *Peripheral manipulation*, ed 2, Newton, MA, 1978, Butterworth-Heinemann.
18. Manske RC, Meschke M, Porter A, et al: A randomized, controlled, single-blinded, comparison of stretching versus stretching and joint mobilization for posterior shoulder tightness measured via internal rotation motion loss. *Sports Health* 2(2):94–100, 2010.
19. Senbursa G, Baltaci G, Atay A: Comparison of conservative treatment with and without manual physical therapy for patients with shoulder impingement syndrome: a prospective, randomized clinical trial. *Knee Surg Sports Traumatol Arthrosc* 15:915–921, 2007.
20. Sran MM, Khan KM, Zhu Q, et al: Failure characteristics of the thoracic spine with a posteroanterior load: investigating the safety of spinal mobilization. *Spine* 29:2382–2388, 2004.
21. Takasaki H, Hall T, Jull G: Immediate and short-term effects of Mulligan's mobilization with movement on knee pain and disability associated with knee osteoarthritis—a prospective case series. *Physiother Theory Pract* 29(2):87–95, 2013.
22. Wooden MJ: Mobilization of the upper extremity. In Donatelli R, Wooden MJ, editors: *Orthopaedic physical therapy*, New York, 1989, Churchill Livingstone.
23. Wright A: Hypoalgesia post-manipulative therapy: a review of a potential neurophysiological mechanism. *Man Ther* 1:11–16, 1995.

REVIEW QUESTIONS

Multiple Choice

1. Which mobilization grade describes a large amplitude motion that occurs at the end of the available range?
   a. I
   b. II
   c. III
   d. IV
2. Which mobilization grades are used for pain relief?
   a. I and II
   b. II and III
   c. III and IV
   d. I and IV
3. What is a normal end-feel for elbow extension?
   a. Soft tissue approximation
   b. Bone-to-bone
   c. Springy
   d. Empty
4. Which of the following is not an accessory joint motion?
   a. Glide
   b. Spin
   c. Lift
   d. Roll
5. At what rate do manually applied joint oscillations typically occur?
   a. 1 to 3 per second
   b. 5 to 7 per second
   c. 10 to 20 per minute
   d. 20 to 40 per minute
6. Which of the following is not considered a relative contraindication for mobilization?
   a. Osteoporosis
   b. Joint pain and hypomobility
   c. Joint hypermobility
   d. Rheumatoid arthritis
7. Which end-feel is described by significant pain and an absence of a mechanical restriction?
   a. Bone-to-bone
   b. Empty
   c. Loose
   d. Capsular
8. Which term refers to the amount of normal looseness found in nonpathologic joint capsules?
   a. Slack
   b. Capsularity
   c. Deformation
   d. Hypermobility
9. Which type of traction involves actual stretching of soft tissues?
   a. Stage I
   b. Stage II
   c. Stage III
   d. Piccolo
10. In which position are the joint capsule and ligaments most relaxed and loose with the maximum amount of joint play?
    a. Functional
    b. Close-packed
    c. Open-packed
    d. Resting
11. Which joint position is best characterized as stable?
    a. Functional
    b. Close-packed
    c. Open-packed
    d. Resting
12. Which arthrokinematic motion is similar to a car wheel sliding on ice when brakes are applied?
    a. Gliding
    b. Spinning
    c. Rolling
    d. Skidding
13. A bucked medial meniscus is an example of which of the following causes of a noncapsular pattern?
    a. Ligamentous adhesions
    b. Internal derangement
    c. Extraarticular lesion
    d. External derangement
14. Terminal knee extension normally results in which type of end-feel?
    a. Empty
    b. Loose
    c. Hard or springy tissue stretch
    d. Bone-to-bone
15. What is the closed-packed position of the glenohumeral joint?
    a. Abduction and lateral rotation
    b. Extension and medial rotation
    c. Flexion and horizontal adduction
    d. Scaption and medial rotation

Short Answer

16. What is the difference between osteokinematics and arthrokinematics?

17. What are the three main types of arthrokinematic movement?
18. What are closed-packed and open-packed positions of a joint?
19. What are three possible causes of noncapsular pattern joint restriction?
20. What does the literature say about the benefits of manual therapy for the hip?

Fill in the Blank

21. When the concave surface is stationary and the convex surface is moving, the gliding movement in the joint occurs in a direction _____________ to the bone movement.
22. When the convex surface is fixed and the concave surface is mobile, the gliding motion occurs in the _____________ direction as the bone movement.
23. _____________ motions, such as hip and shoulder flexion, occur in the cardinal planes of movement such as frontal, sagittal, and transverse.
24. _____________ are passive, skilled manual therapy techniques applied to joints and related soft tissues at varying amplitudes using physiologic motions for therapeutic purposes.
25. Typically, a mobilization grade technique is applied for _____________ seconds only four or five times.

True/False

26. When performing joint ROM, the PTA should encourage the patient to perform all accessory joint motions.
27. The "close-packed" joint position is best used for determining joint stability.
28. The "loose-packed" position is best used for joint mobilization techniques.
29. A patient is being seen immediately after surgery when pain may be significant. If joint mobilization is an appropriate treatment method, it is usually appropriate to use grade I and II mobilizations to help decrease pain.
30. Grade I and II mobilizations are primarily intended to reduce pain as opposed to stretch tissue.

Chapter 16

Biomechanics and Kinesiology

Michael Hales

CHAPTER OUTLINE

LEARNING OBJECTIVES

1. Discuss the basic structure and function of human bone.
2. Define joint architecture and joint movement terminology.
3. Describe functional and structural aspects and the contraction mechanics of skeletal muscle.
4. Describe rhythmic and arrhythmic muscle contraction common with rehabilitation.
5. Define and apply biomechanical concepts in the description of rudimentary movement patterns.
6. Discuss the difference between the kinematics and the kinetics of movement.
7. Identify and discuss the kinematic principles as related to movement in a rehabilitation setting.
8. Discuss the linear and angular kinematics and kinetics of movement, and explain how angular motion translates to linear movements.
9. Describe the differences among the different levers, and explain the concept of mechanical advantage as related to levers.
10. Describe Newton's laws of motion.
11. Identify and discuss the different forces that act on objects and how the forces affect movement.
12. Discuss the concepts of mechanical loading, and describe how loading is associated with different types of injuries.
13. Discuss the principles of mechanical energy.
14. Describe the concept of equilibrium, and identify the factors that contribute to stability.

KEY TERMS

All-or-none
Concentric
Eccentric
Fast-twitch
Force
Force couple
Friction
Inertia
Motor unit
Slow-twitch
Stress
Velocity

The field of kinesiology combines the study of applied human anatomy and physiology with the study of mechanical physics. These combined sciences allow for detailed descriptions of how and why the human body moves the way it does and why a person may or may not have sustained an injury. Understanding the neuromuscular and mechanical factors associated with human movement provides the physical therapy assistant (PTA) with the knowledge and skills necessary for administering rehabilitative techniques correctly and performing patient assistive lifting tasks safely. These kinesiologic descriptions help health professionals to refine their knowledge and their approach to injury rehabilitation as well as to consider new and innovative techniques that may lead to improved rehabilitation processes. This information also provides insight into the mechanical causes of injuries, potentially leading to safer participation as individuals interact with the environment.

A subdiscipline of kinesiology known as biomechanics is the study of the internal and external forces acting on the body and the effects these forces produce. The data obtained from biomechanical research provide a great deal of insight into human movement interactions in fields such as physical and occupational therapy, sports medicine, human factors, prosthetics, orthotics, and ergonomics.[17,55] Clinical biomechanics provides direct measures of human motion, which influence our knowledge of injury mechanics, rehabilitation, treatment, and prevention. This information can directly affect how a PTA rehabilitates a patient, an orthopedist repairs a broken limb or ruptured ligament, an athletic trainer implements modalities for treatment, or a clinician evaluates an individual's gait.[26,29,37]

Kinesiology can provide the health professional with a better understanding and a broadened knowledge of the causes and degrees of severity associated with an injury. To improve on a current rehabilitative technique, repair procedure, or treatment process, the mechanics associated with the causation of the injury must be fully understood. To help the health professional accomplish this task, several factors need to be considered when determining the cause and severity of an injury:[63]

- How much force was applied? (magnitude)
- Where on the body was the force applied? (location)
- Where was the force directed? (direction)
- How long was the force applied? (duration)
- How often was the force applied? (frequency)
- Does the force application vary in magnitude? (variability)
- How quickly is the force applied? (rate)

The major role of a PTA revolves around the causes and the effects of human motion, and it is imperative to have a fundamental understanding of the physiologic and mechanical basis for whole body or segmental movement. Because biomechanics is concerned with the effects of forces on the human body, physiologic and anatomic principles are involved in force production. This chapter offers an overview of the sciences included in understanding human movement with practical applications for the PTA.

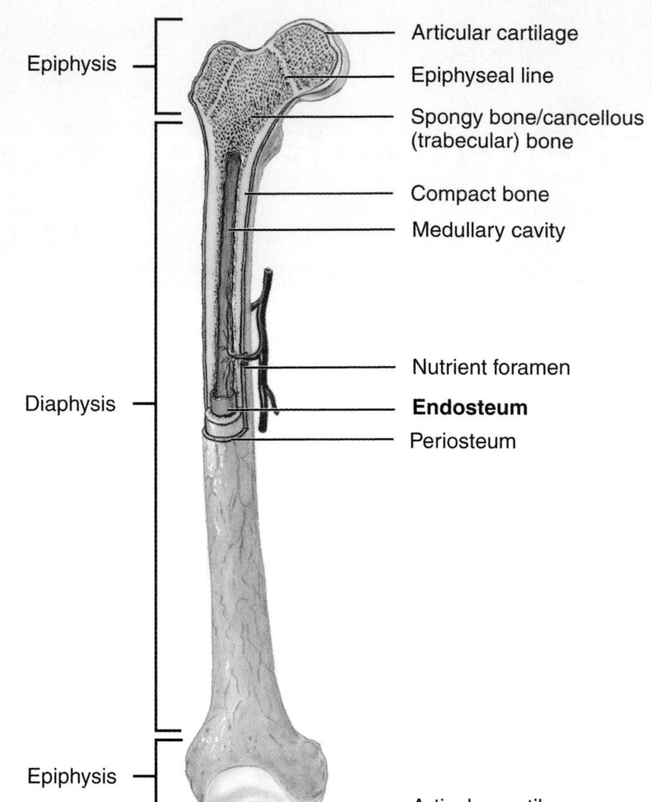

FIG 16-1 Structural components of human bone. *(From Applegate E: The anatomy and physiology learning system, ed 2, Philadelphia, 2000, Saunders.)*

FUNCTIONAL ANATOMY

The skeletal system makes up the framework of the human body, similar to support beams of a building and the chassis of an automobile. These analogies are simplistic and inadequate because these inanimate structures supply structural support only. In addition to a structural role, human bone has a physiologic function. Human bone is a living, dynamic tissue. When the previously mentioned inanimate structures have high loads placed on them, wood beams become stressed and weakened over time, and the chassis or suspension of an automobile may fatigue or fracture. However, living bone has the capability of adapting to large forces by increasing strength and stiffness or the ability to heal a damaged area (i.e., microfractures) resulting from overstress.[1,33,61]

BONE COMPOSITION AND JOINT STRUCTURE

The composition of human bone is designed to fulfill its mechanical and physiologic functions; it is strong but lightweight. A useful analogy for bone is the composite material used to manufacture wheelchair components and joint braces known as carbon fiber reinforced polymer (CFRP), which consists of a carbon fiber matrix cured in an epoxy resin. The final product, CFRP, has mechanical properties that are superior to the properties of its individual components. CFRP, similar to bone, has a high strength-to-weight ratio. Human bone is also the product of several elements (collagen, calcium salts, and water).[1,2,10,14] Individually, these components are not very strong; however, when combined into a single unit, they create a very sturdy but lightweight tissue with the ability to adapt.[14,33,51] Figure 16-1 shows the structural components of human bone where the exterior portion of bone is composed of cortical or trabecular (compact, dense) tissue; the interior portion is composed of cancellous (spongy, latticelike) tissue.[14,49] The fact that bones are a living tissue means that they can hypertrophy owing to load-bearing physical activity or atrophy as a result of immobilization secondary to injury.[51]

The system of joints between the bones is called the *articular system* because the union of bones is an articulation or a *joint*. Anatomic joints may be classified as fibrous, cartilaginous, or synovial. Most joints in the human body articulate, which means they are capable of movement, but they must also provide stability during movement.[23,54,57] The movable joint is known as synovial, which consists of various types of connective tissue that hold and cushion the ends of the bones.[23,27,57] Joints of inanimate objects and structures are simple joints compared with the joints in the human body. This is evident in prostheses research and design because even with all of the

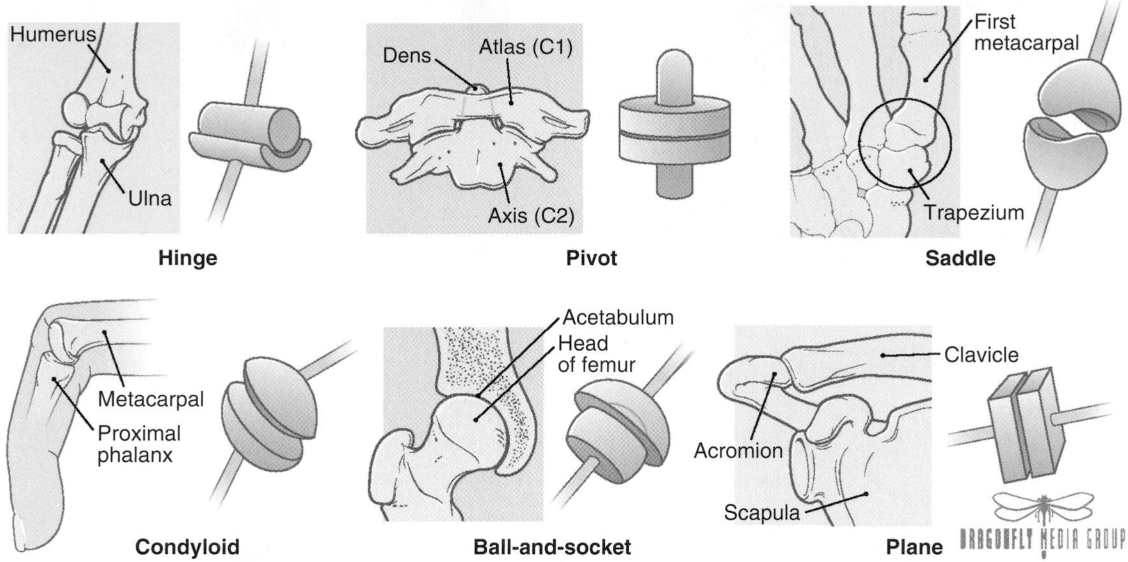

FIG 16-2 Six synovial joint types: hinge, pivot, saddle, condyloid, ball-and-socket, and plane. *(From Hansen J:* Netter's clinical anatomy, *Philadelphia, 2010, Saunders.)*

engineering and medical advances, engineers are still trying to replicate biologic articulations.[34,64] The development of prostheses is progressing rapidly, but replacement joints still do not function as well as natural joints.[25,27] Most of the major joints a PTA needs to be familiar with—shoulder, elbow, knee, ankle, and vertebrae—are examples of synovial joints, which are the focus of the chapter.

Articular cartilage is on the ends of the bones forming the joint. Forming the inner layer of the joint capsule is the synovial membrane. An analogy of a synovial joint capsule is a wheelchair wheel consisting of spokes, rim, and tire.[1] The rubber tire represents the articular cartilage, the composite rim represents the outer surface of bone, and the spokes represent the cross-hatch orientation of collagen fibers. A synovial joint (articulation) can be categorized into one of six different structural types, each especially designed to accommodate the movements of the particular segment of the body (Fig. 16-2).

BOX 16-1 Basic Directional Terms Used to Describe Body Parts or Other Objects in Relation to the Body

- Anterior: Toward the front of the body
- Posterior: Toward the back of the body
- Deep: Toward the inside (core) of the body
- Superficial: Toward the surface (skin) of the body
- Distal: Away from the body or torso
- Proximal: Closer to the body or torso
- Inferior: Toward the feet
- Superior: Toward the head
- Lateral: Away from the midline of the body
- Medial: Toward the midline of the body

REFERENCE TERMINOLOGY

To facilitate the process of describing human movement, standardized terminology has been adopted to identify body positions and directions of motion (Box 16-1). Movements are defined based on a reference or starting position often referred to as the *anatomic position* (Fig. 16-3, *A*), which is a standing position with arms at one's side and palms facing forward. From the anatomic position, three imaginary cardinal planes bisect the body along three dimensions (Fig. 16-3, *B*). The transverse or horizontal plane segments the body into upper and lower parts; the frontal or coronal plane separates the body into front and back parts; and the sagittal or anteroposterior plane divides the body into right and left parts. The planes do not divide the body into equal parts. However, when the segments are equal, the midintersection point of the transverse, frontal, and sagittal planes is referred to as the *center of mass* or *center of gravity*. Although human movement is not restricted to a single plane, most named movements (e.g., flexion and abduction) are described based on the three cardinal planes.

Movements in the transverse plane occur around the longitudinal axis, which runs superiorly-inferiorly while perpendicularly intersecting the transverse plane. These movements include medial and lateral rotation of the leg, thigh, and shoulder; supination and pronation of the forearm; and horizontal abduction and adduction of the shoulder. Movements in the frontal plane occur around the sagittal axis, which runs anteriorly-posteriorly while perpendicularly intersecting the frontal plane. These movements include abduction and adduction of the shoulder and hip, lateral flexion of the neck and trunk, elevation and depression of the shoulder girdle, and inversion and eversion of the foot. Movements in the sagittal plane occur around the frontal axis, which runs from left to right while perpendicularly intersecting the sagittal plane. These movements include flexion and extension of the knee, hip, trunk, elbow, shoulder, and neck and dorsiflexion and plantar flexion of the foot as well as hyperextension movements. A key role of the PTA is to facilitate

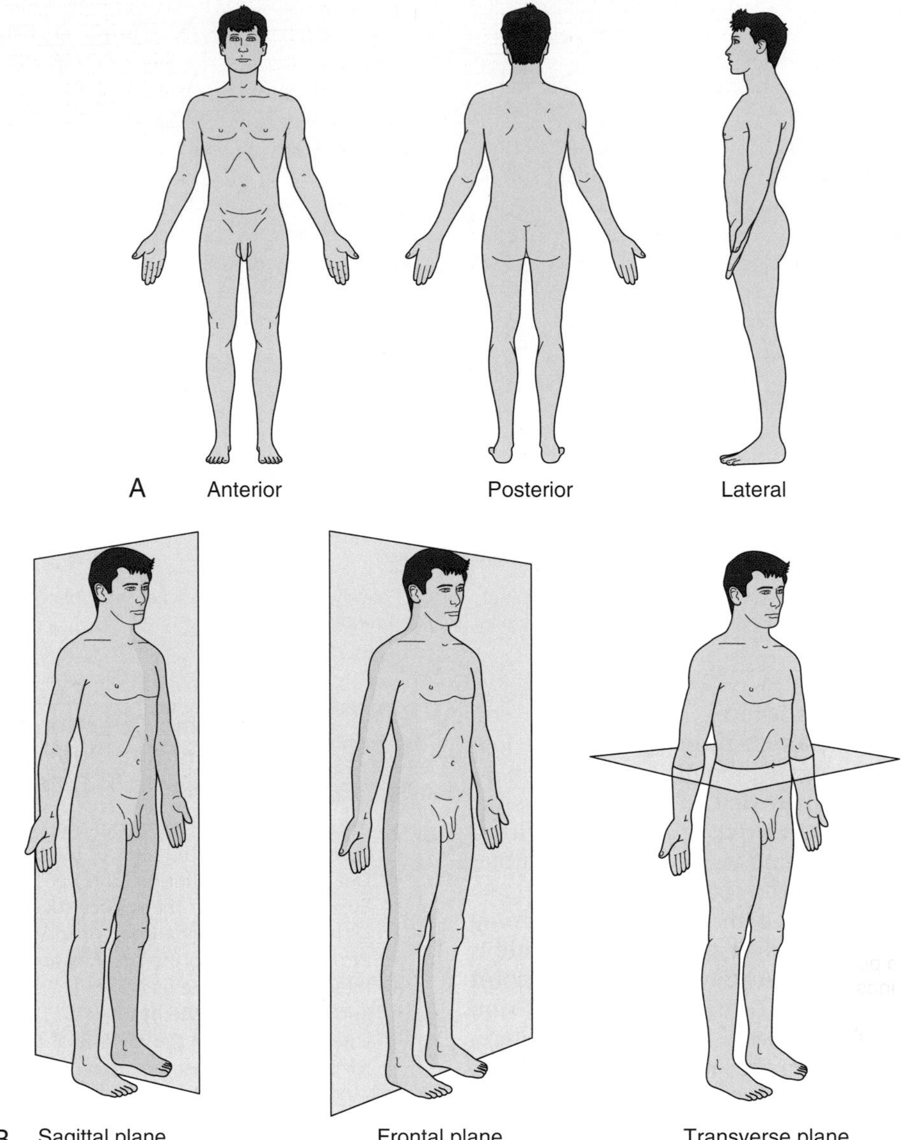

FIG 16-3 **A,** Anatomic reference position for human motion. **B,** Sagittal, frontal, and transverse planes. *(Modified from Cameron MH, Monroe LG:* Physical rehabilitation: evidence-based examination, evaluation, and intervention, *St Louis, 2007, Saunders.)*

patient rehabilitation through the incorporation of various exercises using basic movement patterns. It is important to be familiar with the appropriate terminology for these movements (Fig. 16-4).

Segmental movements are named according to the articulation where the movement occurs and not the segment performing the movement (e.g., hip extension rather than thigh extension).[31] Most movements of the segments occurring at the joint can be categorized according to the plane of movement and the joint's axis of rotation. With the exception of the transverse (horizontal) motions occurring at the shoulder and hip joints, the movement description is defined from the anatomic position.[31] Tables 16-1 through 16-3 list articulations and their movements that occur around the respective axis and its respective plane.

Lastly, when segmental movement is concerned, the joint's axis and plane remain the same regardless of what orientation the body part assumes. For instance, the extension of the elbow occurs around the elbow's mediolateral axis, whether it is extended by the side of the body in the sagittal plane or extended overhead in the frontal plane when the arm is abducted at the shoulder (Fig. 16-5).

STRUCTURE AND FUNCTION OF SKELETAL MUSCLE

What causes these aforementioned segmental movements? In simple terms, movement is influenced by a highly complex tissue with both mechanical and physiologic properties known as muscle. Muscle tissue is one of the most complex structures in the human body. Muscle has four functional properties: irritability, contractility, extensibility, and elasticity.[31] Because muscle tissue is irritable, it responds to stimulation by contracting, or producing force to pull the origin and insertion of a muscle closer together. Muscle can be extended, or stretched to allow nonrestricted joint movement or potential energy storage. The final property of muscle is its elasticity, which gives it the ability to recoil from stretch.

Three different types of muscle tissue are responsible for body movements. They are classified as skeletal, cardiac, and smooth muscles.[36,49] Each type of muscle has some similar characteristics, but they differ in several ways. The contractile process is generally the same in each type of muscle, but rate of contraction, duration of contraction, type of contraction, and purpose of contraction differ greatly.[36] Although cardiac and smooth muscles are essential to life, they are not directly involved in the study of human movement to which the actions of skeletal muscle are of the most importance. This section describes the structure and function of skeletal muscle.

Wrist—sagittal
Flexion
Exercise: wrist curl
Sport: tennis serve
Extension
Exercise: reverse wrist curl
Sport: racquet backhand

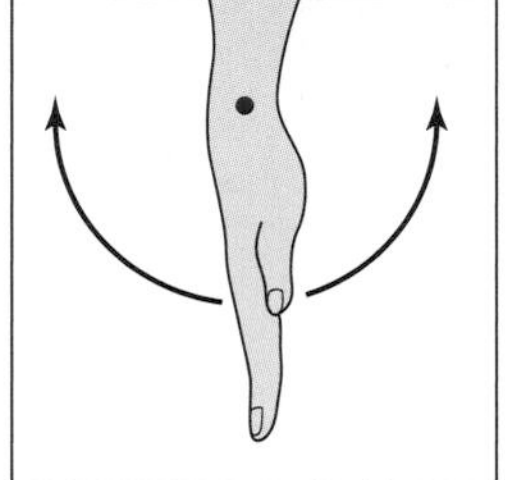

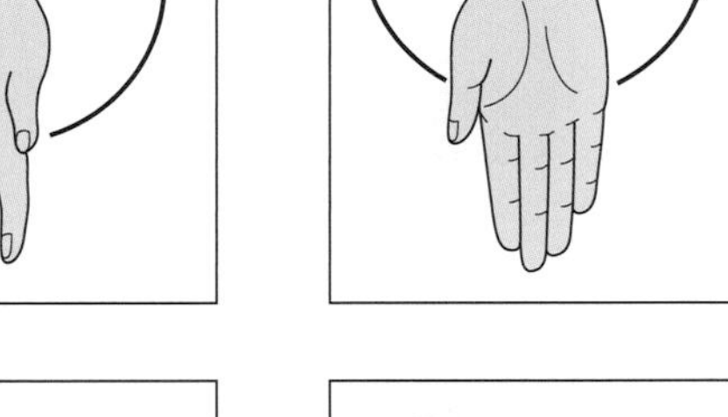

Wrist—frontal
Ulnar deviation
Exercise: specific wrist curl
Sport: baseball batting
Radial deviation
Exercise: specific wrist curl
Sport: golf backswing

Elbow—sagittal
Flexion
Exercise: arm curl
Sport: rowing
Extension
Exercise: triceps pushdown
Sport: boxing jab

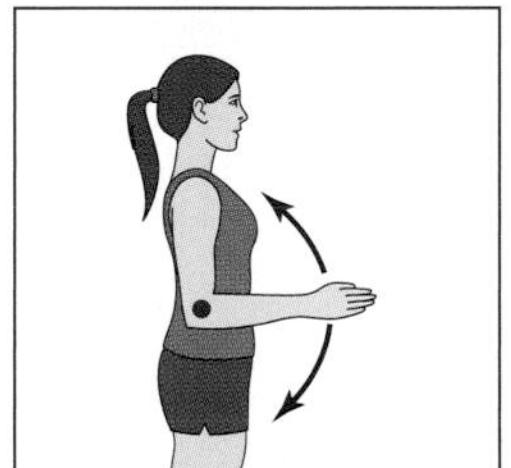

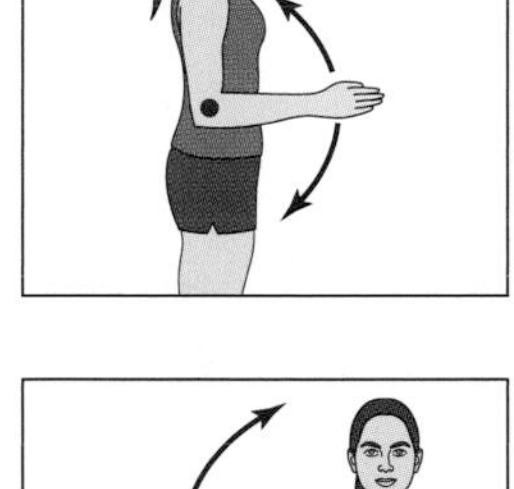

Shoulder—sagittal
Flexion
Exercise: medium-grip military press
Sport: softball pitch
Extension
Exercise: narrow-grip row
Sport: freestyle swimming

Shoulder—frontal
Adduction
Exercise: wide-grip pulldown
Sport: gymnastic rings
Abduction
Exercise: wide-grip military press
Sport: springboard diving

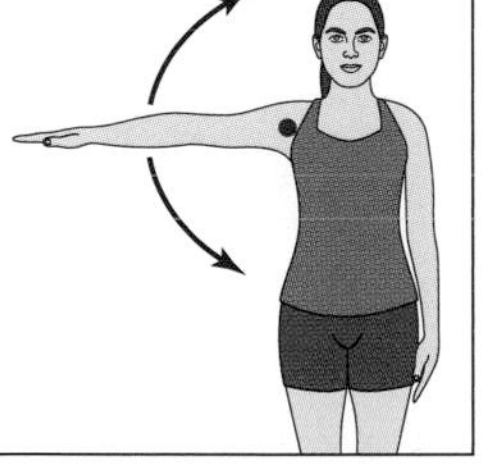

Shoulder—transverse
Internal rotation
Exercise: arm wrestle movement (with dumbbell or cable)
Sport: baseball pitch
External rotation
Exercise: reverse arm wrestle movement
Sport: karate block

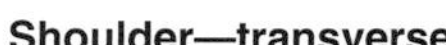

Shoulder—transverse
(upper arm 90° to trunk)
Adduction
Exercise: wide-grip bench press
Sport: boxing hook
Abduction
Exercise: row (elbows high)
Sport: tennis backhand

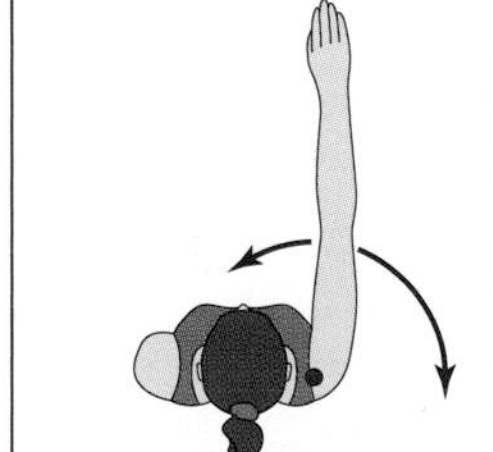

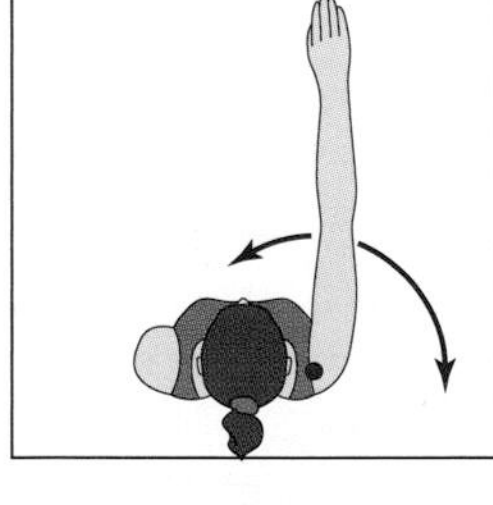

Neck—sagittal
Flexion
Exercise: neck machine
Sport: somersault
Extension
Exercise: neck machine
Sport: wrestling bridge

Neck—transverse
Left rotation
Exercise: neck machine
Sport: wrestling
Right rotation
Exercise: neck machine
Sport: wrestling

Neck—frontal
Left tilt
Exercise: neck machine
Sport: wrestling
Right tilt
Exercise: neck machine
Sport: wrestling

FIG 16-4 Major movements of body segments. *(With permission from Harman EA, Johnson M, Frykman PN: A movement oriented approach to exercise prescription,* NSCA Journal *14(1):47–54, 1992.)*

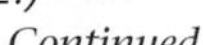

Continued

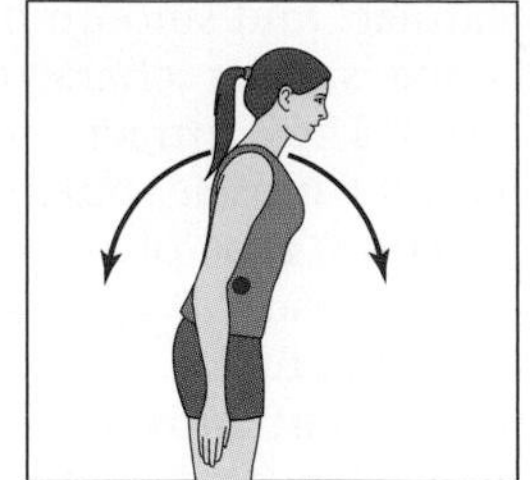
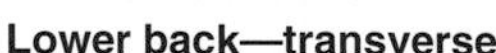
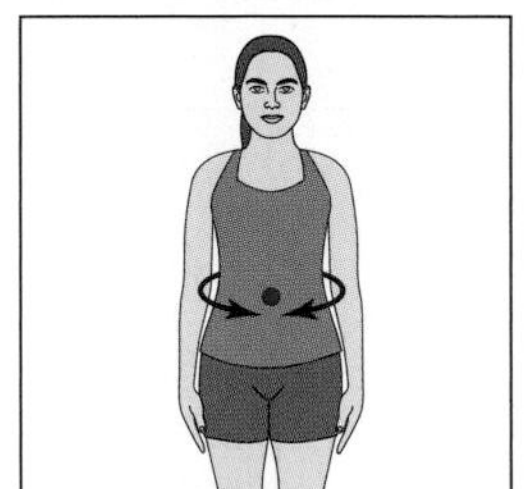
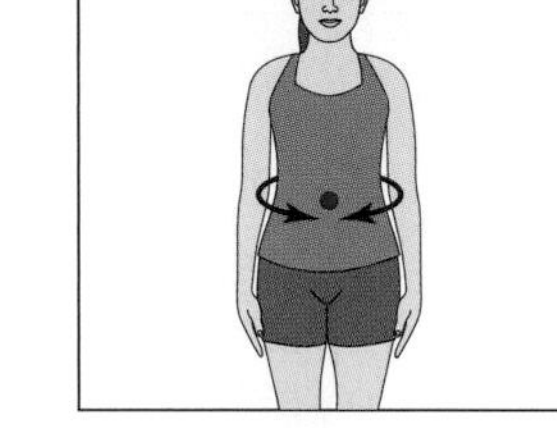
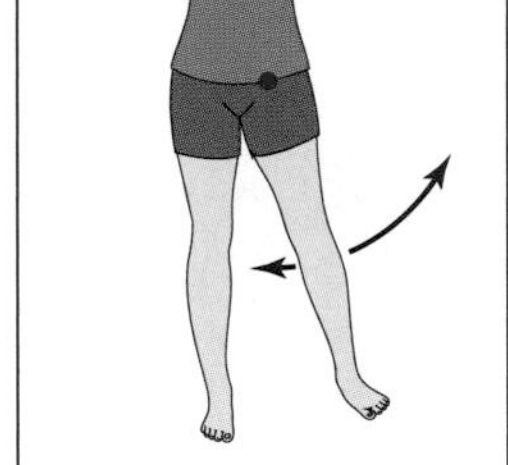
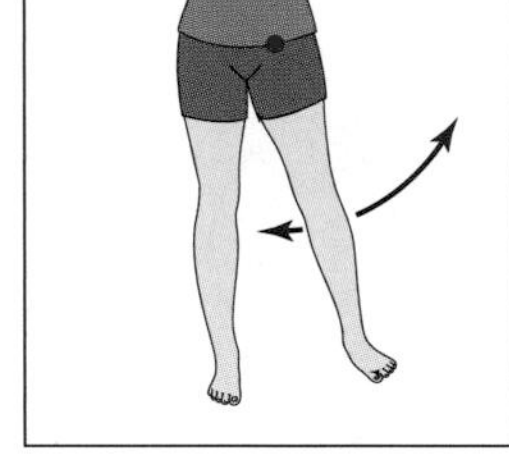
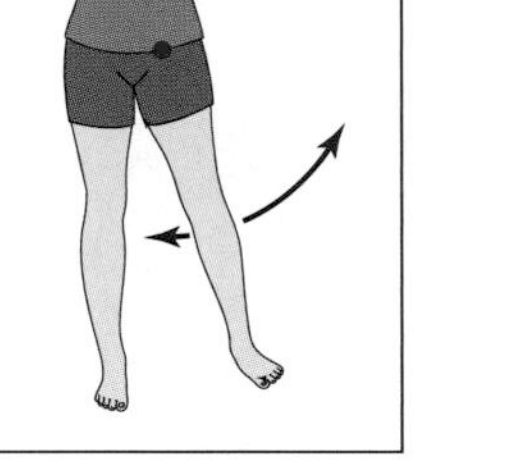
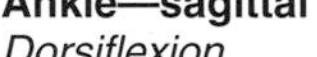
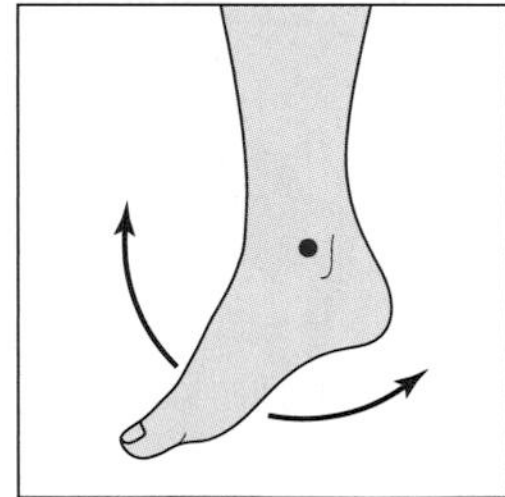

FIG 16-4, cont'd

Skeletal muscles vary in size, ranging in length from less than 1 inch to more than 2 feet.[36,44] Skeletal muscles also vary in shape. Some are long and slender, whereas others are short, round, flat, or fan-shaped. Each muscle is composed of a fiber or fibers (cells). Muscle fibers are the basic units of muscle structure. Each fiber is enclosed by a membrane called the sarcolemma. Underneath the sarcolemma is a plasma membrane, which has the capacity to transmit nerve impulses throughout the fiber.[36] A single muscle fiber contains many long, thin parts called myofibrils arranged in organized bundles. The myofibrils are composed of two contractile proteins: myosin and actin.[43,47,49]

MECHANICAL AND PHYSIOLOGIC ASPECTS OF MUSCLE CONTRACTION

Fibers of a skeletal muscle are organized into **motor units**. Each motor unit consists of a single motor neuron and the muscle fiber or fibers it innervates. The number of fibers in a motor unit can range from a single fiber to

TABLE 16-1 Segmental Movements Occurring Around a Mediolateral Axis and Along a Sagittal Plane

Movement Names	Articulations
Flexion, extension, and hyperextension	Hip, knee, shoulder, elbow, wrist, phalangeal joints, and vertebral column
Dorsiflexion and plantar flexion	Ankle joint

From Kreighbaum E, Barthels KM: *Biomechanics: a qualitative approach for studying human movement,* 4th ed., Boston, MA, 1996, Allyn & Bacon.

TABLE 16-2 Segmental Movements Occurring Around an Anteroposterior Axis and Along a Frontal Plane

Movement Names	Articulations
Lateral flexion	Vertebral column
Abduction and adduction	Shoulder, hip, and metatarsophalangeal joints
Radial and ulnar flexion (deviation)	Wrist joint
Elevation and depression	Sternoclavicular joint

From Kreighbaum E, Barthels KM: *Biomechanics: a qualitative approach for studying human movement,* 4th ed., Boston, MA, 1996, Allyn & Bacon.

TABLE 16-3 Segmental Movements Occurring Around a Longitudinal Axis and Along a Transverse Plane

Movement Names	Articulations
Medial and lateral rotation	Shoulder and hip joints, knee joint at 90° flexion
Pronation and supination	Radioulnar joint
Transverse rotation	Vertebral column
Protraction and retraction	Sternoclavicular joint
Inversion and eversion	Subtalar joint

From Kreighbaum E, Barthels KM: *Biomechanics: a qualitative approach for studying human movement,* 4th ed., Boston, MA, 1996, Allyn & Bacon.

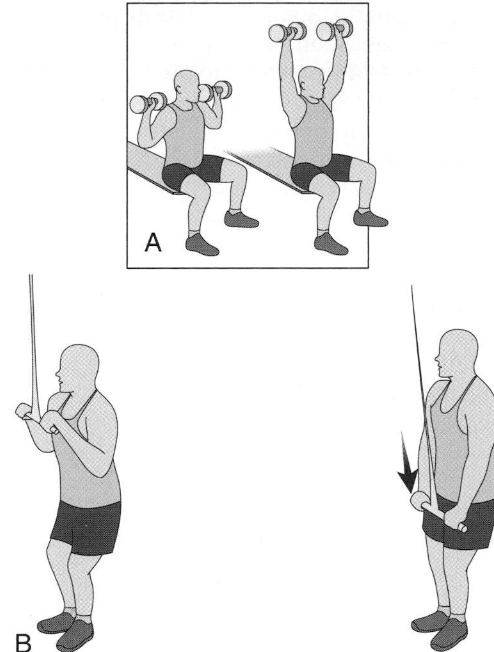

FIG 16-5 Demonstration of elbow extension while **(A)** performing a shoulder press exercise in the frontal plane and **(B)** performing a triceps push-down exercise in the sagittal plane.

Important Concepts

In looking at muscle activity between the upper rectus abdominis (RA) and lower RA during five different exercises (the isometric portion of curl-ups, abdominal muscle lifts, leg raises, and restricted or attempted leg raises and curl-ups), no difference can be found between upper RA and lower RA activity. When comparing the relative amount of muscle activity in the RA while performing the crunch versus a few other common body-weight exercises (yoga boat pose, stability ball crunch, decline bench curl-up, captain's chair crunch, bicycle crunch, side plank, and front plank) and exercises performed with several pieces of abdominal training equipment (Ab Circle Pro, Ab Roller, Ab Lounge, Perfect Sit-Up, Ab Coaster, Ab Rocket, Ab Wheel, and Ab Straps), no exercise showed higher activity in the RA relative to the crunch. Muscle activity of the RA cannot be isolated into upper, middle, or lower sections, but there are certain exercises that have the potential to stimulate the RA muscle more than other abdominal exercises.

hundreds. Muscle contraction begins when a motor neuron transmits an impulse, or action potential, and all of the muscle fibers that it innervates are simultaneously activated and develop force.[11] The extent of control and magnitude of muscle force depend on the number of muscle fibers within each motor unit. Motor units involved in movements requiring a high degree of precision and accuracy (i.e., eye muscle) may have only one fiber per motor neuron.[11,40] In contrast, the quadriceps muscle group, which moves the leg with less precision during walking, may have several hundred muscle fibers per motor neuron.

To understand the excitation-contraction process fully, one must realize an action potential is not capable of directly exciting the muscle fibers. Instead, the motor neuron excites the muscle fiber or fibers that it innervates by chemical transmission. The arrival of the action potential at the motor junction causes a release of a neurotransmitter, acetylcholine, which diffuses across the neuromuscular junction, causing the excitation of the sarcolemma; this initiates the stimulated muscle fibers to contract.[49] The action potential causes calcium to be released into the interior of the muscle fiber, and the contraction continues until the calcium is removed. The presence of calcium allows the myosin and actin to interact, and this causes them to develop tension. If an action potential is strong enough to initiate a contraction, all of the muscle fibers in a motor unit are stimulated and develop force at the same time.[49] Similarly, a stronger action potential cannot produce a stronger contraction. This phenomenon is known as the **all-or-none** principle.[1] It is analogous to pressing a floor selection button in an elevator. When a sufficient amount of pressure is placed on the selector button, the elevator moves; however, pressing the button harder will not cause the elevator to go faster.

A common method is to classify muscle fibers based on twitch time, employing the terms *slow twitch* (type I) and *fast twitch* (type IIA and type IIX).[52,53,58] A **fast-twitch** fiber is one that develops tension and relaxes rapidly and has a short twitch time. In contrast, a **slow-twitch** fiber develops tension and relaxes slowly and has a long twitch time. The fiber types differ with respect to contraction speed, relaxation speed, force production, capillary density, and fiber diameter.[53] The contrast in mechanical characteristics is accompanied by a distinct difference in the ability of the fibers to use energy for muscle contraction and to resist fatigue. It is theorized that motor units are recruited in an orderly manner governed by force production capacity and stimulus threshold. Before a high-threshold motor unit is recruited, all of the motor units below it are recruited sequentially (type I → type IIA → type IIX).[1,49] During the initial stages of resistance exercise used in rehabilitation programs, when loads are relatively light, only slow-twitch muscle fibers are recruited. However, as the patient recovers and is able to lift heavier loads, both slow-twitch and fast-twitch muscle fibers are recruited.

Important Concepts

All humans are born with a predetermined percentage of fast-twitch and slow-twitch muscle fibers (most people are pretty close to half and half). Although a person cannot change the actual number of fast-twitch and slow-twitch muscle fibers they possess, they can improve the function of the muscle fibers they train. For example, if an individual works hard to train his or her fast-twitch muscles but ignores slow-twitch muscles, the fast-twitch fibers will hypertrophy, and the slow-twitch fibers will atrophy. The individual may end up with 65% of muscle mass consisting of fast-twitch fibers and 35% consisting of slow-twitch fibers, but the actual number of each fiber type the individual has will be the same as it was before starting the training program.

If a muscle undergoes a contraction, it is implied to be the primary mover or agonist for the resulting joint movement. For example, if a patient is performing a leg extension exercise to strengthen the quadriceps muscle group, the quadriceps muscle is considered the agonist muscle. The opposing muscle group (hamstrings) is the antagonist.[36,43,44] The agonist and antagonist muscle groups must work in concert with one another to produce a smooth, coordinated, and controlled movement. When the agonist muscle group contracts to produce movement at an articulation, the antagonist must relax to allow full range of motion (ROM) to occur. The coordinated muscle contraction can be classified as either dynamic or static. The two types of dynamic contraction are called concentric and eccentric. When a muscle contracts and shortens, it causes movement of the joint that it crosses—it causes one or both attachments to move closer to the middle of the muscle.[44] This action describes a **concentric** ("moving to the center") muscle contraction. In contrast, when a muscle contracts and lengthens, it causes the attachments to move farther away from the middle of the muscle.[44] This action is described as an **eccentric** ("away from the center") muscle contraction. The third type of muscle contraction is called *isometric*. During an isometric contraction, there is muscular tension, but no noticeable movement (static) occurs between body segments.[44]

RHYTHMIC AND ARRHYTHMIC CONTRACTIONS

Under normal conditions, the contraction of a healthy muscle is smooth and fluid because the responses of the motor units are out of phase with each other, continuously alternating. In contrast, if the activity of the motor units becomes simultaneous in an agonist and an antagonist, rigidity is observed. The types of contractions a PTA may encounter while rehabilitating a patient include contracture, cramps, muscle spasm, and spasticity.

A state of prolonged resistance to passive stretch in a muscle is called *contracture*. Myostatic (stiff muscle) contracture is a condition affecting connective tissues of a muscle or joint that results from immobilization of the muscle. Examples of myostatic contractures occur after a limb has been casted, after a tendon has been severed or detached, or after antagonistic muscles have been paralyzed.[48]

Another type of an abnormal muscle contraction that is observed during exercise or during sleep by individuals experiencing involuntary, sustained, painful contraction is termed *muscle cramp*. The causes of muscle cramps are poorly understood and in many instances are impossible to identify. Cramps may be caused by local fatigue, rapid changes in deep muscle temperature, extreme effort at sustained muscular contraction, and imbalance of ions caused by excessive perspiring. Remedies include rest, warm-up, massage, fluid and electrolyte intake, and passive stretching. A milder version of a muscle cramp is called a *muscle spasm*, which tends to be less severe and more persistent.

Spasticity is a muscle control disorder that is characterized by overly tight or stiff muscles displaying an inability to control muscle contractions. These uncontrollable muscle contractions may persist for a long time and may be very forceful.[35] The PTA may encounter this hyperactive muscle contraction when treating patients with a spinal cord injury. Caution is needed when employing a resistance exercise program with a patient with a spinal cord injury to avoid a serious injury in rehabilitation. Overhead free weight exercises should be avoided in case the muscles in use lose control of their actions.

APPLIED KINESIOLOGY

To facilitate the discussion involving kinesiologic principles, a working understanding of various rudimentary concepts is essential. Following are definitions of some common terms along with their appropriate unit of measure. Most of these terms are discussed in more detail as various biomechanical concepts are introduced.

Mass (m) is the amount of matter an object possesses within its physical boundaries; generally, the denser the material the object comprises, the greater the mass. For example, muscle tissue is denser than fat tissue; two persons of equal size or volume may differ in mass if one is more muscular than the other.

Inertia is the resistance an object offers to a change in its state of motion (**velocity**) or direction of motion and is directly related to its mass. The greater the mass of the object, the more resistance it offers to any attempt at changing its velocity or direction of motion.

Force (F) is a push or pull acting on an object. A force has direction and magnitude, and it is commonly expressed in newtons (N). Forces applied to objects, if sufficient to overcome their inertia, cause them to accelerate in direct proportion to the magnitude of the force.

Friction is created when two objects are in direct contact with one another and a force acts to impede motion of the objects. Frictional force can be increased or decreased by adding substances between the two surfaces, such as the installation of tennis balls on the rear support for walkers. Joint damage (osteoarthritis) caused by chronic exposure to high frictional forces can lead to arthroplasty.

Kinetic energy (KE) is energy by virtue of an object's motion. Joules (J) are the units typically used for KE; however, one may also use newton-meters (N-m), which are equivalent units (i.e., 1 N-m = 1 J). An injury mechanism is predominantly due to the transfer of KE to the body arising from different sources under various conditions: from blunt trauma (impact of an object colliding with the body), penetrating trauma, acceleration/deceleration motion (rapidly moving forward and backward), and crushing weight (high compression forces).

Potential energy is energy generated by virtue of the position or shape of an object. Potential energy may be affected by how much elastic energy is generated by either stretching or compressing the object (e.g., cartilage, tendon, connective tissue) such that if the distorting force is removed, the object recoils to its resting length. The units typically used for potential energy are J; however, one may also use N-m.

Torque (T) is the product of the force and the perpendicular distance from the line of action to the axis point, also called *lever arm length.* Torque is considered a rotary force and more specifically a measure of the ability of a force to cause rotation. Consequently, torque can be increased or decreased easily by altering the length of the moment arm of the force. A **force couple** is formed in situations in which there are two torques that are equal in magnitude but opposite in direction. The resultant action of a force couple is rotation without any translation. Torque is typically expressed in units of N-m.

Work (W) is the product of force and the distance the object moves. If no displacement of the object occurs, even though force may have been applied to the object, no work was done. The unit of measure is N-m or J.

Power (P) is the rate of performing work and can be expressed algebraically as the product of force and displacement over time. If work is accomplished very quickly (i.e., in a very short amount of time), a higher magnitude of power is generated compared with the same amount of work being done over a longer interval of time. Given this explanation, power is work divided by time. Power is expressed in watts (w), and 1 w is equal to 1 J of work per second.

Pressure (p) is a measure of the distribution of a force over a given area (force/area), and it is expressed in newtons per meter^2 (N/m^2). An example of the concept of pressure in a rehabilitation setting is the development of decubitus ulcers that commonly occur in patients with diabetes.[5,56,66] Innovations in shoe design help dissipate the forces applied to the foot over a larger area (e.g., reduced pressure) during locomotion, minimizing soft tissue damage and the incidence of ulceration.[8,15,62]

Momentum is the product of mass and velocity used to determine the outcome of collisions between two objects of mass and to determine the ease with which one can stop or change the direction of travel when velocity is present. A motionless object has no momentum. The unit of measure is kilogram × meters/second (kg × m/sec).

Impulse is the product of the force magnitude and the force application time interval expressed in newton × seconds. The direct relationship between an applied force and the change in momentum it creates is known as the *impulse-momentum principle.* Consider a high force applied to the musculoskeletal system over a very short duration, as is often the case in force-related injuries.

BIOMECHANICAL PRINCIPLES

STATICS AND DYNAMICS

Statics is the branch of mechanics concerned with the analysis of loads (force, torque/moment) on physical systems in static equilibrium. In biomechanics, statics is the study of the body under conditions in which no accelerations or velocity changes are occurring. When acceleration of the body occurs, as is required if a person is to change positions, static conditions would no longer be present. Static conditions are common when considering the immobilization of a joint or when an individual is in traction to immobilize a body segment. A PTA often incorporates proprioceptive neuromuscular facilitation stretching exercises to help a patient regain normal ROM to a joint after injury. During proprioceptive neuromuscular facilitation stretching, a static (isometric) contraction is performed by a patient and health practitioner.

Dynamics is the study of a body segment experiencing accelerations. Body segments increase and decrease in velocity as a particular skill is performed. Varying levels of force are required to produce these accelerations. Depending on the intensity of the exercise, these forces and accelerations may range from very small to very large in magnitude. The legs in walking and running and the arms in wheelchair propulsion are examples of dynamic segments used in performing human activities. A quantified movement analysis can clarify which muscles should be active during a posture or movement in the context of several external forces acting on the body.

LINEAR AND ANGULAR MOTION

Linear motion is the point-to-point, straight-line movement of a body in space. The motion is generally measured in either a two-dimensional or a three-dimensional system depending on the complexity of the activity being monitored. These measures are made in the geometric planes established by the cartesian coordinate system, which are oriented to the human body (local) or Earth (global) or both such that anteroposterior, vertical, and mediolateral measures of motion are described linearly. Forces applied by or on the body in these respective directions lead to accelerations or velocity changes of these body points. Linear forces may be applied by muscles, gravity, the ground, or numerous other animate or inanimate objects.

Angular motion is the measurement of rotation about an axis of a rigid lever and is quantified through the use of a polar coordinate system. This system is generally represented in the human body by body segments; an example is the upper arm rotating about a joint (axis of rotation) such as the shoulder. By tracking over time how the lever, as established by its endpoints (for the upper arm these would be represented by a line connecting the shoulder and elbow), rotates around its proximal joint (the shoulder), one can determine angular positional changes of the lever, rotational velocities of the lever around the joint, and increases and decreases in rotational velocity. These angular measures describe the quality of motion generated angularly by an individual performing an activity of daily living (ADL), occupational activity, or exercise. These angular measures are important because there is a direct link between the quality of angular motion of body segments or levers and the potential for overuse injuries to the subsequent joints. For example, the faster the forearm/racket combination is rotating or extending about the elbow at the instant before impact in a tennis serve, the faster the racket is moving linearly at the moment of impact with the ball. The faster the racket head is moving linearly at impact, the greater the momentum or force imparted to the tennis ball by the athlete. Conversely, because of the high action force and moment, the greater the reaction force and moment imposed on the joints, which could lead to inflammation of the lateral epicondyle (tennis elbow) if poor service mechanics are demonstrated.[30] The rotation of the forearm about the elbow is due in part to the contraction of the muscles (triceps group), which causes acceleration in the direction of elbow extension. The linear force of the triceps tendon pulling on the ulna generates a torque or rotational force. The greater the torque produced by the muscles, the greater the angular acceleration generated, leading to changes in angular velocity that lead to changes in angular position.

KINEMATICS AND KINETICS

Kinematics is the description of human motion in terms of position, velocity, and acceleration. These three variables describe the quality of the motion resulting from forces produced by the muscular system or forces external to the body, such as gravity, other persons, and inanimate objects (e.g., ground, implements). However, the study of kinematics is not concerned with force measurements, and so the magnitude or type of force responsible for generating these human motions is disregarded.

An understanding of kinematic principles is extremely important to PTAs. Analysis of motion can facilitate the determination of the etiology of injury, extent of damage, and assessment of the effectiveness of treatment. Historically, researchers have studied injuries in sport settings, but the same applications are pertinent to nonathletic settings, such as gait analysis of individuals with lower extremity joint injury or joint replacement.[9,13,16,21,42,45] It is imperative for PTAs to be knowledgeable about normal movement patterns from a kinematic perspective to facilitate the recognition of abnormal movements of patients in rehabilitation.

Kinetics is concerned with the forces responsible for maintaining equilibrium and the sources of motion generating the kinematic qualities described earlier. The various forces applied on or by a system can be quantified to determine why a body sustains an injury. This information can lead to very detailed analysis of movement mechanics and injury potential because these forces lead directly to accelerations that cause increases and decreases in velocity, which lead to changes in body position over time.

NEWTON'S LAWS OF MOTION

Much of the basis for kinetics originates from the laws of motion introduced by Sir Isaac Newton (1642-1727) in 1687. Although Newton's theories date back more than 300 years, the basic concepts introduced continue to be used today by biomechanists to provide the explanation for the factors that cause an object to move in a specific manner.[7]

Newton's first law of motion is commonly referred to as the *law of inertia,* which states:

> *"A body remains in a state of rest, or of uniform motion in a straight line, unless it is compelled to change that state by forces impressed on it."*[7]

Inertia of an object describes the reluctance of an object to change its movement pattern—that is, to stay motionless or to move in a linear path unless a force is applied. The amount of inertia an object possesses is related to the mass of the object. As a result, the larger the mass or inertia of an object, the more difficult it is to alter its motion. We can observe the concept of inertia by examining events that occur during car accidents. If an automobile is struck in the rear by another vehicle, the head of the passenger tends to remain at rest momentarily as the body is thrust forward. *Whiplash* is the term used to describe the injury mechanism of the anterior longitudinal ligament.[65] Conversely, when a car strikes an object and is suddenly forced to stop, the passenger continues to move forward because of the person's inertia. This forward motion continues to occur until a force is applied (seat belts and airbags) to counteract the inertia. However, if the passenger is wearing a seat belt but an airbag is either not present or fails to deploy, the head tends to continue moving forward as the body stops. Basilar skull fractures are a common cause of death among race car drivers when their vehicle collides head-on with the race track concrete barrier at extremely high speeds.[37,38]

Newton's second law of motion is commonly referred to as the *law of acceleration,* which states that the change of motion is proportional to the force impressed and is made in the direction of the straight line in which that force is impressed.[7] This law can be expressed algebraically with force (F), mass (m), and acceleration (a):

$$F = m \times a$$

When the equation is rearranged, it yields a useful expression:

$$a = \frac{F}{m}$$

which mathematically illustrates that the acceleration of an object is directly proportional to the force applied and inversely related to mass of the object. Newton's second law is relatively simple with many applications to physical therapy. Because acceleration (motion) is inversely related to mass, basic weight-bearing movements tend to be more challenging for larger patients. In addition, a greater force application is needed for these patients to accomplish said movement. The difficulty in locomotion is compounded if the larger mass of a patient results from too much adipose tissue because adipose tissue does not contribute to force production.

Newton's third law of motion is commonly referred to as the *law of reaction,* which states that to every action there is always opposed an equal reaction, or, the mutual actions of two bodies on each other are always equal and directed to contrary parts.[7] The concept of reaction can be more difficult to visualize than inertia and acceleration, but when a force is applied to an object such as a wall, there is a force opposite in direction and equal in magnitude to the force applied. As the applied force increases, the reaction force likewise increases. From a clinical perspective, reaction forces are of interest during gait analysis. When a patient walks or runs, clinicians may analyze the differences in gait patterns among individuals with varying levels of disability and the subsequent ground reaction forces that occur when the foot strikes the floor. These forces can achieve three times one's body weight during running, and patterns vary based on running style. Physicians and therapists use devices such as orthoses to alter ground reaction force patterns to help minimize foot injuries.[59]

ADVANCED BIOMECHANICAL CONCEPTS

The following advanced concepts highlight several of the major areas that must be considered when evaluating movement skills. These biomechanical principles have direct implications in rehabilitation based on injury causation and level of severity: reaction forces, levers and resistive torque, kinetic link principle, and balance and stability.

REACTION FORCES

Reaction forces are forces applied on a person by a surface with which the person's body is in contact. These forces are applied as an equal and opposite reaction force to the force applied to the surface by the person. The more force generated by the person onto the contact surface, as a result of the person's body weight and musculoskeletal activity, the more force the surface returns to the performer. When analyzing gait abnormalities, ground reaction forces should be measured in relation to a fixed three-dimensional coordinate system oriented at the surface of the platform.[50] The ground reaction force planes of motion are termed *anteroposterior,* which describes forces imposed horizontally directed forward or backward; *mediolateral,* which describes forces generated horizontally side to side; and *vertical,* which describes forces directed upward or downward. In other words, if the person pushes downward on the surface, the surface reacts by pushing upward with equal force. If the person pushes backward on the surface, the surface pushes forward with an equal force. If the person pushes rightward on the surface, the surface pushes leftward with equal force. Other sources for force application are wheelchair pushrims, which are referred to as *pushrim reaction forces.* These multidirectional forces are applied to the hand when in contact with the wheelchair pushrim in an equal and opposite manner. The forces specific to a pushrim are termed *tangential,* which describes forces applied tangent to the pushrim (causes motion); *radial,* which describes forces directed toward the axis of rotation (frictional force); and *mediolateral,* which describes forces directed parallel to the axis of rotation. The forces imposed at the pushrim are transferred to the hand and used to determine subsequent upper extremity joint forces and moments during wheelchair ambulation. Chronic and acute shoulder pain of patients who use manual wheelchairs is one of the foremost issues facing PTAs.[4,6,12]

LEVERS AND RESISTIVE TORQUE

The human body consists of a very poor leverage system when one considers its need to generate large, forceful movements against heavy objects. However, humans are designed with leverage, which allows us to generate high speeds and produce large ROM. In more meaningful terms, because of the structure of the musculoskeletal system with muscle tendon insertion attachment sites occurring very close to the proximal joint of the segment to which they apply force, the human body has very short force lever arms for the muscle to produce torque around the joint. The resistive forces that the muscle must compete against, the weight of a body segment or external object, or both, often have much longer lever arm lengths with which to generate resistive torques. The muscles must be very strong to overcome their poor mechanical leverage when dealing with objects that have great weight or momentum. This is the case when the external object contacts a body segment distal to the body's major torque-producing joints (hip, knee, shoulder, and elbow).

With regard to the ability of the human body to generate speed and ROM, the close attachment of the inserting

Important Concepts

As your journey of learning continues in the area of functional anatomy and kinesiology, you will encounter the mechanical advantage phenomenon. The orientation of most bones and muscles in the human body represent a third-class lever system. The human body is predominantly at a mechanical disadvantage in terms of effort versus load. A small arc of motion at the muscle insertion creates large angular displacement and velocity at a distal segment. Because most human movement is aimed at maximizing angular displacement of a distal segment, the use of third-class levers is the preferred orientation.

A relationship exists between the lever arm distance, distal angular displacement/velocity of a segment, and torque production. The shorter the lever arm of the effort force (decreased mechanical advantage), the greater angular displacement and angular velocity of the distal end of the lever for a given arc of displacement of the effort force; however, with a longer lever arm of the effort force (increased mechanical advantage), there is increased torque production.

tendon to the proximal joint of a segment means that a small amount of muscle shortening through a concentric contraction generates a relatively large rotation of the segment. Were the tendon to attach farther away from the joint, the same amount of muscle shortening would result in a lesser rotation around the joint. When the force production of the muscle is rapid, the large amount of angular displacement generated and the small time in which this displacement occurs means a fast angular velocity for the segment. The linear velocity generated at the end of the lever (i.e., the feet or hands) may be quite large in magnitude.

A lever system includes a fulcrum, which is the point or axis of rotation; an applied force; and a resistance (resistive force). The perpendicular distance from the line of action of the force to the fulcrum is termed the *moment arm of the force* (MF). The perpendicular distance from the line of action of the resistance is termed the *moment arm of the resistance* (MR). A lever may be evaluated based on the computation of its mechanical advantage (MA):

$$MA = \frac{MF}{MR}$$

In a first-class lever, when the fulcrum is located halfway between the point of force and point of resistance on the lever, the MA is equal to 1 (e.g., MF = MR). If the fulcrum is closer to the point of the resistance than the point of force (e.g., MF > MR), the MA becomes greater than 1; a smaller force is necessary to overcome a constant resistance. In the opposite scenario, in which the MF is less than the MR, the MA is less than 1, and a larger force is necessary to move a given resistance. The head tilting backward, initiated by a concentric contraction of the extensor neck muscles (splenius capitis, semispinalis capitis, suboccipital muscles, trapezius) to overcome the resistive force imposed by the weight of the cranium where the fulcrum is the atlantooccipital joint, is an example of a first-class lever system (Fig. 16-6, *A*).

In a second-class lever, the point of resistance is located between the fulcrum and the point of force. The MF is always greater than the MR, yielding a MA greater than 1. This arrangement favors the effort of force because less force is necessary to cause movement of a given resistance. A second-class lever is demonstrated by performing a toe raise exercise. The plantar flexion and dorsiflexion movement can be employed by the PTA to regain ankle ROM after injury or surgery. Resistance can be added to create an exercise designed to strengthen the calf muscles (soleus and gastrocnemius), which represents a second-class lever system (Fig. 16-6, *B*).

In a third-class lever, the point of force is located between the fulcrum and the resistance. The MF always is less than the MR, yielding a MA less than 1. This arrangement favors the effort of resistance because more force is necessary to cause movement of a given resistance. The third-class lever is the more common type of lever found within the human body (Fig. 16-6, *C*). Muscles within the body tend to work under a mechanical disadvantage, resulting in larger internal muscular forces than the mass of the external object (resistance) being moved. Within some joints of the skeletal system, the actual fulcrum point changes through the ROM. Consequently, mechanical advantage and muscle force vary as the length of the moment arm changes. A person performing elbow flexion during a bicep curl exercise depicts a third-class lever system. The olecranon represents the axis of rotation where the biceps muscle group (biceps brachii, brachioradialis, brachialis) exerts a force to overcome the mass of the forearm or any additional resistance held in the hand.

The resistive force, or more specifically the resistive torque, encountered during movements varies based on the length of the resistance arm (moment arm of the resistance). During the performance of a bicep curl exercise, length of the resistance arm is maximized when the elbow is at a 90-degree angle (Fig. 16-7). As the angle increases or decreases, the length of the resistance arm shortens, reducing the magnitude of the resistive torque.[41] Less force is necessary to lift a given resistance when the resistance is closer to the fulcrum (e.g., the resistance arm is reduced). This basic biomechanical principle has numerous applications, including the mechanical function of exercise equipment. Various manufacturers use a pulley system consisting of cam-based pulleys. The unique advantage of a cam compared with a traditional round pulley is the variation in the length of the resistance and force arms during rotation of the pulley. By simply increasing the length of the resistance arm or reducing the length of the force arm, the resistive torque can be increased to provide a variable resistance through the ROM. This relatively simple alteration in design has enhanced the effectiveness of exercise equipment to provide proper loading on muscles throughout the full ROM.

KINETIC LINK PRINCIPLE

The coordination of body movements in sporting activities, occupational skills, or ADL is critical for success. Many terms are used to refer to these coordinated

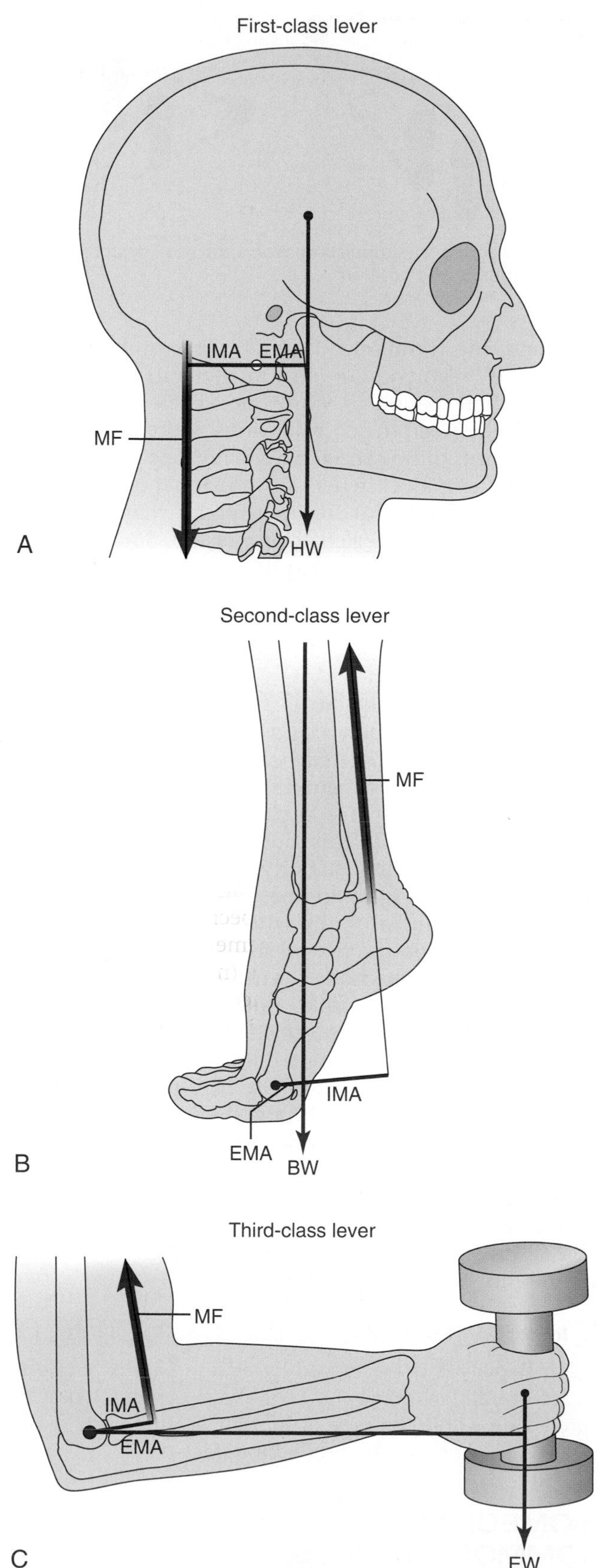

FIG 16-6 Anatomic examples are shown of first-class **(A)**, second-class **(B)**, and third-class **(C)** levers. The muscle activation (depicted in red) is isometric in each case, with no movement occurring at the joint. *(From Neumann DA:* Kinesiology of the musculoskeletal system: foundations for rehabilitation, *ed 2, St Louis, 2010, Mosby.)*

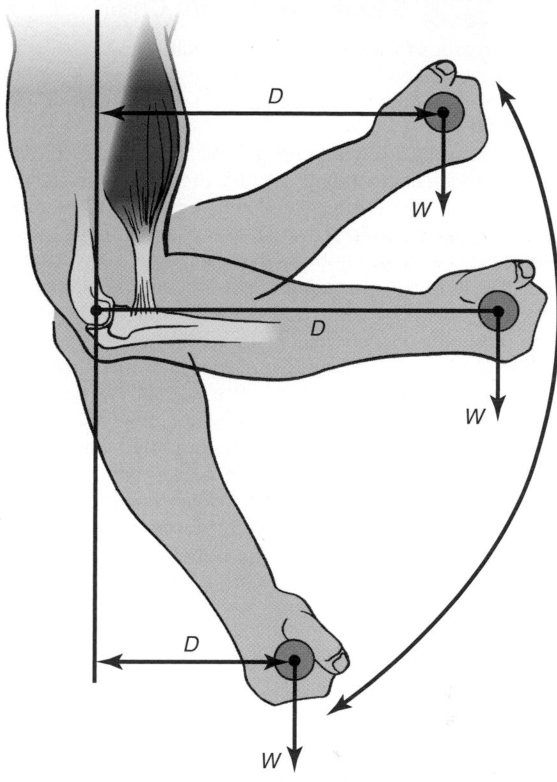

FIG 16-7 Illustration of how changes in the angle at the elbow alter the length of the resistance arm, modifying the resistive torque. *D,* distance; *W,* weight. *(Redrawn from Baechle TR:* Essentials of strength training and conditioning, *ed 3, Champaign, IL, 2008, Human Kinetics.)*

movement patterns, such as "perfect timing," "fluid motion," "natural," and "graceful." Each of these terms means simply that the body's nervous system is finely tuned for stimulating the body's musculature to contract with appropriate intensity or to relax at just the right time to produce the necessary joint rotations required for a successful performance. Without this timing between the nervous and muscular systems, the skeletal system motions that result would be less effective or efficient.

Important Concepts

Kinetic chain shoulder rehabilitation incorporates the kinetic link biomechanical model and proximal-to-distal motor activation patterns with proprioceptive neuromuscular facilitation and closed kinetic chain exercise techniques. This approach focuses on movement patterns rather than isolated muscle exercises. For example, patterns sequentially use the leg, trunk, and scapular musculature to activate weakened shoulder musculature, gain active ROM, and increase strength.

Body segments are connected in more ways than most individuals realize. When there is a perpetual orthopedic problem in one area of the body, chances are the problem is related to another area of the body in some form or fashion. For example, if patients complain their ankles or knees hurt when they walk, it could be linked to an

BOX 16-2 Sequential Kinetic Chain

Common reasons for these issues are as follows:

- Compensation owing to another injury. An example would be putting more weight on one leg to take pressure off of the injured leg.
- Muscular imbalances around a joint. This occurs frequently in the shoulder. In many people, the internal rotators are overdeveloped or overactivated, whereas the external rotators are left weak or underactivated. Many people have muscular imbalances all over the body that can cause many issues.
- Scar tissue buildup or adhesions from previous injury. Most active people have some scar tissue somewhere in the body as a result of a previous injury. The scar tissue can cause a limit in range of motion, causing improper joint mechanics.
- Improper movement patterns. If a person swings a tennis racket incorrectly for long enough, not only will his or her tennis game suffer, but also bad motor patterns or mechanics will quickly develop. In time, the bad motor patterns lead to imbalances of strength and flexibility, pain, injury, and overcompensation patterns. Bad movement patterns can occur in anything a person does, whether it is as simple as walking or as complex as throwing a baseball.

orthopedic issue with their feet. The foot pain could be directly associated with a problem in the calf region. A taut gastrocnemius-soleus muscle group can often lead to problems in the knees, hips, and lower back area. If the pain is ignored, the problem can migrate to the upper back, shoulders, and neck. In a sense, everything in the body is connected; in other words, it is a kinetic chain. When a part of this chain is weak or damaged, it affects other parts of the kinetic chain (Box 16-2).

The kinetic link principle is typically subdivided into two categories. First, the sequential kinetic link principle basically means segmental motions or joint rotations occur in a specific sequence such that time elapses occur between the peak rotational velocities of each involved segment. This coordinated effort typically leads to high velocity or momentum of the last segment involved in the performance. This principle is often observed in sports skills in which the sequential kinetic link is employed for success, and the energy or momentum flows from the core of the body (typically the trunk) distally to the appendages of the body (the leg segments to the foot or the arm segments to the hand). This flow is from the body's more massive segments to its least massive segments. The building of momentum in the bigger, slower segments (trunk and upper legs) of the body leads to effective transference of momentum to the smaller, faster moving segments. In other words, failure to use the trunk appropriately adversely affects the velocity with which a ball is thrown; a club, bat, or racket is swung; or a ball is kicked. Running and wheelchair propulsion demonstrate sequential movement patterns. It is extremely important for individuals with spinal cord injuries to develop core muscle strength because they do not have lower body muscle force contributing to the kinetic chain. For example, wheelchair racing athletes rely on a strong core region in which to transfer momentum generated by the abdominal muscles to the upper extremities.

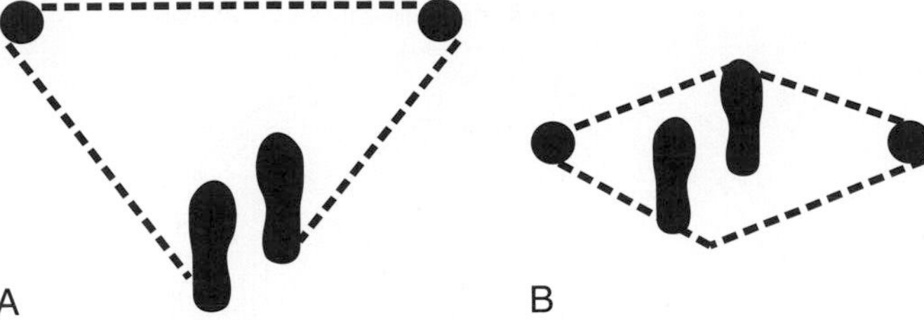

FIG 16-8 Diagram of ambulation with crutches, depicting stable **(A)** and unstable **(B)** positions.

Second, the simultaneous kinetic link principle states that primary segmental or joint movements occur within the same time period in which no visible difference in time exists between the contributions of the involved segments or joints during the activity. This type of movement is generally employed when an individual is required to move objects (or his or her own body) that offer great resistance, such as wheelchair propulsion. Squat lifting is an example of movement requiring force generation by several muscle groups simultaneously. These types of movements generally need high force magnitudes to overcome relatively high inertial conditions.[39]

BALANCE AND STABILITY

Biomechanically, stability and mobility are inversely related. A health professional can apply the principle of balance to provide a patient with an appropriate mix of stability and mobility for a particular activity or skill. Three biomechanical factors directly affect an individual's balance for improving stability: body mass, center of gravity reference height, and base of support area.[3,22] The stability of the human body with respect to the base of support depends on the overall size of the base of support and the height of the body's center of gravity above the base of support. For example, a person recovering from a lower extremity injury may use crutches or a walking cane to relieve the load on the injured limb. The use of crutches also increases the area of the base of support and makes it easier for the user to maintain stability (Fig. 16-8).[46,60] Postural sway is normally under the control of automatic neuromuscular mechanisms that dictate the adequate base of support area. However, these mechanisms are diminished in patients with a muscle atrophy disease or neurologic disorder. The use of crutches would greatly increase the stability of these individuals.[46,60]

Important Concepts

High stability is characterized by a large base of support, a low center of gravity, a centralized center of gravity projection within the base of support, a large body mass, and high friction at the ground interface.

BIOMECHANICS OF COMMON INJURIES

MECHANICAL LOADING

Load is defined as an outside force or group of forces that act on an object. For example, when a patient performs

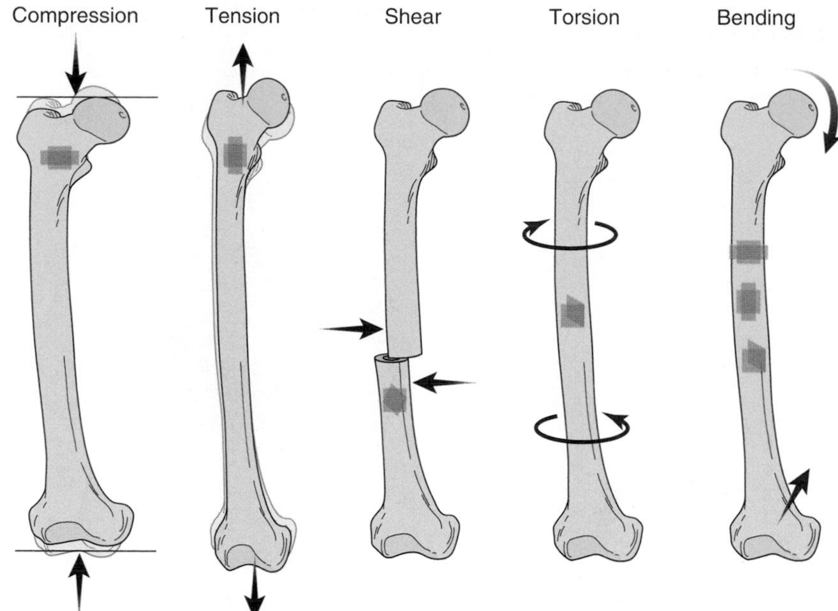

FIG 16-9 Different types of loading. *(Modified from Hamill J, Knutzen KM:* Biomechanical basis of human movement, *Baltimore, 1995, Williams & Wilkins.)*

an exercise with sandbags on the foot, a load is being applied to the muscles that cause knee extension. Although loads apply to the point of contact (e.g., use of compression bandage), other loads are applied away from the point of contact, as described. Depending on the magnitude of the load (**stress**), there is a deformation in the object, termed a *mechanical strain*.

There are three types of stresses: compression, tension, and shear (Fig. 16-9). Compression occurs when two forces or loads are applied toward each other. A common example is the compression stress on the vertebral column during standing while supporting an object (e.g., dumbbell). Excessive compression stress can lead to contusions, fractures, or herniations.[32,39] Tension occurs when two forces or loads are applied in opposite directions. This type of loading is commonly applied to muscles and tendons during stretching activities to improve flexibility.

When the loading exceeds the ability of the object to resist the stress, injuries such as strains, sprains, and avulsion fractures commonly occur.[28] Figure 16-10 illustrates the tension stresses acting on the Achilles tendon during movements of the foot. Injuries associated with tension are more common during activities that use the stretch-shortening cycle most often observed during actions that require fast, quick, change in direction movements. Shear occurs when there are two parallel forces or loads in opposite directions, causing adjacent points on the surface to slide past each other. Injuries such as vertebral disk problems, femoral condyle fractures, and epiphyseal fractures of the distal femur in children occur as a result of shear stress acting on the body.

The resulting action of compression, tension, and shear forces depends on how these forces are distributed, a concept termed *mechanical stress*. Force applied over a smaller surface area results in a greater mechanical stress than force applied over a larger surface area. Given that

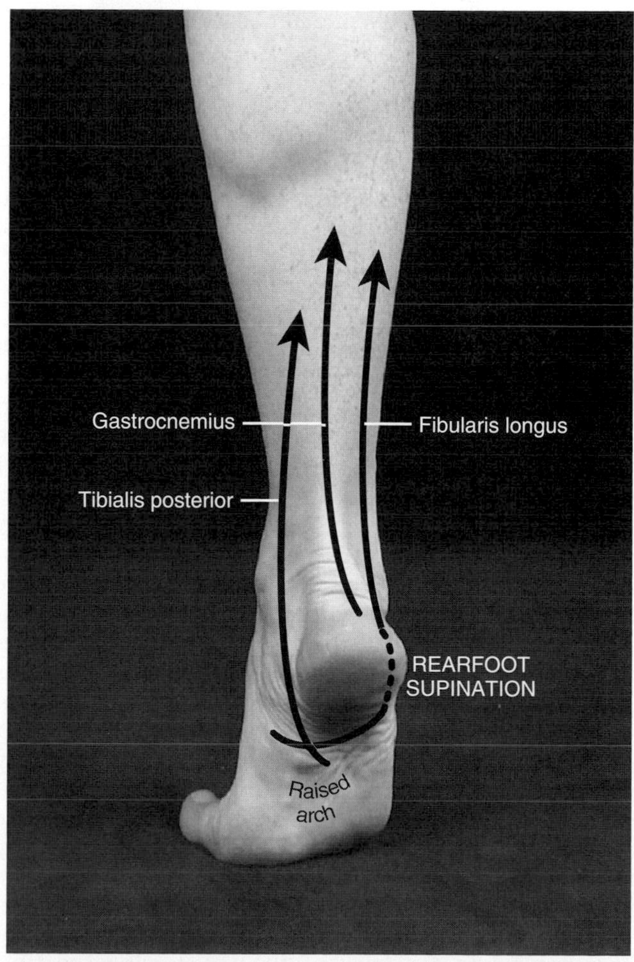

FIG 16-10 Tension stresses acting on the Achilles tendon during foot movements. *(From Neumann DA:* Kinesiology of the musculoskeletal system: foundations for rehabilitation, *ed 2, St Louis, 2010, Mosby.)*

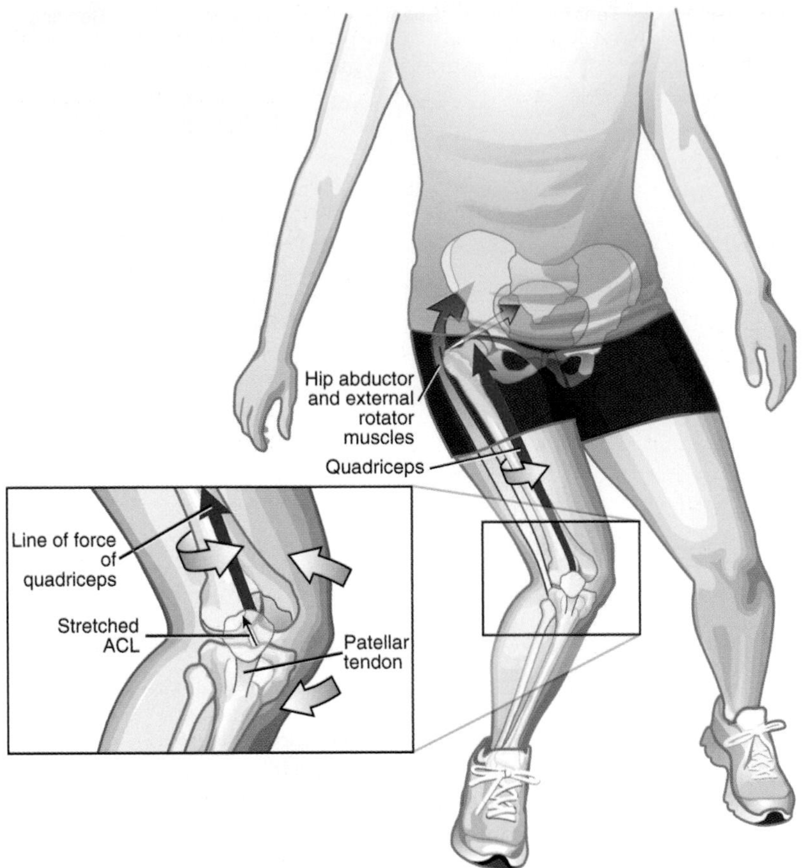

FIG 16-11 Image of a young healthy woman immediately after landing from a jump. The inset on the left shows the increased tension in the anterior cruciate ligament (ACL) and the line of force of the quadriceps muscle. Note the lateral displacement of the patella relative to the intercondylar groove of the femur. *(From Neumann DA:* Kinesiology of the musculoskeletal system: foundations for rehabilitation, *ed 2, St Louis, 2010, Mosby.)*

the lumbar vertebrae typically are more load bearing than the vertebrae in the upper back, one notices that the load-bearing surface area in the lumbar vertebrae is greater than that found in the upper vertebrae.[24] The greater surface area for the thoracic vertebrae translates into a lower mechanical stress for a given load.

Another type of loading on an object, called *bending,* occurs when nonaxial forces are applied, resulting in compressive stress on one side and a tension stress on the other. When an object is forced to twist along the longitudinal axis, a load called *torsion* is produced. Injuries commonly occur because of torsion in activities such as skiing, when a foot is planted and the body begins to twist.[16,21] Another example is an anterior cruciate ligament injury, which commonly occurs during a running activity when one suddenly stops and then turns, causing a deceleration of the lower limb, a forced hyperextension of the knee, or a forced tibial rotation (Fig. 16-11). Other injury mechanisms include an internal rotary force applied to a femur on a fixed weight-bearing tibia, an external rotation force with a valgus (outward) force, or a straight anterior force applied to the back of the leg, forcing the tibia forward relative to the femur.

Deformation or a change in shape can occur when an object is loaded. The load-deformation curve describes the

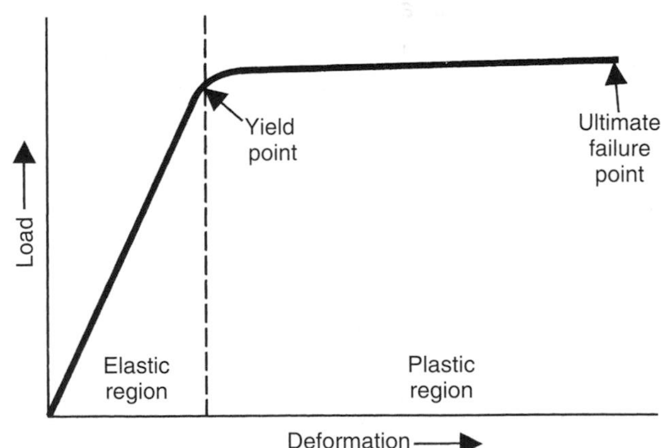

FIG 16-12 Relationship between load and deformation of an object. *(From Hall SJ:* Basic biomechanics, *ed 3, New York, 1999, McGraw-Hill.)*

relationship between the loading and corresponding degree of deformation (Fig. 16-12). Within the elastic region, the object deforms in direct relation to the force and returns to the beginning shape when the force is removed. However, at the elastic limit point, the response becomes plastic, resulting in some degree of permanent deformation, even when the force is removed. Also within the plastic region, excessive loading can result in a point of failure. For a bone, this is the point where a fracture occurs. Although excessive acute loading as described can result in damage to the object, the effect of chronic or repetitive loading that commonly occurs in occupational settings is equally problematic.[55] Repetitive loading can result in microtrauma to the point of stress. If this persists long enough, a chronic wound, termed a *stress-related injury,* may occur.[41]

Another important consideration in predicting injury potential is the rate of loading. This variable reflects how rapidly the load of an external force is transmitted to an internal musculoskeletal tissue. There is a period of time during which muscles are incapable of producing tension to resist forces applied to the body. This period of time, termed *passive loading,* is approximately 50 msec (0.05 second). If a large force is applied to the body such that it reaches a very high magnitude within this 50-msec or passive period, the muscles are unable to resist the force, and other musculoskeletal tissues must assume this role. These other tissues, such as bone, ligaments, cartilage, and tendons, are less capable of enduring these forces. Should the forces be very high in magnitude and occur very rapidly, an acute injury may occur. However, if the force peaks quickly, although not necessarily extremely high in magnitude, overuse injuries to the bone or connective tissues may occur if these forces are applied repetitively, such as in wheelchair propulsion activities. A goal in reducing injury would be to reduce the magnitude of the forces applied to the body or the rate at which they are applied or both.

COMMON MUSCULOSKELETAL INJURIES

Soft Tissue Strains and Sprains

Strain and sprain injuries are usually caused by trauma (slip, fall, collision). Strain refers to an injury to a muscle, occurring when a muscle-tendon unit is stretched or overloaded. Sports that incorporate a running component have a relatively high incidence of soft tissue strains, which are common injuries treated by PTAs. The injury mechanism begins just before ground impact of the foot; the hamstring muscles contract forcefully to halt the knee extension, which occurs at the end of the recovery phase.[28] The action of the hamstrings causes knee flexion to occur, and this continues through the early portions of the ground phase. In combination with the hip extension, this knee flexion serves to reduce the braking force (decelerating force), which occurs when the foot strikes the ground. The braking force is a result of a forward moving foot at initial ground impact, analogous to kicking the ground. Hamstring (semitendinosus, semimembranosus, biceps femoris) muscle group injuries are quite common in running activities.[28] Hamstring injuries, such as strains or ruptures to soft tissues, result when the muscle concentrically contracts while continuing to undergo stretching during heel contact. A non–sport-related soft tissue strain often occurs during slips on surfaces with low coefficient fiction.

Sprain is an injury to a ligament when it is overstretched. The most commonly injured ligaments are located at the ankle, knee, wrist, and low-back region. The purpose of ligaments is to hold the adjacent bones together in a normal alignment and prevent abnormal movements by the bones. However, when too much force is applied to a ligament, such as in a fall, the ligaments can be stretched or torn, leading to an injury. Back pain or injury is a leading cause of disability among warehouse and construction workers. The diagnosis of back sprain (whether lumbar or cervical) implies that the ligamentous and capsular structures connecting the facet joints and vertebrae have been damaged.[24,55]

Rotator Cuff Injury and Shoulder Separation

The primary biomechanical goal of the baseball overhand fastball pitch is to throw a ball at near-maximum horizontal velocity with accuracy. Although there are numerous styles of pitching windups, the delivery phase of the overhand pitch (when the ball is accelerated to the release point) tends to have great similarity.[19] This complex series of body movements is characterized by the sequential nature in which the body segments contribute to the velocity of the ball. Basically, the lower body begins its contribution with the ground contact of the lead foot at the completion of the stride toward home plate. The forces created by the ground contact when combined with the forward moving body cause a rapid rotation of the lower trunk and pelvic area. This rotation is closely followed by the sequential movements of the upper trunk, upper arm, forearm, and hand. When the hand reaches its maximum velocity, the ball is released. The velocity of each successive segment exceeds that of its preceding segment. In other words, these successive segment rotations accept the momentum passed on by the preceding segments and add their momentum before passing it on to the next segment. As momentum builds with each successive segmental contribution, the kinetic energy of the ball increases and reaches a peak at the release point.[18]

One must consider the biomechanical issues associated with shoulder injuries in overhand baseball pitching. As a result of the very high shoulder rotational velocities attained during the acceleration of the ball toward the catcher, the pitcher must create tremendously large deceleration forces to stop this fast shoulder internal rotation. Relatively speaking, the pitcher spends much time building up shoulder internal rotation to throw the ball with high velocity to the batter but must stop this motion in a very short time period to be ready to field his position. This very short time period for deceleration means the torques around the shoulder joint will be quite high.[18,19]

The rotator cuff muscles (supraspinatus, infraspinatus, teres major, and subscapularis) are a group of relatively small muscles that are challenged to maintain shoulder integrity and, particularly, to stop shoulder internal rotation and anterolateral distraction. Because the momentum for the shoulder with regard to both the internal rotation and the anterolateral distraction is high, this muscle group is challenged to the extreme with every ball thrown. With the onset of fatigue and the wear and tear of the forces associated with throwing a large number of pitches, injury to this muscle group occurs frequently.[19] If the injury is severe, it may end a pitcher's career prematurely, similar to a soccer player who dislocates his/her tibiofemoral joint. Another common shoulder injury involves a disruption of the acromioclavicular joint. This joint comprises the collar bone, or clavicle, and the highest portion of the shoulder blade, the acromion of the scapula. These two bones meet on top of the shoulder and form the acromioclavicular joint.[18,22] The most common cause of shoulder separation, or acromioclavicular joint disruption, is a direct fall onto the shoulder. This fall injures the ligaments that provide stability to the joint. The laxity that results allows a degree of separation between the acromion and the clavicle. The degree of separation can range from mild to severe with a noticeable deformity depending on the momentum-impulse relationship. Treatment of this condition can range from conservative management with a period of immobility followed by gentle shoulder strengthening to surgery.

Low-Back Injury

The two most serious leg or squat lifting errors are descending too rapidly and allowing the trunk to flex too far forward during the descent phase. Rapid descent should be avoided because it allows an excessive amount of momentum or kinetic energy to be generated, which the muscles may not be able to overcome when challenged to halt and then reverse this motion. The faster an individual descends, the more muscle force required to reverse this direction. If the person is lifting at a resistance close to his or her maximum or is fatigued, it is likely that at best the ascent phase will not be successfully completed or at worst an injury will occur.[20]

When the individual allows the trunk to flex too far forward, the forces occurring in the low back are greatly increased over the forces associated with a more upright posture. The reason for this is simple. The trunk can be considered a lever with a fulcrum or rotational axis formed in the lumbar area of the vertebral column. When this lever is rotated forward into flexion from a more vertical trunk posture, the line of action of the resistive force of the patient, not to mention the trunk weight itself, is moved from an orientation directly through the vertebral bodies to one very far forward of them.[20]

The shifting of the line of action of the resistive forces to this extreme position causes the torque (force of the weight of the barbell and trunk and head segment multiplied by the distance from this line to the lumbar vertebrae) to increase to very high levels. With the increased torque, the type and magnitudes of forces applied to the cartilaginous vertebral disks, which separate the bony vertebral bodies, are radically different from the forces applied while standing erect. Generally, the anterior portions of two adjacent vertebral bodies (i.e., L4-5) are forced together, a compressive force, while the posterior aspects of the same bones are forced apart by a tensile force (Fig. 16-13).

The cartilaginous or intervertebral disk, which acts as a buffer between these bones, is greatly affected by this condition. The compressive force applied anteriorly forces

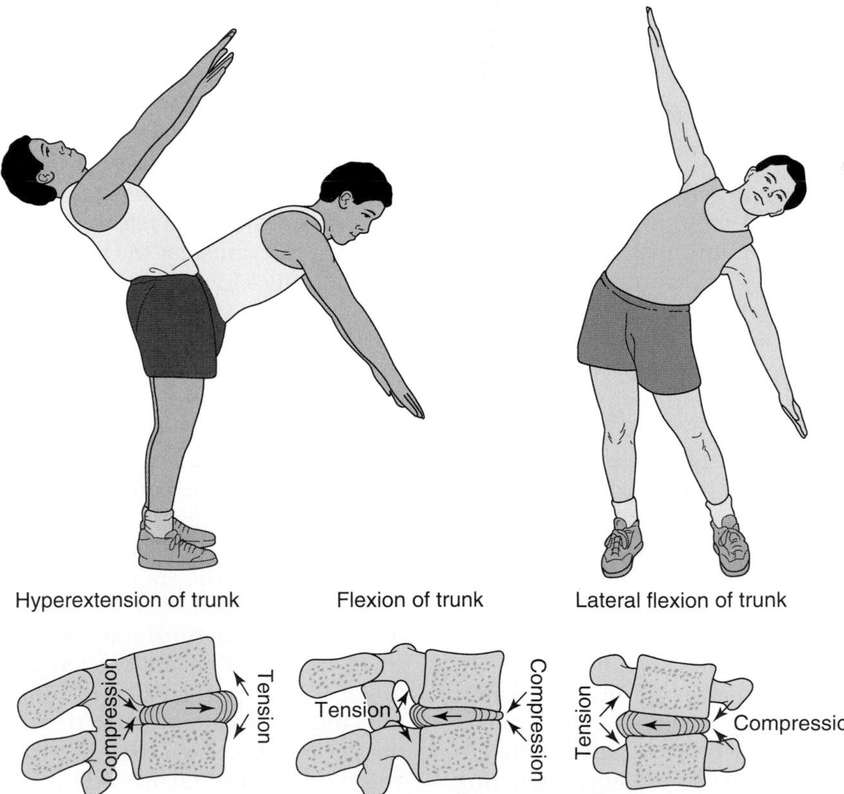

FIG 16-13 Compression and tension stress acting on the vertebrae during trunk motion. *(Modified from Hamill J, Knutzen KM:* Biomechanical basis of human movement, *Baltimore, 1995, Williams & Wilkins.)*

its fluid core posteriorly toward the aspect of the disk that is allowed to bulge by virtue of the gap formed by the tensile force applied to the posterior aspect of the lower vertebral column. If the walls of this disk have been weakened as a result of cumulative trauma from poor biomechanics in lifting and other lumbar-intensive activities, a bulge or rupture of the disk may occur. This occurrence may lead to moderate to severe low back pain and leg pain because nerves are often impinged on by the bulging disk. Surgery is often required to relieve the pain associated with a bulging disk.

SUMMARY

In this chapter, the internal and external forces affecting human movement characteristics were considered along with terminology used to describe injury causation and rehabilitation to the musculoskeletal system. The relationship between mechanical physics and injury was made clear. An understanding was provided of various injury mechanisms that occur to the musculoskeletal system and how these depend on the load characteristics. The chapter concluded with an explanation of specific injuries commonly associated with chronic and acute loading rates.

Kinesiology considers the interaction of the body's anatomic structures and neuromuscular systems with the mechanics of motion as established by the principles of biomechanics. By considering these two important areas, one can effectively evaluate human motion and establish principles on which injuries can be repaired and rehabilitated. A knowledge base in human movement sciences would definitely help the PTA student to understand the complexities involved in basic and advanced physical activities associated with sports, exercise, occupations, physical rehabilitation, and ADL.

GLOSSARY

All-or-none: When exposed to stimuli from the nervous system, each individual muscle fiber in a motor unit contracts either completely or not at all. The strength of the muscle contraction is determined by the number of individual muscle fibers that respond to the stimulus.

Concentric: Contractions that cause the muscle to shorten as it contracts.

Eccentric: Contractions that cause the muscle to lengthen as it contracts.

Fast-twitch: Muscle fibers contract quickly and provide strength and speed, although they also fatigue more quickly.

Force: A push or pull acting on an object.

Force couple: A moment created by equal, noncolinear, parallel but opposite directed forces. The moment created is called a *couple*.

Friction: The result when two objects are in direct contact with one another and a force acts to impede motion of the objects.

Inertia: The resistance an object offers to a change in its velocity or direction of motion, directly related to its mass.

Motor unit: Consists of one motor neuron and all of the muscle fibers that it innervates.

Slow-twitch: Muscle fibers contract slowly and can be used for longer periods of time.

Stress: A force required to maintain the deformation of viscoelastic material. Diminishes with time until equilibrium is reached.

Velocity: A change of position with respect to time. Velocity is also a vector, possessing both speed and direction.

REFERENCES

1. Abernethy B, Hantahan SJ, Kippers V, et al: *The biophysical foundations of human movement*, ed 2, Champaign, IL, 2005, Human Kinetics.
2. Aerssens J, Dequeker J, Mbuyi-Muamba JM: Bone tissue composition: biochemical anatomy of bone. *Clin Rheum* 13(Suppl 1):54–62, 1995.
3. Bloem BR, Steijns JA, Smits-Engelsman BC: An update on falls. *Curr Opin Neurol* 16:15–26, 2003.
4. Boninger ML, Impink BG, Cooper RA, et al: Relation between median and ulnar nerve function and wrist kinematics during wheelchair propulsion. *Arch Phys Med Rehab* 85:1141–1145, 2004.
5. Boulton AJ, Kirsner RS, Vileikyte L: Neuropathic diabetic foot ulcers. *N Engl J Med* 351:48–55, 2004.
6. Burnham RS, May L, Nelson E, et al: Shoulder pain in wheelchair athletes: the role of muscle imbalance. *Am J Sport Med* 21:238–242, 1993.
7. Cajori F: *Sir Isaac Newton's mathematical principles* (translated by Andrew Motte, 1729), Berkeley, CA, 1934, University of California Press.
8. Cavanagh PR, Ulbrecht JS, Caputo GM: New developments in the biomechanics of the diabetic foot. *Diabetes Metab Res Rev* 16(Suppl 1):S6–S10, 2000.
9. Chen CP, Chen MJ, Pei YC, et al: Sagittal plane loading response during gait in different age groups and in people with knee osteoarthritis. *Am J Phys Med Rehabil* 82:307–312, 2003.
10. Chumlea WC, Wisemandle W, Guo SS, Siervogel RM: Relations between frame size and body composition and bone mineral status. *Am J Clin Nutr* 75(6):1012–1016, 2002.
11. Clamann HP: Motor unit recruitment and the gradation of muscle force. *Phys Ther* 73(12):830–843, 1993.
12. Collinger JL, Boninger ML, Koontz AM, et al: Shoulder biomechanics during the push phase of wheelchair propulsion: a multisite study of persons with paraplegia. *Arch Phys Med Rehabil* 89:667–676, 2008.
13. Cooper RA, Quatrano LA, Stanhope SJ, et al: Gait analysis in rehabilitation medicine: a brief report. *Am J Phys Med Rehabil* 78:278–280, 1999.
14. Cowin SC: *Bone mechanics handbook*, ed 2, Boca Raton, FL, 2001, CRC Press.
15. Ctercteko GC, Dhanendran M, Hutton WC: Vertical forces acting on the feet of diabetic patients with neuropathic ulceration. *Br J Surg* 68:608–614, 1981.
16. DeVita P, Hortobagyi T, Barrier J: Gait biomechanics are not normal after anterior cruciate ligament reconstruction and accelerated rehabilitation. *Med Sci Sports Exerc* 30:1481–1488, 1998.
17. di Prampero PE, Narici MV: Muscles in microgravity: from fibres to human motion. *J Biomech* 36:403–412, 2003.
18. Dillman CJ, Fleisig GS, Andrews JR: Biomechanics of pitching with emphasis upon shoulder kinematics. *J Orthop Sports Phys Ther* 18:402–408, 1993.
19. Fleisig GS, Barrentine SW, Escamilla RF, et al: Biomechanics of overhand throwing with implications for injuries. *Sports Med* 21:421–437, 1996.
20. Garg A: Occupational biomechanics and low-back pain. *Occup Med* 7:609–628, 1992.
21. Georgoulis AD, Papadonikolakis A, Papageorgiou CD, et al: Three-dimensional tibiofemoral kinematics of the anterior cruciate ligament-deficient and reconstructed knee during walking. *Am J Sports Med* 31:75–79, 2003.
22. Hart-Hughes S, Quigley P, Bulat T, et al: An interdisciplinary approach to reducing fall risks and falls. *J Rehabil* 70:46–51, 2004.

23. Hettinga DL: Normal joint structures and reaction to injury. *J Orthop Sport Phys Therapy* 1(1):16–22, 1979.
24. Hidalgo JA, Genaidy AM, Huston R, et al: Occupational biomechanics of the neck: a review and recommendations. *J Hum Ergol (Tokyo)* 21:165–181, 1992.
25. Ingham E, Fisher J: Biological reactions to wear debris in total joint replacement. *Proc Inst Mech Eng [H]* 214(1):21–37, 2000.
26. Kejonen P, Kauranen K, Ahsan R, et al: Motion analysis measurements of body movements during standing: association with age and sex. *Int J Rehabil Res* 25:297–304, 2002.
27. Khan IM, Redman SN, Williams R, et al: The development of synovial joints. *Dev Biol* 79:1–36, 2007.
28. Kirkendall DT, Garrett WE, Jr: Clinical perspectives regarding eccentric muscle injury. *Clin Orthop* 403(Suppl):S81–S89, 2002.
29. Koontz AM, Cooper RA, Boninger ML, et al: Shoulder kinematics and kinetics during two speeds of wheelchair propulsion. *J Rehabil Res Dev* 39:635–650, 2002.
30. Kraushaar BS, Nirschl RP: Tendinosis of the elbow (tennis elbow). *J Bone Joint Surg Am* 81:259–278, 1999.
31. Kreighbaum E, Barthels KM: *Biomechanics: A qualitative approach for studying human movement*, ed 3, New York, 1990, Macmillan.
32. Landers JE, Bates BT, DeVita P: Biomechanics of the squat exercise using a modified center of mass bar. *Med Sci Sports Exerc* 18:469–478, 1986.
33. Lanyon LE, Baggott DG: Mechanical function as an influence on the structure and form of bone. *J Bone Joint Surg Br* 58(4):436–443, 1976.
34. Levangie PK, Norkin CC: *Joint structure and function: a comprehensive analysis*, ed 3, Philadelphia, 2001, FA Davis.
35. Lieber RL, Steinman S, Barash IA, Chambers H: Structural and functional changes in spastic skeletal muscle. *Muscle Nerve* 29(5):615–627, 2004.
36. Lieber RL: *Skeletal muscle structure and function: Implications for rehabilitation and sports medicine*, Baltimore, 1992, Williams & Wilkins.
37. McElhaney JH, Hopper RH, Nightingale RW, et al: Mechanisms of basilar skull fracture. *J Neurotrauma* 12:669–678, 1995.
38. McGinnis PM: *Biomechanics of sport and exercise*, Champaign, IL, 1999, Human Kinetics.
39. McLaughlin T, Lardner T, Dillman C: Kinetics of the parallel squat. *Res Q* 49:175–189, 1978.
40. Monti RJ, Roy RR, Edgerton VR: Role of motor unit structure in defining function. *Muscle Nerve* 24(7):646–866, 2001.
41. Nigg BM: *Biomechanics IX-B*, Champaign, IL, 1985, Human Kinetics.
42. Nolan L, Kerrigan DC: Keep on your toes: gait initiation from toe-standing. *J Biomech* 36:393–401, 2003.
43. Nordin M, Frankel VH: *Basic biomechanics of the musculoskeletal system*, ed 3, Philadelphia, 2001, Lippincott Williams & Wilkins.
44. Oatis CA: *Kinesiology: the mechanics of pathomechanics of human movement*, Philadelphia, 2004, Lippincott Williams & Wilkins.
45. Perry J: The use of gait analysis for surgical recommendations in traumatic brain injury. *J Head Trauma Rehabil* 14:116–135, 1999.
46. Piirtola M, Era P: Force platform measurements as predictors of falls among older people—a review. *Gerontology* 52:1–16, 2006.
47. Porter MM, Vandervoort AA, Lexell J: Aging of human muscle: structure, function, and adaptability. *Scand J Med Sci Sports* 5:129–142, 1995.
48. Ranatunga KW: Skeletal muscle stiffness and contracture in children with spastic cerebral palsy. *J Physiol* 589(Pt 11):2665, 2011.
49. Rasch PJ: *Kinesiology and applied anatomy*, ed 7, Malvern, PA, 1989, Lea & Febiger.
50. Riley PO, Kerrigan DC: Torque action of two-joint muscles in the swing period of stiff-legged gait: a forward dynamic model analysis. *J Biomech* 31:835–840, 1998.
51. Rubin CT, Lanyon LE: Regulation of bone formation by applied dynamic loads. *J Bone Joint Surg Am* 66:397–402, 1984.
52. Sieck GC, Prakash YS: Morphological adaptations of neuromuscular junctions depend on fiber type. *Can J Appl Physiol* 22:197–230, 1997.
53. Scott W, Stevens J, Binder-Macleod SA: Human skeletal muscle fiber type classifications. *Phys Ther* 81(11):1810–1816, 2001.
54. Sledge CB: Structure, development and function of joints. *Orthop Clin North Am* 6:619–628, 1975.
55. Stock SR: Workplace ergonomic factors and the development of musculoskeletal disorders of the neck and upper limbs: a meta-analysis. *Am J Ind Med* 19:87–107, 1991.
56. Stokes IA, Faris IB, Hutton WC: The neuropathic ulcer and loads on the foot in diabetic patients. *Acta Orthop Scand* 46:839–847, 1975.
57. Stravino VD: The synovial system. *Am J Phys Med* 51:312–320, 1972.
58. Talmadge RJ, Roy RR, Edgerton VR: Muscle fiber types and function. *Curr Opin Rheumatol* 5:695–705, 1993.
59. Tang SF, Chen CP, Hong WH, et al: Improvement of gait by using orthotic insoles in patients with heel injury who received reconstructive flap operations. *Am J Phys Med Rehabil* 82:350–356, 2003.
60. Thapa PB, Gideon P, Brockman KG, et al: Clinical and biomechanical measures of balance fall predictors in ambulatory nursing home residents. *J Gerontol* 51:239–246, 1996.
61. Van De Graaff KM: *Human anatomy*, ed 6, Boston, 2002, McGraw-Hill.
62. Veves A, Murray HJ, Young MJ, et al: Do high foot pressures lead to ulceration: a prospective study. *Diabetologia* 35:660–663, 1992.
63. Whiting WC, Zernicke RF: *Biomechanics of musculoskeletal injury*, ed 2, Champaign, IL, 2008, Human Kinetics.
64. Wright V, Dowson D, Kerr J: The structure of joints. *Int Rev Connect Tissue Res* 6:105–125, 1973.
65. Yoganandan N, Pintar FA, Klienberger M: Cervical spine vertebral and facet joint kinematics under whiplash. *J Biomech Eng* 120:305–308, 1998.
66. Young MJ, Cavanagh PR, Thomas B, et al: The effect of callus removal on dynamic plantar foot pressures in diabetic patients. *Diabet Med* 9:55–57, 1991.

REVIEW QUESTIONS

Multiple Choice

1. In Which plane would shoulder and hip movement occur when performing a cartwheel?
   a. Sagittal
   b. Frontal
   c. Transverse
   d. Longitudinal
2. Which anatomic plane defines dorsiflexion and plantar flexion?
   a. Sagittal
   b. Frontal
   c. Transverse
   d. Mediolateral
3. What type of muscle contraction is employed by the knee extensors during the ascent (up) phase in the performance of a squat exercise?
   a. Concentric
   b. Eccentric
   c. Isometric
   d. Isokinetic
4. Which of the following terms refers to a numerical representation of a measurable quantity that is defined by direction and magnitude?
   a. Scalar
   b. Mass
   c. Vector
   d. Inertia
   e. All of the above
5. Shoulder abduction occurs around which axis of rotation?
   a. Anteroposterior
   b. Mediolateral
   c. Longitudinal

d. Horizontal
e. Transverse
6. Moving your head so as to say "no" occurs in which plane?
a. Sagittal
b. Frontal
c. Transverse
d. Oblique
e. Mediolateral
7. Which muscle would most likely serve as an antagonist of a flexor muscle?
a. Hyperflexor
b. Adductor
c. Extensor
d. Rotator
e. Abductor
8. A neuron and the muscle fibers it innervates define:
a. A muscle fascicle.
b. A motor unit.
c. A muscle twitch.
d. A muscle spindle.
9. Which of the following is not a property of muscle?
a. Plasticity
b. Irritability
c. Extensibility
d. Contractility
10. The two variables that are used to define momentum are:
a. Velocity and time.
b. Mass and work.
c. Mass and velocity.
d. Velocity and acceleration.
11. A person's inertia would be ________ on earth and on the moon.
a. different
b. the same
c. variable
d. inversely related
12. The product of a force and the time during which it acts defines:
a. Momentum.
b. Velocity.
c. Acceleration.
d. Impulse.
13. The law of _______ shows that if you exert the same force on two objects of different mass, you will get different accelerations (changes in motion).
a. inertia
b. acceleration
c. reaction
d. gravitation
14. The measure of inertia is the quantity called:
a. Mass.
b. Weight.
c. Both a and b.
d. Neither a nor b.
15. The area of biomechanics that describes the effect of motion is:
a. Kinetics.
b. Kinematics.
c. Forces.
d. Gravity.

Short Answer

16. What is the point called where the midtransverse, midfrontal, and midsagittal planes intersect?
17. What is the product of the force magnitude and the force application time interval called?
18. Which lever generally produces the greatest mechanical advantage?
19. Which of Newton's laws of motion describes the relationship among force, mass, and acceleration?
20. What types of injuries commonly occur when tension loading exceeds the ability of the object to resist the stress?

Fill in the Blank

21. The transverse plane divides the body into equal ________.
22. Shoulder abduction occurs in the _________ plane around the ________ axis.
23. _______ is the product of force and distance.
24. _______ and _______ are the contractile proteins found in a muscle fiber.
25. The phenomenon that explains the stimulation of the entire group of muscle fibers within a motor unit is known as the ___________.

True/False

26. Kinematics deals with the description of movements based on alterations in space and time.
27. There is a mechanical relationship between linear and angular motion.
28. When the fulcrum is located somewhere between the point of force and point of resistance, the lever is termed *third class*.
29. Newton's third law is the law of inertia.
30. Pressure is a measure of the distribution of a force over a given area.

Part IV

Management of Orthopedic Patients by Region

This section introduces the physical therapist assistant (PTA) to various musculoskeletal injuries. Each region's area of the body is discussed with specific soft tissue injuries, fractures, and diseases defined. A problem-solving approach is described, and an evidence-based rehabilitation program is provided when available.

A more progressive way to manage rehabilitation is the criterion-based program, or critical mapping. This method, which is also known as *critical treatment pathways,* is "a description of the elements of care to be rendered … for a particular diagnosis. The pathway often takes the form of a chart or care path/care map that can be followed" by the clinician and patient.* Instead of using a timetable for progression, a set of criteria is developed that the patient must meet before progressing to the next phase of rehabilitation. These criteria are based on tissue healing constraints and the patient's individual tolerance to the program. A criterion-based progression fosters close scrutiny of all objective and subjective data concerning the individual's performance.

The components necessary for effective management of orthopedic injuries by the PTA are knowledge of musculoskeletal tissue healing principles, familiarity with various rehabilitation programs, skillful application of rehabilitation techniques, and a fundamental understanding of common and uncommon soft tissue injuries, fractures, and diseases of muscles, bones, and joints. Knowledge of specific indications and contraindications for certain therapeutic interventions also is helpful.

Orthopedic anatomy is not reviewed substantially in this section. Instead, chapters focus on mechanisms of injury, fracture classifications, clinical features of the injury, specific surgical procedures, and rehabilitation programs. The student clinician is strongly encouraged to review comprehensive musculoskeletal anatomy texts along with the study of each body part and disorder.

---

*American Physical Therapy Association guidelines for physical therapists facing changing organizational structures, American Physical Therapy Association Board of Directors, APP 3, 1995.

Chapter 17

Orthopedic Management of the Ankle, Foot, and Toes

Walter Jenkins, Blaise Williams

CHAPTER OUTLINE

LEARNING OBJECTIVES

1. Identify common foot and ankle ligament injuries.
2. Describe intervention methods for common foot and ankle ligament injuries.
3. Identify and describe common lower leg, ankle, and foot tendon injuries.
4. Outline and describe common methods of intervention for lower leg, ankle, and foot injuries.
5. Identify common foot and ankle fractures.
6. Discuss common methods of intervention for foot and ankle fractures.
7. Identify and describe common methods of intervention for toe injuries.
8. Describe common mobilization techniques for the ankle, foot, and toe.

KEY TERMS

Calcaneus fracture
Posterior tibialis tendon
Syndesmosis
Talar tilt test
Talus
Tibial nerve

This chapter introduces the physical therapist assistant (PTA) to injuries affecting the lower leg, ankle, foot, and toes. Repetitive motion injuries (overuse injuries) and traumatic injuries of the lower leg, ankle, and foot are included in this chapter. Specific therapeutic interventions are described in detail for each pathology. When possible, supporting evidence for specific interventions is outlined.

LIGAMENT INJURIES OF THE ANKLE

Injuries to the lateral ligament complex (anterior talofibular ligament, fibulocalcaneal ligament, and posterior talofibular ligament) account for approximately 14% to 25% of all sports-related injuries.[35,65] Inversion ankle sprains are among the most common sports and orthopedic injuries.[32,34,95] Studies report that approximately 95% of all ankle sprains occur to the lateral ligament complex.[96]

Additionally, injuries to associated structures including articular cartilage and the synovial membrane have been identified on arthroscopy in individuals who had recurrent or recalcitrant lateral ankle sprains.[62] Untreated ankle sprains may lead to chronic pain, muscular weakness, and instability.[34] Ankle joint osteoarthritis has been observed in patients with chronic ankle instability.[114]

Important Concepts

Approximately 95% of all ankle sprains occur to the lateral ankle ligaments.

LATERAL LIGAMENT INJURIES (INVERSION ANKLE SPRAINS)

Mechanisms of Injury

Ligament sprains of the lateral aspect of the ankle usually are caused by plantar flexion, inversion, and adduction of the foot and ankle (Fig. 17-1).[101] Large forces are not needed to produce an ankle sprain. Stepping off a curb, stepping into a small hole, or stepping on a rock can produce sudden plantar flexion and inversion motions. During athletic competition, stepping on an opponent's foot is a common occurrence that leads to lateral ligament sprains of the ankle. Most commonly, ankle sprains occur when the foot is in an "unloaded" or non–weight-bearing position before the injury.[110]

Classification of Sprains

Classifying inversion ankle sprains can be difficult and confusing.[101] The standard classification of ligament injuries (e.g., first-degree, second-degree, and third-degree sprains) requires elaboration when applied to inversion ankle sprains, specifically addressing grades, degrees, and descriptive severity of the injury (mild, moderate, or severe). A classification model described by Leach[66] is contrasted with the common standard classification of ankle sprains as a means of comparison and to illustrate the potential for confusion about classification of inversion ankle sprains.

- First-degree sprain: Single ligament rupture.[66] The anterior talofibular ligament is completely torn. In the standard classification of ligament sprains, a complete tear or rupture of a ligament is called a grade III, or third-degree, sprain (Fig. 17-2, *A*).
- Second-degree sprain: Double ligament rupture.[66] The anterior talofibular ligaments and the fibulocalcaneal ligaments are completely torn. The standard classification describes a partially torn single ligament as a grade II sprain (Fig. 17-2, *B*).
- Third-degree sprain: All three lateral ankle ligaments (anterior talofibular, posterior talofibular, and fibulocalcaneal) are completely torn.[66] In the standard classification, a single ligament that is completely torn is defined as a grade III ligament sprain (Fig. 17-2, *C*).

It is essential that the system of classification used to describe the severity or complexity of injury be accepted and understood and not confused with another system or model of classification.

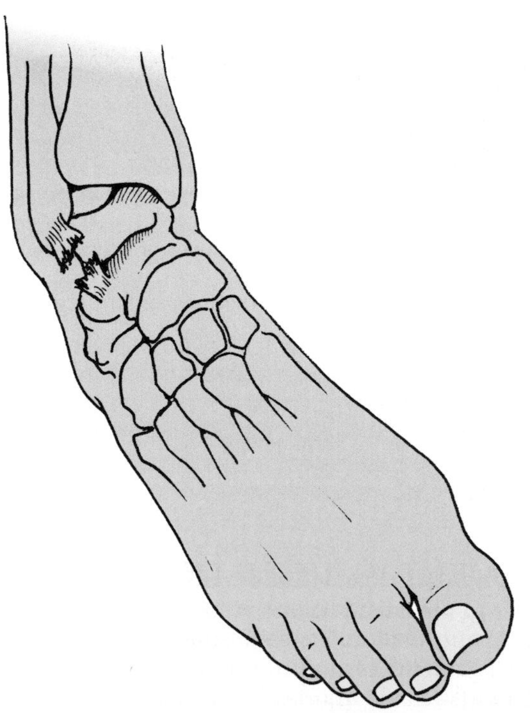

FIG 17-1 Mechanism of injury to the lateral ligament complex of the ankle. Note the motion of plantar flexion, inversion, and adduction of the foot and ankle.

Important Concepts

Use of a classification system to describe severity or complexity of ankle injuries is required to ensure understanding of treatment progression and injury prognosis.

Clinical Examination

The PTA must be aware of the organization and administration of examination procedures used to inspect inversion ankle sprains. Throughout rehabilitation, the PTA must communicate changes in the patient's status relative to initial evaluation data and make safe and appropriate modifications to the existing program based on consultation with the supervising physical therapist (PT).

Testing. Ankle stability tests are used by the PT to identify and quantify the integrity of the lateral ligament complex. Injury to the anterior talofibular ligament can be assessed clinically by performing the anterior drawer test (Fig. 17-3).[101] The patient must be in a relaxed seated or semirecumbent position with the involved leg flexed 90° at the knee and the involved ankle slightly plantar flexed. The PT stabilizes the distal tibia and supports it with one hand, while using the other hand to grasp the calcaneus gently but firmly and attempt to translate or pull the ankle forward. No excessive motion is seen or felt if the ligament is intact. However, the ankle demonstrates excessive forward or anterior motion if the anterior talofibular ligament is torn.

The **talar tilt test** or inversion stress test examines the resistance of the ankle ligament to maximal inversion stress (Fig. 17-4).[101] With the patient in the same position

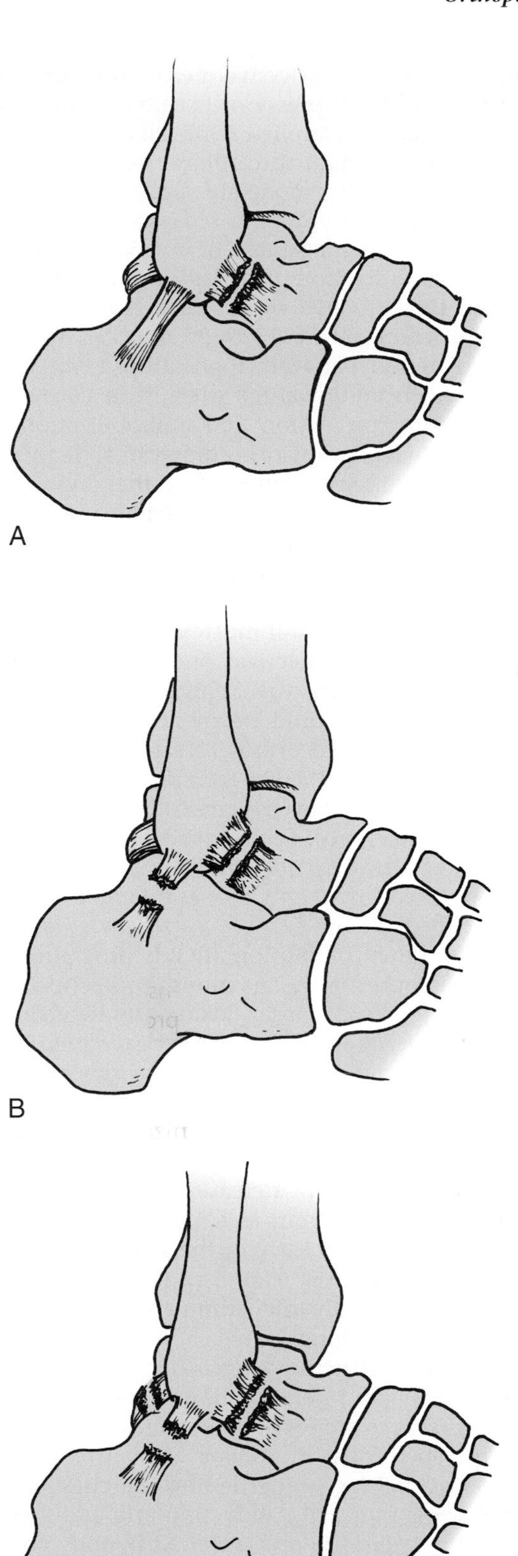

FIG 17-2 First-degree, second-degree, and third-degree sprains. **A,** Tear of the anterior talofibular ligament. **B,** Tears of the anterior talofibular ligament and fibulocalcaneal ligament. **C,** Tears of the anterior talofibular ligament, fibulocalcaneal ligament, and posterior talofibular ligament.

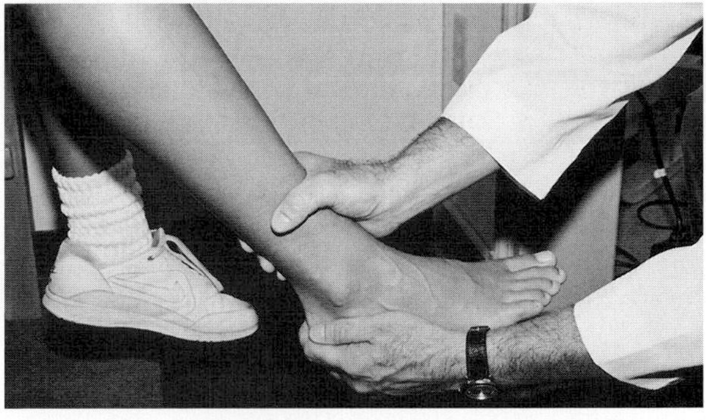

FIG 17-3 Anterior drawer test of the ankle. With the affected foot slightly plantar flexed, the distal tibia is stabilized with one hand, while the other hand grasps the calcaneus and directs an anterior force to manually displace the calcaneus to test the integrity of the anterior talofibular ligament.

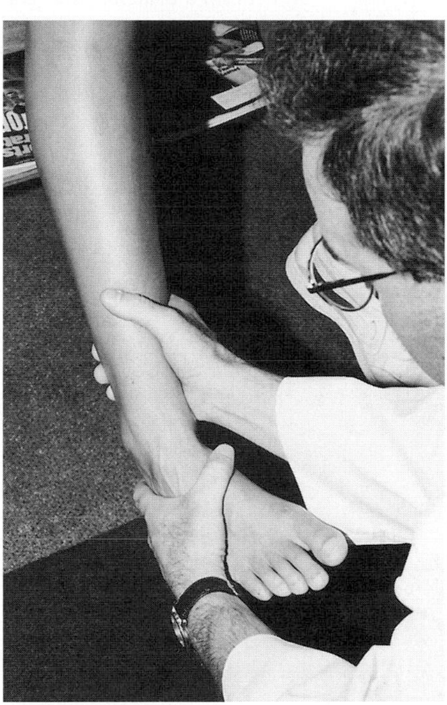

FIG 17-4 Talar tilt test. The distal tibia is stabilized with one hand, while the other hand "tilts" the talus to test the integrity of the lateral ligament complex.

as the anterior drawer test, the ankle is gradually stressed by exertion of constant pressure over the lateral aspect of the foot and ankle, while counter pressure is applied over the inner aspect of the lower leg until maximal inversion is reached.[10] The severity of ligament injury should be graded according to the classification system used by the supervising PT.

Order of Procedures. Table 17-1 outlines the procedure for evaluation of inversion ankle sprains. The mechanism of injury that produces an inversion ankle sprain also may cause other conditions that must be differentiated by the physician[95,101] and PT, such as fracture of the base of the fifth metatarsal, malleolar fractures, osteochondral fractures, osteochondritis dissecans, midfoot ligament sprains, and subluxing peroneal tendons.

TABLE 17-1 Physical Therapist Initial Evaluation Outline for Clinical Assessment of Inversion Ankle Sprains

Order of Assessment	Procedures
History	1. How did the injury happen? 2. Where is the pain located? 3. Did you hear or feel a "pop" or "snap"? 4. Have you had a similar injury previously? If yes, explain.
Observation	1. Note any obvious deformity suggesting a fracture or dislocation. 2. Note the area and degree of swelling. 3. Evaluate complaints of pain. 4. Note any discoloration. 5. Perform a bilateral visual comparison of symmetry.
Palpation*	1. Distal tibia-fibula 2. Lateral ligament complex 3. Medial ligaments–deltoid ligament 4. Base of the fifth metatarsal 5. Peroneal tendons 6. Achilles tendon
Range of motion	1. Active and passive a. Dorsiflexion b. Plantar flexion c. Inversion d. Eversion
Strength	1. Manual muscle testing a. Dorsiflexion b. Plantar flexion c. Inversion d. Eversion
Clinical stability tests	1. Anterior drawer test 2. Talar tilt test

*Always begin palpation by explaining the procedure, then initially performing the procedure on the uninvolved side.

Intervention. The specific rehabilitation program used to treat inversion sprains depends on the severity of sprain (first, second, or third degree). Generally, first-degree and second-degree sprains can be effectively managed nonoperatively with a supervised rehabilitation program.[102]

Initial management of acute inversion ankle sprains calls for rest, ice, compression, and elevation (RICE). *Rest* is a relative term used to define avoidance of unwanted stress; it does not require complete avoidance of all stress. The application of ice, compression, and elevation is directed at minimizing and reducing intense inflammatory response, hemorrhage, swelling, pain, and "cellular metabolism" to provide the most conducive environment for tissue healing.[95]

Important Concepts

Initial management of an acute ankle inversion sprain is rest, ice, compression, and elevation (RICE).

Clinically, the most effective means to reduce swelling are elevation and compression. Elastic compression bandages (Ace wraps) are applied while elevating the injured limb above the heart. A three-phase (phase I, maximum protection; phase II, moderate protection; phase III, minimum protection), criteria-based rehabilitation program is effective for the management of inversion ankle sprains. The maximum-protection phase calls for the RICE program to be used three to five times daily. Application of ice should be encouraged for 15 to 20 minutes, with a 1- to 2-hour rest period between applications. Protecting the torn ligaments from unwanted stress is the cornerstone of this phase. Joint protection and immobilization can be achieved through an array of commercial appliances, tape, casting, and braces; selection is left to the physician or PT. Some physicians choose to use a short-leg walking cast or posterior plaster splint. More commonly, a plastic shell brace with an inflatable air bladder or a leather semirigid ankle support is used. Tape can be used for compression and ligament support, but it must be applied skillfully and reapplied daily to be effective. The ankle must be positioned correctly during the application and use of all support devices. It should be in a neutral position or slightly dorsiflexed and everted for close approximation of the torn ligaments. Weight-bearing status and ambulation with assistive devices are individualized to the patient's pain tolerance. Secondary to improved stability of the ankle during weight bearing, patients are commonly instructed to "weight bear as tolerated" during this phase.

An active range of motion (ROM) program must be used cautiously during the maximum-protection phase. It is imperative to avoid plantar flexion and inversion when instructing patients to perform ROM exercises. Excessive plantar flexion and inversion increase the load on the anterior talofibular and calcaneofibular ligaments leading to a disruption of the healing process in these ligaments.

Motion exercises are important to help reduce pain and swelling as well as help increase function of the joint. However, if certain motions (e.g., plantar flexion or inversion) are employed too early in the rehabilitation period, these "unwanted stresses" can disrupt the normal healing process. Electrical galvanic stimulation also can help reduce pain and swelling.

Isometric strengthening exercises are initiated as soon as the patient's pain tolerance allows. Isometric dorsiflexion and eversion exercises are performed for two or three sets of 10 repetitions, holding each contraction for 10 seconds. Proximal leg-strengthening exercises (leg extension, hamstring curls, hip abduction and adduction, and hip extension exercises) and general full-body conditioning should be encouraged throughout the course of rehabilitation. Clinically, it is vital to view inversion ankle sprains as injuries that affect the whole person, rather than just the injured extremity. Maintaining aerobic fitness and strength during recovery is particularly important in athletes.

The moderate-protection phase can begin when the patient can bear weight on the injured limb without crutches, perform all ROM and isometric exercises without undue complaints of pain, and control the swelling. This

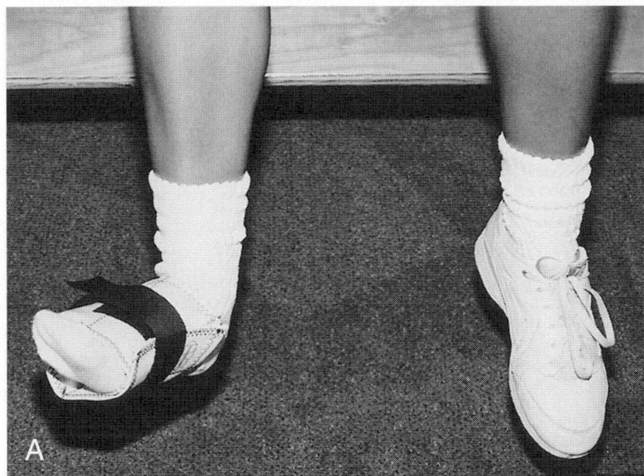

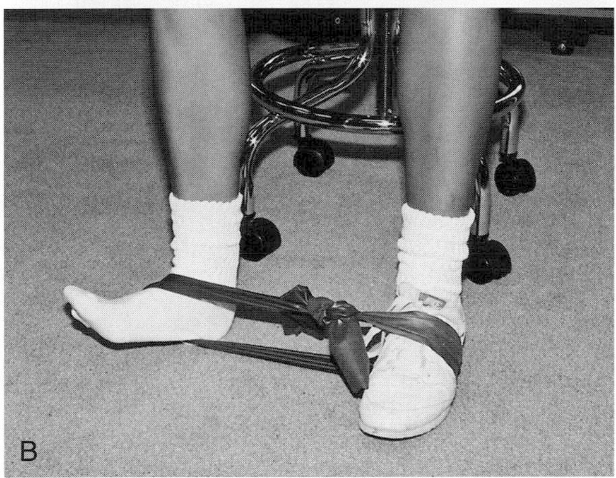

FIG 17-5 **A,** Concentric and eccentric exercise with ankle weights. As the weight is slowly elevated to a position of dorsiflexion and eversion, the patient is encouraged to emphasize the eccentric or lowering phase of the exercise. **B,** TheraBand elastic band resistance for eversion and dorsiflexion.

phase encourages the use of the RICE principle, full weight bearing, and continued ligament support with the use of braces or tape. More progressive exercises are initiated, including concentric and eccentric contractions (Fig. 17-5) (with ankle weights or latex bands), heel cord stretching (Fig. 17-6) (towel stretch, wall stretch, or ProStretch), and standing toe and heel raises.

Gradually and cautiously, inversion and plantar flexion motions are added as pain allows. Stationary bicycling can be initiated with the seat height lowered slightly to encourage a more neutral ankle position instead of a plantar flexion position.

Proprioception exercises are commonly initiated during the moderate-protection phase. Protection of the ligament must be encouraged during these challenging exercises. Balancing on the injured limb on a flat surface is slowly progressed to a balance board and then to a minitrampoline—all excellent exercises that stimulate balance, coordination, and muscular endurance (Fig. 17-7).

The minimum-protection phase can begin when the patient can perform all resistive exercises (ankle weight, TheraBand, and manual resistance) and ambulate without pain or limping and swelling is reduced. Although

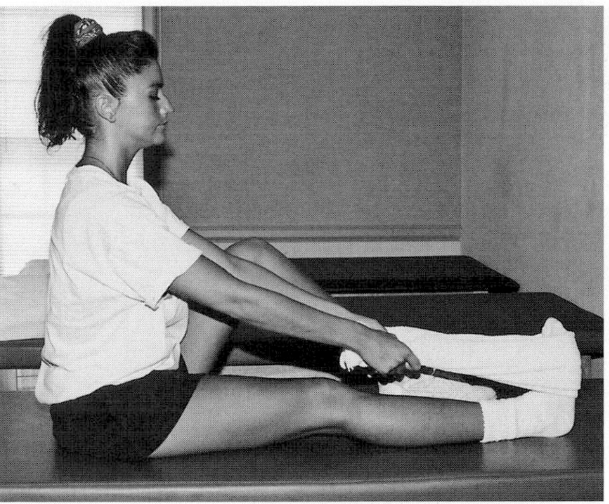

FIG 17-6 Long-seated towel stretch.

proprioception training is commonly used in practice, few articles outlining its effectiveness in rehabilitation exist.[121]

From 4 to 8 weeks after injury, new collagen formation allows almost-normal stresses to be applied (see Chapter 9).[95] At this point, more functional activities are allowed, including straight-line jogging, large figure-of-eight running, jumping drills, and cutting activities.

The minimum-protection phase does not imply removal of all supportive devices. Maturation of the injured ligaments can take 6 to 12 months.[95] It is critical to encourage patient compliance with the use of either tape or a semirigid brace during all running activities.

Box 17-1 outlines a general three-phase rehabilitation program for an inversion ankle sprain. In all instances, if pain, swelling, or irritation persists, the patient is not taken to the next phase until he or she is pain-free in the present phase. The ankle must be securely taped or braced when running, jumping, or otherwise performing aggressive, ballistic motions.

The treatment of grade III ankle sprains (using the standard classification) is controversial.[95,102] At this time, there are few, if any, outcome studies that outline differences in conservative and surgical treatment for acute grade III injuries. Kerkhoffs and colleagues[59] concluded that "there is insufficient evidence available from randomized controlled trials to determine the relative effectiveness of surgical and conservative treatment for acute injuries of the lateral ligament complex of the ankle." Some authors[10,12,109] reported that surgery is needed because "surgical exploration often reveals that the torn ends of the fibulocalcaneal ligament are so widely separated that simple immobilization alone is not sufficient to allow the ligament to heal in a stable position."[10] However, other authors found that "early controlled mobilization (functional treatment) was the method of choice and provided the quickest recovery in ankle mobility and the earliest return to work and physical activity without compromising the late mechanical stability of the ankle."[95] Depending on the physician's choice of treatment, a grade III sprain can be treated either surgically or with early controlled motion and supervised physical therapy. A good to excellent long-term prognosis can be expected in 80% to

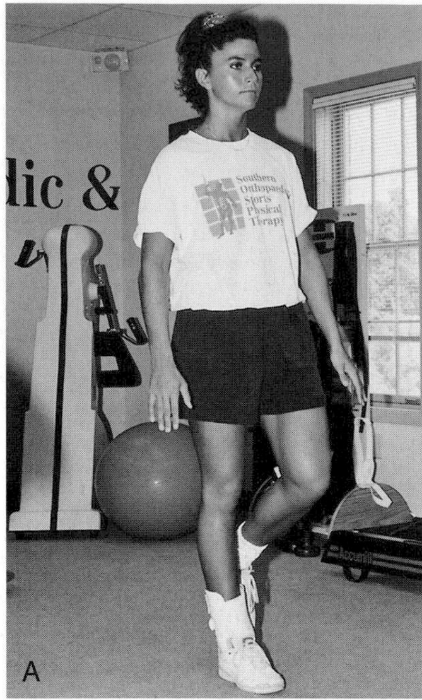
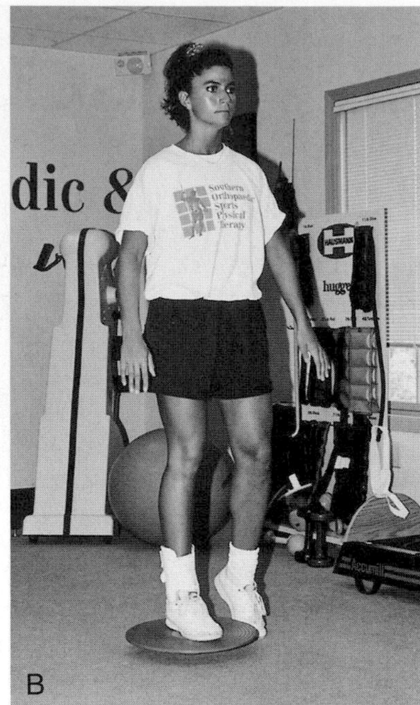
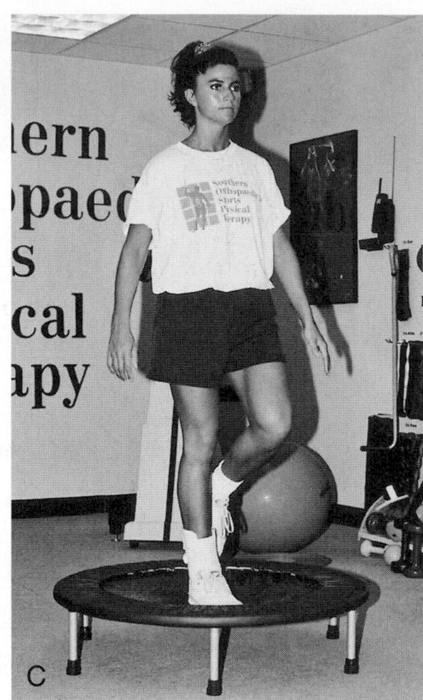

FIG 17-7 **A,** Single-leg standing proprioception and balancing. Note the continued use of external support during the late stage of recovery. **B,** Single-leg standing proprioception and balancing with use of a wobble board or BAPS (Biomechanical Ankle Platform System) board. **C,** Single-leg standing proprioception and balancing on a minitrampoline. The highly unstable surface provides a challenging balance activity.

BOX 17-1 General Three-Phase Intervention Program for Inversion Ankle Sprains

Phase I: Maximum-Protection Phase

1. Rest, ice, compression, and elevation (RICE)
2. Electrical galvanic stimulation (EGS)
3. Weight bearing as tolerated (WBAT)
4. Joint protection (plastic, hinged orthosis, tape, air cast, semi-rigid braces)
5. Active range of motion (dorsiflexion and eversion)
6. Isometric exercises
7. General fitness exercises

Phase II: Moderate-Protection Phase

1. RICE
2. Full weight bearing
3. Concentric and eccentric contractors (bands, ankle weights)
4. Continued joint protection
5. Heel cord stretching
6. Stationary cycling
7. Proprioception exercises
8. General fitness exercises
9. Avoidance of unwanted stresses (inversion and plantar flexion)

Phase III: Minimum-Protection Phase

1. Joint protection during activities
2. Running
3. Jumping
4. Plyometrics
5. Proprioception exercises
6. General fitness exercises
7. Isotonic exercises
8. Isokinetic exercises

90% of patients with grade III ankle sprains regardless of the intervention.[57] However, if inadequate treatment is performed, chronic instability may occur leading to injuries to associated structures.[32] Secondary to the possibility of chronic instability, Ferran and Maffulli[32] proposed that athletes with "acute" grade III injuries be surgically treated.

Generally, joint protection lasts longer with grade III ankle sprains than with grade I and II sprains. When these injuries are treated surgically and postoperative immobilization is used, deleterious effects on muscle, bone, cartilage, tendons, and ligaments can be expected.[1]

DELTOID LIGAMENT SPRAINS (MEDIAL LIGAMENT)

Acute isolated sprains of the deep and superficial layers of the deltoid ligament are rare, occurring in only 3% to 5% of all ankle sprains.[95,96] It is clinically important to recognize that "complete deltoid ligament ruptures occur in combination with ankle fractures."[95]

Important Concepts

Injuries to the medial ligament complex, the deltoid ligament, are far more rare than injuries to the lateral ligament and occur in only 3% to 5% of all ankle sprains.

However, according to Hintermann and co-workers,[46] sprains of the deltoid ligament appear to be more frequent than commonly recognized leading to problems with **posterior tibialis tendon** dysfunction and chronic medial ankle instability. Fractures of the medial or lateral malleolus may cause disruption of the deltoid ligament.[46]

Intervention

Partial tears of the deltoid ligament are managed nonoperatively with physical therapy. Because complete ruptures occur with fractures, many authorities advocate surgical repair and fixation of the fracture fragments.[15,21] However, some authors recommend casting, non–weight bearing for 6 weeks, then progressive weight bearing and physical therapy.[40] In either case, rehabilitation focuses primarily on joint protection and the use of a semirigid orthosis.

The use of ice, compression, and elevation assists with pain and swelling. Progressive strengthening follows a three-phase plan of maximum, moderate, and minimum protection. Isometric exercises, latex rubber band strengthening exercises, active ROM (carefully avoiding unwanted stresses), and progressive weight bearing are added as tolerated. Generally, a total body fitness program can be initiated during cast immobilization and non–weight bearing.

"HIGH" ANKLE SPRAIN OR ANKLE SYNDESMOSIS INJURY

When the ankle is forced into dorsiflexion or rotation with the foot in a weight-bearing position, injury to the ankle **syndesmosis** commonly occurs. This mechanism of injury is prevalent in skiing, football, soccer, and other sport activities.[71] Injury to the structures supporting the ankle syndesmosis, anterior and posterior tibiotalar ligaments, interosseous membrane, interosseous ligament, and deltoid ligament, can result in an unstable distal tibiofibular articulation.[71,89,90,93] Diagnostic testing for "high" ankle sprain includes the external rotation and "squeeze" tests and various forms of diagnostic imaging.

Intervention

Treatment of these injuries may include immobilization, limitation of weight bearing, and surgery.[71,89,93] A conservative approach to treatment and rehabilitation is necessary secondary to weight bearing being disruptive to the healing process for these ligaments. Chronic instability and arthritis commonly occur when this injury is mismanaged.[93]

Important Concepts

An important concept in the treatment of "high" ankle sprains is immobilization and limitation of early weight bearing.

CHRONIC ANKLE LIGAMENT INSTABILITIES

The PTA, as an integral part of the rehabilitation team, must be aware of short-term and long-term complications that may arise from acute or chronic ligament injuries of the ankle. Complications after surgical repair or conservative treatment of ankle sprains are common. Medical advice for ankle sprains is not sought by 55% of patients, and residual symptoms can occur in patients for 18 months.[45] Renstrom and Kannus[95] reported that 10% to 30% of patients have chronic symptoms of weakness, swelling, pain, and joint instability after inversion sprains. There are two types of instabilities associated with chronic ankle sprains: mechanical and functional.

Mechanical Instabilities

Mechanical instability is defined as laxity of the ankle ligaments. With mechanical instabilities, surgery may be necessary to stabilize the ankle joint.[6] The Watson-Jones,[123] Evans,[31] Chrisman-Snook,[18] and Elmslie[18] procedures are common reconstructive surgical procedures used to help stabilize the lateral ligament complex of the ankle. In general, the peroneus brevis muscle is rerouted through a surgically constructed tunnel in the distal fibula (Fig. 17-8, A). The rerouting of the peroneus brevis dynamically stabilizes the lateral aspect of the ankle. Another method used to help stabilize chronic ligament laxity is a delayed anatomic repair of the ligaments. The ligaments are surgically cut, shortened, and reattached to the bone with this method (Fig. 17-8, B). Surgical repair has been gaining popularity among foot and ankle surgeons secondary to the failure of most reconstruction procedures to correct preinjury ankle biomechanics.[47,73]

Ankle arthroscopy has also been gaining popularity among foot and ankle surgeons secondary to the need to identify and treat intraarticular lesions at the time of surgery.[22,62,73] In particular, articular cartilage lesions can be identified and treated with arthroscopy.[14,107]

Intervention. Perhaps secondary to the large number of surgical procedures, the postoperative course of treatment after surgical correction of chronic ankle instability is variable. Commonly, rehabilitation involves some form of ankle immobilization for approximately 2 to 6 weeks depending on the surgeon. Passive dorsiflexion and plantar flexion exercises are begun after immobilization has ended. When reconstructive procedures involving the rerouting of the peroneus brevis tendon are used, active motion is not permitted initially. Restriction of active ROM allows for the reconstruction to stabilize. When tolerated, active ROM exercises begin with careful avoidance of excessive plantar flexion and inversion motions. A general body fitness program is encouraged throughout the period of immobilization. The use of aerobic exercises (stationary bicycle), leg strengthening exercises (leg extensions and hamstring curls), and proprioception exercises is vital throughout rehabilitation.

In primary delayed repair or anatomic reconstruction, the ligament is surgically shortened and reinserted (imbricated). The healing time for ligaments is slightly longer and more tenuous than the healing time for muscle and tendon reconstructions (tenodesis); the period of immobilization may be prolonged. The progression of rehabilitation is the same as with a tenodesis. Active and passive ROM, control of swelling and pain, isometric and manual resistive exercises (being careful to avoid unwanted excessive plantar flexion and inversion motions), TheraBand and isotonic exercises, and isokinetics are used.

Dynamic muscular support is the foundation of various surgical procedures to correct chronic ankle instabilities. Careful and thorough consideration is given to isometric stabilization exercises, TheraBand resistive exercises in all directions, manual resistance, isotonic resistance (with ankle weights), and isokinetic strengthening during the minimal-protective phase. In all cases, full ROM exercises

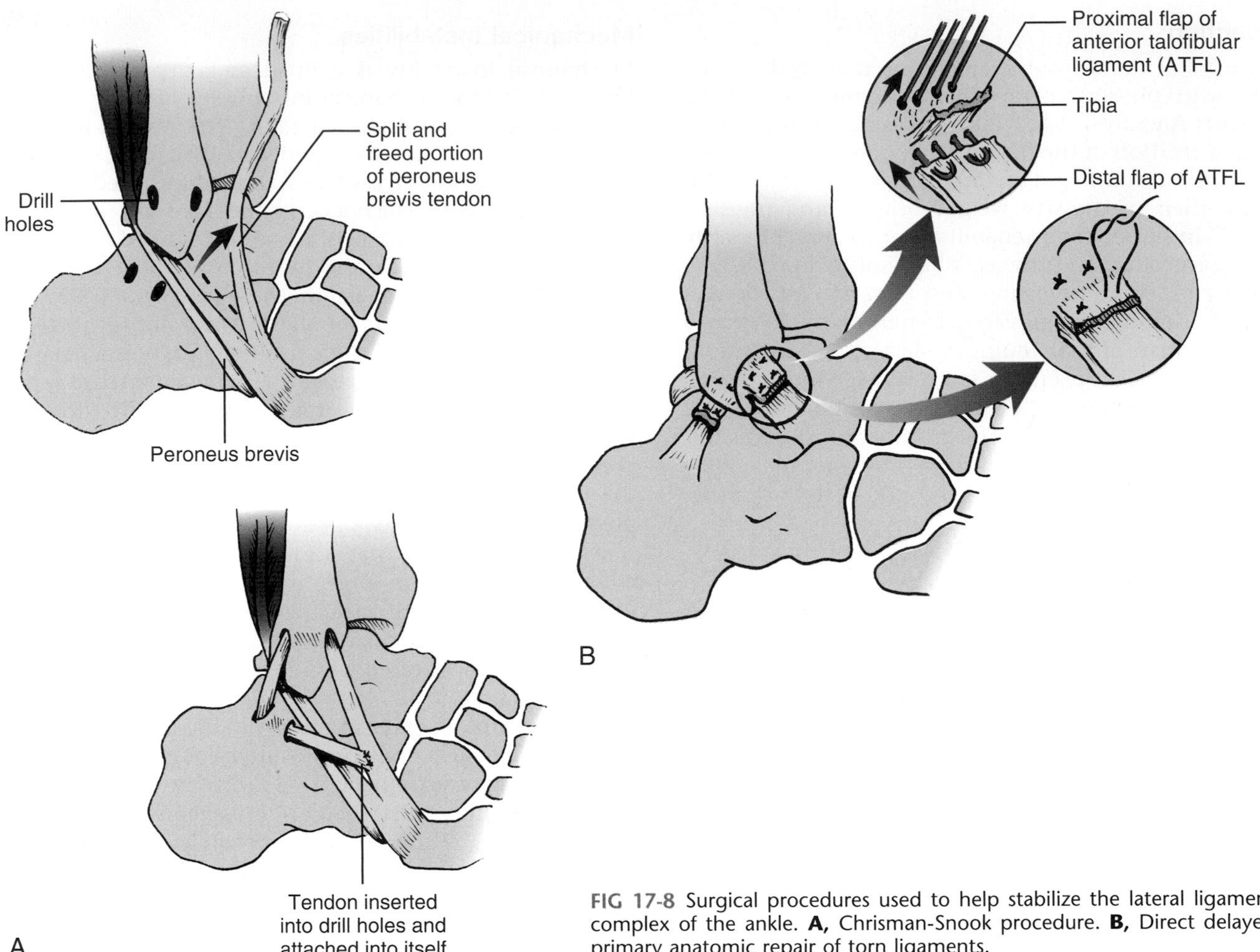

FIG 17-8 Surgical procedures used to help stabilize the lateral ligament complex of the ankle. **A,** Chrisman-Snook procedure. **B,** Direct delayed primary anatomic repair of torn ligaments.

with an emphasis on the eccentric contraction phase of each repetition should be encouraged.

Generally, proprioceptive exercises are used extensively. Single-leg standing exercises, balance board activities, minitrampoline exercises, and heel walking exercises are part of the moderate-protection and minimum-protection phases of rehabilitation. In all cases, joint protection with tape, braces, or a hinged orthosis is a rudimentary but critical principle throughout rehabilitation.

Functional Instabilities

Functional instability refers to a subjective feeling of giving way without affecting ligament laxity. In contrast to mechanical instability, functional instability involves a host of factors, including strength, proprioception, and ligament stability. McVey and associates[80] reported that 40% of patients with lateral ankle instability have functional instability.

Intervention. The primary components of rehabilitation for chronic functional instabilities are closed chain resistance exercises, proprioception maneuvers, dynamic muscular exercises (concentric and eccentric loads), and bracing for support. Single-leg support proprioception exercises with external resistance (Fig. 17-9) provide dynamic support and balance training. Balance board activities, heel-toe walking, and minitrampoline activities are the cornerstones of proprioception exercises for the ankle throughout all phases of rehabilitation for functional ankle instabilities.

SUBLUXING PERONEAL TENDONS

Certain anatomic variations and acute injuries can result in instability of the peroneal tendons and ultimate disability. This injury is classified as acute or chronic. The mechanism of injury involves passive dorsiflexion with the foot slightly everted.[28,76] Acute subluxation of the peroneal tendons can be misdiagnosed as a lateral ankle sprain because of the close anatomic proximity of the tendons to the lateral ligament complex (Fig. 17-10). Patients with peroneal tendon subluxation commonly describe posterior ankle pain and may complain of a popping sensation in the lateral ankle. Active dorsiflexion with eversion of the ankle may reproduce the symptoms.[43]

Important Concepts

A patient with a peroneal subluxation complains of popping and pain in the posterior lateral ankle.

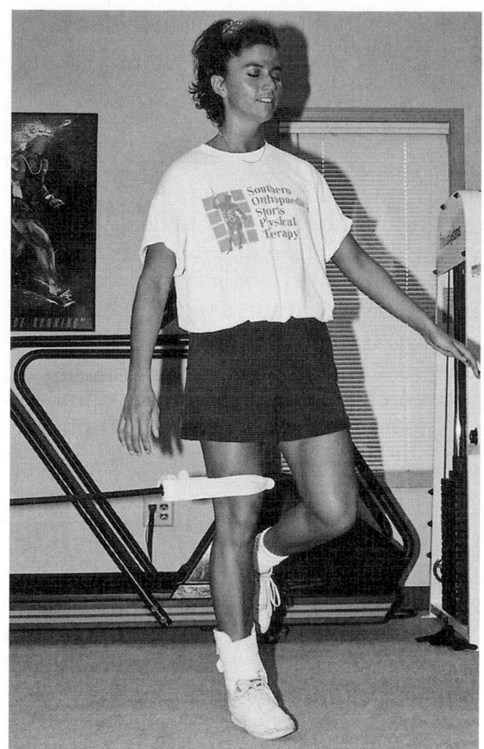

FIG 17-9 Single-leg standing balance and proprioception exercise with the use of elastic cord to stimulate and encourage strength in a weight-bearing closed chain functional position.

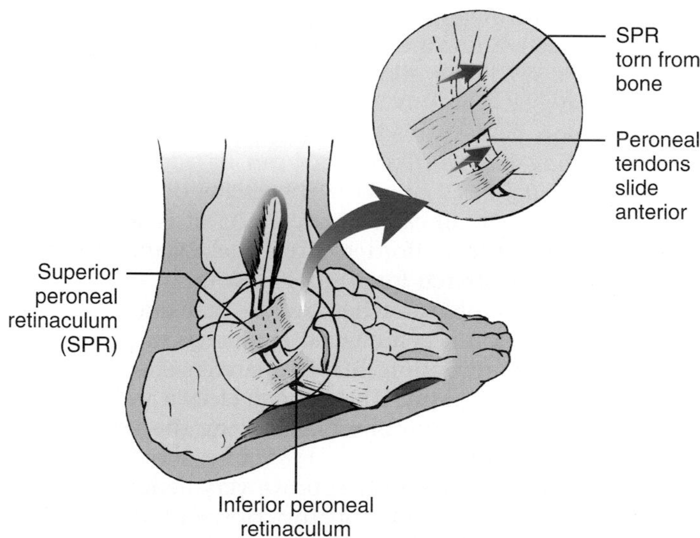

FIG 17-10 Subluxing peroneal tendons. Note anatomic position of the peroneal tendons in relation to the lateral ligament complex of the ankle.

Some patients who experience dislocation of the peroneal tendons have a loose retinaculum (which supports the tendon within the peroneal groove) and may have a very shallow peroneal groove.[33] Acute injuries to the ankle ligaments (grades I, II, and III, using the traditional classification of sprains) may also result in injury to the peroneal retinaculum. Misdiagnosis of an ankle sprain is quite common.[32] When subluxation occurs, the peroneal tendons normally dislocate anteriorly over the lateral malleolus with ankle dorsiflexion.[28,33,76]

INTERVENTION

Acute injuries usually are treated initially with conservative measures, including rigid cast immobilization and non–weight bearing gait for approximately 6 weeks.[33,111] Ferran and colleagues[33] reported that conservative management is successful in approximately 50% of cases. However, patients ultimately require surgical repair to correct the disability in some cases.[58,111] Many authorities still recommend cast immobilization and non–weight bearing for 6 weeks for acute injuries, but operative care is the treatment of choice for cases involving recurrent or chronic subluxing peroneal tendons.[58] Keene[58] described the following five basic types of surgical repair procedures for correction of chronic subluxing peroneal tendons:

- Bone block procedures
- Rerouting procedures
- Periosteal flaps
- Groove deepening procedures
- Tendon slings

Postoperative Interventions

Postoperative care of subluxing peroneal tendons requires excellent communication among the PTA, PT, and surgeon. The exact procedure performed should be explained to the PT, who should articulate the key points of the surgery to the PTA and outline the indications and contraindications for rehabilitation. Usually postoperative care involves the use of immobilization for a few weeks and instruction in weight bearing as tolerated. Keene[58] recommended plantar flexion and dorsiflexion exercises 3 weeks after surgery. Heckman and co-workers[43] suggested that patients remain non–weight bearing for 2 weeks followed by 2 to 4 weeks of immobilization in a cast or walking boot. ROM exercises are commonly initiated at 4 to 6 weeks postoperatively.

While the patient is immobilized, he or she progresses through a general body conditioning program of aerobic exercise and strengthening. After immobilization, active ROM and isometric strengthening exercises are begun. As pain allows, manual resistive and TheraBand strengthening exercises can be added. Care must be taken with extreme dorsiflexion and eversion maneuvers after surgery. Depending on which procedure was used, soft tissue and bone healing constraints must be observed carefully to avoid placing excessive stress on the surgically repaired tissues.

Initially, limited ROM dorsiflexion strengthening exercises should be used. As pain, swelling, and strength improve, greater degrees of dorsiflexion motion can be added. Proprioception exercises on a flat surface can be initiated soon after immobilization ends. Progression to balance board activities and minitrampoline exercises depends on the patient's tolerance. Keene[58] recommended that a running program can begin when ROM has been achieved and the involved limb reaches 80% of the strength of the noninvolved limb.

At first, slow straight-line jogging is attempted. Longer distances are tried if there is no pain, swelling, or complaint of instability. As symptoms allow, sprints can be attempted with careful observation of symptoms.

Plyometric exercises and rapid cutting maneuvers can be included for athletic patients. For example, jumping in place, side-to-side hops, and quick figure-of-eight sprints are progressive functional activities that involve rapid change of direction and ballistic concentric and eccentric open chain and closed chain loading. In most cases, full return to activity can be achieved about 16 weeks after surgery.

ACHILLES TENDINOPATHY

Achilles tendinopathy is an overuse injury resulting from repetitive microtrauma and accumulative overloading of the tendon (Fig. 17-11).[58] The primary feature of Achilles tendinopathy is localized pain at the midportion, distal third, and insertion on the calcaneus. It should be distinguished from other similar posterior foot and ankle disorders, such as retrocalcaneal bursitis (Haglund's deformity).[105]

Many intrinsic and extrinsic factors can lead to Achilles tendinopathy. Decreased vascularity, malalignment of the rearfoot or forefoot, and issues with gastrocnemius-soleus flexibility are common intrinsic factors.[58,105] Extrinsic factors include variations in training, changes in running surface, and poor or inappropriate footwear. The general features of Achilles tendinopathy include soft tissue swelling, pain, and crepitus.

Important Concepts

Extrinsic factors for Achilles tendinopathy include variations in training, changes in running surface, and poor footwear.

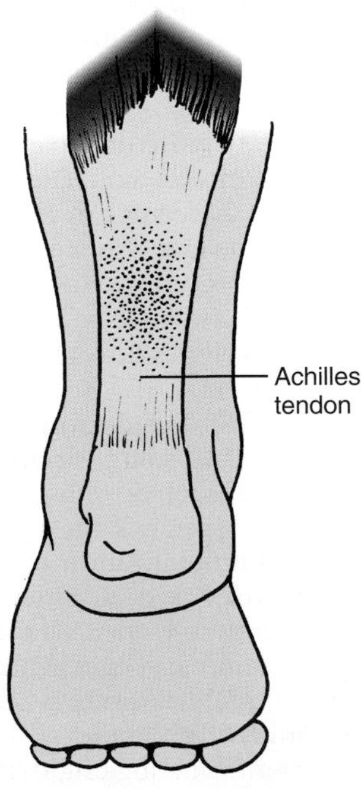

FIG 17-11 Achilles tendinitis.

INTERVENTION

Most cases of Achilles tendinopathy are managed conservatively with various physical agents, oral medications, relative rest, and progressive exercises. Initial management includes the use of ice massage or ice packs for 15 to 20 minutes three to five times daily. The treating physician may prescribe a nonsteroidal antiinflammatory drug (NSAID) to help reduce swelling and pain. All aggravating motions must be stopped. For example, an athletic patient who runs must stop running temporarily until symptoms subside. A program of aerobic exercise using a stationary bicycle or a swimming program can take the place of running. Sometimes a small felt heel-lift can be placed in everyday shoes to help reduce the stress on the tendon. The heel-lift is gradually diminished as symptoms are reduced. It is not advisable to remove the heel-lift support suddenly when symptoms improve because pain and swelling occasionally return.

Ultrasound also can be used to help reduce pain and assist with collagen synthesis.[53] Generally, ultrasound can be used immediately before an exercise program to improve circulation, enhance relaxation of the soft tissues, and reduce pain. Occasionally, phonophoresis (ultrasound used with a topical hydrocortisone cream) is used in cases of severe pain.

Flexibility exercises are used to increase dorsiflexion motion and reduce the effects of scarring in prolonged cases of Achilles tendinopathy. Researchers have pointed out that a lack of dorsiflexion is a common denominator for patients with Achilles tendinopathy.[67]

Initially, active dorsiflexion exercises are used. Towel stretches are gradually added as pain allows. In many cases, it may be helpful to apply ice packs or ice massage to the tendon before stretching and strengthening exercises. Standing heel cord stretches can be added to the flexibility program as soon as towel stretches do not cause pain or swelling. In all cases of stretching, it is advisable to avoid any ballistic motions, to stretch gently and firmly, and to hold each stretch for 10 to 30 seconds.

Standing heel cord stretches can be performed on a small block or with a commercial appliance to produce greater dorsiflexion motion. A soleus stretch is also used for Achilles tendinopathy. The patient faces a wall with the knees touching the wall while keeping the heels on the floor (Fig. 17-12).

Strengthening exercises often prove very beneficial for patients with Achilles tendinopathy. However, most full ROM strengthening and stretching exercises also cause complaints of pain. A safe and effective exercise program focuses initially on limited ROM and submaximal exercises. When the patient can perform all exercises without pain, the next phase of more vigorous exercise can begin.

Curwin and Stanish[24] advocated eccentric strength training exercises for treatment of many types of tendinopathy. When strengthening the gastrocnemius-soleus muscle group, standing heel raises are a preferred form of exercise. The patient is instructed to rise up on the balls of the feet using the uninvolved limb; before descent phase, the patient transfers body weight to the involved limb and slowly lowers using the ipsilateral

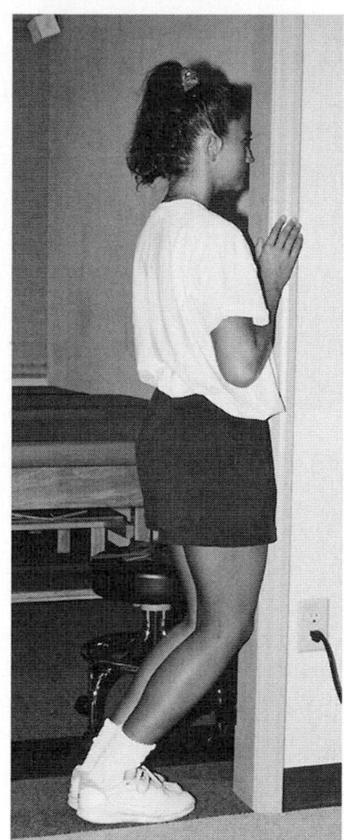

FIG 17-12 Standing soleus stretch. Flexing the knees enhances the stretch to the gastrocnemius-soleus complex.

gastrocnemius-soleus muscle. Several authors strongly advocated the use of eccentric strength training only for Achilles tendinopathy.[3,61] Alfredson and colleagues[3] described excellent clinical outcomes after a 12-week eccentric strength training program for Achilles tendinopathy. In their study, subjects who performed the eccentric program were able to resume running in 12 weeks, whereas subjects who performed a more standard concentric rehabilitation program were unable to return to running during this same time frame. Knobloch[61] reported that "daily eccentric training for Achilles tendinopathy is a safe activity without any evidence of adverse effects in either mid-portion and insertional Achilles tendinopathy."

Important Concepts

A more recent treatment for Achilles tendinopathy includes eccentric exercise.

In some severe cases of Achilles tendinopathy, physicians may prescribe rigid cast immobilization of the ankle for 10 days.[67] The entire program of rehabilitation after cast immobilization progresses at a slightly slower rate because of the loss of ROM and strength associated with immobilization. In all cases of Achilles tendinopathy, the patient is instructed in a general body fitness program. Aerobic exercise can be achieved with an upper body ergometer (UBE), a seated bicycle ergometer with the seat height corrected to prevent plantar flexion, or a swimming program. Upper and lower body stretching and strengthening exercises are encouraged as long as the tendon experiences no undue stress or pain.

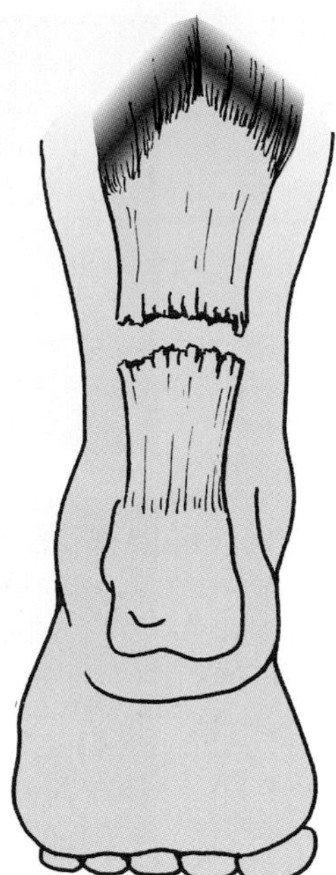

FIG 17-13 Complete rupture of the Achilles tendon.

RUPTURES OF THE ACHILLES TENDON

Complete ruptures of the Achilles tendon can occur with sudden eccentric-concentric contraction of the gastrocnemius-soleus (Fig. 17-13).[105] These ruptures usually involve the area "3 to 4 cm proximal to its insertion on the calcaneus, within the area of decreased vascularity" and occur mostly in men 20 to 50 years old.[58,105] Racquet sports and other activities requiring a deceleration-to-acceleration mechanism are often the mechanism of injury. Approximately 50% of Achilles tendon ruptures are secondary to degenerative changes in the tendon.[105] Corticosteroid injections or fluoroquinolone antibiotics also weaken the tendon and predispose an individual to rupture.[105]

In acute Achilles tendon rupture, palpation reveals a defect or gap in the continuity of the distal third of the tendon. Thompson's test clinically assesses the integrity of the Achilles tendon. To perform this simple test, the patient lies prone on an examining table with the feet extending off the end. The entire lower leg from knee to toes is exposed. The belly of the calf of the uninvolved limb is grasped and squeezed so that the foot plantar flexes. If the tendon is ruptured on the involved limb when the calf is squeezed, no plantar flexion motion results (Fig. 17-14).

INTERVENTION

A ruptured Achilles tendon can be treated surgically or with cast immobilization.[60,105] Nonoperative treatment of Achilles tendon ruptures requires the patient to be immobilized for 8 weeks.[58,60,105] However, with nonoperative treatment, researchers have documented rerupture rates of 8% to 39%.[9,31,55,60] In addition, there is a greater loss of strength, power, and endurance compared with surgically

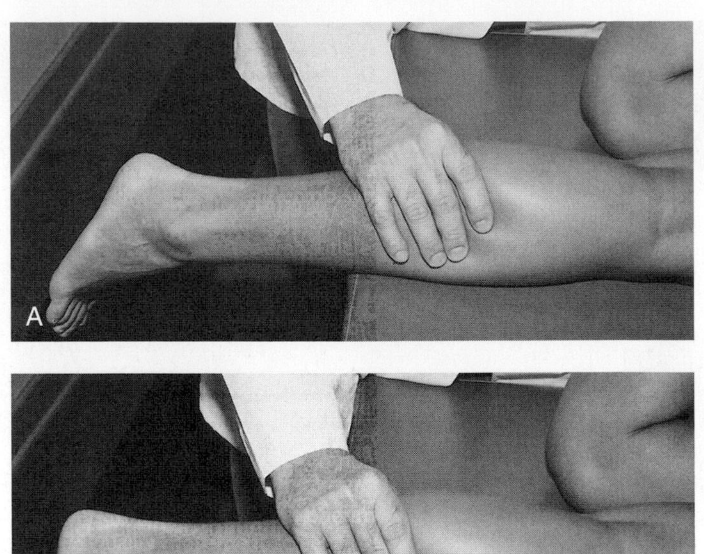

FIG 17-14 Thompson test to confirm or deny the presence of a ruptured Achilles tendon. **A,** A negative Thompson test is demonstrated by observation of plantar flexion of the foot when squeezing the calf. **B,** A positive Thompson test reveals no plantar flexion of the foot when the calf is squeezed.

repaired tendons.[9,52,55,58] Surgically repaired Achilles tendons have a much lower rate of rerupture (0% to 5%), and there is a significant increase in ultimate recovery of muscular strength, power, and endurance.[60] However, Nistor[88] reported only minor differences between surgical and nonsurgical management. Some surgeons prefer nonoperative management because there are fewer complications related to surgery, reduced complaints, no hospitalization, and no significant differences in function compared with surgically treated patients.[88] Numerous surgical techniques are used to repair acute Achilles tendon ruptures, including end-to-end primary repair and direct repair and augmentation with tendon or synthetic grafts.*

The rehabilitation program used after nonoperative immobilization of an Achilles tendon rupture requires the PTA to appreciate the time-dependent nature of tendon healing and plastic and elastic deformation principles (see Chapter 12). Throughout the course of immobilization, the patient should be instructed in a general body conditioning program that does not stress the involved tissues. The muscles of the noninvolved limb (i.e., quadriceps, hamstrings, gastrocnemius-soleus) should be vigorously strengthened along with the thigh and hamstring muscles of the involved limb. Aerobic exercise is also encouraged. Stationary bicycle ergometers using only the uninvolved limb (a toe clip is necessary for single-limb cycling) and UBEs are appropriate and safe cardiovascular fitness tools. When the cast is removed and after the initial evaluation by the PT, the PTA proceeds with thermal agents as indicated. Moist heat can be used before ROM and flexibility exercises. If pain and swelling are present, a cold whirlpool or ice packs with compression can be applied.

Regaining full dorsiflexion and plantar flexion motion is an exceedingly slow process after cast removal. Gentle active dorsiflexion and plantar flexion exercises are initiated immediately. Typically, a small heel-lift is used in everyday shoes to minimize stress on the healing tendon. Because the tendon was not surgically repaired, the process of regaining tensile strength and collagen alignment must be approached cautiously (see Chapter 12). Progressive active motion is an essential component for full return to function. However, if the tendon is stressed too soon or vigorously, it may rerupture. The heel-lift is commonly worn for 3 to 4 weeks and gradually reduced in size to prevent sudden excessive stress on the tendon.[58]

Progressive plantar flexion and dorsiflexion exercises using a latex band are encouraged as pain and motion allow. Proprioception exercises can be employed early, depending on the patient's tolerance. Generally, proprioception exercises begin with the patient in a seated position (Fig. 17-15) and progress as tolerated. If rerupture occurs, it is usually within 4 weeks after immobilization.[58] During this maximum-protection phase, the patient is encouraged to avoid sudden forceful plantar flexion or dorsiflexion motions.

As motion increases gradually, closed chain resistive exercises can be initiated, based on the patient's ROM,

*For more information on these techniques, refer to the articles found in references 2, 16, 30, 37, 44, 48, 50, 51, 56, 58, 60, 63, 64, 72, 92, 103, 104, 112, 113, 117, and 119.

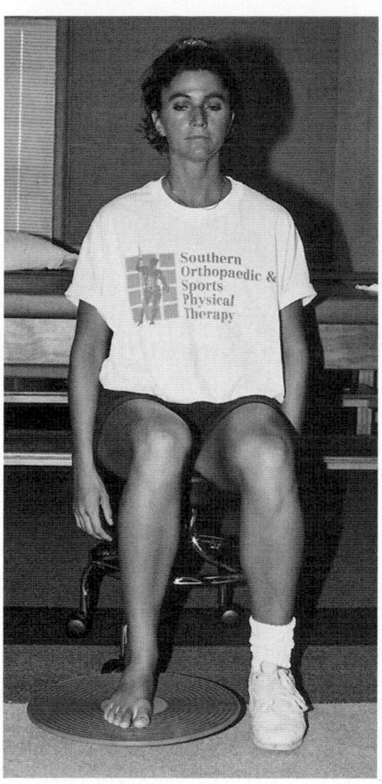

FIG 17-15 Initial proprioception activities can begin in a seated position using a wobble board.

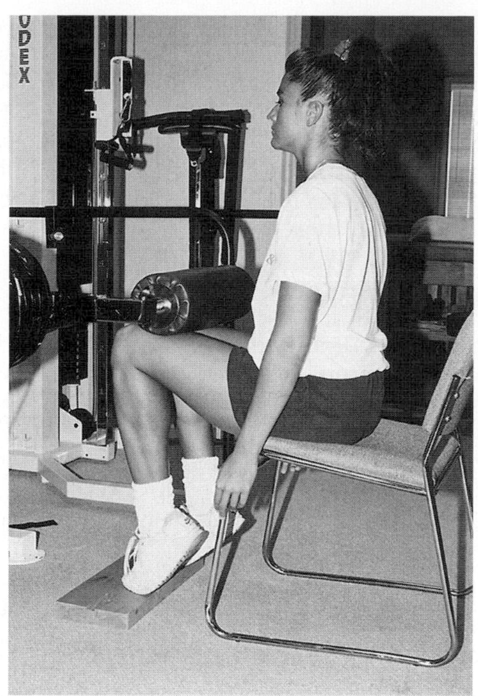

FIG 17-16 Seated heel or calf raises are performed by modifying and adjusting a knee-extension machine with a range-limiting device.

pain tolerance, swelling, and the length of time after cast removal. Seated stationary cycling can be used for aerobic fitness, ROM, and local muscular endurance. The seat must be adjusted to avoid excessive plantar flexion or dorsiflexion. Step-ups can be used (with heel-lift) to encourage weight-bearing eccentric loading.

Weight-bearing plantar flexion can begin gradually after the patient has successfully completed the prescribed program of ROM and strengthening exercises without complications. Standing plantar flexion is initiated without a block to stand on. The patient is instructed to rise up on the toes gradually using primarily the uninvolved limb and then to lower himself or herself using both feet. As strength improves, the patient gradually uses more of the involved limb to rise up on the balls of the feet. Adding a small block of wood on which to rise adds greater dorsiflexion stress and motion. Seated calf raises can be performed by modifying a leg extension machine (Fig. 17-16). The seated position may be more comfortable initially.

The PTA reassesses the patient's ROM, strength, pain, and swelling on a daily basis. Modifications are necessary if the patient is having undue pain with any phase of the program. Daily communication with the PT allows continuous restructuring of the rehabilitation plan based on the patient's needs as assessed by the PTA. Isokinetic testing for plantar flexion, dorsiflexion, ROM, strength, power, and local muscular endurance generally is reserved for the minimal-protection phase. However, isokinetic strengthening exercises can be employed early if done at higher speeds and performed submaximally under limited ROM conditions.

Rehabilitation after surgical repair or reconstruction of the Achilles tendon is variable. Secondary to the numerous procedures available, the timing of the surgery (acute versus chronic), stability of the repair or reconstruction, and intrinsic patient variables, the rehabilitation progression may differ from surgeon to surgeon and from patient to patient. In particular, the surgical variations are numerous, with each variation having differing needs for immobilization and restriction of weight bearing during the immediate postoperative period. Variables such as ROM, weight bearing, and initiation of strength training are determined by the surgeon. Each individual should be rehabilitated independently.*

Generally, rehabilitation after Achilles tendon repair or reconstruction follows a criteria-based rehabilitation program as described previously. After a period of immobilization, a gradual progression of weight bearing and ROM is pursued. Normally, plantar flexion is less restricted than dorsiflexion during the early postoperative period. Strength training can begin 2 to 4 weeks after immobilization.[58]

Secondary to the large differences in Achilles tendon surgery and rehabilitation programs, the return to full activity is also variable. At least one group believed that successful outcomes depend on tendon elongation. Kannas and Renstrom[57] reported that improved outcomes occur when less elongation of the Achilles tendon occurs.

*For more information on these techniques, please refer to the articles found in references 2, 16, 30, 37, 44, 48, 50, 51, 56, 58, 60, 63, 64, 72, 92, 103, 104, 112, 113, 117, and 119.

Symmetric ankle dorsiflexion ROM is a goal of treatment, and increased dorsiflexion beyond the contralateral side is discouraged. Generally, most patients are able to return to full activity within 6 to 9 months. Surgical complications after Achilles tendon repair or reconstruction include sural nerve dysfunction, infection, skin sensitivity, adhesions, rerupture, and tendon necrosis.[60,64] Most patients appear to be satisfied with their results.[2,30,51,60,92]

COMPARTMENT SYNDROMES

Compartment syndromes of the lower leg are defined as either acute or chronic elevated tissue pressure within a closed fascial space, resulting in occlusion of vessels and compromised neuromuscular function.[4,36,97] Acute compartment syndromes of the leg are most commonly associated with tibial fractures, direct trauma to the area, muscle rupture, muscle hypertrophy, and circumferential burns.[65,95] Acute elevated intracompartmental pressure within the lower leg is considered a medical emergency.[36]

Important Concepts

Acute elevated intracompartmental pressure is a medical emergency.

Chronic compartment syndromes also are referred to as exertional compartment syndrome or exercise-induced compartment syndrome. Muscular contractions and exertion have been shown to cause increases in muscle size, leading to increased intracompartmental pressure.[65,95] The result is ischemia and reduced neuromuscular function. To understand this series of events, it is necessary to review pertinent anatomy of the lower leg.

There are four well-defined compartments of the leg, divided by nonyielding fascia.[4,97] The anterior compartment of the lower leg contains the tibialis anterior, anterior tibial artery and vein, and foot and toe extensor muscles. The lateral compartment contains the superficial peroneal nerve and short and long peroneal muscles. The superficial posterior compartment contains the soleus muscle and plantaris and gastrocnemius tendons. The deep posterior compartment contains the posterior tibialis muscle, peroneal artery and vein, **tibial nerve,** and posterior tibial artery and vein. If swelling occurs in one or more of these compartments, reduced capillary blood perfusion results in neurovascular and muscular dysfunction.

Clinical symptoms of acute compartment syndrome include pain, palpable swelling or tenseness, and paresthesias.[4,97] The skin may be warm, shiny, and tense. Passive stretching of the muscles of the lower leg may produce severe pain.

Symptoms of chronic or exertional compartment syndromes include a dull aching pain within the muscle during and after long-term exercise. Paresthesias also may develop as the syndrome progresses. The sections most commonly affected with chronic exercise-induced compartment syndromes are the anterior and deep posterior compartments of the lower leg.

INTERVENTION

Acute compartment syndrome is treated surgically with a fasciotomy.[4,97] When nerve and muscle ischemia lasts longer than 12 hours, severe and irreversible damage occurs.[4] However, if the ischemia can be reduced in less than 4 hours, usually no permanent damage occurs.[4]

A surgical fasciotomy is designed to relieve intracompartmental pressure by opening or releasing the fascial compartment, allowing the pressure to be reduced. The surgical incision is sometimes left open and is managed with sterile dressings.[4] Less invasive techniques such as endoscopy have been used more recently.[126] Immediately after surgery, ice packs and leg elevation are necessary to reduce swelling. Walking as tolerated and active and passive gentle ROM of the ankle and knee are begun 2 days after surgery. Early ROM is crucial to prevent contractures. Treatment with ice and leg elevation is continued after exercise. A general conditioning program can begin with strengthening exercises and aerobic exercises using a single-leg ergometer or UBE. When the patient shows improved motion and reduced pain and swelling, light resistance exercises can begin for the involved leg. Close attention should be paid to foot structure because contractures may develop after surgery resulting in varying levels of equinus deformity in the foot.[115] However, very light resistance should be encouraged because heavy and intense exercise, which leads to muscular hypertrophy, is contraindicated after fasciotomy for acute compartment syndromes. In a review article, Schubert[106] provided a good overview of the rehabilitation guidelines after surgical release of exertional compartment syndromes.

The management of chronic exercise-induced compartment syndromes is similar to management of acute compartment syndromes. However, chronic compartment syndromes do not always represent a surgical emergency. Conservative management includes relative rest, antiinflammatory agents, stretching and strengthening of the involved muscles, and foot orthotic devices (if appropriate).[124] Subcutaneous fasciotomy should be performed only when pain and symptoms affect function. The postoperative management of fasciotomy after chronic compartment syndromes parallels the rehabilitation program outlined for acute compartment syndromes.

ANKLE FRACTURES

The most widely accepted classification of ankle fractures is described by Lauge-Hansen.[79] The organization and classification of ankle fractures frequently involve the direction of force, which results in specific patterns of injury (Fig. 17-17). For example, a Lauge-Hansen pronation-abduction or pronation-lateral rotation injury may result in a malleolar or bimalleolar fracture of the ankle (Fig. 17-18).

Ankle fractures include lateral malleolar fractures, medial malleolar fractures, bimalleolar fractures (combined medial and lateral malleolar fractures), and trimalleolar fractures (bimalleolar fractures plus the posterior margin of the tibia). Although simple malleolar fractures are managed initially with immobilization, many fractures

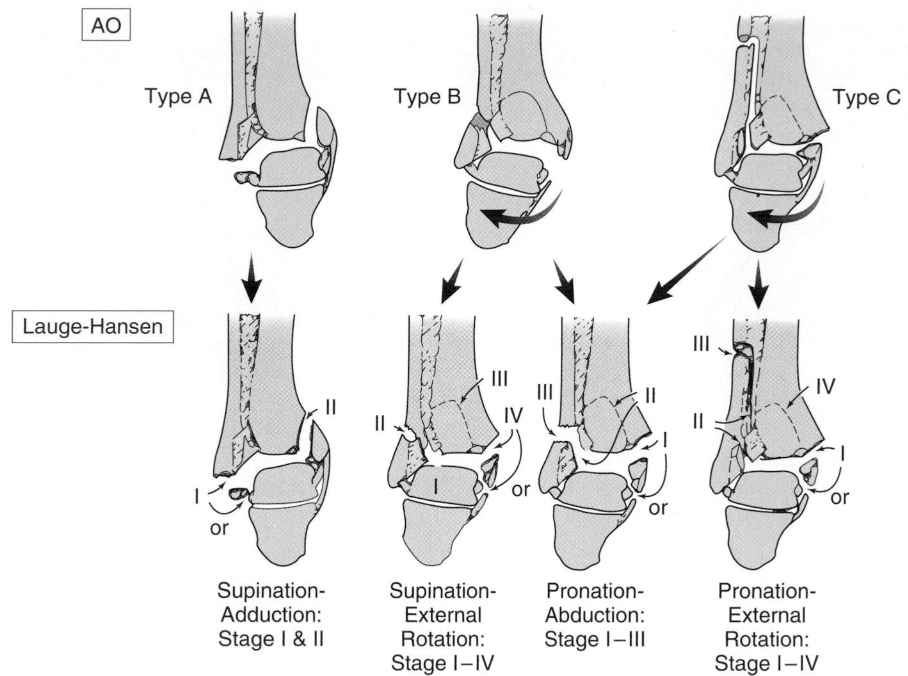

FIG 17-17 AO and Lauge-Hansen classification of ankle fractures. *(Modified from Sangeorzan BJ, Hansen ST: Ankle and foot: trauma. In Poss R, editor:* Orthopaedic knowledge update III, *Park Ridge, IL, 1990, American Academy of Orthopaedic Surgeons.)*

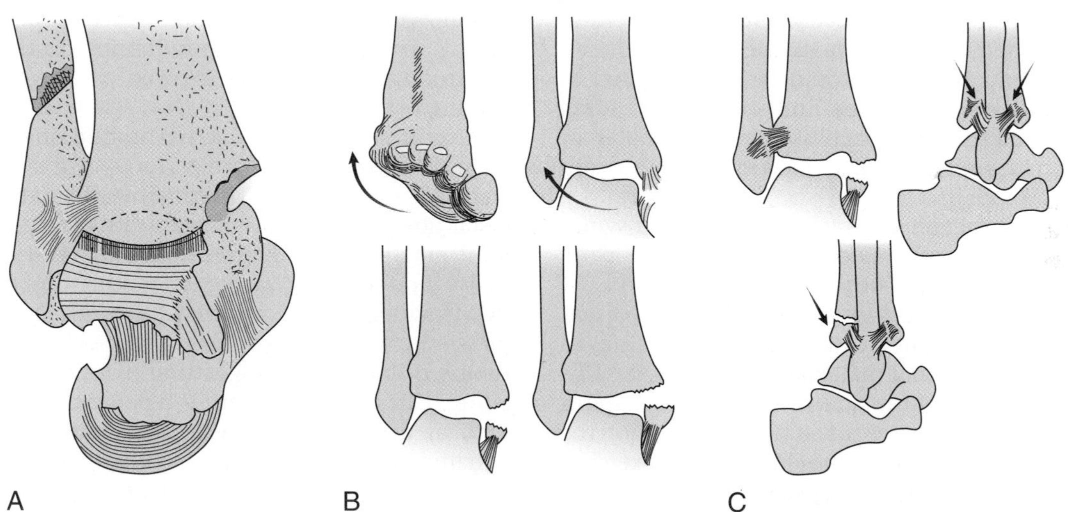

FIG 17-18 **A,** Pronation-lateral rotation injury. **B,** Pronation-abduction injuries. **C,** Pronation-abduction injury. *(Modified from McRae R:* Practical fracture treatment, *ed 3, New York, 1994, Churchill Livingstone.)*

are managed with an open reduction with internal fixation (ORIF) procedure. Typically, these fractures are fixed with various screws and plates to hold the fragments in place (Fig. 17-19).

In many cases of ankle fractures repaired with an ORIF procedure, the patient is in a semirigid postoperative removable splint for 2 weeks. This splint can be removed to allow for active dorsiflexion and plantar flexion ROM exercises; however, this is patient-specific and should be confirmed with the surgeon. Because of the mechanism of injury that caused the malleolar fracture and the position of the internal fixation devices, no inversion or eversion exercises are performed.

A walking cast is applied when the patient achieves full plantar flexion and dorsiflexion ROM. Before casting, the surgical wound must be fully closed, sutures must be removed, infection must be absent, and no drainage must be present. A general full-body conditioning program is prescribed throughout immobilization. Aerobic fitness and strengthening exercises also are advocated. Strengthening of the uninjured limb has shown beneficial crossover results in strength of the injured limb.[120]

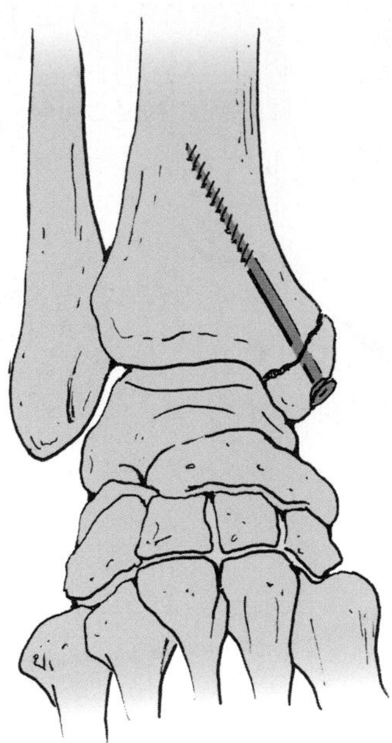

FIG 17-19 Open reduction with internal fixation screw fixation for medial malleolar fracture.

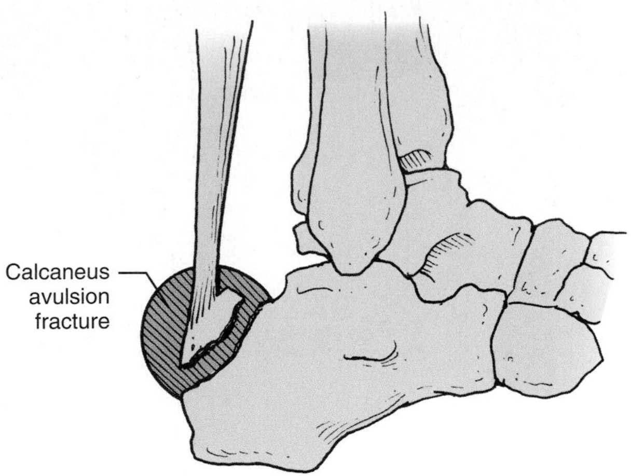

FIG 17-20 Fractured calcaneus type II with avulsion.

ROM exercises, isometric strengthening, stationary cycling, and weight-bearing exercises are begun after the cast is removed. Progressive exercises employ latex rubber tubing or bands, manual resistive exercises, isoinertial/isotonic strengthening, and proprioception exercises. Return to function exercises should be incorporated as soon as the patient is able. Single-limb activities, landing activities, and out of plane activities are examples of important activities used for proprioceptive training and return to activity.

The PTA must be acutely aware of the signs and symptoms of possible hardware loosening (increased pain, swelling, crepitus, and motion) so as to inform the PT swiftly and make all necessary modifications in the present program. For example, after cast removal following an ORIF procedure for a medial malleolar fracture, if the PTA recognized increased swelling and complaints of crepitus when strengthening exercises stressing inversion of the ankle were increased, the PTA should halt the exercises and inform the PT. Weight-bearing status; active, passive, and resisted ROM; and functional progression should be determined by the physician throughout rehabilitation.

Important Concepts

Signs and symptoms of fracture hardware loosening include increased pain, swelling, crepitus, and motion.

DISTAL TIBIA COMPRESSION FRACTURES (PILON FRACTURES)

Distal tibia compression fractures (pilon fractures) occur as a result of vertical or axial loads that "drive" or compress the tibia into the **talus**. The initial management of these injuries usually involves an ORIF procedure, external fixation, or skeletal traction with a calcaneal pin.[79] If the fracture was managed with external fixation, special attention should be given to these individuals because malunion is more common with this type of fixation.[94] Because of the nature of these fractures, weight-bearing activities usually are deferred for 12 or more weeks. Weight bearing creates vertical compression and compromises the natural course of healing needed for a stable outcome. Secondary osteoarthritis is a common complication with severe multifragmented compression fractures.[79] Typically throughout immobilization, a general conditioning program is allowed as long as no weight bearing occurs.

After immobilization, active motion and general ankle strengthening exercises are performed to the patient's tolerance. Care is taken to protect the articular surface of the distal tibia and talus. Also, hardware placed at or near the joint may provide rigid resistance to ROM activities. Initially, non–weight-bearing strengthening exercises and ROM maneuvers are allowed. Progressive loading (compression) can proceed cautiously using latex surgical tubing or bands for long-sitting plantar flexion strengthening. Partial weight bearing repetitive motion activities, such as a stationary bicycle ergometer, can be used to enhance ankle motion and endurance. Weight-bearing activities generally are painful until satisfactory healing has occurred. However, toe-touch weight bearing progressing to partial weight bearing is well tolerated, helps restore proprioception, and assists with healing. Throughout rehabilitation, the physician should determine weight-bearing status; active, passive, and resisted ROM; and functional progression.

CALCANEAL FRACTURES

Calcaneal fractures are intraarticular depression fractures usually caused by falls from a height and resulting in compression of the calcaneus from the talus (Fig. 17-20). McRae[79] described seven common patterns of calcaneal fractures, as follows:

1. Vertical fractures of the calcaneal tuberosity
2. Horizontal fractures
3. Fractures of the sustentaculum tali

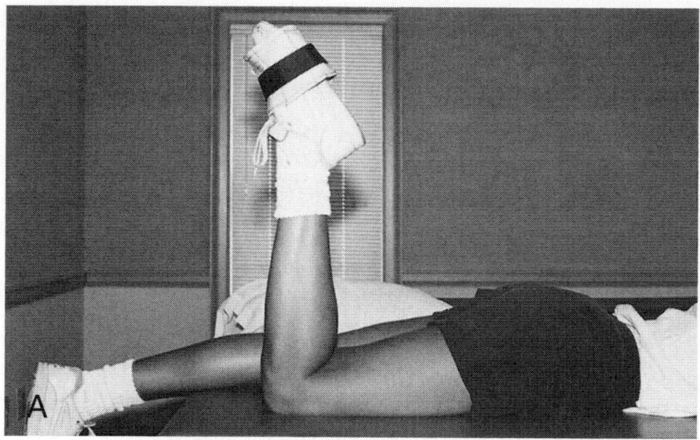

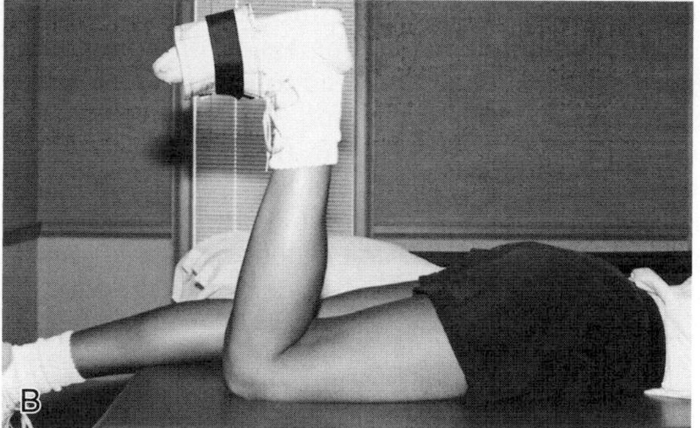

FIG 17-21 Prone gastrocnemius-soleus strengthening. **A,** Starting position with the knee of the affected limb flexed to 90°. **B,** The patient actively plantar flexes the foot against gravity and the applied resistance.

4. Anterior calcaneal fractures
5. Fracture of the body of the calcaneus without involvement of the subtalar joint
6. Calcaneal fractures with lateral displacement and involvement of the subtalar joint
7. Central calcaneus crushing fractures

Each calcaneal fracture type has individual characteristics that allow the physician to determine the treatment options and rehabilitation progression. Conservative (casting) and surgical (ORIF) procedures are used with **calcaneus fractures.**[79] As with all fractures, specific rehabilitation procedures should be cleared by the physician before initiation. When possible, early ROM activity is used in rehabilitation to reduce stiffness and prevent long-term ROM loss. Throughout rehabilitation, the physician should determine weight-bearing status; active, passive, and resisted ROM; and functional progression. Supportive measures to control pain and swelling are used as necessary.

Over the long-term, the cornerstone in recovering from a calcaneal fracture lies in regaining motion and strengthening the plantar flexors. Multiangle isometric plantar flexion can be initiated and progressed to full ROM manual resistance dorsiflexion and plantar flexion. The use of latex rubber tubing and bands for plantar flexion in a long-seated position is an appropriate and challenging calf strengthening exercise during the moderate-protection phase of rehabilitation. Strengthening of the soleus can be achieved by having the patient lie prone with the affected leg flexed 90° at the knee and placing ankle weights around the foot of the affected leg (Fig. 17-21).

Gait examination and retraining are necessary in these patients because initial contact during gait is compromised. Patients are more likely to load on the midfoot or forefoot at initial contact. Training of a normal heel-strike pattern on soft surfaces may be necessary to avoid long-term gait deviations.

FRACTURES OF THE TALUS

The talus can be fractured by falling from a height and landing on the foot in a crouched position.[79] This mechanism produces an axial compression load between the talus and calcaneus. There are four classifications of talar fractures, as follows:[79]

- Type I: Talar neck fracture without displacement
- Type II: Talar fracture with subtalar subluxation (the incidence of avascular necrosis is 50%)[79]
- Type III: Talar fracture with further subtalar subluxation (the incidence of avascular necrosis is 85%)[79]
- Type IV: The talar head dislocates from the navicular in association with a type III injury

These fractures can be treated with closed reduction and cast immobilization or with an ORIF procedure. To allow for proper healing, these fractures require 3 months of non–weight bearing. The rehabilitation program can proceed during this immobilization period with single-leg stationary cycling, aerobic training, UBE, or contralateral limb strengthening. Strengthening exercises include knee extension and hamstring curl maneuvers and non–weight-bearing hip abduction, adduction, flexion, and extension. Usually the patient is immobilized in a posterior splint that can be removed for exercise periods. ROM exercises and supportive measures for pain and swelling control can be used during the maximum-protection phase of the rehabilitation program. Osteoarthritis is a common long-term complication with talar fractures because of the duration of immobilization and non–weight-bearing status. As with all fractures, the physician should determine weight-bearing status; active, passive, and resisted ROM; and functional progression throughout rehabilitation.

STRESS FRACTURES OF THE FOOT AND ANKLE

A stress fracture is a partial or complete fracture of bone caused by unrelenting stress and force that do not allow for osteoblastic repair of bone and cause accelerated bone resorption. Common sites for stress fractures in the foot and ankle are the metatarsals, lateral malleolus, os calcis, navicular, and sesamoid.

Clinically, pain is the predominant feature of a stress fracture. The pain usually increases with activity and subsides with rest. The incidence of stress fractures in the foot and ankle is partly related to participation in demanding physical activity. If stress and forces are applied to bone and are not removed to allow the bone to repair, osteoclast activity overtakes the rate of osteoblast activity, and stress fractures occur.

The development of stress fractures can be viewed in part as resulting from a linear progression or continuum of excessive external forces that lead to intrinsic reactions of muscle, bone, and periosteum. For example, with increased muscular forces resulting from continued and excessive use (marathon running, recreational jogging, aerobic dance, or occupations that require standing or walking all day), there is an associated increased rate of bone remodeling around the area of increased stress.[108] If the stress is not removed, this increase in bone remodeling is followed by a greater rate of bone resorption. If the stress continues, the bone eventually responds by developing microfractures, periosteal inflammation, and resultant stress fractures.[108] If further stress occurs and the bone and soft tissues are not allowed to recover fully and heal properly, the development of linear fractures and ultimately displaced fractures can occur.[108]

Certain stress fractures pose a greater risk of delayed union, nonunion, and displacement than others.[77] The base or proximal diaphysis of the fifth metatarsal is described as "no man's land" and is "at risk" for delayed union or nonunion after a stress fracture.[77,95] Usually, when conservative relative rest has failed to arrest symptoms of pain, complete rigid cast immobilization is indicated for 6 to 8 weeks.[77,95,96] Other stress fractures termed at risk[23] are tarsal navicular fracture, sesamoid fractures, and all intraarticular fractures.

Not-at-risk[77] stress fractures of the foot and ankle can be effectively rehabilitated with activity modification; relative rest; therapeutic agents to relieve pain and swelling; and specific leg, ankle, and foot stretching and strengthening exercises. Low-impact aerobic exercise is useful in athletic patients who are extremely active. For example, instead of running, the patient can use a stationary cycle, recumbent cycle, or elliptical trainer or run in a non–weight-bearing manner under water.

For stress fractures of the foot and ankle that are at risk (fifth metatarsal, navicular sesamoids, and intraarticular fractures),[77] more caution is necessary during the advancement of closed chain activities to protect the healing bone from unwanted forces. With at-risk stress fractures, some form of external support can be used to brace the area. Usually some type of bracing, padding, casting, or orthosis is applied to control stress and forces to the healing bone.[77] The application of therapeutic exercises must be approached cautiously. Submaximal isometric exercises are encouraged initially. Active ROM and light concentric and eccentric loads are added as pain allows. Vertical compressive loads and shearing forces (i.e., jumping, running, cutting) are strictly prohibited to allow proper healing. Modifications in aerobic activity and general physical conditioning can allow the patient to continue to participate in strenuous physical conditioning, provided that no stress is applied to the healing tissues. The initiation of closed chain functional activities must be deferred until radiographic confirmation by the physician documents stable bone healing.

MEDIAL TIBIAL STRESS SYNDROME

Musculoskeletal overuse injuries of the lower leg involving the distal third of the posterior medial border of the tibia have historically been referred to as *shin splints*. This term has no place in orthopedic management and should be discarded as a nonspecific term used to describe any pain occurring in the lower leg.[4] A more precise and descriptive term is *medial tibial stress syndrome* (MTSS), which describes pain over the distal and middle thirds of the tibia along the posterior medial border.[10] Differential diagnosis by the physician and PT includes stress fractures of the tibia and fibula, ischemic disorders, and deep compartment syndromes of the lower leg.

The predominant feature of MTSS is tenderness over the distal, posteromedial tibia.[83] Traditionally, many different structures are thought to cause these symptoms. Musculotendinous inflammation; periosteal inflammation of the muscle-tendon-bone interface at the posterior medial border of the tibia; and injury to the tibia bone, the posterior tibialis muscle, and the medial origin of the soleus muscle have been identified as primary sources of pain in patients with MTSS.[4,7,26,81] More recent work has noted that a primary source of symptoms with MTSS is the tibial bone.[75,83]

Several studies have attempted to determine the etiology of MTSS.[8,29,49,83,118,127] Intrinsic factors for MTSS include overpronation of the foot, female sex, high body mass index, hip ROM loss (internal and external rotation), and ankle ROM loss (dorsiflexion). Hubbard and associates[49] reported that a previous history of MTSS, previous history of stress fracture, and less than 5 years of experience in a sport predispose an athlete to MTSS. Runners, basketball players, volleyball players, tennis players, and military recruits have a greater incidence of MTSS.[29,83] Diagnosis of MTSS is primarily made on physical examination, but diagnostic imaging including plain film radiographs, bone scans, dual-energy x-ray absorptiometry scans, and magnetic resonance imaging is also used.[75,83]

Because pain is the predominant feature of MTSS, it is helpful to classify and describe the severity of pain related to the patient's ability to perform activities.[54] Grade I describes pain that is experienced after activities. Grade II describes pain felt during and after activities that does not affect the performance of activities. Grade III pain is felt before, during, and after activities and affects the patient's ability to perform activities. Grade IV pain is so significant that no activities can even be attempted.

In general, grade I pain refers to muscle soreness and minor soft tissue inflammation. Grade II pain is viewed as a mild or moderate soft tissue inflammation. Grade III pain involves significant soft tissue inflammation and bone microfractures. Grade IV pain defines an actual stress fracture.

A patient experiencing minor pain (grade I) typically describes transient muscle soreness and general tenderness after activities. Treatment generally consists of ice packs or ice massage, physician-prescribed NSAIDs, rest, and gradual stretching and strengthening exercises for the entire lower leg. However, treatment of MTSS is highly individualized and specifically related to the comprehensive evaluation performed by the PT. If the PT determines that the patient demonstrates excessive foot pronation, custom-molded orthotics may be prescribed to relieve stress. External cold therapy (ice packs or ice massage in conjunction with stretching and strengthening exercises), or cryokinetics, usually is advocated as a means to control pain and swelling and encourage motion and function. Relative rest is prescribed in most cases of MTSS. Instead of complete rest and immobilization, the patient's activity level is modified to accommodate his or her complaints of pain and dysfunction. For example, a patient who is an avid jogger may be encouraged to jog in a pool instead. If a UBE is available, the patient can still actively perform aerobic conditioning activities without the associated stress on the lower leg.

There is evidence to support the use of relative rest, foot orthotic devices, and stretching to improve symptoms in patients with MTSS.[83,118] However, a multimodal approach using mechanical and therapeutic approaches appears to be most beneficial with this disorder.[29]

PLANTAR FASCIITIS (HEEL SPUR SYNDROME)

Chronic inflammation of the plantar aponeurosis, with or without an associated calcaneal heel spur, is called plantar fasciitis (Fig. 17-22). Leach and co-workers[68] described plantar fasciitis as repetitive microtrauma leading to injury, attempted repair, and chronic inflammation. Brody[13] described plantar fasciitis as an "inflammatory reaction due to chronic traction on the plantar aponeurosis (fascia) at its insertion into the calcaneus."

Although most authors and clinicians believe this pathology is an inflammation of the plantar fascia, several authors describe this disorder as a "plantar fasciopathy" or "plantar fasciosis."[70,98] These authors believe that the pathology can be degenerative as well as inflammatory in nature depending on the chronicity of the pathology. The same issue has been discussed with other overuse tendon injuries.

Patients with plantar fasciitis frequently complain of pain along the medial border of the calcaneus on the plantar surface. Many patients report that pain is worse in the morning when the foot contacts the floor in getting out of bed. Palpation of the plantar fascia usually reveals tenderness at the medial tuberosity of the os calcis or throughout the entire course of the fascia.[4] Palpation is performed with the toes flexed, which reduces tension on the fascia, or with the toes extended, which increases tension on the fascia.[11] Dorsiflexion of the ankle may also provoke symptoms.[17]

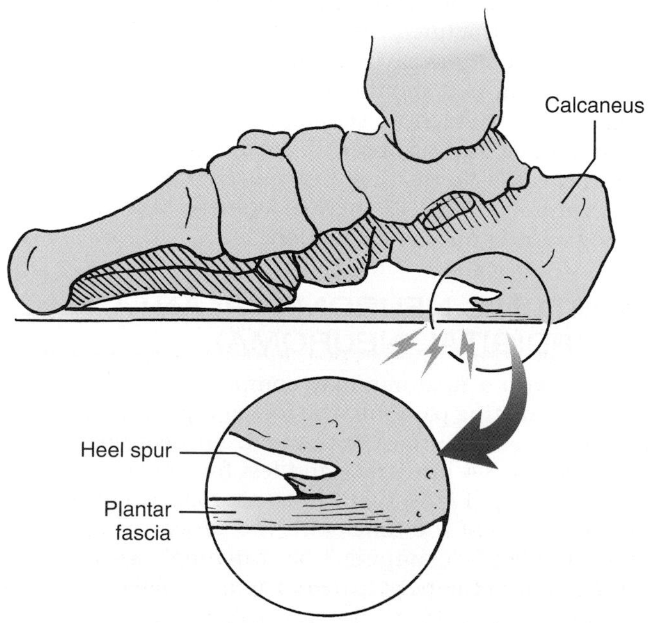

FIG 17-22 Plantar fasciitis with heel spur.

INTERVENTION

Many patients respond well to conservative physical therapy procedures.[86,98] Relative rest, stretching, manual therapy, exercise, iontophoresis, arch taping, and foot orthotic devices have been shown to improve symptoms and function in patients with plantar fasciitis.* A specific physical therapy approach where the clinician treats impairments, functional limitations, and disabilities with interventions designed to improve each item observed in the examination appears to have the greatest impact on patients with plantar fasciitis.[78]

Specifically addressing ROM deficits at the ankle joint (dorsiflexion) with manual therapy and stretching exercises appears to be helpful in these patients. If indicated, both the gastrocnemius and the soleus muscles should be stretched. However, if stretching of the gastrocnemius or soleus is painful in the area of the plantar fascia, the clinician may want to decrease this activity.[17] In the author's experience, if arch taping is helpful in reducing symptoms, use of an over-the-counter foot orthotic device may be helpful. Custom-made foot orthotic devices may also be used in selected patients. In particular, patients who have a large arch deformity and did not respond favorably to an over-the-counter device may be good candidates for a custom-made foot orthosis.

Strength training for the musculature in the foot and lower leg may be indicated if specific weaknesses are observed during the examination. Inversion, eversion, dorsiflexion, or plantar flexion strength training is necessary when weakness occurs. Strength training for the intrinsic musculature in the foot may also be necessary. Activities such as toe curls, picking up marbles with the toes, or gripping a towel can be used to strengthen the foot intrinsic musculature (Fig. 17-23).

In more severe cases, the physician may inject a local steroid to help decrease pain and swelling. Because many patients complain that the most severe pain is in the morning, some physicians and PTs prescribe night splints to stretch the Achilles tendon and the plantar fascia. In an athletic population, plantar fasciitis occurs from running and competitive sports participation. During recovery from plantar fasciitis, it is imperative to maintain aerobic fitness and general body strength. Aerobic exercises can be performed without weight bearing in a pool or with a UBE to decrease repetitive loading on the plantar fascia. Stationary cycling is an excellent alternative.

Extracorporeal shock wave therapy has been used for several years to assist in the healing process in patients

*For more information on these techniques, please refer to the articles found in references 5, 20, 27, 69, 78, 85, 91, 99, 122, and 128.

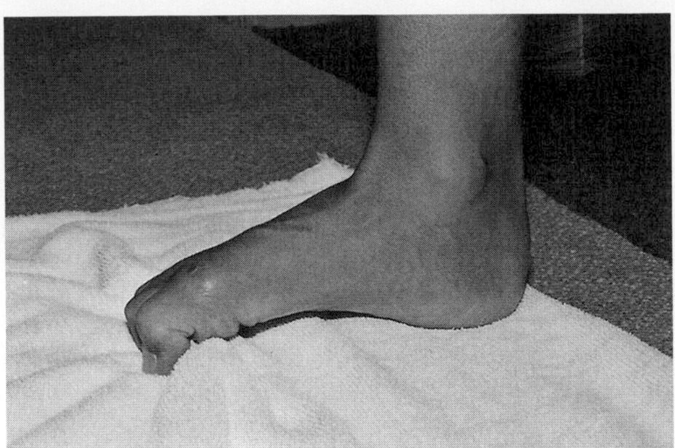

FIG 17-23 Resistive toe curls are performed by gripping a towel.

with plantar fasciitis. This modality attempts to break up adhesions and improve soft tissue extensibility of the plantar fascia. Several authors have shown good results with this form of treatment.[98,116,122]

With some patients who do not respond to conservative therapy, the physician may decide to correct the problem surgically. Surgical options include plantar fascia release (fasciotomy) and partial plantar fascia release. Rompe[98] described that conservative management is the first and best option and should last approximately 6 months before other forms of treatment. If conservative management fails, surgery is the next option.

ARCH DEFORMITIES (PES PLANUS AND PES CAVUS)

Pes planus (flatfoot) is a congenital or acquired deformity of the foot where the medial longitudinal arch of the foot is reduced, causing the medial border of the foot to contact the ground when a person is standing.[74] The usual cause of acquired pes planus is muscular weakness, laxity of ligaments that support the medial longitudinal arch, paralysis, or a pronated foot.[74] Pes planus deformity can be classified as mild, moderate, or severe.[84]

During the initial evaluation, the PT measures the degree of rearfoot and forefoot alignment in non–weight bearing. The rearfoot alignment is defined as the longitudinal bisection of the calcaneus relative to the long axis of the lower leg, and the forefoot alignment is defined as the metatarsal alignment relative to the perpendicular of the longitudinal bisection of the calcaneus. If the plantar surface of the distal segment is medial relative to the proximal segment, this is defined as a varus alignment. If the plantar surface of the distal segment is lateral relative to the proximal segment, this is defined as a valgus alignment. In addition, the PT assesses the deformity in a weight-bearing position.[96] With a rigid pes planus deformity, the foot appears to have an abnormally low arch in weight-bearing and non–weight-bearing positions.[96] With a flexible pes planus deformity, the foot appears to have a normal arch in a non–weight-bearing position, but an abnormally low or flat arch in weight bearing.

No specific therapeutic interventions are necessary if there is no associated pain or dysfunction. However, because the area is a terminal component of the closed kinetic chain during weight bearing (the arch can affect the knee, hip, and spine in a closed kinetic chain), treatment that is specific to the arch may be indicated if associated pain and dysfunction are experienced in other joints along the kinetic chain. For example, pes planus can affect the normal neutral-to-pronation sequence of the foot during the gait cycle. Because the foot is already pronated (with pes planus), the reduced normalized motion from neutral to pronation is affected during gait. The knee and other joints along the kinetic chain must compensate for this reduced motion. If pain and resultant dysfunction occur in one or more of these associated joints, corrective action is necessary to place the foot in a more neutral position to enhance the normal physiologic motion of the entire kinetic chain. Injuries common to those with pes planus occur more often to medial soft tissue structures of the knee.[125]

The use of a custom-fabricated foot orthotic device is usually indicated to create a more normal mechanical arch. Materials used to fabricate foot orthotic devices include cork, leather, rubber, foam, felt, and plastic.[19] The rationale for the use of a custom-molded foot orthotic device to correct a symptomatic pes planus is supported in the literature.[25] Successful treatment of other lower extremity injuries commonly attributed to pes planus have been documented.[39] However, individual consideration should be given to each patient for prescription foot orthoses because lower extremity overuse injuries are always multifactorial.[87]

Pes cavus describes an abnormally high arch.[74,95] Pes cavus usually is a result of neurogenic pathologic processes, muscle imbalances, and congenital abnormalities; medial and lateral longitudinal arches can be affected. Clinically, patients may complain of painful calluses beneath the metatarsal heads because of the mechanical friction and pressure that occur with metatarsal heads. Osteoarthritic changes are common in the tarsal area because of the altered biomechanics of the foot. Mechanical compensation at proximal joints in the lower extremity is also common with injuries being more common to lateral bony structure of the foot and lower leg.[125]

Treatment for pes cavus is much more challenging than for pes planus and should be focused on pain and shock attenuation. Evidence supports the effectiveness of custom-made foot orthoses for treatment of pain related to pes cavus.[42] No treatment is indicated if no symptoms exist, although the PT may document this deformity during a lower quarter evaluation.

MORTON'S NEUROMA (PLANTAR INTERDIGITAL NEUROMA)

Patients with a neuroma may complain of diffuse, occasionally radiating pain into the toes and proximally to the dorsal or plantar surface of the foot.[23] A neuroma usually occurs at the 3-4 interspace and less frequently at the 2-3 interspace (Fig. 17-24).[82] Morton's neuroma occurs bilaterally only 15% of the time, with the patient complaining of a "burning," "cramping," or "catching" sensation.[23,82] A painful mass can be palpated in approximately one third of cases.[82]

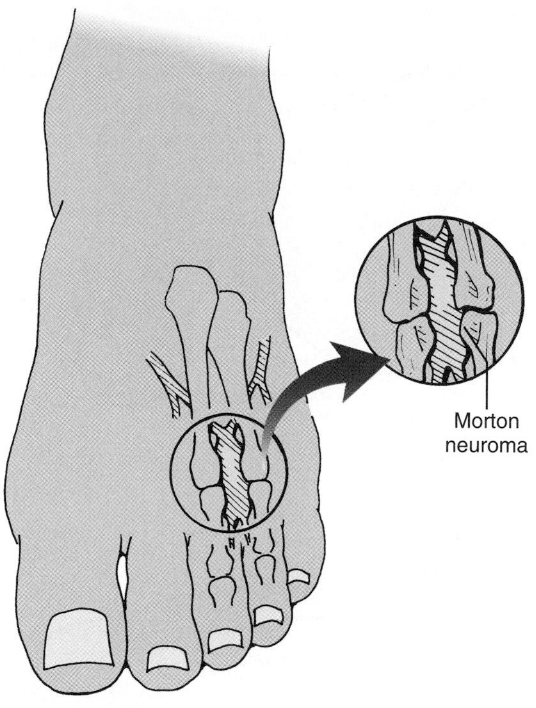

FIG 17-24 Morton's neuroma.

INTERVENTION

Conservative care calls for the use of a metatarsal pad; change of footwear to a wider, softer shoe; and local corticosteroid injections. Surgical excision of the neuroma may be necessary when all attempts at conservative care fail to relieve pain. Success of the surgical technique is around 83%.[41]

Postoperative physical therapy care involves early active motion of the involved metatarsophalangeal (MTP) joint to limit stiffness and fibrosis. Postoperative care dictates that the patient be weight bearing as tolerated and progressed to full weight bearing as pain allows. Compression bandages are used with elastic tape to assist with swelling and pain management. Generally, physical therapy care begins 2 to 3 weeks after surgery, when the sutures are removed. However, patients typically are encouraged to perform active ankle, foot, and knee ROM exercises during the early healing phase before physical therapy is begun. Patients are likely to need a molded foot orthotic device after surgery. This device may be advanced to a custom-molded device if the mechanics and morphology of the foot dictate.

Thermal agents used to reduce swelling and pain include whirlpool baths and cryotherapy. In addition, ultrasound can be used under water in conjunction with active motion exercises to improve circulation, reduce tissue congestion, and improve motion. Active ROM exercises include ankle motion in all directions, knee flexion and extension, and specific toe extension exercises with toe curls and splaying of the toes as tolerated. Occasionally, passive mobilization of the metatarsals may be needed to avoid the development of movement limitations. Strengthening exercises can be initiated as soon as the pain allows.

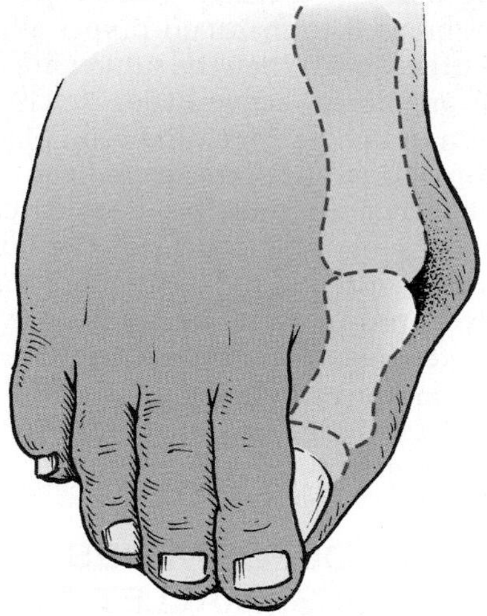

FIG 17-25 Hallux valgus.

All strengthening exercises for the ankle and knee are included with specific intrinsic foot strengthening exercises. Resistive toe curls can begin as an open kinetic chain exercise and progress to a closed kinetic chain exercise as strength and patient tolerance allow.

HALLUX VALGUS

Hallux valgus is a lateral or valgus deviation of the great toe with soft tissue and bony deformity (Fig. 17-25). This condition can be exacerbated by improper footwear (narrow toe box), and associated pain often can be relieved by modifying or changing poor footwear. Examination should include assessment of the deformity in a standing position, which often accentuates the deformity,[23,82] and measurement of the hallux valgus angle (normal is $<15°$) to determine the degree of deformity and angle of deviation. Hallux valgus is often associated with hallux rigidus. First MTP joint extension ROM should also be assessed. It has also been suggested that abnormal pronation and a lack of dorsiflexion are associated with the development of hallux valgus.[38,100]

Management options include conservative care and operative procedures. Initial care is supportive, with a change in footwear to include a wider toe box (this alone can significantly reduce symptoms), over-the-counter or custom-made foot orthotic devices, or pads to dissipate stress and relieve pain. Modifications in activity may reduce symptoms profoundly. In an athlete, changing from running activities to swimming or bicycling can reduce pain caused by the repetitive pounding of running. Ultimately, activity modification alone is not enough to eliminate pain related to hallux valgus.

Many surgical options are available, depending on the severity of the deformity. General physical therapy management of postoperative bunionectomy is designed to reduce pain and swelling, improve first MTP joint ROM, and increase strength to enable a return to normal daily activities. Initially after surgery, the patient wears a hard-soled shoe, progressing to walking boot and then to shoes with a wide or open toe box. Gauze padding and toe spacers may be used to maintain proper alignment after the surgical procedure. When the sutures are removed and the wounds are closed, active ROM exercises for flexion and extension of the great toe can begin. Manual resistive toe extension and toe flexion exercises can begin as pain allows. Gait mechanics must be reviewed carefully, and correct walking must be encouraged after bunionectomy. Weight-bearing patterns and restrictions of movement usually affect proper gait mechanics, especially the strength, power, and motion needed for toe-off. Restoration of joint motion and stability as well as toe flexion and extension strength forms the foundation of the rehabilitation program.

LESSER TOE DEFORMITIES (HAMMER TOES, MALLET TOES, AND CLAW TOES)

Three distinct types of lesser toe deformities are hammer toes, mallet toes, and claw toes (Fig. 17-26). All three deformities are worsened by wearing improper shoes (narrow toe box). Hammer toe (see Fig. 17-26, A) is characterized by deformity of the MTP joint, proximal interphalangeal (PIP) joint, and distal interphalangeal (DIP) joint. The MTP joint is in either neutral position or extension. The PIP joint is held in flexion with the DIP joint in either flexion or extension. Mallet toe (see Fig. 17-26, B) is characterized by a neutral MTP joint, a neutral PIP joint, and a flexed DIP joint. Claw toes (see Fig. 17-26, C) often are associated with neuromuscular disease and are similar in appearance to hammer toes. Claw toes are distinguished by MTP hyperextension, PIP flexion, and DIP flexion. This deformity usually results from "simultaneous contraction of the extensors and flexors."[82]

The physician or PT determines if the lesser toe deformity is either rigid (fixed) or flexible. Flexible deformities usually are correctable with conservative, passive measures, whereas fixed deformities may require surgery.

INTERVENTION

Nonoperative conservative care of lesser toe deformities focuses on modifying activities that exacerbate pain; changing footwear to a wider, softer toe box (to avoid pressure and the occurrence of soft or hard callus formation over bony prominences); padding areas subjected to blistering and corn formation; and using supportive measures to reduce pain and swelling (e.g., over-the-counter or custom-molded foot orthotic devices). Ultrasound, stretching exercises for the toes, and foot and ankle strengthening exercises may help reduce pain and swelling.

Surgical repair is reserved for fixed or rigid deformities, although some flexible deformities also require operation. Typically, sutures and pins are removed about 3 weeks after surgery.[23] The patient is weight bearing as tolerated initially, with a progression to full weight bearing as pain allows. The affected extremity is held in a rigid-solid, open-toe postsurgical boot to protect the repair from unwanted excessive flexion and extension of the toes.

For approximately 6 weeks after surgery, taping, padding, and protecting the repair are emphasized before progressing to weight bearing toe-off proper gait mechanics. This time is necessary to protect the surgical repair and to allow for the healing of bone and tendons (tenotomies are done for flexible lesser toe deformities). Throughout the rehabilitation program, from the immediate postoperative period until discharge, strength, flexibility, and aerobic fitness are maintained. The affected extremity may be strengthened with open chain resistive exercises (knee extension and leg curls), and aerobic fitness can be achieved with a stationary bicycle ergometer with the seat height lowered to maintain a neutral ankle position at the bottom of the pedal stroke. If the patient cannot operate the bicycle in this fashion, the opposite, uninvolved

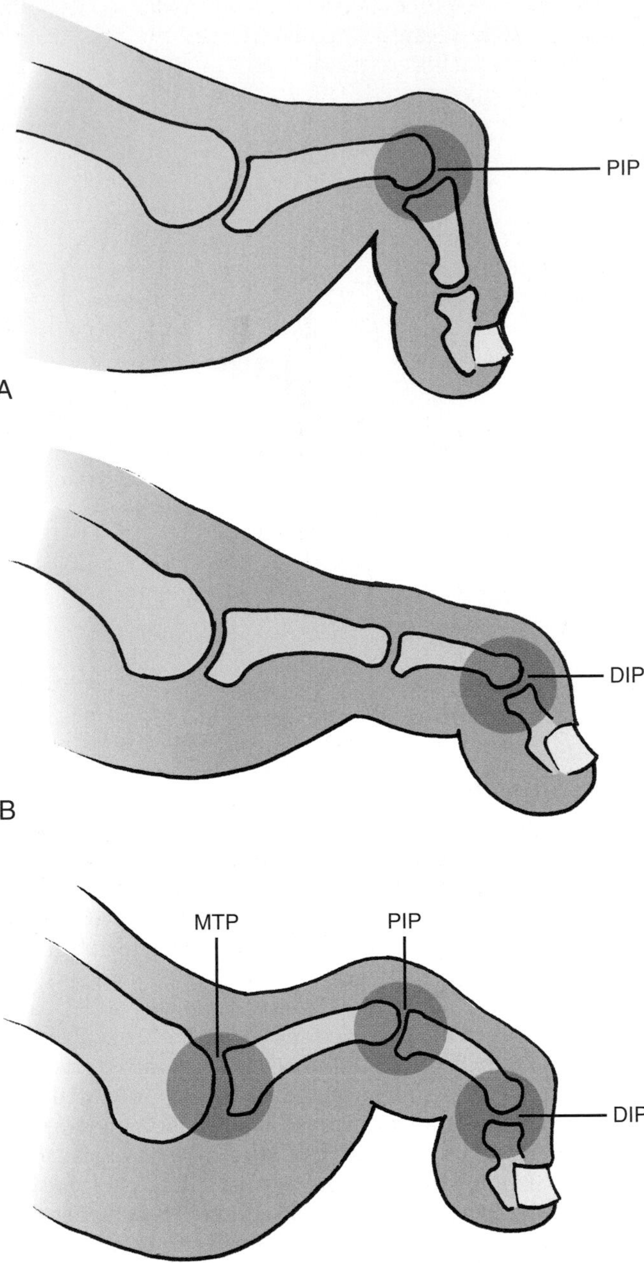

FIG 17-26 Lesser toe deformities. **A,** Hammer toe. **B,** Mallet toe. **C,** Claw toe.

extremity can be used alone (single-leg pedaling) using toe clips. A UBE also can be an effective aerobic conditioning tool during rehabilitation.

When the pins and sutures are removed at 3 weeks, physical therapy management can begin. Ultrasound, active ROM, and gentle stretching and strengthening exercises (open chain progressing to closed chain toe curls with a towel or marbles) can be employed. The toes must be protected from unwanted stress throughout the maximum-protection phase (6 to 8 weeks after surgery) of rehabilitation. Coughlin[23] recommended avoiding all running activities for 9 to 12 weeks after surgery to allow for proper healing.

COMMON MOBILIZATION TECHNIQUES FOR THE ANKLE, FOOT, AND TOES

Limitations of movement resulting from fibrosis after trauma, surgery, or disease of the foot, ankle, or toes frequently require specific mobilization procedures to regain normal joint function. Mobilization techniques typically are used in conjunction with thermal modalities to control pain and swelling and aid in relaxation; these modalities include hot packs, ultrasound, whirlpool baths, and ice packs. Active and passive exercises, specific stretching exercises, strengthening exercises (open chain progressing to closed chain), and proprioception tasks help the patient regain balance, coordination, and function. The choice of mobilization technique, direction of application, grades, amplitude of force, velocity, oscillations, and distractions is made by the PT based on the specific pathologic condition involved, tissue healing constraints, and overall appropriateness with regard to the short-term and long-term goals of the rehabilitation program.

The following techniques are general procedures used for various specific joint limitations. These techniques can be modified by the PT depending on the specific nature of the limitations involved. This list is not intended to be a comprehensive review of all techniques for each joint of the ankle, foot, and toes. These methods are commonly used, easily practiced, effective procedures for treating a host of joint limitations. The delegation of selected mobilization techniques to be used by the PTA is entirely at the discretion of the PT, and peripheral joint mobilization is not universally accepted as a routine domain of practice of the PTA. Information concerning peripheral joint mobilization has been provided as a means to stimulate the PTA's awareness of the rationale for improving motion and for the reduction of pain as identified and prescribed by the PT.

ANKLE MOBILIZATION

Anterior and posterior glides are best performed with the patient in a supine or "long-sitting" position with the lower leg firmly and comfortably supported. For anterior glide of the calcaneus, the hand position, stabilization, and direction of force are similar to those for the anterior drawer test for ligament stability testing of the anterior talofibular ligament. One hand should be placed firmly on the distal anterior surface of the tibia and fibula. The application hand should be used to "cup" the calcaneus firmly and provide an anterior-directed force (Fig. 17-27).

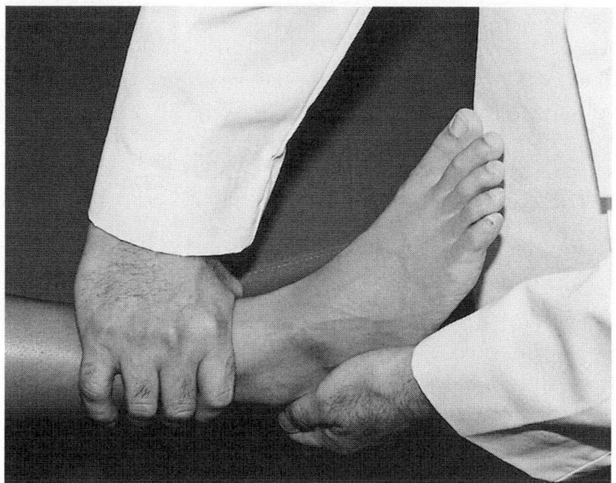

FIG 17-27 Anterior glide of the calcaneus.

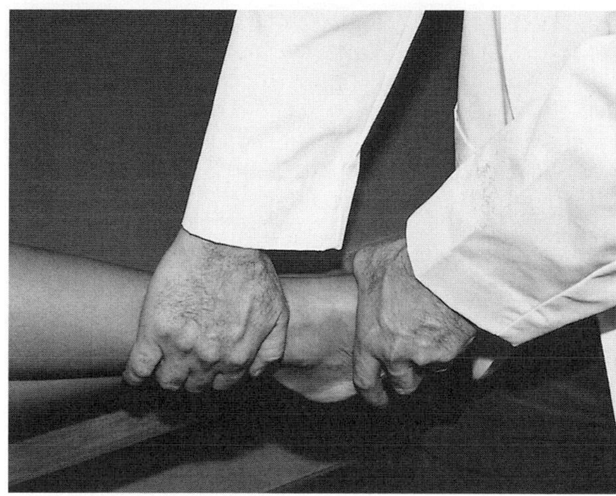

FIG 17-28 Posterior glide of the talus.

The posterior glide technique is performed with the patient in the same position as the anterior glide. The distal tibia and fibula should be stabilized with the palm of one hand. The application hand should be placed on the dorsal surface of the talus to provide a posterior-directed force (Fig. 17-28).

Traction is achieved through long-axis distraction of the talus caudally from the tibia and fibula. The patient can be supine or prone with the lower leg firmly and comfortably supported. The dorsal surface of the talus should be firmly grasped with the open palm of one hand, while the other hand is used to grasp and cup the calcaneus firmly. The force should be applied simultaneously with both hands along the long axis of the tibia and fibula (Fig. 17-29), effectively distracting the talus from the mortise.

METATARSAL MOBILIZATION

Distal metatarsal glides are performed while the patient is supine with the lower leg supported. The hand, thumb, and fingers of one hand should be used to stabilize the ray of the second metatarsal, while the hand, thumb, and

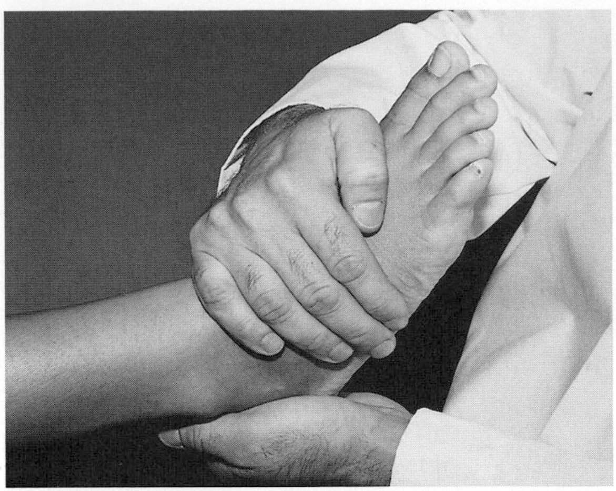

FIG 17-29 Long-axis distraction of the talus.

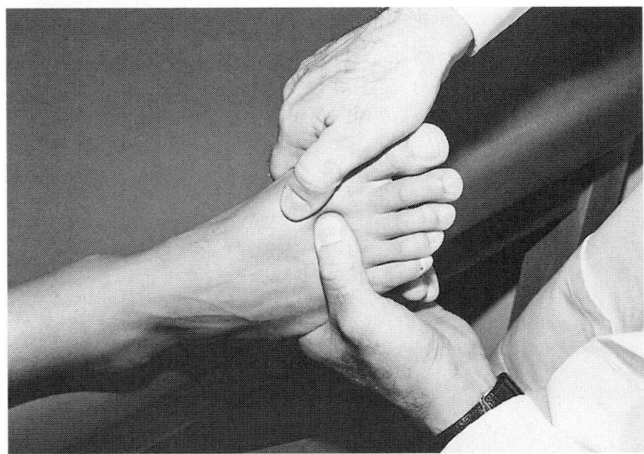

FIG 17-30 Distal metatarsal anterior-posterior glides.

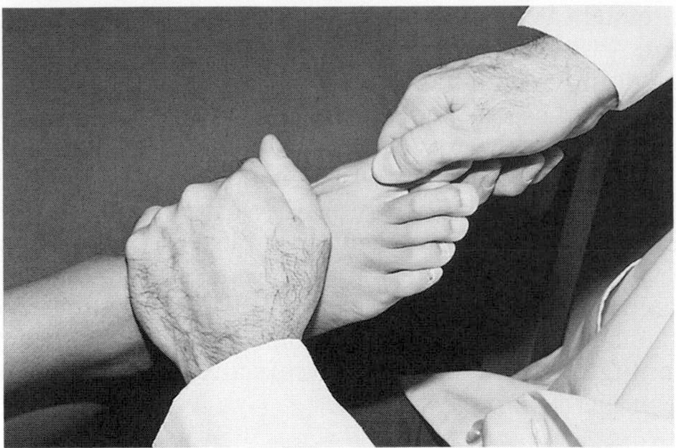

FIG 17-31 Long-axis proximal interphalangeal distraction.

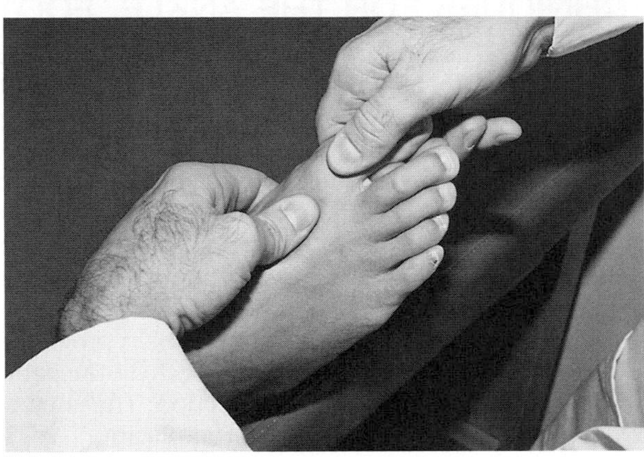

FIG 17-32 Proximal interphalangeal plantar and dorsal glides.

fingers of the application hand firmly grasp the first ray at the metatarsal head. Force should be applied in a plantar and dorsal direction (Fig. 17-30).

PROXIMAL INTERPHALANGEAL JOINT MOBILIZATION

Long-axis distraction of the PIP joint is achieved by stabilizing the affected metatarsal ray with one hand, while using the application hand to grasp the affected phalanx firmly. The thumb and fingers apply long-axis traction (distraction) (Fig. 17-31).

Plantar and dorsal PIP glides are performed with the patient supine and the lower leg supported. One hand should be used to grasp the first metatarsal ray firmly at the metatarsal head. The thumb of the stabilizing hand must be placed on the dorsal surface of the metatarsal head. The application hand should be used to grasp the proximal phalanx and apply a plantar and dorsal force while stabilizing the metatarsal head (Fig. 17-32).

GLOSSARY

Calcaneus fracture: A fracture that locks the subtalar joint in inversion when it heals in a varus position, creating a rigid transverse tarsal joint.

Posterior tibialis tendon: Rupture results in planovalgus, or "flatfoot."

Syndesmosis: Ligaments responsible for maintaining stability of the distal tibiofibular articulation.

Talar tilt test: Tests integrity of anterior talofibular ligament and calcaneofibular ligament; both must be disrupted for a positive tilt.

Talus: No muscle attachment origin or insertion; has a tenuous blood supply.

Tibial nerve: Passes behind the medial malleolus.

REFERENCES

1. Akeson WH, Amiel D, Abel MF, et al: Effects of immobilization on joints. *Clin Orthop Relat Res* 219:28–37, 1987.
2. Aktas S, Kocaoglu B: Open versus minimal invasive repair with Achillon device. *Foot Ankle Int* 30:391–397, 2009.
3. Alfredson H, Pietila T, Jonsson P, et al: Heavy-load eccentric calf muscle training for the treatment of chronic Achilles tendinosis. *Am J Sports Med* 26:360–366, 1998.
4. Andrish JT: The leg. In DeLee JD, Drez D, editors: *Orthopaedic sports medicine: principles and practice*, vol 2, Philadelphia, 1994, Saunders.
5. Baldassin V, Gomes CR, Beraldo PS: Effectiveness of prefabricated and customized foot orthoses made from low-cost foam for noncomplicated plantar fasciitis: a randomized controlled trial. *Arch Phys Med Rehabil* 90:701–706, 2009.
6. Baumhauer JF, O'Brien T: Surgical consideration in the treatment of ankle instability. *J Athl Train* 37:458–462, 2002.
7. Beck BR, Osternig LR: Medial tibial stress syndrome. The location of muscles in the leg to symptoms. *J Bone Joint Surg Am* 76:1057–1061, 1994.

8. Bennett JE, Reinking MF, Pluemer B, et al: Factors contributing to the development of medial tibial stress syndrome. *J Orthop Sports Phys Ther* 31:504–510, 2001.
9. Beskin JL, Sanders RA, Hunter SC, et al: Surgical repair of Achilles tendon ruptures. *Am J Sports Med* 15:1–8, 1987.
10. Black HM, Brand RL: Injuries of the foot and ankle. In Scott NW, Nisonson B, Nicholas J, editors: *Principles of sports medicine*, Baltimore, 1984, Williams & Wilkins.
11. Bordelon RL: Heel pain. In DeLee JD, Drez D, editors: *Orthopaedic sports medicine: principles and practice*, vol 2, Philadelphia, 1994, Saunders.
12. Brand RL, Collins MDF, Templeton T: Surgical repair of ruptured lateral ankle ligaments. *Am J Sports Med* 9:40–44, 1981.
13. Brody DM: Running injuries: prevention and management. *Clin Symp* 39:1–36, 1987.
14. Calder JD, Sexton SA, Pearce CJ: Return to training and playing after posterior ankle arthroscopy for posterior in elite professional soccer. *Am J Sports Med* 38:120, 2010.
15. Canale ST: Ankle injuries. In Crenshaw AH, editor: *Campbell's operative orthopaedics*, vol 3, 7th ed, St Louis, 1987, Mosby.
16. Ceccarelli F, Berti L, Giuriati L, et al: Percutaneous and minimally invasive techniques of Achilles tendon repair. *Clin Orthop Relat Res* 458:188–193, 2007.
17. Cheung JT, Zhang M, An KN: Effect of Achilles tendon loading on plantar fascia tension in the standing foot. *Clin Biomech* 21:194–203, 2006.
18. Chrisman OD, Snook G: Reconstruction of lateral ligament tears of the ankle: an experimental study and clinical evaluation of seven patients treated by a new modification of the Elmslie procedure. *J Bone Joint Surg Am* 51:904–912, 1969.
19. Clanton TO: Sport shoes, insoles and orthoses. In DeLee JD, Drez D, editors: *Orthopaedic sports medicine: principles and practice*, vol 2, Philadelphia, 1994, Saunders.
20. Cleland JA, Abbott JH, Kidd MO, et al: Manual physical therapy and exercise versus electrophysical agents and exercise in the management of plantar heel pain: a multicenter randomized clinical trial. *J Orthop Sports Phys Ther* 39:573–585, 2009.
21. Conrad JJ, Tannin AH: Trauma to the ankle. In Jahss MH, editor: *Disorders of the foot*, Philadelphia, 1982, Saunders.
22. Corte-Real NM, Moreira RM: Arthroscopic repair of chronic lateral ankle instability. *Foot Ankle Int* 30:213–217, 2009.
23. Coughlin MJ: Conditions of the forefoot. In DeLee JD, Drez D, editors: *Orthopaedic sports medicine: principles and practice*, vol 2, Philadelphia, 1994, Saunders.
24. Curwin S, Stanish W: *Tendinitis: its etiology and treatment*, Lexington, MA, 1984, Callamore Press.
25. D'Ambrosia RD: Orthotic devices in running injuries. *Clin Sports Med* 4:611–618, 1985.
26. Detmer DE: Chronic shin splints. Classification and management of medial tibial stress syndrome. *Sports Med* 3:436–446, 1986.
27. Digiovanni BF, Nawoczenski DA, Malay DP, et al: Plantar fascia-specific stretching exercise improves outcomes in patients with chronic plantar fasciitis: a prospective clinical trial with two-year follow-up. *J Bone Joint Surg Am* 88:1775–1781, 2006.
28. Eckert WR, David EA: Acute rupture of the peroneal retinaculum. *J Bone Joint Surg Am* 58:670–673, 1976.
29. Edwards PH, Wright ML, Hartman JF: A practical approach for the differential diagnosis of chronic leg pain in the athlete. *Am J Sports Med* 33:1241–1249, 2005.
30. El Shewy MT, El Barbbary HM, Abdel-Ghani H: Repair of chronic rupture of the Achilles tendon using 2 intratendinous flaps from the proximal gastrocnemius-soleus complex. *Am J Sports Med* 37:1570–1577, 2009.
31. Evans DL: Recurrent instability of the ankle: a method of surgical treatment. *Proc R Soc Med* 46:343–344, 1953.
32. Ferran NA, Maffulli N: Epidemiology of sprains of the lateral ankle ligament complex. *Foot Ankle Clin* 11:659–662, 2006.
33. Ferran NA, Oliva R, Maffulli N: Recurrent subluxation of the peroneal tendons. *Sports Med* 36:839–846, 2006.
34. Ferran NA, Oliva R, Maffulli N: Ankle instability. *Sports Med Arthrosc* 17:139–145, 2009.
35. Fong DT, Chan YY, Mok KM, et al: Understanding acute ankle ligamentous sprain injury in sports. *Sports Med Arthrosc Rehabil Ther Technol* 30:1–14, 2009.
36. Frink M, Hildebrand F, Krettek C, et al: Compartment syndrome of the lower leg and foot. *Clin Orthop Relat Res* 468:940–950, 2010.
37. Gigante A, Moschini A, Verdenelli A, et al: Open versus percutaneous repair in the treatment of acute Achilles tendon rupture: a randomized prospective study. *Knee Surg Sports Traumatol Arthrosc* 16:204–209, 2008.
38. Glasoe WM, Nuckley DJ, Ludewig PM: Hallux valgus and the 1st metatarsal arch segment: a theoretical biomechanical perspective. *Phys Ther* 90:110–120, 2010.
39. Gross ML, Napoli RC: Treatment of lower extremity injuries with orthotic shoe inserts. An overview. *Sports Med* 15:66–70, 1993.
40. Harper MC: The deltoid ligament: an evaluation of need for surgical repair. *Clin Orthop Relat Res* 226:156–168, 1988.
41. Hassouna H, Singh D: Morton's metatarsalgia: pathogenesis, aetiology and current management. *Acta Orthop Belg* 71:646–655, 2005.
42. Hawke F, Burns J, Radford JA, et al: Custom-made foot orthoses for the treatment of foot pain. *Cochrane Database Syst Rev* (3):CD006801, 2008.
43. Heckman DS, Gluck GS, Parekh SG: Tendon disorders of the foot and ankle, part 1: peroneal tendon disorders. *Am J Sports Med* 37:614–625, 2009.
44. Herbort M, Haber A, Zantop T, et al: Biomechanical comparison of the primary stability of suturing Achilles tendon rupture: a cadaver study of Bunnell and Kessler techniques under cyclic loading conditions. *Arch Orthop Trauma Surg* 128:1273–1277, 2008.
45. Hertel J: Functional anatomy, pathomechanics, and pathophysiology of lateral ankle instability. *J Athl Train* 37:364–375, 2002.
46. Hintermann B, Knupp M, Pagenstert GI: Deltoid ligament injuries: diagnosis and management. *Foot Ankle Clin* 11:625–637, 2006.
47. Hintermann B, Renggli P: Anatomic reconstruction of the lateral ligaments of the ankle using a plantaris tendon graft in the treatment of chronic ankle joint instability. *Orthopade* 28:778–784, 1999.
48. Hohendorff B, Siepen W, Staub L: Treatment of acute Achilles tendon rupture: fibrin glue versus fibrin glue augmented with the plantaris longus tendon. *J Foot Ankle Surg* 48:439–446, 2009.
49. Hubbard TJ, Carpenter EM, Cordova ML: Contributing factors to medial tibial stress syndrome: a prospective investigation. *Med Sci Sports Exerc* 41:490–496, 2009.
50. Huffard B, O'Loughlin PF, Wright T, et al: Achilles tendon repair: Achillon system vs. Krackow suture: an anatomic in vitro biomechanical study. *Clin Biomech* 23:1158–1164, 2008.
51. Ibrahim SA: Surgical treatment of chronic Achilles tendon rupture. *J Foot Ankle Surg* 48:340–346, 2009.
52. Inglis AE, Sculco TP: Surgical repair of ruptures of the tendon Achilles. *Clin Orthop Relat Res* 156:160–168, 1981.
53. Jackson BA, Schwane JA, Starcher BC: Effect of ultrasound therapy on the repair of Achilles tendon injuries in rats. *Med Sci Sports Exerc* 23:171–176, 1991.
54. Jackson DW: Shin-splints: an update. *Phys Sports Med* 6:101–161, 1978.
55. Jacobs D, Martens M, Van Audekercke R, et al: Comparison of conservative and operative treatment of Achilles tendon rupture. *Am J Sports Med* 6:107–111, 1978.
56. Kangas J, Pajala A, Ohtonen P, et al: Achilles tendon elongation after rupture repair: a randomized comparison of 2 postoperative regimens. *Am J Sports Med* 35:59–64, 2007.
57. Kannus P, Renstrom P: Current concepts review: treatment of acute tears of the lateral ligaments of the ankle. *J Bone Joint Surg Am* 73:305–312, 1991.
58. Keene JS: Tendon injuries of the foot and ankle. In DeLee JD, Drez D, editors: *Orthopaedic sports medicine: principles and practice*, vol 2, Philadelphia, 1994, Saunders.
59. Kerkhoffs GM, Handoll HH, deBie R, et al: Surgical versus conservative treatment for acute injuries of the lateral ligament complex of the ankle in adults. *Cochrane Database Syst Rev* (2):CD000380, 2007.
60. Khan RJ, Fick DP, Keogh A, et al: Interventions for treating acute Achilles tendon ruptures. *Cochrane Database Syst Rev* (9):CD003674, 2010.

61. Knobloch K: Eccentric training in Achilles tendinopathy: is it harmful to tendon microcirculation? *Br J Sports Med* 41:e2, 2007.
62. Komenda GA, Ferkel RD: Arthroscopic findings associate with the unstable ankle. *Foot Ankle Int* 20:708–713, 1999.
63. Labib SA, Rolf R, Dacus R, et al: The "Giftbox" repair of the Achilles tendon: a modification of the Krackow technique. *Foot Ankle Int* 30:410–414, 2009.
64. Lansdaal JR, Goslings JC, Reichart M, et al: The results of 163 Achilles tendon ruptures treated by a minimally invasive surgical technique and functional aftertreatment. *Injury* 38:839–844, 2007.
65. Lassiter TE, Malone TR, Garrett W: Injury to the lateral ligaments of the ankle. *Orthop Clin North Am* 20:629–640, 1989.
66. Leach R: Acute ankle sprains: vigorous treatment for best results. *J Musculoskelet Med* 1:68–76, 1983.
67. Leach RE, James S, Wasilewski S: Achilles tendinitis. *Am J Sports Med* 9:23–98, 1981.
68. Leach RE, Seavey MS, Salter DK: Results of surgery in athletes with plantar fasciitis. *Foot Ankle* 7:161–356, 1986.
69. Lee SY, McKeon P, Hertel J: Does the use of orthoses improve self-reported pain and function measures in patients with plantar fasciitis? A meta-analysis. *Phys Ther Sport* 10:12–18, 2009.
70. Lemont H, Ammirati KM, Usen N: Plantar fasciitis: a degenerative process (fasciosis) without inflammation. *J Am Podiatr Med Assoc* 93:234–237, 2003.
71. Lin CF, Gross ML, Weinhold P: Ankle syndesmosis injuries: anatomy, biomechanics, mechanism of injury, and clinical guidelines for diagnosis and intervention. *J Orthop Sports Phys Ther* 36:372–384, 2006.
72. Maffulli N, Ajis A: Management of chronic ruptures of the Achilles tendon. *J Bone Joint Surg Am* 90:348–1360, 2008.
73. Maffulli N, Ferran NA: Management of acute and chronic ankle instability. *J Am Acad Orthop Surg* 16:608–615, 2008.
74. Magee DJ: Lower leg, ankle and foot. In *Orthopaedic physical assessment*, 2nd ed, Philadelphia, 1992, Saunders.
75. Magnusson HI, Ahlborg HG, Karlsson C, et al: Low regional tibial bone density in athletes with medial tibial stress syndrome normalizes after recovery from symptoms. *Am J Sports Med* 31:596–600, 2003.
76. Marti R: Dislocation of the peroneal tendons. *Am J Sports Med* 5:19–22, 1977.
77. McBryde A: Stress fractures of the foot and ankle. In DeLee JD, Drez D, editors: *Orthopaedic sports medicine: principles and practice*, vol 2, Philadelphia, 1994, Saunders.
78. McPoil TG, Martin RL, Cornwall MW, et al: Heel pain-plantar fasciitis: clinical practice guidelines linked to the international classification of function, disability, and health from the Orthopaedic Section of the American Physical Therapy Association. *J Orthop Sports Phys Ther* 38:A1–A18, 2008.
79. McRae R: *Practical fracture treatment*, New York, 1994, Churchill Livingstone.
80. McVey ED, Palmieri RM, Docherty CL, et al: Arthrogenic muscle inhibition in the leg muscles of subjects exhibiting functional ankle instability. *Foot Ankle Int* 26:1055–1061, 2005.
81. Michael RH, Holder LE: The soleus syndrome: a cause of medial tibial stress (shin splints). *Am J Sports Med* 13:27–94, 1985.
82. Miller M: *Review of orthopaedics*, Philadelphia, 1992, Saunders.
83. Moen MH, Tol JL, Weir A, et al: Medial tibial stress syndrome: a critical review. *Sports Med* 39:523–546, 2009.
84. Myerson MS: Injuries to the forefoot and toes. In Jahss MH, editor: *Disorders of the foot and ankle: medical and surgical management*, vol 2, 2nd ed, Philadelphia, 1991, Saunders.
85. Nawoczneski DA, Janisse DJ: Foot orthoses in rehabilitation—what's new. *Clin Sports Med* 23:157–167, 2004.
86. Neufeld SK, Cerrato R: Plantar fasciitis: evaluation and treatment. *J Am Acad Orthop Surg* 16:338–346, 2008.
87. Nigg BM, Nurse MA, Stefanyshyn DJ: Shoe inserts and orthotics for sport and physical activities. *Med Sci Sports Exerc* 31:S421–S428, 1999.
88. Nistor L: Surgical and nonsurgical treatment of Achilles tendon rupture. *J Bone Joint Surg Am* 63:394–399, 1981.
89. Norkus SA, Floyd RT: The anatomy and mechanisms of syndesmotic ankle sprains. *J Athl Train* 36:68–73, 2001.
90. Nussbaum ED, Hosea TM, Sieler SD, et al: Prospective evaluation of syndesmotic ankle sprains without diastasis. *Am J Sports Med* 29:31–35, 2001.
91. Osborne HR, Allison GT: Treatment of plantar fasciitis by LowDye taping and iontophoresis: short term results of a double blinded, randomized, placebo controlled clinical trial of dexamethasone and acetic acid. *Br J Sports Med* 40:545–549, 2006.
92. Pajala A, Kangas J, Siira P, et al: Augmented compared with nonaugmented surgical repair of a fresh total Achilles tendon rupture. A prospective randomized study. *J Bone Joint Surg Am* 91:1092–1100, 2009.
93. Porter DA: Evaluation and treatment of ankle syndesmosis injuries. *Instr Course Lect* 58:575–581, 2009.
94. Pugh KJ, Wolinsky PR, McAndrew MP, et al: Tibial pilon fractures: a comparison of treatment methods. *J Trauma* 47:937–941, 1999.
95. Renstrom PA, Kannus P: Injuries of the foot and ankle. In DeLee JD, Drez D, editors: *Orthopaedic sports medicine: principles and practice*, vol 2, Philadelphia, 1994, Saunders.
96. Riddle DL: Foot and ankle. In Richardson JK, Iglarsh ZA, editors: *Clinical orthopaedic physical therapy*, Philadelphia, 1994, Saunders.
97. Riehl R: Rehabilitation of lower leg injuries. In Prentice WE, editor: *Rehabilitation techniques in sports medicine*, 2nd ed, St Louis, 1994, Mosby.
98. Rompe JD: Plantar fasciopathy. *Sports Med Arthrosc* 17:100–104, 2009.
99. Roos E, Engstrom M, Soderberg B: Foot orthoses for the treatment of plantar fasciitis. *Foot Ankle Int* 27:606–611, 2006.
100. Ross FD: The relationship of abnormal foot pronation to hallux abductor valgus—a pilot study. *Prosthet Orthot Int* 10:72–78, 1986.
101. Safran MR, Benedetti RS, Bartolozzi AR, III, et al: Lateral ankle sprains: a comprehensive review: part 1: etiology, pathomechanics, histopathogenesis, and diagnosis. *Med Sci Sports Exerc* 31 (7 Suppl):S429–S437, 1999.
102. Safran MR, Zachazewski JE, Benedetti RS, et al: Lateral ankle sprains: a comprehensive review: part 2: treatment and rehabilitation with an emphasis on the athlete. *Med Sci Sports Exerc* 31 (7 Suppl):S438–S447, 1999.
103. Sanchez M, Anitua E, Azofra J, et al: comparison of surgically repaired Achilles tendon tears using platelet-rich fibrin matrices. *Am J Sports Med* 35:245–251, 2007.
104. Saxena A, Muffulli N, Nguyen A, et al: Wound complications from surgeries pertaining to the Achilles tendon: an analysis of 219 surgeries. *J Am Podiatr Med Assoc* 98:95–101, 2008.
105. Schepsis AA, Jones H, Haas AL: Achilles tendon disorders in athletes. *Am J Sports Med* 30:287–305, 2002.
106. Schubert AG: Exertional compartment syndrome: a review of the literature and proposed rehabilitation guidelines following surgical release. *Int J Sports Phys Ther* 6:126–141, 2011.
107. Smyth NA, Murawski CD, Levine DS, et al: Hindfoot arthroscopic surgery for posterior ankle impingement: a systematic surgical approach and case series. *Am J Sports Med* 41:1869–1876, 2013.
108. Stanitski CL, McMaster JH, Scranton PE, et al: On the nature of stress fractures. *Am J Sports Med* 6:391–396, 1978.
109. Staples OS: Ruptures of the fibular collateral ligaments of the ankle: results study of immediate surgical treatment. *J Bone Joint Surg Am* 57:101–107, 1975.
110. Stormont DM, Morrey BF, An K-N, et al: Stability of the loaded ankle. *Am J Sports Med* 13:295–300, 1985.
111. Stover CN, Bryan D: Traumatic dislocation of peroneal tendons. *Am J Surg* 103:180–186, 1962.
112. Suchak AA, Bostick GP, Beaupre LA, et al: The influence of early weight-bearing compared with non-weight-bearing after surgical repair of the Achilles tendon. *J Bone Joint Surg Am* 90:1876–1883, 2008.
113. Suchak AA, Spooner C, Reid DC, et al: Postoperative rehabilitation protocols for Achilles tendon rupture: a meta-analysis. *Clin Orthop Relat Res* 445:216–221, 2006.
114. Suqimoto K, Takakura Y, Okahashi K, et al: Chondral injuries of the ankle with recurrent lateral instability: an arthroscopic study. *J Bone Joint Surg Am* 91:99–106, 2009.

115. Thati S, Carlson C, Maskill JD, et al: Tibial compartment syndrome and the cavovarus foot. *Foot Ankle Clin* 13:275–305, 2008.
116. Toomey EP: Plantar heel pain. *Foot Ankle Clin* 14:229–245, 2009.
117. Twaddke BC, Poon P: Early motion for Achilles tendon ruptures: is surgery important? A randomized, prospective study. *Am J Sports Med* 35:2033–2038, 2007.
118. Tweed JL, Campbell JA, Avil SJ: Biomechanical risk factors in the development of medial tibial stress syndrome in distance runners. *J Am Podiatr Med Assoc* 98:436–444, 2008.
119. Uchiyama E, Nomura A, Takeda Y, et al: A modified operation for Achilles tendon ruptures. *Am J Sports Med* 35:1739–1743, 2007.
120. Uh BS, Beynnon BD, Helie BV, et al: The benefit of a single-leg strength training program for the muscles around the untrained ankle. *Am J Sports Med* 28:568–573, 2000.
121. Valovich McLeod TC: The effectiveness of balance training programs on reducing the incidence of ankle sprains in adolescent athletes. *J Sports Rehabil* 17:316–323, 2008.
122. Wang CJ, Wang FS, Yang KD, et al: Long-term results of extracorporeal shockwave treatment for plantar fasciitis. *Am J Sports Med* 34:592–596, 2006.
123. Watson-Jones R: Recurrent forward dislocation of the ankle joint. *J Bone Joint Surg Br* 34:519, 1952.
124. Wilder RP, Sethi S: Overuse injuries: tendinopathies, stress fractures, compartment syndrome, and shin splints. *Clin Sports Med* 23:55–81, 2004.
125. Williams DS, 3rd, McClay IS, Hamill J: Arch structure and injury patterns in runners. *Clin Biomech* 16:341–347, 2001.
126. Wittstein J, Moorman CT, 3rd, Levin LS: Endoscopic compartment release for chronic exertional compartment syndrome. *J Surg Orthop Adv* 17:119–121, 2008.
127. Yates B, White S: The incidence and risk factors in the development of medial tibial stress syndrome among naval recruits. *Am J Sports Med* 32:772–780, 2004.
128. Young B, Walker Strunce J, Boyles R: A combined treatment approach emphasizing impairment-based manual physical therapy for plantar heel pain: a case series. *J Orthop Sports Phys Ther* 34:725–733, 2004.

REVIEW QUESTIONS

Multiple Choice

1. Which of the following statements regarding injuries to the lateral ligament complex is true?
   a. Of all ankle sprains, 80% are to lateral ligaments.
   b. Injuries to the lateral ligament complex rarely become recurrent or chronic.
   c. These injuries always include the deltoid ligament.
   d. Injuries to the lateral ligament complex account for 25% of all sports-related injuries.
2. A first-degree ankle sprain:
   a. Exhibits injuries to both the anterior talofibular and the posterior talofibular ligaments.
   b. Has severe swelling in the ankle and lower leg.
   c. Completely injures the anterior talofibular ligament.
   d. None of the above
3. The talar tilt test is performed for which ankle ligament?
   a. Calcaneofibular ligament
   b. Posterior talofibular ligament
   c. Anterior talofibular ligament
   d. All of the above
4. The anterior drawer test is done for which ankle ligament?
   a. Calcaneofibular ligament
   b. Posterior talofibular ligament
   c. Anterior talofibular ligament
   d. All of the above
5. Which degree of ankle ligament injury typically can be treated conservatively?
   a. First degree
   b. Second degree
   c. Third degree
   d. a and b
   e. All of the above
6. Taping an ankle for an inversion sprain should place the ankle in which position?
   a. Dorsiflexion and eversion
   b. Dorsiflexion and inversion
   c. Plantar flexion and eversion
   d. Plantar flexion and inversion
7. Which of the following positions places undue stress on the anterior talofibular ligament?
   a. Dorsiflexion and eversion
   b. Dorsiflexion and inversion
   c. Plantar flexion and eversion
   d. Plantar flexion and inversion
8. What is the length of time it takes for full maturation of an injured ligament?
   a. 4 to 8 weeks
   b. 8 to 12 weeks
   c. 3 to 6 months
   d. 6 to 12 months
9. Which of the following statements regarding injury to the medial ankle ligament is true?
   a. The medial ankle ligament includes calcaneofibular ligament when severe.
   b. It occurs in up to 80% of all ankle ligament injuries.
   c. Medial ankle ligaments rarely cause acute functional instability.
   d. Medial ankle ligaments can also cause fractures of the medial or lateral malleolus.
10. A "high ankle sprain" occurs when:
   a. The ankle is plantar flexed and rotated.
   b. The anterior and posterior talofibular ligaments are disrupted.
   c. The ankle is dorsiflexed and rotated.
   d. The ankle is in a non–weight bearing position.
11. Chronic instabilities in the ankle create which of the following symptoms?
   a. Weakness
   b. Swelling
   c. Pain
   d. Instability
   e. All of the above
12. Which of the following statements about subluxing peroneal tendons is true?
   a. The mechanism of injury involves dorsiflexion and inversion.
   b. The condition is easily misdiagnosed as lateral ligament injury.
   c. The injury is described as anterior medial snapping
   d. None of the above
13. Acute management of subluxing peroneal tendons includes:
   a. Immediate weight bearing.

b. Immediate full ROM for ankle.
c. Plyometrics off a 4-inch box.
d. Immobilization in rigid cast.

14. Which of the following statements regarding Achilles tendinopathy is true?
    a. Achilles tendinopathy occurs secondary to repetitive macrotrauma.
    b. It causes pain at the musculotendinous junction of Achilles.
    c. It can be caused by increased vascularity in the insertion site.
    d. Achilles tendinopathy occurs secondary to chronic overload.
15. Which of the following statements regarding compartment syndrome of the lower leg is true?
    a. Chronic muscle atrophy in the lower leg can cause compartment syndrome.
    b. There are three major compartments in the lower leg that can become inflamed.
    c. The tibial nerve is contained in the lateral compartment.
    d. The lateral compartment contains the peroneal nerves.

Short Answer

16. Name and describe the classification system for lateral ankle ligament injuries.
17. Describe three common lower leg or foot injuries that require non–weight-bearing status and give an estimate for each injury regarding prognosis for return to unrestricted activity.
18. Name and describe the classification system for ankle fractures.
19. Describe signs and symptoms of lower leg stress fractures.
20. List the various forms of modalities that could be used in treating plantar fasciitis, and describe why each might be used and indications and contraindications for each.

Fill in the Blank

21. A "high ankle" sprain also injures the tibiofibular ____________.
22. Ankle ____________ is a surgical treatment used to identify and treat intraarticular lesions.
23. A tendon reconstruction at the ankle is known as a ____________.
24. After surgery to repair subluxing peroneal tendons, limited __________________ is prescribed for 2 to 4 weeks.
25. A patient with severe Achilles tendinopathy has a lack of ankle ____________.

True/False

26. An inversion ankle sprain injures the deltoid ligament.
27. Treatment of grade III ankle sprains is controversial.
28. Repetitive ankle sprains can result in chronic ankle instability.
29. A syndesmotic injury is treated most aggressively of all ankle ligament injuries.
30. Surgically shortening a ligament is termed imbrication.

Chapter 18

Orthopedic Management of the Knee

John T. Cavanaugh, Jessica Hettler, Victoria Moran, Pawel Wawrzyniak

CHAPTER OUTLINE

LEARNING OBJECTIVES

1. Identify common ligament injuries of the knee joint.
2. Understand the etiology and evaluation of ligamentous knee injuries.
3. Discuss general rehabilitation guidelines for nonoperative and postoperative management of common knee ligament injuries.
4. Identify and evaluate meniscal injuries of the knee.
5. Discuss general rehabilitation guidelines for nonoperative and postoperative management of meniscal injuries.
6. Discuss general rehabilitation guidelines for nonoperative and postoperative management of articular cartilage injuries.
7. Discuss common methods of evaluation and nonoperative and postoperative management of patellofemoral disease of the knee.
8. Identify and evaluate common fractures, including patella, supracondylar femur, and proximal tibia.
9. Discuss general rehabilitation guidelines for fractures around the knee.
10. Discuss general rehabilitation guidelines for postoperative management of total knee replacements.

KEY TERMS

Active quadriceps drawer test
Closed kinetic chain (CKC) exercises
Lachman test
Modified Thomas test
Osteochondral allograft
Thessaly test
Timed Up and Go (TUG) test

Pathologic knee conditions are among the most frequent diagnoses seen in outpatient rehabilitation clinics. The role of the physical therapy assistant (PTA) is to progress the patient safely through a course of rehabilitation and assist the patient in achieving his or her goals. Prerequisites for the PTA to be successful include having a set of sound rehabilitation principles, understanding and applying a good knowledge of the basic sciences, appreciating the mechanism of injury of the various knee pathologies, respecting the body's natural healing response, and following a criteria-based functional progression of rehabilitation. This chapter discusses these fundamentals as they pertain to knee ligamentous injuries, articular cartilage and meniscus lesions, patellofemoral disorders, fractures around the knee joint, and arthritis including management with total knee arthroplasty (TKA).

REHABILITATION PRINCIPLES

1. Apply a working knowledge of the basic sciences to the rehabilitation program; this should include anatomy, function, and biomechanics of the knee joint as well as the pathophysiology of knee joint injuries. A thorough understanding of the mechanism of injury can assist in formulating a comprehensive assessment. An appreciation of the processes of inflammation and tissue healing is invaluable to advance the patient safely through the rehabilitative course and ultimately return the patient to the desired level of activity.
2. Adopt a team approach. For a successful outcome after injury or surgery, the physician, physical therapist (PT), PTA, and patient must be responsible and work together. Communication among the team members is vital. The physician has the responsibility of ascertaining the proper diagnosis based on patient history, clinical examination, and diagnostic information from evaluative procedures (e.g., radiographs, magnetic resonance imaging [MRI], knee ligament arthrometer recordings) The physician may also be responsible for performing the proper surgical procedure and directing the postoperative rehabilitation program. The PT and PTA responsible for the rehabilitation program should be aware of the most current therapeutic approaches, based on clinical evidence, in rehabilitating each specific condition a patient has. The patient has an important role as well. The patient should adhere to the advice given by the physician, PT, or PTA. This includes compliance to prescribed home therapeutic exercises and recommended activity modifications in the patient's daily routine. In today's managed care environment, patient compliance is essential for a successful outcome.
3. Adhere to the rules of rehabilitation as described by Gray.[80]
   a. Create a safe environment. The PTA should use his or her knowledge of the basic sciences to ensure that a prescribed exercise or activity does not compromise the healing response of a specific structure. Examples include maintaining weight-bearing precautions after a surgical procedure, using an underwater treadmill (Fig. 18-1) to unload the knee during gait training, or limiting the arc of motion on a progressive resistance machine (e.g., leg press, knee extension) during strengthening interventions. The PTA should use the most appropriate kinetic chain environment throughout the rehabilitative course. In the lower extremity, during **closed kinetic chain (CKC) exercises** or activities, the distal segment (foot) is relatively fixed, which results in simultaneous movement of all other joints. Cocontraction of agonist and antagonist muscles during these CKC activities provides joint stabilization by decreasing shear forces acting on the knee.[150] Wojtys and colleagues[213] reported that the dynamic coactivation of the quadriceps and hamstrings can reduce tibial translation by 200%, decrease internal and external rotation by 80%, and enhance knee stiffness by two to four times. CKC activities also facilitate the integration of proprioceptive feedback coming from mechanoreceptors in the ligaments, tendons, and joint capsule.[180] Open kinetic chain (OKC) exercises use isolated joint and muscle function. Motion during OKC exercises is uniplanar, and the load is unnatural and sometimes abnormal.[80] During OKC knee exercises, as resistive force is applied to the distal tibia, tibiofemoral shear forces are maximized.[21,88,102,121] Patellofemoral joint reaction stress is less during CKC exercise than during OKC resistive exercises when the range of motion (ROM) is restricted to approximately 0° to 50°.[91,181]

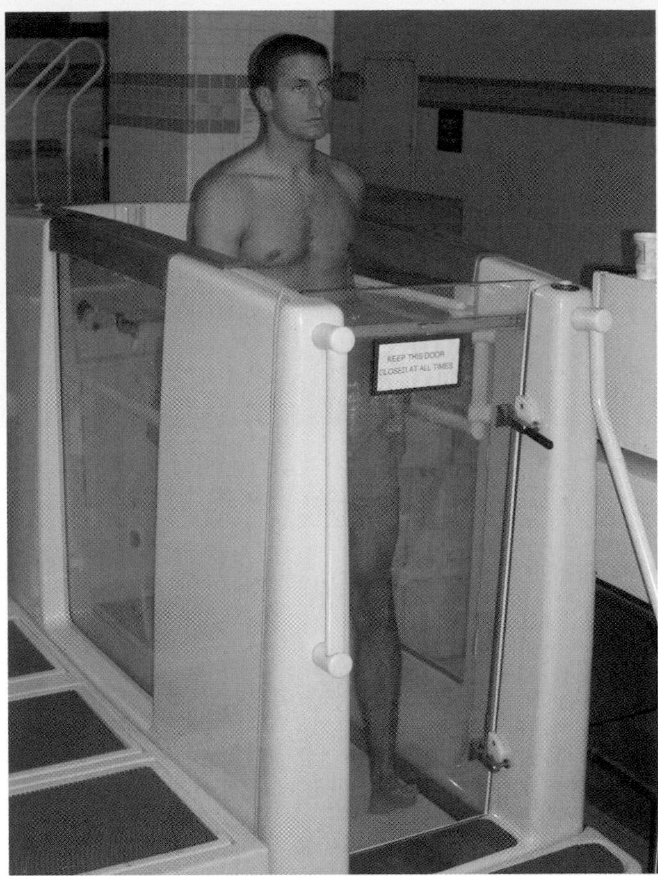

FIG 18-1 Underwater treadmill.

OKC exercises can be used for isolated training of the quadriceps and hamstrings and to identify muscular deficits (i.e., isokinetic testing). Regardless of which kinetic chain is used, the PTA should ensure that the exercise or activity is performed in a pain-free and crepitus-free ROM.

b. Do not hurt the patient. Incorporate exercises and activities that are pain-free. Gains in ROM, strength, and flexibility can best be achieved in this manner. Modifications can be made by adapting pain-free arcs of motion on strengthening equipment and in functional activities. It is also important to emphasize to the patient not to have "the patient hurt the patient." The PTA should encourage the patient to modify his or her activity level. This recommendation can be particularly valuable in the early phases of rehabilitation when ROM and lower extremity strength are lacking to meet the demands of activities of daily living (ADL).

c. Be aggressive without breaking rules 1 and 2. The PT or PTA can be aggressive as long as a safe environment is maintained and the patient does not complain of knee pain during the exercise or activity. A safe and expeditious outcome can be achieved.

4. Follow a functional progression. A functional progression was defined by Kegerreis[105] as an ordered sequence of activities enabling the acquisition or reacquisition of skills required for the safe, effective performance of athletic endeavors. To ensure a safe progression, criteria need to be established whereby the patient demonstrates the mastery of a simple activity before advancing to more demanding activity. In rehabilitating the knee after injury or surgery, it is recommended that the PTA adhere to the following functional progression:
   - Develop quadriceps control and progress ROM
   - Establish a normal gait pattern
   - Demonstrate the ability to ascend normal steps
   - Demonstrate the ability to descend normal steps
   - Initiate a running program (if appropriate)
   - Initiate a plyometric, sport-specific training program (if appropriate)
5. Follow an assessment-based guideline. Modern rehabilitation programs should follow a plan that is not as structured as previous protocols. Protocols based on timetables can accelerate a program too quickly for a patient whose progress is delayed or can hold back a patient who is progressing very well. Rehabilitation specialists should combine their understanding of the basic sciences with an ongoing assessment of the patient to "guide" the patient through the rehabilitative course. These guidelines should incorporate flexible time frames in the progression to allow for individualization (e.g., "week 4 to 6, discontinue crutches when a nonantalgic gait is demonstrated" versus "week 5, discontinue crutches for ambulation"). Continual reassessment of the patient is vital to ensure a consistent and safe progression of the program. Too rapid a progression in therapy or normal functional ADL is demonstrated by increased effusion and pain. Therapeutic exercise programs often must be modified based on changes in subjective and objective findings.

KNEE LIGAMENT REHABILITATION

ANTERIOR CRUCIATE LIGAMENT INJURY

The anterior cruciate ligament (ACL) is a commonly injured knee ligament; nearly 200,000 ACL injuries are reported annually in the United States.[122,134] Most of these injuries occur during sports activities that involve rapid change of direction and jumping, such as in soccer, basketball, or football. The ACL functions as the primary stabilizer for resisting anterior translation of the tibia on the femur and serves to control knee hyperextension. The ACL has a secondary responsibility as a stabilizer in resisting internal and external rotation and varus and valgus stress.[137] The pathomechanics of ACL injury include contact and noncontact mechanisms, with noncontact mechanisms accounting for up to 78% of all ACL injuries.[100,146] The typical mechanism of injury is deceleration and rotation with the foot planted.

Important Concepts

The ACL is the primary stabilizer for resisting anterior translation of the tibia on the femur and a secondary stabilizer in rotations and varus and valgus stress.

The literature supports a higher incidence of ACL injuries among female athletes.[68,117,124,154] Malone and colleagues[124] reported that female collegiate basketball players were eight times more likely to sustain an ACL injury than their male counterparts. This phenomenon is related to intrinsic and extrinsic factors. Women usually exhibit a wider pelvis, increased flexibility, less developed thigh musculature, decreased strength, increased genu valgum, and increased external tibial torsion compared with men.[83,107,202] Women have demonstrated diminished muscular force, an increased dependence on the quadriceps muscles for stability, a longer time to develop force, and a longer neuromuscular response time. Women also exhibit greater ROM, increased genu recurvatum, and increased joint laxity.[20,94]

Clinical Evaluation

After an acute injury, an examination by an orthopedic physician is warranted. The **Lachman test** (Fig. 18-2) has been universally recognized as the most specific test in assessing the integrity of the ACL.[188] The test assesses the amount of anterior tibial translation and the quality of the endpoint. The anterior drawer test (Fig. 18-3), although less sensitive, can also be performed to assess ACL laxity at a higher knee flexion angle.[191] A pivot shift test, although more difficult to perform, can assess anterolateral rotational instability.[77] The PTA should be competent in assessing knee ligament stability during the rehabilitation period so as to report any significant findings in laxity to the supervising PT or physician.

MRI is routinely ordered to confirm an ACL tear diagnosis and to identify any associated ligament, meniscal, or chondral injury (Fig. 18-4). A KT1000 knee ligament arthrometer may be used to quantify the difference in laxity compared with the noninvolved knee (Fig. 18-5). Based on these findings, the orthopedist and patient discuss and agree on a course of intervention.

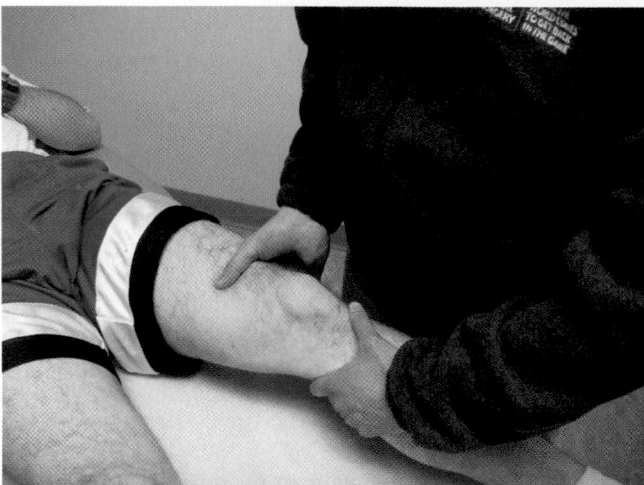

FIG 18-2 Lachman test. With the knee stabilized in a 25° to 30° angle, the clinician attempts to displace the tibia anteriorly. The amount of excursion and quality of the endpoint versus the contralateral knee can assess the laxity of the ACL.

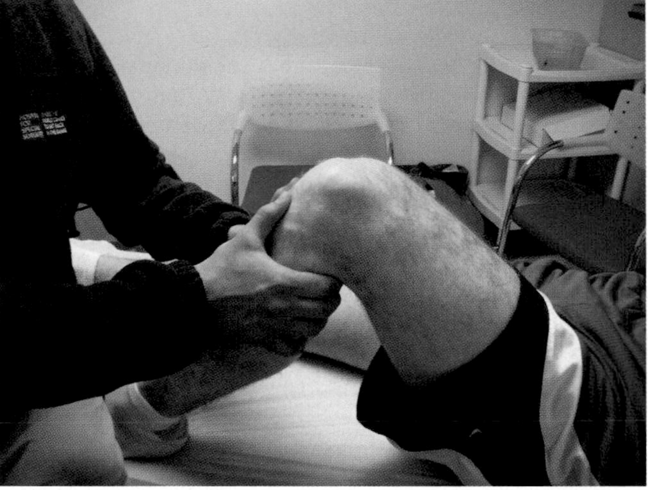

FIG 18-3 Anterior drawer test. With the knee flexed to 90°, the clinician attempts to provide an anteriorly directed force on the tibia. The amount of excursion and quality of the endpoint versus the contralateral knee can assess the laxity of the ACL.

Important Concepts

The Lachman test is recognized as the most specific test in assessing integrity of the ACL. The anterior drawer test is less sensitive compared with the Lachman test.

Conservative Management

Everyone who sustains an ACL injury does not require surgery. A conservative approach to treatment may be elected if the patient has an isolated ACL tear and has a sedentary lifestyle or does not have the time or motivation to commit to a postoperative rehabilitation program. The patient will also need to alter his or her sports activity level by avoiding athletic activities involving rapid deceleration and pivoting. Buss and colleagues[30] reported satisfactory results with conservative management in a group of selected patients older than 30 years with sedentary occupations and low athletic demands.

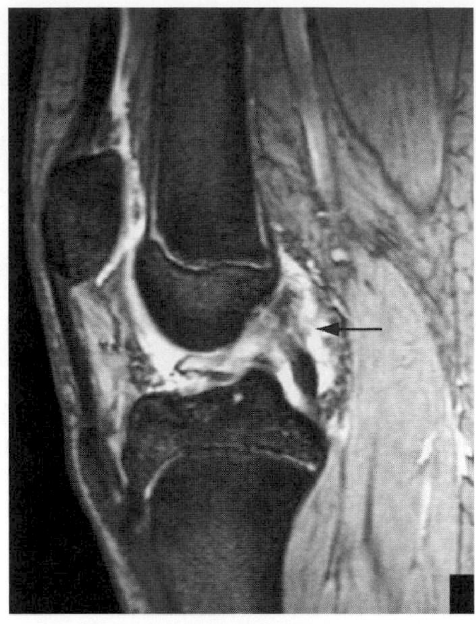

FIG 18-4 MRI of an ACL tear.

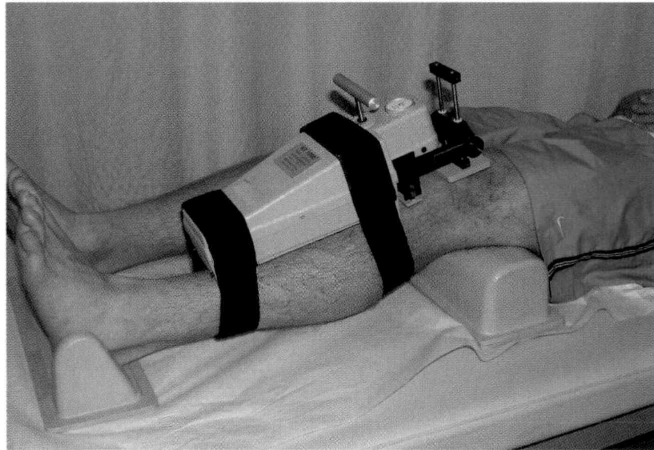

FIG 18-5 KT1000 knee ligament arthrometer (MEDmetric Corp, San Diego, CA).

In the early period after an acute ACL injury, symptoms of pain, swelling, and instability and loss of motion and muscular control are expected. The main focus of the rehabilitation program should be directed toward protecting the knee from further trauma and treating these symptoms.

A safe environment can be created by unloading the knee using weight bearing as tolerated strategy. Crutches can be discarded when a nonantalgic gait is demonstrated. Cryotherapy, compression, and electrical stimulation (transcutaneous electrical nerve stimulation) may prove beneficial in treating pain and swelling. Therapeutic exercises such as quadriceps setting, straight leg raise (SLR), and ROM (active, active-assistive) exercises can facilitate quadriceps control and improve motion. Proximal strengthening to include the hip and core musculature is introduced to meet better the demands placed on the lower extremity in the weeks and months that follow.

Should a concomitant medial collateral ligament (MCL) or lateral collateral ligament injury be present, a hinged knee brace is used to protect the ligament from excessive valgus and varus forces during ADL.

As inflammation subsides and ROM improves, lower extremity strengthening is advanced using CKC and OKC exercises. CKC exercises afford a more functional approach to develop strength and endurance of the lower extremity musculature: Examples include squats, leg press, dead lifts, and step-ups. CKC activities decrease tibiofemoral shear and minimize patellofemoral stress.[91,210,216] During CKC exercises, the involved extremity is loaded, more functionally stimulating the neuromuscular system addressing the component of proprioception training in the rehabilitation program.

Important Concepts

Examples of CKC exercise include squats, leg press, dead lifts, and step-ups.

Adequate proprioception is a precursor of good balance and adequate function.[193] Mizuta co-workers[135] demonstrated increased postural sway in functionally unstable ACL-deficient knees compared with normal and functionally stable ACL-deficient knees. Proprioception training is advanced when appropriate to include perturbation training (Fig. 18-6). The goal of these interventions is to stimulate reflex muscle activation. Training the reflex pathways with perturbations has been shown to decrease response time and develop reactive strategies to unexpected joint load.[34,39,71,142]

Important Concepts

Training the reflex pathways with perturbation exercises has been shown to decrease response time and develop reactive strategies to unexpected joint load.

OKC exercises can be beneficial for isolated quadriceps and hamstring strengthening. OKC extensions (Fig. 18-7) with progressive resistance should be carefully monitored and discontinued should complaints of patellofemoral joint pain or crepitus or both occur. If an isokinetic device is available, isokinetic strengthening for quadriceps and hamstrings can be used.

A functional progression, as described earlier, is followed monitoring the patient's symptoms throughout the rehabilitative course. Return to sport criteria include full ROM, negative complaints of knee instability, and the lack of apprehension with sport-specific movements. In addition, the patient should demonstrate 90% limb symmetry for quadriceps and hamstring muscle strength as measured isokinetically, 90% limb symmetry for lower extremity power as measured with a functional hop test, and symmetric unilateral functional movement without deviation (e.g., step-down and single-leg squat).

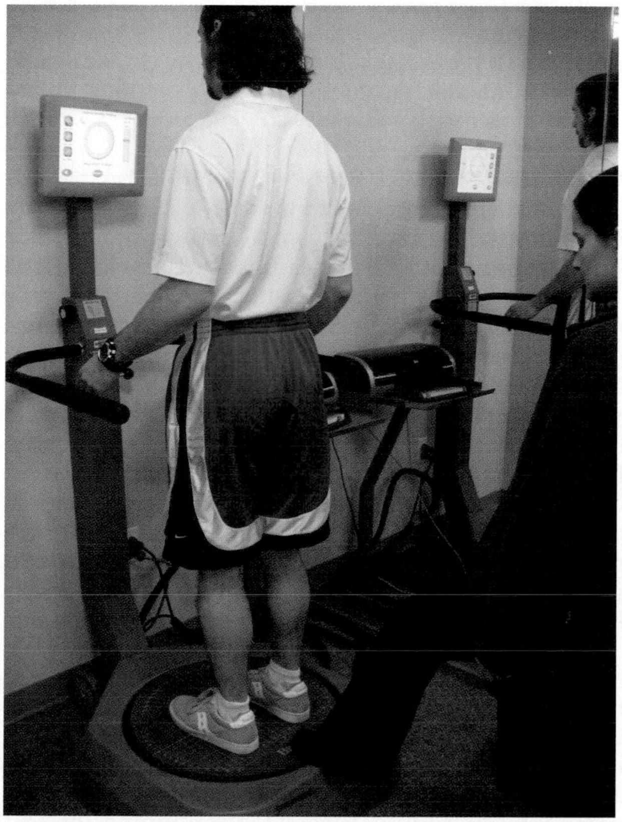

FIG 18-6 Perturbations on the Biodex Balance System (Biodex Medical Systems Inc, Shirley, NY). The clinician applies unanticipated linear and angular destabilizing forces as the patient attempts to maintain balance.

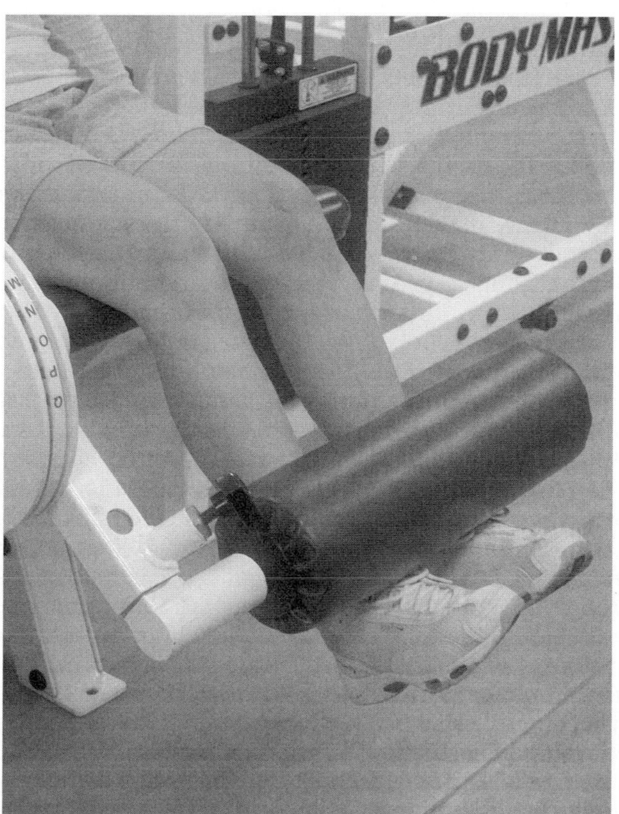

FIG 18-7 OKC knee extension bilaterally. *(From Hospital for Special Surgery, et al:* Postsurgical rehabilitation guidelines for the orthopedic clinician, *St Louis, 2006, Mosby.)*

Important Concepts

OKC exercises are beneficial for isolating the quadriceps and hamstring muscles.

Many physicians may prescribe a functional knee brace for patients with ACL deficiency to wear during sport activity. This practice is controversial because these braces have not been shown to control tibial translation at functional loads.[18,212] However, bracing may enhance proprioception. Lephart and associates[115] demonstrated increased joint position sense with the application of a neoprene sleeve. Bracing may stimulate cutaneous sensory receptors and enhance conscious or subconscious awareness of the knee's position sense.

Surgical Management

Surgical intervention for ACL injuries has changed dramatically over the past few decades. Strict postoperative protocols that dictated periods of prolonged immobilization, bracing with limited ROM, and non–weight-bearing (NWB) ambulation have been replaced by more aggressive criteria-based guidelines in which immediate motion and weight bearing are the norm. Surgical procedures such as primary repair of the ACL with or without augmentation have been replaced by less invasive, arthroscopically assisted techniques. Surgical reconstructions using high-strength grafts, isometric placement, and improved fixation methods have created conditions for the rehabilitation team to adopt a more accelerated treatment continuum. Several graft choices are available to reconstruct the ACL, including autogenous central-third bone–patellar tendon–bone, semitendinosus-gracilis, quadriceps tendon, or Achilles tendon allografts.

It is common practice to delay surgery until the inflammation subsides and ROM, muscle function, and gait are restored.[128,176,202] Shelbourne and colleagues[176] reported that delaying surgery until ROM was restored decreased the incidence of postoperative arthrofibrosis. These authors also reported that quadriceps muscle strength returns more quickly when reconstructive surgery is delayed longer than 21 days.[174] Rehabilitation may take several weeks to achieve preoperative goals. Patients should be evaluated on an individual basis. Patient education is emphasized during the preoperative period so as to prepare the patient better physically and mentally for the demanding rehabilitation program that follows surgery. Instruction and subsequent independence in a postoperative exercise program prevents complications from developing in the immediate postoperative period. Postoperative exercises include passive extension with a towel rolled up under the heel, quadriceps setting, SLR with a postoperative brace locked at 0°, and an active assistive knee flexion/extension ROM (Fig. 18-8). The patient is instructed in self patellar mobilizations to prevent a postoperative contracture from developing. The patient is measured for a postoperative brace and instructed in its management (i.e., donning and doffing). The patient is also measured for crutches and is gait trained using partial weight bearing (PWB) for ambulation with the postoperative brace locked at 0°.

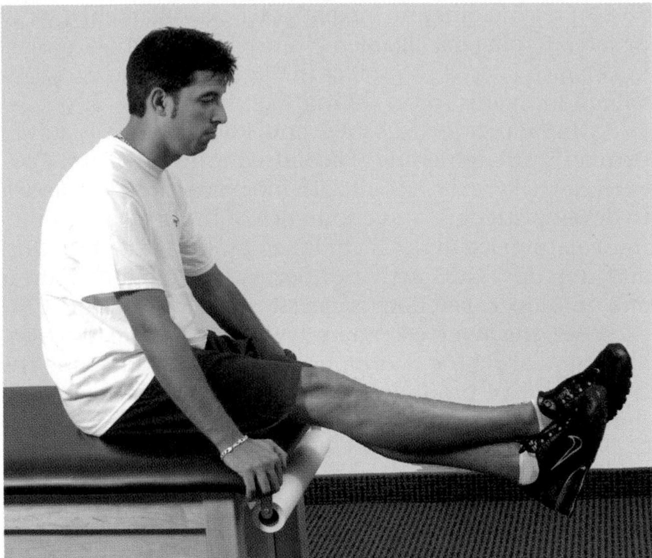

FIG 18-8 AAROM. Supporting the involved leg with the contralateral leg, the patient flexes the involved knee to the point of a gentle stretch. The patient then extends the involved knee with the assistance of the noninvolved leg. *(From Noyes FR:* Noyes' knee disorders: surgery, rehabilitation, clinical outcomes, *Philadelphia, 2010, Saunders.)*

Important Concepts

Graft choices for ACL reconstruction include autogenous central-third bone–patellar–bone, semitendinosus-gracilis, quadriceps tendon, and Achilles tendon allografts.

Immediate Postoperative Rehabilitation

The immediate postoperative phase after ACL reconstruction is designed primarily to protect the graft substitute, while encouraging ROM and muscle reeducation (Table 18-1). The PT and PTA must consider ACL biology throughout the postoperative rehabilitation program. The graft substitute is at its strongest at the time of reconstruction. Over time, the graft undergoes periods of necrosis, revascularization, and remodeling. Graft strength decreases during the period of necrosis and gradually increases as the graft revascularizes and remodels. Animal studies reported that graft strength and stiffness are 30% to 50% of the native ACL 1 year after surgery.[46,61] Histologic studies in humans demonstrated earlier changes in revascularization and remodeling in reconstructed grafts than were previously reported.[65,169]

Contemporary postoperative ACL reconstruction rehabilitation is characterized by early mobilization to minimize the deleterious effects of immobilization, such as articular cartilage degeneration, excessive adverse collagen formation, and pain.[2,144,170] Isometric graft placement allows for immediate motion without imposing adverse loads. Achieving full passive extension during the first 2 postoperative weeks is crucial for a noncomplicated recovery because loss of extension after ACL reconstruction results in an abnormal gait, increased patellofemoral

TABLE 18-1 Anterior Cruciate Ligament Reconstruction Rehabilitation Guidelines: Immediate Postoperative Phase

GOALS	• Emphasis on full passive extension • Control postoperative pain/swelling • ROM 0° → 125° • Prevent quadriceps inhibition • Restore normal gait pattern (nonantalgic) without assistive device • Ascend 8-inch stairs with good control without pain • Independence in home therapeutic exercise program
PRECAUTIONS	• Avoid active knee extension 40° → 0° • Avoid ambulation without brace locked at 0° until quadriceps control is demonstrated • Avoid heat application • Avoid prolonged standing/walking
TREATMENT STRATEGIES	• Towel extensions, prone hangs • Quadriceps reeducation (quadriceps sets with EMS or EMG) • Progressive weight bearing: PWB → WBAT (patella tendon) with brace locked at 0° with crutches • Ambulation with open brace on demonstration of quadriceps control • Brace changed to physician preference (e.g., OTS brace, patellar sleeve) • Patellar mobilization • Active flexion/active-assisted extension 90° → 0° exercise • SLRs (all planes) → PRE • Brace locked at 0° initially for SLR (supine) • Short crank ergometry → standard ergometry • Hip progressive resisted exercises • Proprioception activities (bilateral → unilateral weight bearing) • Leg press (bilateral/80° → 0° arc) (if ROM >90°) • Initiate FSU program • Minisquats/weight shifts • Hamstring/calf flexibility exercises • Core strengthening • Upper extremity cardiovascular exercises as tolerated • Cryotherapy • Home therapeutic exercise program: evaluation based • Emphasize patient compliance to home therapeutic exercise program and weight bearing precautions/progression
CRITERIA FOR ADVANCEMENT	• ROM 0° → 125° • Normal gait pattern • Demonstrate ability to ascend 8-inch step • Good patellar mobility

EMG, electromyography; *EMS,* electrical muscle stimulation; *FSU,* forward step-up; *PRE,* progressive resistive exercise; *PWB,* partial weight bearing; *ROM,* range of motion; *SLR,* straight leg raise; *WBAT,* weight bearing as tolerated.

symptoms, and quadriceps weakness. To achieve this goal, the patient is instructed to sit or lie with a towel under the heel, allowing gravity to apply a low-load prolonged stretch into extension (Fig. 18-9). Bracing is locked at 0° for ambulation and sleeping. These activities engage the graft in the intercondylar notch to avoid creating an interval during which notch scarring or arthrofibrosis can occur. To promote gains in flexion, the patient is instructed to perform an active flexion/active-assistive extension exercise several times per day. A continuous passive motion (CPM) machine is recommended for home use if the patient has difficulty attaining flexion ROM. Numerous outcome studies demonstrated no adverse effects when an immediate motion program was initiated after ACL reconstruction with various graft substitutes.[8,13,33,144,175]

Advanced fixation techniques, such as cancellous screw bone-to-bone fixation, allow for immediate postoperative weight bearing. The patient is initially instructed to use a postoperative brace locked at 0° for ambulation. Patients are instructed to begin with PWB (50%) with crutches and to progress weight-bearing status gradually to weight bearing as tolerated (WBAT) as ROM and lower extremity muscle strength demonstrate improvement. ACL reconstruction outcome studies using an accelerated weight-bearing program demonstrated excellent results and decreased complications.[13,14,138,175]

Additional goals in the first phase include controlling postoperative effusion and quadriceps reeducation. The two are closely related. Spencer and colleagues[178] demonstrated a quadriceps inhibition in the presence of knee joint effusion. Mechanoreceptors in the joint capsule respond to changes in tension and inhibit motor nerves supplying the quadriceps muscles. Controlling postoperative effusion leads to decreased quadriceps inhibition and results in a faster return of muscle function. A commercial cold wrap device (Fig. 18-10) is recommended for 20 to 30 minutes several times per day in the early postoperative course. After suture removal, ice packs may be used directly for improved cooling. Quadriceps setting with a small towel under the knee provides a high-quality, pain-free

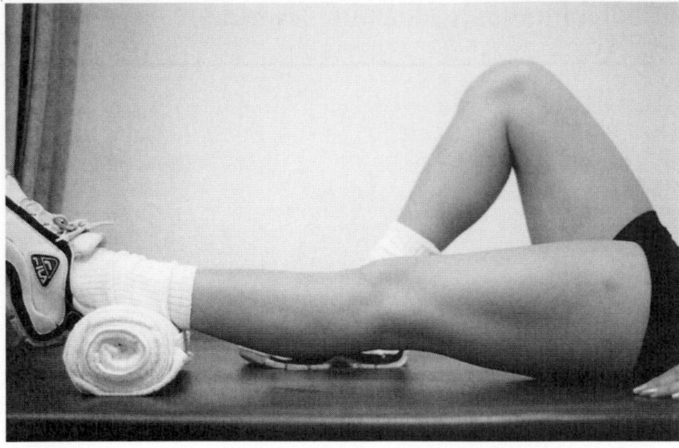

FIG 18-9 Towel extensions. Low-load prolonged stretch being applied at the knee to facilitate the return of full knee extension. *(From Maxey L, Magnusson J:* Rehabilitation for the postsurgical orthopedic patient, *ed 3, St Louis, 2013, Mosby.)*

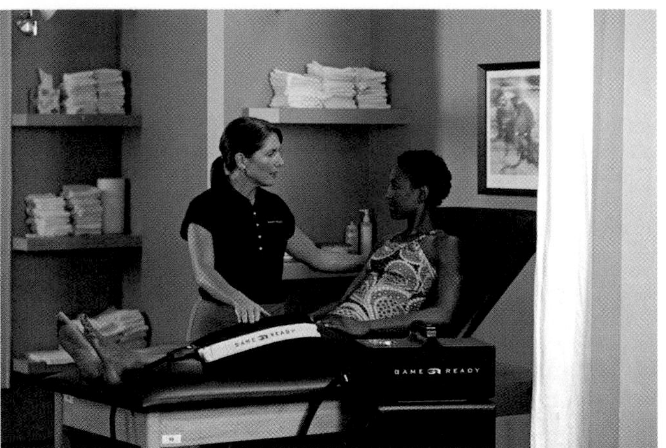

FIG 18-10 Game Ready commercial ice machine (Coolsystems Corporation, Berkeley, CA). *(From Noyes FR:* Noyes' knee disorders: surgery, rehabilitation, clinical outcomes, *Philadelphia, 2010, Saunders.)*

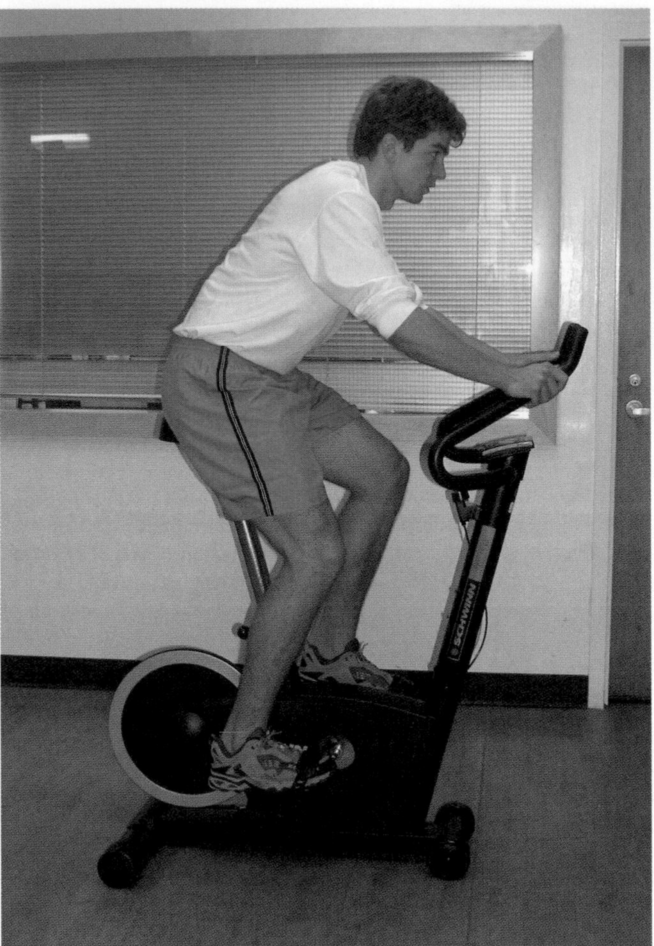

FIG 18-11 Short crank bicycle.

exercise for quadriceps reeducation. If a patient has difficulty eliciting a quadriceps contraction, a biofeedback unit or an electrical muscle stimulator can be used in conjunction with the quadriceps-setting exercise to facilitate quadriceps reeducation better. The literature supports the use of this modality.[58,63,118] SLR is performed with the postoperative brace locked at 0° until sufficient quadriceps control is demonstrated, as evidenced by ability to perform a SLR without pain or quadriceps lag. Patellar mobilization should be performed by the PT or PTA to assist in reestablishing normal patellar mobility. Superior mobility of the patella is required for complete knee extension. Inferior glide of the patella is necessary for full unrestricted knee flexion.[76] Hamstring and calf stretching is introduced to enhance flexibility. When ROM reaches 80°, a short-crank ergometer (Fig. 18-11) can be used to develop strength, ROM, and cardiovascular conditioning.[171] Proximal (hip and core) strengthening is initiated using mat exercises and a progressive resistive exercise regimen (e.g., cuff weights, isotonic exercise machines). Progressive weight bearing and early neuromuscular training are encouraged.

After surgery, afferent information is altered, which results in a disruption in the pathway between the patient's center of gravity and base of support.[39,50] This phenomenon contributes to balance deficits after ACL reconstruction.[98,153,177] Improving neuromuscular reaction time to imposed loads enhances dynamic stabilization around the knee and protects the static reconstructed tissue from overstress or reinjury.[99]

A rocker board proprioception device or dynamic balance system can be used as soon as the patient achieves 50% weight-bearing status. Balance activities are increased progressively to include unilateral weight bearing, use of multiplanar support surfaces, and perturbation training. Activities should attempt to eliminate or alter sensory information from the visual, vestibular, and somatosensory systems so as to challenge the other systems. Altering vision by having the patient close the eyes or catch and throw a ball while balancing more specifically challenges the somatosensory system.

When the patient demonstrates improved quadriceps control by demonstrating a pain-free SLR without a lag, the postoperative brace is opened 0° to 50° to allow for sufficient knee motion for level gait. Weight bearing is progressed as tolerated using crutches until a normal gait pattern without assistive device is demonstrated. An underwater treadmill system may be used to unload the

TABLE 18-2 Anterior Cruciate Ligament Reconstruction Rehabilitation Guidelines: Return to Function Phase

GOALS	• ROM 0° → WNL • Restore normal patellar mobility • Ascend and descend 8-inch stairs with good control without pain • >75% limb symmetry on isokinetic testing (quadriceps/hamstrings average peak torque and total work) • Ability to run short distance symptom-free
PRECAUTIONS	• Avoid descending stairs reciprocally until adequate quadriceps control and lower extremity alignment • Avoid pain with therapeutic exercise and functional activities
TREATMENT STRATEGIES	• Standard ergometry • Leg press (90° → 0° arc) • AAROM exercises • Squats (PRE) • Treadmill retrograde (progressive incline) • Proprioception training: unilateral weight-bearing activities/unstable surface/perturbations • Initiate FSD program • Stair climber/elliptical machine • Quadriceps/hamstring/calf flexibility exercises • Hip/hamstring PRE • If full ROM: PRE knee extension to 40° at 12 weeks, full arc at 16 weeks (monitor for crepitus/pain) including isokinetic training • Initiate running program (treadmill) • Controlled agility activities • Isokinetic test at 16 weeks • Soft tissue massage/foam rolling (if indicated) • Patellar mobilization • Home therapeutic exercise program: evaluation based
CRITERIA FOR ADVANCEMENT	• ROM 0° → WNL • Restore normal patellar mobility • Ascend and descend 8-inch stairs with good control without pain • ≥75% limb symmetry on isokinetic testing (quadriceps/hamstrings average peak torque and total work) • Ability to run short distance symptom-free

AAROM, active-assisted range of motion; *FSD,* forward step-down; *PRE,* progressive resistive exercise; *ROM,* range of motion; *WNL,* within normal limits.

involved extremity for ambulation training during this progression. Walking in chest-deep water results in a 60% to 75% reduction in weight bearing, whereas walking in waist-deep water results in a 40% to 50% reduction in weight bearing.[16,85]

As ROM and strength improve, additional CKC exercises such as squatting and leg press are introduced into the program. CKC exercises are used predominantly for strengthening in this phase because these activities have been shown to minimize stress to the ACL.[88,121,148,204,213,216] Lutz and colleagues[121] calculated lower posterior shear force (the resisting force to anterior drawer) during a squat than during OKC knee extension at all angles. As ROM improves to 110° to 115°, cycling is advanced to a standard 170-mm ergometer. Fleming and colleagues[72] demonstrated relatively low ACL peak strain values in vivo during stationary cycling. Compliance with prescribed home therapeutic exercise and with modification in ADL is emphasized.

Return to Function Phase

The next phase of rehabilitation, the return to function phase, after ACL reconstruction is designed to return the patient to normal ADL (Table 18-2). ROM continues to be addressed with the goal of achieving full symmetric ROM at the end of this phase. Strengthening and balance activities are progressed with the expectation of having the patient demonstrate the ability to ascend and descend normal stairs reciprocally without pain or movement deviation.

Unilateral CKC exercises such as contralateral hip abduction (Fig. 18-12) and extension with resistive bands and graduated forward step-ups are introduced during this phase. As ROM and strength improve, a forward step-down progression program is introduced (step heights of 4, 6, and 8 inches) (Fig. 18-13). Retrograde treadmill ambulation on a progressive percentage incline is used to facilitate quadriceps strengthening (Fig. 18-14).[185] At 3 months postoperatively, isotonic knee extensions in a 90° to 40° arc may be implemented with patellofemoral symptoms monitored. Advanced neuromuscular training activities are added, including lateral agility activities, dynamic balance activities on less stable surfaces (e.g., foam rollers, rocker boards), and perturbation training. Quadriceps stretching is first introduced in a supine position and later in a prone position as ROM demonstrates improvement.

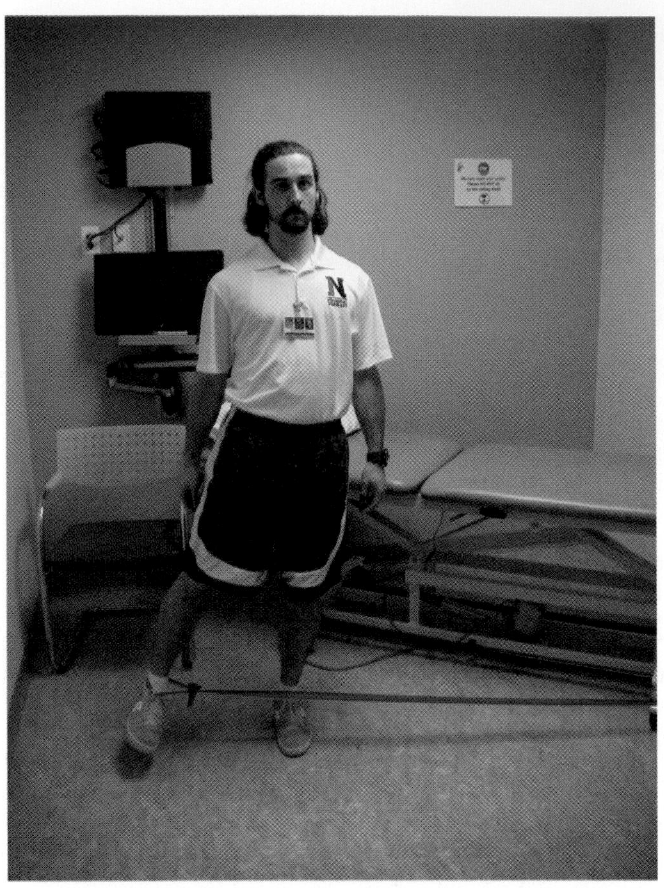

FIG 18-12 Contralateral abduction with TheraBand.

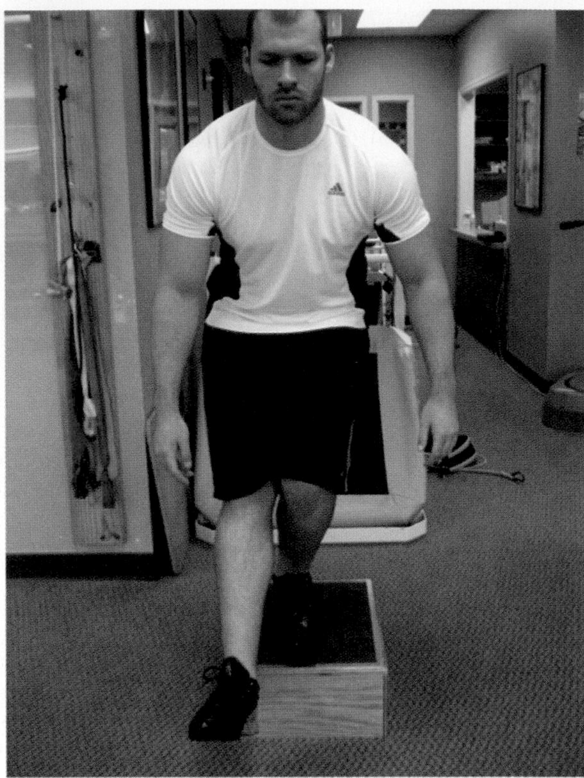

FIG 18-13 Step-down exercise on a 6-inch step. Patient steps down from a step in a slow and controlled manner, leading with the noninvolved extremity. Deviations from limb alignment and subjective complaints from the patient are considered before progressing to a higher step. *(From Noyes FR:* Noyes' knee disorders: surgery, rehabilitation, clinical outcomes, *Philadelphia, 2010, Saunders.)*

Return to Sport Phase

The final phase of rehabilitation, the return to sport phase, begins at approximately 4 months postoperatively when the goals of the return to function phase are met (Table 18-3). Therapeutic exercise is concentrated on strengthening to prepare the lower extremity for the demands placed on it during athletic activity. CKC and OKC exercises are progressed via a progressive resistance exercise (PRE) approach. OKC knee extensions are performed isotonically and isokinetically in a 90° to 0° arc of movement while monitoring any patellofemoral symptoms. Backward running precedes forward running because retrograde running has been shown to generate lower patellofemoral joint compression forces than forward running.[73] Advanced sport-specific activities such as deceleration training and plyometrics are added as appropriate to meet the athlete's sport-specific requirements.

Plyometrics has been defined as a quick, powerful movement involving prestretching the muscle and activating the stretch-shortening cycle to produce a subsequently stronger concentric contraction.[194] Plyometric training should follow a functional progression, with the components of speed, intensity, load, volume, and frequency monitored and advanced accordingly. Activities should begin with simple drills and advance to more complex exercises (e.g., double leg in-place jumping versus box drills [Fig. 18-15]).

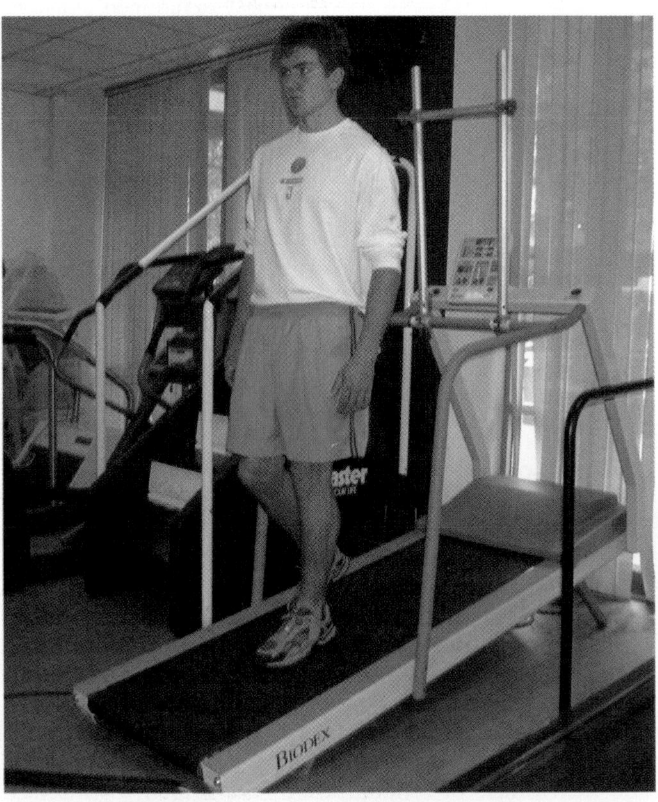

FIG 18-14 Retrograde treadmill ambulation.

TABLE 18-3 Anterior Cruciate Ligament Reconstruction Rehabilitation Guidelines: Return to Sport Phase

GOALS	• ≥90% limb symmetry on isokinetic testing (quadriceps/hamstrings average peak torque and total work) • Hop test ≥90% limb symmetry • Symmetric quality movement screen • Lack of apprehension with sport-specific movements • Maximize strength and flexibility to meet demands of sport activity
PRECAUTIONS	• Avoid pain with therapeutic exercise and functional activities • Avoid sport activity until adequate strength development and physician clearance
TREATMENT STRATEGIES	• Progress running program • Continue lower extremity strengthening (PRE) and flexibility programs • Advance agility program/sport-specific program • Plyometric program • Isotonic knee extension (full arc/no pain or crepitus) • Isokinetic training (fast → moderate velocities) • Proprioception training: unilateral weight-bearing activities/unstable surface/perturbations • KT1000 knee ligament arthrometer examination at 6 months • Isokinetic test • Functional (hop) test • Quality movement screen • Home therapeutic exercise program: evaluation based
CRITERIA FOR ADVANCEMENT: RETURN TO SPORTS	• ≥90% limb symmetry on isokinetic testing (quadriceps/hamstrings average peak torque and total work) • Hop test ≥ 90% limb symmetry • Symmetric quality movement screen • Lack of apprehension with sport-specific movements • Physician clearance

PRE, progressive resistive exercise.

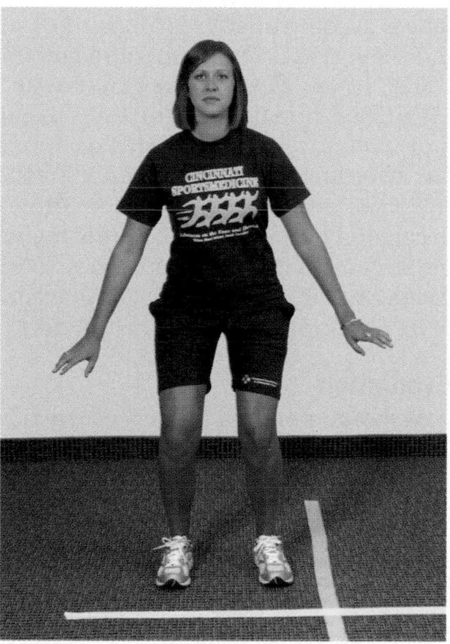

FIG 18-15 Plyometric four-quadrant exercise. Plyometric bilateral jumps in a "+" pattern. The patient jumps and lands into each quadrant continuously. Four jumps clockwise are followed by four jumps counterclockwise. *(From Noyes FR:* Noyes' knee disorders: surgery, rehabilitation, clinical outcomes, *Philadelphia, 2010, Saunders.)*

Quantitative and qualitative assessments of strength, power, and movement are needed to determine best an athlete's ability to return to sport after ACL reconstruction. Isokinetic testing of the knee involves assessment of the quadriceps and hamstring muscles during a testing procedure in which velocity is constant and resistance is variable and accommodating. Isokinetic testing has been shown to be reliable and valid.[67,155] Data interpretation from the testing can include among other parameters peak torque, peak torque-to-body weight ratio, total work, average power, quadriceps-to-hamstring ratio, and force decay rate.

Functional testing allows a more functional approach to strength assessment by using a CKC environment during measurement. Functional testing links specific components of function with the actual task and provides evidence to prove functional status. Observation during testing can assist the PT or PTA in ascertaining the athlete's apprehension or lack thereof in performing a functional task. Functional tests include vertical jump and hop tests. Daniel and associates[53] introduced the one-legged hop test for distance in 1982. Barber and colleagues[12] described four hop tests to assess lower extremity functional limitations: single-legged hop for distance, timed hop, triple hop for distance, and crossover triple hop for distance (Fig. 18-16). Normal limb symmetry was identified as limb values within 85% of one another for men and women regardless of limb dominance or sports activity level. The single-legged hop for time and the crossover hop have been reported to be the most sensitive and best indicators of function.[143] A quality movement assessment measures strength throughout the entire kinetic chain. The clinician can look to assess unilateral movement during such tasks as a step-down, single-leg squat, and lateral landing from a jump. Limb control, asymmetries, and apprehension are observed and documented.

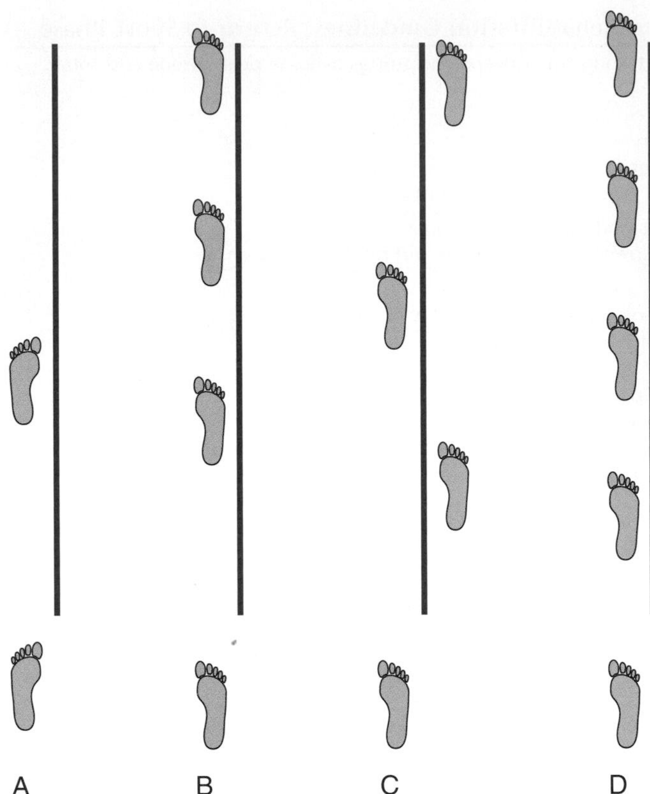

FIG 18-16 Hop tests. **A,** Single-leg hop for distance. **B,** Triple hop for distance. **C,** Crossover hop test. **D,** Timed 10-m hop test.

The data gathered from all of the aforementioned assessments are shared with the referring orthopedic surgeon, who ultimately makes the final decision on the patient's ability to resume athletic activities. Bracing of the reconstructed knee for sport activity is directed by the surgeon. Although controversial, some surgeons recommend bracing for sports activity for the first year after reconstruction.

POSTERIOR CRUCIATE LIGAMENT INJURY

The posterior cruciate ligament (PCL) functions as the primary restraint to posterior displacement of the tibia relative to the femur.[31] PCL injuries are less frequent than ACL injuries. Injury to the PCL accounts for approximately 3% of all knee injuries in the general population.[134] In patients who present to trauma centers with knee injuries, the incidence has reported to be 37%.[66] Isolated PCL injuries may occur at a rate of 40%.[45] The most frequent mechanism of injury in isolated PCL tears is a direct blow on the anterior tibia with the knee flexed position[103] (e.g., motor vehicle accidents involving the knee hitting the dashboard).

> **Important Concepts**
>
> The PCL functions as a primary restraint to posterior displacement of the tibia relative to the femur.

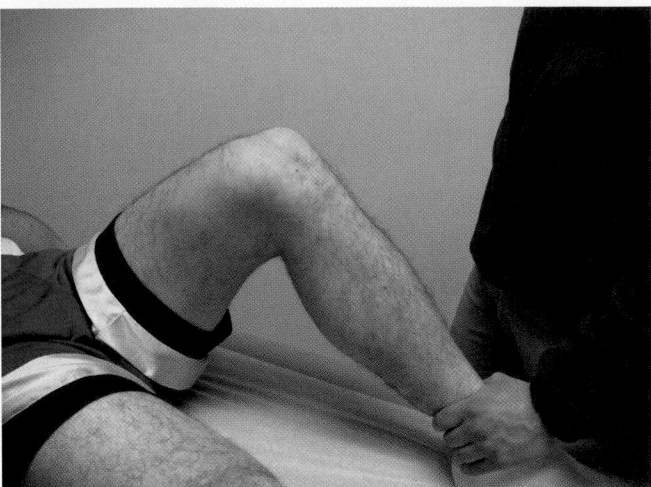

FIG 18-17 Active quadriceps drawer test. With the knee flexed to 70° and the clinician stabilizing the ankle on the table, the patient straightens the knee using the quadriceps muscle. Anterior translation of the tibia is consistent with a positive test.

Management of isolated PCL injury depends on the orthopedic surgeon's preference. The literature reported successful outcomes in patients treated without surgery who subsequently developed excellent quadriceps strength.[51,57,74,152,187] Other long-term follow-up studies of PCL injuries treated conservatively demonstrated degenerative changes accompanied by pain in the patellofemoral joint and the medial compartment of the tibiofemoral joint.[7,45,192] PCL injury is often associated with concomitant pathology. Additional knee structures may be injured as a result of hyperextension, hyperflexion, or rotational mechanisms associated with valgus/varus stress.[51,103] These injuries tend to be treated surgically more often than not. Whether reconstruction of the PCL alters the natural history of the PCL-deficient knee continues to be studied. Clinical results after PCL reconstruction have not been as predictable as results after ACL reconstruction.[7]

Clinical Evaluation

The clinician should obtain a proper history including an accurate description of the mechanism of injury. Reports of trauma to the front of the knee in a flexed position often correlate with the positive signs of a subsequent knee laxity examination. The most common and accurate test for a PCL injury is the posterior drawer test.[31] Other supporting tests include the Godfrey posterior sag test[208] and the **active quadriceps drawer test** (Fig. 18-17).[54] Patients often first present with an effusion, a flexion ROM deficit, and an antalgic gait.

Conservative Management

The rehabilitation program immediately after PCL injury is dedicated to combating the effects of inflammation and quadriceps inhibition. The patient is often allowed to ambulate WBAT with crutches with an open brace limited to a 0° to 60° ROM. Cryotherapy, compression, and activity modification are emphasized to assist in meeting this goal. Quadriceps setting and SLR are initiated early to prevent loss of quadriceps control and to minimize atrophy. Electrical stimulation may be used to facilitate quadriceps reeducation. Therapeutic interventions to regain ROM are introduced gradually. As ROM, gait, and quadriceps control normalize, the patient enters a more aggressive strengthening period of the rehabilitation program. The PT or PTA should take note of the forces generated during select exercises. Strengthening exercises such as OKC isometrics at multiple angles and CKC squats and leg presses are incorporated inside a 0° to 60° ROM. Wilk[201] demonstrated increased posterior forces with OKC knee extension, CKC squat, and leg press at flexion angles greater than 60°. Lutz and colleagues[121] demonstrated posterior shear forces during a CKC squat exercise, but the forces were significantly less than forces produced during OKC knee flexion. Isolated OKC hamstring strengthening is avoided. Toutoungi and associates[189] calculated that peak PCL loads occur at approximately 90° of knee flexion during isokinetic and isometric flexion exercise, and that these loads may exceed four times the body weight. The clinician should pay careful attention to the patellofemoral joint during a strengthening program. Loaded arcs of motion that produce pain or crepitus should be avoided. Functional activities such as step-ups, step-downs, and running are advanced using a progression similar to that described earlier in the section on ACL injury. Neuromuscular control activities inside a CKC are used to aid in the development of dynamic stability. Functional bracing for sports may be used at the physician's direction.

Important Concepts

Peak PCL loads occur at 90 degrees of flexion and exceed four times body weight.

Postoperative Rehabilitation

Rehabilitation after PCL reconstruction needs to consider biomechanical properties of the ligament and the altered biomechanics inherent in a PCL-deficient knee. Rehabilitation guidelines must consider graft selection, fixation, and surgical technique. Communication between the surgeon and PT and PTA is vital. Common graft choices include autogenous patellar tendon, and Achilles tendon allograft. A transtibial fixation split Achilles tendon allograft PCL reconstruction performed using an all arthroscopic technique allows for excellent tibial fixation with a bone block and sufficient soft tissue for two femoral bundles (Fig. 18-18). Additional structural involvement identified during surgery has a direct effect on program design and progression.

During the immediate postoperative period, the involved knee is placed in a postoperative brace locked at 0° of extension for ambulation. Weight bearing with crutches is begun with toe-touch weight bearing (TTWB) and advanced to PWB over the first 6 weeks.[36] The brace is kept locked for ambulation during this period to minimize posterior tibial shear forces created by hamstring activation. ROM exercises are performed sitting, initially to 70° of flexion and advancing to 90° during this phase.

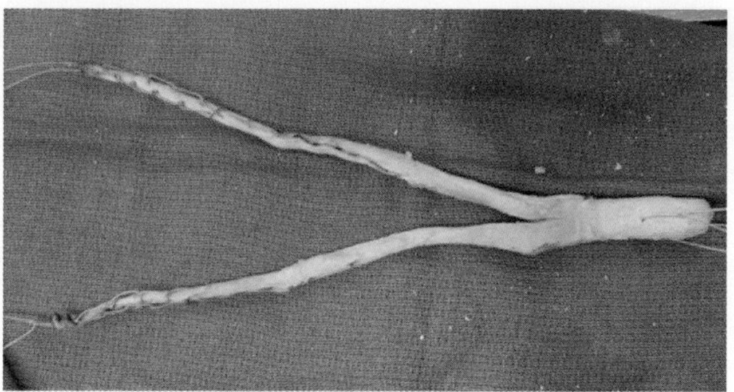

FIG 18-18 Split Achilles tendon allograft prepared for passage. *(From Kim HM, Stannard JP: How I manage the multiple-ligament injured (dislocated) knee,* Oper Tech Sports Med *19[1]:42-50, 2011.)*

The patient is taught to passively flex the involved knee with the support of the noninvolved extremity (eccentric quadriceps contraction). The knee is extended active assistively to 0° via concentric contractions of bilateral quadriceps muscles. Failure to achieve full passive extension is seldom a complication after PCL reconstructive surgery, but it must be addressed, and full extension must be achieved in the early postoperative period to ensure proper patellofemoral mechanics.

PCL reconstructive surgery with a concomitant MCL repair requires a more aggressive approach in addressing ROM. Injury to the medial capsule may accelerate the healing response and cause a greater propensity for motion restriction, arthrofibrosis, and development of a flexion contracture.

Patellar mobilization is crucial to improve patellar mobility in this early postoperative period because flexion is restricted to protect the graft substitute. Quadriceps reeducation using electrical stimulation or biofeedback can be helpful in preventing quadriceps inhibition and atrophy. OKC multiple-angle quadriceps isometric exercises inside a 60° to 30° arc of motion are used bilaterally with submaximal effort. As ROM improves, CKC leg press is introduced inside a 60° to 0° arc of motion. When ROM achieves 80° of flexion, short-crank ergometry is begun. At 6 weeks postoperatively, the postoperative brace is changed to an off-the-shelf PCL brace. ROM and weight bearing are gradually progressed with the goals of a normalized gait and 120° of knee flexion attained by 8 weeks. The rehabilitation program should advance via the functional progression outlined earlier. Resisted isolated hamstring strengthening exercises, whether isotonic or isokinetic, are avoided. Return to sports is anticipated between 8 and 12 months postoperatively and is based on the individual athlete's sport, level of participation, and medical clearance. Postoperative PCL rehabilitation guidelines are outlined in Table 18-4.

MEDIAL COLLATERAL LIGAMENT INJURY

The MCL is the most injured ligament in the knee[134] and is the primary restraint to abduction of the knee.[200] It is also a restraint to external rotation of the tibia on the femur.[137] Scriber and Matheny[172] reported that MCL injury

TABLE 18-4 Posterior Cruciate Ligament Reconstruction: Postoperative Guidelines

POSTOPERATIVE PHASE I (POD 1-21)	
Goals	• Emphasis on full passive extension • Control postoperative pain/swelling • ROM 0° → 70° • Prevent quadriceps inhibition • Improve patellar mobility • Independence in home therapeutic exercise program
Precautions	• Avoid active knee flexion • Avoid heat application • Maintain prescribed weight-bearing status • Avoid ambulation without brace locked at 0°
Treatment Strategies	• Towel extensions, prone hangs • Quadriceps reeducation (quadriceps sets with EMS or EMG) • Gait: TTWB with brace locked at 0° with crutches • Patellar mobilization • Active-assisted knee extension/passive flexion exercise (ROM 0° → 70°) • SLRs (supine/prone) with brace locked at 0° • Hip progressive resisted exercises • Quadriceps (OKC) isometrics at 60° (bilateral) • Cardiovascular exercises (e.g., UBE, Airdyne) as tolerated • Cryotherapy • Emphasize patient compliance to home therapeutic exercise program and weight-bearing precautions
Criteria for Advancement	• ROM 0° → 70° • Ability to SLR without quadriceps lag • Improved patellar mobility
POSTOPERATIVE PHASE II (WEEK 3-6)	
Goals	• ROM 0° → 90° • Good patellar mobility • Minimize swelling • Progressive weight bearing: TTWB → PWB (75%)
Precautions	• Avoid exceeding ROM and weight-bearing limitations • Avoid active knee flexion • Avoid pain with therapeutic exercise and functional activities
Treatment Strategies	• Continue therapeutic exercises and modalities as in phase I • Progressive weight bearing: TTWB → PWB (75%) with crutches (brace locked at 0°) • Active-assisted knee extension/passive flexion (ROM 90° → 0°) • SLRs (all planes)/progressive resistance • Multiple-angle quadriceps isometrics (ROM 60° → 20°) • Leg press (ROM 60° → 0° arc) (bilaterally) • Proximal (hip) strengthening PREs • Proprioception training (bilateral weight bearing) • Hamstring/calf flexibility exercises • Short crank ergometry
Criteria for Advancement	• ROM 0° → 90° • Ability to bear 75% weight on involved extremity • Continued improvement in patellar mobility and proximal strength
POSTOPERATIVE PHASE III (WEEK 6-12)	
Goals	• ROM 0° → 120° • Restore normal gait • Demonstrate ability to ascend 8-inch stairs with good leg control without pain • Demonstrate ability to descend 6-inch stairs with good leg control without pain • Improve ADL endurance • Improve lower extremity flexibility • Protect patellofemoral joint
Precautions	• Avoid exceeding ROM limitations in therapeutic exercises • Avoid resistive knee flexion exercises • Avoid pain with therapeutic exercise and functional activities • Monitor activity level (prolonged standing/walking)

TABLE 18-4 Posterior Cruciate Ligament Reconstruction: Postoperative Guidelines—cont'd

Treatment Strategies	• Discontinue crutches when gait is nonantalgic (week 6-8) • Brace changed to physician preference (e.g., OTS brace, patellar sleeve, Unloader brace) • Standard ergometry (if knee ROM >115°) • Leg press/minisquats (ROM 60° → 0° arc) • AAROM exercises • Proprioception training: prop board/foam/contralateral CKC exercises (elastic band) • Initiate FSU program (week 6-8) • Step machine (week 6-8) • Underwater treadmill system/pool (gait training) • Retrograde treadmill ambulation • Active knee extension: PRE (OKC) 60 → 0° *(monitor patellar symptoms)* • *No* active (OKC) hamstring exercises • Initiate step-down program when appropriate
Criteria for Advancement	• ROM 0° → 120° • Normal gait pattern • Demonstrate ability to ascend 8-inch step • Demonstrate ability to descend 6-inch step • Functional progression pending knee ligament arthrometer examination and functional assessment
POSTOPERATIVE PHASE IV (WEEK 12-20)	
Goals	• Restore full ROM • Demonstrate ability to descend 8-inch stairs with good leg control without pain • Improve ADL endurance • Improve lower extremity flexibility • Protect patellofemoral joint
Precautions	• Avoid descending stairs reciprocally until adequate quadriceps control and lower extremity alignment • Avoid resistive knee flexion exercises • Avoid pain with therapeutic exercise and functional activities • Monitor activity level (prolonged standing/walking)
Treatment Strategies	• Leg press/squats (ROM 80° → 0° arc) • AAROM exercises • Proprioception training: proprioception board/foam/contralateral CKC exercises (elastic band)/ perturbations • Lunges • Agility exercises (sport cord) • Retrograde treadmill running • Quadriceps stretching • Active knee extension: PRE (OKC) to (ROM 80° → 0°) *(monitor patella symptoms)* • *No* active (OKC) hamstring exercises
Criteria for Advancement	• ROM to WNL • Demonstrate ability to descend 8-inch step with good leg control without pain • Functional progression pending functional assessment • Improved flexibility to meet demands of running and sport-specific activities
POSTOPERATIVE PHASE V (WEEK 20-26)	
Goals	• Initiate forward running program • Hop test ≥75% limb symmetry • Isokinetic test ≥75% limb symmetry • Improve ADL endurance • Improve lower extremity flexibility • Protect patellofemoral joint
Precautions	• Avoid pain with therapeutic exercise and functional activities • Avoid sport activity until adequate strength development and physician clearance
Treatment Strategies	• Start forward running (if descend 8inch step satisfactory) • Continue lower extremity strengthening, flexibility, proprioceptive, and agility programs • Initiate plyometric program (if sufficient strength base) • Isokinetic training/test (Full arc) • Functional hop test • Knee ligament arthrometer examination at 6 months
Criteria for Advancement	• Symptom-free running • Hop test ≥75% limb symmetry • Isokinetic test ≥75% limb symmetry • Functional progression pending knee ligament arthrometer examination and functional assessment

Continued

TABLE 18-4 Posterior Cruciate Ligament Reconstruction: Postoperative Guidelines—cont'd

POSTOPERATIVE PHASE VI (WEEK 26 TO RETURN TO SPORT)	
Goals	• Lack of apprehension with sport-specific movements • Maximize strength and flexibility to meet demands of individual's sport activity • Hop test ≥ 90% limb symmetry • Isokinetic test ≥ 90% limb symmetry • Quality movement screen
Precautions	• Avoid pain with therapeutic exercise and functional activities • Avoid sport activity until adequate strength development and physician clearance
Treatment Strategies	• Continue lower extremity strengthening, flexibility, proprioceptive, and agility programs • Advance plyometric program • Advance agility program/sport-specific program • Isokinetic/functional/balance testing • Monitor patient's activity level throughout course of rehabilitation • Reassess patient's complaints (i.e., pain/swelling) daily and adjust program accordingly • Encourage compliance to home therapeutic exercise program
Criteria for Discharge	• Hop test ≥90% limb symmetry • Isokinetic test ≥90% limb symmetry • Quality movement screen • Lack of apprehension with sport-specific movements • Flexibility to accepted levels for sport performance • Independence with gym program for maintenance and progression of therapeutic exercise program at discharge

ADL, activities of daily living; *AAROM,* active-assisted range of motion; *CKC,* closed kinetic chain; *EMG,* electromyography; *EMS,* electrical muscle stimulation; *FSU,* forward step-up; *OKC,* open kinetic chain; *POD,* postoperative day; *PRE,* progressive resistive exercise; *PWB,* partial weight bearing; *ROM,* range of motion; *SLR,* straight leg raise; *TTWB,* toe-touch weight bearing; *UBE,* upper body ergometer; *WNL,* within normal limits.

was the most common knee injury sustained (40% of the total) in an 18-year survey of a college football program. The most common mechanism of injury is a laterally applied valgus force to the knee with the foot fixed to the ground. The most common site for MCL injury is at the femoral insertion; such injuries account for approximately 65% of all MCL sprains.[190]

Important Concepts

The MCL is the primary restraint to abduction of the knee and secondary restraint to external rotation of the tibia on the femur.

Management of MCL injury begins with evaluation. The grade of MCL injury is ascertained by the amount of laxity demonstrated on valgus stress testing. Grade 1 sprains manifest with a firm endpoint with no change in laxity compared with the contralateral knee. Grade 2 injuries represent a partial tear of the ligament and manifest with increased laxity. A firm endpoint is maintained when tested at 30° of knee flexion. Grade 3 injuries suggest a complete tear of the MCL and manifest with significant laxity and no endpoint when tested in full extension. The grade 3 injury is consistent with injury to the medial joint capsule and to the cruciate ligaments.[96]

Isolated MCL injuries seldom require surgery. Clinical studies demonstrated no significant improvement in function or stability in patients who were treated operatively compared with patients treated conservatively.[69,95,195] Residual laxity may persist with grade 3 injuries treated nonoperatively.

The PTA needs to incorporate an understanding of the soft tissue healing process while advancing a patient with MCL injury through rehabilitation. The PTA should be sure to apply the correct therapeutic intervention (i.e., correct modality or exercise) at the right time so as not to disrupt or overload healing tissue.

Grade 1 injuries are treated symptomatically. Acute management includes the use of cryotherapy and compression to aid in controlling pain and localized swelling. Early ROM exercise, early weight bearing, and quadriceps reeducation are encouraged. As inflammatory symptoms subside, aggressive strengthening (OKC and CKC) and flexibility programs are introduced. The patient is advanced to higher level functional activities (e.g., running, plyometrics) in preparation for a return to sports via a functional progression. The athlete may return to sports on meeting standard criteria in 1 to 2 weeks. A functional brace is seldom required.

Grade 2 and 3 injuries are treated more conservatively. These injuries require use of a hinged rehabilitation brace to protect the injured MCL from harmful stresses during collagen synthesis and the remodeling or maturation phases of healing. After a grade 2 MCL injury, crutches are used, with WBAT for the first 2 weeks or whenever a normal gait pattern is demonstrated. ROM and strengthening (OKC and CKC) exercises are performed avoiding valgus or rotational loads. A functional progression of therapeutic exercise is implemented with the demands of the athlete's sport and position in that sport taken into consideration. The athlete may return to sport participation on meeting the return to sports criteria 3 to 5 weeks after injury. The athlete is encouraged to don a functional knee brace for the remainder of the sports season.

Grade 3 injuries require a prolonged immobilization period. A hinged rehabilitation brace is worn and crutches are used for 6 weeks to protect the healing ligament from valgus and inherent forces. Weight bearing is limited to

PWB (25%) for the first 3 weeks after injury and then progressively advanced as tolerated. At 6 weeks after injury, a smaller double-hinged brace is used for ADLs. The patient is advanced via a functional progression and returns to normal activities as rehabilitative criteria are met. For an athlete, a grade 3 MCL sprain is usually a season-ending injury because healing and rehabilitation require 2 to 3 months.

MENISCUS INJURIES

Injuries to the meniscus are very common among professional and amateur athletes and are one of the most common indications for knee surgery.[90] Hede and co-workers[87] reported the mean annual incidence of meniscus tears as 9.0 in male subjects and 4.2 in female subjects per 10,000 subjects. Tears were found to be more common in the third, fourth, and fifth decades of life.

The meniscus functions in load bearing, load transmission, shock absorption, joint stability, joint lubrication, and joint congruity.[112,116,209] The menisci consist of approximately 75% type I collagen.[78] Most of the collagen fibers are oriented circumferentially to resist tensile forces and contain hoop stresses, which are generated while weight bearing.[70] Radially oriented "ties" hold circumferential fibers together and provide resistance to shear.[47] The most peripheral 20% to 30% of the medial meniscus and the peripheral 10% to 25% of the lateral meniscus receive a rich blood supply from the medial and lateral genicular arteries.[6] The menisci occupy 60% of the contact area between the tibial and femoral cartilage surfaces and transmit 50% of the joint compressive forces in full extension and approximately 85% of the load in 90° of extension.[1] The lateral meniscus picks up 70% of the load transmitted across the lateral compartment, whereas the medial meniscus and articular cartilage share the load across the medial compartment.[197]

The meniscus can be injured from either mechanical or biochemical (degenerative) causes.[199] Noncontact forces are the most frequent mechanism of injury to the menisci.[116] These stresses result from a sudden acceleration or deceleration in conjunction with a change of direction (rotation force) that traps the menisci between the tibia and femur resulting in a tear. Contact injuries involving ligamentous pathology (ACL or MCL or both) can displace the meniscus from its peripheral attachments and result in a tear. Degenerative meniscal lesions are common in older individuals, as the menisci become stiffer and less compliant with age.[89] The most common types of meniscal tears are vertical longitudinal, oblique, degenerative, radial, and horizontal.[183]

Meniscal lesions manifest with various clinical symptoms, such as pain, effusion, locking, and persistent focal joint line tenderness. Displaced tears, such as bucket-handle tears, can produce locking and "giving way" episodes. Nondisplaced tears can alter meniscus mobility and produce abnormal traction stresses on the capsule and synovium, which result in pain and swelling.[55]

Meniscal tears may be treated conservatively based on location within the meniscus, type of lesion, and associated symptoms. Surgical options include meniscectomy (partial or total), meniscal repair, or meniscus transplantation. Meniscal tear pattern, geometry, site, vascularity, size, stability, tissue viability or quality, and associated pathology all are taken into account when determining whether to resect or repair a meniscal lesion.[173] It has been well demonstrated that meniscal excision leads to articular cartilage degeneration,[3,64,101] and it has been generally recognized that the amount of meniscal tissue removed should be minimized, repaired, or replaced.[123,149,166]

> **Important Concepts**
>
> Meniscus symptoms include pain, effusion, locking, and persistent focal joint line tenderness.

CLINICAL EVALUATION

A comprehensive evaluation sets the baseline from which progress is measured, particularly in a patient being treated conservatively. Observing this examination, the PTA can better appreciate the patient's presentation, which directly affects their subsequent treatment. A comprehensive history reveals the mechanism of injury, how the injury was initially managed, medical diagnosis including work-up (e.g., radiographs, MRI), surgery date, and post-surgical management. MRI has been proven to be a valuable diagnostic tool not only for identifying meniscal lesions but also for recognizing associated meniscal cysts, capsular detachments, ligament insufficiencies, and articular cartilage lesions.[133,158]

Observations document patient's weight-bearing status, gait deviations, joint effusion, muscle atrophy, and joint alignment. Attention to the patient's subjective complaints is extremely valuable because reports of pain (location and description), lack of mobility, and weakness have a direct effect on the progression of a rehabilitation program. The physical examination should document available active range of motion (AROM) and passive range of motion (PROM). Girth measurements should be taken above, at, and below each knee joint for comparison to assess muscle atrophy or swelling and effusion. Palpation in particular joint line tenderness is a valuable component of the evaluation of a patient with a meniscal lesion. Eren[62] demonstrated that joint line tenderness as a test for lateral meniscal tears was 96% accurate, 89% sensitive, and 97% specific.

Manual muscle testing may reveal a proximal or distal weakness or muscle imbalance. Quadriceps testing often is inappropriate in the immediate postinjury or postoperative setting. Neurovascular integrity should be evaluated. Assessment of patellar tracking and orientation where appropriate can provide valuable information when quadriceps strengthening exercises are implemented at a later date. Flexibility assessment is important because tight muscles about one joint can alter forces at another joint. Gait evaluation (when applicable) can be useful in assessing the patient's biomechanical profile.

> **Important Concepts**
>
> Joint line tenderness for lateral meniscus tears is 96% accurate, 89% sensitive, and 97% specific.

For a patient with meniscal pathology who is conservatively managed, provocative testing can be performed to identify meniscal injury further. These tests attempt to capture a torn meniscal fragment while placing the meniscus under physiologic loads. The Steinman test[164] is performed with the patient in a seated position, knees hanging comfortably at a 90° angle. The examiner grabs the foot of the involved extremity and sharply rotates the lower leg internally and externally. Apley's compression test[5] is performed with the patient in a prone position with the involved knee positioned in 90° of flexion. The clinician attempts to provide a compressive force through the long axis of the tibia, while internally and externally rotating the tibia on the femur. Pain elicited on these tests to either the medial or the lateral aspect of the knee is consistent with a positive test. The McMurray test[129] is performed to identify posterior horn tears of the menisci. The test is performed with the patient in the supine position with the knee fully flexed and externally rotated. The clinician holds the patient's knee with one hand and the foot and ankle with the other. While palpating the knee, the clinician applies a valgus stress as the knee is extended. The procedure is repeated with a varus stress with internal rotation.

Complaints of pain, discomfort over the posterior medial or lateral joint lines, snapping, or locking are indicative of a positive test. The **Thessaly test**[104] uses dynamic reproduction of load transmission in the knee joint. The clinician supports the patient by holding his or her outstretched hands while the patient stands flatfooted on the floor. The patient rotates his or her knee and body, internally and externally, three times, keeping the knee in slight flexion (5°). The same procedure is carried out with the knee flexed at 20° (Fig. 18-19). Patients with suspected meniscal tears experience medial or lateral joint line discomfort and may have a sense of locking or catching.

The clinical evaluation includes defining goals and forming a treatment plan to meet these goals. The information gathered should be reviewed with the patient. Realistic goals should be discussed and established by the patient, physician, PT, and PTA.

CONSERVATIVE REHABILITATION

When a meniscal injury is treated conservatively, the referring physician should discuss with the PT and PTA the prognosis for the patient. Concomitant pathology (e.g., degenerative joint disease, chondromalacia, ligament deficiency, chondral injury) should be discussed and considered as well. Such findings prolong the rehabilitation period and alter the time frame for meeting expected goals.

Cryotherapy, quadriceps setting, SLR in multiple planes, progressive WBAT, gait training with crutches, active-assisted range of motion (AAROM) exercises, and flexibility exercises are early post-traumatic treatment strategies. The patient is progressed via a functional progression as outlined earlier in this chapter. The aforementioned "rules of rehabilitation" should be followed. The PTA should ensure that an adequate strength base in the presence of full ROM is present before advancing to high-level activities such as plyometrics and sport-specific training.

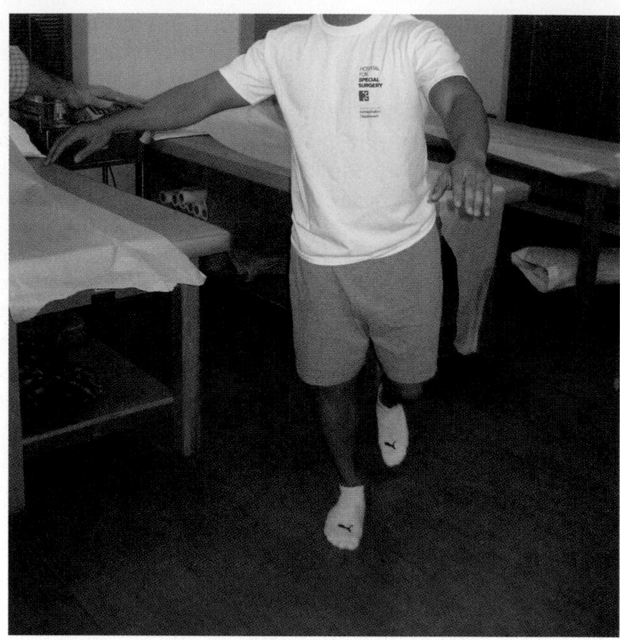

FIG 18-19 Thessaly test.

REHABILITATION AFTER PARTIAL MENISCECTOMY

Early proper intervention after surgery is vital in ensuring a fast and safe recovery. The PTA needs to encourage the patient to monitor load and volume of activity in the days after surgery. Postoperative effusion and pain are controlled by encouraging the patient to use axillary or Lofstrand crutches. A progressive weight-bearing gait is advised. Crutches can be discontinued when the patient develops a more normal, nonantalgic gait. Cold and compression is applied postsurgically using a commercial cryotherapy device. Nonsteroidal antiinflammatory drugs are recommended by some surgeons. Rasmussen and colleagues[162] reported on 120 patients randomly assigned to either naproxen twice a day or placebo for 10 days after arthroscopy. At 20 days after surgery, patients in the naproxen group had less effusion and pain and more ROM and walking activity.

Quadriceps setting and SLR in multiple planes are encouraged immediately after surgery to regain motor control and inhibit atrophy. AROM and AAROM exercises are started to improve motion. On achieving approximately 85° knee flexion, a short-crank ergometer can be introduced. As knee flexion ROM approaches 110°, the patient can be progressed to a standard ergometer.

The rehabilitation program is advanced in a similar fashion following the criteria-based functional progression as described earlier in this chapter. Objective testing should demonstrate near-symmetry with the noninvolved lower extremity before a return to sport activity.

REHABILITATION AFTER MENISCAL REPAIR

The postoperative management of a meniscal repair is more conservative compared with management after partial meniscectomy to allow for successful meniscal healing. Rehabilitation guidelines are controversial and differ among surgeons.[11,49,56,165] Discrepancies exist in the amount of weight bearing and knee flexion allowed in the early postoperative time frame and the time frame for return to sports activity. Programs should be individualized to the type of surgical procedure performed, the type of meniscal tear repaired, and the basic science information that is currently available. Information from the surgeon regarding the classification of the tear, anatomic site of the repair (vascular versus nonvascular), and location within the meniscus (anterior or posterior) directly affects the postoperative regimen.

The rehabilitation guideline at our institution after meniscal repair routinely provides for a strict protection phase for 4 to 6 weeks postoperatively (Table 18-5). ROM is restricted to a 0° to 90° arc of motion. Walker and Erkman[197] demonstrated that progressive knee flexion subjects the menisci to greater stress. WBAT is allowed with a postoperative brace locked at 0° of extension. Weight bearing in conjunction with tibiofemoral rotation during knee flexion could produce shear forces capable of compromising meniscal healing. Weight bearing is limited to TTWB for radial or more complex repairs. During this phase, AROM and AAROM exercises along with isometric exercises are used inside the prescribed protected ROM. After the prescribed protection phase, the patient is advanced in a fashion similar to that described earlier. However, running and sports activity are not recommended until at least 4 months postoperatively.[35,49]

TABLE 18-5 Meniscal Repair Rehabilitation Guideline

POSTOPERATIVE PHASE I (WEEK 0-6)	
Goals	• Emphasis on full passive extension • Control postoperative pain/swelling • ROM → 90° flexion • Regain quadriceps control • Independence in home therapeutic exercise program
Precautions	• Avoid active knee flexion • Avoid ambulation without brace locked at 0° before 4 weeks • Avoid prolonged standing/walking
Treatment Strategies	• Towel extensions, prone hangs • Quadriceps reeducation (quadriceps sets with EMS or EMG) • Progressive weight bearing: PWB → WBAT with brace locked at 0° with crutches • TTWB for complex or radial tears • Patellar mobilization • Active-assisted flexion/extension 90° → 0° exercise • SLRs (all planes) • Hip progressive resisted exercises • Proprioception board (bilateral weight bearing) • Aquatic therapy: pool ambulation or underwater treadmill (week 4-6) • Short crank ergometry (if ROM >85°) • Leg press (bilateral/60° → 0° arc) (if ROM >85°) • OKC quadriceps isometrics (submaximal/bilateral at 60°) (if ROM >85°) • Upper extremity cardiovascular exercises as tolerated • Hamstring and calf stretching • Cryotherapy • Emphasize patient compliance to home therapeutic exercise program and weight bearing and ROM precautions/progression
Criteria for Advancement	• Ability to SLR without quadriceps lag • ROM 0° → 90° • Demonstrate unilateral (involved extremity) weight bearing without pain
POSTOPERATIVE PHASE 2 (WEEK 6-14)	
Goals	• Restore full ROM • Restore normal gait (nonantalgic) • Demonstrate ability to ascend and descend 8-inch stairs with good leg control without pain • Improve ADL endurance • Improve lower extremity flexibility • Independence in home therapeutic exercise program
Precautions	• Avoid descending stairs reciprocally until adequate quadriceps control and lower extremity alignment • Avoid pain with therapeutic exercise and functional activities • Avoid running and sport activity

Continued

TABLE 18-5 Meniscal Repair Rehabilitation Guideline—cont'd

Treatment Strategies	• Progressive weight bearing/WBAT with crutches/cane (brace opened 0° → 60°), if good quadriceps control (good quadriceps set/ability to SLR without lag or pain) • Aquatic therapy: pool ambulation or underwater treadmill • Discontinue crutches/cane when gait is nonantalgic • Brace changed to physician preference (e.g., Unloader brace, patellar sleeve) • AAROM exercises • Patellar mobilization • SLRs (all planes) with weights • Proximal progressive resisted exercises • Neuromuscular training (bilateral → unilateral support) • Balance apparatus, foam surface, perturbations • Short crank ergometry → standard ergometry (if knee ROM >115°) • Leg press (bilateral/eccentric/unilateral progression) • Squat program (PRE) 0° → 60° • OKC quadriceps isotonics (pain-free arc of motion) • Initiate FSU and FSD programs • Stair climber • Retrograde treadmill ambulation • Quadriceps stretching • Elliptical machine • Upper extremity cardiovascular exercises as tolerated • Cryotherapy • Emphasize patient compliance to home therapeutic exercise program
Criteria for Advancement	• ROM to WNL • Ability to descend 8-inch stairs with good leg control without pain
POSTOPERATIVE PHASE 3 (WEEK 14-22)	
Goals	• Demonstrate ability to run pain-free • Maximize strength and flexibility to meet demands of ADL • Hop test ≥90% limb symmetry • Isokinetic test >90% limb symmetry • Quality movement screen • Lack of apprehension with sport-specific movements • Flexibility to accepted levels of sport performance • Independence with gym program for maintenance and progression of therapeutic exercise program at discharge
Precautions	• Avoid pain with therapeutic exercise and functional activities • Avoid sport activity until adequate strength development and physician clearance
Treatment Strategies	• Progress squat program <90° flexion • Lunges • Retrograde treadmill running • Start forward running (treadmill) program at 4 months postoperatively if 8-inch step down satisfactory • Continue lower extremity strengthening and flexibility programs • Agility program/sport-specific program (sport cord) • Start plyometric program when sufficient strength base demonstrated • Isotonic knee flexion/extension (arc free of pain and crepitus) • Isokinetic training (fast → moderate → slow velocities) • Functional testing (hop test) • Isokinetic testing • Home therapeutic exercise program: evaluation based
Criteria for Advancement	• Symptom-free running and sport-specific agility • Hop test ≥90% limb symmetry • Isokinetic test >90% limb symmetry • Quality movement screen • Lack of apprehension with sport-specific movements • Flexibility to accepted levels of sport performance • Independence with gym program for maintenance and progression of therapeutic exercise program at discharge

AAROM, active-assistive range of motion; *ADL,* activities of daily living; *EMG,* electromyography; *EMS,* electrical muscle stimulation; *FSD,* forward step-down; *FSU,* forward step-up; *OKC,* open kinetic chain; *PRE,* progressive resistive exercise; *PWB,* partial weight bearing; *ROM,* range of motion; *SLR,* straight leg raise; *TTWB,* toe-touch weight bearing; *WBAT,* weight bearing as tolerated.

Important Concepts

Postoperative management of meniscal repair is more conservative compared with postoperative management of partial meniscectomy.

REHABILITATION AFTER MENISCAL TRANSPLANTATION

In 1984, Milachowski introduced the meniscal transplantation procedure to address symptomatic meniscal deficiency.[132] The procedure has evolved into a primarily arthroscopic technique in which a cadaveric meniscus is inserted into a meniscus-deficient knee (Fig. 18-20). Ideal candidates for this procedure are patients whose knees are normally aligned and stable and demonstrate few degenerative changes.

Rehabilitation guidelines after meniscal transplantation are similar to guidelines used after a complex meniscal repair.[38] Ambulation is limited to TTWB using crutches for the first 4 postoperative weeks. The involved knee is maintained in full extension using a double upright hinged brace locked at 0° for the first 6 weeks. Gradual progressive weight bearing is encouraged during postoperative weeks 4 to 6. ROM exercises are begun immediately postoperatively. Full extension is encouraged, with flexion limited to 90° for the first 6 weeks. Isometric and isotonic strengthening exercises for the involved lower extremity, including quadriceps setting and SLR in multiple planes, are initiated immediately postoperatively and advanced accordingly during the early maximal protection phase. At 6 weeks postoperatively, the hinged brace is opened to 60° of flexion to allow for normal knee flexion during gait. Crutch use is discontinued as gait is normalized and quadriceps control is established. ROM is advanced as tolerated after 6 weeks. CKC exercises are initiated with flexion and weight-bearing limitations at week 4 and advanced accordingly. Squatting to more than 90° and hyperflexion are discouraged for the first 6 months after surgery.

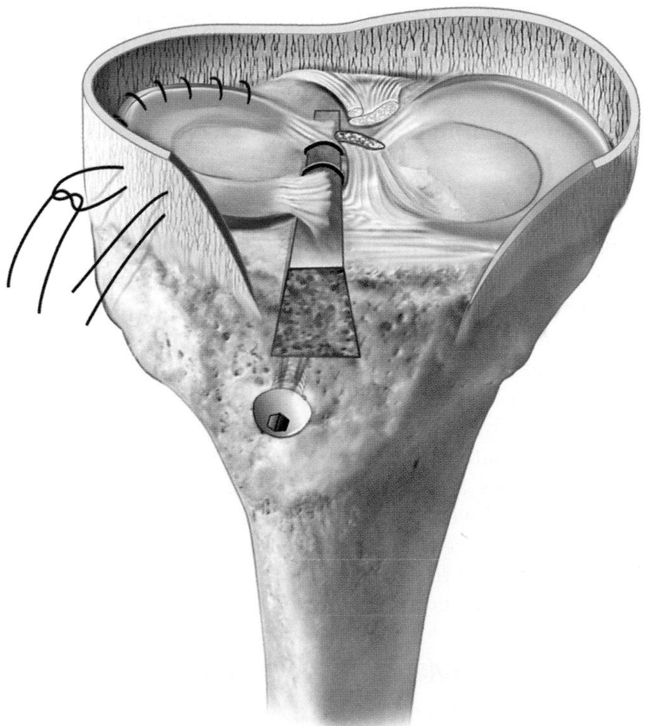

FIG 18-20 Medial meniscal allograft. Two bone plugs, one to the anterior horn and another to the posterior horn, are inserted in their respective tibial tunnels while sutures along the rim hold the graft in place. *(From Noyes FR:* Noyes' knee disorders: surgery, rehabilitation, clinical outcomes, *Philadelphia, 2010, Saunders.)*

The rehabilitation program is advanced over the course of several months to restore full knee ROM; develop muscle strength, power, and endurance; and reestablish flexibility and balance. These goals are pursued to assist the patient in meeting the demands of functional daily activities and low-demand sports participation. Return to recreational sports such as running, doubles tennis, skiing, and golf are allowed 9 to 12 months after surgery if appropriate criteria have been met. High-load activities involving cutting, jumping, and pivoting are not recommended after meniscal transplantation at the present time.[167]

ARTICULAR CARTILAGE INJURIES

Articular cartilage plays a vital role in the function of the musculoskeletal system by allowing nearly frictionless motion to occur between the articular surfaces of synovial joints.[27] During the course of a lifetime, articular cartilage endures high compressive and shear forces inherent to ADL and sports participation.

Mechanisms of injury at the knee include direct trauma, indirect impact loading, or torsional loading. Abnormal unloading at the knee joint can also be detrimental to articular cartilage. If deprived of the mechanical stimulus of load, cartilage becomes less stiff and is more vulnerable to injury.[151,196] Articular cartilage is avascular and aneural and has a minimal potential to regenerate after injury.[125] Articular cartilage may become problematic resulting in pain, mechanical symptoms, and effusion, which can interfere in an individual's normal ADL and participation in sports activity.

SURGICAL MANAGEMENT

Management of these lesions continues to this day to be a significant challenge for orthopedic surgeons, PTs, and PTAs. Modern operative procedures include the following:

1. Arthroscopic débridement or chondroplasty.[40] This procedure removes mechanical impediments to motion, reduces delamination, and improves joint surface congruency.
2. Marrow stimulation techniques such as abrasion arthroplasty or microfracture procedure.[40,179,207] With the microfracture technique, vascular channels are created by puncturing several holes into the subchondral bone beneath the lesion (Fig. 18-21). The result is the formation of a fibrin clot, which over time formulates into fibrocartilage.
3. Osteochondral autograft transplantation.[84] The articular cartilage lesion is filled using osteochondral plugs taken from NWB regions of the knee (Fig. 18-22).

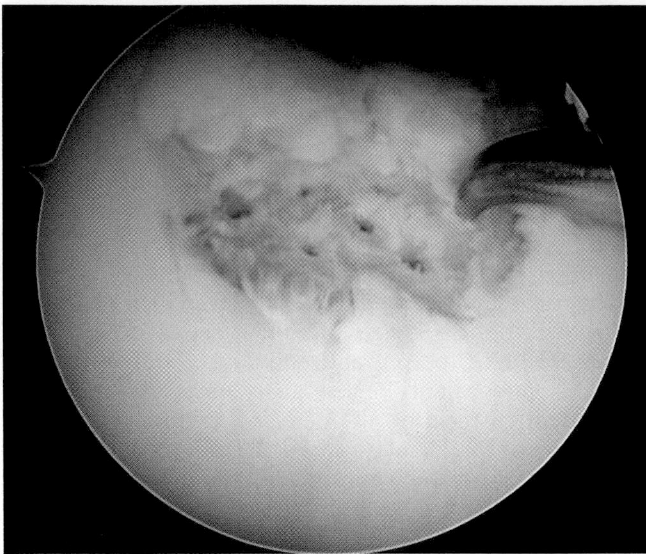

FIG 18-21 Microfracture awls penetrate the subchondral plate to stimulate the marrow elements and to allow access of the marrow elements to the bony surface. *(From Brown T, Cui Q, Mihalko WM, et al, editors:* Arthritis and arthroplasty: the knee, *Philadelphia, 2009, Saunders.)*

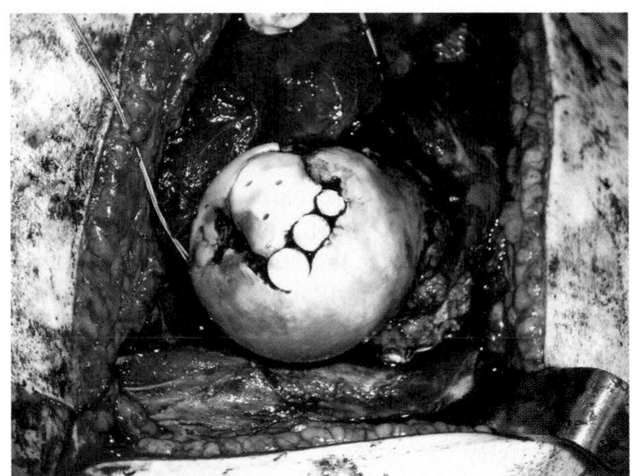

FIG 18-22 A demonstration of the osteochondral autograft transfer system procedure, with multiple cylindrical grafts in place. *(From Sekiya JK, Safran M, Ranawat AS:* Techniques in hip arthroscopy and joint preservation surgery, *Philadelphia, 2011, Saunders.)*

4. **Osteochondral allograft** transplantation.[28] Allograft transplantation is used routinely in first-stage procedures where the lesion is large or as a second-stage procedure after prior failed procedures. The lesion is resurfaced with a size-matched whole tissue allograft containing viable cells in its cartilage layer.
5. Autologous chondrocyte transplantation.[79] In this two-stage procedure, a chondrocyte biopsy specimen is cultured for several weeks and then reimplanted in the lesion under a periosteal or collagen patch.
6. Allograft cartilage transplantation (DeNovo NT).[186] The lesion is filled with minced pieces of juvenile cartilage held together with fibrin glue.

POSTOPERATIVE REHABILITATION

Rehabilitation after any of the above-listed procedures is individually determined because the type and location of each articular cartilage lesion differ. For example, femoral condyle lesions are commonly found in the area that contacts the tibia between 30° and 70° of flexion.[168] The PT and PTA should communicate with the surgeon to ascertain the size and location of the defect. Therapeutic exercises can be implemented that do not hinder the healing process by producing a shear or compressive force.

Research supports early controlled motion after articular cartilage injury.[26,170,182] Suh and colleagues[182] demonstrated that joint motion after articular cartilage injury may facilitate healing as long as shear forces are minimized. A CPM machine is often prescribed in the early postoperative period.

Weight bearing may be restricted depending on the surgical procedure performed. For femoral condyle lesions, WBAT with crutches may be allowed immediately after arthroscopic débridement; TTWB to PWB, after an osteochondral autograft procedure; PWB to WBAT, after osteochondral allograft surgery; and NWB to TTWB, after microfracture and autologous chondrocyte transplantation.[37] A more liberal approach to weight bearing is taken with patellofemoral lesions. When advancement of weight bearing is deemed therapeutic, a progressive weight-bearing approach is recommended. Weight bearing may be advanced using a deweighting system (Fig. 18-23), pool, or underwater treadmill.

Prolonged periods of restricted weight bearing after several of these procedures result in significant muscular atrophy, particularly of the quadriceps muscles. Proper strengthening interventions are important in restoring normal function. The PT and PTA should avoid exercises that induce shear in conjunction with compression forces in the range in which the healing defect is articulating with the opposing joint surface.

Quadriceps sets, SLR with progressive resistance, stationary cycling, and multiple-angle quadriceps and hamstring isometric exercises are recommended in the early postoperative period. Limited arc isotonic quadriceps strengthening exercises are later initiated inside a safe, crepitus-free, pain-free arc of motion. Low resistance with high repetitions is recommended. CKC exercises such as leg press are initiated bilaterally, progressing to eccentric training. Unilateral balance, strengthening, and functional activities are initiated when a sufficient strength base has been developed. Rehabilitation after articular cartilage surgery is a long and tedious process. The PTA should encourage the patient to be compliant throughout the rehabilitation course.

PATELLOFEMORAL PATHOLOGIC CONDITIONS

This section addresses the etiology of patellofemoral conditions, physical examination, nonoperative rehabilitation, and operative management and rehabilitation for proximal and distal realignments and articular cartilage procedures. As noted earlier, it is important that PTAs have

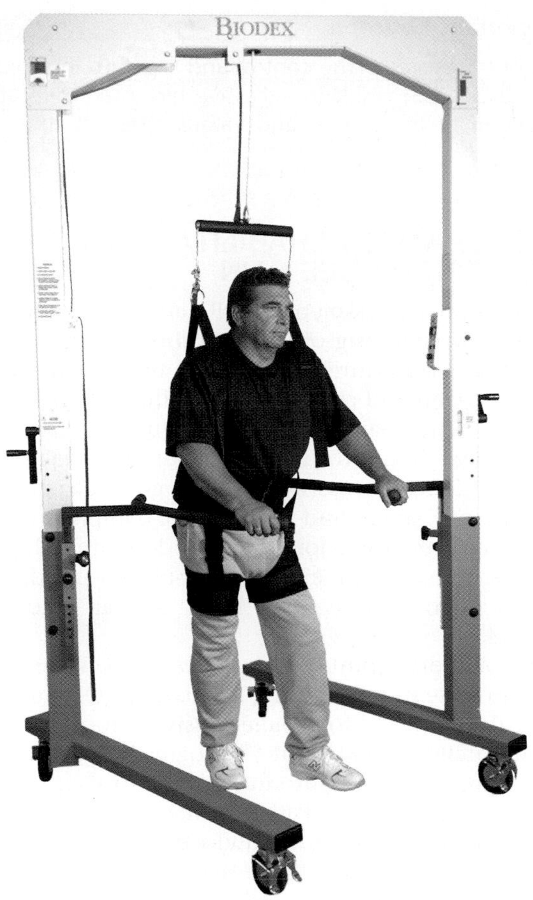

FIG 18-23 Biodex deweighting system (Biodex Medical Systems, Shirley, NY).

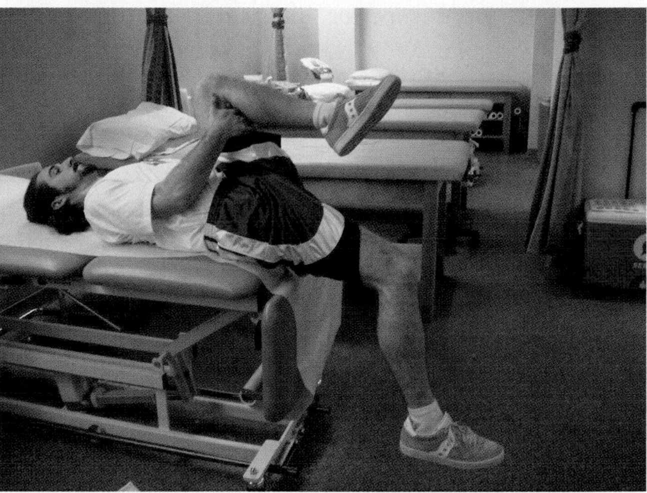

FIG 18-24 Modified Thomas test. The patient is supine with both knees against the chest and the buttocks near the edge of the table. The patient slowly lowers one leg until it is fully relaxed or until there is excessive spinal movement into lordosis or pelvic tilting. Positive findings are (1) lack of hip extension (iliopsoas tightness), (2) knee flexion less than 80° (rectus femoris tightness), and (3) external rotation of hip (iliotibial band tightness).

Important Concepts

PFPS may include anterior knee pain, fat pad syndrome, patellofemoral arthritis, chondromalacia, and anterior knee pain.

a good understanding of the anatomy and biomechanics of the lower extremity before implementing concepts into patient care. The operative management and rehabilitation overview should assist in understanding of criteria-based progression for this population.

Patellofemoral pain syndrome (PFPS) is a challenging condition to define. Patellar pain diagnoses include anterior knee pain, fat pad syndrome, patellofemoral arthritis, chondromalacia, and anterior knee pain.[184] PFPS affects a wide age range from active young athletes to elderly adults, but the cause and underlying pathology may be different. The common finding among all patients is pain around the patella. Potential causes for PFPS include bony malalignment, muscular imbalances, poor proprioception, and overloading of the patellofemoral joint.[139,184] Common complaints include pain with activities such as ascending and descending stairs, walking uphill, squatting motions, and prolonged sitting.[159] One pearl to understanding PFPS is to realize that most cases are chronic and have been progressively worsening over time. The PTA should educate clients on having patience and commitment to selected interventions to see changes and the benefit of physical therapy over the course of their treatment.

PHYSICAL EXAMINATION

Physical examination of the entire lower extremity chain (core to the floor) is important. The PT and PTA should look at mobility (joint and soft tissue) above and below the knee, isolated muscular strength, flexibility, posture, and static and dynamic alignment. To treat these patients effectively, one must uncover the source or pain and the cause of pain, which can be accomplished with a thorough examination.

Joint Mobility

The PT and PTA should assess the patient's ROM for hip, knee, and ankle to obtain a general understanding on joint limitations above and below the affected area. This understanding may help in determining the potential cause of imbalances and pain at the knee.

Flexibility

The PT and PTA should assess general lower extremity flexibility for hamstring (active hamstring test), hip flexor and quadriceps length (**modified Thomas test**) (Fig. 18-24), and gastrocnemius-soleus complex (measure active dorsiflexion with knee extended [gastrocnemius] and flexed at 90° [soleus]).

Posture and Static Alignment

Factors associated with PFPS include femoral anteversion, genu valgum, genu recurvatum, quadriceps Q angle, tibia varum, and rearfoot pronation.[184] The Q angle is the angle from the anterior superior iliac spine to the patellar tendon. Normative values are between 10° and 15° with knee extended. Differences are seen between men and women because of increased pelvic width in women.[81] Less correlation has been seen between high static Q angle measurements and PFPS, but it may play a role when symptoms are present.

The PT and PTA should assess patellar alignment and mobility bilaterally. Patellar alignment can display as baja, alta, or tilt (lateral). Lateral tilt can be due to restriction in the lateral retinaculum and muscular tightness in quadriceps and iliotibial band. Patellar mobility is assessed in a relaxed state in full extension. When passively mobilized to the left and right, the patella should move approximately 1 cm medially and laterally. Motion beyond 1 cm laterally may indicate possible subluxation or instability.[75,203]

Overall implications of malalignment and instability can lead to increased contact pressures across the patellofemoral joint and result in cartilage wearing and pain over time.[81,203] Compressive forces across the patellofemoral joint increase from the inferior to the superior pole as flexion angles are increased.[184]

Muscle Strength and Dynamic Movement Patterns

A critical part of assessment of PFPS involves observation of a patient's movement patterns. A few movement patterns to assess include gait, squat, single-leg balance, and step-down activity. It is best to observe lower extremity kinematics when the joint is clearly visible (best with patient wearing shorts).

Gait

Patients with patellofemoral pain or dysfunction may display a lack of eccentric quadriceps control (quadriceps avoidance) and present with hyperextension with loading of the affected leg. Hyperextension is used as a pseudostability of the capsule. The effects of this altered gait mechanism cause quadriceps weakness, increased loading forces on the tibiofemoral joint, and possible impingement of the fat pad.[136]

Squat, Single-Leg Stance, and Step-Down

Throughout these movement patterns, it is important to assess movement strategies. Addressing alignment problems including pelvic and foot position can help in determining muscular imbalances, neuromuscular control, and soft tissue and joint mobility restrictions. Common alterations with squatting include knee strategy (initiation of motion with knee flexion), increased trunk fold, and excessive dorsiflexion at the ankles. These all result in excessive loading of the patellofemoral joint secondary to collapse in the kinetic chain.[136]

It is important to address rotational control of the lower extremity by assessing pelvic and hip control. Hip and pelvic control is facilitated by activation of the gluteus medius and maximus. Lack of rotational control and strength in these muscles can result in excessive hip internal rotation, adduction of the femur, and valgus stress on the knee joint. Restoring strength, coordination, and endurance can assist in improved kinematics and reduction of knee pain.[136]

Important Concepts

Lack of transverse plane control and strength in proximal hip muscles can result in excessive hip internal rotation, adduction of the femur, and valgus stress on the knee joint.

NONOPERATIVE REHABILITATION OF ANTERIOR KNEE PAIN

After the initial assessment, the PT and PTA should have a better understanding of the contributing factors: quadriceps weakness and imbalances, soft tissue tightness and restrictions, hip and core weakness, altered foot kinematics, and kinetic chain failure with dynamic movements. The clinician should focus on addressing the factors that can easily change to assist in overall goals of pain relief, improved mechanics, and reduction of compressive forces on the patellofemoral joint. When designing the treatment program, the PT and PTA should be mindful that postural alignment is the basis for all movement patterns.[211]

Patellofemoral joint stress increases as knee flexion angles increase in CKC during a squat. The optimal angle of knee flexion is 60° to avoid excessive compressive loads on the patellofemoral joint.[198] Progression to unilateral loading requires good neuromuscular control and strength throughout the chain. Patients may display ipsilateral trunk lean secondary to hip abduction weakness, which leads to the ground reaction force passing lateral to the knee as it moves closer to the hip joint center.[139] This change in force results in valgus stress at the knee. Another deficit may be seen in the transverse and frontal plane with gluteus medius weakness. Delayed or short duration activation of the gluteus medius results in increased hip internal rotation and adduction. The hip musculature must work to contract eccentrically while loading to prevent compensation in the transverse and frontal planes.[10,15,139]

Basic principles of rehabilitation of patellofemoral pathology are reducing swelling and pain, restoring mobility and flexibility, reeducating and enhancing proper muscle recruitment, enhancing neuromuscular control, strengthening and fostering proper mechanics and gait, and functionally retraining for activity.[205] A challenging component of patellofemoral rehabilitation is ensuring patient understanding of the condition and setting realistic goals. A case series by Mascal and colleagues[127] demonstrated 3 months or more of rehabilitation for achievement of results. Patients commonly struggle with number of repetitions of specific exercises because of weakness and fatigue. The clinician should gradually build up the number of repetitions per set over duration of time. The frequency in exercise prescription is important for muscle recovery as well. A helpful tool for patients is to give cues and feedback during performance of specific exercises. Use of consistent verbal cues and visual feedback through use of mirrors or replay of videotape fosters proper lower limb alignment with weight-bearing activities in the facility and at home.

Addressing the "core to the floor" is a systematic way to begin treatment. It is important to achieve stable proximal attachment sites for hip abductors and lateral rotators because this assists in minimizing trunk flexion and contralateral pelvic drop in the frontal plane. Activation of specific muscles should be initiated in NWB positions to ensure proper sequence of firing: abdominals, gluteals, and quadriceps.[127] Use of a blood pressure cuff for feedback of spinal position in hook lying position (Fig. 18-25) can assist in fostering motor learning and muscle recruitment for lower extremity movement patterns. When a stable core is found, dynamic NWB movements may occur with alternating hip and knee motions coupled and further challenged with opposite upper extremity movement.[127] Progression toward side planks and forward planks can continue to challenge core stability with transverse abdominals and gluteus medius activation.

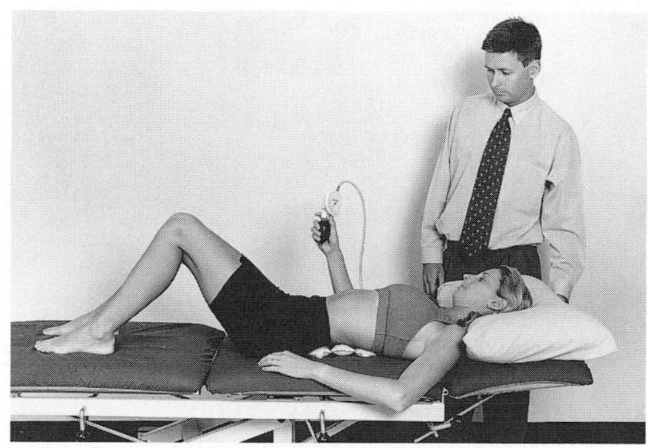

FIG 18-25 Hook lying blood pressure cuff feedback for spinal position. *(From Cameron MH, Monroe LG:* Physical rehabilitation: evidence-based examination, evaluation, and intervention, *St Louis, 2007, Saunders.)*

Two exercises that have been shown to optimize gluteus medius and maximus activation are clamshells and side-lying hip abduction.[59,206] Clamshells (Fig. 18-26) must be performed with the pelvis in neutral to achieve isolated gluteus maximus and medius motions. A variation to increase gluteus medius activation is seen with increased hip flexion angle.[206] Side-lying hip abduction (Fig. 18-27) also focuses on activation of gluteus medius and tensor fascia lata activity.[59]

The clinician should progress patients with bilateral loading exercises before unilateral loading. Activities such as squatting can be initiated on a leg press (Fig. 18-28). Band or tubing may be used as a subtle reminder for input to activate hip lateral rotators and abductors to maintain proper alignment. Using less tension is better to foster body awareness and muscle recruitment. Progression to body-weight loading with squatting (Fig. 18-29) adds the forces of gravity to joint movement. The PTA should avoid having the patient squat deeper than 90° of flexion so as to mimic the functional activity of sit to stand. This modification avoids excessive patellofemoral loading. As the patient progresses, maintains form, and has no complaints of pain, external loads can be applied to progress functional strength building and progression to unilateral activity.[198]

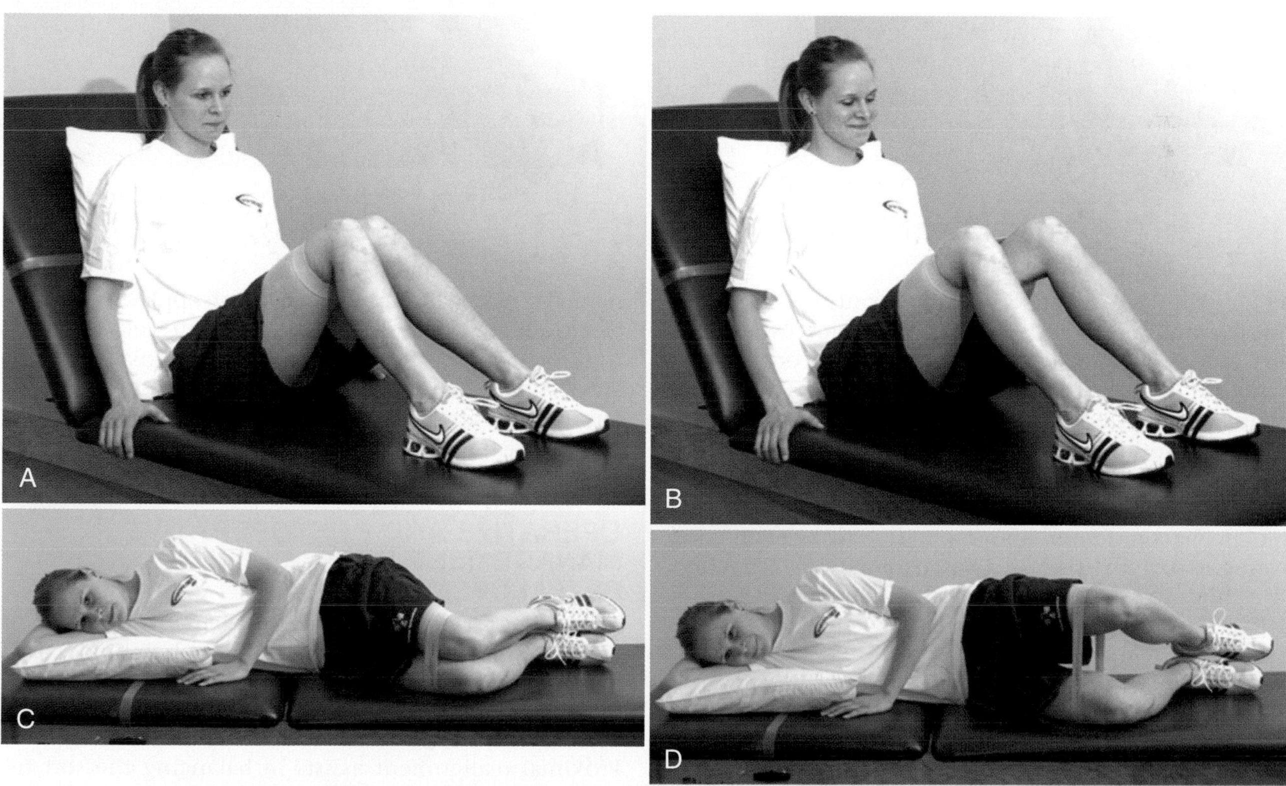

FIG 18-26 The clamshell exercise is performed in either the long sitting (**A** and **B**) or the side-lying (**C** and **D**) position. *(From Noyes FR:* Noyes' knee disorders: surgery, rehabilitation, clinical outcomes, *Philadelphia, 2010, Saunders.)*

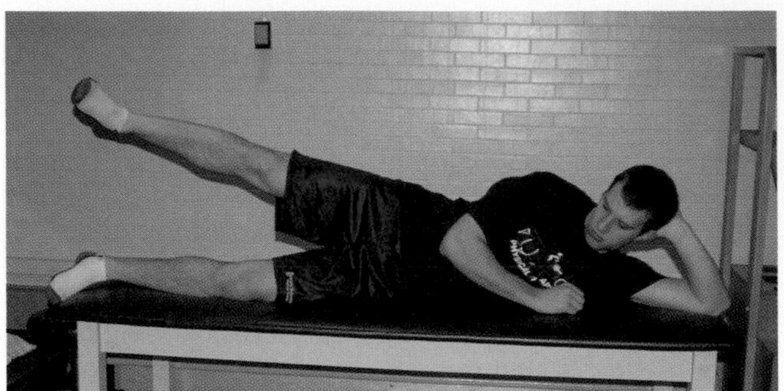

FIG 18-27 Side-lying hip abduction. *(From Sekiya JK, Safran M, Ranawat AS:* Techniques in hip arthroscopy and joint preservation surgery, *Philadelphia, 2011, Saunders.)*

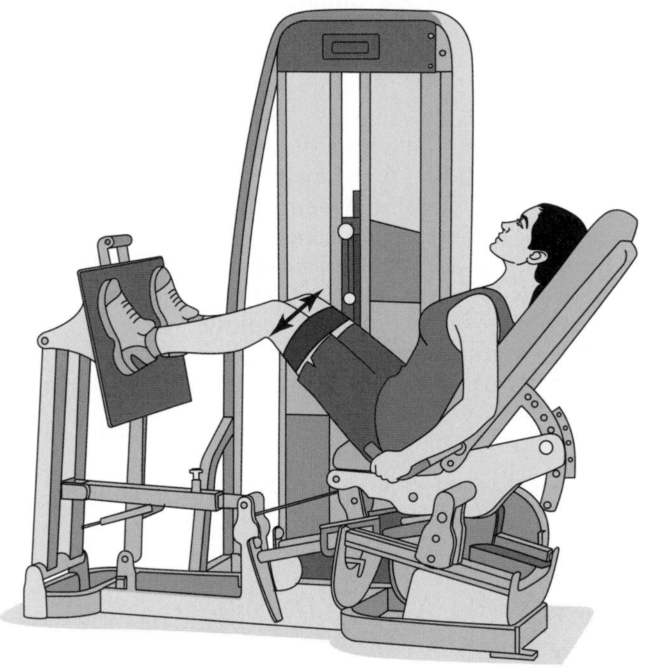

FIG 18-28 Leg press with exercise band.

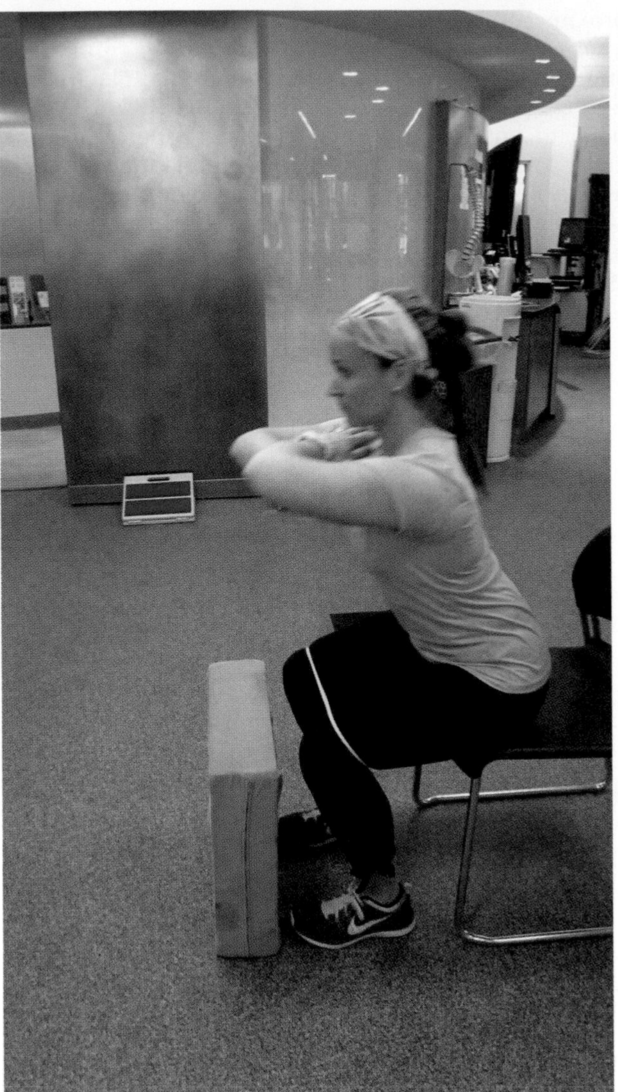

FIG 18-29 Body-weight squatting (lateral view).

Progression to unilateral loading continues to challenge the activation and endurance of gluteus medius. Exercises include monster walks (Fig. 18-30), contralateral hip motion (see Fig. 18-12), and lawnmowers (Fig. 18-31). Carrying an additional load on the contralateral side has been shown to increase gluteus medius activation on the ipsilateral side.[127,206] With these selected exercises, it is important for the core to remain activated to facilitate a stable pelvis on femur and maintain an overall good movement pattern strategy. Gluteus maximus activation is also important during unilateral loading and has been identified in exercises including single-leg squat (Fig. 18-32) and single-leg dead lift.[59]

Additionally, PTs may suggest bracing or taping for a patellofemoral condition. Lun and colleagues[120] found that bracing did not improve symptoms of PFPS more quickly when added to a home exercise program. Taping may also serve as a therapeutic tool for patients with patellar pain. Over the years, different types of taping have been developed from standard McConnell taping to the newer Kinesio Taping. The goal of applying tape is to create a mechanical shift of the patella to centralize it into the trochlea groove.[52] In a 2011 study, Dolak and associates[60] stated that tape may have more of a neuromuscular effect when applied in a corrective manner. Taping (Fig. 18-33) assists in the short-term to allow patients to perform exercises in a pain-free manner.

OPERATIVE AND POSTOPERATIVE MANAGEMENT FOR PATELLOFEMORAL PAIN

Guidelines for postoperative management should be individualized for each patient, and the rehabilitative course should be advanced via a criteria-based approach.

Proximal Realignment

Proximal realignment assists in balancing the soft tissue of the lateral retinaculum or the medial retinaculum (including medial patellofemoral ligament) or vastus medialis oblique. The medial patellofemoral ligament is

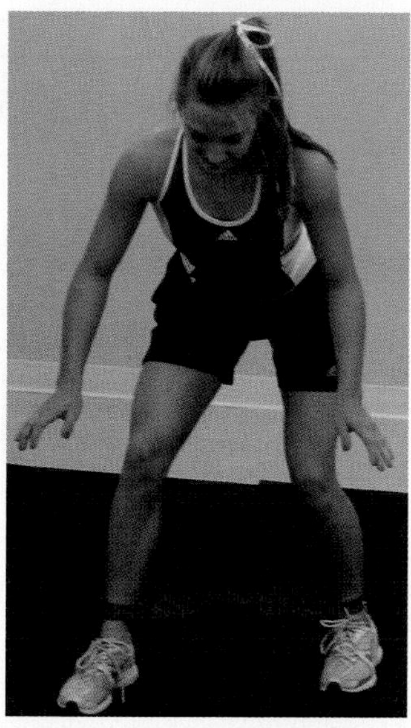

FIG 18-30 Monster walks. *(From Miller MD, Thompson SR:* DeLee & Drez's orthopaedic sports medicine, *ed 3, Philadelphia, 2009, Saunders.)*

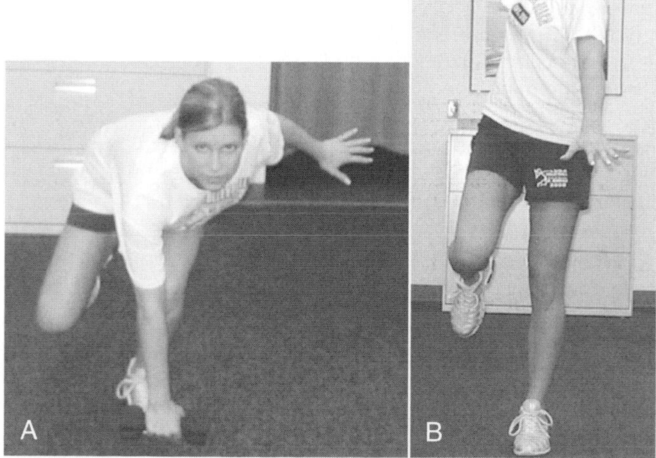

FIG 18-31 Lawnmowers. **A,** Starting position. **B,** Ending position. *(From Manske RC:* Postsurgical orthopedic sports rehabilitation: knee & shoulder, *St Louis, 2006, Mosby.)*

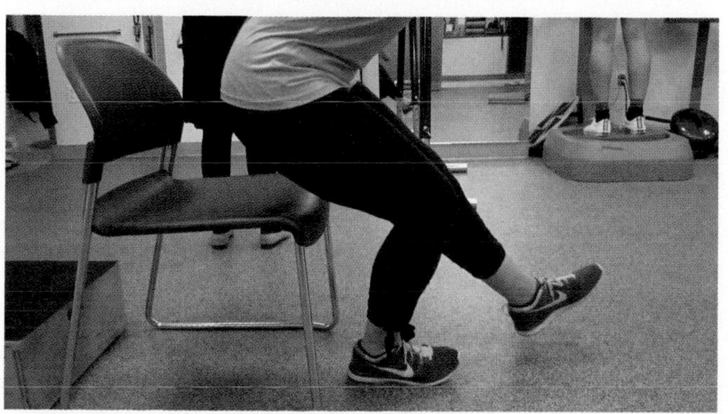

FIG 18-32 Single-leg squat.

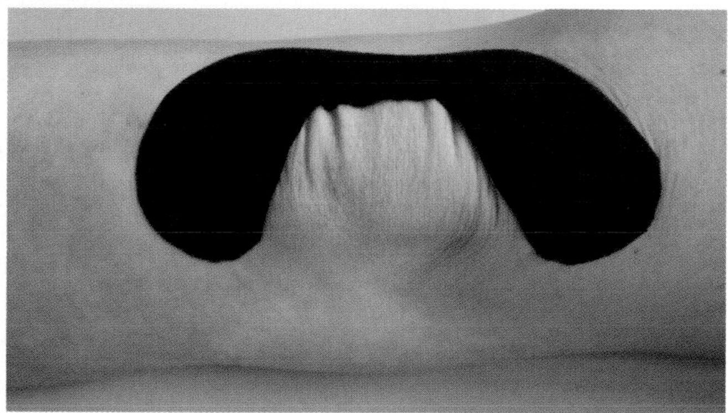

FIG 18-33 Kinesio Taping for patellar stabilization.

the main medial restraint for lateral displacement of the patella.[4] Reconstruction of this ligament fixates a tissue graft to the adductor tubercle in which tension is set based on alignment of the patella into the trochlea. Additionally, a lateral retinacular release may be performed at the time of realignment. See Table 18-6 for proximal realignment guidelines.

Phase 1: Respect Healing, Range of Motion, and Weight Bearing (0 to 6 Weeks). During phase 1 of rehabilitation, it is important to try to return the joint to homeostasis without disruption of the repair. Interventions should focus on reducing pain, reducing inflammation and joint effusion, and minimizing quadriceps inhibition. Quadriceps inhibition affects the proprioceptive abilities of the joint and provides a suboptimal environment for articular cartilage healing. Cryotherapy is an important part of this phase.

Range of Motion Parameters. ROM parameters are 0° to 60° (0 to 4 weeks postoperatively), with advancement to 90° knee flexion (4 to 6 weeks postoperatively). AAROM and PROM in sitting are used at this time. Maintaining knee

TABLE 18-6 Proximal Realignment

PHASE I
Respect Healing, ROM, Weight Bearing (0-6 Weeks)
	• Cryotherapy: reduce inflammation and joint effusion
	• ROM parameters: AAROM/PROM
	  • 0° → 60° (0-4 weeks)
	  • 0° → 90° (4-6 weeks)
	• Patellar mobility: medial
	• Flexibility: gastrocnemius-soleus
	• Quadriceps reeducation: home E-Stim unit
	• Weight bearing: progressing WBAT with crutches and brace locked at 0° extension (0-6 weeks); wean crutches, brace remains
	• Strengthening: proximal and distal to knee in NWB positions

Criteria for Advancement	• Good quadriceps contraction • Maintain knee extension with SLR • AAROM/PROM 0° → 90° • Controlled pain and swelling

PHASE II
Functional Gait, ROM, Strength (7-12 weeks)
	• Gait training: transition to functional brace
	  • Crutches: normalization of gait
	• ROM: 0° → 110° (8 weeks)
	  • Short crank: 0° → 80°
	  • Standard upright bicycle: 115° flexion
	• Strength/balance
	  • Neuromuscular control (bilateral → unilateral)
	  • CKC exercises: quadriceps, gluteals, core, gastrocnemius-soleus
	• Flexibility: quadriceps, hamstring, gastrocnemius-soleus

Criteria for Advancement	• Functional ROM • Normal gait • Controlled pelvic and knee stability in SLS
PHASE III **Advanced Strengthening and Endurance (13-17 Weeks)**	• Full ROM • Normal patellar mobility • Progressive strengthening • Flexibility: 2-joint hip flexors and posterior chain • Cross-training for cardiovascular endurance • Elliptical used after performing good 6-inch FSU

PHASE IV
Functional Return to Sport (18-25 Weeks)
	• Understand demands of sport
	• Low impact: cardiovascular endurance training
	• High impact
	  • Plyometric progression (bilateral → unilateral)
	  • Running progression
	• Testing: isokinetic testing and single-leg hop test (>85% limb symmetry)

AAROM, active-assistive range of motion; *CKC,* closed kinetic chain; *FSU,* forward step-up; *NWB,* non–weight bearing; *PROM,* passive range of motion; *ROM,* range of motion; *SLS,* single-leg stance; *WBAT,* weight bearing at tolerated.

extension at 0° can be done with the knee extended and the heel on a towel roll.

Patellar Mobilization and Flexibility. Patellar mobilization should be initiated in the medial direction. Stretching of the gastrocnemius-soleus complex can be started as needed.

Quadriceps Reeducation. Initiation of quadriceps activation is a crucial part of the rehabilitative process. Submaximal activation is initiated with a towel roll under the knee for tactile feedback and minimizing fat pad irritation. Home electrical stimulation units (E-Stim) may be used to assist with reeducation and patient compliance.

Weight-Bearing Guidelines. A progressive weight bearing is used as tolerated (WBAT) with crutches and brace locked in extension for the initial 6 weeks. As the patient is able to tolerate and accept loading without pain and swelling, he or she may wean off the crutches while maintaining the knee brace locked in extension. Balance and proprioceptive double-limb exercises are initiated as weight-bearing tolerance improves later in phase 1.

Proximal and Distal Strengthening. Exercises to target hip external rotators, gluteals, and gastrocnemius-soleus are emphasized in NWB positions. To progress to phase 2, the patient must demonstrate good quadriceps contraction, maintain knee extension with SLR, achieve ROM 0° to 90°, and exhibit controlled pain and swelling.

Phase 2: Functional Gait, Range of Motion, and Strength (Weeks 7 to 12)

Gait Training. The patient is transitioned into a functional brace and remains at WBAT. Crutches are reintroduced to assist with normalization of gait. It is important to avoid hyperextension of the knee during the gait cycle. This quadriceps avoidance gait pattern may be due to quadriceps weakness, hip weakness, soft tissue tightness above or below the knee, or lack of neuromuscular control. It is important to identify and treat the causative factors. Use of retro treadmill (see Fig. 18-10) walking focuses on eccentric quadriceps control and loading to allow for shock absorption.

Range of Motion Progression. Patients need to maintain 0° knee extension and progress flexion toward 110° by postoperative week 8. When 85° to 90° of knee flexion is achieved, a short crank (90-mm) cycle can be used. Advancement toward full knee flexion occurs from postoperative weeks 8 to 12. ROM at 115° or greater allows for progression of standard upright cycling. Patellar mobilization continues and the patient can be educated in techniques to complete independently at home.

Strengthening and Balance Training. CKC is used for progression of functional exercises. Exercises should focus on gluteals, core musculature, quadriceps, and gastrocnemius-soleus. Activities include (but are not limited to) leg press, calf raises and step-up progression. The focus should be on quality of movement and maintaining proper alignment during dynamic movement. Progression from bilateral to unilateral balance along with additional challenges of surface changes or perturbations can be used to challenge the patient.

Flexibility. Reassessment is necessary to maintain balance between flexibility and strength. Flexibility allows for proper alignment and avoids compensatory mechanisms and increased loading forces on the patellofemoral joint during functional movements. To progress safely to phase 3, functional ROM, normal gait, and controlled pelvic and knee stability in single-leg stance should be achieved.

Phase 3: Advanced Strengthening and Endurance (Weeks 13 to 17). The PTA should monitor the patient to ensure that he or she is maintaining full ROM and patellar mobility, so as to build strength successfully during this phase. Flexibility focuses on two-joint hip flexors and the posterior chain. Static stretching and foam rolling are two ways to work on flexibility daily. Strengthening progresses to activities including eccentric leg press and squatting and step-down progressions. The use of resistance bands with loading activities such as retro walking and sidestepping, can assist in facilitating dynamic balance. Cross-training is also important to assist in cardiovascular endurance. Patients should demonstrate a good 6-inch forward step-up before advancing to using the elliptical trainer.

Phase 4: Functional Return to Sport (Weeks 18 to 25). The PT and PTA should understand the demands of the sport in which the patient will return to participation. If activity is low impact, focus should be placed on cardiovascular training. If the activity is higher level, involving running, cutting, and jumping, maintaining a strict strengthening program and integration of plyometrics is important to reintegrate the patient safely. Double-limb plyometrics are initiated before advancing to single-leg bounding and jumping. The patient should be able to maintain stability, alignment, and symmetry throughout the kinetic chain. During these activities, progression to running can be initiated. When initiating running, the PTA should increase running time gradually. Deceleration drills and change-of-direction drills can be implemented to advance and prepare the patient for the demands of his or her sport.

Testing for strength and criteria for return to sports include isokinetic testing and single-leg hop tests. Patients should display greater than 85% limb symmetry for safe reintegration to high-demand sports.

Distal Realignment

The distal realignment procedure is an osteotomy of the tibial tubercle with transfer of the tubercle medially, anteriorly, anteromedially, or distally. The tibial tubercle is fixated with two cortical bone screws. Complications can be due to fixation, fracture, wound healing, and deep vein thrombosis.[43] Lateral retinacular release is commonly performed in conjunction with this procedure. See Table 18-7 for distal realignment guidelines.

Important Concepts

A distal realignment is an osteotomy of the tibial tubercle with transfer of the tubercle medially, anteriorly, anteromedially, or distally.

Phase 1: Respect Healing, Range of Motion, and Weight Bearing (0 to 6 Weeks). ROM should be focused on 0° to 60° for the first 2 weeks and progressed to 0° to 90° by week 6. Short crank ergometry can be used as 85° to 90° of flexion is achieved.

Time frames for the phases are longer because of weight-bearing progression and risk of fracture. Patients are NWB for 6 weeks with the brace locked at 0° of extension. At a 6-week postoperative follow-up appointment with the surgeon, an x-ray is taken to check for bony healing. Should sufficient healing be demonstrated, weight bearing is progressed to WBAT with crutches.

Phase 2: Functional Gait, Range of Motion, and Strength (7 to 14 Weeks). Until postoperative week 8, ambulation is completed with the brace locked at 0° knee extension. Gait training with an assistive device then takes place without the brace to focus on a normal heel-to-toe gait pattern. Use of aquatic therapy to focus on gait training and progression offloading is advised. Retrograde ambulation can also be used for gait training as ground reaction forces are absorbed by calf muscles.

ROM is progressed at week 8 to flexion of 120°. A standard upright bicycle for motion can be used at this time. Progressive resistive exercises are performed in NWB positions as the patient is gradually increasing load during this time. Use of band, ankle weights, and machines is beneficial for progressive loading and strengthening.

Phase 3: Advanced Strengthening and Endurance (15 to 22 Weeks) and Phase 4: Functional Return

TABLE 18-7 Distal Realignment

PHASE I
Respect Healing, ROM, Weight Bearing (0-6 Weeks)
	• Cryotherapy: reduce inflammation and joint effusion
	• ROM parameters: AAROM/PROM
	  • 0° → 60° (0-2 weeks)
	  • 0° → 90° (by 6 weeks)
	  • Short crank: 0° → 80°
	• Quadriceps reeducation: home E-Stim unit
	• Patellar mobility: cephalad direction
	• Flexibility: hamstring, gastrocnemius-soleus
	• Proximal and distal strengthening: NWB
	• Weight bearing: NWB (0-6 weeks) with brace locked in 0° extension
	• X-ray to check bony healing → WBAT with crutches

Criteria for Advancement	• Radiographic evidence of adequate healing • Good quadriceps activation • Good patellar mobility • AAROM/PROM 0° → 90°

PHASE II
Functional Gait, ROM, Strength (7-14 weeks)
	• Weight bearing: focus on normalization 8 weeks with brace locked in 0° extension
	• Crutches needed without brace for ambulation
	• ROM parameters: (AAROM/PROM)
	  • 0° → 120° (8 weeks)
	  • Standard upright bicycle used
	• Patellar mobility: cephalad and medially
	• Quadriceps strengthening
	  • Isometric
	  • Leg press: bilateral (monitor arc)
	  • OKC: knee extension (monitor arc)
	  • FSU progression
	• Flexibility: AROM knee flexion with hip extension
	• Advanced proximal strengthening: CKC
	• Balance and proprioception
	  • Bilaterally → unilaterally
	  • Change surfaces for challenge

Criteria for Advancement	• Normal gait • Ability to support and control knee in SLS • Ability to perform 8-inch FSU • Good postural alignment with SLS

PHASE III
Advanced Strengthening and Endurance (15-22 Weeks)
	• ROM: maintain extension
	  • Progress to full flexion (wall slides)
	• Normalize gait
	• Quadriceps strengthening
	  • FSU progression
	  • Eccentric leg press
	  • FSD progression
	  • Squat progression
	• Advanced proximal strengthening: functional activities
	• Balance: SLS → dynamic activities
	• Cross-training: elliptical machine, bicycle, stair climber

Criteria for Advancement	• ROM WNL • Normalized gait • Controlled knee in dynamic SLS • Descend 8-inch step: good control and alignment
PHASE IV **Functional Return to Sport (36-44 Weeks)**	• Understand demands of sport • Maintain functional strengthening and balance program • Plyometric progression • Initiate running program • Cutting and deceleration drills • Monitor volume and symptom provocation • Testing: isokinetic testing and single-leg hop test (>85% limb symmetry)

AAROM, active-assistive range of motion; *AROM*, active range of motion; *CKC*, closed kinetic chain; *FSU*, forward step-up; *NWB*, non–weight bearing; *OKC*, open kinetic chain; *PROM*, passive range of motion; *ROM*, range of motion; *SLS*, single-leg stance; *WBAT*, weight bearing at tolerated; *WNL*, within normal limits.

to Sport (36 to 44 Weeks). A functional strengthening phase should remain in place for a minimum of 8 weeks. Because of risk of fracture, progression to higher level activities is dependent on surgeon clearance. Return to sport can be expected 9 to 12 months after surgery.

KNEE FRACTURES

PATELLAR FRACTURES

Patellar fractures represent 1% of all skeletal injuries and are most prevalent among adults 20 to 50 years old.[23] Two major mechanisms of injury are direct or indirect trauma to the knee. In the case of direct trauma, the patella may be fractured by a direct blow during the fall onto the knee or when the knee hits the dashboard in the motor vehicle accident. Direct trauma often produces comminuted or stellate fracture with little displacement of fragments and may produce chondral injury to the distal femur or patella owing to the proximity of the patella with the posterior part of the distal femur. Indirect trauma results from excessive tension through the extensor mechanism, such as an abrupt quadriceps contraction or an unexpected quick flexion of the knee against a fully contracted quadriceps. This indirect mechanism of injury usually causes an avulsion of the inferior or superior pole of the patella or a transverse fracture (Fig. 18-34).

Patients with patellar fracture present with pain, swelling, and tenderness at the knee; there may be a palpable defect in the patella as well. Inability of the patient to extend the knee fully usually indicates an associated injury to the extensor mechanism. Patients report a feeling of instability in the knee while attempting to walk.[23] Patellar fractures are mostly classified as either undisplaced or displaced and by their morphologic fracture pattern as stellate, comminuted, transverse, vertical, polar, or osteochondral type.

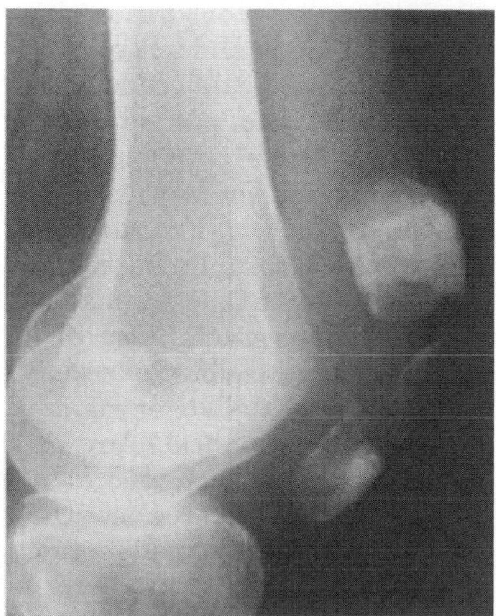

FIG 18-34 Transverse patellar fracture with displacement. *(From Eiff MP, Hatch RL, Calmbach WL:* Fracture management for primary care, *ed 2, Philadelphia, 2003, Saunders.)*

Nonoperative Management

Indications for nonoperative management of patellar fractures are based on fragment displacement of less than 3 mm or less than 2 mm of articular incongruity in which extensor mechanism remains intact.[19] Other relative indications for nonoperative management include patients with medical conditions in which anesthesia would be contraindicated or patients with severe osteopenia in which stable internal fixation would be impossible. Pritchett[160] reported on a series of 18 patients with significant medical comorbidities who presented with patellar fracture with greater than 1 cm of displacement. At 2-year follow-up, 12 patients reported satisfactory outcomes with nonoperative management, which included knee immobilization with splint and early full weight bearing. Braun and associates[25] reported on a larger series of 40 nonoperatively managed patellar fractures with intact extensor mechanism and less than 1 mm of fracture displacement. Nonoperative management consisted of long-leg splinting with PWB and physical therapy. At an average follow-up of 30.5 months, 80% of patients reported no pain with ADL, and 90% had full ROM. According to these reports, good to excellent results can be expected with nonoperative management of minimally displaced fractures with intact extensor mechanism. In general, rehabilitation management of patellar fractures largely depends on physical examination and physician recommendations for progression of weight bearing. Typically, the treatment of choice for nondisplaced patellar fractures is WBAT using a knee immobilizer or hinged brace locked at 0° of extension.

Important Concepts

Nonoperative management can be expected to have good to excellent results for minimally displaced patellar fractures.

The rehabilitation plan for each patient should be individualized and follow a criteria-based progression rather than following strict protocols. In the acute phase of rehabilitation, the use of modalities such as cryotherapy becomes important to reduce edema and quadriceps inhibition and modulate pain. It has been reported that 10 mL of fluid in the knee can induce quadriceps inhibition.[214] Isometric quadriceps exercises are initiated. Electrical stimulation can be used if the patient cannot produce a voluntary quadriceps contraction (Fig. 18-35). It is essential to educate the patient that the prescribed exercises should be performed without any pain to progress to more advanced exercises. SLR is started with the brace locked in extension. When the patient can demonstrate a pain-free SLR without a quadriceps lag, he or she can progress to SLR without the brace. The patient should be educated on a home exercise program emphasizing the importance of maintaining full extension at the knee. Prolonged stretching into knee extension with a towel under the ankle can assist in preventing a knee flexion contracture. Additional early exercises include gluteal isometrics, ankle plantar flexion isotonic exercises with elastic tubing, and

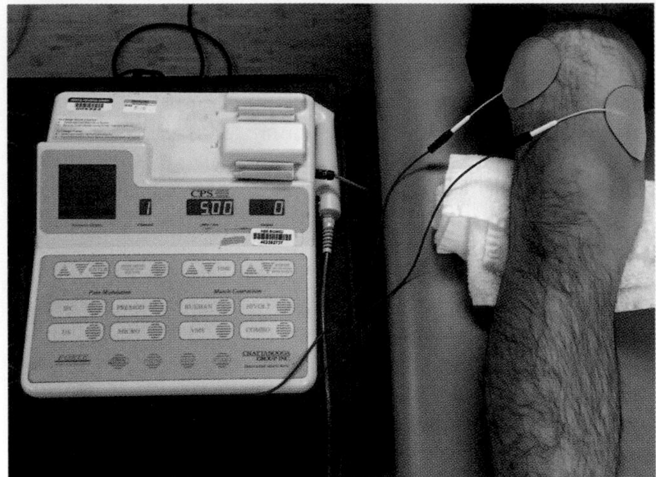

FIG 18-35 Electrical stimulation to facilitate quadriceps contraction.

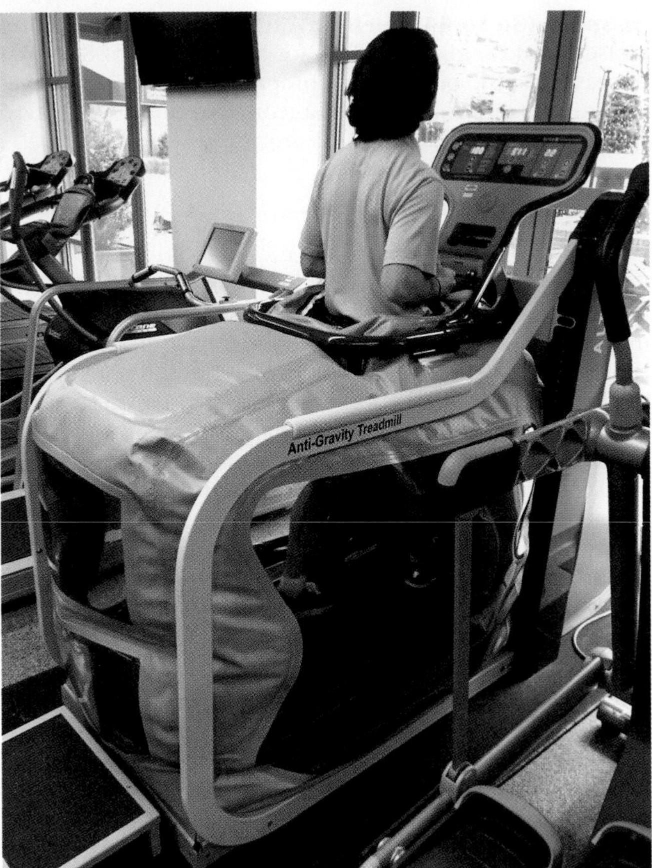

FIG 18-36 Gait training with decreased weight bearing using the AlterG® Anti-Gravity Treadmill® (AlterG® Inc, Fremont, CA).

gastrocnemius stretching in long sit position. Patient education should also emphasize the use of cryotherapy at home. On radiographic evidence of healing, AAROM of the knee is initiated with the patient using the contralateral leg for support. At this stage, the PT or PTA can begin gentle patellar glides to prevent knee stiffness.

As the patient demonstrates adequate quadriceps strength by performing SLR without a lag, the patient's knee brace can be unlocked for ambulation with crutches. Crutches should be used until the patient can demonstrate a normal gait cycle. The knee brace can be discontinued on physician recommendation. If available, the use an underwater treadmill or an AlterG® Anti-Gravity Treadmill® (Fig. 18-36) during this period can assist in facilitating a normal gait. A short crank stationary bicycle can be used to facilitate knee ROM when the patient can demonstrate 85° of knee flexion without pain. As the patient progresses to 110° of knee flexion, a standard stationary bicycle can be used.

When achieving 120° of knee flexion, a leg press machine can be introduced to facilitate lower extremity strengthening. At approximately 6 weeks, if the patient has achieved full ROM, isometric quadriceps exercise at 45° to 60° of knee flexion can be initiated.[108] A graduated forward step-up program can be initiated. The patient can be progressed to more advanced exercises such as OKC isotonic knee extension exercise inside a pain-free, crepitus-free arc of motion and forward step-downs.

Proprioception exercises can be initiated with bilateral standing on an unstable surface and progressing to unilateral balance activities. If available, a commercial balance system such as the Biodex Balance System SD (Fig. 18-37) can be used for improving the patient's balance. As the patient follows a criteria-based progression, it is important to monitor s signs and symptoms, especially anterior knee pain with weight-bearing exercises such as a step-up or step-down. At approximately 3 months, the patient can start with a running progression program as long as the following criteria are met: full AROM and adequate strength demonstrated by being able to perform an 8-inch step-down without compensatory patterns. For an athlete, sport-specific and plyometric activities can be gradually introduced to prepare for a safe return to the sport. The PTA needs to educate the patient on adequate rest days between strength training and plyometric training days to avoid overuse injuries.

Before an athlete can return to his or her sport, the following criteria should be met: a functional hop test greater than an 85% limb symmetry, an isokinetic test demonstrating less than 10% quadriceps and hamstring deficits, and a lack of apprehension with sport-specific movements. A qualitative screening of functional movement should also demonstrate symmetry with the contralateral extremity.

Operative Management

Disruption of the extensor mechanism with loss of active knee extension is the most common indication for surgery.[131] Patellar fractures with greater than 3 mm of fragment displacement or greater than 2 mm of articular incongruity are indications for surgical management.[19] Additional surgical considerations include intraarticular loose bodies and osteochondral fracture. The preferred surgical intervention for most patellar fractures is open reduction with internal fixation. Regardless of the choice of surgical intervention, the goal is to achieve a stable fixation with restoration of normal anatomy and restoration of functional extensor mechanism.[131] At the present time, the most common method of fixation is the tension band wiring technique which uses longitudinal Kirschner wires and stainless steel wire that is looped in a figure-of-eight pattern over the anterior patella (Fig. 18-38). The purpose of the tension band wire fixation is to function as a stress-sharing device that converts tensile forces generated by the quadriceps muscle as it contracts and pulls on the patella into compressive forces at the fracture site of the patella as the wire tightens.[19,108]

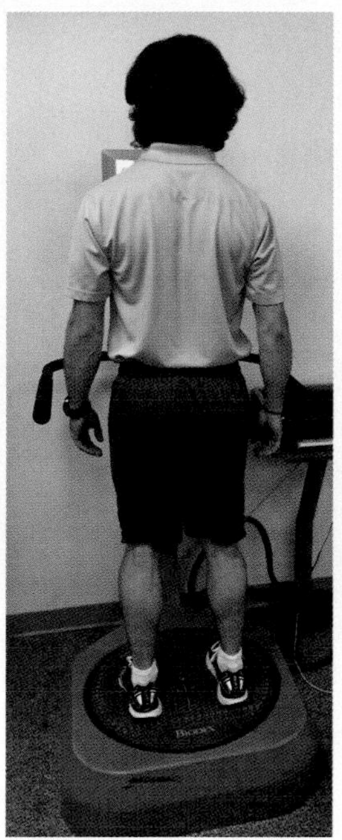

FIG 18-37 Proprioception training with visual feedback using the Biodex Balance System SD (Biodex Medical Systems Inc, Shirley, NY).

Postoperative Rehabilitation

During the progression of the patient's rehabilitation, it is essential to consider physiologic healing after surgery as well as having the patient meet certain criteria before advancing to the next stage of rehabilitation. Within the first week, patient can start with gentle AAROM of the knee using the contralateral leg for support. Depending on surgeon's guidelines, a CPM machine can used within a certain ROM set by the surgeon. WBAT is allowed on crutches with a knee immobilizer or hinged knee brace locked at 0° extension for 4 to 6 weeks. As mentioned in the previous section on nonoperative management, distal ankle ROM and gluteal isometrics can be initiated. At the end of 4 weeks, the patient can start with quadriceps isometric exercises and progress to SLR. The rehabilitation program is progressed in a similar fashion as described in the previous section.

SUPRACONDYLAR FEMUR FRACTURES

Supracondylar femur fractures are relatively uncommon, accounting for about 6% of all femur fractures.[147] This type of injury occurs in young adults usually as a result of high-energy trauma and in elderly adults as a result of minor falls. Especially in cases of high-energy trauma, disruption of vascular structures or other associated injuries can occur with this type of fracture. Supracondylar fractures are

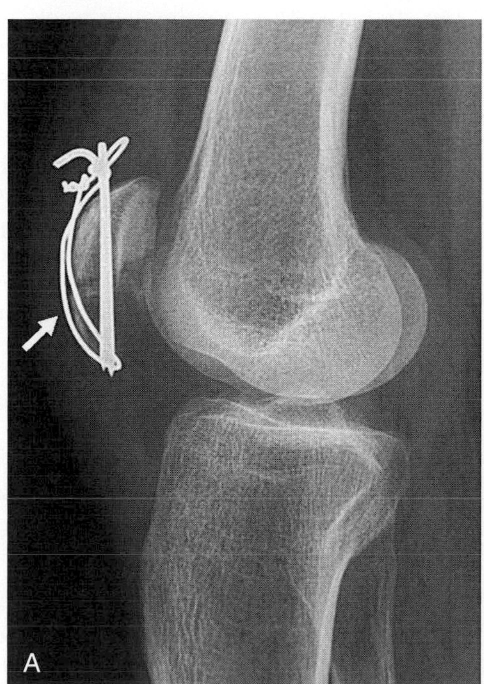

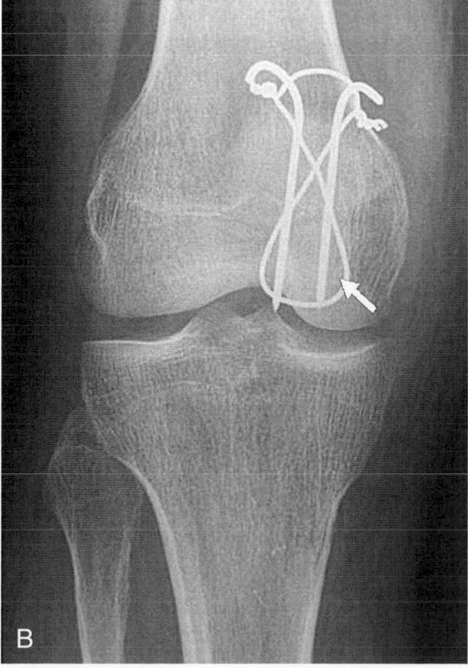

FIG 18-38 **A** and **B,** Tension band wiring fixation using Kirschner wires for transverse patellar fracture. The tension band tightens to prevent fragment separation as the quadriceps muscle attempts to distract the fracture fragments. *(From Stanton I, White LM, Satchithananda K, et al: The postoperative patellofemoral joint: expected radiological appearances and complications,* Curr Probl Diagn Radiol *35[2]:55-64, 2006.)*

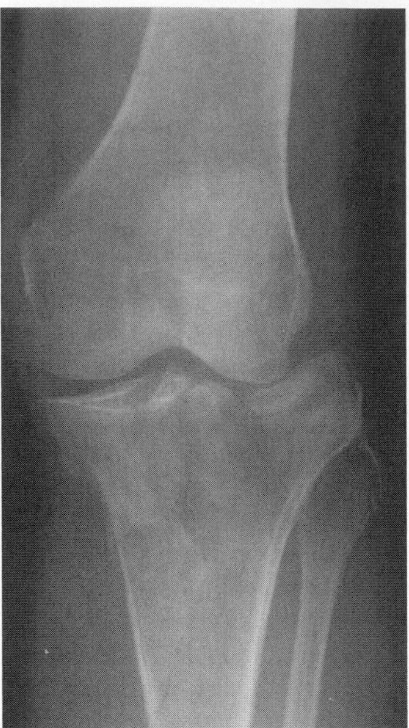

FIG 18-39 Type C (bicondylar) tibial plateau fracture. *(From Mills WJ, Nork SE: Open reduction and internal fixation of high-energy tibial plateau fractures,* Orthop Clin North Am *33[1]:177-198, 2002.)*

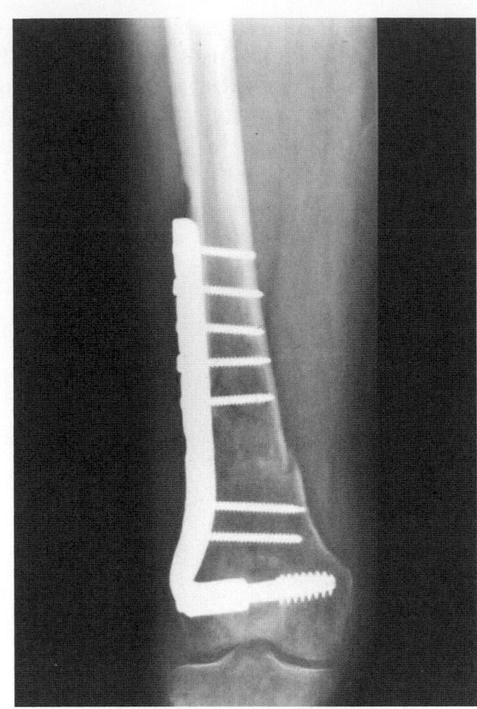

FIG 18-40 Supracondylar fracture of distal femur treated with locking plate with screws. *(From Scott WN:* Insall & Scott surgery of the knee, *ed 5, Philadelphia, 2012, Churchill Livingstone.)*

classified by Müller's AO classification system, which is widely accepted and useful in determining treatment and prognosis. This system classifies fractures into extraarticular (type A), unicondylar (type B), and bicondylar (type C). Each type A through C contains subtypes 1 through 3, and as the number increases, the severity of the fracture increases.[109] A series of radiographs is usually obtained to determine the fracture AO classification based on pattern and location of the fracture (Fig. 18-39).

Nonoperative Management

Nonoperative management is indicated for incomplete or nondisplaced fractures. Also, nonoperative treatment is indicated for elderly patients who present with stable impacted fractures and have medical comorbidities such as severe osteopenia.

Typically, nondisplaced fractures are placed in a hinge brace with PWB. In cases of displaced supracondylar femur fractures in which surgery is contraindicated, skeletal traction for 6 to 12 weeks is followed by a period of bracing. Complications associated with nonoperative treatment include knee stiffness, varus alignment, and internal rotation deformity.[109]

Operative Management

Open reduction and internal fixation is the most common method of treatment for displaced supracondylar femur fractures (Fig. 18-40). Regardless of fixation device, stability is essential for early knee mobilization and prevention of knee stiffness.

Postoperative Rehabilitation

Postoperatively, the patient is NWB for ambulation with crutches for 12 weeks.[147] Within the first week, the patient can start AAROM at the knee from 0° to 60° and gradually progress to 90°. PROM by the PT or PTA should be avoided. Distal ROM at the ankle is encouraged to prevent stiffness, and gluteal isometric exercises are prescribed to maintain hip strength. At approximately week 2, the patient can start with quadriceps isometrics progressing to SLRs in multiple planes as tolerated. Within 4 to 8 weeks, a radiograph should show signs of fracture stability by callus formation. The patient can then progress from AAROM to AROM beyond 90°. Distal flexibility at the ankle is maintained with gastrocnemius stretching.

At 12 to 16 weeks, following radiographic evidence of fracture stability, a weight-bearing progression is initiated: TTWB to WBAT. Crutches are discontinued on demonstration of a normal gait pattern. Stengthening and proprioceptive training are progressed in a similar fashion as decribed earlier. Typically, patients are not permitted to participate in sports or repetitive high-load activities such as running for the first 6 months after surgery. Patients should be educated on modifiying their activity and performing low-impact exercises such as stationary cycling or swimming to maintain their fitness.

TIBIAL PLATEAU FRACTURES

Tibial plateau fractures are common in high-impact sports such as downhill skiing or soccer.[111] Also, these fractures often occur in motor vehicle accidents as a result of high-energy trauma. Typically, tibial plateau fractures occur as a result of varus or valgus forces in combination with axial loading. This type of fracture involves the metaphysis of the tibia and the articular surface. Tibial plateau fractures were classified by Schatzker into types I through VI with ascending number representing increase in the level of severity.[48] Usually, younger individuals with strong metaphyseal bone sustain a type I fracture, whereas elderly individuals with poor bone quality are more likely to sustain a more complex fracture.

Nonoperative Management

Nonsurgical treatment is recommended for fractures without displacement or minimal displacement. Displaced lateral tibial plateau fractures with varus or valgus instability not exceeding 10° at any point in the arc of knee motion are considered stable without the need for surgical management.[110] In addition, patients with severely comminuted fractures or patients who have contraindications for surgery can be managed nonsurgically. Patients are placed in an hinged knee orthosis locked in extension with NWB ambulation on the affected extremity. Depending on fracture stability on diagnostic imaging, AAROM from 0° to 60° within the first week can be initiated and increased to 90° of knee flexion after the first week. PROM or valgus/varus stresses to the knee should be avoided during ROM exercises. Isometric gluteal exercises and gentle active ankle motion can start within the first week. At week 2, the patient can begin isometric quadriceps exercise as long as he or she has no pain at the fracture site. The goal is to achieve 90° of knee flexion by 4 weeks after the injury.[147] The PTA should communicate any delay in ROM to the PT and referring physician.

Within the first couple of weeks, patient education should emphasize the importance of cryotherapy and adherence to ROM exercises and NWB status on the injured leg. Within 6 to 8 weeks, based on radiographic examination of fracture healing, the patient can be progressed to PWB. Full weight bearing is allowed at 12 weeks. At 10 to 12 weeks, the patient progresses to gentle resistive quadriceps exercises such as bilateral leg press and knee extension isometric exercises at 60° of knee flexion. A strengthening and return to activity progression as descibed earlier is followed monitoring patient symptoms during exercise and activities.

Operative Management

Open reduction with internal fixation is indicated for fractures with displacement or greater than 3 mm of articular depression. Other indications are fractures with greater than 10° of varus or valgus instability, posterior wedge fractures, fractures associated with trapped menisci, and fractures involving the medial plateau.[110] The goal of surgical management is stabilization and reduction of the fracture and restoration of articular surface and repair or reposition of the meniscus. Choice of surgical fixation largely depends on the type and location of fracture and any other associated injuries to the knee. Usually, surgical technique requires bone graft for restoration of the underlying metaphyseal bone and placement of a buttress plate with screws to maintain the reduction (Fig. 18-41).[110]

Postoperative Rehabilitation

Early AAROM can begin within 1 to 2 weeks after surgery from 0° to 40° of flexion with progression to 90° of knee flexion within the first 2 weeks.[48] A stationary short crank bicycle can be used for ROM gains with later progession to a standard crank bicycle when the patient achieves 110° of knee flexion. PROM to the knee by the PT or PTA is typically avoided for the first 8 weeks. As mentioned in the section on nonoperative management, cryotherapy and patient education regarding NWB status are important elements in the early phase of rehabilitation.

For ambulation, patients are NWB for 6 to 8 weeks and progressed to PWB in a hinged brace locked in extension.

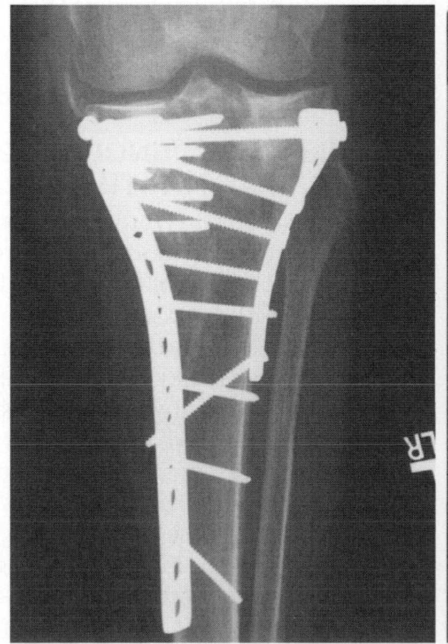

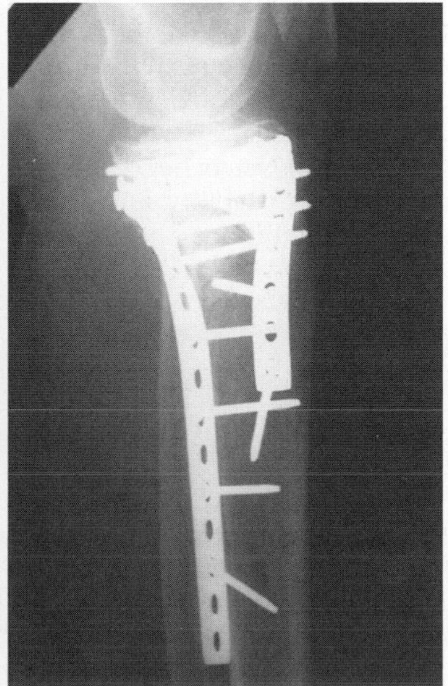

FIG 18-41 Tibial plateau fracture with buttress plate and screw fixation. *(From Mills WJ, Nork SE: Open reduction and internal fixation of high-energy tibial plateau fractures,* Orthop Clin North Am *33[1]:177-198, 2002.)*

Typically, the fracture line begins to disappear on radiographs secondary to callus formation, which can facilitate the surgeon's decision for the patient to start weight bearing. Strengthening exercises follow the progression as indicated in nonoperative management, starting with quadriceps isometric, ankle isotonic, and distal ROM exercises. As the patient progresses to PWB, CKC exercises such as bilateral leg press within 0° to 60° are permitted. Proprioception exercises are initiated as the patient begins weight bearing on an unstable surface.

When the patient becomes full weight bearing at approximately 12 weeks and is weaned off the assistive device, a similar strengthening and return to activity progression as described earlier is followed. The PTA should monitor the patient for any signs or symptoms in the knee during weight-bearing exercises. At 6 months to 1 year, the patient can progress to low-impact sports activities. Kraus and colleagues[111] surveyed 89 consecutive patients with surgical fixation of tibial plateau fracture and found that 88.8% engaged in sports at the time of injury. At 1 year postoperatively, only 62.9% returned to sport activities. At 4 years postoperatively, 73% of patients had returned to low-impact sports, but not at their preinjury sports activity. It is important for the PTA to educate patients on activity modification as they return to participation in sports.

HIGH TIBIAL OSTEOTOMY

High tibial osteotomy (HTO) is an effective surgical method for patients younger than 60 years with symptomatic medial compartment knee arthrosis associated with a varus knee alignment.[215] In the presence of less common lateral compartment arthritis, varus-producing HTO or varus-producing distal femoral osteotomy may be performed. The goal of valgus-producing HTO is to unload an arthritic medial compartment by creating a wedge to redistribute the compressive loads more evenly across the joint. HTO is the preferred treatment of choice for a more active individual who would otherwise be restricted from certain sports participation after a TKA procedure. However, long-term studies indicate that HTO postpones a TKA for only about 7 to 10 years.[215] Osteochondritis dissecans, osteonecrosis, posterolateral instability, and chondral resurfacing are other knee conditions that can be managed by HTO.

Important Concepts

HTO is used to unload an arthritic medial compartment by creating a wedge to redistribute compressive loads more evenly across the joint.

TTWB is premitted early postoperatively with the brace locked in extension for 4 weeks.[145] Within the first couple of days after surgery, the patient can start quadriceps isometric and active ankle exercises and progress to SLR when tolerated. Use of modalities such as cryotherapy and electrical stimulation becomes important in the early postoperative phase to decrease edema and facilitate quadriceps activation, respectively. Knee AAROM can start immediately and progress from 0° to 110°. Passive extension and patellar mobilization are emphasized. The patient should gradually achieve 135° of knee flexion by 4 weeks. At 6 weeks, weight bearing is progressed to PWB (50%) if radiographs show evidence of healing at the osteotomy site. As the patient demonstrates good quadriceps strength, the knee brace can be unlocked for ambulation. At 8 weeks postoperatively, the patient is permitted full weight bearing without an assitive device when a normal gait is demonstrated. At this stage, strengthening and proprioceptive training follow a similar progression as mentioned earlier in this section. However, the progression to running is typically started around 6 months postoperatively.[145] Routinely, return to sport activity occurs between 9 and 12 months postoperatively.

TOTAL KNEE ARTHROPLASTY

According to the Healthcare Costs and Utilization Project, more than 687,000 TKAs are performed each year in the United States.[9] The primary disease conditions leading to TKA are osteoarthritis and rheumatoid arthritis. Osteoarthritis is a common condition that affects the U.S. population. According to the Centers for Disease Control and Prevention, by 2030, 67 million (25%) adults 18 years old or older, with women more prevalent than men, will have been given a diagnosis of arthritis by a physician. An estimated 37% (25 million) of adults with arthritis will report limitation in daily functional activities because of arthritis by 2030. Daily functional activities are described as grasping, reaching, sitting, carrying, stairs, pushing, walking, standing stooping, and bending. Statistics from the Centers for Disease Control and Prevention indicate 8 million people with arthritis are limited in daily functional activities reporting severe limitations in ability to stoop, bend, or kneel, and 6 million cannot walk ¼ mile. It is predicted that over the next few decades the number of TKA surgeries will increase exponentially because of the aging population and increased demands. This situation represents a big socioeconomic burden that costs the United States approximately $128 billion annually.[41,42]

CAUSES, INCIDENCE, AND RISK FACTORS OF KNEE ARTHRITIS

Several risk factors categorized as general or modifiable causes increase the incidence of osteoarthritis in people. The biggest modifiable risk factor for the development and progression of osteoarthritis is obesity. Obesity continues to increase in the United States at a rapid rate. Obese adults are four times more likely to develop knee osteoarthritis than normal-weight adults.[9,41] Approximately 35% of adults with osteoarthritis diagnosed by a physician are obese compared with only 21% of adults without arthritis.[41,42] Being overweight increases the risk of osteoarthritis in the knee because of extra weight on the joints, which causes more wear and tear leading to destruction and loss of cartilage and resulting in osteoarthritis. Cartilage is flexible connective tissue found in many areas in the body including the joints between bones. It cushions bones at the joints and allows bones to glide over one another. If the cartilage breaks down and wears away, the bones rub together as occurs with osteoarthritis. This rubbing causes pain, swelling, and stiffness. Bony spurs or extra bone may form around the joint. The ligaments and muscles around the joint become weaker and stiffer. Patients with osteoarthritis experience the following impairments: decreased knee ROM, pain, swelling, decreased knee strength (especially quadriceps), decreased balance, decreased proprioception, and gait deviations.[92,93]

The general causes of osteoarthritis are the normal aging process, which tends to be hereditary, and fractures and other joint injuries including injuries to the cartilage and ligaments. Jobs that involve kneeling or squatting for more than an hour a day put one at the highest risk, and jobs that involve lifting, climbing stairs, or walking also put one at risk. Playing sports that involve direct impact on the joint (e.g., football), twisting (e.g., basketball or soccer), or throwing also increase the risk of arthritis. Bleeding disorders such as hemophilia and avascular necrosis and other types of arthritis, such as chronic gout, pseudogout, or rheumatoid arthritis, can also increase the risk of osteoarthritis.[22,92,93,163]

SURGICAL OVERVIEW

The indication for TKA is to relieve pain associated with osteoarthritis. People who have failed conservative approaches, such as the use of nonsteroidal antiinflammatory drugs, injections, activity modification, use of an assistive device to unload the joint, and physical therapy, are good candidates for TKA.[126] Osteoarthritis is diagnosed by a physician based on radiographs showing decreased joint space within the knee. Clinical impairments are considered loss of knee ROM, poor quadriceps strength, and antalgic gait, which lead to functional impairments of poor negotiation of steps and difficulty with squatting and kneeling and performing ADLs. Contraindications for TKA are active infection, incompetent extensor mechanism, compromised vascularity, recurvatum deformity secondary to muscle weakness, neurologic disruption affecting muscles of the knee, and a painless well-functioning arthrodesis.[126]

Surgical techniques and design for TKAs have improved and advanced over the years. Implants are smaller, lighter, more dynamic, and gender-specific. The entire knee can be replaced or a part of the knee, such as the lateral side, medial side, or patella. High flexible prostheses and minimally invasive surgery are among the most current technologic advances in TKA. Standard TKA designs allow for bicondylar surface replacement, with either a posterior cruciate–retaining or a posterior cruciate–substituting design.[97] Other prosthetic designs are either constrained or semiconstrained providing varying degrees of freedom and different levels of stability.[29] Most commonly, titanium alloy is used for the tibial and femoral components, and the tibial tray and patellar button are made of polyethylene (Fig. 18-42).

For joint exposure, a midline or parapatellar incision is made. The knee extensor mechanism is cut with tendon release. Osteotomies of the proximal tibia, distal femur, anterior and posterior aspect of the femoral condyles, and retropatellar surface are performed.[119] Usually the ACL is resected to provide joint exposure. The PCL is resected if the surgeon prefers a posterior cruciate–substituting design or if degenerative osteophytes have caused damage. The medial and lateral ligaments are preserved. To achieve optimal varus or valgus alignment, the anatomic positions of the lateral and medial ligaments may be surgically altered. If a knee flexion contracture is found, posterior osteophytes may be removed and the capsule released.[82] The soft tissue is balanced, and a trial reduction is performed; stability and alignment are checked in knee flexion and extension.[97,119] When the optimal alignment is achieved, the implant is cemented with methyl methacrylate to fixate the implant. Cemented prostheses have proven to have a higher survival rate over 10 to 12 years of follow-up. Depending on the facility, local femoral or saphenous nerve blocks can be used. Epidural anesthesia is commonly used. Pain is controlled by a patient-controlled analgesia pump via an epidural catheter and oral medication.[161] The most common surgical complications after TKA are infection, loosening of hardware, knee instability, and high international normalized ratio (international normalized ratio values can range from 2.0 to 4.0 based on the surgeon's preference).[24,161]

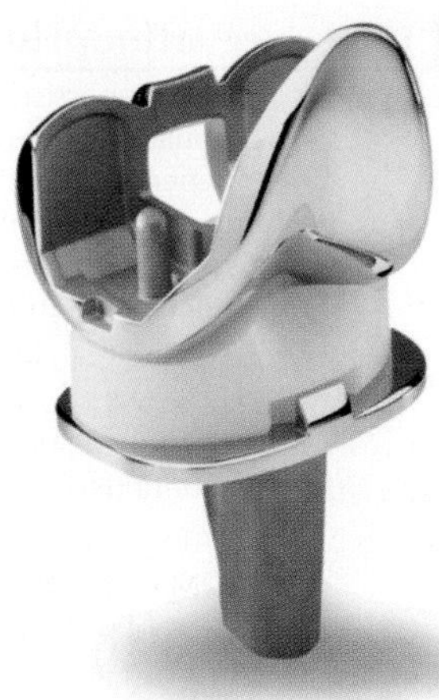

FIG 18-42 Zimmer NextGen LPS-Flex Mobile and LPS Mobile Bearing Knees (Zimmer Inc, Warsaw, IN).

REHABILITATION

Preoperative rehabilitation is an imperative part of patient success and outcomes after TKA. Preoperative measurements and function are strong predictors of postoperative TKA outcomes. The progressive nature of osteoarthritis leads to quadriceps inhibition and atrophy. It has been observed that there is a 20% weakness of the quadriceps and hamstrings in patients with osteoarthritis of the knee.[130] Preoperative rehabilitation interventions should strive to optimize ROM, strength, and flexibility.

The goals of rehabilitation after TKA are to maximize ROM, relieve pain, restore soft tissue balance, maximize strength, normalize gait, restore proprioception and balance, and maximize function. It is essential to educate the patient before surgery on appropriate exercises, activity modification, use of modalities (cryotherapy), proper use of an assistive device to help normalize gait and to unload the affected knee, and psychosocial support. The

TABLE 18-8 Total Knee Arthroplasty Rehabilitation Guidelines: Acute Phase (Postoperative Day 1 to Week 2)

GOALS	• Transfer unassisted
	• Ambulate with appropriate device on level surfaces and negotiate stairs unassisted
	• Independent with home exercises
	• Improve AROM/AAROM
	  • Active flexion ≥80° (sitting)
	  • Active extension <10° (supine)

NOTES	• Avoid prolonged sitting, standing, and walking • Pain should not increase with exercises or walking • Monitor swelling • Discontinue CPM when 90° knee flexion achieved over consecutive days
ACUTE PHASE	• WBAT • PROM knee extension with towel roll under heel (10-15 minutes, 4-6 times a day) • Use of CPM POD 1 from −5° knee extension → 60° knee flexion to increase as tolerated (4-6 hours daily) • Transfer training • Gait training with assistive device, WBAT with Jordan brace for safety to prevent knee from buckling (femoral nerve blocks decrease quadriceps activation) • Cryotherapy • NMES for use with quadriceps weakness to elicit contraction of muscles • Quadriceps sets • Hamstring isometrics • Ankle pumps • Gluteal sets • AROM knee flexion/extension • Calf/hamstring stretch • Stair stretch

AAROM, active-assistive range of motion; *AROM,* active range of motion; *CPM,* continuous passive motion; *NMES,* neuromuscular electrical stimulation; *POD,* postoperative day; *PROM,* passive range of motion; *WBAT,* weight bearing as tolerated

patient should be instructed in an individualized home exercise program. The program should address ROM, muscle strengthening, stretching, gait corrections, balance, proprioception training, and cardiovascular exercises for endurance. The patient's expectations and goals should be considered when developing a postoperative rehabilitation program.

Certain precautions should be taken during the rehabilitation phases after TKA. Patients are usually prescribed anticoagulants such as warfarin (Coumadin) to prevent blood clots. The PTA should also observe for increased drainage from the incision site and notify the surgeon accordingly. If the patient had epidural analgesia or a femoral nerve block, it is important that the patient's sensation and motor control be reassessed daily. This assessment is particularly vital in the first 24 to 48 hours after surgery because deficits can affect the patient's functional performance and objective measures.[24,32,161]

Acute Phase (Postoperative Day 1 to Week 2)

The goals of rehabilitation initially following TKA are to decrease pain and swelling, improve knee ROM of flexion/extension as well as patellar mobility, perform safe unassisted transfers, improve ambulation with an appropriate assistive device, restore function, and achieve independence in a home exercise program (Table 18-8). It is important not to overstress the new prosthesis or overdo exercises. Prolonged sitting, standing, and walking should be avoided. During this phase, it is important to initiate exercises such as quadriceps, hamstring, and gluteal isometrics; ankle pumps; supine heel slides (Fig. 18-43); and seated knee AAROM flexion/extension (Fig. 18-44).

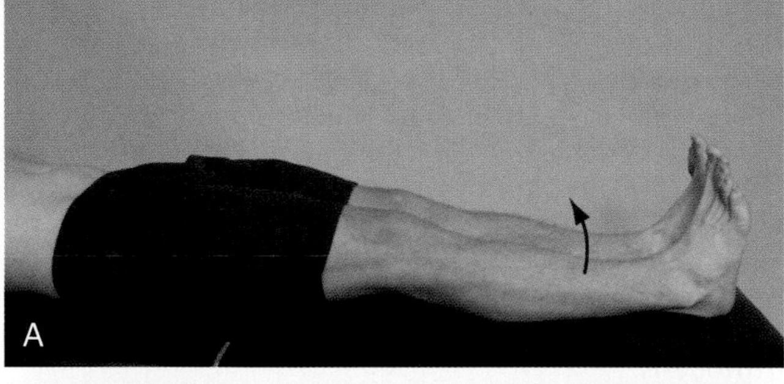

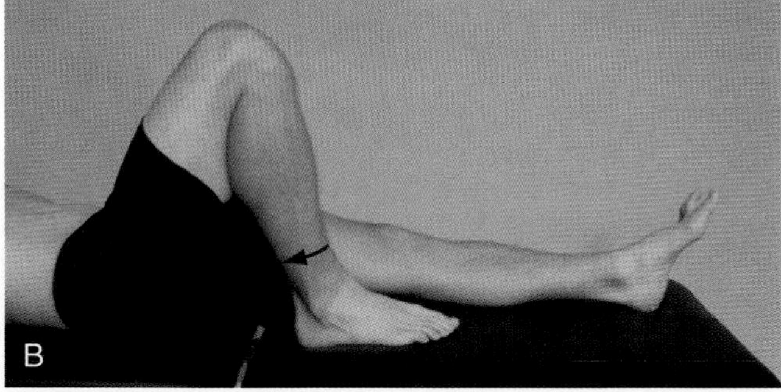

FIG 18-43 Supine heel slides to increase knee flexion and extension ROM. **A,** Extension. **B,** Flexion. *(From Magee DJ, Sueki D:* Orthopedic physical assessment atlas and video, *St Louis, 2011, Saunders.)*

If adequate quadriceps strength (no quadriceps lag) is demonstrated, active assisted SLRs are introduced. If there is diminished quadriceps activation, neuromuscular electrical stimulation can be used to help facilitate quadriceps contraction.[156] A towel roll can be used under the ankle of

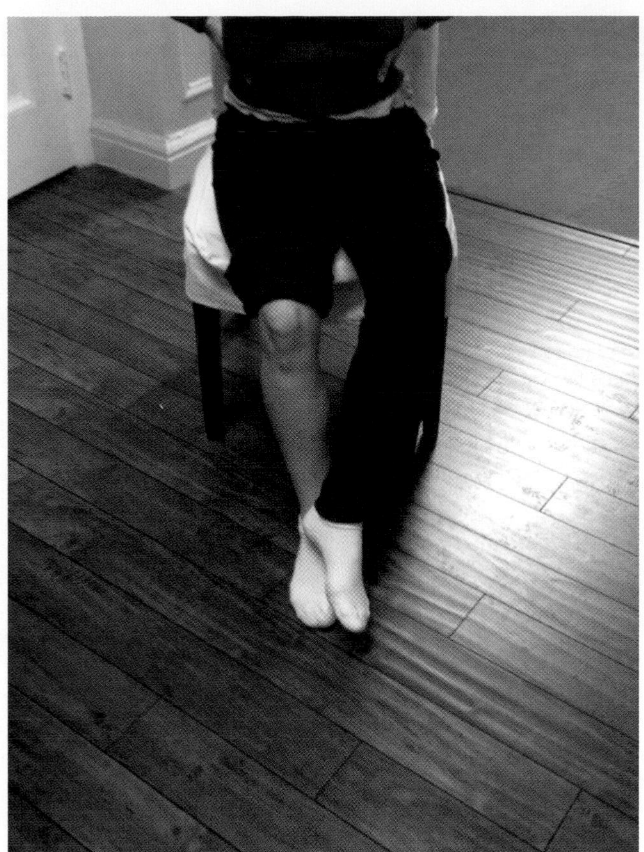

FIG 18-44 Seated active-assisted knee flexion and extension to increase knee ROM.

the involved leg to promote passive knee extension. It is important to ensure there is no increase in pain or swelling as exercises are initiated and progressed.

To improve ROM, a CPM machine may be used. The available ROM of the CPM machine is gradually progressed as tolerated by the patient. There should not be any increased pain or swelling with use. The CPM is used until 90° of knee flexion has been consistently maintained over consecutive days or until the patient is discharged from the hospital. The use of a CPM machine helps facilitate knee ROM postoperatively, but there is no statistically significant difference between use of a CPM machine versus physical therapy exercises alone.[17,113] Cryotherapy should be used to control pain and swelling.

Postoperative Phase 2 (Weeks 2 to 8)

The second phase of rehabilitation after TKA continues to focus on increasing ROM, decreasing swelling, improving strength, improving gait and ambulation, promoting independence in functional activities, and performing the home exercise program independently (Table 18-9). It is important at this time to maximize knee ROM to prevent arthrofibrosis. As ROM and strength improve, swelling should decrease. Patellar mobility is incorporated at this point using superior and inferior glides and lateral medial tilts to restore patellar motion. On achieving 90° of knee flexion, a short crank (90-mm) bicycle can be used to facilitate gains in ROM, overall conditioning, and lower extremity strength.[171]

Gastrocnemius muscle stretching during this phase is incorporated to promote knee extension. Therapeutic exercises to strengthen the involved extremity include OKC exercises such as SLR in multiple planes, proximal hip strengthening (hip abduction, adduction, flexion, and extension) using a multiaxial hip machine, and core stability exercises. CKC exercises include leg press with bilateral lower extremities and wall squats with a therapeutic ball behind the back (short arc angle) (Fig. 18-45). When full extension is achieved, standing terminal knee extension can be used with a TheraBand behind the involved knee for resistance. A progressive step-up program (2-, 4-, and 6-inch step) (Fig. 18-46) is introduced when improved quadriceps strength and ROM greater than 83° of knee flexion is demonstrated.[114] The PTA should continue to focus on normalizing gait with or without an assistive device. Using a treadmill for retro walking helps improve gait, knee extension, balance, and weight bearing to bilateral lower extremities.[44] To improve balance and proprioception, the PTA can incorporate bilateral progressing to unilateral lower extremity balance activities, with devices such as wobble boards and the Biodex Balance System. Hydrotherapy can be therapeutic by unloading the knee joint and improving strength, ROM, and gait.

The PTA can use functional testing to obtain objective data on progress of balance and postural control. Examples include the **Timed Up and Go (TUG) test** (Fig. 18-47)[157] and the 6 Minute Walk Test (6MWT).[140] The TUG test measures the time to rise from an arm chair, walk 3 m, turn around, and return to sitting in the same chair without physical assistance. The minimal detectable change for the TUG test 1.5 months after TKA is 2.49 seconds.[106] The 6MWT measures the total distance walked by an individual over 6 minutes. The minimal detectable change associated with the 90% confidence interval for the 6MWT is 6.34 m in patients 1.5 months after TKA.[106]

Postoperative Phase 3 (Weeks 9 to 16)

The PTA should continue to focus on knee ROM and lower extremity strengthening (Table 18-10). At least 125° of knee flexion is expected for a full recovery. The knee requires 93° of flexion for stair sitting and 106° to tie shoes.[114] Achieving functional strength, especially of the quadriceps, hamstrings, gluteals, and core musculature, is an expected goal during this phase. Adequate quadriceps strength and knee ROM is required to ascend and descend 6- to 8-inch steps using a reciprocal gait pattern and to transfer from a sit to stand from a standardized height surface without difficulty. A normalized reciprocal gait with symmetric weight bearing and heel to toe off pattern should be established. The patient continues to perform advanced functional activities such as squatting and ascending and descending 6- to 8-inch steps in a functional progression (see Figs. 18-5 and 18-6). A quadriceps stretching program can be used to help achieve optimal knee ROM. Strengthening and balance exercises are progressed from bilateral to unilateral.

Balance and proprioception exercises can be progressed from static to dynamic bilateral exercises to more advanced

TABLE 18-9 Postoperative Total Knee Arthroplasty Rehabilitation: Phase 2 (Weeks 2 to 8)

GOALS	• Knee flexion ROM >105°, extension 0° • Minimize swelling • Ascend 4-inch step • Independent home exercise program • Normalize gait with/without assistive device
NOTES	• Avoid ambulation with antalgic gait • Avoid pain • Avoid prolonged sitting/standing • Avoid negotiating stairs until strength and ROM achieved • Activity modification
POSTOPERATIVE TKA REHABILITATION PHASE 2 (WEEKS 2-8)	• AAROM: heel slides, wall slides, seated assisted knee flexion/extension • Short crank bicycle (90 mm): knee flexion ROM must be 90° • Regular bicycle if ≥110° of knee flexion ROM • Patellar mobilization • Cryotherapy • NMES: improve quadriceps activation • Core stability/strengthening exercises • SLR: all planes • Bridges: TheraBand/ball • Clamshells with TheraBand • Leg press/wall slides with ball • FSU: 2- to 4-inch • Multiaxial hip machine • Standing hip abduction/extension with TheraBand • Terminal knee extension • Balance/proprioception training: unilateral stance, bilateral dynamic activities • Gait training with/without assistive device: heel strike to toe off, symmetric weight bearing on bilateral lower extremities, underwater treadmill to help unload joint and normalize gait (Aquaciser)

AAROM, active-assisted range of motion; *FSU,* forward step-up; *NMES,* neuromuscular electrical stimulation; *ROM,* range of motion; *SLR,* straight leg raise; *TKA,* total knee arthroplasty.

unilateral static and dynamic exercises. The PTA should monitor any reports of pain and swelling with any of these exercises. The functional tests performed during phase 3 can be readministered during this phase to document improvement objectively. According to Newton,[141] a TUG score of 15 seconds or less signified an independent level of function in older adults. The use of a hydrotherapy program decreases weight-bearing forces on the affected limb based on the water level.[85] The higher the water, the more it reduces the weight-bearing forces. The hydrotherapy program can be progressed initially from exercises in chest-height water to waist-height water to challenge the patient. The use of the pool allows implementation of more advanced exercises with less risk of swelling and pain based on the buoyancy of the water.

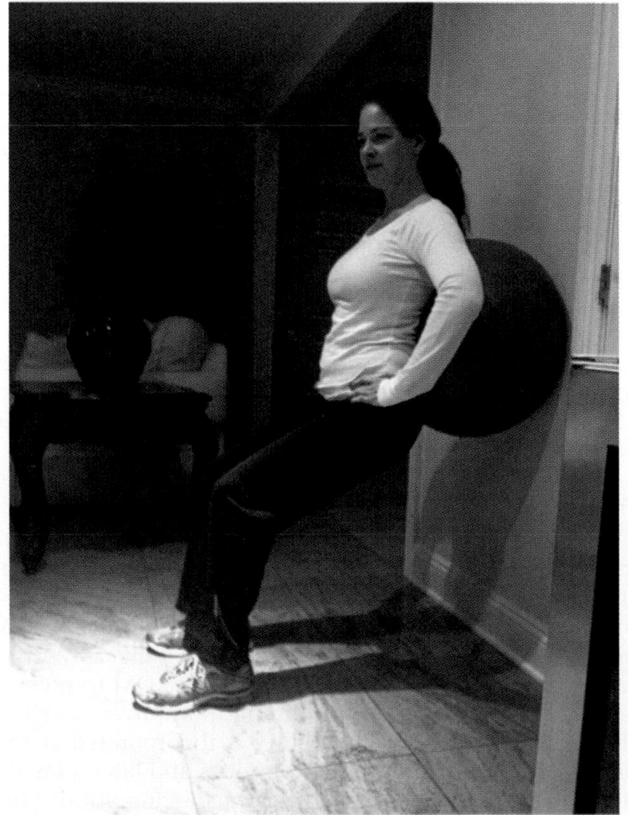

FIG 18-45 CKC wall squat with therapeutic ball behind the back in a short arc angle to improve quadriceps strength.

Postoperative Phase 4 (16 Weeks to Return to Sport)

It is important to note the athletic activity level of the patient before surgery. Patients who newly participate in sporting activities after joint replacement put themselves at higher risk for injury. Return to athletic or higher demand activity is based on surgeon approval. Criteria to return the patient safely back to athletic activity include patient education, implant fixation, high-demand versus low-demand activities, and the SAID (specific adaptations to impose demands) principle. A functional progression of exercises should continue to be followed in this

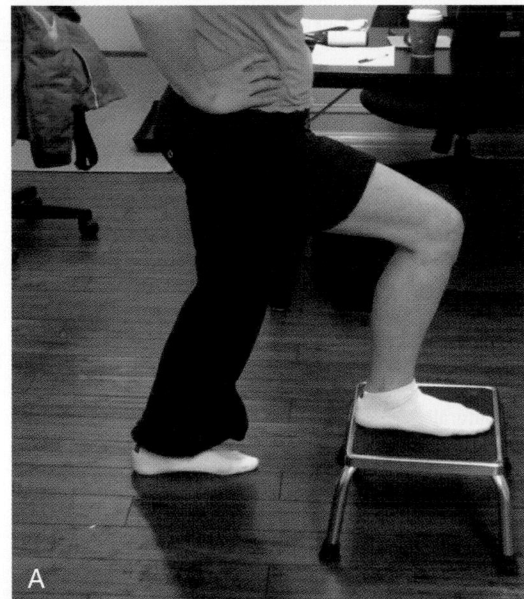

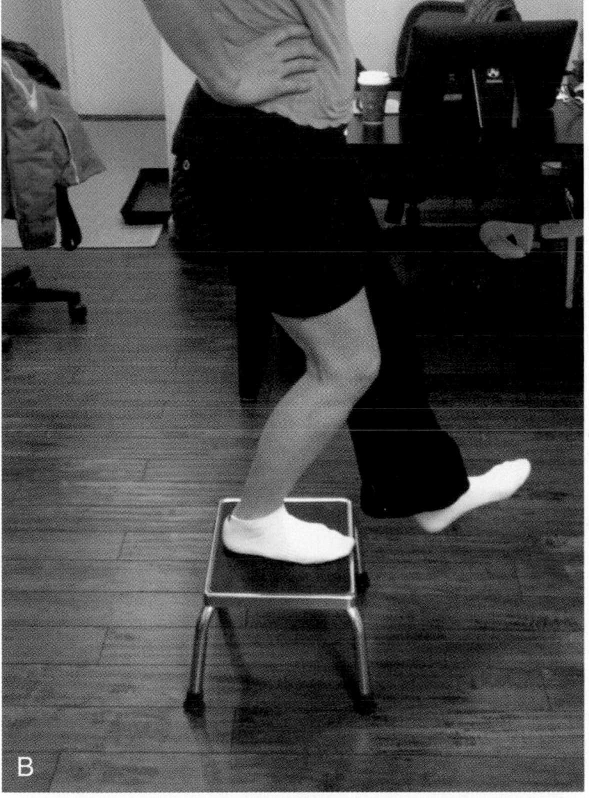

FIG 18-46 Progressive step-up/step-down program using an 8-inch step to improve strength of quadriceps. **A,** The patient steps up onto the step with the involved leg. **B,** The patient slowly steps down with the uninvolved leg leading with the heel and controlling the motion with the involved lower extremity.

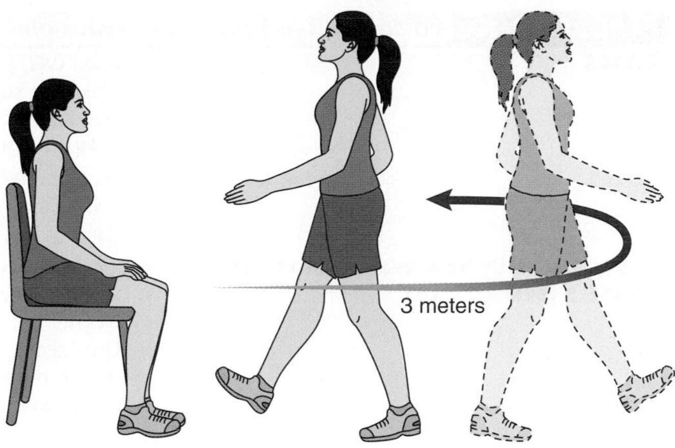

FIG 18-47 TUG test. The patient arises from a standard arm chair, walks 3 m, turns around, and returns to sitting in the same chair without assistance.

advanced stage of rehabilitation (Table 18-11). This progression entails strengthening exercises progressing from bilateral to unilateral lower extremity activities such as squats and leg press. Adequate eccentric strength and single-leg stability should be demonstrated (e.g., demonstration of the ability to descend an 8-inch step without pain with good lower extremity control). Balance exercises are progressed to unilateral on unstable surfaces. An example is single-leg stance on foam at cable column performing scapular retraction with a single-leg squat. The patient should not have any pain or apprehension with sport-specific activity. Adequate warmup and cool down periods should be implemented. Cardiovascular training can be addressed for endurance. Limb symmetry can be measured to identify deficits. The use of a commercial balance device can measure single-leg balance. Isokinetic testing can be used to measure quadriceps and hamstring strength. Meeting the adequate criteria of the surgeon can result in discharge from physical therapy and return to athletic activity.

Popular sports such as golf and tennis can be resumed. Precautions need to be addressed when returning to play. For golf, caution should be used with rotational forces when the patient swings a club and getting in and out of bunkers. Care should be taken on wet grounds to reduce risk of falls. For tennis, caution should be used when accelerating and decelerating on the court. Care should be taken with rotational movements at ball contact because excessive rotational or axial forces can high load the implant. It is important that the patient is aware of the effects of excessive wear and tear on the prosthetic implant. Patients who participate in athletic activity after joint replacement are at increased risk for prosthetic loosening, instability and dislocations, and periprosthetic fracture.[24] Healy and colleagues[86] reviewed the orthopedic literature and surveyed members of the Hip Society and Knee Society for their recommendations on return to athletic activity after TKA. The 1999 Knee Society survey rated athletic activities they allowed after TKA as "with experience," "no opinion," or "not recommended." Athletic activities allowed after TKA included stationary bicycling, low-impact aerobics, bowling, golfing, dancing, horseback riding, croquet, walking, and swimming. Activities allowed with experience included cross country skiing, doubles tennis, hiking, and road bicycling.

TABLE 18-10 Postoperative Total Knee Arthroplasty Rehabilitation Phase 3 (Weeks 9 to 16)

GOALS	• ROM WFL (>115°) • Maximize strength quadriceps, hamstrings, core • Negotiating steps: FSU 6- and 8-inch steps; FSD 4-, 6-, and 8-inch steps • Independent with ADL
NOTES	• Avoid swelling • Avoid pain • No running, jumping unless physician approval
POSTOPERATIVE TKA REHABILITATION PHASE 3 (WEEKS 9-16)	• Patellar mobilization • Soft tissue scar mobilization • Bicycle • Quadriceps stretching • Hamstring stretching • Leg press eccentric progression to unilateral • Bridges on ball: bilateral/unilateral • Core stabilizing/strengthening exercises • Hip PREs • Ball/wall squats with medicine ball • FSU 6- and 8-inch steps • FSD 4-, 6-, and 8-inch steps • Retro treadmill on incline • Balance/proprioception: from bilateral lower extremity to unilateral lower extremity

ADL, activities of daily living; *FSD,* forward step-down; *FSU,* forward step-up; *PRE,* progressive resistive exercise; *ROM,* range of motion; *TKA,* total knee arthroplasty; *WFL,* within functional limits.

TABLE 18-11 Postoperative Total Knee Arthroplasty Rehabilitation Phase 4 (Weeks ≥16)

GOALS	• ROM WFL (>115°) • Full-strength quadriceps, hamstrings, core • Negotiating steps: FSU 6- and 8-inch steps, FSD 6- and 8-inch steps • Good mechanics for sport-specific activities
NOTES	• Avoid swelling • Avoid pain • No running, jumping unless physician approval
POSTOPERATIVE TKA REHABILITATION PHASE 4 (WEEKS 9 TO ≥16)	• Bicycle/elliptical • Quadriceps stretching • Hamstring stretching • Leg press eccentric/unilateral • Bridges on ball unilateral • Core stabilizing/strengthening exercises (planks 60 seconds) • Hip PREs • FSU 6- and 8-inch steps • FSD 6- and 8-inch steps • Balance/proprioception: from bilateral lower extremity to unilateral lower extremity on unstable surface • Sport-specific training

FSD, forward step-down; *FSU,* forward step-up; *PRE,* progressive resistive exercise; *ROM,* range of motion; *TKA,* total knee arthroplasty; *WFL,* within functional limits.

GLOSSARY

Active quadriceps drawer test: A test that assesses the integrity of the posterior cruciate ligament.

Closed kinetic chain (CKC) exercises: In the lower extremity, physical exercises performed where the foot is relatively fixed, which results in simultaneous movement of all other joints.

Lachman test: A test that assesses the amount of anterior tibial translation and the quality of the endpoint; universally recognized as the most specific test in assessing the integrity of the ACL.

Modified Thomas test: A test that assesses general lower extremity flexibility of hip flexors and quadriceps length.

Osteochondral allograft: One of several types of cartilage transplant procedures used in the treatment of individuals with symptomatic, disabling cartilage injury or disease.

Thessaly test: A dynamic reproduction of load transmission in the knee joint, performed at 5° and 20° of flexion.

Timed Up and Go (TUG) test: A test that is used to assess a person's mobility; measures the time to rise from an arm chair, walk 3 m, turn around, and return to sitting in the same chair without physical assistance.

REFERENCES

1. Ahmed AM, Burke DL: In-vitro measurement of static pressure distribution in synovial joints—Part I: Tibial surface of the knee. *J Biomech Eng* 105(3):216–225, 1983.
2. Akeson WH, Woo SL-Y, Amiel D: The connective tissue response to immobilization: biomechanical changes in periarticular connective tissue of the immobilized rabbit knee. *Clin Orthop* 93:356–362, 1973.
3. Allen PR, Denham RA, Swan AV: Late degenerative changes after meniscectomy. Factors affecting the knee after operation. *J Bone Joint Surg Br* 66(5):666–671, 1984.
4. Amis AA, Firer P, Mountney J, et al: Anatomy and biomechanics of the medial patellofemoral ligament. *Knee* 10(3):215–220, 2003.
5. Apley AG: The diagnosis of meniscus injuries. *J Bone Joint Surg* 29:78–84, 1947.
6. Arnoczky SP, Warren RF: Microvasculature of the human meniscus. *Am J Sports Med* 10(2):90–95, 1982.
7. Bach BR, Jr: Graft selection for posterior cruciate ligament surgery. *Oper Tech Sports Med* 1:104–109, 1993.
8. Bach BR, Levy ME, Bojchuk J, et al: Single-incision endoscopic anterior cruciate ligament reconstruction using patellar tendon autograft. Minimum two-year follow-up evaluation. *Am J Sports Med* 26(1):30–40, 1998.
9. Bade MJ, Stevens-Lapsley JE: Early high-intensity rehabilitation following total knee arthroplasty improves outcomes. *J Orthop Sports Phys Ther* 41:932–941, 2011.
10. Baldon RD, Serrao FV, Silva RS, et al: Effects of functional stabilization training on pain, function, and lower extremity biomechanics in women with patellofemoral pain: a randomized clinical trial. *J Orthop Sports Phys Ther* 44(4):240–249, 2014.
11. Barber FA: Accelerated rehabilitation for meniscus repairs. *Arthroscopy* 10:206–210, 1994.
12. Barber SD, Noyes FR, Mangine RE, et al: Quantitative assessment of functional limitations in normal and anterior cruciate ligament deficient knees. *Clin Orthop* 255:204–214, 1990.
13. Barber-Westin SD, Noyes FR: The effect of rehabilitation and return to activity on anterior-posterior knee displacements after anterior cruciate ligament reconstruction. *Am J Sports Med* 21(2):264–270, 1993.
14. Barber-Westin SD, Noyes FR, Heckmann TP, et al: The effect of exercise and rehabilitation on anterior-posterior knee displacements after anterior cruciate ligament reconstruction. *Am J Sports Med* 27(1):84–93, 1999.
15. Barton CJ, Lack S, Malliaras P, et al: Gluteal muscle activity and patellofemoral pain syndrome: a systematic review. *Br J Sports Med* 47:207–214, 2013.
16. Bates A, Hanson N: The principles and properties of water. In *Aquatic Exercise Therapy*, Philadelphia, 1996, Saunders.
17. Beaupre LA, Davies DM, Jones CA, et al: Exercise combined with continuous passive motion or slide board therapy compared with exercise only: a randomized controlled trial of patients following total knee arthroplasty. *Phys Ther* 81:1029–1037, 2001.
18. Beck C, Drez D, Young J, et al: Instrumented testing of functional knee braces. *Am J Sports Med* 14:253–256, 1986.
19. Bedi A, Karunakar MA: Patella fractures and extensor mechanism injuries. In Rockwood CA, Bucholz RW, Court-Brown CM, et al, editors: *Rockwood and Green's fractures in adults*, vol 2, ed 7, Philadelphia, 2010, Lippincott Williams & Wilkins.
20. Bell DG, Jacobs I: Electro-mechanical response times and rate of force development in males and females. *Med Sci Sports Exerc* 18:31–36, 1986.
21. Beynnon BD, Fleming BC, Johnson RJ, et al: Anterior cruciate ligament strain behavior during rehabilitation exercises in vivo. *Am J Sports Med* 23(1):24–34, 1995.
22. Bijlsma JW, Berenbaum F, Lafeber FP: Osteoarthritis: an update with relevance for clinical practice. *Lancet* 377:2115–2126, 2011.
23. Bostorm A: Fracture of the patella. A study of 422 patellar fractures. *Acta Orthop Scand Suppl* 143:1–80, 1972.
24. Brander V, Stulberg SD: Rehabilitation after hip and knee replacement an experience and evidence based approach to care. *Am J Phys Med Rehabil* 85:S98–S118, 2006.
25. Braun W, Wiedemann M, Rutter A, et al: Indications and results of nonoperative treatment of patellar fractures. *Clin Orthop Relat Res* 289:197–201, 1993.
26. Buckwalter JA: Effects of early motion on healing musculoskeletal tissues. *Hand Clin* 12:13–24, 1996.
27. Buckwalter JA, Mankin HJ: Articular cartilage I: tissue design and chondrocyte-matrix interactions. *J Bone Joint Surg Am* 79(4):600–611, 1997.
28. Bugbee WD, Convery FR: Osteochondral allograft transplantation. *Clin Sports Med* 18(1):67–75, 1999.
29. Burke D, O'Flynn H: Primary total knee arthroplasty. In Chapman M, editor: *Chapman's orthopedic surgery*, Philadelphia, 2001, Lippincott Williams & Wilkins.
30. Buss DD, Min R, Skyhar M, et al: Nonoperative treatment of acute anterior cruciate ligament injuries in a selected group of patients. *Am J Sports Med* 23(2):160–165, 1995.
31. Butler DL, Noyes FR, Grood ES: Ligamentous restraints to anterior-posterior drawer in the human knee. A biomechanical study. *J Bone Joint Surg Am* 62(2):259–270, 1980.
32. Cahill JB, Kosman LM: Total knee arthroplasty. In Cioppa-Mosca J, Cahill JB, Cavanaugh JT, et al, editors: *Postsurgical rehabilitation guidelines for the orthopedic clinician*, St Louis, 2006, Mosby, pp 17–28.
33. Callaway GH, Nicholas SJ, Cavanaugh JT, et al: Hamstring augmentation versus patella tendon reconstruction of acute anterior cruciate ligament disruption: a randomized prospective study. Presented at: Annual meeting of the American Academy of Orthopaedic Surgeons, New Orleans, LA, February 1994.
34. Caraffa A, Cerulli G, Proietti M, et al: Prevention of anterior cruciate ligament injuries in soccer: a prospective controlled study of proprioceptive training. *Knee Surg Sports Traumatol Arthrosc* 4(1):19–21, 1995.
35. Cavanaugh JT: Rehabilitation following meniscal surgery. In Engle RP, editor: *Knee ligament rehabilitation*, New York, 1991, Churchill Livingstone, pp 59–69.
36. Cavanaugh JT: Posterior cruciate ligament reconstruction. In Cioppa-Mosca J, Cahill JB, Cavanaugh JT, et al, editors: *Postsurgical rehabilitation guidelines for the orthopedic clinician*, St Louis, 2006, Mosby, pp 439–452.
37. Cavanaugh JT: Rehabilitation strategies following articular cartilage surgery in the knee. In Williams RJ, editor: *Strategies in cartilage repair*, Totowa, NJ, 2007, Humana Press, pp 341–369.
38. Cavanaugh JT: Meniscal rehabilitation. In Manske RC, editor: *Current concepts in evaluation, examination and rehabilitation of the knee*, Indianapolis, IN, 2011, Sports Physical Therapy Association.
39. Cavanaugh JT, Moy RJ: Balance and postoperative lower extremity joint reconstruction. *Orthop Phys Ther Clin North Am* 11(1):75–99, 2002.
40. Cavanaugh JT: Sgaglione NA. Rehabilitation after articular cartilage repair: chondroplasty, abrasion arthroplasty, microfracture. In Manske R, editor: *Rehabilitation for the post surgical sports patient: knee and shoulder*, St Louis, 2006, Mosby, pp 365–382.
41. Centers for Disease Control and Prevention: Prevalence of disabilities and associated health conditions—United States, 1991-1992. *MMWR Morb Mortal Wkly Rep* 43:730–739, 1994.
42. Cheng YJ, Hootman M, Murphy LB, et al: Prevalence of doctor-diagnosed arthritis and arthritis-attributable activity limitation—United States, 2007-2009. *MMWR Morb Mortal Wkly Rep* 59(39):1261–1265, 2010.
43. Chiaia T, Cronin T: Proximal and distal realignment. In Cioppa-Mosca J, Cahill JB, Cavanaugh JT, editors: *Postsurgical rehabilitation guidelines for the orthopedic clinician*, St. Louis, 2006, Mosby, pp 407–424.
44. Cipriani D, Armstrong CW, Gaul S: Backward walking at three levels of treadmill inclination: an electromyographic and kinematic analysis. *J Orthop Sports Phys Ther* 22(3):95–102, 1995.
45. Clancy WG, Jr: Repair and reconstruction of the posterior cruciate ligament. In Chapman MW, editor: *Operative orthopaedics*, Philadelphia, 1988, Lippincott, pp 1651–1666.
46. Clancy WG, Narechania RG, Rosenberg TD, et al: Anterior and posterior cruciate ligament reconstructions in rhesus monkeys. *J Bone Joint Surg Am* 63:1270–1284, 1981.

47. Cole BJ, Carter TR, Rodeo SA: Allograft meniscal transplantation: background, technique and results. *J Bone Joint Surg Am* 84(7):1236–1250, 2002.
48. Cole P, Levy B, Watson T, et al: Tibial plateau fractures. In Browner BD, Jupiter JB, Krettek C, et al, editors: *Skeletal trauma*, Philadelphia, 2009, Saunders, pp 2276–2277.
49. Cooper DE, Arnoczky SP, Warren RF: Meniscal repair. *Clin Sports Med* 10(3):529–548, 1991.
50. Corrigan JP, Cashman WF, Brady MP: Proprioception in the cruciate deficient knee. *J Bone Joint Surg Br* 74:247–250, 1992.
51. Cross MJ, Powell JF: Long-term follow-up of posterior cruciate ligament rupture: a study of 116 cases. *Am J Sports Med* 12:292–297, 1984.
52. Crossley K, Bennell K, Green S, et al: A systematic review of physical interventions for patellofemoral pain syndrome. *Clin J Sport Med* 11:103–110, 2001.
53. Daniel DM, Malcolm L, Stone ML, et al: Quantification of knee stability and function. *Contemp Orthop* 5:83–91, 1982.
54. Daniel DM, Stone ML, Barnett P, et al: Use of the quadriceps active test to diagnose posterior cruciate-ligament disruption and measure posterior laxity of the knee. *J Bone Joint Surg Am* 70(3):386–391, 1988.
55. DeHaven KE: Injuries to the menisci of the knee. In Nicholas JA, Hershmann EB, editors: *The lower extremity and spine in sports medicine*, St Louis, 1986, Mosby, p 905.
56. DeHaven KE, Lohrer WA, Lovelock JE: Long term results of open meniscal repair. *Am J Sports Med* 23:524–530, 1995.
57. Dejour H, Walsh G, Peyrot J, et al: The natural history of rupture of the PCL. *J Orthop Surg* 2:112–120, 1988.
58. Delitto A, Rose SJ, McKowen JM: Electrical stimulation versus voluntary exercise in strengthening thigh musculature after anterior cruciate ligament reconstructive surgery. *Phys Ther* 68:660–663, 1988.
59. DiStephano LJ, Blackburn JT, Marshall SW, et al: Gluteal muscle activation during common therapeutic exercises. *J Orthop Sports Phys Ther* 39(7):532–540, 2009.
60. Dolak KL, Silkman C, McKeon JM, et al: Hip strengthening prior to functional exercises reduces pain sooner than quadriceps strengthening in females with patellofemoral pain syndrome: a randomized clinical trial. *J Orthop Sports Phys Ther* 41(8):560–571, 2011.
61. Drez DJ, DeLee J, Holden JP, et al: Anterior cruciate ligament reconstruction using bone-patella tendon-bone allografts. A biological and biomechanical evaluation in goats. *Am J Sports Med* 19:256–263, 1991.
62. Eren OT: The accuracy of joint line tenderness by physical examination in the diagnosis of meniscal tears. *Arthroscopy* 19(8): 850–854, 2003.
63. Eriksson E, Haggmark T: Comparison of isometric muscle training and electrical stimulation supplementing isometric muscle training in the recovery after major knee ligament surgery. *Am J Sports Med* 7:169–171, 1979.
64. Fairbank TJ: Knee joint changes after meniscectomy. *J Bone Joint Surg Br* 30(4):664–670, 1948.
65. Falcoiero RP, DiStefano VJ, Cook TM: Revascularization and ligamentization of autogenous anterior cruciate ligament grafts in humans. *Arthroscopy* 14(2):197–205, 1998.
66. Fanelli GC: Posterior cruciate ligament injuries in trauma patients. *Arthroscopy* 9:291–294, 1993.
67. Farrell M, Richards JG: Analysis of the reliability and validity of the kinetic communicator device. *Med Sci Sports Exerc* 18(1):44–49, 1986.
68. Ferretti A, Papandrea P, Contedica F, et al: Knee ligament injuries in volleyball players. *Am J Sports Med* 20:203–207, 1992.
69. Fetto JF, Marshall JL: Medial collateral ligament injuries of the knee: a rationale for treatment. *Clin Orthop Relat Res* 132:206–218, 1978.
70. Fithian DC, Kelly MA: Material properties and structure-function relationships in the menisci. *Clin Orthop Relat Res* 252:19–31, 1990.
71. Fitzgerald GK, Axe MJ, Snyder-Mackler L: The efficacy of perturbation training in nonoperative anterior cruciate ligament rehabilitation programs for physical active individuals. *Phys Ther* 80(2):128–140, 2000.
72. Fleming BC, Beynnon BD, Renstrom PA, et al: The strain behavior of the anterior cruciate ligament during bicycling. *Am J Sports Med* 26(1):109–118, 1998.
73. Flynn TW, Soutas-Little RW: Patellofemoral joint compressive forces in forward and backward running. *J Orthop Sports Phys Ther* 21(5):277–282, 1995.
74. Fowler PJ: Messieh SS: Isolated posterior cruciate ligament injuries in athletes. *Am J Sports Med* 15:553–557, 1987.
75. Fulkerson JP, editor: *Disorders of the patellofemoral joint*, ed 3, Baltimore, 1997, Williams & Wilkins.
76. Fulkerson JP, Hungerford D: *Disorders of the patellofemoral joint*, ed 2, Baltimore, 1990, Williams & Wilkins.
77. Galway RD, Beaupre A, MacIntosh DL: Pivot shift: a clinical sign of symptomatic anterior cruciate insufficiency. *J Bone Joint Surg Br* 54:763–764, 1972.
78. Ghosh P, Taylor TK: The knee joint meniscus. A fibrocartilage of some distinction. *Clin Orthop Relat Res* 224:52–63, 1987.
79. Gillogly SD, Voight M, Blackburn T: Treatment of articular cartilage defects of the knee with autologous chondrocyte implantation. *J Orthop Sports Phys Ther* 28:241–251, 1998.
80. Gray G: Successful strategies for closed chain testing and rehabilitation. Presented at: Chain Research Seminar, May 1989.
81. Grelsamar RP, Klein JR: The biomechanics of the patellofemoral joint. *J Orthop Sports Phys Ther* 28(5):286–298, 1998.
82. Guyton J: Arthroplasty of ankle and knee. In Canale T, editor: *Campbell's operative orthopaedics*, St Louis, 1998, Mosby, pp 232–295.
83. Hakkinen K: Force production characteristics of leg extensor, trunk flexor and extensor muscles in male and female basketball players. *J Sports Med Phys Fitness* 31:225–231, 1991.
84. Hangody L: Fules P: Autologous osteochondral mosaicplasty for the treatment of full thickness defects of weight-bearing joints: ten years of experimental and clinical experience. *J Bone Joint Surg Am* 85:25–32, 2003.
85. Harrison RA, Hilman M, Bulstrode S: Loading of the lower limb when walking partially immersed: implications for clinical practice. *Physiotherapy* 78:164, 1992.
86. Healy WL, Iorio R, Lemos MJ: Athletic activity after total knee arthroplasty. *Am J Sports Med* 29(3):377–388, 2001.
87. Hede A, Jensen DB, Blyme P, et al: Epidemiology of meniscal lesions in the knee: 1,215 open operations in Copenhagen 1982-84. *Acta Orthop Scand* 5:435–437, 1990.
88. Henning CE, Lynch MA, Glick KR: An in vivo strain gauge study of elongation of the anterior cruciate ligament. *Am J Sports Med* 13:22–26, 1985.
89. Hough AL, Webber RJ: Pathology of the meniscs. *Clin Orthop Relat Res* 252:32–40, 1990.
90. Howell GED: Clinical presentation of the knee. In Bulstrode CJK, Buckwalter J, Carr A, et al, editors: *Oxford textbook of orthopedics and trauma*, vol 2, New York, 2002, Oxford University Press, pp 1108–1113.
91. Hungerford DS, Barry M: Biomechanics of the patellofemoral joint. *Clin Orthop Relat Res* 144:9–15, 1979.
92. Hunter DJ: In the clinic: osteoarthritis. *Ann Intern Med* 147(3):ITC8-1–ITC8-16, 2007.
93. Hunter DJ, Lo GH: The management of osteoarthritis: an overview and call to appropriate conservative treatment. *Med Clin North Am* 93:127–143, 2009.
94. Huston LJ, Wojtys EM: Neuromuscular performance characteristics in elite female athletes. *Am J Sports Med* 24:427–436, 1996.
95. Indelicato PA: Nonoperative management of complete tears of the medial collateral ligament. *Orthop Rev* 18:947–952, 1989.
96. Inoue M, McGurk-Burleson E, Hollis JM, et al: Treatment of the medial collateral ligament injury. I. The importance of anterior cruciate ligament on the varus-valgus knee laxity. *Am J Sports Med* 15(1):15–21, 1987.
97. Insall JN: Surgical approaches to the knee. In Insall JN, Scott WN, editors: *Surgery of the knee*, New York, 1984, Churchill Livingstone, pp 41–54.
98. Jerosch J, Schaffer C, Prymka M: Proprioceptive abilities of surgically and conservatively treated knee joints with injuries of the cruciate ligament. *Unfallchirurg* 101(1):26–31, 1998.

99. Johansson H, Sjolander P, Soojka P: Activity in receptor afferents from the anterior cruciate ligament evokes reflex effects on fusimotor neurones. *Neurosci Res* 8:54–59, 1990.
100. Johnson RJ: The anterior cruciate ligament problem. *Clin Orthop Relat Res* 172:14–18, 1983.
101. Jorgensen U, Sonne-Holm S, Lauridsen F, Rosenklint A: Long-term follow-up of meniscectomy in athletes. A prospective longitudinal study. *J Bone Joint Surg Br* 69(1):80–83, 1987.
102. Jurist KA, Otis JC: Anteroposterior tibiofemoral displacements during isometric extension efforts. *Am J Sports Med* 13:254–258, 1985.
103. Kannus P, Bergfeld J, Jarvinen M, et al: Injuries to the posterior cruciate ligament of the knee. *Sports Med* 12(2):110–131, 1981.
104. Karachalios T, Hantes M, Zibis AH, et al: Diagnostic accuracy of a new clinical test (the Thessaly test) for early detection of meniscal tears. *J Bone Joint Surg Am* 87:955–962, 2005.
105. Kegerreis S: The construction and implementation of a functional progression as a component of athletic rehabilitation. *J Orthop Sports Phys Ther* 5:14–19, 1983.
106. Kennedy DM, Stratford PW, Wessel J, et al: Assessing stability and change of four performance measures: a longitudinal study evaluating outcome following total hip and knee arthroplasty. *BMC Musculoskeletal Disord* 6:3, 2005.
107. Komi PV, Karlsson J: Skeletal, muscle fiber types, enzyme activities and physical performance in young males and females. *Acta Physiol Scand* 103:210–218, 1978.
108. Kram DA, Hoppenfeld S, Murthy VL: Patellar fractures. In Hoppenfeld S, Murthy VL, editors: *Treatment and rehabilitation of fractures*, Philadelphia, 2000, Lippincott Williams & Wilkins, pp 334–344.
109. Kram DA, Hoppenfeld S, Murthy VL: Supracondylar femur fractures. In Hoppenfeld S, Murthy VL, editors: *Treatment and rehabilitation of fractures*, Philadelphia, 2000, Lippincott Williams & Wilkins, pp 320–331.
110. Kram DA, Murthy VL: Tibial plateau fractures. In Hoppenfeld S, Murthy VL, editors: *Treatment and rehabilitation of fractures*, Philadelphia, 2000, Lippincott Williams & Wilkins, pp 346–360.
111. Kraus TM, Martetschlager F, Muller D, et al: Return to sports activity after tibial plateau fractures. *Am J Sports Med* 20(10):1–8, 2012.
112. Kurosawa H, Fukubayashi T, Nakajima H: Load-bearing mode of the knee joint: physical behavior of the knee joint with or without menisci. *Clin Orthop Relat Res* 149:283–290, 1980.
113. Lachiewicz P: The role of continuous passive motion after total knee arthroplasty. *Clin Orthop Relat Res* 380:144–150, 2000.
114. Laubenthal KN, Schmidt GL, Kettlekamp DB: A quantitative analysis of knee motion during activities of daily living. *Phys Ther* 52:34–42, 1972.
115. Lephart SM, Kocher MS, Fu FH, et al: Proprioception following anterior cruciate ligament reconstruction. *J Sport Rehabil* 1:188–196, 1992.
116. Levy IM, Torzilli PA, Warren RF: The effect of medial meniscectomy on anterior-posterior motion of the knee. *J Bone Joint Surg Am* 64(6):883–888, 1982.
117. Lindenfeld TN, Schmitt DJ, Hendy MD, et al: Incidence of injury in indoor soccer. *Am J Sports Med* 22:364–371, 1994.
118. Lossing I, Gremby G, Johnson T: Effects of electrical muscle stimulation combined with voluntary contractions after knee ligament surgery. *Med Sci Sports Exerc* 20:2093–2098, 1988.
119. Lotke P: Primary total knees: standardized principles and techniques. In Lotke P, editor: *Knee arthroplasty*, New York, 1995, Raven Press, pp 65–92.
120. Lun VM, Wiley JP, Meeuwisse WH, et al: Effectiveness of patellar bracing for treatment of patellofemoral pain syndrome. *Clin J Sport Med* 15:235–240, 2005.
121. Lutz GE, Palmitier RA, An KN, et al: Comparison of tibiofemoral joint forces during open kinetic chain and closed kinetic chain exercises. *J Bone Joint Surg Am* 75:732–739, 1993.
122. Lyman S, Koulouvaris P, Sherman S, et al: Epidemiology of anterior cruciate ligament reconstruction: trends, readmissions, and subsequent knee surgery. *J Bone Joint Surg Am* 91:2321–2328, 2009.
123. Macnicol MF, Thomas NP: The knee after meniscectomy. *J Bone Joint Surg Br* 82:157–159, 2000.
124. Malone TR, Handaker WT, Garrett WE, et al: Relationship of sex to anterior cruciate ligament injuries in intercollegiate basketball players. *J South Orthop Assoc* 2:36–39, 1993.
125. Mankin HJ: The response of articular cartilage to mechanical injury. *J Bone Joint Surg Am* 64:460–466, 1982.
126. Martin SD, Scott RD, Thornhill TS: Current concepts of total knee arthroplasty. *J Orthop Sports Phys Ther* 28:252–261, 1998.
127. Mascal CL, Landel RL, Powers C: Management of patellofemoral pain targeting hip, pelvis, and trunk muscle function: 2 case reports. *J Orthop Sports Phys Ther* 33(11):647–660, 2003.
128. McHugh MP, Tyler TF, Gleim GW, et al: Preoperative indicators of motion loss and weakness following anterior cruciate ligament reconstruction. *J Orthop Sports Phys Ther* 27(6):407–411, 1998.
129. McMurray TP: The semilunar cartilages. *Br J Surg* 29:407–414, 1942.
130. Meier W, Mizner R, Marcus R, et al: Total knee arthroplasty: muscle impairments, functional limitations, and recommended rehabilitation approaches. *J Orthop Sports Phys Ther* 38:246–256, 2008.
131. Melvin JS, Mehta S: Patellar fractures in adults. *J Am Acad Orthop Surg* 19:198–207, 2011.
132. Milachowski KA, Weismeier K, Wirth CJ: Homologous meniscus transplantation. Experimental and clinical results. *Int Orthop* 13(1):1–11, 1989.
133. Miller GK: A prospective study comparing the accuracy of the clinical diagnosis of meniscus tear with magnetic resonance imaging and its effect on clinical outcome. *Arthroscopy* 12(4):406–413, 1996.
134. Miyasaka KC, Daniel DM, Stone ML, et al: The incidence of knee ligament injuries in the general population. *Am J Knee Surg* 4:3–8, 1991.
135. Mizuta H, Shiraishi M, Kubota K, et al: A stabilometric technique for evaluation of functional instability in the anterior cruciate ligament deficient knee. *Clin J Sport Med* 2:235–239, 1992.
136. Monson J, Arendt EA: Rehabilitative protocols for select patellofemoral procedures and nonoperative management schemes. *Sports Med Arthrosc Rev* 20(3):136–144, 2012.
137. Muller W: *The knee*, New York, 1982, Springer-Verlag.
138. Muneta T, Sekiya I, Ogiuchi T, et al: Effects of aggressive early rehabilitation on the outcome of anterior cruciate ligament reconstruction with multi-strand semitendinosus tendon. *Int Orthop* 22(6):352–356, 1998.
139. Nakagawa TH, Moriya ET, Maciel CD, et al: Trunk, pelvis, hip, and knee kinematics, hip strength, and gluteal muscle activation during a single-leg squat in males and females with and without patellofemoral pain syndrome. *J Orthop Sports Phys Ther* 42(6):491–501, 2012.
140. Nalke B: A simple field test for the assessment of physical fitness. *Rep Civ Aeromed Res Inst US* (53):1–8, 1963.
141. Newton R: Balance screening of an inner city older adult population. *Arch Phys Med Rehabil* 78(6):587–591, 1997.
142. Nichols TR: A biomechanical perspective on spinal mechanisms of coordinated muscular actions: an architecture principle. *Acta Anat (Basel)* 151:1–13, 1994.
143. Noyes FR, Barber SD, Mangine RE: Abnormal lower limb symmetry determined by function hop tests after anterior cruciate ligament rupture. *Am J Sports Med* 19(5):513–518, 1991.
144. Noyes FR, Mangine RE, Barber S: Early knee motion after open and arthroscopic ACL reconstruction. *Am J Sports Med* 15(2):149–160, 1987.
145. Noyes FR, Mayfield W, Barber-Westin SD, et al: Opening wedge high tibial osteotomy: an operative technique and rehabilitation program to decrease complications and promote early union and function. *Am J Sports Med* 34(8):1262–1273, 2006.
146. Noyes FR, Mooar PA, Matthews DS, et al: The symptomatic anterior cruciate-deficient knee. Part 1. The long term functional disability in athletically active individuals. *J Bone Joint Surg Am* 65:154–162, 1983.
147. Obakponovwe O, Kallala R, Stavrou P, et al: The management of distal femoral fractures: a literature review. *Orthop Trauma* 26(3):176–183, 2012.

148. Ohkoshi Y, Yasuda K, Kaneda K, et al: Biomechanical analysis of rehabilitation in the standing position. *Am J Sports Med* 19(6):605–611, 1991.
149. Packer JD, Rodeo SA: Meniscal allograft transplantation. *Clin Sports Med* 28(2):259–283, 2009.
150. Palmitier RA, An KN, Scott SG, et al: Kinetic chain exercises in knee rehabilitation. *Sports Med* 11:402–413, 1991.
151. Palmoski MJ, Colyer RA, Brandt KD: Joint motion in the absence of normal loading does not maintain normal articular cartilage. *Arthritis Rheum* 23(3):325–334, 1980.
152. Parolie JM, Bergfeld JA: Long-term results of nonoperative treatment of isolated posterior cruciate ligament injuries in the athlete. *Am J Sports Med* 14(1):35–38, 1986.
153. Paterno MV, Gelb ID, Hewett TE, et al: The return of neuromuscular coordination after anterior cruciate ligament reconstruction. *J Orthop Sports Phys Ther* 27(1):96, 1998. (abstract).
154. Pearl AJ: *The female athlete*, Champaign, IL, 1993, Human Kinetics Publishing.
155. Perrin DH: Reliability of isokinetic measures. *Athlet Train* 23:319–321, 1986.
156. Petersen S, Snyder-Mackler L: The use of neuromuscular electrical stimulation to improve activation deficits in a patient with chronic quadriceps strength impairments following total knee arthroplasty. *J Orthop Sports Phys Ther* 36:678–685, 2006.
157. Podsiadlo D, Richardson S: The timed "Up and Go": a test of basic functional mobility for frail elderly persons. *J Am Geriatr Soc* 39:142–148, 1991.
158. Polly DW, Callaghan JJ, Sikes RA, et al: The accuracy of selective magnetic resonance imaging compared with the findings of arthroscopy of the knee. *J Bone Joint Surg Am* 70(2):192–198, 1988.
159. Powers CM: Rehabilitation of patellofemoral joint disorders: a critical review. *J Orthop Sports Phys Ther* 28(5):345–354, 1998.
160. Pritchett JW: Nonoperative treatment of widely displaced patella fractures. *Am J Knee Surg* 10(3):145–148, 1997.
161. Ranawat CS, Ranawat AS, Mehta A: Total knee arthroplasty rehabilitation protocol what makes the difference? *J Arthroplasty* 18:27–30, 2003.
162. Rasmussen S, Thomsen S, Matsen SN, et al: The clinical effect of naproxen sodium after arthroscopy of the knee: a randomized, double-blind, prospective study. *Arthroscopy* 9(4):375–380, 1993.
163. Richmond J, Hunter D, Irrgang J, et al: Treatment of osteoarthritis of the knee (nonarthroplasty). *J Am Acad Orthop Surg* 17:591–6000, 2009.
164. Ricklin P, Ruttiman A, del Buono MS: *Meniscal lesions: practical problems of clinical diagnosis, arthrography, and therapy*, Orlando, FL, 1971, Grune & Stratton.
165. Rispoli DM, Miller MD: Options in meniscal repair. *Clin Sports Med* 18:77–91, 1999.
166. Rockborn P, Messner K: Long-term results of meniscus repair and meniscectomy: a 13-year functional and radiographic follow-up study. *Knee Surg Sports Traumatol Arthrosc* 8:2–10, 2000.
167. Rodeo SA: Meniscal allografts—where do we stand? *Am J Sports Med* 29(2):246–261, 2001.
168. Rosenberg TD, Paulos LE, Parker RD, et al: The forty-five degree posteroanterior flexion weight bearing radiograph of the knee. *J Bone Joint Surg Am* 70(10):1479–1483, 1988.
169. Rougraff BT, Shelbourne KD: Early histologic appearance of human patella tendon autografts used for anterior cruciate ligament reconstruction. *Knee Surg Sports Traumatol Arthrosc* 7(1):9–14, 1999.
170. Salter RH, Simmonds DF, Malcolm BW, et al: The biological effect of continuous passive motion on healing of full-thickness defects in articular cartilage. *J Bone Joint Surg Am* 62(8):1232–1251, 1980.
171. Schwartz RE, Asnis PD, Cavanaugh JT, et al: Short crank cycle ergometry. *J Orthop Sports Phys Ther* 13:95, 1991.
172. Scriber K, Matheny M: Knee injuries in college football: an 18-year report. *Athletic Train* 25(3):233–236, 1990.
173. Sgaglione NA, Steadman JR, Shaffer B, et al: Current concepts in meniscus surgery: resection to replacement. *Arthroscopy* 19(Suppl 1):161–188, 2003.
174. Shelbourne KD, Foulk AD: Timing of surgery in acute anterior cruciate ligament tears on the return of quadriceps muscle strength after reconstruction using an autogenous patella tendon graft. *Am J Sports Med* 23:686–689, 1995.
175. Shelbourne KD, Nitz P: Accelerated rehabilitation after anterior cruciate ligament reconstruction. *Am J Sports Med* 18(3):292–299, 1990.
176. Shelbourne KD, Wilckens JH, Mollabaashy A, et al: Arthrofibrosis in acute anterior cruciate ligament reconstruction: the effect of timing of reconstruction and rehabilitation. *Am J Sports Med* 9:332–336, 1991.
177. Shiraishi M, Mizuta H, Kubota K, et al: Stabilometric assessment in the anterior cruciate ligament reconstructed knee. *Clin J Sport Med* 6(1):32–39, 1996.
178. Spencer JD, Hayes KC, Alexander LJ: Knee joint effusion and quadriceps inhibition in man. *Arch Phys Med Rehabil* 65(4):171–177, 1984.
179. Steadman JR, Briggs KK, Rodrigo JJ, et al: Outcomes of microfracture for traumatic chondral defects of the knee: average 11-year follow-up. *Arthroscopy* 19:477–484, 2003.
180. Steindler A: *Kinesiology of the human body under normal and pathological conditions*, Springfield, IL, 1977, Charles C Thomas.
181. Steinkamp LA, Dillingham MF, Markel MD, et al: Biomechanical considerations in patellofemoral joint rehabilitation. *Am J Sports Med* 21:438–444, 1993.
182. Suh J, Aroen A, Mozzonigro T, et al: Injury and repair of articular cartilage: related scientific issues. *Oper Tech Orthop* 7(4):270–278, 1997.
183. Swenson TM, Harner CD: Knee ligament and meniscal injuries. Current concepts. *Orthop Clin North Am* 26(3):529–546, 1995.
184. Thomee R, Augustsson J, Karlsson J: Patellofemoral pain syndrome: a review of current issues. *Sports Med* 28(4):245–262, 1999.
185. Threlkeld AJ, Jorn TS, Wojtowicz GM: Kinematics, ground reaction force and muscle balance produced by backward running. *J Orthop Sports Phys Ther* 11(2):56–63, 1989.
186. Tompkins M, Adkisson HD, Bonner KF, et al: Allograft. *Oper Tech Sports Med* 21:82–89, 2013.
187. Torg JS, Barton TM: Natural history of the posterior cruciate deficient knee. *Clin Orthop Relat Res* 246:208–216, 1989.
188. Torg JS, Conrad W, Kalen V: Clinical diagnosis of anterior cruciate ligament instability in the athlete. *Am J Sports Med* 4:84–93, 1976.
189. Toutoungi DE, Lu TW, Leardini A, et al: Cruciate ligament forces in the human knee during rehabilitation exercises. *Clin Biomech (Bristol, Avon)* 15(3):176–187, 2000.
190. Tria A, Klein KS: *An illustrated guide to the knee*, New York, 1991, Churchill Livingstone.
191. Turek SL: The knee. In Turek SL, editor: *Orthopaedics—principles and their application*, vol 2, ed 4, Philadelphia, 1984, Lippincott, pp 1397–1401.
192. Van Dommelen BA, Fowler PJ: Anatomy of the posterior cruciate ligament. A review. *Am J Sports Med* 17:24–29, 1989.
193. Voight M, Blackburn T: Proprioception and balance training and testing following injury. In Ellenbecker TS, editor: *Knee ligament rehabilitation*, New York, 2000, Churchill Livingstone, pp 361–385.
194. Voight M, Tippett S: Plyometric exercise in rehabilitation. In Prentice WE, editor: *Rehabilitation techniques in sports medicine*, ed 3, New York, 1999, McGraw-Hill, pp 157–169.
195. Wagner UA, Gotzen L, Buhr T: Treatment of isolated medial ligament lesions of the knee joint. *Orthopade* 18(4):315–319, 1989.
196. Walker JM: Pathomechanics and classification of cartilage lesions, facilitation of repair. *J Orthop Sports Phys Ther* 28(4):216–231, 1998.
197. Walker PS, Erkman MJ: The role of the menisci in force transmission across the knee. *Clin Orthop Relat Res* 109:184–192, 1975.
198. Wallace DA, Salem GJ, Salinas R, et al: Patellofemoral joint kinetics while squatting with and without an external load. *J Orthop Sports Phys Ther* 32(4):141–148, 2002.
199. Warren RF, Marshall JL: Injuries of the anterior cruciate ligament and medial collateral ligament of the knee. *Clin Orthop Relat Res* 136:191–197, 1978.
200. Warren RF, Marshall JL, Girgis F: The prime static stabilizer of the medial side of the knee. *J Bone Joint Surg Am* 56(4):665–674, 1974.

201. Wilk KE: Rehabilitation of isolated and combined posterior cruciate ligament injuries. *Clin Sports Med* 13(3):649–677, 1994.
202. Wilk KE, Arrigo C, Andrews JR, et al: Rehabilitation after anterior cruciate ligament reconstruction in the female athlete. *J Athl Train* 34(2):177–193, 1999.
203. Wilk KE, Davies GJ, Mangine RE, et al: Patellofemoral disorders: a classification system and clinical guidelines for nonoperative rehabilitation. *J Orthop Sports Phys Ther* 28(5):307–322, 1998.
204. Wilk KE, Escamilla RF, Fleisig GS, et al: A comparison of tibiofemoral joint forces and electromyographic activity during open and closed kinetic chain exercises. *Am J Sports Med* 24(4):518–527, 1996.
205. Wilk KE, Reinhold MM: Principles of patellofemoral rehabilitation. *Sports Med Arthrosc Rev.* 9(4):325–336, 2001.
206. Willcox EL, Burden AM: The influences of varying hip angle and pelvis position on muscle recruitment patterns of the hip Abductor muscles during the clam exercise. *J Orthop Sports Phys Ther* 43(5):325–331, 2013.
207. Williams RJ, 3rd, Harnly HW: Microfracture: indications, technique, and results. *Instr Course Lect* 56:419–428, 2007.
208. Wind WM, Jr, Bergeld JA, Parker RD: Evaluation and treatment of posterior cruciate ligaments. *Am J Sports Med* 32:1765–1775, 2004.
209. Wirth CJ, Peters G: Meniscus injuries of the knee joint: pathophysiology and treatment principles. In *Baillière's Clinical Orthopedics*, London, 1997, Baillière Tindall, pp 123–144.
210. Witvrouw E, Lysens R, Bellemans J, et al: Open versus closed kinetic chain exercises for patellofemoral pain: a prospective, randomized study. *Am J Sports Med* 28(5):687–694, 2000.
211. Witvrouw E, Werner S, Mikkelsen C, et al: Clinical classification of patellofemoral pain syndrome: guidelines for non-operative treatment. *Knee Surg Sports Traumatol Arthrosc* 13:122–130, 2005.
212. Wojtys EM, Loubert PV, Samson SY, et al: Use of a knee brace for control of tibial translation and rotation. A comparison in cadaver of available models. *J Bone Joint Surg Am* 72:1323–1329, 1990.
213. Wojtys EM, Wylie BB, Huston LJ: The effects of muscle fatigue on neuromuscular function and anterior tibial translation in healthy knees. *Am J Sports Med* 24:615–621, 1996.
214. Wood L, Ferrell WR, Baxendale RH: Pressures in normal and acutely distended human knee joints and effects on quadriceps maximal voluntary contractions. *Q J Exp Physiol* 73:305–314, 1988.
215. Wright JM, Crockett HC, Slawski DP, et al: High tibial osteotomy. *J Am Acad Orthop Surg* 13:279–289, 2005.
216. Yack HJ, Collins CE, Whieldon TJ: Comparison of closed and open kinetic chain exercise in the anterior cruciate ligament-deficient knee. *Am J Sports Med* 21(1):49–54, 1993.

REVIEW QUESTIONS

Multiple Choice

1. Which of the following is the correct order of functional progression for rehabilitation of a knee after injury or surgery?
   a. Normal gait pattern, descend steps, ascend steps, develop quadriceps control, initiate running program
   b. Develop quadriceps control, normal gait pattern, ascend steps, descend steps, initiate running program
   c. Develop quadriceps control, normal gait pattern, descend steps, ascend steps, initiate running program
   d. Normal gait pattern, develop quadriceps control, ascend steps, descend steps, initiate running program
2. After an acute knee injury, what test is universally recognized as the most specific test to assess the integrity of the ACL?
   a. Anterior drawer test
   b. Lachman test
   c. Posterior drawer test
   d. Pivot shift test
3. What is the most important goal for the patient to achieve in the first 2 postoperative weeks after ACL reconstruction surgery?
   a. Normalize gait
   b. AROM to 90° knee flexion
   c. Full passive knee extension
   d. SLR without quadriceps lag
4. What is a safe and recommended ROM for CKC strengthening exercise such as the leg press in the early stages of rehabilitation after PCL reconstruction?
   a. 60° to 0°
   b. 60° to 30°
   c. 0° to 90°
   d. Not recommended
5. A 28-year-old man sustained a right tibial plateau fracture during a skiing accident. The patient is unable to achieve ROM of 90° of knee flexion at the end of 4 weeks of rehabilitation. As a PTA, what is your next step in the plan of care?
   a. Communicate any delay in ROM to PT and referring physician
   b. Begin aggressive PROM
   c. Continue with the current treatment plan for another 2 weeks
   d. Begin a standard crank stationary bicycle
6. A 19-year-old college football player sustained a grade II MCL knee injury during a collegiate game in the middle of the season. What is the approximate time frame for this athlete to return to play?
   a. Unable to return for the season, and surgery is necessary
   b. 3 to 5 weeks
   c. 1 to 2 weeks
   d. 2 months
7. A 21-year-old patient underwent open reduction with internal fixation for a displaced supracondylar fracture. What are the criteria for progression of knee ROM exercises beyond 90°?
   a. Normal gait pattern
   b. Radiographic evidence of fracture stability
   c. SLR without quadriceps lag
   d. Set time frame by a protocol
8. The weight-bearing status after a microfracture procedure is usually:
   a. Weight bearing as tolerated.
   b. PWB.
   c. No weight-bearing restrictions.
   d. NWB or TTWB
9. Approximately how much should the patella move passively?
   a. 2 cm laterally and 1 cm medially
   b. 2 cm laterally and medially
   c. 1 cm laterally and 2 cm medially
   d. 1 cm medially and laterally
10. Proximal realignment for patellofemoral alignment consists of:
    a. Balancing of the soft tissues of the lateral or medial retinaculum including the medial patellofemoral ligament or vastus medialis oblique.

b. Realignment of the patellar tendon, fat pad removal, and medial alignment of the retinaculum.
c. Soft tissue balancing, release of the lateral and medial retinaculum, and bursectomy.
d. Excision of the patella fat pads and lateral patellofemoral ligament fixation.

11. A distal realignment procedure is an osteotomy of the tibial tubercle with transfer of the tubercle:
    a. Laterally, anterolaterally, or distally.
    b. Inferiorly, anteromedially, and proximally.
    c. Superiorly, posteromedially, and distally.
    d. Medially, anteriorly, anteromedially, or distally.
12. The medial patellofemoral ligament is the main medial restraint for:
    a. Medial displacement of the patella.
    b. Lateral displacement of the patella.
    c. Inferior and lateral displacement of the patella.
    d. Medial and superior displacement of the patella.
13. What are the most commonly used prosthetic knee components today for TKA?
    a. Copper alloy tibial and femoral components with tibial tray and patella button made of plastic
    b. Titanium alloy tibial and femoral components with tibial tray and patella button made of polyethylene
    c. Ceramic tibial and femoral components with tibial tray and patella button made of plastic
    d. Chromium cobalt alloy tibial and femoral components with tibial tray and plastic patella
14. Which of the following is true regarding the required knee ROM needed to perform the listed functional activities?
    a. 114° of knee flexion for stairs and sitting, 130° of knee flexion to tie shoes
    b. 93° of knee flexion for stairs and sitting, 106° of knee flexion to tie shoes
    c. 38° of knee flexion for stairs and sitting, 76° of knee flexion to tie shoes
    d. 70° of knee flexion for sitting and stairs, 83° of knee flexion to tie shoes
15. Which criteria are required for return to sport after TKA?
    a. Patient's skill of the sport, ability to squat full body weight, ability to jog for 45 minutes
    b. Return to sport is not allowed after TKA
    c. Age of patient, gender, type of implant, low-demand activity only
    d. Patient education, surgeon approval, implant fixation, high-demand versus low-demand activities, specific adaptation to imposed demand

Short Answer

16. List one common subjective complaint associated with PFPS.
17. List two common surgical complications after TKA.
18. List two main goals during the early phase of rehabilitation after TKA.
19. List three rules of rehabilitation as described by Gray.
20. What are the two most sensitive functional tests for return to sport after ACL reconstruction?

Fill in the Blank

21. The goal of taping the knee is to create a mechanical shift of the patella to centralize it into the ________________.
22. During isokinetic testing of the knee, the velocity is ________________, and resistance is ________________.
23. MCL is the primary restraint to ________________ rotation of the knee.
24. The goal of valgus producing HTO is to unload the ________________ compartment of the arthritic knee.
25. The menisci consist of approximately ____% of type I collagen.

True/False

26. Articular cartilage becomes less stiff and more vulnerable to injury if a mechanical stimulus of a load is applied.
27. Compressive forces across the patellofemoral joint increase from the inferior to superior pole as flexion angles of the knee are increased.
28. One of the biggest modifiable risk factors for osteoarthritis is the aging process.
29. Isolated OKC hamstring strengthening exercises are typically prescribed after PCL injury.
30. Patellar fractures with greater than 3 mm of fragment displacement require surgical management.

Chapter 19

Orthopedic Management of the Hip and Pelvis

Michael P. Reiman

CHAPTER OUTLINE

LEARNING OBJECTIVES

1. Identify common hip fractures.
2. Outline and discuss common methods of management and rehabilitation of common hip fractures.
3. Outline and describe common methods of management and rehabilitation after hip arthroplasty.
4. Identify and describe common soft tissue injuries of the hip.
5. Outline and describe common methods of management and rehabilitation of soft tissue injuries of the hip.
6. Identify common fractures of the pelvis and hip.
7. Outline and describe methods of management and rehabilitation for fractures of the pelvis and acetabulum.
8. Describe common mobilization techniques for the hip.

KEY TERMS

Comminuted fracture
Delayed union
Displaced fracture
Hip osteoarthritis
Malunion
Nonunion avascular necrosis
Osteitis pubis
Osteonecrosis
Pubalgia
Simple fracture

The practicing physical therapist assistant (PTA) is exposed to many orthopedic problems involving the hip and pelvis. This chapter focuses attention on the more common classifications, management, and rehabilitation of hip fractures, joint reconstructive surgery (total hip arthroplasty), rehabilitation after hip replacement, and management of various pelvic fractures and soft tissue injuries of the hip.

ANATOMY

The hip joint, similar to the shoulder joint, is a traditional ball and socket–type joint. Also similar to the shoulder, the hip is a large synovial joint proximal to the spine that affects the remainder of the distal extremity. However, in contrast to the shoulder, the hip is a primary weight-bearing joint that is structurally aligned to tolerate large amounts of force and is an extremely stable joint.

Important Concepts

Reasons for increased stability in the hip joint compared with a similar ball and socket joint (shoulder) include that it is a weight-bearing joint, the orientation of the acetabulum, the limited mobility, and the stability of the ligaments in the hip.

The hip joint is composed of the femur articulating with the pelvis. The pelvis is composed of three bones: the ilium, ischium, and pubis. The junction of these bones is the articulating surface of the hip, called the *acetabulum*.

The acetabulum is concave and articulates with the convex femoral head. The acetabulum faces lateral, inferior, and anterior. It is deepened by the acetabular labrum. Additionally, a fat pad is located in the fossa of the acetabulum. The articulating surface of the acetabulum is a horseshoe-shaped surface called the *lunate surface*.

Because of the orientation and the depth of the acetabulum, the fact that the hip is a weight-bearing joint, and the strength of the ligaments surrounding the hip, this joint is extremely stable. The primary ligaments stabilizing this joint are the iliofemoral, pubofemoral, and ischiofemoral ligaments. Although the ligaments are each selectively tightened in various ranges of motion, they all are collectively tightened in hip extension. The closed packed position of the hip includes hip extension, abduction, and internal rotation. The open packed position is traditionally described as approximately 30° flexion, 30° abduction, and 20° external rotation. Although debated, the described capsular pattern of the hip is flexion, abduction, internal rotation more restricted than extension, adduction, and external rotation.

There are several bursae around the hip. The superficial and deep trochanteric bursae are located laterally. The ischial bursa is located between the ischial tuberosity and the hamstrings tendon. The iliopsoas and iliopectineal bursae are located anterior to the iliopsoas muscle on the anterior surface of the hip joint. The three most commonly affected bursae described for bursitis in the hip joint are the trochanteric, ischial, and iliofemoral bursae.

There are several muscles surrounding the hip. The primary hip flexors include the psoas, iliacus, sartorius, and rectus femoris. The primary hip extensors are the gluteus maximus, hamstring muscles (biceps femoris, semitendinosus, semimembranosus), and adductor magnus. The primary hip abductors include the gluteus medius and minimus and the tensor fascia lata. Hip adduction primary movers include the adductor longus, adductor brevis, adductor magnus, gracilis, and pectineus. Primary hip external rotators include the gluteus maximus, piriformis, obturator internus, superior and inferior gemellus, quadratus femoris, and sartorius. It is generally believed that there are no primary hip internal rotators. Secondary hip internal rotators include the gluteus medius and minimus, tensor fascia lata, adductor longus, and adductor brevis.

KINESIOLOGY

Hip motion is based on the traditional concave on convex or convex on concave principles. The primary motions at the hip joint are flexion, extension, abduction, adduction, external rotation, and internal rotation. Unique to the hip is the fact that these motions can be accomplished via traditional descriptions (femur moving on pelvis—convex moving on concave; pelvis moving on fixed femur—concave moving on convex). These motions are described in detail with respect to the traditional description further on.

Important Concepts

The hip joint has arthrokinematic movements of convex on concave and concave on convex movement depending on the stable and moving surface.

Hip flexion is accomplished by the femur moving in the sagittal plane. Normal hip flexion is approximately 140° with the knee bent. With flexion and extension, the femur stays relatively fixed in the center of the joint. However, some posterior glide of the femur is likely necessary for flexion.

Hip extension is also in the sagittal plane. Range of motion (ROM) for hip extension is approximately 20° with a small amount of anterior femoral glide likely necessary.

Hip abduction and adduction occur in the frontal plane. The ROM for abduction is 40°, whereas adduction is 25° beyond the neutral position. The femoral head glides inferiorly with abduction and superiorly with adduction.

Hip external and internal rotation occurs in the transverse plane. The normal amount of ROM for both motions is commonly described as 45°. The femoral head glides anteriorly for external rotation and posteriorly for internal rotation.

HIP FRACTURES

The clinical significance of hip fractures is reflected in the annual rate of fractures and the financial burden to the economy that hip fractures produce.[10,17] Goldstein[10] stated that more than 300,000 fractures occur annually with an associated cost of $10 billion. Other authorities[4,17] report that 267,000 fractures occur annually, with a price tag of $33.8 billion.[4] Although fractures in general occur to all age groups, hip fractures are most common among elderly women.[4,16,17] Hip fractures in women can be attributed in part to the higher incidence of osteoporosis in this group[16]; with regard to age, hip fractures represent the most common acute orthopedic injury in the geriatric population.[17]

The classification of hip fractures is clinically significant for the PTA because the severity and location of the fracture profoundly affect surgical management and physical therapy interventions. The vascular supply to the femoral head and neck may be significantly compromised with certain fracture patterns and levels of severity (Fig. 19-1).[16] LeVeau stated, "The extent of the supply of blood to the head of the femur determines remodeling and healing after femoral neck fracture or hip dislocation."[16]

Generally, hip fractures can be classified by location and described by severity (**simple** or **comminuted**).[9] Fractures of the hip can be located in the following areas:

- Extracapsular or intertrochanteric[9,10,21] (Fig. 19-2, *A*)
- Femoral neck or subcapital areas[11] (intracapsular) (Fig. 19-2, *B*)
- Proximal femoral shaft or subtrochanteric areas (Fig. 19-2, *C*)[11]

Secondary to the location and severity of hip fracture, the most significant complication is related to **osteonecrosis** and the loss of blood supply to the femoral head leading to avascular necrosis. Gross and associates affirmed, "any fracture of the neck (femoral) can disrupt this tenuous blood supply. As a result, there is an exceedingly high incidence of avascular necrosis of the femoral head after hip fractures."[11] LeVeau stated, "avascular necrosis may

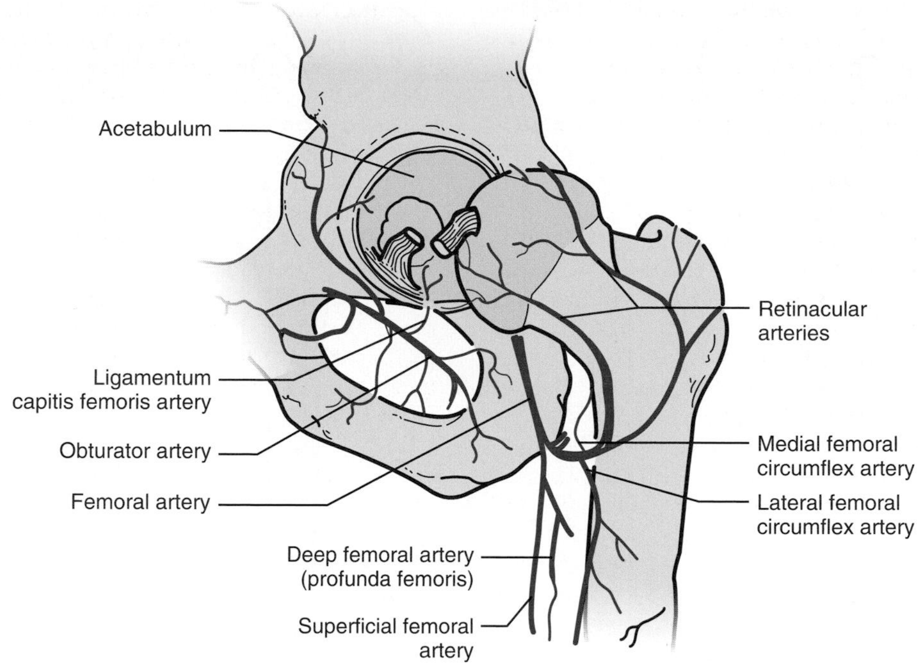

FIG 19-1 Vascular supply to the femoral head and neck. *(Modified from Richardson JK, Iglarsch JK, editors:* Clinical orthopedic physical therapy, *Philadelphia, 1994, Saunders.)*

occur after hip fracture in about 65% to 85% of the patients."[16]

Three main clinical complications are noted with subtrochanteric fractures: **malunion, delayed union,** and **nonunion avascular necrosis.**[18] Two factors associated with malunion and nonunion of subtrochanteric hip fractures are as follows:

- The subtrochanteric area of the proximal femur is cortical bone, which has a decreased blood supply.
- The subtrochanteric area is prone to large biomechanical stresses that can lead to loosening of various fixation devices.[18] This complication must be considered by the PTA when treating patients with this type of fracture.

Many options are available to treat hip fractures. The choice of treatment depends on the patient's age, location of the fracture, quality of bone, severity of the fracture (simple, **displaced,** or comminuted), activity level of the patient, associated soft tissue injuries, and specific goals for the patient's return to activity. Generally, hip fractures are managed surgically with open reduction with internal fixation (ORIF) that secures the fracture fragments with various rods, nails, pins, screws, and plates.[9,10,17] Some hip fractures can be managed conservatively with bed rest, traction, and protected weight bearing.[18] For example, in a fractured greater trochanter in which the displaced fracture fragment is less than 1 cm (as evaluated by the physician radiographically), the treatment could be bed rest for several days, ROM exercises, and limited weight bearing for 4 weeks.[18]

With an isolated lesser trochanteric fracture (most common in adolescents), the physician bases treatment on the amount of fragment displacement. If the fracture is displaced more than 2 cm, the physician could perform ORIF; if the fragments are in closer apposition, the physician may elect rest, protected weight bearing, and limited exercise for 3 to 4 weeks.[18] Figure 19-3 depicts common fixation devices used to secure fracture fragments with ORIF.

While treating patients with hip fractures, the PTA must be aware that venous thrombosis is a potentially critical complication after hip surgery. Without prophylactic medications to minimize thrombosis, statistics show that 40% to 90% of patients develop this condition after hip surgery.[18] Venous thrombosis is the most common complication after hip fracture in elderly patients.[18]

Hip fractures and dislocations can occur in combination and as isolated events. Usually hip dislocations are either anterior or posterior (Fig. 19-4). Isolated hip dislocations generally are treated conservatively with bed rest, traction, and protected limited weight bearing for up to 12 weeks.[18] For example, with an anterior hip dislocation, bed rest with traction is prescribed, with specific precautions to avoid extreme hip abduction and external rotation to prevent redislocation. Usually protected weight bearing is allowed when the patient can achieve painless hip ROM around 3 to 4 weeks after the incident.[18] Conversely, an isolated posterior hip dislocation is treated with bed rest and traction in abduction with precautions to prevent hip abduction, flexion, and internal rotation to protect the joint from redislocation.[18]

REHABILITATION AFTER HIP FRACTURES

The patient's overall preoperative physical and mental condition is a predictor of postoperative success. Patients with major cardiovascular or pulmonary disease processes, obesity, osteoporosis, dementia, or poor upper body strength are at increased risk for postoperative complications. Overall,

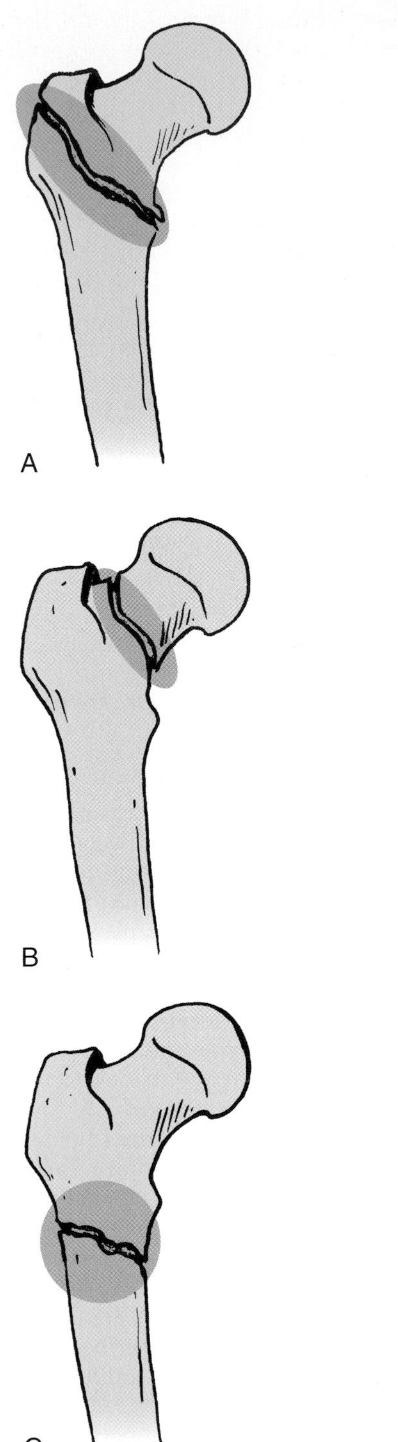

FIG 19-2 **A,** Intertrochanteric hip fracture. **B,** Femoral neck fracture. **C,** Subtrochanteric hip fracture.

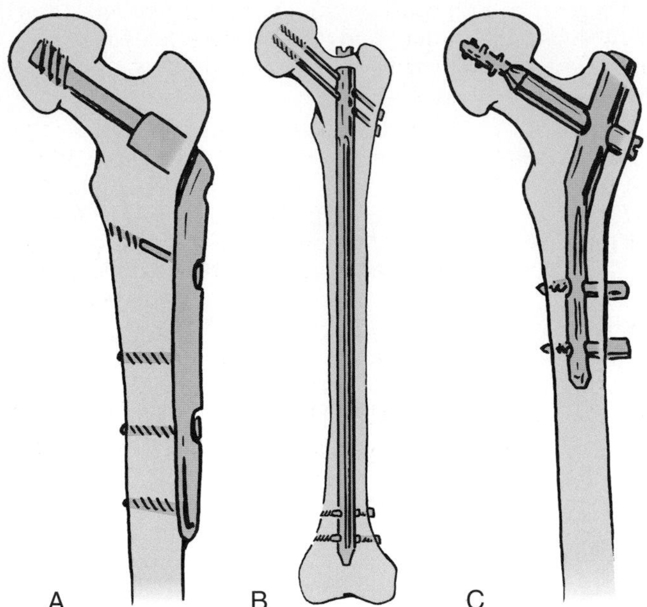

FIG 19-3 Methods of internal fixation for hip fractures. **A,** Screws and sideplate. **B,** Rod. **C,** Nails.

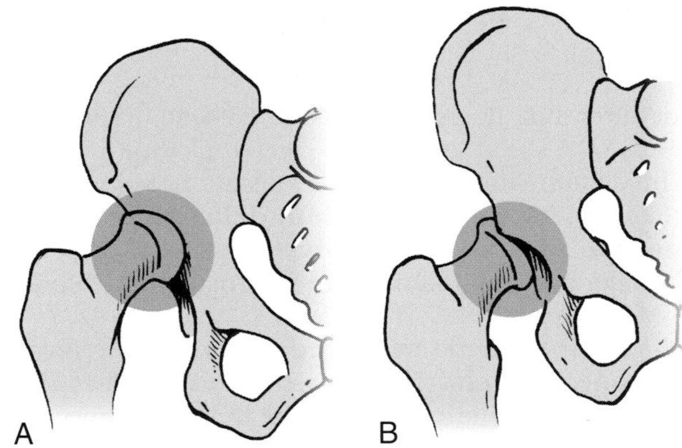

FIG 19-4 Dislocation of the hip. **A,** Anterior dislocation. **B,** Posterior dislocation.

mortality rates of 20% after 1 year, 50% at 3 years, 60% at 6 years, and 77% after 10 years have been reported.[7]

Although the overall goal of rehabilitation is to restore patients to preinjury level, this may not be realistic. Only 20% to 35% of patients regain their preinjury level of independence. Institutionalized care is required for more than 1 year after surgery in 15% to 40% of patients. Many patients (50% to 83%) require devices to assist with ambulation.[14]

A rehabilitation program used to treat hip fractures is highly individualized. The nature of the fracture type, classification, location, and method of internal fixation (if any) are considered, and the treatment program is adjusted to the patient's ability to cope with specific identified criteria. These criteria are established by the physical therapist (PT) and carried out by the PTA.

The progression from maximum to minimum protection closely follows the rate of bone healing. However, other factors are considered in safely and effectively providing an environment for the return to functional activities. In the maximum-protection phase of recovery (1 to 21 days postoperatively),[9] the fracture site is protected; pain and swelling are reduced; and isometric exercises, gentle protected ROM, and limited weight bearing begin.[9,16]

The general goals of recovery are to increase muscular strength specific to the surgery, improve overall conditioning, increase ROM of the affected hip, enhance aerobic fitness, increase local muscular endurance, reduce pain and swelling, reestablish normalized gait mechanics, and protect the healing structures from internal and external forces that can impede healing.[9,16] The exercises used during the maximum-protection phase include active ankle pumps for both lower extremities, isometric quadriceps sets, gluteal sets, heel slides, hip abduction and adduction, and supine internal and external hip rotation. These exercises must be done at submaximal levels at first and then made progressively more difficult according to the patient's tolerance.

Goldstein[9] identified a few major complications that occur, particularly during the maximum-protection phase of recovery. Generally, no combined diagonal or rotary forces are used in exercises during this phase. Hardware loosening and delayed healing may occur if increased torque is placed through the healing fracture site by excessive forces.[9] No active straight leg raises or supine hip bridges should be performed during the first 6 to 8 weeks after surgery. Goldstein stated, "The power generated by the massive hip muscles is so great during those exercises that there is a danger of displacing the fractured segments."[9] In addition to rudimentary isometric quadriceps sets, gluteal sets, ankle pumps, and gentle hip motion exercises, authorities advocate adding the exercises described in Figure 19-5 progressively during the first 3 weeks after surgery,[9] although I do not advocate exercise number 3 (forward bending of trunk) and exercise number 12 (hip extension in prone).

Important Concepts

Postoperative rehabilitation for a patient with a fracture must be individualized to the patient with specific consideration of multiple variables. The maximum-protection phase of exercises must initially be implemented at submaximal levels.

Early protected weight bearing is encouraged soon after surgery. Generally, touchdown weight bearing (TDWB) or partial weight bearing (PWB) is allowed by the second day postoperatively. Weight-bearing status increases as dictated by the rate of bone healing (>8 to 12 weeks), which should be verified radiographically by the physician. Avoiding torque through the affected limb during standing minimizes loosening of the fixation device.

More demanding exercises are added as the bone and associated soft tissues heal. Closed chain functional exercises are added as full weight bearing (FWB) is achieved. Partial wall squats and step-ups are usually initiated to regain concentric and eccentric muscle control of the quadriceps and hip extensors. A restorator or bike ergometer can be used during the early recovery phase if the patient can tolerate sitting and depending on restrictions about hip flexion, ROM, and precautions.

The moderate-protection phase, defined as 3 to 6 weeks after surgery,[9] provides for more challenging exercises directed at regaining hip and knee motion; improving quadriceps and hamstring strength; and increasing strength to the hip extensors, abductors, and adductors. Standing four-position hip strengthening can be achieved initially without any resistance until a proper pattern of movement is achieved. Advancing this exercise can be accomplished using a cable system (Fig. 19-6), lower levels of bands, or ankle weights. Limited ROM leg presses can be initiated during this phase as well.

The late healing phase (after 6 to 8 weeks) is characterized by normalized gait mechanics and reduced use of assistive devices for ambulation. A treadmill can be used, with step cadence and stride length adjusted, to enhance gait and provide a stimulus for greater hip and quadriceps strength.

More advanced hip strengthening exercises can be added cautiously for more active patients. A stair stepper stimulates hip extension strength and local muscular endurance, but extreme caution must be used when initiating various open and closed chain exercises after surgery for hip fractures. A fine line must be followed to avoid excessive forces (e.g., straight leg raises or hip bridges), torque, and weight bearing, while stimulating hip and knee motion and improving strength and function.

PROXIMAL FEMORAL OSTEOTOMY

Intertrochanteric osteotomy may be performed when degenerative joint disease (DJD) is extensive and results in hip pain associated with subchondral bone erosion, articular cartilage fibrillation and fissuring, and hip joint incongruity.[15] The goal of this surgical procedure is to reduce pain and improve function related to advanced osteoarthritis (OA) by surgically changing the femoral neck-shaft angle so that healthy cartilage is exposed, "improving joint surface congruity."[15] Figure 19-7 illustrates this procedure and shows the changed neck-shaft angle relationship, reduced ligamentous and muscular tension, and improved joint articulation occurring after surgery.[15]

REHABILITATION AFTER PROXIMAL FEMORAL INTERTROCHANTERIC OSTEOTOMY

Because a proximal femoral intertrochanteric osteotomy is performed to reduce symptoms related to advanced OA (DJD) of the hip, the rehabilitation program must focus on joint protection principles (unloading forces through the hip) and postsurgical bone healing precautions. During the maximum-protection phase of recovery, avoiding unwanted forces, managing pain (with thermal agents or pain medication), using protected weight bearing (to unload the hip from repetitive articular cartilage destruction), restoring hip motion, and improving strength are stressed. Quadriceps-setting exercises, gluteal sets, ankle pumps, and gentle active hip ROM exercises are allowed from the first day after surgery.

Weight-bearing status is highly individualized but generally is progressed according to the rate and quality of bone healing. Typically, a walker or crutches reduces compressive loads through the hip during TDWB, PWB, and non–weight bearing (NWB) gait techniques. In most cases, protected weight bearing is strictly enforced for 8 to 12 weeks after this procedure.[15]

The contralateral hip, bilateral knee joints, and spine are targets of joint protection related to OA. The PTA must fully understand that the whole person—not just the affected joint—should be addressed during all phases of recovery. In keeping with joint protection, when the surgical incision has healed and the patient is allowed PWB status, an underwater treadmill or unweighting device can be useful to enhance normalized gait mechanics in a protected weight-bearing environment. The buoyancy of the water allows reduced compressive loads through the hip.

When radiographic evidence suggests secure bone healing, more challenging and intense strengthening exercises are added gradually. Isotonic knee extensions; leg curls; and standing hip abduction, adduction, flexion, and extension motions are strengthened through use of a cable system or wall pulleys, lighter band resistances, and ankle weights. As with rehabilitation after a hip fracture, the PTA must recognize the advantages and disadvantages of these different therapeutic modalities. A major disadvantage of resistive bands or tubing is that the resistance increases as the range of the movement increases. This increased resistance is a disadvantage to most muscle groups in the hip joint with these types of exercises because the length-tension relationship of a muscle demonstrates maximal

Sitting

1. Knee extension (kicking)
   Slowly extend knee fully, hold for 1 second, and return slowly to flexed position under control.

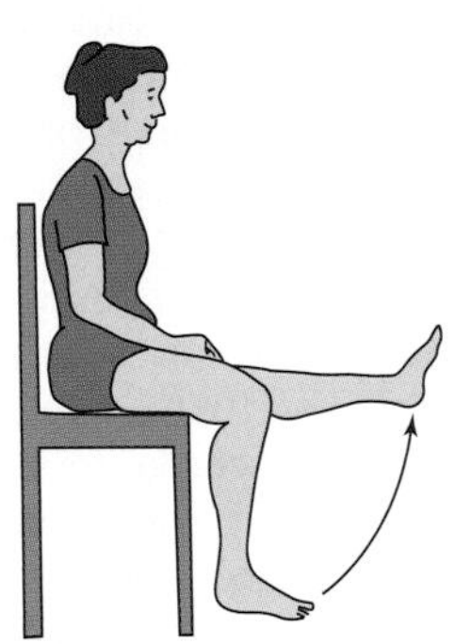

2. Hip flexion (marching)
   Lift alternate knees to chest, as if slowly marching in place while sitting.

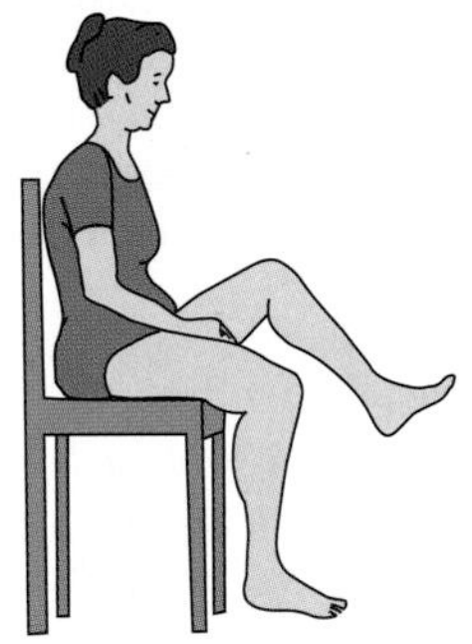

3. Forward bending of trunk
   Slowly reach hands down along the insides of the legs. Stop at the first pulling sensation. Return slowly to erect posture.

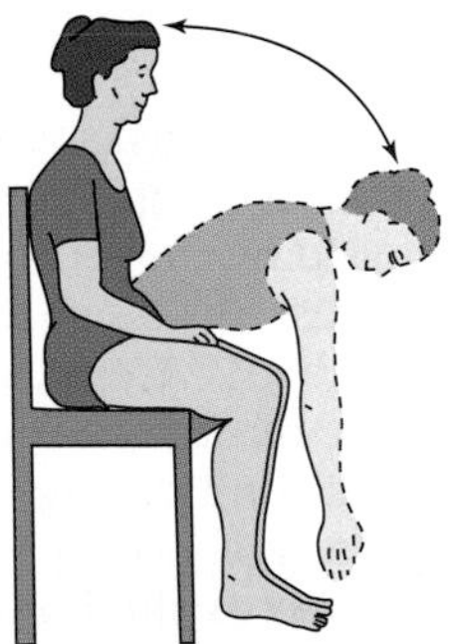

4. Armchair push-ups
   While seated, place hands on armrests (or push-up blocks) and extend both elbows, lifting torso from chair seat. Feet should be placed on floor for balance, support, and assist.

Supine Lying

5. Hip rotations
   With hips slightly abducted and knees extended, slowly roll legs in and out.

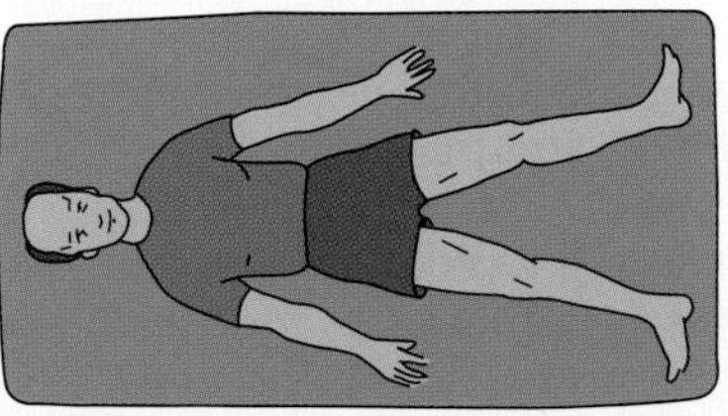

FIG 19-5 Progressive hip exercises are employed during the first 3 to 4 weeks after surgery. *(Adapted from Goldstein T:* Geriatric orthopaedics: rehabilitative management of common problems, *ed 2, Austin, TX, 1999, PRO-ED, Inc. Adapted with permission.)*

6. Heel slides
   Slide heel along mat toward the buttocks and slowly return to original position.

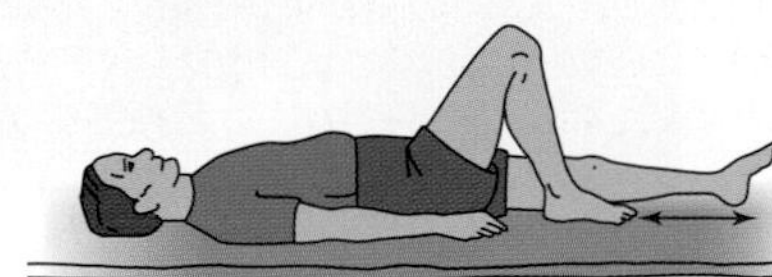

7. Knee to chest
   Flex hip, bringing knee toward the chest, and slowly return limb to extended position.

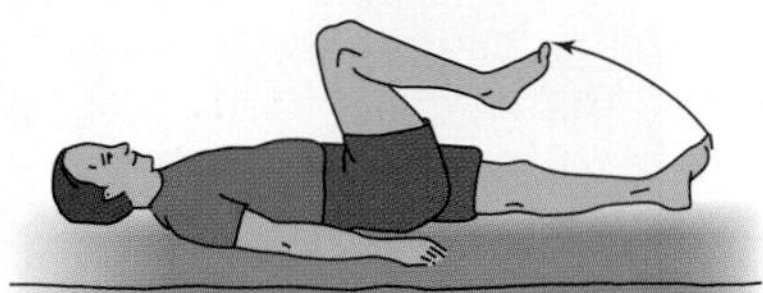

8. Hip abduction/adduction
   Slowly spread legs apart and pull them together, keeping the knees extended and the toes pointed upward.

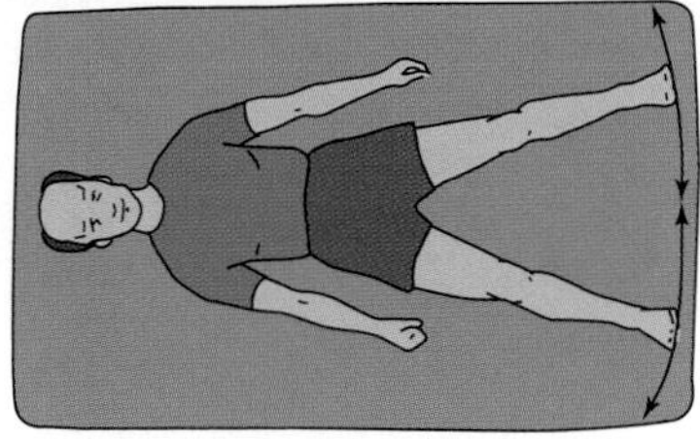

9. Terminal knee extension
   While supine with towel roll under knee, slowly contract the thigh muscles to bring knee into straightened position.

Prone Lying

10. Hip flexor stretch
    Lie prone for up to 20 minutes daily. Place pillow or bolster under ankles for comfort.

11. Knee flexion
    Flex knee and bring heel toward buttocks. Return to extended position.

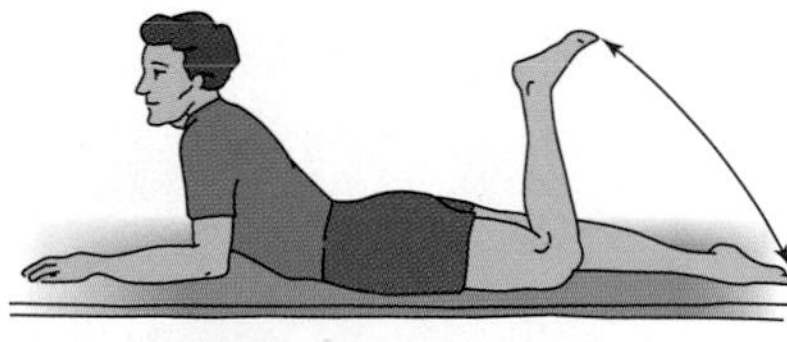

12. Hip extension
    With knee flexed to 90°, lift knee slightly off mat without rotating pelvis and slowly lower knee to mat.

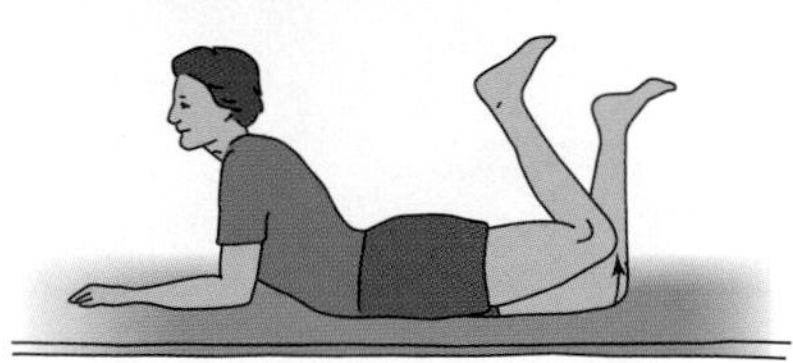

FIG 19-5, cont'd

strength at approximately 80% to 120% of its resting length. At the very end range of these motions, the hip musculature is potentially actively insufficient and is required to resist the resistance band at its maximal resistance. The length-tension relationships between the resistance modality (resistive band or tubing) and the muscle do not match up in many cases. These same exercises can be performed in shortened ranges. The PTA must be cognizant as to the most favorable way to match up these length-tension relationships.

Extreme caution must be used with closed chain strengthening exercises. Minimizing joint compressive loads, which may contribute to articular cartilage degeneration, is the cornerstone in the long-term care of patients with severe OA. Functional weight-bearing exercises must be added judiciously and without increased pain.

A limited ROM leg press exercise can be used as the first closed chain activity. This exercise may allow the PTA to increase the resistance load systematically, while still using lower loads than the patient would encounter with FWB

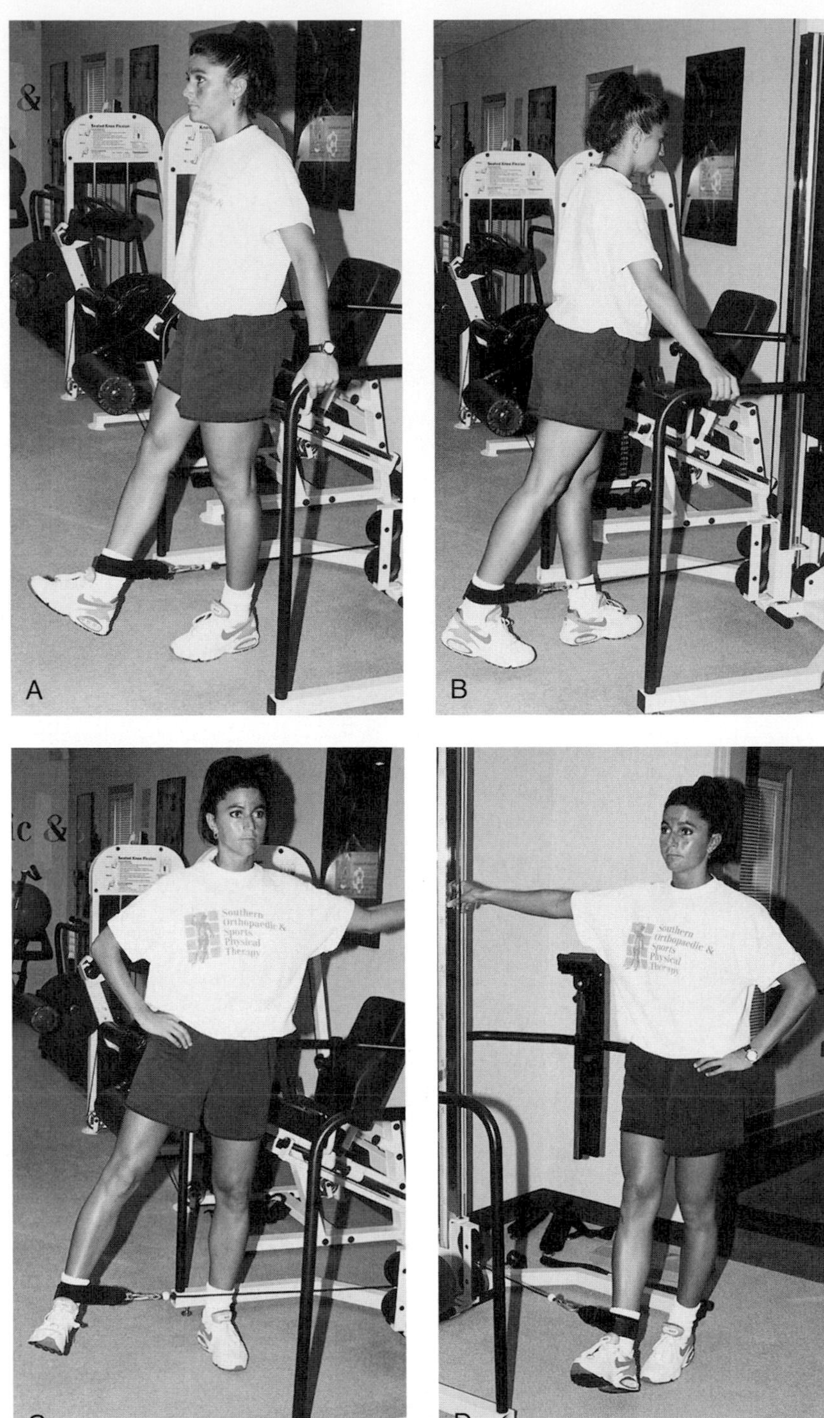

FIG 19-6 Standing four-way hip strengthening exercises using a cable column system. **A,** Hip flexion straight leg raise. **B,** Hip extension. **C,** Hip abduction. **D,** Hip adduction.

status. The compressive loads would also be systematically increased. As healing progresses, mini-step-ups, short-arc wall squats, and treadmill walking are added. A general conditioning program that encourages weight control, specifically using aerobic exercise (unloaded, upper body ergometer, or recumbent or semirecumbent stationary cycle ergometer), strengthening (minimizing joint compressive loads and shearing joint motions), and flexibility should be implemented as soon as the patient can tolerate these activities.

HEMIARTHROPLASTY OF THE HIP

For femoral head osteonecrosis or severe femoral head fractures, hemiarthroplasty is used to eliminate pain and improve function. This procedure replaces the damaged

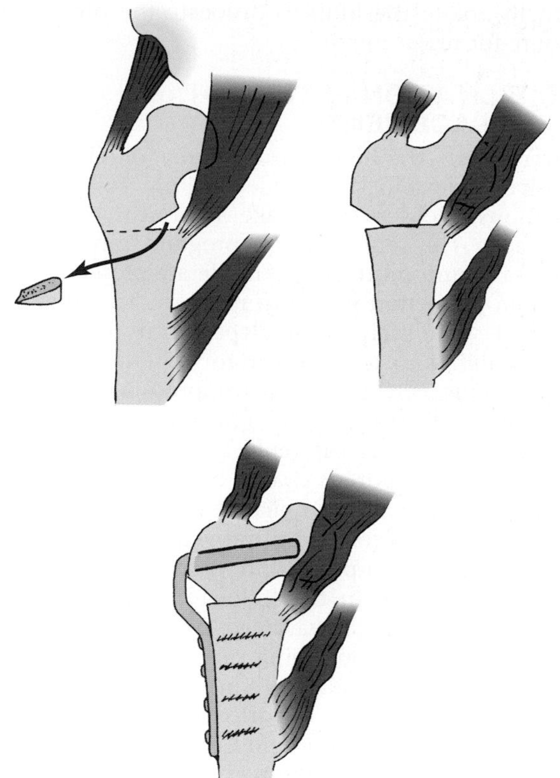

FIG 19-7 Proximal femoral osteotomy.

femoral head with a bipolar prosthesis. Because hemiarthroplasty requires a normal acetabular surface,[15,22] it is rarely used to treat arthritis.[22] This is considered a conservative procedure[15] compared with total hip replacement (THR). Hemiarthroplasty can be converted at a later date to THR if symptoms persist and the joint degenerates.[22] Bipolar refers to two separate snap-fit components of one femoral prosthetic unit. A bipolar prosthesis is usually a large-diameter femoral head component that snap-fits snugly onto a smaller diameter femoral head, which is part of the total prosthetic unit.[9,15] A unipolar femoral prosthesis is a self-contained femoral head and shaft without additional components. The bipolar prosthesis usually produces less wear caused by friction and reduced impact loading of the acetabulum.[20]

FIXATION OF PROSTHETIC HIP COMPONENTS

The method of fixation of various prosthetic components directly affects the short-term and long-term course of rehabilitation after hip arthroplasty. Femoral and acetabular components usually can be secured to the bone with a cement, polymethyl methacrylate, which is not actually an adhesive, but rather provides a strong interference fit between the prosthesis and the bone.[20] Alternatively, the components can be secured with a noncemented biologic tissue ingrowth prosthesis. Miller[22] recommended that cemented femoral stems be used only for patients older than 65 years and that noncemented prostheses be used for younger patients. Weight-bearing precautions are related to the specific type of fixation procedure used to secure the prosthesis. Weight bearing generally is deferred for longer periods of time with a noncemented biologic tissue fit prosthesis so that the bone can grow into the porous-coated femoral stem. Weight bearing with cemented devices can progress at a slightly faster rate. However, in either case, rotational forces (torque) must be avoided to minimize the loosening of components.

TOTAL HIP REPLACEMENT

Total hip arthroplasty (THR) involves replacing both the femoral head and the acetabulum, as contrasted with a hemiarthroplasty, which replaces only the femoral head. Indications for THR include the following:

- Rheumatoid arthritis
- OA (femoral head and acetabulum)
- Osteonecrosis
- Fractures
- Juvenile rheumatoid arthritis (the most common indication for THR in adolescents)[20]
- Pain
- Reduced ambulation
- Significant alterations in activities of daily living[22]

Before discussing rehabilitation procedures, this chapter reviews pertinent complications and component designs related to THR because these issues influence specific physical therapy interventions and precautions.

Surgeons must select a proper femoral head size for each patient. In theory, a large-diameter femoral head may provide for greater ROM and inherent stability.[20,22] This makes sense because greater forces are necessary to dislocate a large-diameter head from the acetabulum. In practice, large-diameter femoral head components do not reduce the incidence of dislocation after surgery. The most commonly used head size is moderate (26 to 28 mm) rather than overly large (32 mm).[20,22]

One of the most common complications related to THR, using a noncemented femoral stem component, is persistent thigh pain with an antalgic gait (painful limp gait) pattern. This thigh pain may last for 1 or 2 years after surgery and is reported in approximately 20% of all patients with this fixation type.[20,22]

The most significant complication after THR, with the highest mortality, is thromboembolic disease.[20] The entire rehabilitation team (e.g., PT, PTA, physician) must be concerned with this complication and monitor for this continually. Although many of the signs of thromboembolic disease after THR are the same as with any other lower extremity injury or surgery, some specific signs after THR are localized tenderness and swelling along the distribution of the deep venous system of the hip, specifically the femoral vein along the anterior thigh.

Because the method of fixation is directly related to the initiation and progression of weight bearing after surgery with uncemented components, some authorities recommend TDWB on the second day postoperatively, gradually progressing to FWB by 8 weeks postoperatively.[9] With a cemented (polymethyl methacrylate) prosthesis, Goldstein[9] suggested TDWB 2 days after surgery, progressing to

FWB by the third week postoperatively. These timetables for weight bearing are directed by the biologic rate of bone healing and the wishes of the physician and are applied under the direction of the PT. A cemented component generally allows earlier ROM and weight bearing than an uncemented prosthesis.

The occurrence of loosening of components has been estimated to be 10% to 40% by 10 years postoperatively.[22] Loosening is more common among younger, more active patients; obese patients; patients with rheumatoid arthritis; and patients with previous hip surgery.[22] The PTA must be aware of these factors when treating patients with THR and recognize the increased potential for component loosening.

Postoperative dislocation of the hip after THR is another clinically significant complication with an occurrence of 1% to 4%.[22] These dislocations are multifactorial, requiring an awareness of the basic concepts of hardware design, fixation procedures, and surgical approaches and patient compliance with specific total hip precautions to avoid dislocation. The most immediate concern during recovery from THR is teaching and reinforcing precautions to the patient, nursing staff, family, and other caregivers.

The PTA also should be familiar with the surgical approach used to gain exposure to the hip. Universal total hip precautions are intended to avoid the exact position the surgeon used to expose and dislocate the hip to carry out the procedure. Usually these precautions are as follows:

- Avoid hip adduction. This is usually accomplished by using an abduction wedge or pillow.
- Avoid hip internal rotation. The affected limb can be supported medially with pillows or a wedge to maintain the limb in neutral or slight external rotation.
- Avoid hip flexion greater than 90°.
- Avoid the combination (simultaneous performance) of hip flexion, internal rotation, and adduction for 4 months after surgery.[9]

The preceding precautions apply when a posterior (Fig. 19-8), posterolateral, or lateral approach is used. If an anterior surgical approach is used, combined hip extension and external rotation should be avoided.[9] This variation is needed because the surgeon had to extend and externally rotate the limb to dislocate the hip and gain exposure for replacement.

REHABILITATION AFTER TOTAL HIP REPLACEMENT

Recovery from the significant trauma of THR requires extensive bone and soft tissue healing. Following THR precautions, recovery may take 4 months or longer in some cases. The rehabilitation program can be divided into maximum-protection, moderate-protection, and minimum-protection phases of recovery. The time frames associated with each phase depend on the individual patient's ability to achieve certain criteria of improved motion (being careful not to compromise THR precautions), increased strength, weight-bearing status (taking into account whether the replacement has been secured with cement or a porous-coated biologic ingrowth component), reduced pain, compliance with THR precautions, bed mobility, transfers, and improved confidence.

In the maximum-protection phase of recovery, the patient is instructed in the following exercises: bilateral ankle pumps, isometric quadriceps sets, gluteal isometrics, and active knee flexion (being careful to avoid excessive hip flexion). The contralateral limb can be exercised with active straight leg raises, quadriceps sets, hamstring sets, ankle pumps, and full knee and hip mobility exercises. To ensure primary healing, all universal hip precautions must be enforced (avoid hip flexion, adduction, and internal rotation with a posterior, posterolateral, or lateral surgical approach, and avoid hip extension and external rotation with an anterior approach). In addition, the patient should be strongly cautioned to avoid the following positions and actions (Fig. 19-9), as outlined by LeVeau[16]:

- Do not sit in low chairs.
- Do not cross your legs.
- Do not sleep on your side.
- Do not bend forward at your hip (causes excessive hip flexion).
- Do not squat.

Transfer training and bed mobility must be addressed immediately after surgery. The affected limb should be maintained in a stable, secure position during all transfers

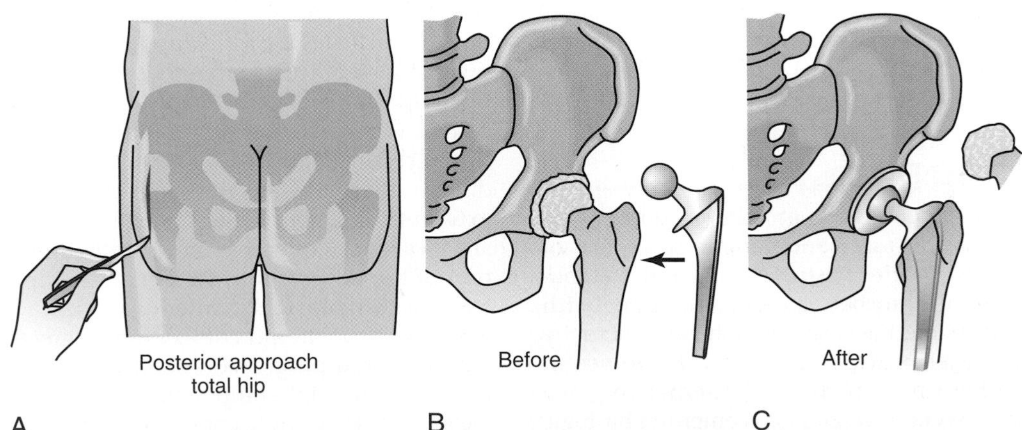

FIG 19-8 Posterior approach for total hip arthroplasty procedure. *(From Cameron MH, Monroe LG: Physical rehabilitation: evidence-based examination, evaluation, and intervention, St Louis, 2007, Saunders.)*

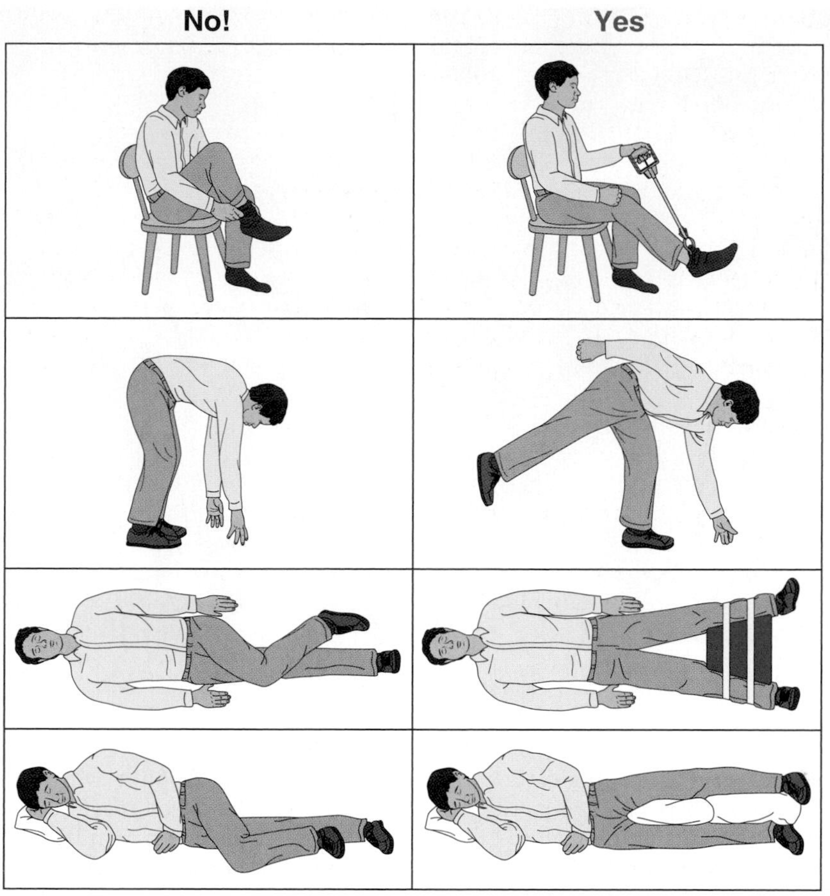

FIG 19-9 Positions to be avoided and recommended alternatives after total hip arthroplasty. *(From Cameron MH, Monroe LG:* Physical rehabilitation: evidence-based examination, evaluation, and intervention, *St Louis, 2007, Saunders.)*

from bed to commode or wheelchair. A raised toilet seat is a basic requirement during the early phase of recovery. In addition, a raised and rigid (although padded) seat cushion is necessary to eliminate the sling effect of the wheelchair seat, which places the hip in an internally rotated position.[9]

The use of crutches or a walker is advocated for TDWB or PWB, depending on how the prosthesis is secured. A cemented prosthesis requires TDWB on the second day after surgery, with the patient gradually progressing to FWB by 3 weeks. A patient with an uncemented THR can begin with PWB, and the patient can progress to FWB 8 weeks after surgery.

The moderate-protection phase can begin when the patient has demonstrated improved quadriceps control, active knee flexion, reduced pain, compliance with all precautions and exercises, independent bed mobility and transfers, and improved gait (with necessary weight-bearing precautions). Moderate protection does not imply reduced THR precautions in any way. During this phase, more challenging exercises are added to approximate functional activities more closely. Light resistance exercises for quadriceps strengthening in a semirecumbent position and elastic tubing also can be used to strengthen the hamstrings and hip extensors in a semirecumbent or seat-elevated position (Fig. 19-10). Standing exercises

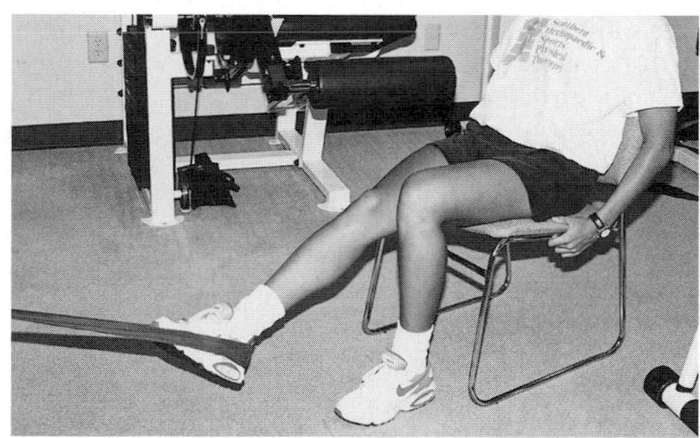

FIG 19-10 Seated hamstring strengthening using an elastic band.

stress active hip motion (straight-plane motions, no combined rotational forces, THR precautions strictly enforced) and strengthening.

To enhance aerobic fitness, a recumbent bucket-seat bicycle ergometer or an upper body ergometer can be used. Increases in weight bearing are added as determined by component fixation, tissue healing constraints, and the wishes of the physician. Closed chain functional activities begin 3 to 8 weeks postoperatively[10] for cemented prostheses, with increased weight bearing orders by the physician. These activities can include sit-to-stand exercises

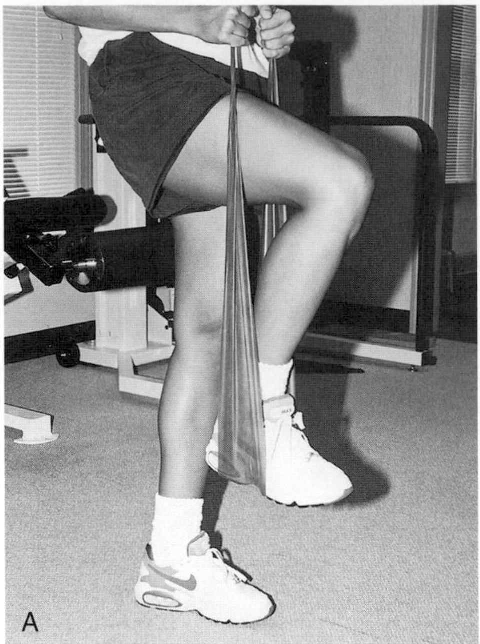

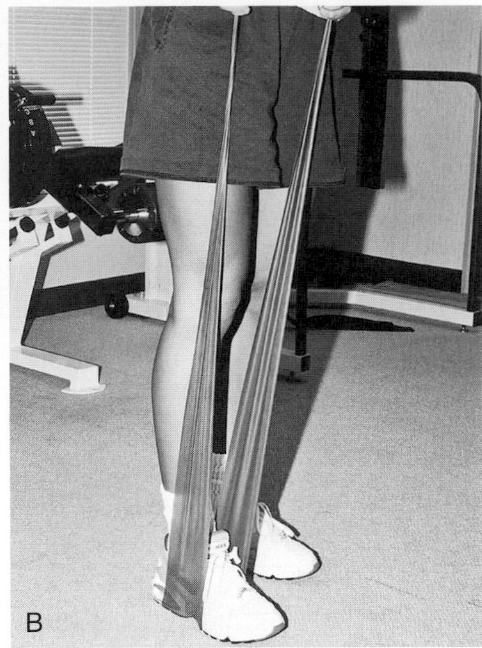

FIG 19-11 Standing hip and knee extension press-down using an elastic band. **A,** Starting position. **B,** Finish.

with an elevated seat, partial supported knee bends (for concentric and eccentric quadriceps control), weight-shifting exercises, treadmill walking, mini-step-ups, and standing resisted hip and knee extension (Fig. 19-11). For an uncemented prosthesis, closed chain functional activities are deferred for 2 or 3 weeks longer than for cemented prostheses. However, standing straight-plane resistance exercises (hip extension, adduction, abduction, and flexion) are allowed between 3 and 8 weeks postoperatively.

The minimum-protection phase of recovery is initiated 12 to 16 weeks after surgery. Depending on individual cases, the physician may elect to discontinue THR precautions during this phase. A great deal of soft tissue and bone healing must occur and muscular strength must improve dynamic stability before THR precautions are relaxed.

The minimum-protection phase is classically characterized by a return to normalized gait patterns without assistive devices and by instruction in balance, coordination, proprioception, and advanced closed chain functional activities that duplicate the patient's specific activities of daily living. Most patients recover most of their hip motion during the first year after surgery.[20] At this phase of recovery (approximately 4 months after surgery), the patient may still demonstrate decreased motion and must be reassured that more time is needed before assessing the ultimate degree of hip motion attainable.

While addressing proprioception, coordination, and balance after either knee or hip replacement (single-leg standing, eyes open and eyes closed, single-leg standing on a minitrampoline or balance board), the PTA must recognize that certain afferent neural input mechanoreceptors (type I, Ruffini; type II, pacinian; types III and IV, free nerve endings) will be lost because of the removal of the articulating joint surfaces. However, the joint capsule surrounding the joint replacement remains essentially intact and well supplied with mechanoreceptor feedback organs, which can be retrained and enhanced via appropriately applied weight-shifting activities, balance board exercises, and closed chain functional strengthening exercises.

Returning to higher level activities, including sport activity, should be discussed with the physician, PT, PTA, and patient as a team. Multiple factors should be considered, including presurgical activity level, experience in the activity or sport to which the patient wants to return, strength, balance, proprioception, and mobility status. Activities and their level of recommendation are listed in Box 19-1.

Important Concepts

Rehabilitation after THR must be individualized to the patient and type of surgical procedure performed.

HIP LABRAL TEAR AND REPAIR

Diagnosis and treatment of labral tear in the hip are still relatively new, and the investigation regarding conservative and postsurgical intervention is limited. Postsurgical protocols are quite variable. It is highly recommended that the rehabilitation team (e.g., PT, PTA) have excellent communication among themselves and with the physician and nursing staff. It is imperative that the rehabilitation team follow the postsurgical instructions and guidelines. These guidelines and protocols might be variable for various reasons (e.g., physician, patient, surgical procedure). Additionally, the surgical procedure may involve more than labral resection or repair. Osteoplasty (reshaping or removal of bone off the femoral head or acetabular rim) also may have been performed. As with all surgical procedures, the rehabilitation team must

BOX 19-1 Activity after Total Hip Arthroplasty

Recommended/Allowed	Allowed with Experience	Not Recommended	No Conclusion
• Stationary biking	• Low-impact aerobics	• High-impact aerobics	• Jazz dancing
• Croquet	• Road biking	• Baseball/softball	• Square dancing
• Ballroom dancing	• Bowling	• Basketball	• Fencing
• Golf	• Canoeing	• Football	• Ice skating
• Horseshoes	• Hiking	• Gymnastics	• Roller or inline skating
• Shooting	• Horseback riding	• Handball	• Rowing
• Shuffleboard	• Cross-country skiing	• Hockey	• Speed walking
• Swimming		• Jogging	• Downhill skiing
• Doubles tennis		• Lacrosse	• Stationary skiing machine
• Walking		• Racquetball	• Weight lifting
		• Squash	• Weight machines
		• Rock climbing	
		• Soccer	
		• Singles tennis	
		• Volleyball	

From Healy WL, Iorio R, Lemos M: Athletic activity after total joint replacement, *Am J Sports Med* 29:377–388, 2001.

clearly understand all of the variables that can influence the patient's outcome.

Very general guidelines are presented here owing to the above-mentioned concerns. In general, a patient with a labral resection can be progressed more quickly than a patient undergoing labral repair. Weight-bearing restrictions (although quite variable) are generally less limiting as well. The rehabilitation team must consider the portions of the hip stressed with gait. Normally, the toe-off and initial swing phase of gait require end-range hip extension. A patient with hip pain or a postsurgical patient may be unable to achieve extension past neutral or even to neutral. The PT and PTA must consider how this affects the patient's gait pattern and whether extension past neutral is indicated.

It has generally been described with all patients after hip surgery that it is important to avoid deep groin pinching pain with ROM, especially flexion. The theoretical basis for this restriction is the avoidance of soft tissue impingement and increasing inflammation or potentially stressing the surgical area.

Hip extension and external rotation are usually restricted for the patient after hip labral repair. These motions biomechanically stress the anterior portion of the labrum. If the patient has a posterior labral repair (generally less common), the motions of hip flexion and internal rotation are more likely to be restricted by the physician. The location and size of the labral repair affect the postsurgical restrictions. The importance of communication with the physician and PT is stressed.

Unless contraindicated, for most types of hip labral surgeries, gentle isometric exercises are generally initiated within the first week after surgery. The ROM should not be stressed when performing these exercises, especially for patients with labral repair. When indicated, isotonic hip exercises should be initiated in pain-free ROM that does not compromise the surgical procedure. As with all postsurgical cases, initiation of these exercises requires submaximal effort initially and progression of required patient effort as indicated.

Conservative intervention for a patient with labral tear depends on the patient's impairments. Communication with the supervising PT is necessary to appreciate the extent of these impairments fully. Generally, it is expected that the patient may have some gluteal weakness and potential limits or pain with some movements of the hip. If these impairments are due to joint mobility restrictions, it is suggested that the appropriate joint mobilization described later in this chapter be used. If these impairments are more related to soft tissue, the appropriate stretches should be employed.

HIP OSTEOARTHRITIS

Hip osteoarthritis is defined as the focal loss of articular cartilage with variable subchondral bone reaction. The prevalence of OA ranges from 7% to 25% in adults 55 years old and older in the white European population.[24] Although specific characteristics of hip OA have not always correlated with radiographic features, joint pain and functional impairment seem consistent.

Intervention goals for hip OA include relieving symptoms, minimizing disability, and reducing the risk of disease progression. Additional goals are education, modification of activities, maintenance of ROM if possible, instruction on proper diet and weight control, proper footwear, and the use of an assistive device if appropriate. Conservative interventions that have demonstrated success in patients with hip OA include gait and balance training, manual therapy techniques, and systematically progressed therapeutic strengthening.[2]

Functional, gait, and balance training is recommended to address impairments of proprioception, balance, and strength, all of which are commonly found in individuals with lower extremity arthritis. Assistive devices, such as canes, crutches, and walkers, can be used by patients with hip OA to improve function associated with weight-bearing activities.

Clinicians should consider the use of manual therapy procedures to provide short-term pain relief and improve hip mobility and function in patients with mild hip OA. Distractive techniques are particularly helpful to patients with hip OA. Manual therapy techniques were also found to be superior in terms of pain relief and improvement in function compared with therapeutic exercise in all patients with hip OA except patients with highly limited function, high pain levels, and limited ROM.[13]

It is also recommended that clinicians should consider the use of flexibility, strengthening, and endurance exercises in patients with hip OA. The psoas muscle group should be assessed for lack of flexibility, and the gluteus medius should be assessed for weakness. Appropriately designed rehabilitation programs by the PT should be implemented. Strengthening of the weak gluteal muscles is addressed later in this chapter.

Important Concepts

Manual therapy has demonstrated favorable results in patients with hip OA.

LEGG-CALVÉ-PERTHES DISEASE

In 1910, three researchers identified a hip condition that usually affects children between the ages of 4 and 8 years (the range is 2 to 12 years of age with the most common age being 6 years).[3] This condition, which is referred to as *Legg-Calvé-Perthes disease* or *coxa plana,* is characterized as a noninflammatory, self-limiting (can heal spontaneously with or without specific treatment) syndrome in which the femoral head becomes flattened at the weight-bearing surface[11] as a result of disruption of the blood supply (avascular necrosis) to the femoral head in the growing child.[11,16] The long-term complications of the flattened femoral head lead to an incongruous joint surface and advanced DJD (Fig. 19-12).[11,16,19]

Throughout the management of this disease, the primary focus is on maintaining the femoral head within the confines of the acetabulum, regaining motion, and reducing pain and dysfunction.[11,16,19] In the acute or maximum-protection phase, reducing pain and dysfunction is generally accomplished using physician-prescribed nonsteroidal antiinflammatory drugs (NSAIDs), bed rest, and traction to take the load off the hip and restore motion in abduction.

Keeping the femoral head seated within the acetabulum can be accomplished using an abduction orthosis (Fig. 19-13).[11,16] To aid healing and reduce unwanted stress on the affected hip, the abduction orthosis can be worn up to 2 years.[16] During this time, the brace can be removed for short periods each day to exercise the limb and attend to personal hygiene.[16] With the brace removed, the patient must maintain hip abduction during ROM exercises for the knee (flexion and extension), internal rotation of the hip, quadriceps strengthening, hip abduction, and hip extension strengthening exercises (gluteus medius and gluteus maximus).[16]

Surgical versus conservative intervention is controversial because there is a lack of agreement on the benefit of surgical intervention versus conservative care. Patient prognosis is much improved if there is no collapse of the femoral head.

PUBALGIA

Pubalgia is a collective term for all disorders causing chronic pain in the region of the pubic tubercle and the inguinal region. Although typically resulting from athletic involvement, it can be present in other individuals. Pubalgia is often characterized by lower abdominal pain with exertion and minimal to no pain at rest. A unilateral presentation can be noted, although bilateral involvement is also possible. Identification of the contributing dysfunction is imperative in this wide-ranging condition.

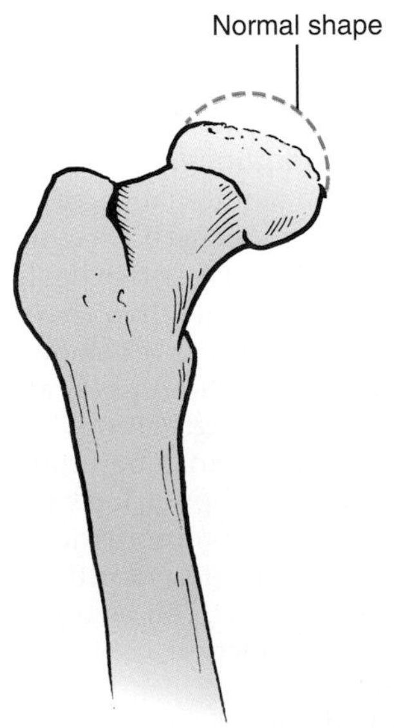

FIG 19-12 Legg-Calvé-Perthes disease.

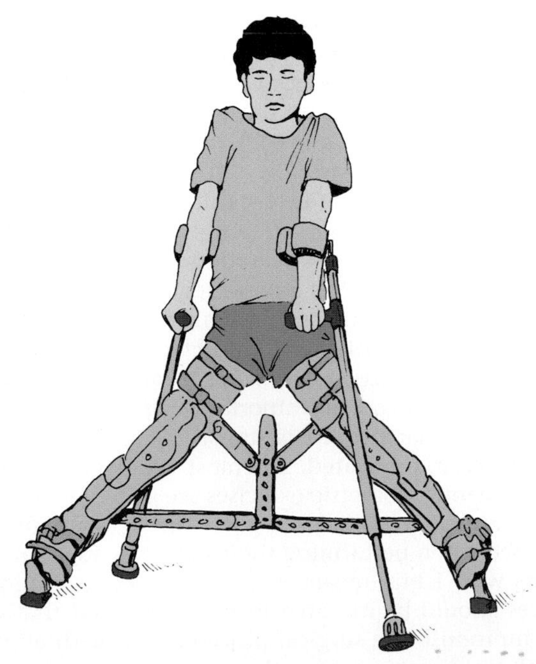
FIG 19-13 An abduction orthosis can be used during treatment of Legg-Calvé-Perthes disease to help maintain the femoral head seated within the acetabulum.

Arthrokinematic dysfunction of the pubic joint, sacroiliac joint dysfunction, and muscle imbalances all are potential contributing factors to this dysfunction. Typically, stretching of traditionally tight muscle groups (psoas major and adductor muscle group) with strengthening of traditionally weaker muscles (gluteal muscles) is indicated as long as it is pain-free. Specific examples of gluteal strengthening exercises are given later in the chapter.

OSTEITIS PUBIS

Osteitis pubis is often part of the necessary differential diagnosis for pubalgia. These two dysfunctions are often confused. Osteitis pubis is characterized by pain and bony erosion of the symphysis pubis. The bony erosion is often a much later finding and can complicate early diagnosis. These patients generally present with pain over the pubic area that radiates laterally across the anterior hip, which is usually aggravated by striding, kicking, or pivoting.

Examination findings include tenderness over the symphysis and proximal adductors, pain with adduction against resistance, and restricted hip rotation with pelvic obliquity and sacroiliac dysfunction.[8] A bone scan of the area may assist in differential diagnosis of this dysfunction versus pubalgia and athletic pubalgia (sports hernia).

Treatment is traditionally conservative, without any advantages to surgical intervention. Treatment is aimed at addressing the primary dysfunction, whether it is muscle imbalance, joint mobility dysfunction, or some other cause. Similar to pubalgia, the treatment approach must be systematic and address the problem areas with consideration of progression principles.

SOFT TISSUE INJURIES OF THE HIP

BURSITIS

Trochanteric bursitis is a common soft tissue injury affecting the hip in active individuals. The greater trochanter of the femur is most commonly affected. The trochanteric bursa may become irritated and inflamed because of excessive compression and repeated friction as the iliotibial band (ITB) snaps over the bursa while lying superior to the greater trochanter (Fig. 19-14).

Treatment for greater trochanteric bursitis is centered on relieving pain and inflammation while addressing the underlying cause of the condition. Rest, ice, and antiinflammatory medications are commonly used first to arrest the symptoms of pain and swelling. Any specific motions or activities (e.g., running) that may exacerbate the pain must be modified or eliminated. Intervention for this condition primarily consists of removal of the causative factors; stretching the soft tissues of the lateral thigh (especially the tensor fascia lata and ITB); and focusing on the flexibility of the external rotators, quadriceps, and hip flexors. Strengthening of the hip abductors is essential, as is establishing a muscular balance between the hip abductors and adductors. Stretching is thought to be essential for reducing the compression and friction from the ITB over the greater trochanter.

Specific strengthening exercises include quadriceps strengthening, hamstring curls, hip extension exercises (partial squats, leg press), and the previously mentioned hip abduction exercises. Aerobic fitness can be maintained using a stationary cycle (although this is typically painful in this condition), upper body ergometer, treadmill, or stair climber (if not painful). In all cases, the ROM must be modified to limit hip and knee motion and avoid repeated snapping of the ITB over the trochanter. Ultrasound and hydrotherapy also may be useful during the acute phase of recovery.

Two other areas of bursitis commonly affecting the hip are ischial bursitis and iliopectineal bursitis. Ischial bursitis (Fig. 19-15) has also been termed *Weaver's bottom* and is characterized by pain over the ischial tuberosity underlying the gluteus maximus. It can be caused by direct contusion of the ischial tuberosity or extended periods of sitting.[11,23] Occasionally, this condition can mimic a hamstring strain at the origin of the muscle at the ischial tuberosity.[11,23] This condition tends to affect thinner people and cyclists. Management is similar to other forms of bursitis and includes rest from the aggravating activity, ice packs, NSAIDs, and a judiciously applied program of stretching exercises that do not aggravate the symptoms. Generally, hamstring stretches are encouraged along with quadriceps-strengthening exercises. Unique to this particular bursitis is the use of a padded seat cushion as an

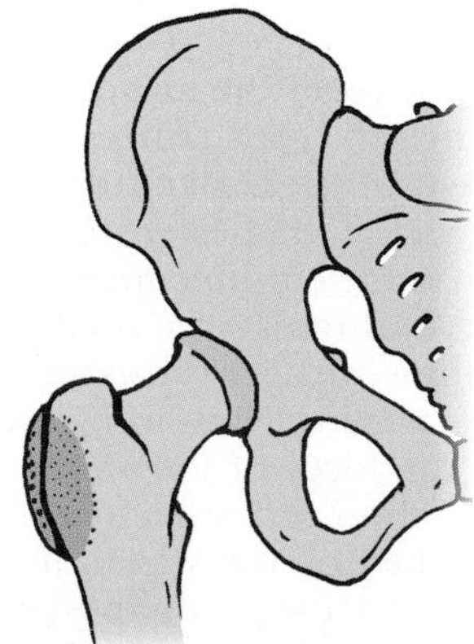

FIG 19-14 Greater trochanteric bursitis.

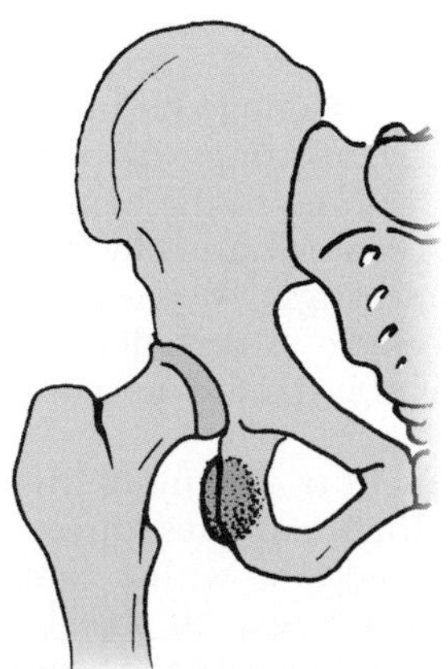

FIG 19-15 Ischial bursitis.

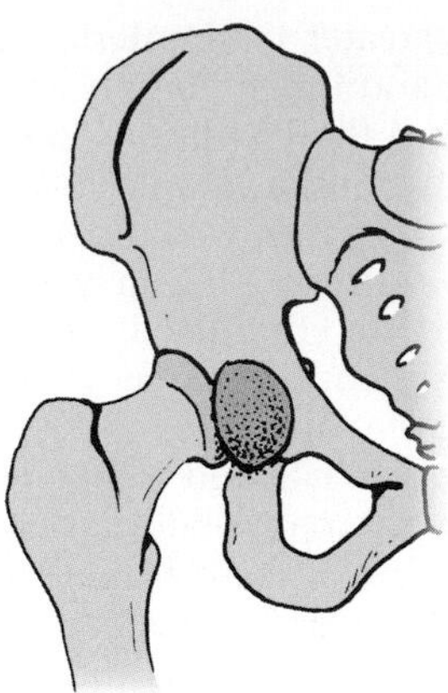

FIG 19-16 Iliopectineal bursitis.

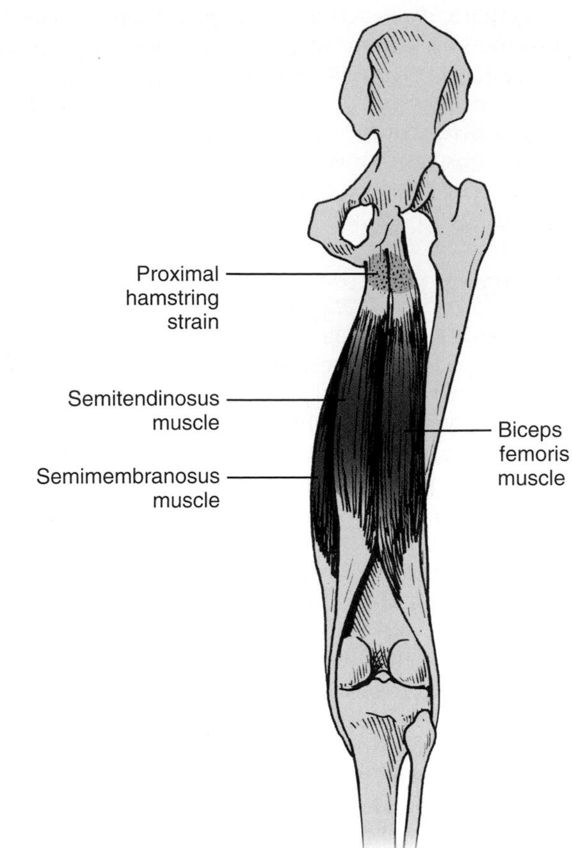

FIG 19-17 Anatomy of posterior thigh musculature. Note proximal hamstring strain just inferior to the origin at the ischial tuberosity.

intervention method because of the bursa location. Occasionally, conservative care fails, and the physician may elect to inject the area with corticosteroids.[11]

Iliopectineal bursitis is characterized by either local tenderness over the iliopsoas muscle and tendon or diffuse radiating pain into the anterior thigh (Fig. 19-16).[23] Because the iliopectineal bursa lies deep to the tendon of the iliopsoas muscle, tightness of the iliopsoas alone and in conjunction with excessive hip extension can cause compression and frictional wear of the iliopectineal bursa. Pain may also be noted with passive hip flexion and adduction at the end range. Specific care centers on reducing pain and irritation using a program of rest; ice; antiinflammatory medications; and physical therapy interventions such as thermal agents, stretching, and strengthening exercises.

In some cases of iliopectineal bursitis, stretching the tight iliopsoas muscle group increases pain over the bursa. Stretching of the psoas muscle perhaps should be deferred in cases where pain is exacerbated by such activity. The use of ice, hydrotherapy, ultrasound, and physician-prescribed NSAIDs can minimize the pain and allow for the initiation of quadriceps-strengthening exercises, hamstring stretches, ITB stretches, hip adductor stretches, and the beginning of an aerobic fitness program, as long as the symptoms do not increase. Specific stretching of the iliopsoas is indicated when initial healing has occurred, and the acute inflammatory process is arrested.

MUSCLE STRAINS

Most acute injuries affecting the hip are musculotendinous strains of the hamstrings, iliopsoas, adductors, and rectus femoris.[11,23] Injuries to the hamstrings at the origin (ischial tuberosity) can be caused by sudden, forceful contraction of the hamstrings or by decelerating the lower leg against the concentric contraction of the quadriceps during running as the hamstrings contract eccentrically (Fig. 19-17).

Initial management of the injury involves the application of cold packs for 20 minutes, three to five times daily. Wrapping the affected limb with a compression bandage also can help relieve stress on the limb. Motions that produce pain and interfere with the healing process should be avoided. Two motions should not be attempted during the acute or maximum-protection phase of recovery: full knee extension combined with forward trunk flexion and full leg flexion.[3,4]

The use of crutches may be indicated during this phase to limit stress on the hamstrings. The PTA can significantly aid the patient in coping with a difficult problem during the early recovery phase. Sleeping may be extraordinarily painful. The PTA should counsel the patient to sleep supine with pillows under both knees to support the injured limb and to reduce passive nocturnal stretching by placing the hamstrings in a relaxed position. As pain and swelling are reduced, active knee extension and leg flexion are encouraged (if the patient remains pain-free) to help influence the direction of immature collagen fibers. The PTA must recall the intrinsic nature of muscle and tendon healing time constraints and avoid the temptation to encourage an aggressive stretching program for the hamstrings during the early maximum-protection phase of recovery. Sufficient time must be allowed for the torn tissue to scar and reorganize itself before subjecting the fragile immature collagen to excessive tensile loads that may impede healing. However, flexibility must be addressed and is the focus of long-term recovery during the moderate-protection and minimum-protection phases of recovery, as defined by the significance of the injury; the patient's ability to achieve improved motion, strength, and pain-free gait; the physician's wishes; and the PT's direction.

Strength training proceeds according to the patient's individual situation and is strongly influenced by muscle and tendon healing constraints. Initially, isometric quadriceps sets and submaximal multiangle hamstring sets can be done as pain allows. Progressive strengthening can be achieved with prone manual resistive leg curls, ankle weights, or sitting resistance band leg curls. The last-mentioned exercise strongly encourages slow eccentric hamstring muscle contractions. An excellent, dynamic, and fun exercise to perform is scooting with a rolling adjustable-height stool. This exercise encourages knee flexion against resistance at various controllable speeds. Supine hip bridges can be added as function increases. Depending on the patient's requirements, closed kinetic chain and higher functional demand exercises can be systematically implemented to allow individuals such as athletes a gradual return to their sport. The specific time frames for these different phases of the rehabilitation continuum must be determined with a team approach including the physician, PT, PTA, and patient.

An adductor muscle strain is termed a *groin pull.* A classic program of protection, ice, compression bandaging, crutches, and protected weight bearing during the acute or maximum-protection phase should be followed. As with other muscle and tendon strains, early aggressive stretching should be avoided. When pain subsides, active hip flexion, gentle hip abduction and adduction motion, and knee ROM exercises should begin. Specific hip abduction stretching can be initiated, instructing the patient to perform the seated butterfly stretch, with a strong caution to proceed slowly without pain. Some authorities suggest waiting 3 to 6 weeks before instructing the patient in progressive resistance exercises.[11] However, resistance exercises can begin earlier, depending on the severity of the strain. To strengthen the hip adductors specifically, submaximal isometrics (Fig. 19-18) can give way to proximally placed resistance in various positions (Fig. 19-19).

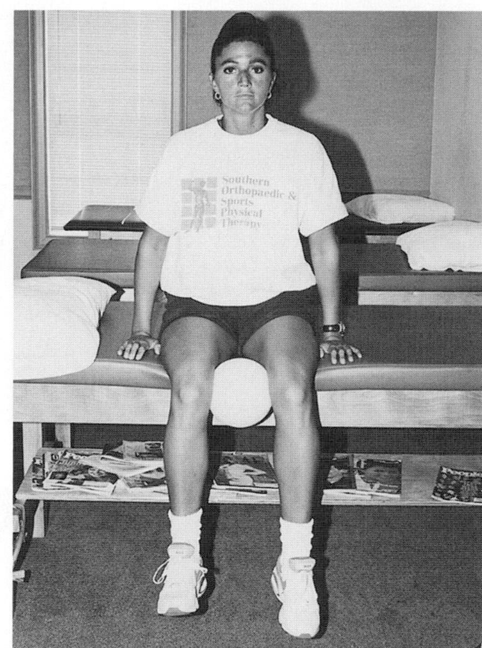

FIG 19-18 Seated hip adduction isometrics.

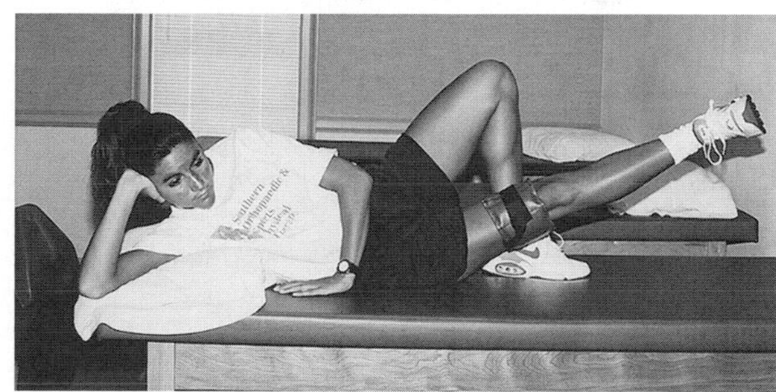

FIG 19-19 Side-lying hip adduction concentric and eccentric contractions. Note the proximally placed resistance.

Progression to more dynamic strengthening exercises depends on the specific goals established by the patient and PT. For example, in a young athletic population of patients eager to return to sports activities, a slide board can be an effective tool to introduce dynamic hip adduction and abduction motions (Fig. 19-20).

An iliopsoas muscle strain also is referred to as a *hip flexor pull.* This injury can occur from sudden, forceful extreme hip extension or by forced hip flexion against resistance.[23] A standard program of protection, rest, ice, and compression bandages with crutches and limited weight bearing is encouraged in the acute phase. Sleeping comfort can be enhanced by sleeping supine with pillows under the knees to reduce hip extension. Gentle, active hip flexion and extension exercises are begun when the initial healing phase has ended and the patient no longer complains of pain. A prolonged period of time may be needed to avoid hip extension (e.g., push-off during gait running or hip extension past neutral) and encourage healing. Gentle active stretching of the hip flexors can begin with the patient supine and the nonaffected knee and hip flexed. In addition, a hurdler's stretch can be initiated when the patient demonstrates improved hip extension motion without pain. The PTA should strongly encourage the patient to perform these stretches in a slow, static fashion without pain. Very close supervision is needed to guard against any ballistic, forceful, or violent motions that could impede healing and reinjure the affected limb.

Also, as previously mentioned with other conditions, correction of muscle imbalance and joint dysfunctions (as identified by the PT) need to be addressed. Antagonistic muscle group strengthening (gluteal muscles in this case) is necessary to maintain the newly gained flexibility achieved with stretching of the affected muscle. Some specific gluteal strengthening exercises with corresponding electromyographic percentage of maximal volitional contraction (values ± standard deviation) for the gluteus maximus and medius are as follows:

- Side-lying hip abduction (gluteus medius, 42% ± 23%).[1] Patient lies on contralateral side with shoulder, hip, and ipsilateral heel in contact with wall. Patient lifts ipsilateral lower extremity 6 to 12 inches in frontal plane, while keeping contact with wall throughout the motion (Fig. 19-21, *A*). As the patient increases strength and requires less stabilization, he or she can move away

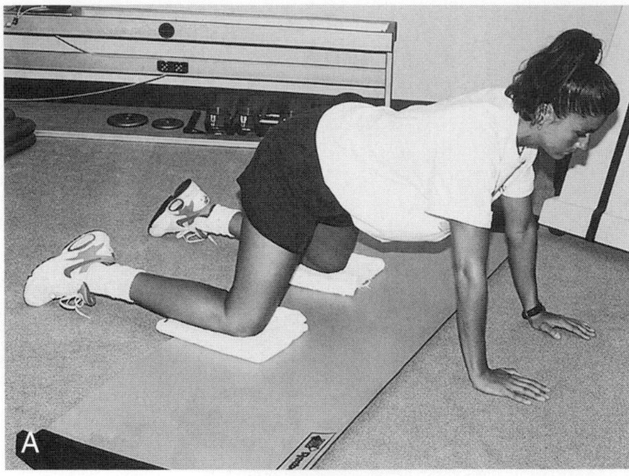

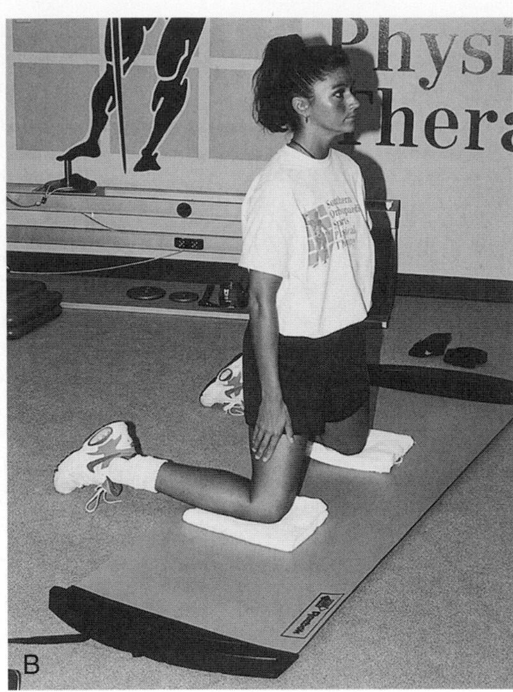

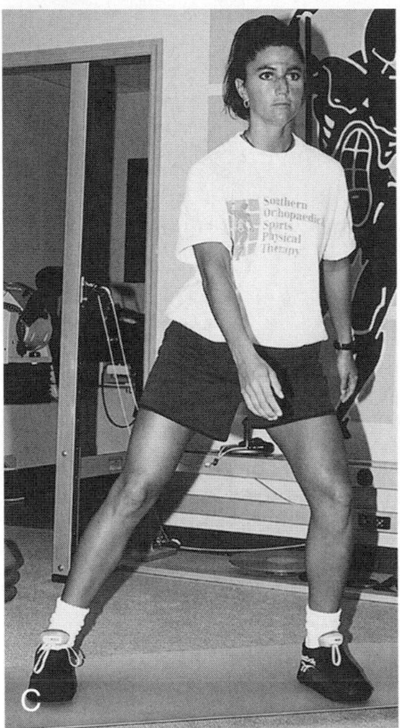

FIG 19-20 Progressive slide board activities for dynamic closed chain hip abduction and adduction. **A,** On hands and knees for support; the patient slowly abducts and adducts both hips. **B,** Kneeling position is slightly more challenging. **C,** Standing position.

from wall to perform this exercise as the PTA monitors compensation of abducting anterior to frontal plane.

- Side bridge (gluteus medius, 74% ± 30%).[5] Patient lies on ipsilateral side with ipsilateral forearm directly below shoulder and lifts bilateral hips off table as demonstrated (Fig. 19-21, *B*).
- Bilateral lower extremity bridge (gluteus medius, 28% ± 17%; gluteus maximus, 27% ± 13%; hamstrings, 35% ± 21%).[5,6] Patient lies supine with bilateral feet flat on table. Patient lifts bilateral hips off table to neutral spine position (Fig. 19-21, *C*).
- Single lower extremity bridge (gluteus medius, 47% ± 24%).[5] Patient starting position as with bilateral bridge exercise. Patient lifts contralateral lower extremity with knee extended as patient lifts bilateral hips with ipsilateral lower extremity to neutral spine position (Fig. 19-21, *D*).
- Standing hip abduction without weight (gluteus medius, 33 ± 23%).[1] Patient stands on contralateral lower extremity and abducts ipsilateral lower extremity 6 to 12 inches (Fig. 19-21, *E*).

Important Concepts

When implementing muscle performance exercises, the PTA must be cognizant of the muscle force produced by the muscle during specific exercises.

MUSCLE CONTUSIONS

The most common contusion affecting the hip and pelvis involves the subcutaneous tissues of the iliac crest and is commonly termed a *hip pointer*.[12] Typically, this injury can occur in one of two ways:

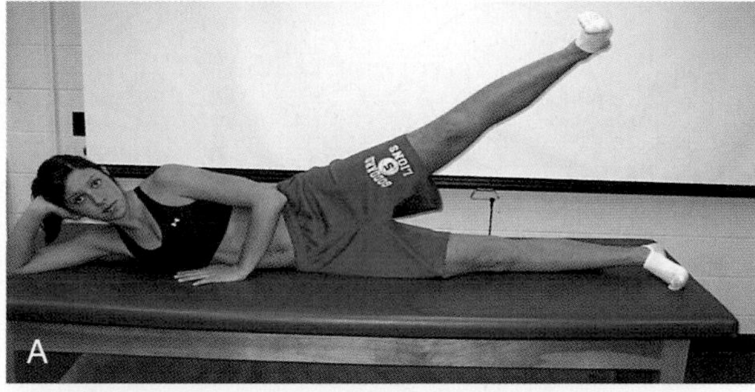

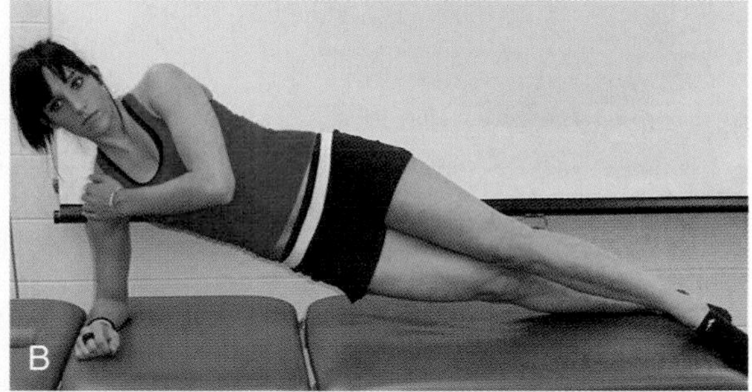

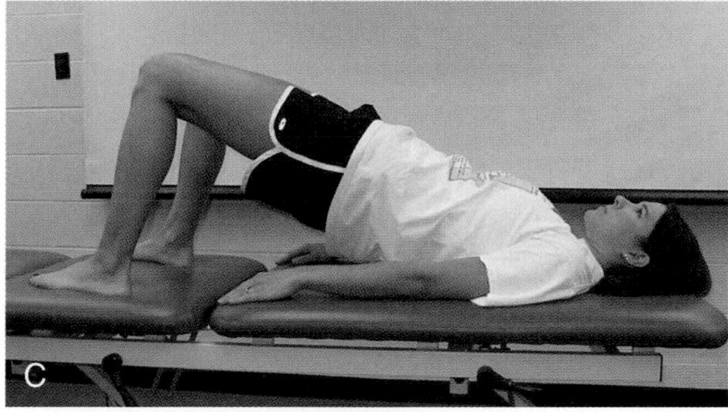

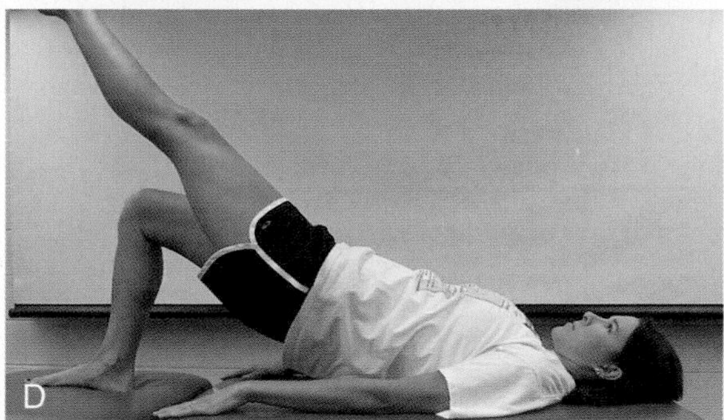

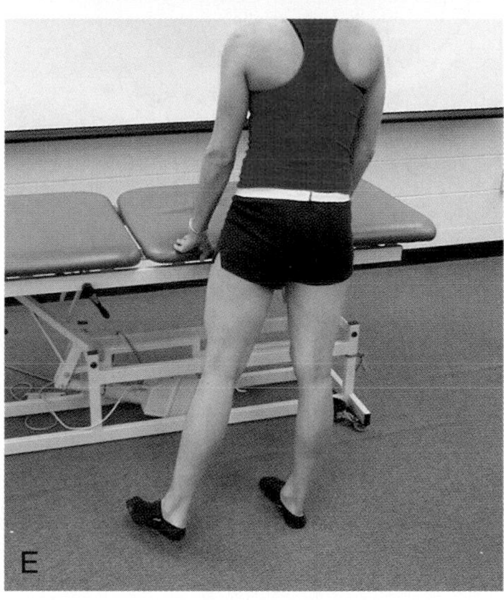

FIG 19-21 **A,** Side-lying hip abduction. **B,** Side bridge. **C,** Bilateral lower extremity bridge. **D,** Single lower extremity bridge. **E,** Standing hip abduction.

1. The iliac crest is contused by direct contact from an external force or falling on the exposed iliac crest.
2. There is a sudden forceful contraction or overstretching of the muscles attached to the iliac crest.[12] This seemingly minor injury can be severe, causing extreme pain and dysfunction.

First, the patient is treated with protection, rest, ice, gentle compression wraps, crutches, and PWB. Initial soft tissue healing must proceed without delay, so extreme caution is warranted to guard against unwanted forces or stress to the affected area. Stretching and strengthening of the affected hip can begin when soft tissue healing has progressed and pain is controlled. Usually in the moderate-protection phase, ultrasound, hydrotherapy, electrical stimulation, phonophoresis, or iontophoresis can be used at the discretion of the physician and PT to help control pain and swelling.

FRACTURES OF THE PELVIS AND ACETABULUM

General principles dealing with pelvic fractures and their classification with acetabular fractures dramatically show the PTA the extensive and potentially life-threatening nature of these injuries.[11,21,22] This discussion outlines the profound complications that may occur with pelvic fractures, giving the PTA a better understanding of the long-term rehabilitation needed in many cases of severe fractures.

The most basic classification of pelvic fractures refers to the injury as either stable or unstable.[11,21,22] Stable fractures

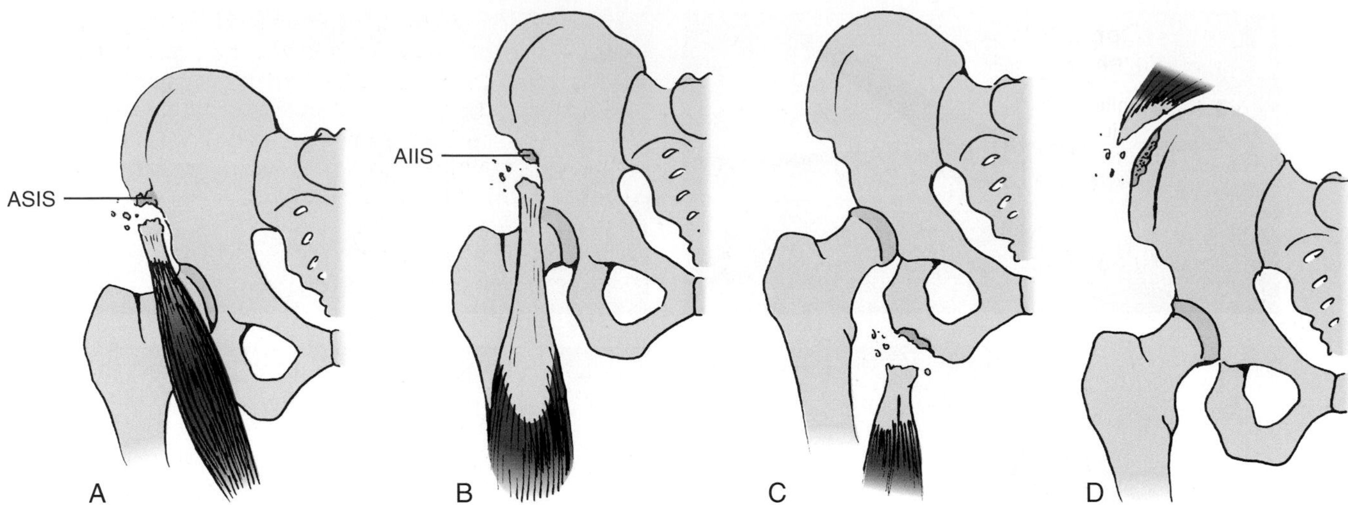

FIG 19-22 **A,** Avulsion fracture of anterior superior iliac spine. **B,** Avulsion fracture of anterior inferior iliac spine. **C,** Avulsion fracture of ischial tuberosity. **D,** Avulsion fracture of iliac crest.

include avulsion-type fractures of the anterior superior iliac spine, anterior inferior iliac spine, ischial tuberosity, and iliac crest (Fig. 19-22).[11,21] Avulsion fractures of the pelvis can be treated conservatively with rest, protected weight bearing, crutches, and avoidance of premature stretching and resistive exercises, which may delay bony union (usually within 6 weeks).[11]

McRae[21] advocated ORIF with avulsion fractures of the ischial tuberosity and fragment separation greater than 2 cm, stating, "Non-union is an appreciable risk, and if this occurs there may be problems with chronic pain and disability." Usually avulsion fractures of the ischial tuberosity can be treated with rest, keeping the hip extended and externally rotated to avoid continued stress on the healing bone and enforcing protected weight bearing for approximately 6 weeks.[21] When secure bone healing has been established, the PT may direct the assistant to carry out a gentle, progressive flexibility program to regain hip flexion. Strengthening exercises are added when the physician confirms radiographic evidence of secure union of the avulsion.

Other stable pelvic fractures include fractures of the superior pubic ramus, superior and inferior pubic rami on one side, and ilium (Fig. 19-23).[21] In general, stable fractures of the pelvis are treated nonsurgically with protection, bed rest (2 to 3 weeks),[21] and progressive motion and exercise when stable bone union has been confirmed.

Unstable pelvic fractures usually can be defined as either rotationally unstable but vertically stable or rotationally and vertically unstable.[21] These severe injuries can be treated with an external fixator, ORIF, or extended convalescence including bed rest.[11,21,22] The PTA must be aware of complications after unstable pelvic fractures that can influence the time to begin rehabilitation procedures and can require protracted periods of recovery before physical therapy interventions. Box 19-2 outlines complications associated with these potentially life-threatening injuries.

The rehabilitation program employed after pelvic fractures is individualized and specific to the type and severity of fracture and the methods used to stabilize the fracture (ORIF, external fixator, and long-term convalescence). Because of the fragile hemodynamic nature of significant pelvic fractures, weight bearing of any kind is deferred for 8 weeks or longer.[21]

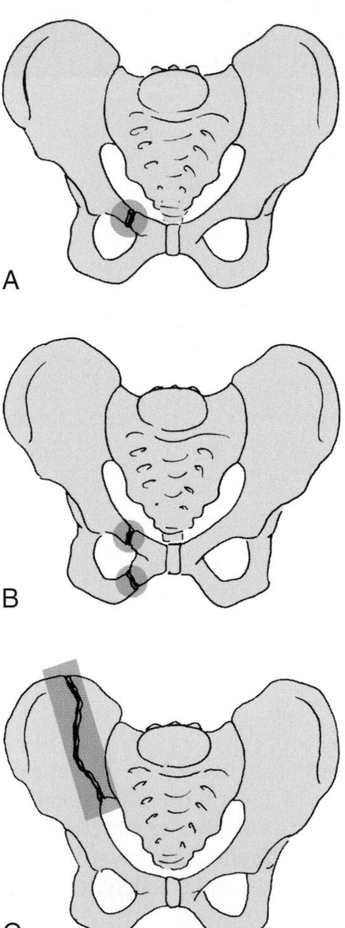

FIG 19-23 **A,** Fracture of superior pubic ramus. **B,** Fracture of superior and inferior pubic ramus on one side. **C,** Fracture of ilium.

BOX 19-2 Complications after Pelvic Fractures

1. Hemorrhage (significant blood loss, shock)
2. Gastrointestinal injury
3. Diaphragm rupture
4. Bony malunion (limb length shortening)
5. Nonunion
6. Neurologic damage
7. Degenerative joint disease
8. Infection (sepsis)

From Miller M: Adult reconstruction and sports medicine. In *Review of orthopaedics,* Philadelphia, 1992, Saunders; McRae R: *Practical fracture treatment,* ed 3, New York, 1994, Churchill Livingstone.

Initially, the patient may be introduced to the vertical position using a tilt table. Pulse, respiration, and blood pressure are carefully monitored by the PTA as directed by the PT. Postural hypotension can be adequately addressed by gradually increasing the duration of elevation by small increments under the PT's direction. Maintenance of joint mobility is addressed early after surgery and during long periods of immobilization.

Active bilateral upper extremity ROM begins as soon as the patient's condition is stable. Lower extremity motion is limited to bilateral ankle pumps, gentle knee motion, and limited hip motion, depending on the nature of the fracture, fixation techniques used, stabilization of visceral damage (if any), and direction of the physician and PT. The most significant clinical features associated with pelvic fractures are the potentially life-threatening complications, which can be acute or arise during early recovery or just after the acute phase of the injury. The PTA must closely supervise all vital signs before, during, and after all rehabilitation procedures. When the physician has determined that the fracture site is stable and healed and the patient is medically stable, the PT may direct the PTA to follow a gradual program of general strength and fitness (a high priority with all patients requiring protracted periods of immobilization), quadriceps strengthening, hip motion, gait training, bed mobility, and transfer training.

Fractures of the pelvis also can involve the acetabulum. The acetabulum has an articular cartilage surface that allows for articulation between the femoral head and acetabulum. Care of this area is extremely important because the hip joint is a major weight-bearing structure.

The classification system used to identify specific patterns of acetabular fractures is defined by Loth[18] as the Letournel classification model (Fig. 19-24). Generally, these fractures are treated according to the severity of the fracture, usually with ORIF or conservatively with bed rest and traction to reduce compression of the joint.[21] Conservative management of acetabular fractures is reserved for severely fragmented acetabular floor fractures in which surgery cannot realign the fragments for anatomic reconstruction of the articular surface.[21] ORIF is used to stabilize the fracture in all other cases.[18]

Protected weight bearing is encouraged for 8 to 10 weeks; in cases of nonsurgical management, weight bearing is permitted at 9 weeks. A lower extremity strength program is initiated immediately after surgery and involves ankle motion, quadriceps sets, hamstring sets, gentle submaximal gluteal sets, and active knee and hip motion. As with all fractures, as bone healing progresses and the patient achieves individualized criteria (e.g., strength, motion, reduced pain, minimal swelling, increased weight bearing, and normalized gait), the rehabilitation program can be advanced, gradually incorporating more challenging functional exercises.

The PTA must remember the nature of specific acetabular fractures because these fractures involve articular cartilage and bone. The initiation of closed chain functional activities, which naturally require vertical loads, may be deferred for longer periods to allow for appropriate articular cartilage healing. If premature loads are directed through the weight-bearing surface of the affected articular cartilage of the acetabulum, delayed union may result.

Important Concepts

With all injuries and dysfunctions of the hip and their rehabilitation, the PTA must understand the indications, contraindications, and precautions for each exercise implemented. Constant communication with the supervising PT, patient, and physician is required.

COMMON MOBILIZATION TECHNIQUES FOR THE HIP

Reduced motion secondary to pain and fibrosis after fractures, soft tissue injuries, and various hip arthroplasty techniques may warrant mobilization in conjunction with thermal agents, strengthening, stretching, and functional activities. The techniques presented here are identified by the PT as appropriate techniques to use based on pathology, the presence of pain, or defined limitations of movement. As with all mobilization techniques, the PT selects which techniques to use and the direction of force, amplitude, grades, velocity, and distractions (see Chapter 15).

Most important, patient comfort and compliance with relaxation before and throughout the treatment are of paramount concern. Before each treatment session, the patient should be placed in the most comfortable position with attention paid to supporting the affected limb. The application of thermal agents (e.g., hot packs or ultrasound) to the affected limb and surrounding structures may be helpful to compose and relax the patient before treatment. If the patient has physician-prescribed pain medications or muscle relaxants, it may be helpful to consult with the PT to suggest that the patient take these medications in a timely fashion before treatment to enhance relaxation further.

Other general rules of mobilization for the hip joint that should be implemented include the following:

- Warming of the tissues and body through exercise is advisable.
- Both the patient and the PTA must be in the correct position, relaxed, and at ease.

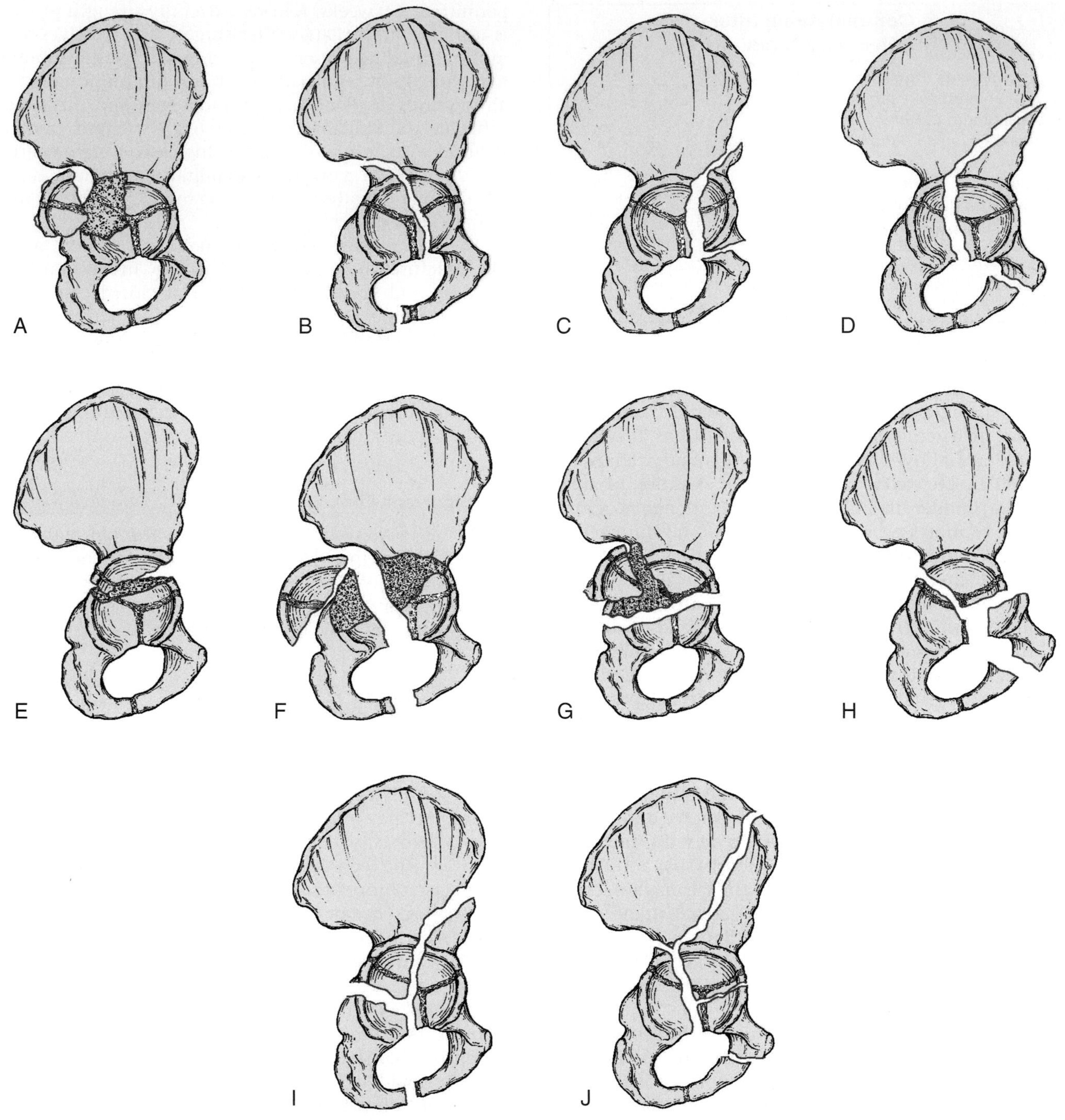

FIG 19-24 Letournel classification of acetabular fractures. Simple: posterior wall **(A)**, posterior column **(B)**, anterior wall **(C)**, anterior column **(D)**, transverse **(E)**. Combined: posterior column and posterior wall **(F)**, transverse and posterior wall **(G)**, T-shaped **(H)**, anterior column and posterior hemitransverse **(I)**, both columns **(J)**. *(From Green N, Swiontkowski M:* Skeletal trauma in children, *ed 4, Philadelphia, 2009, Saunders.)*

- All techniques must be modified to suit both PTA and the patient.
- Whenever possible, the patient's body weight should serve as a means of stabilization to prevent unwanted movement.
- Hand placement for mobilization should be as close to the joint as possible, with a firm but comfortable grasp.
- Visualizing the joint surface, its direction, and contour can assist the PTA in correctly performing the technique.
- Whenever possible on hip joint mobilizations, the forearms should be positioned in line with the direction of the mobilization force to be applied.
- The PTA must use the minimum of force consistent with achieving the objective.

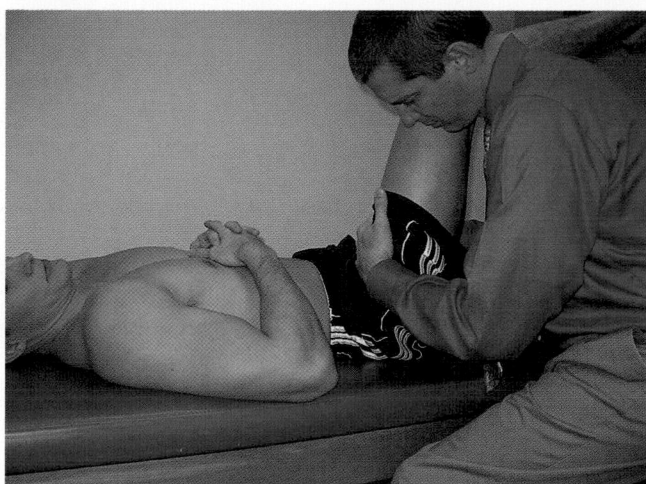

FIG 19-25 Distraction.

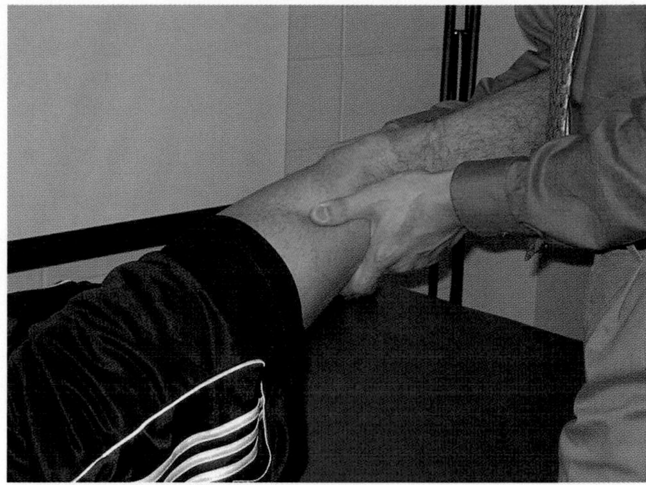

FIG 19-26 Inferior glide (long-axis distraction).

- Signs of overmobilization are:
  - Increase in pain.
  - Increase in swelling.
  - Decrease in mobility.

DISTRACTION

- *Patient position:* Supine with the leg positioned over the clinician's shoulder, hip in resting position.
- *PTA position:* Standing to side of the leg to be mobilized facing the patient's hip.
- *Stabilization:* The rest of the body on the table serves as stabilizing force. A belt may be wrapped around the patient's pelvis and the treatment table to help stabilize the pelvis.
- *Mobilization:* Position both hands on anterior and medial surfaces of the proximal thigh. Both hands move the femoral head away from the acetabulum at a 90° angle.
- *Direction of force:* Impart a caudal/inferior and lateral force to the hip joint by leaning back away from the patient (Fig. 19-25).
- *Suggestions:*
  - Maintain mobilizing and stabilizing hand as proximal to hip joint as possible.
  - Hip joint is positioned in as close to the resting position as possible if conservative techniques are indicated. Approximating restricted ROM can be used if more aggressive techniques are indicated by PT.

INFERIOR GLIDE (LONG-AXIS DISTRACTION)

- *Patient position:* Supine on table, lumbar spine side-bent away from side to be mobilized.
- *PTA position:* Standing at the patient's foot facing the patient's hip.
- *Stabilization:* The rest of the body on the table serves as stabilizing force, especially with the lumbar spine side-bent away. A belt may be wrapped around the patient's pelvis and the treatment table to help stabilize the pelvis.
- *Mobilization:* Grab patient's leg proximal to the knee (supracondylar ridges of femur) with both hands. Distraction force in caudal direction imposed via both hands. PTA can lean back and use entire body for more aggressive mobilization if prescribed by PT.
- *Direction of force:* Directly inferior and along longitudinal axis from hip joint imparted via PTA body leaning back.
  - The result is distraction of the head of the femur away from the acetabulum (Fig. 19-26).

POSTERIOR GLIDE

- *Patient position:* Supine with arms relaxed. Patient's dysfunctional side is flexed so that the foot is placed on the table just lateral to the noninvolved knee.
- *PTA position:* Standing on side opposite of dysfunction, directly facing the patient.
- *Stabilization:* Patient resting on table serves as stabilization. The dysfunctional lower extremity is placed in a position of flexion, adduction, and internal rotation such that the foot is placed on the table as stated under "Patient position."
- *Mobilization:* PTA places bilateral hands on top of the knee on the dysfunctional side.
- *Direction of force:* Mobilization is imparted to the posterolateral hip and capsule through the long axis of the femur. Mobilization force is via PTA's body through his or her hands (Fig. 19-27).
- *Suggestions:*
  - This technique can be progressed by adding more flexion, adduction, or internal rotation, eventually crossing mobilizing foot over other lower extremity.
  - Maintain good body mechanics to improve mobilization force.
  - Place a towel under ilium for greater posterior hip stretch.

ANTERIOR GLIDE IN FLEXION, ABDUCTION, AND EXTERNAL ROTATION

- *Patient position:* Prone on table with dysfunctional hip in a position of flexion, abduction, and external rotation.
- *PTA position:* Standing on side of dysfunction. Contact the proximal femur just distal to greater trochanter.

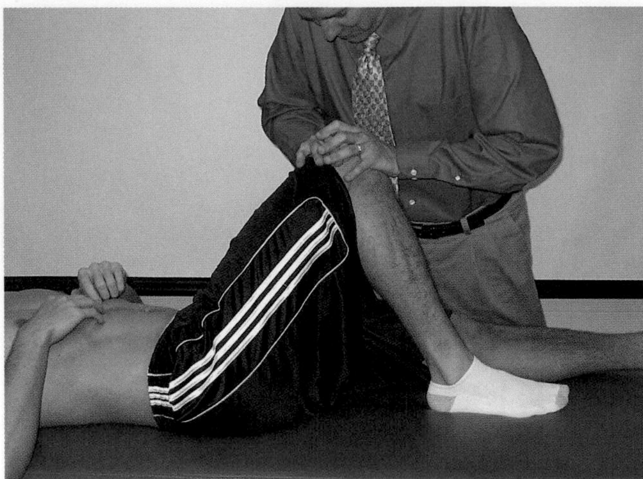

FIG 19-27 Posterior glide.

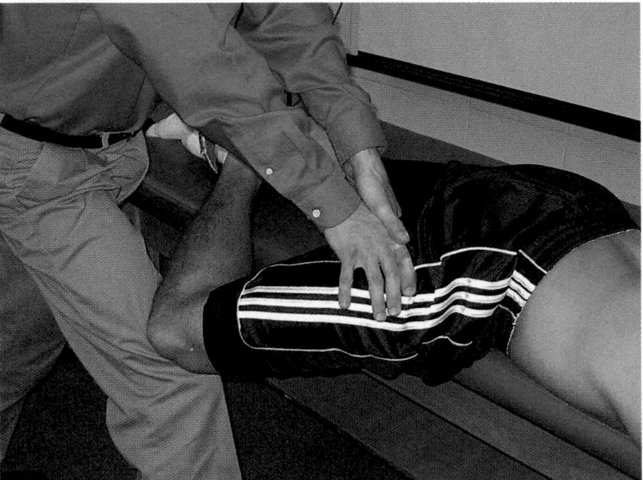

FIG 19-28 Anterior glide in flexion, abduction, and external rotation.

- *Stabilization:* Patient's body resting on table serves as stabilizing force. A belt may be wrapped around patient's pelvis and treatment table to help stabilize pelvis.
- *Mobilization:* Mobilizing force is imparted to hip through the proximal femur using passive accessory glides from posterior to anterior.
- *Direction of force:* Passive accessory glides imparted from posterior to anterior (Fig. 19-28). Direction may also be imparted anterior-medial depending on direction of restriction. Consider joint surface with mobilization.
- *Suggestions:*
  - Maintain mobilizing and stabilizing hand as proximal to hip joint as possible.
  - Maintain mobilizing elbow in full extension to use entire body as mobilizing force in contrast to using only mobilizing upper extremity.

Important Concepts

As with exercise, the PTA must clearly understand the need, indications, contraindications, and precautions when implementing manual therapy techniques on a patient. Careful and constant communication with the supervising PT is necessary.

GLOSSARY

Comminuted fracture: A fracture with more than two fracture fragments.

Delayed union: Complication of subtrochanteric fractures characterized by any time that a fracture fails to unite in a normal time frame.

Displaced fracture: Any fracture in which there is loss of contact between surfaces.

Hip osteoarthritis: The focal loss of articular cartilage with variable subchondral bone reaction.

Malunion: Complication of subtrochanteric fractures characterized by a fracture in which successful union has occurred, but a degree of angular or rotary deformity exists.

Nonunion avascular necrosis: Complication of subtrochanteric fractures characterized by when blood supply to bone or segment of bone is compromised, leading to bone death.

Osteitis pubis: A disorder characterized by pain and bony erosion of the symphysis pubis.

Osteonecrosis: Subchondral bone necrosis secondary to vascular insufficiency.

Pubalgia: Term referring to all disorders causing chronic pain in the region of the pubic tubercle and inguinal region.

Simple fracture: A fracture in which the skin and soft tissues overlying the skin are intact.

REFERENCES

1. Bolgla L, Uhl TL: Electromyographic analysis of hip rehabilitation exercises in a group of healthy subjects. *J Orthop Sport Phys Ther* 35(8):487–494, 2005.
2. Cibulka MT, White DM, Woehrle J: Hip pain and mobility deficits—hip osteoarthritis: clinical practice guidelines. *J Orthop Sports Phys Ther* 39(4):A1–A25, 2009.
3. Corrigan B, Maitland GD: The hip. In *Practical orthopaedic medicine*, Newton, MA, 1992, Butterworth-Heinemann.
4. Cummings SR, Nevitt MC: A hypothesis: the causes of hip fractures. *J Gerontol* 44:M107–M111, 1989.
5. Ekstrom R, Donatelli R, Carp K: Electromyographical analysis of core trunk, hip, and thigh muscles during 9 rehabilitation exercises. *J Orthop Sport Phys Ther* 37(12):754–762, 2007.
6. Ekstrom RA, Osborn RW, Hauer PL: Surface electromyographic analysis of the low back muscles during rehabilitation exercises. *J Orthop Sports Phys Ther* 38(12):736–745, 2008.
7. Elmerson S, Zetterberg C, Andersson G: Ten-year survival after fractures of the proximal end of the femur. *Gerontology* 34:186–191, 1988.
8. Fricker PA, Taunton JE, Ammann W: Osteitis pubis in athletes. Infection, inflammation or injury? *Sports Med* 12:266–279, 1991.
9. Goldstein TS: Treatment of common problems of the hip joint. In Goldstein TS, Lewis CB, editors: *Geriatric orthopaedics: rehabilitative management of common problems*, Gaithersburg, MD, 1991, Aspen Publishers.
10. Goldstein TS: The adult and geriatric hip. In *Continuing education course notes*, Boston, 1994, Quest Seminars.
11. Gross ML, Nasser S, Finnerman GAM: Hip and pelvis. In DeLee JC, Drez D, editors: *Orthopaedic sports medicine: principles and practice*, vol 2, Philadelphia, 1994, Saunders.
12. Henry JH: The hip. In Scott WN, Nisonson B, Nicholas JA, editors: *Principles of sports medicine*, Baltimore, 1984, Williams & Wilkins.
13. Hoeksma HL, Dekker J, Ronday HK, et al: Comparison of manual therapy and exercise therapy in osteoarthritis of the hip: a randomized clinical trial. *Arthritis Rheum* 51:722–729, 2004.
14. Jette AM, Harris BA, Cleary PD, Campion EW: Functional recovery after hip fractures. *Arch Phys Med Rehabil* 68:735–740, 1987.
15. Kozinn SC, Wilson PD: Adult hip disease and total hip replacement. *Clin Symp* 39(5):1–32, 1987.

16. LeVeau B: Hip. In Richardson JK, Iglarsh ZA, editors: *Clinical orthopaedic physical therapy*, Philadelphia, 1994, Saunders.
17. Lewis CB, Bottomley JM: Orthopaedic treatment considerations. In *Geriatric physical therapy: a clinical approach*, New York, 1994, Appleton & Lange.
18. Loth TS: Lower extremity. In *Orthopedic boards review*, St Louis, 1993, Mosby.
19. MacEwen GD, Bunnell WP, Ramsey PL: The hip. In Lovell WW, Winter RB, editors: *Pediatric orthopaedics*, Philadelphia, 1986, Lippincott.
20. McDonald D, et al: Total joint reconstruction. In *Orthopedic boards review*, St Louis, 1993, Mosby.
21. McRae R: *Practical fracture treatment*, ed 3, New York, 1994, Churchill Livingstone.
22. Miller M: Adult reconstruction and sports medicine. In *Review of orthopaedics*, Philadelphia, 1992, Saunders.
23. Saudek CE: The hip. In Gould JA, editor: *Orthopaedic and sports physical therapy*, ed 2, St Louis, 1990, Mosby.
24. Tepper S, Hochberg MC: Factors associated with hip osteoarthritis: data from the first National Health and Nutrition Examination Survey (NHANES-I). *Am J Epidemiol* 137:1081–1088, 1993.

REVIEW QUESTIONS

Multiple Choice

1. With hip flexion, the normal ROM is:
   a. 150°.
   b. 140°.
   c. 110°.
   d. 90°.
2. Hip extension normal ROM is:
   a. 5°.
   b. 10°.
   c. 15°.
   d. 20°.
3. Hip internal and external rotation ROM normally is:
   a. 15°.
   b. 25°.
   c. 35°.
   d. 45°.
4. Hip abduction normal ROM is:
   a. 20°.
   b. 30°.
   c. 40°.
   d. 50°.
5. Hip adduction normal ROM is:
   a. 20°.
   b. 25°.
   c. 30°.
   d. 15°.
6. Hip flexion motion requires the femoral head to glide a slight amount in the direction of:
   a. Anterior glide.
   b. Posterior glide.
   c. Superior glide.
   d. Inferior glide.
7. Hip extension motion requires the femoral head to glide a slight amount in the direction of:
   a. Anterior glide.
   b. Posterior glide.
   c. Superior glide.
   d. Inferior glide.
8. Hip internal rotation requires the femoral head to glide in the direction of:
   a. Anterior glide.
   b. Posterior glide.
   c. Superior glide.
   d. Inferior glide.
9. Hip external rotation requires the femoral head to glide in the direction of:
   a. Anterior glide.
   b. Posterior glide.
   c. Superior glide.
   d. Inferior glide.
10. Hip abduction requires the femoral head to glide in the direction of:
   a. Anterior glide.
   b. Posterior glide.
   c. Superior glide.
   d. Inferior glide.
11. Hip adduction requires the femoral head to glide in the direction of:
   a. Anterior glide.
   b. Posterior glide.
   c. Superior glide.
   d. Inferior glide.
12. Which of the following is a primary hip flexor muscle?
   a. Psoas
   b. Gluteus maximus
   c. Gluteus medius
   d. There are none
13. Which of the following is a primary hip extensor muscle?
   a. Psoas
   b. Gluteus maximus
   c. Gluteus medius
   d. There are none
14. Which of the following is a primary hip abductor?
   a. Psoas
   b. Gluteus maximus
   c. Gluteus medius
   d. There are none
15. Which of the following is a primary hip internal rotator?
   a. Psoas
   b. Gluteus maximus
   c. Gluteus medius
   d. There are none

Short Answer

16. Name the type of injury in the following figure.

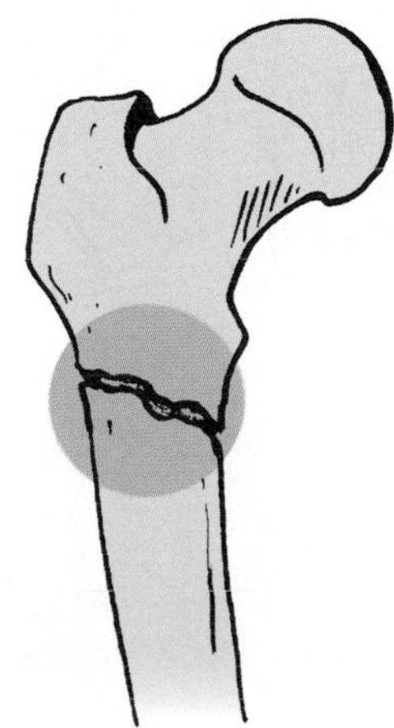

17. Name the type of injury in the following figure.

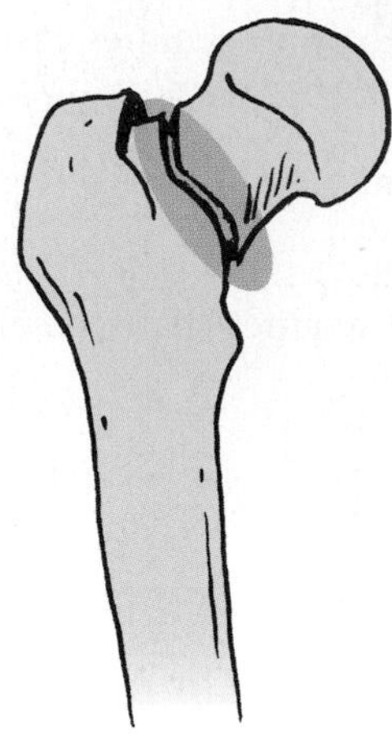

18. Name the type of injury in the following figure.

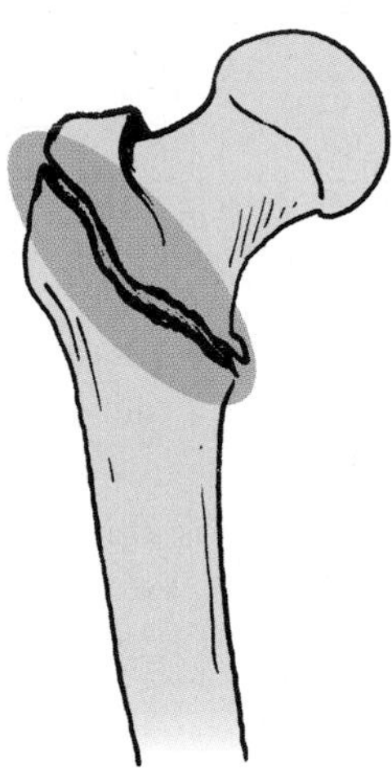

19. Name the soft tissue injury in the following figure.

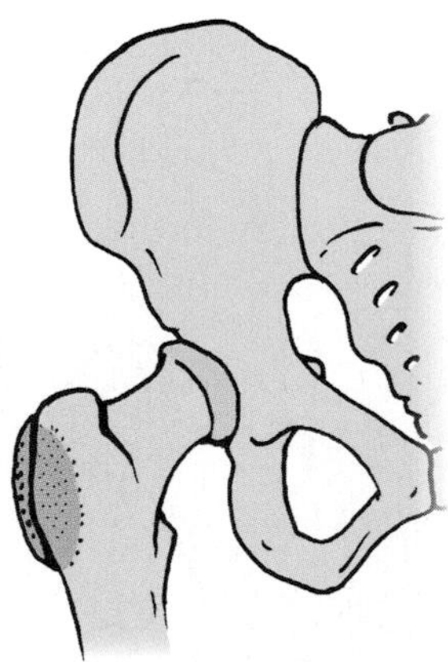

20. Name the soft tissue injury in the following figure.

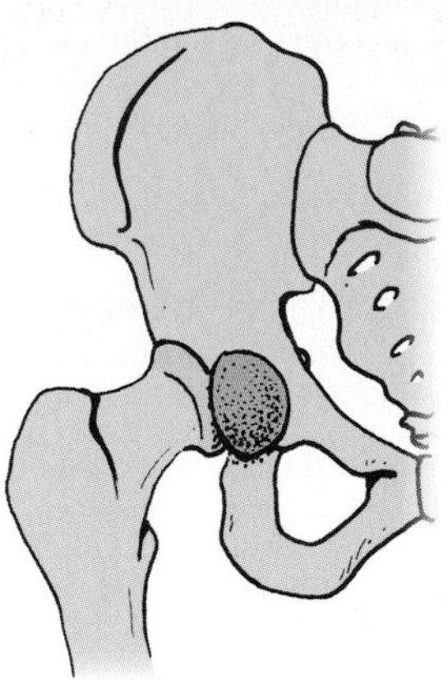

Fill in the Blank

21. A patient with restrictions of no hip flexion and no adduction past neutral likely had a _____________ approach for a THR.
22. Another commonly restricted motion for the approach identified in Question 28 is hip _____________.
23. Manual therapy for a patient with hip _____________ has shown favorable results.
24. For the patient complaining of lateral hip pain, the _____________ bursa is most likely involved.
25. The long-term complications of a flattened femoral head lead to an incongruous joint surface and advanced _____________.

True/False

26. Hip fractures represent the most common acute orthopedic injury in the geriatric population.
27. The subtrochanteric area of the hip is prone to large biomechanical stresses, which can lead to loosening of various internal fixation devices.
28. The performance of hip flexion, internal rotation, and adduction should be avoided for up to 4 months after THR surgery.
29. It is appropriate to encourage full knee extension after a hamstring strain during the first 3 weeks after injury.
30. Unstable pelvic fractures generally are defined as either rotationally unstable but vertically stable or rotationally and vertically unstable.

Chapter 20

Orthopedic Management of the Lumbar, Thoracic, and Cervical Spine

Cheryl Sparks, Joseph Kelly, Gary A. Shankman

CHAPTER OUTLINE

LEARNING OBJECTIVES

1. Outline and describe basic mechanics of the lumbar spine.
2. Discuss and apply the principles of fundamental mechanics of lifting.
3. Identify common sprains and strains of the lumbar spine.
4. Discuss common methods of management and rehabilitation of lumbar spine sprains and strains.
5. Identify and describe injuries to the lumbar intervertebral disk.
6. Define and describe methods of quantifying back strength.
7. Define and describe components of the back school model.
8. Define ergonomic and functional capacity evaluations.
9. Define spinal stenosis and describe methods of management and rehabilitation.
10. Define and contrast the terms *spondylolysis* and *spondylolisthesis*.
11. Describe methods of management and rehabilitation for spondylolysis and spondylolisthesis.
12. Identify common lumbar and thoracic spine fractures.
13. Define kyphosis, lordosis, and scoliosis.
14. Identify and describe methods of management and rehabilitation for kyphosis and scoliosis.
15. Identify and describe common cervical spine injuries, and discuss methods of management and rehabilitation.

KEY TERMS

Annulus
Directional preference
Disk
Disk protrusion
Extruded disk
Herniated nucleus pulposus (HNP)
Kyphosis
Lordosis
Nucleus pulposus
Radiculopathy
Scoliosis
Sequestrated disk
Spine stabilization
Thoracic inlet syndrome
Treatment-based classification (TBC)

In an age when health care expenditures are a concern for many, back pain continues to cost billions of dollars in intervention and lost labor.[43,46] It is imperative that the physical therapist assistant (PTA) possess a sound understanding of the anatomy and appropriate management of patients with various spinal disorders. In this chapter, the PTA is introduced to overall symptoms and effective intervention strategies for some of the more prevalent diagnoses affecting the spine.

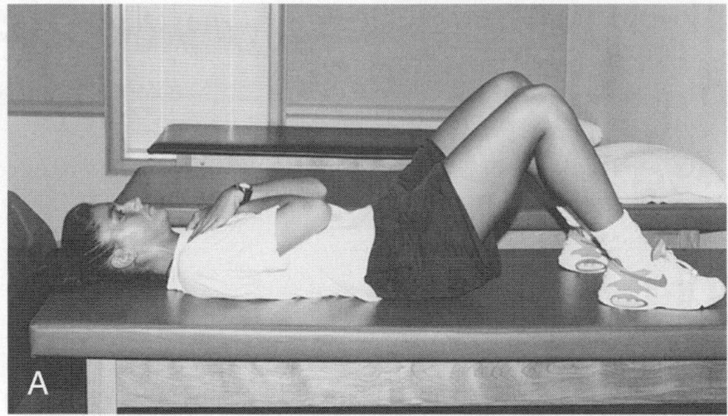

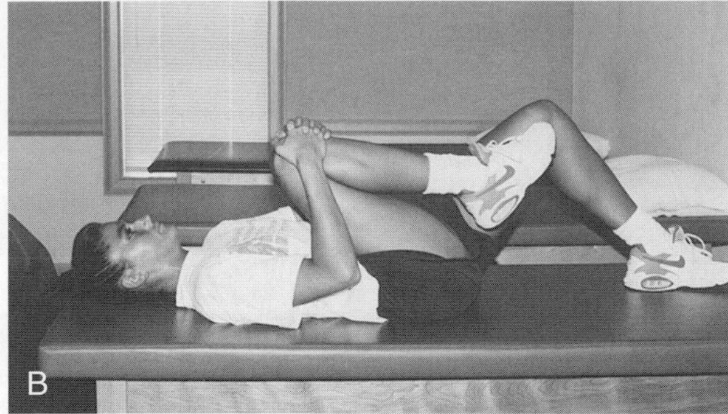

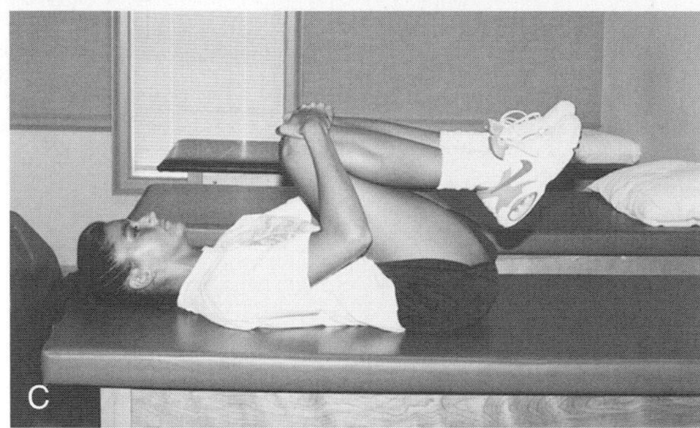

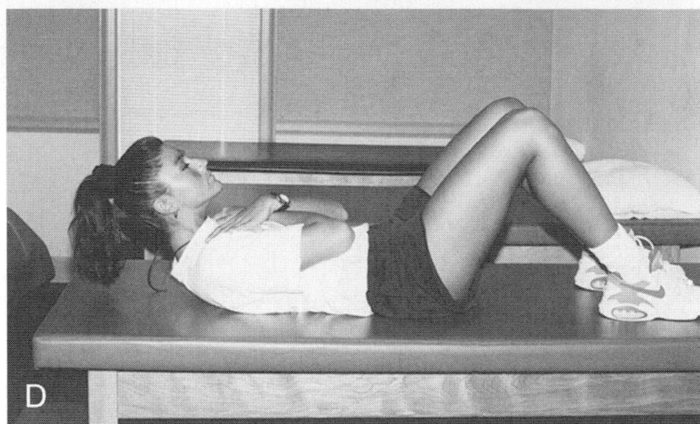

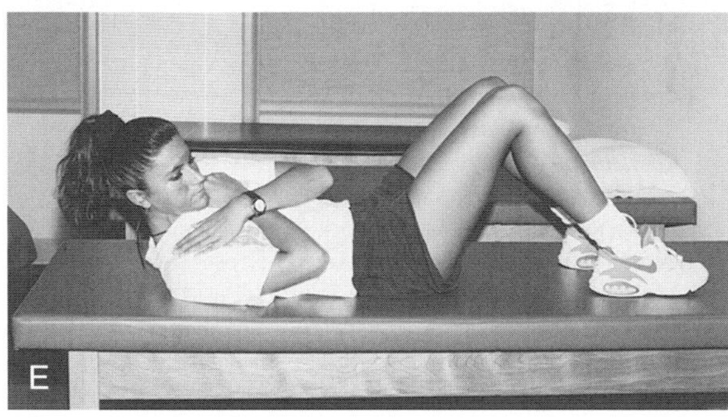

FIG 20-1 Williams flexion exercises. **A,** Pelvic tilt. **B,** Single knee to chest. **C,** Double knee to chest. **D,** Partial direct sit-ups. **E,** Partial oblique sit-ups.

LUMBAR SPINE

Perhaps no other medical condition draws as much attention from researchers and clinicians as the identification and management of lumbar spine injuries. The primary cause of disability in middle-aged working class adults is related to low-back pain and accounts for approximately $50 billion in health care costs annually in the United States.[26,43,46] Lumbar spine injuries are also to blame for millions of lost work days per year in the United States and internationally. The rate of disability from injuries to the low back was estimated over a 10-year period to be 14 times greater than the rate of population growth for that same period.[1,15] Overall, lumbar spine injuries are the second leading cause of all physician visits in the United States, and the prevalence of low-back pain in the population is close to that of the common cold.[1,5,8,16,17,43]

Historically, absolute bed rest, medications, thermal agents (e.g., hot packs or ultrasound), and a series of rudimentary lumbar flexion exercises (e.g., pelvic tilts, single knee-to-chest, double knee-to-chest, and partial direct and oblique sit-ups) (Fig. 20-1) were the components of a typical protocol for lumbar sprains, strains, and disk-related pathologic conditions. It is now widely accepted that active rest and resumption of function have a significant impact on improving long-term outcomes.[20,24]

Important Concept

Overall, lumbar spine injuries are the second leading cause of all physician visits in the United States, and the prevalence of low-back pain in the population is close to that of the common cold.[1,5,8,16,17,43]

BASIC MECHANICS

The spine comprises 33 bones, which increase in size caudally. There are five regions: cervical, thoracic, lumbar, sacral, and coccyx. Components of the axial skeleton include osseous (bony) and nonosseous structures. Osseous structures include the vertebrae, and nonosseous structures include the intervertebral disks and the surrounding ligaments. Together these make up the normal spinal curves that define posture. These curves function to absorb shock and balance the center of gravity. The typical spinal vertebra has two portions: the body, which assists in weight bearing, and the vertebral arch, which protects the spinal cord. There are also facet joints, or zygapophyseal joints, which guide range of motion (ROM) in the spine. These joints are plane joints, which glide relative to one another. The inferior aspect of the superior facet joint articulates with the superior aspect of the inferior facet joint. ROM is determined by the orientation of the facet joint. For example, in the cervical spine, the facet joints are more horizontal in alignment, which allows for increased rotation. In the lumbar spine, the joints have a vertical orientation, which allows for flexion and extension.

Important Concept

The inferior aspect of the superior facet joint articulates with the superior aspect of the inferior facet joint. ROM is determined by the orientation of the facet joint.

In the adult spine, there are 23 intervertebral disks found in between the vertebral bodies (Fig. 20-2). The outer wall of the **disk** is the **annulus** and comprises 12 to 18 concentrically arranged rings of fibroelastic cartilage.[30,57] Contained within the annulus is the **nucleus pulposus**. Nuclear material is a mucopolysaccharide gel[30] that transmits forces, equalizes stress, and promotes movement.[56] The annulus provides stability, enhanced movement between vertebral bodies, and minimal shock absorption. The greater portion of shock absorption comes from the vertebral body.[57,66] The intervertebral disk is largely avascular and aneural. The vascular supply to the disk is provided by diffusion from the vertebral bodies above and below the disk.[14,30,50,57] The outer one third of the annulus is said to be innervated along with the facet joint capsule and exiting nerve roots.[14] When injured, without an intense vascular response, the disk has a limited capacity to heal and repair. In addition, degenerative changes occur within the disk as a normal process of aging throughout the life span.

A popular theoretical model describes the fluid mechanics of the disk (nucleus pulposus) influenced by the motion of the lumbar vertebral segments. McKenzie[50] described flexion and extension motion of the spine as having clinically significant effects on the direction of movement of the nucleus (Fig. 20-3, *A*). The theoretical model proposes when positional changes occur in the lumbar spine, from

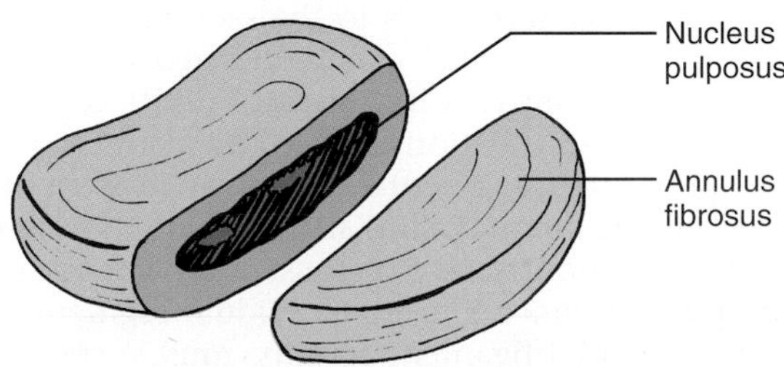

FIG 20-2 Intervertebral disk.

flexion to extension, the nucleus moves anteriorly (Fig. 20-3, *B*).[50] Conversely, when the spine moves from extension to full flexion, the nucleus tends to displace or move posteriorly (Fig. 20-3, *C*). It is necessary to understand fully the individual nature of each injury and avoid or enhance certain motions and postures as directed by the physical therapist (PT).

Important Concept

When injured, without an intense vascular response, the disk has a limited capacity to heal and repair.

The amount of motion in the spine is primarily determined by the size of the vertebral body and the disk. Ligaments, fascia, and musculature assist in restricting certain movements. The direction of motion is determined by the orientation of the facets. Spinal motions include flexion, extension, lateral flexion (side bending), and rotation.

The lumbar spine is composed of five anterior convex and posterior concave segments that produce the recognizable lordotic curve. Normal **lordosis** is increased with spinal extension and reduced with spinal flexion. The lumbar spine serves to support the weight of the upper body and dissipate compressive loads with minimal production of muscular torque. As a result, significant forces are transmitted through the intervertebral disk during certain motions. Allman[1] described lumbar motion and postural alterations as producing significant pressure within the disk (intradiscal pressure). The compressive forces that influence intradiscal pressure are as follows[1]:

- Standing: Disk pressure is equal to 100% of body weight.
- Supine: Disk pressure is less than 25% of body weight.
- Side-lying: Disk pressure is less than 75% of body weight.
- Standing and bending forward: Disk pressure is approximately 150% of body weight.
- Supine with both knees flexed: Disk pressure is less than 35% of body weight.
- Seated in a flexed position: Disk pressure is approximately 85% of body weight.
- Bending forward in a flexed posture and lifting: Disk pressure is close to 275% of body weight.

Intradiscal pressure also can be expressed in terms of pressure or load measured within the intervertebral lumbar disk. Cailliet[9] reported that isometric abdominal sets produce approximately 110 kg of pressure within the disk, whereas walking produces 85 kg; sitting, 100 kg; and bilateral straight leg raises in supine position, 120 kg; lifting with a flexed torso and knees held straight produces an astounding 340 kg of intradiscal pressure. This information may help clarify the rationale for protective postures, lifting protocols, and appropriate body mechanics as well as prescribed exercises for specific lumbar spine conditions. The PTA is encouraged to review thoroughly the anatomic relationships among the lumbar vertebral bodies, disks, spinal canal, and nerve roots.

Muscle Strains

Spinal musculature includes the dorsally located superficial and deep paravertebral muscles. Deep paravertebral

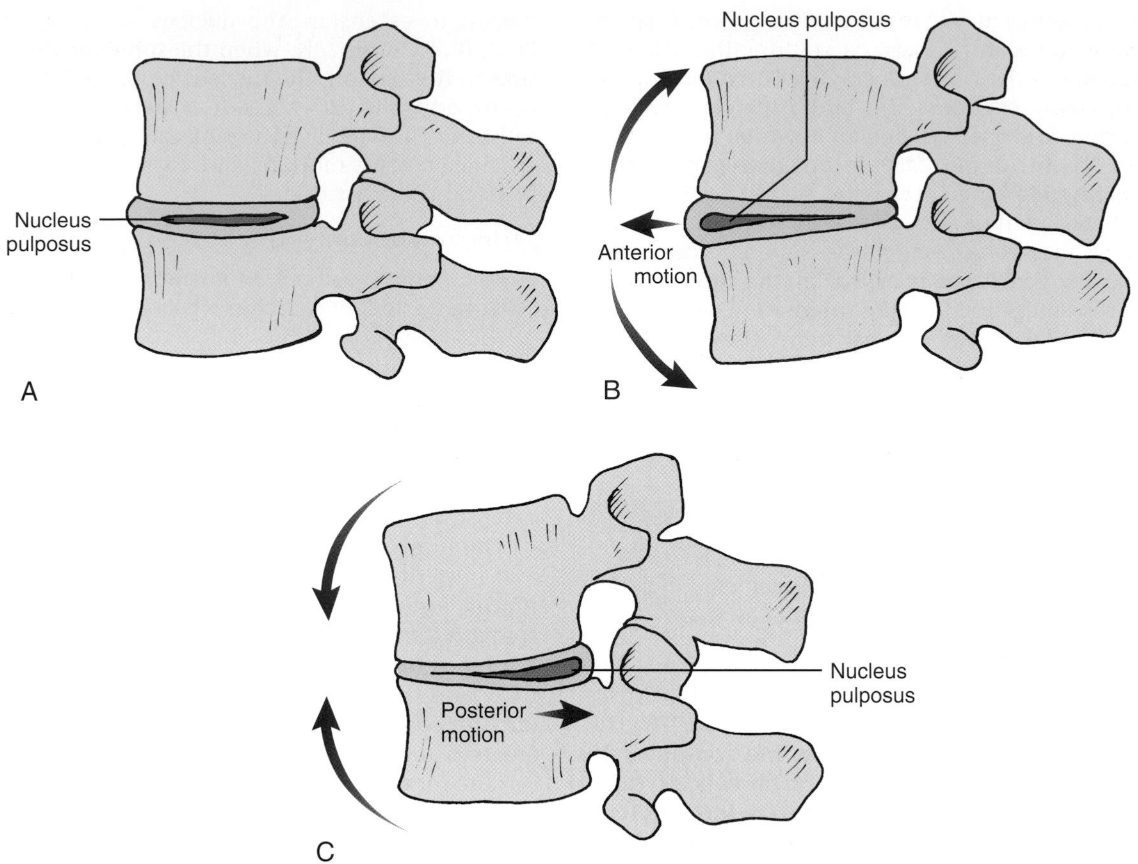

FIG 20-3 Movement of the nucleus pulposus. **A,** Stasis. **B,** Spinal flexion to extension. **C,** Spinal flexion to extension.

muscles include the semispinalis, splenius, multifidi, rotatores, interspinales, and intertransversarii. The more superficially located muscles include iliocostalis, longissimus, and spinalis. Anteriorly positioned are the rectus abdominis, the internal and external obliques, and the transversus abdominis. Injury to the muscles of the lumbar spine can be caused by sudden, violent contraction (e.g., attempting to lift a heavy object), rapid stretching, combined lumbar extension and rotation (torque), eccentric loading, and repetitive overuse resulting in microscopic damage to the muscle.

Although some authorities[27] point out that most low-back–related dysfunction results from soft tissue injury, many other structures can potentially be involved (e.g., ligaments, disk, nerve tissue, bone), and often the exact pathoanatomic cause of pain is elusive. However, the function of the lumbar spine musculature is to contribute to dynamic stability.[56] Panjabi and co-workers[56] identified the need for specific low-back strengthening to reduce injury and "to stabilize the spine within its normal physiologic motions."

Muscle strains of the lumbar spine are common, and general treatment goals are as follows[63]: reduce or eliminate inflammation (pain and swelling), restore muscle strength and control, restore flexibility, enhance cardiorespiratory fitness, restore function, and protect the affected area from further injury through education and supervised practice of proper lifting mechanics.

Ligament Sprains

Ligamentous support to the lumbar spine consists of the anterior longitudinal ligament (ALL), the posterior longitudinal ligament (PLL), the ligamentum flavum, the interspinous ligament, and the supraspinous ligament. The ALL runs anteriorly along the vertebral body blending with the annulus of the disk to reinforce it anterolaterally. The PLL runs posteriorly along the vertebral body within the vertebral canal. It is more narrow and weaker than the ALL and offers little in terms of substantial support. The ligamentum flavum lies within the vertebral canal and connects the lamina on the vertebral arch of adjacent vertebrae. The interspinous ligament lies between the spinous processes. It is well developed in the lumbar spine but weaker than the ALL, PLL, and ligamentum flavum. The supraspinous ligament attaches the tip of a spinous process to the next spinous process, traveling from the seventh cervical vertebra (C7) to the sacrum.

These spinal ligaments[70] can be injured by a sudden violent force or from repeated stress. The PT conducts a comprehensive examination of the patient to confirm or deny the presence of segmental instability (hypermobility resulting from ligament sprain) and evaluate the degree of pain with or without active or passive movement of the lumbar spine in general or in individual segments.[1,5] In addition to isolated ligament sprains, muscle strains can be superimposed, making the identification of specific single-ligament sprains exceedingly difficult. The management of lumbar ligament sprains parallels the care of muscle strains. Each patient has specific, identified impairments and goals that must be addressed individually through the initial evaluation performed by the PT. The PTA, under the direction of the PT, must identify which specific positions are contraindicated by carefully reviewing the initial evaluation data. The short-term and long-term goals for recovery from lumbar strains and sprains emphasize protecting the spine from unwanted forces and positions.

Radiculopathy

Radiculopathy is defined as mechanical compression or inflammation of a nerve root that causes neurologic symptoms in the lower extremities. Radiculopathy can be caused by encroachment on the spinal nerve root by osteophytes or a large disk herniation. Symptoms include pain, numbness, tingling, weakness, burning, and paresthesias. This condition is frequently referred to as *sciatica* or a *pinched nerve*. However, a true radiculopathy consists of more than just pain and paresthesia; it often involves a change in reflexes, strength loss in a myotomal distribution, and sensory loss in a dermatomal distribution, which is identified by the PT during the initial examination.

Radiating pain into one or both lower extremities could signify nerve root compression from an adjacent herniated intervertebral disk. A sensitive test for nerve root compression or disk herniation requires the patient to be supine while the symptomatic leg is raised passively with the knee completely extended. This is called a *straight leg raise test*. When the uninvolved, or asymptomatic, lower extremity is tested in the same manner, this is called a *crossed straight leg raise test*. The crossed straight leg raise test has been found to be highly specific for disk herniation. These tests are considered positive only if radicular pain is increased or reproduced.[21] Any positive findings noted during the initial examination performed by the PT should be confirmed or denied.[63]

Important Concept

True radiculopathy consists of more than just pain and paresthesia; it often involves a change in reflexes, strength loss in a myotomal distribution, and sensory loss in a dermatomal distribution, which is identified by the PT during the initial examination.

LUMBAR INTERVERTEBRAL DISK PATHOLOGIES

Various terms are used to describe injuries to the disk. Although "slipped disk" is a common expression used to describe various ailments of the low back among the general population, a disk does not "slip" from within its confines between the vertebral bodies. Also incorrectly applied are the terms *disk bulge* and ***herniated nucleus pulposus (HNP)***. These terms are frequently used interchangeably. To clarify, a HNP can be defined by specific nomenclature to describe the injury more precisely. Miller[52] described the three categories of HNP as protruded, extruded, and sequestrated. In a **disk protrusion**, the nucleus bulges against an intact annulus (Fig. 20-4, *A*); this would more closely resemble the layperson's disk bulge terminology. An **extruded disk** is characterized by the nucleus extending through the annulus, but the nuclear material remains confined by the PLL (Fig. 20-4, *B*). Finally, in a **sequestrated disk**, the nucleus is free within the canal (Fig. 20-4, *C*).

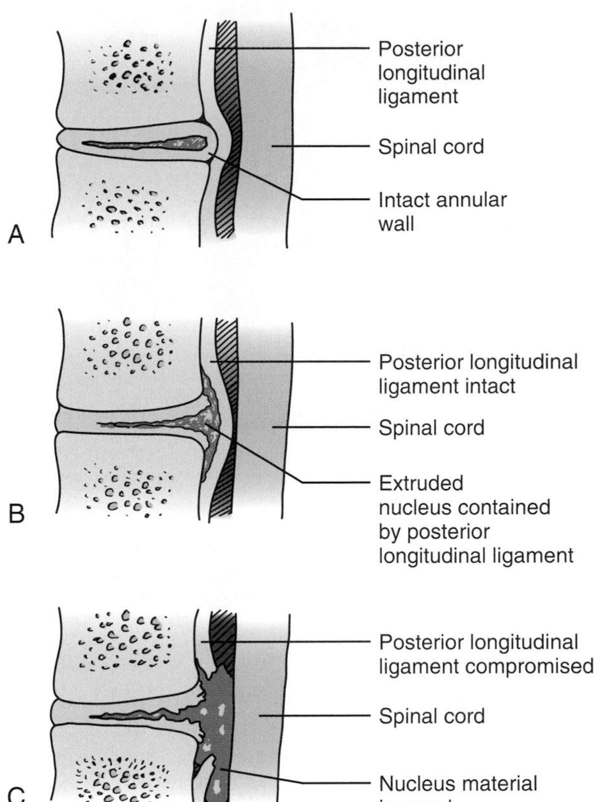

FIG 20-4 Three categories of herniated nucleus pulposus. **A,** Disk protrusion. The nucleus bulges against an intact annulus. **B,** Extruded disk. The nucleus extends through the annulus; however, the nuclear material remains confined by the posterior longitudinal ligament. **C,** Sequestrated disk. The nucleus is free within the spinal canal.

Macnab[47] offered the following variation of this classification model:

- Disk protrusion
  - Type I: Peripheral annular bulge
  - Type II: Localized annular bulge
- Disk herniation
  - Type I: Prolapsed intervertebral disk
  - Type II: Extruded intervertebral disk
  - Type III: Sequestrated intervertebral disk

In a disk protrusion, the annular fibers are intact, although the annulus bulges. A prolapsed disk has the nucleus contained only by the outer fibers of the bulging annulus.

Regardless of the exact nature of the injury, a HNP remains primarily a disease of young to middle-aged adults.[52] Common age-related degenerative changes that occur within the disk include decreased hydration, with a decreased water content from 70% to 88% by the third decade; biochemical changes in the glycosaminoglycans of the nucleus; and increases in collagen. As a result, these changes make disk herniations rare in elderly people.[52,57]

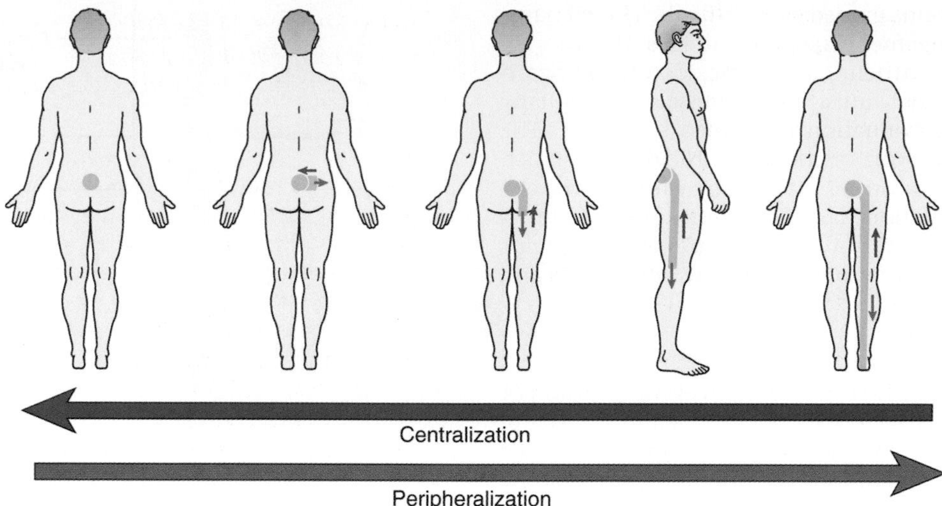

FIG 20-5 Centralization of pain is the progressive retreat of the most distal extent of referred or radicular pain toward the lumbar midline. Peripheralization of pain moves in the opposite direction. *(From Magee DJ:* Orthopedic physical assessment, *ed 5, St Louis, 2008, Saunders.)*

When examining a patient who exhibits radicular signs, the PT confirms or denies the presence of peripheralization or centralization phenomena by observing a **directional preference.**[42,50] These conditions identified during the initial examination are defined by Kisner and Colby[42] as follows: "When repeating the forward-bending test, the symptoms increase or peripheralize. Peripheralization means the symptoms are experienced further down the leg." Centralization is defined by McKenzie[50] as "the phenomenon whereby, as a result of the performance of certain repeated movements or the adoption of certain positions, radiating pain originating from the spine and referred distally, is made to move away from the periphery and toward the mid-line of the spine" (Fig. 20-5). The evaluation data obtained by the PT regarding the presence of a directional preference is essential in determining treatment.

Spondylolysis and Spondylolisthesis

Spondylolysis is a bony defect (stress fracture or fracture) in the pars interarticularis of the posterior elements of the spine (Fig. 20-6, *A*).[8,9,15,21,52,57,63] Spondylolisthesis describes a forward slippage of one superior vertebra over an inferior vertebra (usually L4-L5 and L5-S1)[18,21] as a result of instability caused by the bilateral defect in the pars interarticularis (Fig. 20-6, *B*).[8,9,15,21,52,57,63] There are specific classification types and degrees of slippage or "migration" of the vertebrae in the disease process of spondylolisthesis.[21] Five types, or classifications, have been identified, as follows:[8,21,52]

- Type I: Congenital or dysplastic. Results from a "congenital malformation of the sacrum or neural arch of L5, which allows forward slippage of L5 on the sacrum."[8] Most common in children.
- Type II: Isthmic spondylolisthesis. The most common type, affecting persons 5 to 50 years old.[52] Usually a result of mechanical stress that causes a stress fracture at the pars interarticularis.[21,52]

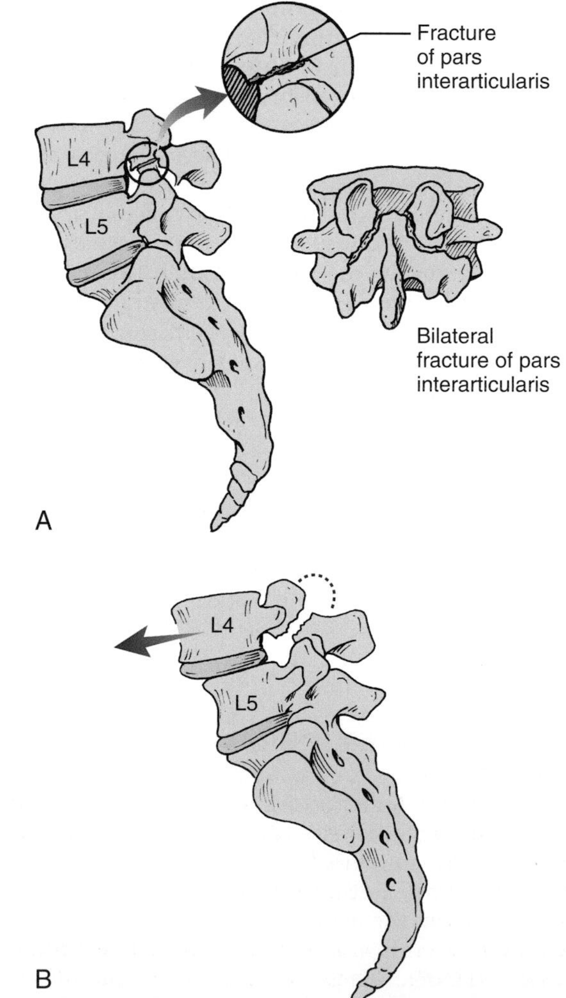

FIG 20-6 Spondylolysis and spondylolisthesis. **A,** Spondylolysis. Fracture of pars interarticularis of the posterior elements of the spine. **B,** Spondylolisthesis. The resultant forward slippage of a superior vertebra over an inferior vertebra.

- Type III: Degenerative spondylolisthesis. Most commonly affects the older population. Characterized by a loss of ligament integrity (or stability) that results in forward slippage of the vertebrae. Generally associated with the normal aging process.[8]
- Type IV: Traumatic spondylolisthesis. Caused by trauma that produces an acute fracture of the pars interarticularis. Casting is the most appropriate form of treatment.[8] This type usually affects young patients because of their generally high levels of physical activity.[52]
- Type V: Pathologic spondylolisthesis. Characterized by bone tumors that affect the pars interarticularis.

The degree or grade of slippage is determined radiographically by the examining physician and is defined as the amount of forward displacement of the superior vertebrae over the inferior vertebrae, as follows:[8,15,52]

- Grade I: 0 to 25%
- Grade II: 25% to 50%
- Grade III: 50% to 75%
- Grade IV: 75% to 100%

Important Concept

Spondylolysis is a bony defect (stress fracture or fracture) in the pars interarticularis of the posterior elements of the spine.[8,9,15,21,52,57,63] Spondylolisthesis describes a forward slippage of one superior vertebra over an inferior vertebra (usually L4-L5 and L5-S1)[18,21] as a result of instability caused by the bilateral defect in the pars interarticularis.[8,9,15,21,52,57,63]

The cause of the defect in the pars interarticularis is in part a congenital weakness in this area. In addition, the pars interarticularis is subjected to high levels of mechanical stress.[65,66] Authorities have also suggested that the primary initial cause of the most common type of spondylolisthesis (isthmic) is fatigue fracture of the pars interarticularis.[66]

Patients primarily report pain with extremes of lumbar motion, especially extension. The pain generally follows the belt line.[37] During examination, the PT also may identify a palpable step-off between the affected lumbar vertebrae (usually L4-L5) because of the forward slippage.[15]

The management of spondylolisthesis is dictated by symptoms and the degree of vertebral slippage (grades I to IV). For example, an adult with isthmic spondylolisthesis of radiographically determined grade I (0 to 25% slippage) may not experience significant symptoms with activity or extremes of lumbar extension. Treatment is aimed at preventing any progression to grade II (25% to 50% slippage); this usually is accomplished by instructing the patient to avoid ballistic lumbar extension and vertical loading while seated or standing so as to minimize anteriorly directed shearing forces on the spine. In addition, abdominal strengthening exercises, neutral **spine stabilization** exercises (controlled lumbar extension strengthening, isometrics, and rectus and oblique abdominal strengthening while in the neutral spine position), and stretching exercises for the trunk and lower extremities are encouraged.

Important Concept

The management of spondylolisthesis is dictated by symptoms and the degree of vertebral slippage (grades I to IV).

The patient may require more specific attention when there is a greater degree of slippage with significant symptoms. Generally, pain and muscle spasm are addressed with physician-prescribed analgesics, muscle relaxants, nonsteroidal antiinflammatory drugs (NSAIDs), and agents (heat, ice, ultrasound, and electrical stimulation) to alleviate acute pain and swelling. If the pain is related to a fatigue fracture of the pars interarticularis, initial treatment focuses on managing stress to the fracture site using a lumbosacral corset or orthosis, which reduces anterior shearing forces through the fracture site and allows for bone healing.[21,37]

The cornerstone in the care of spondylolisthesis is application of abdominal and paravertebral muscle strengthening exercises to provide dynamic support for the spine during activity and avoidance of extreme lumbar extension. A young active patient must modify activities that directly influence the course of this disease. For example, weightlifting without proper precaution can contribute significantly to the occurrence of spondylolysis.[19]

Important Concept

The cornerstone in the care of spondylolisthesis is application of abdominal and paravertebral muscle strengthening exercises to provide dynamic support for the spine during activity and avoidance of extreme lumbar extension.

Surgery is rarely performed and usually is reserved for patients with radicular symptoms and high-grade slippage (grades III or IV), which compresses the nerve roots and causes neurologic signs.[8,52] The type of surgery advocated in these cases is a decompression laminectomy (to reduce compression of the nerve roots) with fusion to stabilize the vertebral segments.[8,52]

Rehabilitation after surgery for spondylolisthesis is deferred until solid bony union is determined radiographically. The patient is usually in a lumbosacral orthosis that does not permit lumbar extension. During immobilization, the patient can ambulate as tolerated and perform rudimentary ROM and strengthening exercises for the upper and lower extremities (ankle pumps, quadriceps sets, and knee ROM). When bone healing is confirmed, a gradually progressive program of abdominal strengthening (from isometrics to concentric and eccentric abdominal contractions), lumbar ROM (avoiding dynamic, ballistic, and extreme lumbar extension), general conditioning, and a progressive return to function is advocated.[8,52]

Lumbar Spondylosis

Spondylosis is defined as osteoarthritis of the spine. Radiographic findings may include bone spurs and osteophytes and fusing of adjacent levels in advanced stages. It is also referred to as *degenerative joint disease*. Spondylosis is a

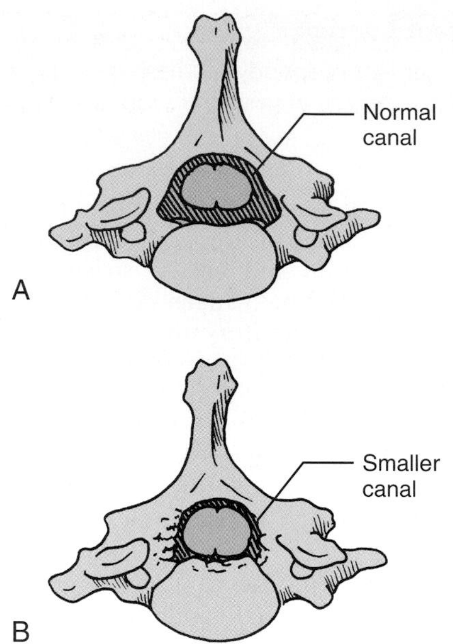

FIG 20-7 Lumbar spinal stenosis. **A,** Normal. **B,** Stenotic spine. The narrow diameter of the spinal canal can lead to constriction and compression of nerve roots.

degenerative process associated with aging. It can also be associated with decrease in disk height or degenerative disk disease. This degenerative process may lead to encroachment on the nerve roots and resultant neurologic symptoms.

Spinal Stenosis

Lumbar spinal stenosis is defined as a narrowing of the spinal canal, which constricts and compresses nerve roots (Fig. 20-7).[52] This gives rise to symptoms of neurogenic or spinal claudication, as follows:

1. Radicular ache into the thigh and less frequently into the calf[8]
2. Paresthesias into the lower extremity[29]
3. Disturbances in motor function[29]

This condition occurs in male patients "twice as often as females"[52] and typically is observed in adults during late middle age and older.[29,52]

Lumbar spinal stenosis is most commonly acquired as a result of degenerative arthritic changes that encroach on the diameter of the canal, producing nerve root compression.[52] A patient with stenosis frequently complains of pain and increased symptoms with lumbar extension. Extension of the lumbar spine in a patient with stenosis further compresses the spinal canal, increasing pain and paresthesias.[15,29,52]

During ambulation and gait training, an elderly patient typically demonstrates a forward-flexed trunk posture when using a walker. Under careful observation and questioning, the patient may reveal that leaning forward feels better and reduces back and leg pain. The role of the PTA is to educate the patient continually, reinforcing appropriate postures, body mechanics, and lifting techniques. Sitting and sleeping changes, general physical conditioning, and weight management programs are also addressed and have been identified as important adjuncts in the overall management of patients with spinal stenosis.[52] Whitman and colleagues[64] demonstrated that subjects with spinal stenosis experienced greater improvements in pain and recovery at 6 weeks with manual therapy, exercise, and walking than subjects who performed routine flexion exercises and walking. The physical therapy team should work together to provide the appropriate manual intervention followed by specific exercise and a walking program for the best management of patients with spinal stenosis.

LUMBAR SPINE FRACTURES

Fractures of the lumbar vertebrae generally occur after a profound traumatic event and can be classified according to the forces that produce the fracture. Compression, flexion, extension, flexion-distraction, flexion-rotation, and lateral flexion are forces that produce fractures.[52] Lumbar spine fractures also can be described in terms that graphically depict a specific fracture deformity, including crush, wedge, burst, shear, slice, and teardrop fractures.[52]

Perhaps the most clinically relevant spine fracture for the PTA to consider is the vertebral compression fracture. Vertebral compression fractures are the most common osteoporosis-related spinal fracture with approximately 700,000 occurring per year, and the prevalence of vertebral compression fractures increases with age.[15,29,44]

Important Concept

Vertebral compression fractures are the most common osteoporosis-related spinal fracture with approximately 700,000 occurring per year, and the prevalence of vertebral compression fractures increases with age.[15,29,44]

Many benign activities can produce compression fractures in elderly patients with osteoporosis.[8,44] Care must be taken to ensure that no rapid deceleration occurs when an elderly patient transfers to a bedside commode or any other hard surface. This seemingly trivial activity frequently causes multilevel compression fractures in patients with osteoporosis. Compression fractures produce symptoms ranging from acute local pain to essentially no signs at all.[44] Subtle complaints of pain caused by typical daily activities, such as bending, lifting, or rising from a chair, must be viewed with a high level of suspicion in elderly patients.[44]

Treatment of compression fractures focuses on relief of pain; authorities[29,44] advocate activity modification, physician-prescribed analgesics, NSAIDs, heat, ice, massage, and electrical stimulation to control pain, swelling, and associated muscle spasm. During the acute and subacute phases of recovery, a patient with compression fractures must avoid thoracic or lumbar flexion activities.[29] Repeated trunk flexion is contraindicated because it creates an anterior wedging of the vertebral bodies, producing greater stress and compression at the fracture site.[29] Appropriate exercise progression should target the muscles supporting or attached to the affected bone, and they are determined by the PT. Exercises should be combined with postural correction, scapular stabilization, and improving weight-bearing patterns, strength, balance, and flexibility.

Important Concept

During the acute and subacute phases of recovery following a spine compression fracture, a patient must avoid thoracic or lumbar flexion activities.[29] Repeated trunk flexion is contraindicated because it creates an anterior wedging of the vertebral bodies, producing greater stress and compression at the fracture site.[29]

Compression fracture prevention education programs, especially in patients with osteoporosis, should focus on implementing an exercise program designed to increase strength, flexibility, and bone density as well as improve balance, posture, and body mechanics to help maintain bone mass. Other preventive measures include identifying potential hazards in the home, selecting appropriate assistive devices, and general patient education.

Treatment-Based Classification

Rehabilitation of the lumbar spine is focused toward impairments rather than labeling pathoanatomic findings. As a result, when a patient experiences low-back pain, the evaluating PT assimilates information from the patient history, examination, and current best evidence and classifies the patient into the most appropriate category. The rehabilitation plan includes a multimodal approach that categorizes patients based on their overall symptoms and response to a specific intervention. This system has been identified as **treatment-based classification (TBC)**.[6]

The TBC system consists of subgroupings that the patient moves fluidly in and out of during the course of care. The interventions within these categories include manual therapy and exercise,[12,22] specific exercise for directional preference,[7,64] traction,[24,25] neuromuscular reeducation and stabilization exercise,[34,53,55] aerobic exercise, and recommendations to stay active. PTs use their findings from the clinical examination to match the patient with the most appropriate intervention. Research has shown that patients managed with this systematic approach experience significant decreases in pain and disability.[6,24] For the PTA, it is important to be aware of the categories along with exercise and educational concerns within each.

Important Concept

The Treatment-Based Classification system consists of subgroupings that the patient moves fluidly in and out of during the course of care. The interventions within these categories include manual therapy and exercise,[12,22] specific exercise for directional preference,[7,64] traction,[24,25] neuromuscular reeducation and stabilization exercise,[34,53,55] aerobic exercise, and recommendations to stay active.

Some patients with acute or chronic low-back pain benefit from first restoring mobility in the spine, and these patients initially are placed in the manual therapy and exercise category. The PT addresses any segments that need to be mobilized before initiating an exercise program for the patient. Early exercises are chosen to enhance the restoration of normal movement in the lumbar spine and include pelvic rocking and abdominal bracing. Patients with short duration of symptoms (<2 or 3 weeks), no symptoms distal to the knee, and low fear avoidance behaviors are expected to experience a 50% reduction in disability in 1 to 2 weeks on the Oswestry Disability Index.[12,22] However, the PT may choose to progress the patient gradually based on the presence of elevated fear avoidance beliefs noted on the Fear Avoidance Beliefs Questionnaire.[28]

Patients with more chronic or recurring symptoms of low-back pain are managed with neuromuscular reeducation and stabilization exercise. These patients often present with an average straight leg raise greater than 91° and the presence of aberrant motions. Exercises focus on recruitment and control of the multifidi, transversus abdominis, internal and external obliques, and gluteal muscles. With this strategy, patients can also be expected to achieve a 50% reduction in disability on the Oswestry Disability Index in 8 weeks.[34]

In the presence of a directional preference, the patient experiences a centralization phenomenon where distal lower extremity symptoms and low-back pain are lessened with repeated movements in a particular direction. The symptoms become more centrally located with certain motions. An example of a repeated movement or prone progression is shown in Figure 20-8. Research has shown that the adoption of the appropriate exercise program based on the patient's directional preference allows for less pain and disability for up to 6 months.[7] Occasionally, patients with distal lower extremity symptoms and neurologic signs do not demonstrate centralization with movement testing. In such cases, patients may benefit from mechanical traction in addition to specific exercises.[24]

The PTA should be cognizant of any new reports of changes or worsening in patients' signs and symptoms and report these findings immediately to the evaluating PT. Changes may include worsening or peripheralization of symptoms into the lower extremity, the presence of night pain, changes in bowel or bladder activity, and saddle anesthesia.

Invasive Management

When conservative physical therapy (including active rest, medications, exercise, and postural correction) fails to bring significant relief from symptoms, the physician may offer several invasive procedures. For some patients whose persistent radicular pain (sciatica) cannot be controlled by conservative measures, the physician may prescribe an epidural steroid injection to relieve symptoms.[21,52] These injections are given only to relieve pain and reduce inflammation and are not intended as a curative procedure to correct any neurologic deficits.

Patients may undergo surgery in the presence of a large disk herniation. As described by Miller[52] and Eismont and Kitchel,[21] the most common procedure is a laminotomy with a decompression diskectomy. In this procedure, the physician gains exposure to the herniated disk by cutting into the lamina and removing all nonviable disk material, decompressing the affected nerve root (Fig. 20-9). Although some patients report good or excellent results with this

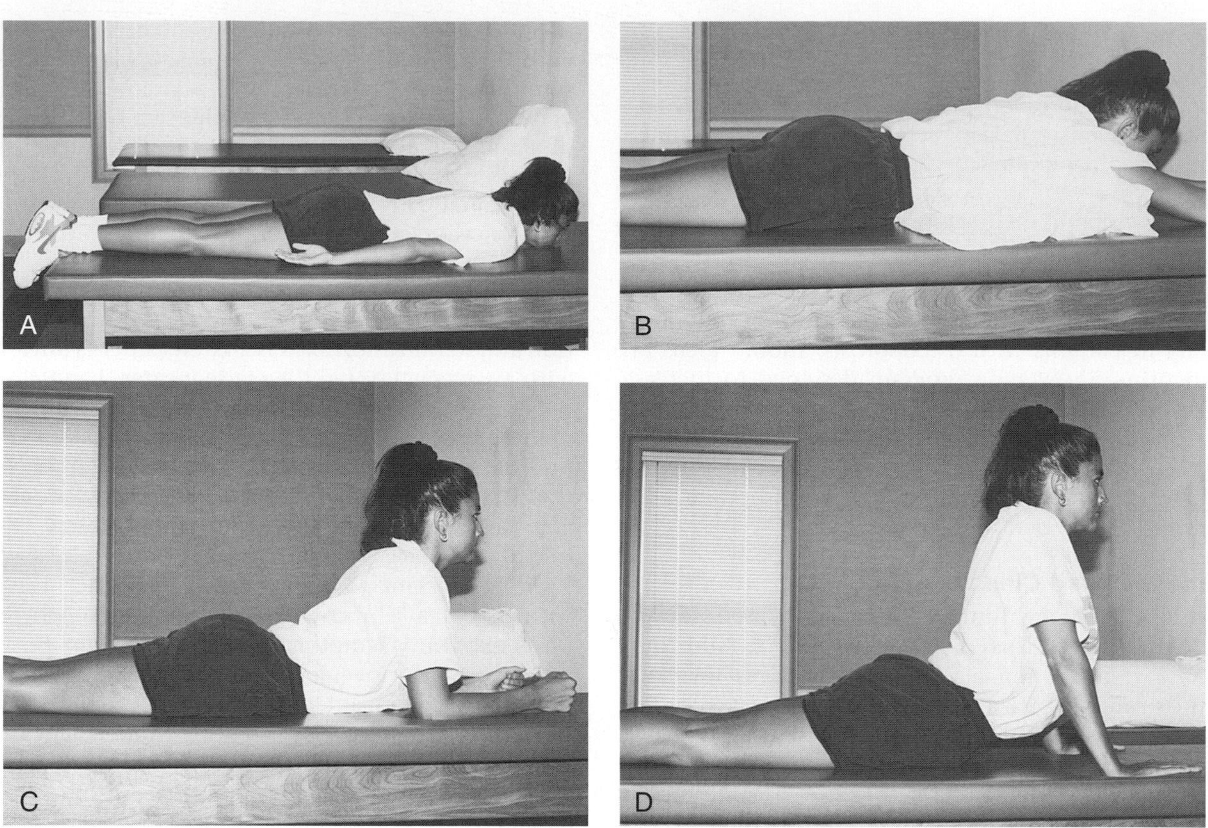

FIG 20-8 Passive prone extension sequence. **A,** Patient lying prone without pillow for support. **B,** Patient prone with pillow under the chest for mild thoracic and lumbar extension. **C,** Patient propped up on elbows for improved extension. **D,** Patient prone with elbows extended for maximum extension.

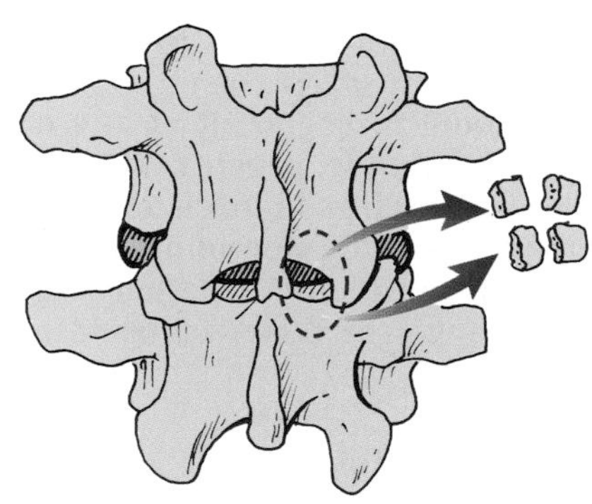

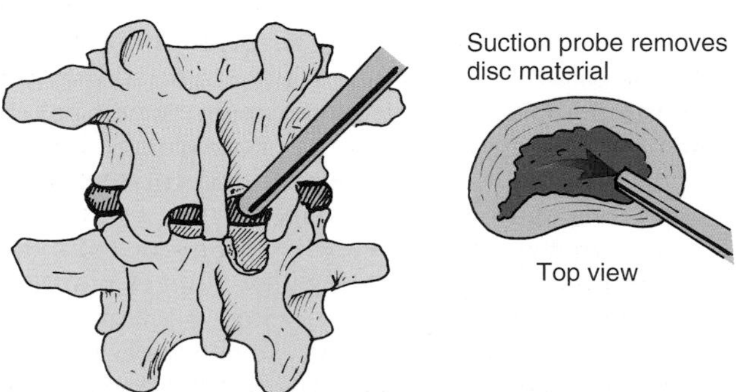

FIG 20-9 Laminotomy with decompression diskectomy.

surgical procedure, 30% of these patients may have significant back pain at long-term follow-up.[18,52] Other invasive procedures exist, such as microsurgical diskectomy and automated percutaneous diskectomy.

Rehabilitation after any surgical procedure is highly patient-specific and directly related to the data obtained at the initial postoperative physical therapy evaluation. Generally, recovery closely parallels the criteria established with conservative management including neuromuscular reeducation and stabilization exercise. However, extensive surgical exposure is necessary to perform a laminotomy with diskectomy, and tissue healing constraints influence recovery.

After surgery, the patient is taught bed mobility and transfer training using the log-roll technique to move from a supine to sitting position. Ambulation with a walker or crutches is generally allowed 1 day after surgery. Ambulation distance and endurance activities are increased according to each patient's ability. Rudimentary bed exercises can be performed the day after surgery and include active ankle pumps, gentle hip and knee flexion, and isometric exercises (quadriceps and gluteals). The PT guides the PTA concerning whether the postoperative patient can perform any isometric exercises. The PTA must instruct the patient in and reinforce proper breathing techniques if isometric exercises are done. The Valsalva maneuver is strictly avoided during all exercises.

For the first 3 days after surgery, the patient is limited to sitting for no more than 1 hour at a time and must maintain proper spinal position with no flexion.[10] The PTA continually reinforces and encourages proper posture during the first week of recovery. The patient should be cautioned to avoid forward bending and trunk rotation.

More demanding and functionally relevant activities that do not stress the surgical site are added gradually. Transfers from supine to sitting and from sitting to standing must be demonstrated by the patient and observed by the clinician to be safe, efficient, and free from all unwanted stress. Throughout the first week, exercises can progress to include functional closed chain activities while maintaining proper neutral spine positioning.

When initial wound healing is complete and pain is decreased, a more accelerated program of strengthening can begin. ROM is encouraged gradually as soon as the patient can tolerate these motions. Gentle active extension exercises and pelvic tilts (which promote pelvic motion, control, and limited-motion lumbar spine flexion and extension) begin early in the recovery phase.

The patient must achieve increased motion, controlled pain, improved endurance, and sufficient strength before beginning a general conditioning program after surgery. A longer recovery period is needed to allow for proper soft tissue healing, bone healing, and control of inflammation and pain before subjecting the affected area to stress. From 3 to 5 weeks after surgery, the goals of recovery are identified as restored lumbar motion, normalized upper and lower extremity strength, improved aerobic fitness, and decreased pain and swelling.[10]

Progressive functional exercises can be added as the patient achieves these criteria. Exercises include treadmill walking, balance activities, isotonic strengthening exercises, general flexibility exercises, and cardiovascular conditioning (via upper body ergometer, recumbent cycle ergometer, treadmill, stair climber, and cross-country ski machine).

FUNDAMENTAL MECHANICS OF LIFTING

Forces and stresses related to lifting, sitting, standing, walking, sleeping, and twisting are common to all activities of daily living (ADL). O'Sullivan and colleagues[54] identified a novel concept to instruct patients in proper lifting mechanics, listing the "five L's" of lifting: load, lever, lordosis, legs, and lungs.

The *load* to be lifted is central to all concepts of lifting mechanics. The amount of weight to be hoisted should be appropriate for the task and for the individual attempting to lift it. The *lever* refers to keeping the object as close to the body as is functionally possible throughout the lift. If the object is held away from the body, the increased force (intradiscal pressure and muscle strain) may strain the lumbar spine. *Lordosis* refers to maintaining a normal anatomic lordotic curve while lifting any object. Teaching the patient (and PTA) to lift with the *legs* is basic to all lifting procedures. The muscles of the legs should be conditioned to participate fully during the lifting of any object from the floor. If the legs are not used fully, the muscles of the back may be necessary to absorb increased stress. The *lungs* refer to the use of proper breathing techniques during lifting. The Valsalva maneuver (closed glottis during attempted expiration) should be avoided, and instruction should be given on exhaling during the actual lift.

Important Concept

Teaching the patient (and PTA) to lift with the *legs* is basic to all lifting procedures. The muscles of the legs should be conditioned to participate fully during the lifting of any object from the floor. If the legs are not used fully, the muscles of the back may be necessary to absorb increased stress.

Kaiser and co-workers[41] identified a lumbar stabilization model comparing two lumbar spine postures during lifting. In the first posture (tested electromyographically), the starting position is characterized by a posterior pelvic tilt. The abdominal muscles are in a shortened position, the lumbar paravertebral muscles show no electromyographic activity, the posterior ligaments and posterior annular wall are stretched, the knees are in a position of decreased leverage, and the patient's center of gravity is posterior to the base of support (Fig. 20-10, *A*).[14] In the second posture, the patient's lumbar lordosis is maintained during the lift. The abdominal muscles are in their normal anatomic length, the paravertebral muscles are contracted, the posterior ligaments are relaxed, the knees are in an optimal leverage position, and the patient's center of gravity is over the base of support (Fig. 20-10, *B*).

PREVENTION AND EDUCATION FOR BACK DYSFUNCTION: THE BACK SCHOOL MODEL

Although understanding and managing low-back dysfunction is the focus of this section, prevention of lumbar spine injuries also is pertinent to this discussion because the PTA is frequently directed to participate in and to carry out community-based back injury prevention programs under the supervision and direction of a PT. These education programs are commonly referred to as *back schools* and are designed to provide an understanding of anatomy, causes of back pain, lifting mechanics, posture, self-care for back pain, exercise, nutrition (weight management), ergonomics (which involves lifting, posture, general body mechanics, job modifications, and work site protection and redesign to minimize back injury), and stress reduction for high-risk patients and the population at large.

Patients with a history of back pain often are identified as ideal candidates to participate in these programs. Also, persons at risk (identified by job responsibilities, repetitive lifting, overweight condition, poor posture, poor body mechanics, relative weakness, and poor general physical conditioning) may be referred to these programs.

Many back schools involve a 1- or 2-hour class (consisting of lectures, slides, demonstration, and participation) each week for 4 to 6 weeks. Each session or class builds on the previous lecture to convey the principles seen in spinal anatomy, causes of back dysfunction, risk factors, posture, body mechanics, and treatment approaches.[1] Back schools can be based in outpatient physical therapy clinics, hospitals, industrial health clinics, wellness programs at work, or community fitness centers. In every case, the program should be under the direction and supervision of a PT, physician, or both.

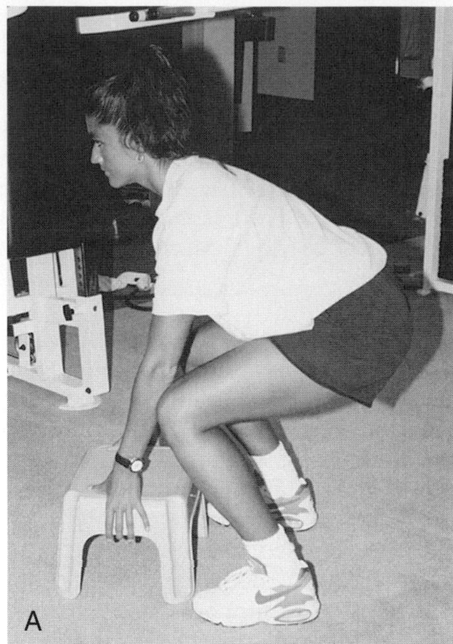

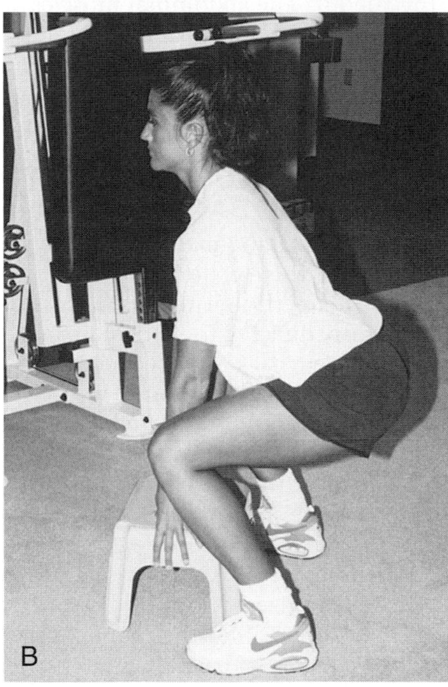

FIG 20-10 Lifting postures. **A,** Flat back lifting position. **B,** Lifting with lumbar lordosis maintained.

Allman[1] identified the outline in Table 20-1 as an appropriate general back school program. The curriculum clarifies the rudimentary concepts of education and prevention for a wide variety of back-related problems. The PTA who presents this information must be given specific information, evaluation data, indications, and contraindications for each patient participating in the back school program. In this way, all phases of recovery and prevention can be individualized for each patient.

Most recently in a systematic review of completed research, Martimo and colleagues[49] concluded that the evidence to support back school programs is lacking. The effectiveness of a back school program in preventing pain, injury, and dysfunction is still under scrutiny. Despite this lack of evidence, there is still value in patient education by the PT and PTA. Future studies may provide evidence that back school programs prevent further injury.

ERGONOMICS AND FUNCTIONAL CAPACITY EVALUATIONS

In concert with back injury prevention through education and in accordance with the back school model is the concept of ergonomics and the implementation of functional capacity evaluations (FCEs), which are also referred to as *physical capacity assessments,* related to physical stress job analysis. The term *ergonomics* refers to a quantifiable system of job or ADL modification (or redesign) that allows for continued productivity while reducing work-related physical stress. As with the back school model, a FCE may require the PTA to prepare the evaluation area; set up all necessary testing equipment; and assist the PT with the collection, documentation, and storage of data. The implementation of a FCE is highly specific to the individual's job task. The goal is to identify risk factors associated with a particular job or activity and quantify the physical capacity of the individual being asked to perform the specific task to reduce the risk of back injury. In most cases, a FCE is administered to a patient recovering from a back injury before returning to the job. A FCE also can be used as a screening tool to acquire data related to preemployment risk assessment and management of back injuries. Certain job or activity risk factors have been identified that directly relate to the FCE.[33] A few ergonomic risk factors were outlined by Hebert as follows[33]:

- How much weight you lift
- How often you lift
- How low you bend to lift the load
- How high you lift the load
- How far you carry the load
- How far you twist with the load
- How far you reach with the load
- How long you sit at your job
- What the specific design of your seat is
- If there is sustained or repeated bending, twisting, or reaching

Hundreds of factors may be related to job tasks. Each item to be tested in the FCE must be quantifiable and reproducible to enable the PT to make recommendations for reducing the risk of back injury. General testing parameters may be divided into categories that attempt to duplicate the requirements of the task to be performed while evaluating the patient's physiologic responses and assessing his or her physical abilities to carry out the task.

Authorities[61] advocate a multiphase testing procedure that identifies the various components of a FCE, as shown in Table 20-2. Within each FCE, the aerobic endpoint (heart rate exceeds 85% of maximum heart rate) and biomechanical analysis of the patient's lifting-risk posture is assessed. In each section of the test, the parameters evaluated are performed directly as they relate to the specific job or task in question.

TABLE 20-1 Appropriate General Back School Program

Education Topics	Components of Education Topics
Introduction to back dysfunction	Primary purpose is to increase the patient's awareness of back care, posture, and body mechanics.
Basic spinal anatomy and physiology: Causes of back pain and dysfunction	1. Sprains and strains 2. Disk injuries (herniated nucleus pulposus) 3. Spinal stenosis 4. Spondylolisthesis
Risk factors associated with back injury	1. Poor general conditioning 2. Poor posture 3. Poor body mechanics and poor lifting style 4. Repetitive heavy lifting 5. Long-term sitting and driving 6. Stress (emotional)
Posture positioning and general body mechanics	1. Sitting 2. Sleeping 3. Standing 4. Lifting 5. ADL, job assessment, and recreational activities
Treatment approaches	1. Ice or heat 2. Stretching 3. Posture changes 4. Back support 5. Conditioning
General physical conditioning	1. Warm-up. Patients are introduced to the concept of a general warm-up preceding any physical activity. 2. Aerobic fitness. Patients are introduced to the methods, equipment, and implementation of general and specific endurance activities to improve cardiovascular fitness and control body weight. 3. Anaerobic power. Activities are outlined that develop intense physical effort of short duration. 4. Strength. Patients are instructed in methods to improve general body strength and specific lumbar extension strength exercises. 5. Flexibility. Patients are introduced to the philosophy, design, and implementation of daily, full-body stretching exercises with specific emphasis on the trunk and lower extremities. 6. Nutrition. Direct attention is focused on reducing the number of calories consumed by overweight individuals. Usually this education is conducted by a registered dietitian. 7. Relaxation techniques, stress reduction, and recreational activities are explored.

ADL, Activities of daily living
From Allman FL: Back school program. In: *Introduction to back injuries,* Atlanta, 1990, The Atlanta Sports Medicine Clinic.

TABLE 20-2 Testing Procedure That Identifies the Components of a Functional Capacity Evaluation

Testing	Procedure
Musculoskeletal profile	1. Blood pressure 2. Posture 3. Gait 4. Balance 5. ROM 6. Neurologic (reflexes) 7. Sensory 8. Muscle strength
Functional abilities screening	1. Push-pull 2. Dynamic lifting 3. Gross mobility 4. Hand strength (grip dynamometer) 5. Sitting and standing

ROM, range of motion.
From U.S. Physical Therapy: Work site partners, functional capacity evaluation system, industrial rehabilitation solutions, Houston, TX, 1994, USPT System Manual.

THORACIC SPINE

THORACIC SPINE MUSCLE INJURIES

Soft tissue injuries of the thoracic spine usually involve some type of direct contact (contusion during athletic activities) or indirect overstretching or contraction of the thoracic muscles. Muscle contusions and strains of the thoracic spine occur primarily in younger active patients. The primary focus of management for these self-limiting injuries is the control of pain and swelling. Generally, ice is applied directly over the involved area during the acute stage of injury. Physician-prescribed analgesics, NSAIDs, moist heat applications, ultrasound, electrical stimulation, and massage are used judiciously to help control pain. When pain has been effectively limited, the patient is allowed to participate in active ROM activities and strengthening exercises. The PTA may instruct the patient to perform seated, postural awareness exercises that focus on thoracic extension and scapular retraction.

Prone thoracic and lumbar extension exercises are employed based on patient tolerance. These involve a

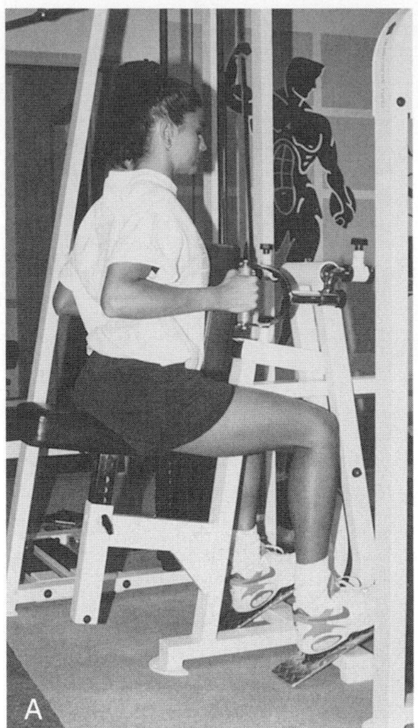

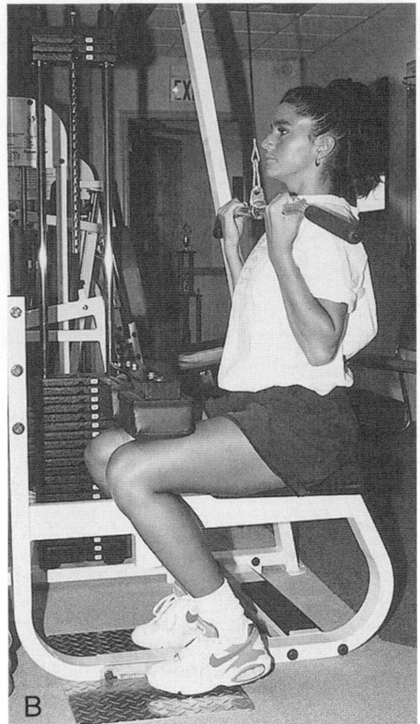

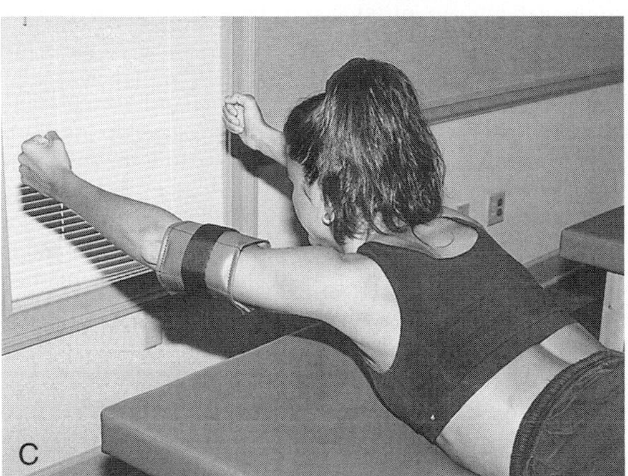

FIG 20-11 Scapular and thoracic extension strengthening. **A,** Seated rowing machine to encourage scapular retraction. **B,** Latissimus bar pull-down in front. **C,** Prone lumbar and thoracic extension with scapular retraction using cuff weights. Notice the proximal placement of the resistance. As strength increases, resistance can be moved to the patient's hands.

three-position progression from hands at the sides, to hands behind the head, to arms fully extended while performing prone thoracic and lumbar extension. As pain is reduced and strength increases, the patient can begin isotonic strengthening exercises that focus on the scapular and thoracic spine muscles (Fig. 20-11).

THORACIC DISK INJURIES

Thoracic disk herniations are rare (<0.3% of the population) and affect men and women equally from the fourth through the sixth decades.[8] The most common segments affected are between the ninth and twelfth thoracic vertebrae.[8]

The type of treatment employed for thoracic disk herniations depends on whether the disk is herniated laterally or centrally.[8,21] A large central disk prolapse may produce symptoms of "spastic paraparesis, increased deep tendon reflexes, and a positive Babinski response."[21] However, lateral thoracic disk protrusions can produce signs more consistent with nerve root compression.

The PTA is exposed to conservative care and postsurgical recovery after thoracic spine disk herniations. Less severe lateral disk herniations can be treated effectively with periods of active rest, analgesics, modalities to control pain and swelling, and epidural injections. More severe central disk herniations, involving progressive neurologic deficits, must be treated surgically to decompress the neurologic impingement.[8,21] Recovery after thoracic decompression closely follows the time necessary for healing of bone and soft tissue with extensive periods of supportive bracing to protect the affected spine from unwanted forces; a progressive regimen of active motion, strengthening, and endurance activities; and a return to function with specific limitations delineated within the protocol developed by the surgeon and PT.

KYPHOSIS

Kyphosis is defined as an increase in the thoracic posterior convexity that is manifested by a rounded-back (and protracted scapulae) posture. Kyphosis can be subdivided into congenital, neuromuscular, and postural categories.[21] Osteoporosis, which can lead to multilevel thoracic compression fractures, causes anterior wedging of the involved segments and creates the kyphotic curvature. The causes of pain associated with an increased thoracic convexity have been identified as stress originating from the PLLs, muscle fatigue resulting from stretched and weakened erector spinae and rhomboid muscle groups, and various postural and neurologic syndromes.[42]

Important Concept

Kyphosis is defined as an increase in the thoracic posterior convexity that is manifested by a rounded-back (and protracted scapulae) posture. Kyphosis can be subdivided into congenital, neuromuscular, and postural categories.[21]

The treatment of kyphosis depends on the degree of curvature, which is determined radiographically by the treating physician; any associated disk involvement; and the severity of symptoms.[5] In advanced cases of postural kyphosis with profound curvature and significant symptoms, the patient may require supportive bracing of the thorax to minimize the compression associated with anterior wedging of the vertebral bodies. With less severe kyphosis, the PTA plays a critical role in patient education, postural awareness, and application of specific exercises simultaneously to stretch the anterior shoulder and pectorals and strengthen the thoracic extension muscles.

To strengthen the scapular retractors, rhomboids, middle trapezius, and erector spinae of the thoracic region effectively, a sufficient degree of freedom of movement in these areas is needed. Generally, the anterior shoulder muscles and pectorals are shortened and relatively weak in response to the increased thoracic convexity. To provide the needed stimulus for full ROM strengthening, the anterior aspect of the thorax also must be addressed. Stretching the anterior shoulder muscles can be done actively by the patient and passively, where the clinician provides the stretching. An effective active assisted stretch can be performed with the patient facing the corner of a room or standing in an open doorway. Both of the patient's hands are placed in a comfortable position on either side of the doorway, and the patient slowly leans forward, providing a slow, static stretch to the pectorals and anterior shoulder. This position can be held for a prolonged stretch and usually is performed for multiple sets.

A passive stretch also can be employed with the patient in a seated position. With both of the patient's hands placed behind his or her head, the PTA stands behind the patient and grasps both elbows. The PTA delivers a slow, posteriorly directed stretch to the pectorals and anterior shoulder muscles. To be effective, stretching must be performed consistently each day. The patient must perform stretches two or three times daily as part of a home exercise program. In addition to stretching the thorax, posterior thoracic strengthening must be addressed. The patient performs seated active scapular retraction exercises with an emphasis on maintaining an isometric contraction, or set, of the scapular muscles with each repetition.

As described, the patient does the three-progression prone thoracic extension exercises. In addition, the patient performs scapular adduction while lying prone with both arms held straight at 90°. Both arms are elevated while adducting the scapulae and holding the contracted position isometrically for 10 seconds.[42] This position can be modified slightly by having the patient hold weights while performing scapular adduction with both elbows flexed, creating more of a prone rowing motion.

The patient must perform stretching and strengthening exercises daily as part of a home program. As the patient's motion improves and where posterior scapular strength increases, isotonic resistance exercises should be encouraged to a greater degree to provide increased stimulus for strengthening. In the home program, latex tubing or a TheraBand can be used in a seated rowing position to enhance scapular adduction. Commercially available isotonic rowing machines effectively provide greater resistance for the scapular muscles.

When treating postural kyphosis, the home exercise program must be carried out faithfully, and the patient must develop an acute postural awareness at home and work. If the patient performs tasks at work that contribute to a rounded-shoulder position, modifications of these tasks is necessary. In many cases, the cause of poor thoracic posture is an inefficient workstation arrangement in which the patient must maintain poor posture to perform tasks such as typing, writing, assembly work, or computer data entry. A simple adjustment in the height of the workstation so that it is closer to and centered midline with the patient encourages a more erect thoracic spine. The total care of the patient focuses on symptomatic pain relief using physician-prescribed analgesics; thermal agents; massage; and a comprehensive program of stretching, strengthening, education, and work site modifications.

SCOLIOSIS

Scoliosis can be identified as any lateral curvature of the cervical, thoracic, or lumbar spine.[42] Scoliosis usually is idiopathic (cause unknown), but it also can result from neuromuscular causes or can be related to degenerative disease, osteoporosis, trauma, and postsurgical factors.[52] Kisner and Colby[42] identified the incidence of idiopathic scoliosis as 75% to 85% of all recognized types of scoliosis. Generally, scoliosis can be recognized as either structural or nonstructural.[42]

Important Concept

Scoliosis can be identified as any lateral curvature of the cervical, thoracic, or lumbar spine.[42] Scoliosis usually is idiopathic (cause unknown), but it also can result from neuromuscular causes or can be related to degenerative disease, osteoporosis, trauma, and postsurgical factors.[52]

Structural scoliosis is defined as an "irreversible lateral curve of the spine with fixed rotation of the vertebrae."[42]

During the initial evaluation of structural scoliosis, the PT observes whether the identified lateral curve decreases with forward trunk flexion. If not, structural idiopathic scoliosis is not corrected by changes in the patient's position or during active voluntary activities.[42] Nonstructural scoliosis is classified as reversible, wherein the lateral curve dissipates with positional changes. In either case, pain is the foremost presenting feature of scoliosis,[52] although cosmesis is a great concern. Other complaints involve decreased cardiopulmonary function (usually with thoracic curves >65°) and neurologic symptoms associated with spinal stenosis.[52]

In the nonoperative management of idiopathic scoliosis, the PTA primarily instructs the patient about therapeutic exercises outlined and prescribed by the PT. Scoliosis treatment involves stretching and strengthening, similar to kyphosis treatment. Exercise by itself does not halt the progression or correct scoliosis.[42] The effective use of therapeutic exercise is intended primarily to improve spinal motion, increase muscle strength, and reduce back pain.[42]

Important Concept

The effective use of therapeutic exercise in the treatment of scoliosis is intended primarily to improve spinal motion, increase muscle strength, and reduce back pain.[42]

Bracing has been advocated in addition to exercises in the treatment of scoliosis.[42,52] Bracing is intended to halt progression of the curve and not correct cosmetic deformity.[52] Perhaps the most commonly used brace for scoliosis is the Milwaukee brace.[42,52] This brace is generally worn 23 or 24 hours a day.[42] However, Miller[52] suggested that part-time brace wearing is as effective as the traditional long-term application.

A fundamental principle in managing idiopathic scoliosis is stretching of the tight muscles on the concave side of the curve, while strengthening the muscles on the convex side of the curve. In addition, trunk axial elongation (stretching vertically) is important throughout exercise. As stated in the section on kyphosis, some freedom of motion must be available for strengthening exercises to be effective.

Stretching exercises directed toward the concavity must address all of the spinal muscles. A right thoracic convexity results in a left lower thoracic concavity and associated right lumbar concavity with left lumbar convexity (Fig. 20-12). Strengthening exercises are performed for all of the muscles affected on the convex side of each lateral curve.

Various stretching exercises can be performed in the prone, side-lying, or heel-sitting position.[42] In the prone position, the patient places both hands behind his or her head while tilting the thorax away from the concave side of the curve (Fig. 20-13, *A*). In another prone stretching exercise, the patient reaches overhead and extends the arm on the concave side, effectively stretching the thoracic concavity (Fig. 20-13, *B*).

In the heel-sitting position, the patient places both hands forward and flat while emphasizing long-axis stretching. The lateral stretching component of this exercise is accomplished by having the patient slowly stretch both arms laterally away from the concave side of the curve (Fig. 20-14).

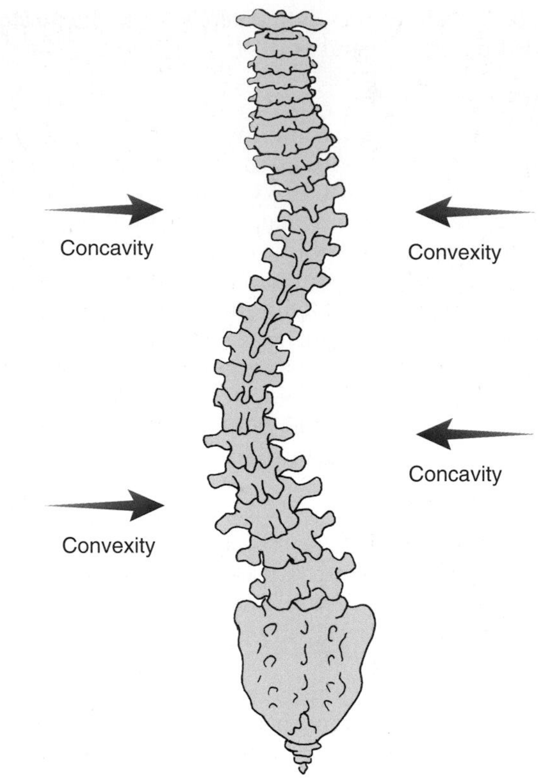

FIG 20-12 Scoliosis. A right thoracic convexity results in a left lower thoracic concavity and an associated right lumbar concavity with left lumbar convexity.

Static stretching also can be performed with the patient lying on his or her side. A small, soft rolled pillow or towel is placed directly under the apex of the thoracic convex curve to support and stabilize the pelvis. For an advanced progression of side-lying stretching, the patient lies over the apex bolster toward the end of a treatment table (Fig. 20-15).

As alluded to earlier, trunk elongation (axial stretching) also is an effective stretching procedure used to treat scoliosis. Standing, the patient faces a wall and attempts to "walk up the wall" with both hands. The patient must reach as high as possible with both hands. A more progressive form of trunk elongation is to have the patient hang by both arms from an overhead bar.

Strengthening the thoracic and lumbar spine toward the convex side focuses on thoracic and lumbar extension strength and specific lateral strengthening maneuvers. Prone thoracic and lumbar spine active exercises were outlined and described in the preceding section. These exercises are effective when used early to enhance thoracic strength.

Specific lateral strengthening can proceed with the patient in a side-lying position on the concave side of the curve. The PTA stabilizes the trunk and then has the patient lift the trunk up toward the convex side of the curve (Fig. 20-16). This exercise can be viewed as a side-lying sit-up.

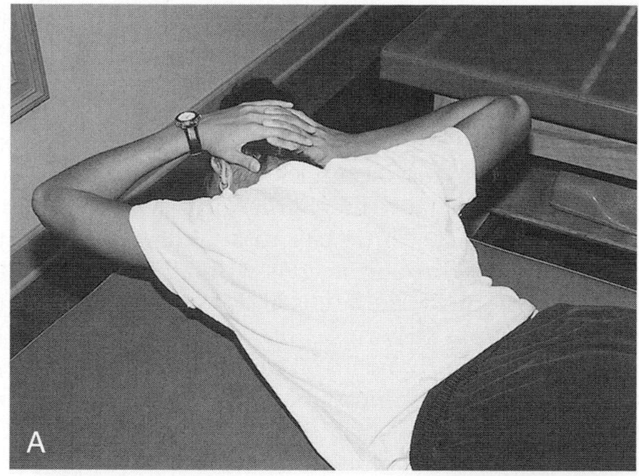

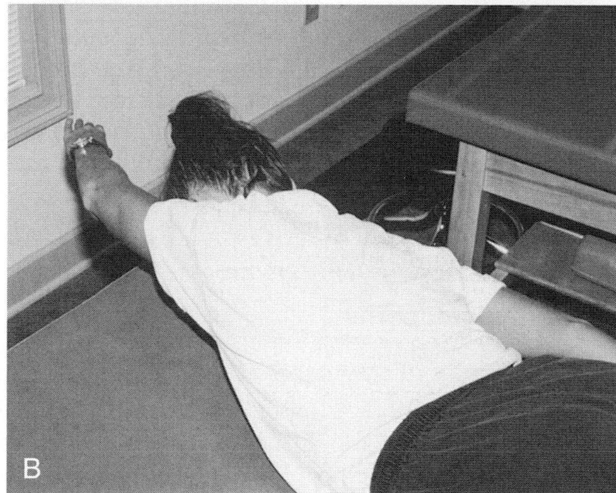

FIG 20-13 Stretching exercises. **A,** Prone lateral trunk tilt. **B,** Prone lateral trunk tilt with arm stretch.

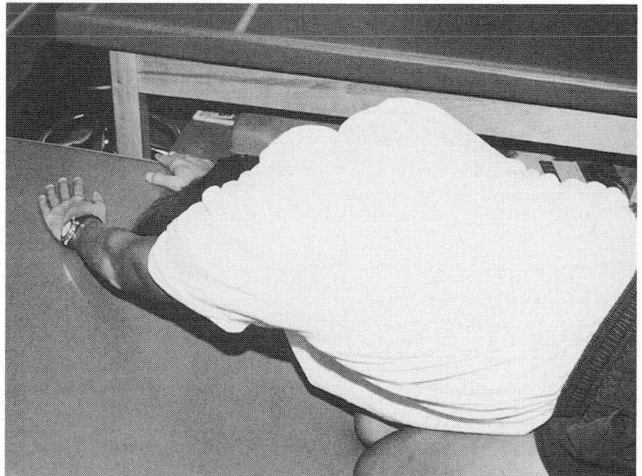

FIG 20-14 Heel-sitting lateral trunk stretch with long-axis stretch and lateral stretch of both arms.

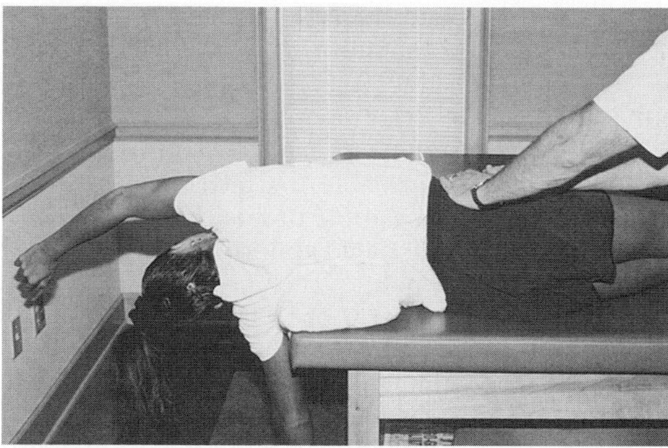

FIG 20-15 Side-lying apex stretch over the end of a table.

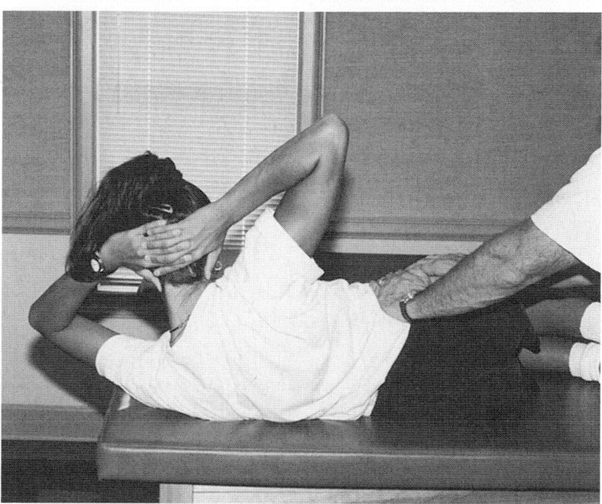

FIG 20-16 Side-lying lateral trunk sit-up.

Discussion so far has focused on a few rudimentary stretching and strengthening exercises for mild to moderate idiopathic scoliosis. An outline of surgical procedures to correct severe scoliosis is presented now. Surgery is reserved for severe symptomatic curves more than 50° to 60°.[52] Curves of this magnitude can be improved by approximately 50% with surgery.[42] The exact surgical procedure performed depends on many factors. A spinal fusion with or without Harrington rod instrumentation[42] is designed to elongate and stabilize the spine and reduce pain and improve appearance. Physical therapy after spinal fusion for advanced, severe scoliosis requires extensive convalescence, the application of a postoperative brace, and limited activity for several weeks after surgery, depending on the protocol designed by the surgeon and PT in collaboration.[42]

CERVICAL SPINE

Neck pain is thought to affect 66% of the population at least once in an individual's lifetime.[45] The economic burden of neck pain in the form of lost wages, cost of treatment, and workers' compensation is high. This cost is second only to low-back pain.[67] Individuals who experience an episode of neck pain may develop symptoms lasting more than 6 months.[4] Patients with neck pain are frequently seen in outpatient physical therapy. Jette and associates[38] reported 25% of an outpatient physical therapy caseload is represented by patients with neck pain. Women are affected by neck pain more frequently than men.[67]

The most profound and catastrophic cervical spine injury is a fracture dislocation resulting in quadriplegia. The description of these spinal injuries is beyond the scope of this chapter. When an evaluation is completed and a cervical spine fracture or spinal cord compression (myelopathy) is ruled out, nerve root involvement or nonspecific mechanical neck pain is often diagnosed in patients with neck pain. The pathoanatomic cause for neck pain is not identifiable for most patients seen in physical therapy.[3] In a sample of healthy people without neck pain, 19% demonstrated abnormalities with imaging studies.[2] These abnormalities included disk protrusion or extrusion and impingement of the nerve root and spinal cord. The significant prevalence of abnormal findings on magnetic resonance imaging in asymptomatic individuals can lead to medical misdiagnosis.

The evaluating PT identifies impairments in muscle, connective tissue, and nerves. As identified and explained in the section on the lumbar spine, rehabilitation of the cervical spine is focused on impairments. This section identifies various soft tissue and bony injuries of the cervical spine common to orthopedic physical therapy. General rehabilitation ideas are included with these pathoanatomic findings.

WHIPLASH ASSOCIATED DISORDER: ACUTE SPRAINS AND STRAINS

Muscular strains of the cervical spine are common among young athletes and in association with motor vehicle accidents with flexion/extension, lateral flexion, and acceleration/deceleration "whiplash"-type injuries.[60,68] Numerous impairments, stemming from bony and soft tissue injury, can be classified as whiplash associated disorder.[59] The U.S. annual cost associated with whiplash associated disorder is $29 billion.[67] The muscles that can be involved in cervical strains are the sternocleidomastoid, trapezius, scalenes, erectors, rhomboids, and levator scapulae.[68] The mechanism of injury producing cervical strains and sprains varies but includes hyperflexion, rotation, and lateral flexion of the head and cervical spine.[60]

Forces usually are great enough with automobile accidents that ligament injuries occur in conjunction with muscle strains. Experimental studies performed by Stratton and Bryan[60] demonstrated a wide range of tissue damage with hyperextension-type automobile injuries, as follows:

1. Tearing of sternocleidomastoid muscle
2. Tearing of longissimus coli muscle
3. Pharyngeal edema
4. Tearing of ALL
5. Separation of cartilaginous end plate of the intervertebral disk

Similar types of injuries occur with hyperflexion injuries as a result of automobile accidents[60]:

1. Tears of the posterior cervical muscles
2. Tears of the ligamentum nuchae
3. Tears of the PLL
4. Intervertebral disk injury

The treatment of traumatic cervical spine sprains and strains is symptomatic during the acute stage of recovery. Patients may present with neck pain and referred upper extremity pain. The treating physician usually prescribes a course of analgesics, NSAIDs, or muscle relaxants; rest; and agents to control pain and swelling (heat, cold, ultrasound, and electrical stimulation). The healing constraints of muscle and ligament tissues differ; both must be addressed throughout recovery.

After initial pain and swelling are controlled, the patient may be introduced to a series of active ROM exercises, cervical isometric strengthening exercises, and education in cervical posture mechanics. Initial ROM exercises must be approached cautiously to avoid reproducing the motion that caused the injury. As with all soft tissue injuries, attention must be focused on protection of the affected area while striving to prevent further injury. For example, if the mechanism of cervical sprain and strain was hyperflexion, care must be directed at avoiding the end range of head and neck flexion. Gentle active ROM exercises can proceed after moist heat application for 20 minutes to enhance muscle relaxation, relieve pain, and stimulate greater mobility. Full recovery from acute sprains and strains of the cervical spine involves the elimination of pain and swelling initially, appropriate rest from any aggravating positions, protection from unwanted stress, the return of normal cervical spine ROM, enhanced muscle strength through isometric stabilization exercises, work site modifications, and postural awareness activities (axial extension-retraction exercises).

Cervical Radiculopathy

Cervical radiculopathy is defined as mechanical compression or inflammation of a nerve root that causes neurologic symptoms into the upper extremities. The most common causes of radiculopathy are cervical disk herniation, spondylosis, and osteophytes.[62] The symptoms of peripheral pain, radicular signs, local cervical pain, and scapular pain are consistent with the symptoms of disk herniations observed in the lumbar spine.[60]

Important Concept

Cervical radiculopathy is defined as mechanical compression or inflammation of a nerve root that causes neurologic symptoms into the upper extremities.

As with lumbar disk herniations, the initial goals are to relieve symptoms, reduce pain and swelling, control muscle spasm, and work toward centralizing the symptoms. Iglarsh and Snyder-Mackler[36] defined improvement as "a decrease in the extent or intensity of the peripheral symptoms." The specific exercises for patients with cervical disk herniation must be identified carefully by the physician and PT. When the appropriate subgrouping of treatment is recognized, the PT organizes a comprehensive plan of pain relief, motion, strength, and postural education activities for the PTA to follow and apply.[11]

Cervical Spondylosis

In contrast to cervical disk herniations, cervical spondylosis involves chronic rather than acute degenerative disk, which results from "wear and tear on the weight-bearing structures of the cervical spine."[60] The symptoms are characteristic of spinal cord compression (myelopathy) or nerve root compression with radicular signs.[52] Cervical spondylosis is seen most often during the fourth and fifth decades of life and characteristically affects men more than women at the C5-C6 and C6-C7 segments.[52] Sustained impact loading and repetitive microtrauma[60] are causative factors that can produce cervical cord impingement, nerve root impingement, osteophytes, bone sclerosis, loss of cervical lordosis, and central or posterolateral disk herniations.[52,60]

Initial physical therapy interventions focus on pain relief with the evaluation of thermal and electrical agents, physician-prescribed analgesics, and rest from aggravating positions. As with the evaluation of other disk conditions, the PT provides a comprehensive evaluation to determine accurately which motions cause pain and radicular symptoms and which motions relieve pain. From this detailed initial evaluation, the PT outlines and describes specific exercises consistent with these findings. In some cases, traction is an effective tool to minimize joint compressive loads and reduce cord compression or nerve root irritation.[52,58] The PT determines if mechanical traction or manual cervical traction is more appropriate. Isometric cervical spine stabilization exercises (four-way isometrics) and ROM exercises are initiated when pain has been reduced; the appropriateness of these activities is determined by the PT.

When cord compression (myelopathy) progresses and radicular pain persists, the physician can use various surgical interventions. Miller[52] described an anterior cervical spine approach to accomplish a diskectomy and fusion or a posterior approach for a foraminotomy or multilevel laminectomy to relieve cord or root compression. Because cervical spondylosis is a chronic degenerative condition, long-term care involves protection from inappropriate and unwanted forces and instruction in cervical posture mechanics, flexibility exercises, and strengthening activities.

Cervical Facet Syndrome

The cervical facet joint is another possible source of neck pain.[51] Symptoms include posterior neck stiffness, pain with cervical extension or rotation, cervicogenic headaches, and possible pain referral into the shoulder and scapula.[69] Degenerative changes to the cervical facet and surrounding soft tissue may cause this radiation. It is estimated that facet involvement affects 54% to 60% of patients with chronic neck pain.[48] Appropriate interventions identified by the PT include pain control, ROM, and exercise.

Thoracic Inlet Syndrome

Some texts address thoracic inlet syndrome when addressing the shoulder.[70] Because of the anatomic proximity of the structures involved, this condition is discussed within the context of the cervical spine. Authorities point out that the term *thoracic inlet syndrome* is a more precise and anatomically accurate term used to describe compression of vascular or neurologic tissues as they exit the "superior triangle opening of the thorax" (Fig. 20-17).[60,70] (This syndrome has been commonly called *outlet syndrome* in the past.) Specifically, the most probable neurovascular factors involved with thoracic inlet syndrome are proximal compression of the subclavian artery and vein and the brachial plexus.[60] Many structures can cause compression of these tissues. Foremost is the presence of a cervical rib, a shortened or hypertrophied anterior scalene muscle, or malunion of the clavicle and subluxed first thoracic rib.[32,60,70] Symptoms of this condition include radicular signs of pain, numbness, tingling, weakness, and skin and temperature changes consistent with neurovascular tissue compression.[32,60,70]

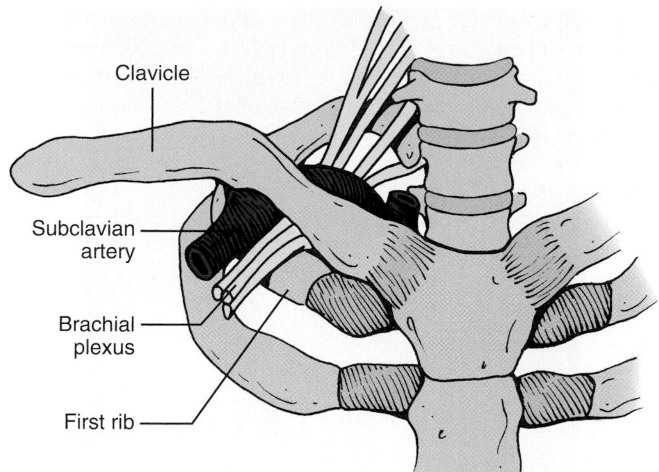

FIG 20-17 Thoracic inlet syndrome. Note proximal compression of the subclavian artery and vein and brachial plexus.

Typically, physical therapy management addresses specifically defined limitations of movement and affected bony or soft tissues during the initial evaluation performed by the PT. An individualized comprehensive program of stretching, strengthening, and education can begin when the PT has determined which specific tissues are affected and has identified any underlying causes of postural variations.

Soft tissue stretching focuses on the anterior scalene muscles. The patient is instructed to laterally flex and extend the head to the opposite side of the shortened muscle (Fig. 20-18). Thoracic kyphosis tends to accentuate the symptoms of thoracic inlet syndrome, so pectoral stretching (facing an open doorway with hands on either side and leaning forward) and thoracic extension mobility and strengthening exercises are used specifically to address muscle weakness and soft tissue restrictions. A host of clinically applicable thoracic extension mobility exercises can be used. Examples include seated scapular retraction, prone scapular and thoracic extension, and seated rowing activities with elastic tubing.

In addition to stretching and strengthening exercises, cervical posture correction is needed; poor cervical posture is a common problem in the workplace.[32] To address the forward head posture and tight anterior neck muscles, the patient can perform axial extension or cervical retraction stretching exercises. The effective management of thoracic inlet syndrome focuses on specific stretching of affected muscles, thoracic mobility, and extension strengthening as well as education concerning proper cervical spine alignment and the performance of cervical retraction exercises.

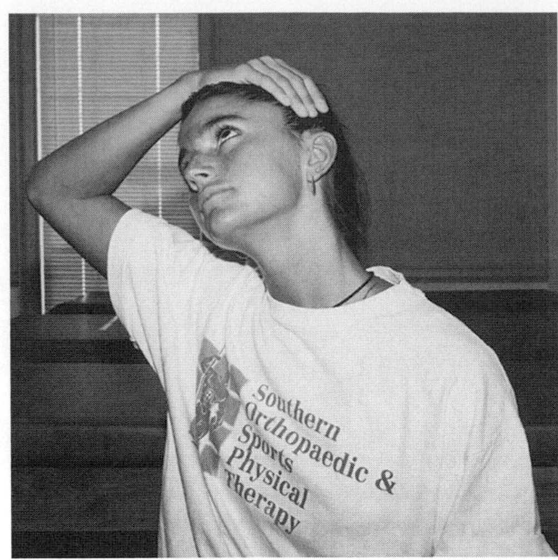

FIG 20-18 Stretching of the anterior scalene muscles by laterally flexing and extending the head toward the opposite side of the shortened muscle. Note the gentle overpressure provided by the hand.

TREATMENT-BASED CLASSIFICATION: CERVICAL SPINE

Effective management of the cervical spine requires a multimodal treatment approach. The cervical spine TBC system assimilates information from the patient history and physical examination to classify the patient for the most appropriate treatment subgroup.[13,23] The five subgroups are labeled mobility, centralization, exercise and conditioning, pain control, and headache. As explained earlier, the patient moves fluidly in and out of these subgroupings throughout the duration of care. Preliminary research identified that patients experienced improved outcomes when matched to interventions of their treatment subgroup.[23]

The cervical region is the most mobile region of the spine. Impairments in ROM in one vertebral level change the motion in adjacent levels. The restoration of mobility in the cervical spine may be the first subgrouping chosen by the PT after the initial evaluation. Interventions include mobilization, active ROM, passive ROM, and manipulation of the thoracic spine.[23] The PT initiates exercise in the form of ROM, strength, and conditioning with the PTA. Research suggests that patients treated with manual therapy and exercise experience a clinically important reduction in pain.[31,35]

Important Concept

Research suggests that patients with cervical spine injuries treated with manual therapy and exercise experience a clinically important reduction in pain.[31,35]

An important practical matter to consider when instructing patients to perform cervical ROM exercises is how to stabilize the trunk and shoulders. With muscle and ligament damage, the long-term effect of healing is fibrous tissue contraction, which results in stiffness, restriction, and limitation of motion.[68] To direct the stretch to the affected area effectively, the surrounding structures must be supported and stabilized. For example, if a patient with a lateral flexion injury that results in muscle and ligament damage is instructed to stretch gently laterally away from the side of the injury, the opposite shoulder would elevate (because of the shortened tissues) if the shoulders are not stabilized, rendering the stretch ineffective. To stabilize the shoulder, the patient should perform the stretch while seated and use both hands to grasp under the seat. No shoulder elevation occurs when the patient attempts to stretch the head and neck laterally with the arms fully extended and secured under the seat.

Strengthening and conditioning exercise for the neck and upper quarter include the deep neck flexors. Prevailing theory suggests that stability of the cervical spine is dependent on deep neck flexor strength.[39] Jull and co-workers[40] reported retraining the deep cervical flexors in conjunction with manual therapy to the cervicothoracic spine can effectively decrease neck pain and headache with results being maintained at 1-year follow-up.[15] Precise instruction by the PTA for retraining deep cervical flexors is very important for improved patient function.

Treatment of the deep neck flexors begins with the patient in the supine position. This exercise is designed to recruit the deep neck flexor muscles while avoiding cocontraction of superficial neck flexors. Instruction is given to the patient to keep his or her mouth closed and to nod the head gently, performing a chin tuck. The patient holds this contraction for 10 seconds while the PTA observes for superficial muscle substitution (sternocleidomastoid). Progression of this contraction may occur when the patient is able to contract sufficiently without substitution. To increase intensity, the patient is instructed to perform the contraction and then slightly raise his or her head off the supporting surface. Attention is again focused on substitution of superficial muscles. A neutral spine position should be reinforced with cueing. The goal is to progress to an inclined position and then more functional positions with increasing control and strength.

Initial strengthening of the cervical spine may also include isometric stabilization exercises. Submaximal contractions and precise techniques are important and must be carefully explained and demonstrated to the patient. For isometric stabilization exercises, the patient performs a series of four-way isometrics in an anatomically neutral cervical spine position. The four-position isometric exercises are forward flexion, lateral flexion (right and left), and extension. In preparing to perform these exercises, the patient must demonstrate the ability to hold his or her head and neck in midline without excessive rotation, lateral flexion, forward flexion, or extension malalignment.

To begin, the patient should sit before a mirror to get visual feedback while maintaining proper head and neck alignment. The proper execution of the first isometric position of forward flexion should be explained and demonstrated. With one hand placed on the midline of the forehead (the patient must bring the hand into the described position and not rotate the head toward the hand), the patient should direct a posterior force to the forehead with the hand while resisting head and neck flexion, stimulating isometric strengthening of the

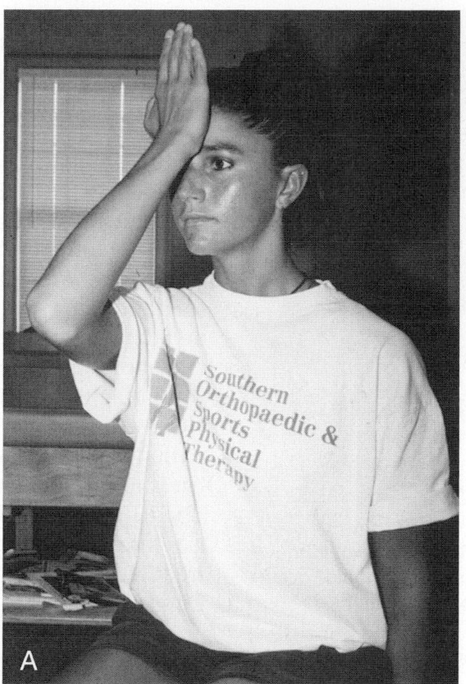

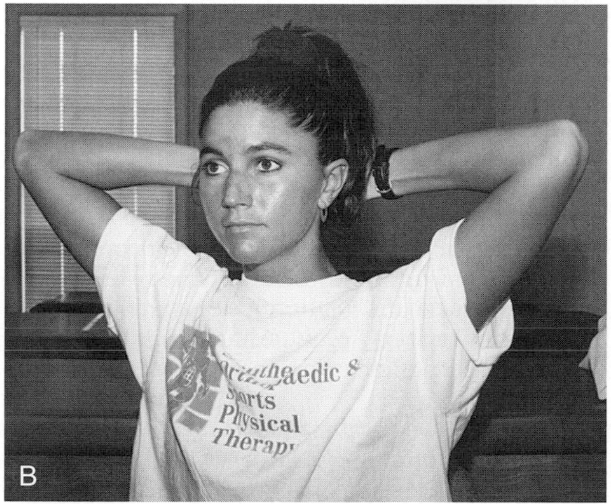

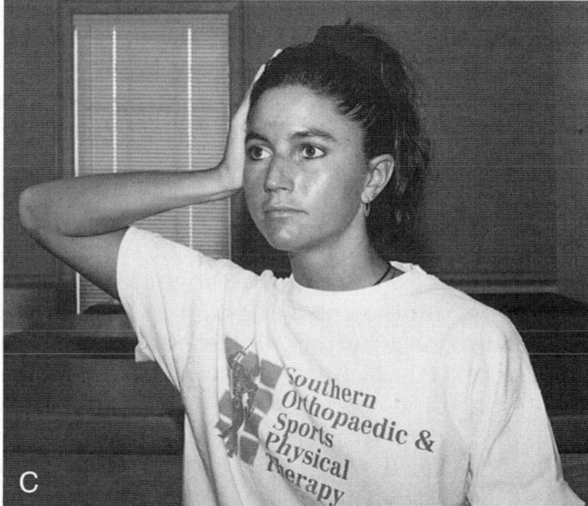

FIG 20-19 Cervical isometrics. **A,** For forward flexion (notice the head must remain in midline and not be allowed to rotate). **B,** For head and neck extension. **C,** For lateral flexion.

anterior cervical muscles. The patient should gradually and slowly build the resistance using the rule of 10's (gradually initiate isometrics with 2-second submaximal contraction, then hold for 6 seconds, then slowly reduce for 2 seconds) rather than suddenly applying maximal force (Fig. 20-19, *A*).

The patient should use both hands to support the occiput for the second position. The patient should maintain the head and neck in the anatomic midline position and not allow the head to flex forward. The patient should be encouraged to apply an anteriorly directed force gradually with both hands while resisting extension of the head. This position effectively strengthens the head and neck extensor group (Fig. 20-19, *B*).

The next position is lateral flexion. While the PTA observes proper head and neck alignment in the mirror, the patient should bring one hand to the side of the head but not allow the head to rotate or laterally flex to meet the hand. The patient should apply lateral pressure while resisting this force. This position is repeated on the opposite side. In each position, no head or neck motion must occur. Usually the patient carries out a series of two to three sets of 10-second isometric exercises two to three times daily. As strength improves, the patient gradually increases the intensity, but sudden or ballistic contractions should be avoided (Fig. 20-19, *C*).

Educating the patient about cervical spine postural mechanics is as important as the actual management of any physical dysfunction. One of the most commonly recognized postural malalignment syndromes affecting the cervical spine is a forward head posture. Typically, this posture is characterized by a loss of flexion in the upper cervical spine region and a loss of extension in the lower cervical spine. The patient should perform axial extension

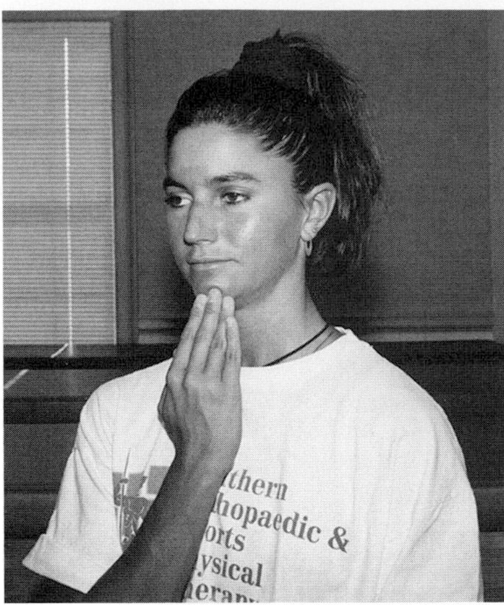

FIG 20-20 Axial extension–cervical retraction. The head should move directly posterior. No head or cervical extension should occur. Attempt to produce a double chin without head or neck flexion.

or cervical retraction exercises. The PT determines which exercises are appropriate for each patient and identifies which patients are candidates for specific axial-extension exercises.

The PT may determine that the patient responds to repeated movements in a specific directional preference. A centralization phenomenon may occur where distal symptoms in the upper quarter decrease or abolish, and symptoms increase or manifest near the central location of the cervical spine. The patient often responds to repeated retraction exercises in supine and sitting positions. Retraction exercises require the patient to be able to demonstrate a midline neutral position. The patient should sit in front of a mirror initially to perform this exercise correctly. The patient should imagine that his or her head is resting on a conveyor belt. The patient must be able to align the ears with the shoulders and move the head straight back on the conveyor belt (Fig. 20-20). If done correctly, a "double chin" is produced as the patient moves the head back. If done incorrectly, the head and neck move into extension. The patient should be encouraged to perform this exercise at home for multiple sets throughout the day or as prescribed by the PT.

The centralization subgroup includes repeated movements and a cotreatment technique with the PT. The PT may request the assistance of the PTA to perform a passive upper extremity movement on the patient while the PT mobilizes the cervical spine. The upper extremity movement follows the upper limb neurodynamic tension test for the median nerve. The PT instructs regarding the direction of the passive movement and the static position to mobilize the nervous system.

UPPER LIMB NEURODYNAMIC TENSION TEST A: MEDIAN NERVE BIAS

The upper limb tension test is assessed by placing the patient in the following positions:

- Supine position
- Scapular depression
- Shoulder abduction
- Forearm supination; wrist and finger extension
- Shoulder lateral rotation
- Elbow extension
- Contralateral/ipsilateral cervical side-bending

Impairments in ROM and strength are frequently accompanied by pain. Pain control subgrouping includes patients with high pain and disability scores noted on outcome measures. These patients may have been involved in a traumatic event or report very recent onset of symptoms. In many cases, these patients present with poor tolerance to interventions and possibly elevated fear avoidance beliefs noted on the Fear Avoidance Beliefs Questionnaire.[28]

Managing these patients requires patient reassurance. Gentle active ROM should be encouraged within the patient's pain tolerance. ROM for adjacent regions such as the shoulder and thoracic spine should also be included. The PT addresses appropriate activity modification, which is reinforced by the PTA. Often these patients require more frequent collaboration with the PT for progression of interventions.

MOBILIZATION OF THE LUMBAR, THORACIC, AND CERVICAL SPINE

Although peripheral joint mobilization is covered in this text, axial skeleton mobilization techniques for the lumbar, thoracic, and cervical spine are not addressed. The extraordinarily complex arrangement and intimate anatomic relationship between vertebral segments and surrounding neurovascular structures require intense, exhaustive study and precise application of techniques after detailed training and clinical practice to be safe, effective, and efficient. The scope of the PTA's training is not consistent with the demanding working knowledge of neurovascular anatomy, biomechanics, and pathophysiology of the lumbar, thoracic, and cervical spine needed to provide mobilization techniques to these areas.

GLOSSARY

Annulus: The outer wall of a vertebral disk. It is composed of 12 to 18 concentrically arranged rings of fibroelastic cartilage.

Directional preference: During repetitive movements into spinal flexion or extension, a patient's symptoms either centralize or peripheralize. Patients with a directional preference have symptoms that centralize with a movement into their directional preference. Patients with a directional preference are thought to have a more favorable prognosis than patients who do not.

Disk: The plate of fibrocartilage between the bodies of adjacent vertebrae.

Disk protrusion: Condition in which nucleus bulges against an intact annulus.

Extruded disk: Condition characterized by nucleus extending through the annulus, but nuclear material remains confined by the posterior longitudinal ligament.

Herniated nucleus pulposus (HNP): A specific type of disk bulge that is further subdivided into protrusion, extrusion, and sequestration.

Kyphosis: An increase in the thoracic posterior convexity that is manifested by a rounded back (and protracted scapulae) posture.

Lordosis: The maintenance of a normal anatomic lordotic curve while lifting any object.

Nucleus pulposus: The fiber (or substance or gel) contained within the annulus.

Radiculopathy: Mechanical compression or inflammation of a nerve root that causes neurologic symptoms into the lower extremities. It can be caused by encroachment on the spinal nerve root by osteophytes or a large disk herniation. Symptoms include pain, numbness, tingling, weakness, burning, or paresthesias.

Scoliosis: A disorder defined as any lateral curvature of the cervical, thoracic, or lumbar spine. It can be classified as structural or nonstructural.[41]

Sequestrated disk: A condition in which the nucleus has breached the confines of the annulus and is free within the spinal canal.

Spine stabilization: Exercises performed to strengthen muscles in the trunk to provide dynamic stabilization of the spinal segments.

Thoracic inlet syndrome: A term used to describe compression of vascular or neurologic tissues as they exit the superior triangle opening of the thorax. This syndrome has been commonly called *outlet syndrome* in the past.

Treatment-based classification (TBC): A multimodal rehabilitation plan that categorizes patients based on their overall symptoms and response to a specific intervention.

REFERENCES

1. Allman FL: Back school program. In *Introduction to back injuries*, Atlanta, GA, 1990, The Atlanta Sports Medicine Clinic.
2. Boden SD, McCowin PR, Davis DO, et al: Abnormal magnetic resonance scans of the cervical spine in asymptomatic subjects. A prospective investigation. *J Bone Joint Surg Am* 72(8):1178–1184, 1990.
3. Borghouts JA, Koes BW, Bouter LM: The clinical course of prognostic factors of non-specific neck pain: a systematic review. *Pain* 77:1–13, 1998.
4. Bovim G, Schrader H, Sand T: Neck pain in the general population. *Spine (Phila Pa 1976)* 19:1307–1309, 1994.
5. Brashear HR, Raney RB: Affections of the spine and thorax. In *Handbook of orthopaedic surgery*, ed 10, St Louis, 1986, Mosby.
6. Brennan GP, Fritz JM, Hunter SJ, et al: Identifying subgroups of patients with acute/subacute "nonspecific" low back pain: results of a randomized clinical trial. *Spine (Phila Pa 1976)* 31(6):623–631, 2006.
7. Browder DA, Childs JD, Cleland JA, et al: Effectiveness of an extension-oriented treatment approach in a subgroup of subjects with low back pain: a randomized clinical trial. *Phys Ther* 87(12):1608–1618, 2007.
8. Burkus JK: Spine. In Loth T, editor: *Orthopaedic boards review*, St Louis, 1993, Mosby.
9. Cailliet R: *Low back pain syndrome*, ed 3, Philadelphia, 1981, FA Davis.
10. Chappuis JL, Johnson GD, Gines AM: *A source guide for spine care*, Atlanta, GA, 1994, Greater Atlanta Spine Center.
11. Childs JD, Cleland JA, Elliott JM, et al: Neck pain: clinical practice guidelines linked to the International Classification of Functioning, Disability and Health from the Orthopedic section of the American Physical Therapy Association. *J Orthop Sports Phys Ther* 38(9):A1–A34, 2008.
12. Childs JD, Fritz JM, Flynn T, et al: Validation of a clinical prediction rule to identify patients with low back pain likely to benefit from spinal manipulation: a validation study. *Ann Intern Med* 141(12):920–928, 2004.
13. Childs JD, Fritz Piva SR, Whitman JM: Proposal of a classification system for patients with neck pain. *J Orthop Sports Phys Ther* 34(11):686–696, 2004.
14. Delitto RS, Rose SJ, Apts DW: An electromyographic analysis of two techniques for squat lifting. *Phys Ther* 67(9):1329–1334, 1987.
15. DeRosa C, Porterfield JA: Lumbar spine and pelvis. In Richardson JK, Iglarsh ZA, editors: *Clinical orthopaedic physical therapy*, Philadelphia, 1994, Saunders.
16. Deyo RA, Gray DT, Kreuter W, et al: United States trends in lumbar fusion surgery for degenerative conditions. *Spine (Phila Pa 1976)* 30:1441–1445, 2005.
17. Deyo RA, Phillips WR: Low back pain: a primary care challenge. *Spine (Phila Pa 1976)* 21:2826–2832, 1996.
18. Dietrich N, Kurowski P: The importance of mechanical factors in the etiology of spondylolysis: a model analysis of loads and stresses in the human lumbar spine. *Spine (Phila Pa 1976)* 10:541–632, 1985.
19. Duda M: Elite lifters at risk of spondylolysis. *Phys Sports Med* 15:107–158, 1987.
20. Ehrmann-Feldman D, Rossignol M, Abenhaim L, et al: Physician referral to physical therapy in a cohort of workers compensated for low back pain. *Phys Ther* 76(2):150–156, 1996.
21. Eismont FJ, Kitchel SH: Thoracolumbar spine. In DeLee JC, Drez D, editors: *Orthopaedic sports medicine: principles and practice*, vol 2, Philadelphia, 1994, Saunders.
22. Flynn T, Fritz J, Whitman J, et al: A clinical prediction rule for classifying patients with low back pain who demonstrate short-term improvement with spinal manipulation. *Spine (Phila Pa 1976)* 27(24):2835–2843, 2002.
23. Fritz JM, Brennan GP: Preliminary classification of a proposed treatment based classification system for patients receiving physical therapy interventions for neck pain. *Phys Ther* 87(5):513–524, 2007.
24. Fritz J, Delitto A, Erhard RE: Comparison of classification-based physical therapy with therapy based on clinical practice guidelines for patients with acute low back pain: a randomized clinical trial. *Spine (Phila Pa 1976)* 28(13):1363–1371, 2003.
25. Fritz JM, Lindsay W, Matheson JW, et al: Is there a subgroup of patients with low back pain likely to benefit from mechanical traction? Results of a randomized clinical trial and subgrouping analysis. *Spine (Phila Pa 1976)* 32(26):E793–E800, 2007.
26. Frymoyer JW: Predicting disability from low back pain. *Clin Orthop Relat Res* 279:101–109, 1992.
27. Fulton M: *Lower-back pain: a new solution for an old problem*, Rolling Meadows, IL, 1992, MedX.
28. George SZ, Fritz JM, Bialosky JE, et al: The effect of a fear-avoidance-based physical therapy intervention for patients with acute low back pain: results of a randomized clinical trial. *Spine (Phila Pa 1976)* 28(23):2551–2560, 2003.
29. Goldstein TS: Treatment of common problems of the spine. In Lewis CB, editor: *Geriatric orthopaedics: rehabilitative management of common problems*, Gaithersburg, MD, 1991, Aspen.
30. Gould JA: The spine. In Gould JA, Davies G, editors: *Orthopedic and sports physical therapy*, ed 2, St Louis, 1990, Mosby.
31. Gross AR, Hoving JL, Haines TA, et al: A Cochrane review of manipulation and mobilization for mechanical neck disorders. *Spine (Phila Pa 1976)* 29(14):1541–1548, 2004.
32. Hebert LA: *The neck-arm-hand book*, Greenville, MA, 1989, IMPACC.
33. Hebert LA: *Your back for life*, Greenville, MA, 1993, IMPACC.
34. Hicks GE, Fritz JM, Delitto A, et al: Preliminary development of a clinical prediction rule for determining which patients with low back pain will respond to a stabilization program. *Spine (Phila Pa 1976)* 86:1753–1762, 2005.
35. Hoving JL, Koes BW, de Vet HC, et al: Manual therapy, physical therapy or continued care by a general practitioner for patients with neck pain. A randomized controlled trial. *Ann Intern Med* 136(10):713–722, 2002.
36. Iglarsh ZA, Snyder-Mackler L: Temporomandibular joint and the cervical spine. In Richardson JK, Iglarsh ZA, editors: *Clinical orthopaedic physical therapy*, Philadelphia, 1994, Saunders.
37. Jackson DW: Low back pain in young athletes: evaluation of stress reaction and discogenic problems. *Am J Sports Med* 7:366–664, 1979.

38. Jette AM, Smith K, Haley SM, et al: Physical therapy episodes of care for patients with low back pain. *Phys Ther* 76:924–935, 1996.
39. Jull G: *Management of cervicogenic headaches. Physical therapy of the cervical and thoracic spine*, St Louis, 2002, Churchill Livingstone.
40. Jull G, Trott P, Potter H, et al: A randomized controlled trial of exercise and manipulative therapy for cervicogenic headache. *Spine (Phila Pa 1976)* 27(17):1835–1843, 2002.
41. Kaiser RK, Rose SJ, Apts DW: *An electromyographic analysis of two techniques for squat lifting*, St Louis, Washington University School of Medicine, Applied Kinesiology Laboratory, Program in Physical Therapy, 1992.
42. Kisner C, Colby LA, editors: *Therapeutic exercise foundations and techniques*, ed 2, Philadelphia, 1989, FA Davis.
43. Knight M, Stewart-Brown S, Fletcher L: Estimating health needs: the impact of a check-list of conditions and quality of life measurement on health information derived from community surveys. *J Public Health Med* 23:179–186, 2001.
44. Lewis CB, Bottomley JM: Orthopaedic treatment considerations. In *Geriatric physical therapy: a clinical approach*, New York, 1994, Appleton & Lange.
45. Linton SJ, Hellsing AL, Hallden K: A population based study of spinal pain among 35-45 year old individuals. Prevalence, sick leave and health care use. *Spine (Phila Pa 1976)* 23(13):1457–1463, 1998.
46. Luo X, Pietrobon R, Sun SX, et al: Estimates and patterns of direct health care expenditures among individuals with back pain in the United States. *Spine (Phila Pa 1976)* 29:79–86, 2004.
47. Macnab I: *Backache*, Baltimore, 1977, Williams & Wilkins.
48. Manchikanti L, Boswell MV, Singh V, et al: Prevalence of facet joint pain in chronic spinal pain of cervical, thoracic, and lumbar regions. *BMC Musculoskelet Disord* 5:15, 2004.
49. Martimo KP, Verbeek J, Karppinen J, et al: Effect of training and lifting equipment for preventing back pain in lifting and handling: a systematic review. *BMJ* 336(7641):429–431, 2008.
50. McKenzie RA: *The lumbar spine: mechanical diagnosis and therapy*, Waikanae, New Zealand, 1981, Orthopedic Physical Therapy Products.
51. McLain RF: Mechanoreceptor endings in human cervical facet joints. *Iowa Orthop J* 13:149–154, 1993.
52. Miller MD, editor: *Review of orthopaedics*, Philadelphia, 1992, Saunders.
53. Niemisto L, Lahtinen-Suopanki T, Rissanen P, et al: A randomized trial of combined manipulation, stabilizing exercises, and physician consultation compared to physician consultation alone for chronic low back pain. *Spine (Phila Pa 1976)* 28(19):2185–2191, 2003.
54. O'Sullivan JJ, Ellis JJ, Makofsky HW: The five "L's" of lifting. *Phys Ther Forum* 10(14):3–6, 1991.
55. O'Sullivan PB, Twomey LT, Allison GT: Evaluation of specific stabilizing exercise in the treatment of chronic low back pain with radiologic diagnosis of spondylolysis or spondylolisthesis. *Spine (Phila Pa 1976)* 22:2959–2967, 1997.
56. Panjabi M, Abumi K, Duranceau J, et al: Spinal stability and intersegmental muscle forces. A biochemical model. *Spine (Phila Pa 1976)* 14(2):194–200, 1989.
57. Paris SV: *The spine: etiology and treatment of dysfunction including joint manipulation*, Atlanta, GA, 1979, Course Notes.
58. Raney NH, Petersen EJ, Smith TA, et al: Development of a clinical prediction rule to identify patients with neck pain likely to benefit from cervical traction and exercise. *Eur Spine J* 18(3):382–391, 2009.
59. Spitzer WO, Skovron ML, Salmi LR, et al: Scientific monograph of the Quebec Task Force on Whiplash-Associated Disorders: redefining "whiplash" and its management. *Spine (Phila Pa 1976)* 20(Suppl 8):1S–73S, 1995.
60. Stratton SA, Bryan JM: Dysfunction, evaluation and treatment of the cervical spine and thoracic inlet. In Donatelli R, Wooden MJ, editors: *Orthopaedic physical therapy*, New York, 1989, Churchill-Livingstone.
61. U.S. Physical Therapy: *Work site partners, functional capacity evaluation system, industrial rehabilitation solutions*, Houston, TX, 1994, USPT System Manual.
62. Wainner RS, Gill H: Diagnosis and nonoperative management of cervical radiculopathy. *J Orthop Sports Phys Ther* 30:728–744, 2000.
63. Watkins RG, Dillin WH: Lumbar spine injury in the athlete. *Clin Sports Med* 9:419–448, 1990.
64. Whitman JM, Flynn T, Fritz JM: Nonsurgical management of patients with lumbar spinal stenosis: a literature review and a case series of three patients managed with physical therapy. *Phys Med Rehabil Clin N Am* 15(1):77–101, 2003.
65. Wiltse LL: Spondylolisthesis in children. *Clin Orthop* 21:156–163, 1957.
66. Wiltse LL, Widell EH, Jackson DW: Fatigue fracture: the basic lesion in isthmic spondylolisthesis. *J Bone Joint Surg Am* 57:17–22, 1975.
67. Wright A, Mayer TG, Gatchel RJ: Outcomes of disabling cervical spine disorders in compensation injuries. A prospective comparison to tertiary rehabilitation response for chronic lumbar spinal disorders. *Spine (Phila Pa 1976)* 24(2):178–183, 1999.
68. Wroble RR, Albright JP: Neck and low back injuries in wrestling. *Clin Sports Med* 5(2):295–325, 1986.
69. Wyatt LH: Facet syndrome in the cervical spine. *J Am Chiropr Assoc* 47(3):27–28, 2010.
70. Yahara ML: Shoulder. In Richardson JK, Iglarsh ZA, editors: *Clinical orthopaedic physical therapy*, Philadelphia, 1994, Saunders.

REVIEW QUESTIONS

Multiple Choice

1. Which of the following statements about the spine is true?
   a. The spine has 20 intervertebral disks.
   b. The greatest portion of shock absorption comes from the disk.
   c. The annulus provides some stability.
   d. The disk is highly vascularized.
2. Which of the following statements about intradiscal pressure is true?
   a. Standing pressure is 75% of body weight.
   b. Supine pressure is less than 25% of body weight.
   c. Bending forward creates pressure in excess of 350% of body weight.
   d. Bending forward creates pressure in excess of 500% of body weight.
3. Which spinal ligament runs anterior along the vertebral body?
   a. ALL
   b. PLL
   c. Ligamentum flavum
   d. Supraspinous ligament
4. At what level would a spondylolisthesis that has 0% to 25% anterior slipping be graded?
   a. Grade I
   b. Grade II
   c. Grade III
   d. Grade IV
5. Which of the following describes a condition in which referred pain symptoms distally move more toward the spine?
   a. Slipped disk
   b. Extruded disk
   c. Directional preference
   d. Centralization
6. A patient with a spondylolisthesis would most often complain of pain with which spinal motion?
   a. Flexion
   b. Extension
   c. Side bending
   d. Rotation

7. Which of the following conditions is caused by a progressive narrowing of the spinal canal that constricts and compresses nerve roots?
   a. Spondylolisthesis
   b. Spondylolysis
   c. Radiculopathy
   d. Stenosis
8. Which of the following statements regarding spinal fractures is true?
   a. There is a decreased incidence with increased age.
   b. Spinal fracture occurs after traumatic event.
   c. All spinal motions could produces fractures.
   d. Greater bone density increases fracture risk.
9. In which of the following conditions is there an increase in the thoracic posterior convexity?
   a. Kyphosis
   b. Lordosis
   c. Scoliosis
   d. Concavity
10. Treatment of acute cervical spine whiplash injuries includes:
    a. Aggressive passive ROM
    b. Strict immobilization
    c. Gentle active ROM
    d. Resisted isotonics
11. Which of the following is most likely not a cause of cervical radiculopathy into the hands and fingers?
    a. Disk herniation
    b. Spondylosis
    c. Osteophytes
    d. Facet hypertrophy
12. Intradiscal pressures are increased most during which of the following activities?
    a. Sitting
    b. Walking
    c. Bilateral leg raise
    d. Lifting with flexed torso and knees straight
13. Using the traditional theoretical model to describe fluid mechanics of the disk, when a person bends forward, which way does the nucleus pulposus move?
    a. Backward
    b. Forward
    c. Left
    d. Right
14. The greatest amount of shock absorption of the lumbar segments comes from which of the following tissues?
    a. Disk
    b. Annulus
    c. Nucleus pulposus
    d. Vertebral body
15. Which of the following terms refers to a condition in which the nucleus bulges against an intact annulus?
    a. Protrusion
    b. Extrusion
    c. Prolapse
    d. Sequestration

Short Answer

16. Match the following list of percentages relating to intradiscal pressure with the appropriate and corresponding body position.

100%	Supine (knees flexed)
75%	Standing
35%	Bending forward
25%	Side-lying
275%	Supine

17. List the "five L's" of lifting, as described by O'Sullivan, Ellis, and Makofsky.
18. Describe the causes and symptoms of radiculopathy.
19. What are the differences between protruded, extruded, and sequestrated discs?
20. Explain the methods of treatment for kyphosis.

Fill in the Blank

21. ____________ is the mechanical compression or inflammation of a nerve root that causes neurologic symptoms in the lower extremities.
22. ____________ is the forward slippage of one superior vertebra over an inferior vertebra, whereas ____________ is a bony defect in the pars interarticularis of the posterior elements of the spine.
23. Thoracic disk herniations occur in ____________% of the population.
24. ____________ is the most commonly used brace for scoliosis.
25. The ____________ is the outer wall of a vertebral disk that is composed of 12 to 18 concentrically arranged rings of fibroelastic cartilage.

True/False

26. The intervertebral lumbar disk is essentially avascular and aneural except for the periphery of the annulus, which is innervated.
27. Manual muscle testing is the most effective way to quantify lumbar muscle strength and performance.
28. Lumbar extension exercises are advocated for spondylolisthesis.
29. With nonstructural scoliosis, positional changes result in a decrease in the curvature.
30. Axial stretching (trunk elongation) is not advocated for the treatment of scoliosis.

Chapter 21

Orthopedic Management of the Shoulder

Terry Trundle

CHAPTER OUTLINE

LEARNING OBJECTIVES

1. Identify and describe methods, management, and rehabilitation for subacromial rotator cuff impingement.
2. Identify and describe methods of management and rehabilitation for tears of the rotator cuff.
3. Describe methods of management and rehabilitation for glenohumeral instability.
4. Discuss methods of management and rehabilitation for adhesive capsulitis.
5. Identify and describe common injuries of the acromioclavicular joint.
6. Describe common methods of management and rehabilitation for injuries of the acromioclavicular joint.
7. Identify and describe common fractures of the scapula, clavicle, and proximal humerus.
8. Outline and describe methods of management and rehabilitation of fractures around the shoulder.
9. Describe methods of management and rehabilitation after shoulder arthroplasty.
10. Describe common manual exercise techniques for the shoulder.

KEY TERMS

Acromioplasty
Bankart lesion
Glenohumeral joint
Hawkins-Kennedy test
Hill-Sachs lesion
Neer impingement test
Primary shoulder impingement
Scapular dyskinesis
Secondary shoulder impingement

This chapter introduces common injuries, treatment, and rehabilitation procedures related to the **glenohumeral joint**, acromioclavicular (AC) joint, scapula, and proximal humerus. The shoulder is the most mobile of all joints with multiple planes of motion. This anatomic complex is made up of three main components: bones, joints, and passive stabilizing structures. Bones include the humerus, clavicle, and scapula. Joints include glenohumeral, AC, sternoclavicular, and scapulothoracic articulation. Passive stabilizers are the labrum, superior glenohumeral ligament, middle glenohumeral ligament, inferior glenohumeral ligament, and capsule. Muscles provide dynamic support and stability. The shoulder is made up of more than 18 major muscles that directly or indirectly provide mobility and stability of the entire shoulder complex (Table 21-1).

Because of the complexity of the shoulder and surrounding tissues, the physical therapist assistant (PTA) is strongly encouraged to review pertinent anatomy and kinesiology of the glenohumeral, AC, and scapulothoracic joints. The PTA should review the mechanisms of tissue healing because these principles clarify tissue healing concepts and reinforce the need for early protected motion after injury, immobilization, and recovery of strength and function of the shoulder complex. This chapter focuses on the recognition of certain orthopedic injuries and rehabilitation procedures used to reduce pain and swelling, improve motion, restore strength and endurance, and return the patient to normal function.

TABLE 21-1 Kinesiology

Muscle	Action	Innervation	Attachments
Supraspinatus	Abduction and elevation of humerus	C4-C5-C6	Medial two thirds of supraspinous fossa of scapula to greater tubercle of humerus
Subscapularis	Internal rotation of humerus	C5-C6-C7	Subscapular fossa to lesser tubercle of humerus
Infraspinatus	External rotation of humerus	C4-C6 suprascapular	Suprascapular fossa to middle facet of greater tuberosity of humerus
Teres minor	External rotation of humerus	C5-C6 axillary	Lateral border of scapula to lowermost of three facets on humerus
Trapezius	Elevation of scapula and stabilization of scapulothoracic motion	Spinal accessory for motor innervation and C3-C4 sensory	Superior nuchal line of occipital bone, external occipital protuberance, and ligamentum nuchae and spinal processes of C7-T12
Serratus anterior	Abduction and lateral tilt of scapula	C5-C6-C7-C8	Outer surface and superior borders of upper eight to nine ribs to medial borders of scapula
Levator scapulae	Elevation and downward rotation of scapula	C3-C4-C5	Transverse processes of first four cervical vertebrae to medial border of scapula
Rhomboids	Downward rotation adduction and elevation of scapula	C4-C5	Spinous processes of fourth to fifth thoracic vertebrae to medial border of scapula
Teres major	Internal rotation of humerus	C5-C7 lower subscapular	Dorsal aspect of inferior angle of scapula to medial lip of bicipital groove
Latissimus dorsi	Retraction of shoulder girdle and strong extensor of humerus	C6-C8 thoracodorsal	Supraspinous ligament of lower six thoracic vertebrae and thoracolumbar fascia, posterior iliac crest, and lower four ribs with small slip to inferior angle of scapula
Deltoid	Flexion, abduction, and extension of humerus	C5-C6 axillary	Deltoid tuberosity to clavicle, acromion, and spine of scapula
Pectoralis major	Adductor and internal rotator of humerus	C5-C6 clavicular portion C7-T1 sternal portion	Sternum and clavicle to lateral lip of bicipital groove

SUBACROMIAL ROTATOR CUFF IMPINGEMENT

A common cause of shoulder pain and dysfunction in laborers, athletes, and individuals who repetitively lift overhead is subacromial rotator cuff impingement. In this disorder, the tendons of the rotator cuff are crowded, buttressed, or compressed under the coracoacromial arch, resulting in mechanical wear, stress, and friction.[20,23,26] Clinically, the distinction must be made between primary and secondary impingement because there are important differences in treatment related to the specific cause of impingement.[33] **Primary shoulder impingement** refers to mechanical compression of the rotator cuff tendons, primarily the supraspinatus tendon, as they pass under the coracoacromial ligament between the acromion and coracoid process.

Important Concepts

Clinically, the distinction must be made between primary and secondary impingement because there are important differences in treatment related to the specific cause of impingement.

Secondary shoulder impingement is related to glenohumeral instability that creates a reduced subacromial space because the humeral head elevates and minimizes the area under the coracoacromial ligament.[23] This mechanical instability is the result of impairment of muscle coordination and weakness of the scapular stabilizers.

Age-related degenerative changes also can result in a decreased subacromial margin between the rotator cuff and coracoacromial arch. Bony osteophyte formation can occupy space under the anteroinferior surface of the acromion, which consequently reduces the available space. A reduction in available space in the shoulder is known as *anatomic crowding*. The supraspinatus tendon is the most common structure involved with rotator cuff impingement; the vascularity of the supraspinatus tendon is causative.[23] An area just proximal to the insertion on the greater tuberosity is hypovascular and is commonly referred to as a *watershed zone, critical zone,* or *critical portion*. This area of relatively transient hypovascularity occurs with repeated arm motions from abduction to adduction, which compromises the blood supply to the area. The combination of reduced blood supply to the supraspinatus tendon and mechanical wear, stress, and friction as a result of repeated overhead motions can lead to primary impingement, supraspinatus tendinitis, and ultimately tears within the rotator cuff.[30]

The various stages of rotator cuff impingement are related to age and degenerative changes in the cuff itself. Neer[36] identified three specific stages of impingement (tendinitis):

- Stage I: Occurs in younger patients (usually <25 years old) but can occur at any age. Clinical features are edema and hemorrhage. Pain is worse with shoulder abduction greater than 90°. It is essentially a reversible lesion that responds to conservative physical therapy interventions.[37]

- Stage II: Fibrosis and tendinitis stage, which usually affects patients between the ages of 25 and 40 years.[2] It is classified as irreversible because of long-term repeated stress, wherein the supraspinatus tendon, biceps tendon, and subacromial bursa become fibrotic. Pain is the predominant feature and occurs with daily activities; it frequently causes the patient difficulty at night.
- Stage III: Affects patients older than 40 years. It is characterized by tendon degeneration, rotator cuff tears, and rotator cuff ruptures. It is usually associated with a long history of repeated shoulder pain and dysfunction and significant muscle weakness and atrophy.

Various clinical tests can be used to identify the presence of pain related to specific maneuvers of the shoulder. During the initial evaluation performed by the physical therapist (PT), tests are used to elicit impingement signs. One of these is the **Neer impingement test**, in which pain is reported while the shoulder is passively taken through elevation with internal rotation. This test elicits impingement secondary to compression of the rotator cuff against the coracoacromial arch.[11] The **Hawkins-Kennedy test** is performed by passively elevating the shoulder to 90° in the scapular plane with internal rotation over pressure (Fig. 21-1). In most cases, elevation of more than 80° or 90° elicits pain. Exercise and all activities that require the shoulder to elevate or abduct past 80° or 90° must be strictly avoided until all symptoms of pain have been eliminated.

Important Concepts

The Hawkins-Kennedy test is performed by passively elevating the shoulder to 90° in the scapular plane with internal rotation over pressure. In most cases, elevation of more than 80° or 90° elicits pain. Exercise and all activities that require the shoulder to elevate or abduct past 80° or 90° must be strictly avoided until all symptoms of pain have been eliminated.

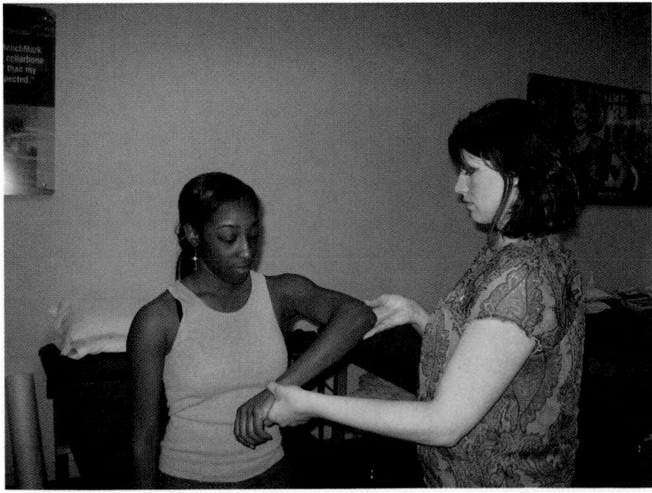

FIG 21-1 The Hawkins-Kennedy impingement test demonstrates the impingement sign by forcibly medially rotating the proximal humerus when the arm is forward flexed to 90°.

REHABILITATION OF PRIMARY AND SECONDARY ROTATOR CUFF IMPINGEMENT

Kamkar and colleagues[23] identified scapular weakness as leading to "functional scapular instability," which affects scapular position during activities that cause a "relative decrease in the subacromial space." This secondary impingement requires the scapulothoracic muscles to be strengthened and stabilized before specific rotator cuff weakness can be addressed. The scapula thoracic articulation is known to many clinicians as the true core of the upper extremity. To stabilize the humeral head effectively so that it does not migrate superiorly, causing "winging" or "tipping," the scapular muscles (serratus anterior; upper, middle, and lower trapezius; levator scapulae; and rhomboid muscles) must be strengthened.[20,23] If the supraspinatus is overworked trying to stabilize the humeral head, it is unable to function effectively to depress the humeral head. The resultant upward movement decreases the subacromial space and irritates the subacromial soft tissues, perpetuating the impingement process.[19]

The initial evaluation performed by the PT is crucial in determining which exercises are to be performed to help stabilize the scapula and which should be avoided initially to reduce rotator cuff irritation with glenohumeral instability or superior migration of the humeral head.[41] One of the assessments needed in the treatment of impingement is to rule out **scapular dyskinesis**. The normal position of the scapula is symmetric mounted on the rib cage. Any alteration of normal position affects the pathology of the glenohumeral joint.[44] The static examination of the scapulothoracic positions has been described by Kibler.[14,44] Type 1 scapula position is referred to as an anterior tilting, which means the inferior angle of the scapula is asymmetric. Internal rotated scapula type 2 is noted by the observation of the medial border being asymmetric. The type 3 scapula position is known as the elevated scapula with asymmetric alignment of the superior glide appearance of the AC joint.

Important Concepts

Normal position of the scapula is symmetric mounted on the rib cage. Any alteration of normal position affects the pathology of the glenohumeral joint.

Scapular stabilization exercises are only one component of a successful rehabilitation program.[8,13] In general, a comprehensive rehabilitation program to address rotator cuff impingement, rotator cuff tendinitis (supraspinatus tendinitis), and degenerative tears of the rotator cuff tendons includes modification of activities, local and systemic methods to control pain and swelling (nonsteroidal antiinflammatory drugs [NSAIDs], corticosteroid injections, ice, ultrasound, iontophoresis, phonophoresis), stretching and strengthening exercises, and a return to normal function after reevaluation by the PT and with continued maintenance of protective positions and general conditioning.

The nonoperative treatment of impingement and symptomatic rotator cuff tears focuses on a three-phase, criterion-based rehabilitation program. The three phases of rehabilitation are as follows: phase I, prefunctional; phase II, return to function; and phase III, return to activity. Phase I, prefunctional, concentrates on relief of symptoms and initiating exercises to improve or maintain motion. Because impingement symptoms are usually worsened with overhead activities, the patient must modify activities of daily living (ADL) and all other motions that may place the shoulder at or above 80° to 90° elevation. Home activities that require modification include cleaning hard-to-reach places and painting overhead. Work site tasks that must be adapted include heavy overhead lifting, manual labor, reaching, and climbing. Sporting activities such as tennis, golf, swimming, and baseball also must be modified to avoid impingement. The key to remember in each case is modification, not elimination, of compromising activities. For example, for a recreational tennis player, overhead serving should be avoided, but all other ground strokes may be able to be maintained. For household activities and work site modifications, rearrangement and advanced planning of overhead tasks may be all that is needed to minimize the aggravating position of elevation greater than 80° or 90°. The PTA must constantly reinforce the concept of protective positioning and should encourage compliance throughout the course of rehabilitation.

In addition to activity modification, management of pain and swelling can be achieved with various physician-prescribed oral NSAIDs and physical therapy agents. Usually ice packs, ultrasound, iontophoresis or phonophoresis, and infrared laser application are used to help control symptoms.

Throughout phase I, stretching exercises are performed to increase blood flow and contractility and improve range of motion (ROM). The PTA must pay particular attention to performing all stretching activities because many generalized shoulder stretches involve full forward shoulder elevation and abduction maneuvers. All phase I stretching should encourage nonballistic, slow, controlled, pain-free motion at less than 80° to 90° of elevation. Capsular mobility has been shown to be very helpful in increasing motion and preparing the surrounding muscles to assist in shoulder elevation in all planes of motion.[29,35,41] However, once symptoms are managed, the patient can perform all stretches involving elevation and abduction if these stretches do not produce symptoms. Depending on the initial evaluation data gathered by the PT, the patient may be instructed in two specific stretches that are suggested to be effective in addressing posterior capsular tightness. Shoulder adduction across the chest (cross-body stretching) and internal shoulder rotation are used cautiously to improve posterior capsular tightness and overcome the limitations on motion of internal rotation of the shoulder. The effective use of the sleeper stretch to increase posterior capsular mobility has been reported.[3,27] The sleeper stretch involves lying on the affected shoulder at 90° of abduction with neutral positioning of the trunk. The shoulder is slowly placed into internal rotation to place a stretch to the posterior capsule. This position may be tolerated well by younger or athletic patients (Fig. 21-2).[25] Older patients with impingement may find this position uncomfortable, and the modified sleeper stretch may be effective for posterior capsular stretching.[44] This stretch involves allowing the patient to open up the trunk by rotating posteriorly 30° and placing the shoulder at a lower angle of abduction to allow a more comfortable start position of posterior capsular stretch. The angle of the glenohumeral joint is placed at 60° of abduction and progressed to angles of 70°, 80°, and back to 90° based on tolerance over time.[44] Each stretch is held for 30 seconds, and the number of repetitions is determined by the PTA (Fig. 21-3). The concept of anterior capsular mobility has been presented as important for shoulder mobility to treat or prevent impingement while regaining horizontal abduction to prepare for triplane overhead motion.[28]

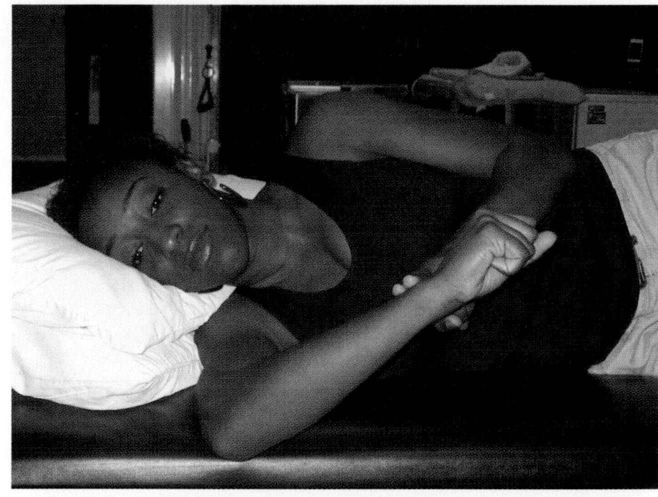

FIG 21-2 Sleeper stretch.

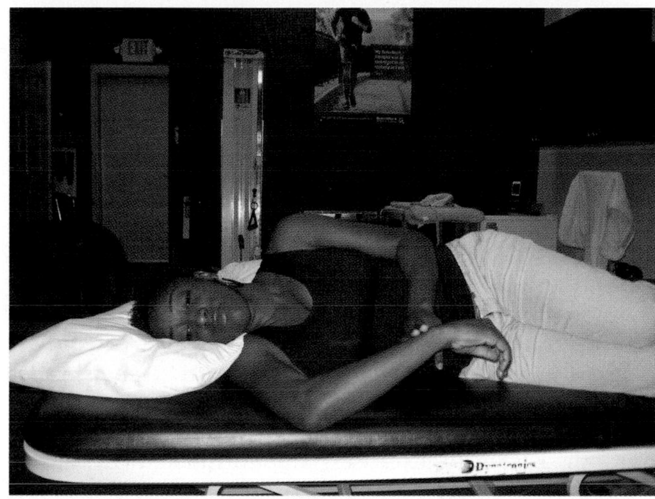

FIG 21-3 Modified sleeper stretch.

Important Concepts

The sleeper stretch involves lying on the affected shoulder at 90° of abduction with neutral positioning of the trunk. The shoulder is slowly placed into internal rotation to place a stretch to the posterior capsule.

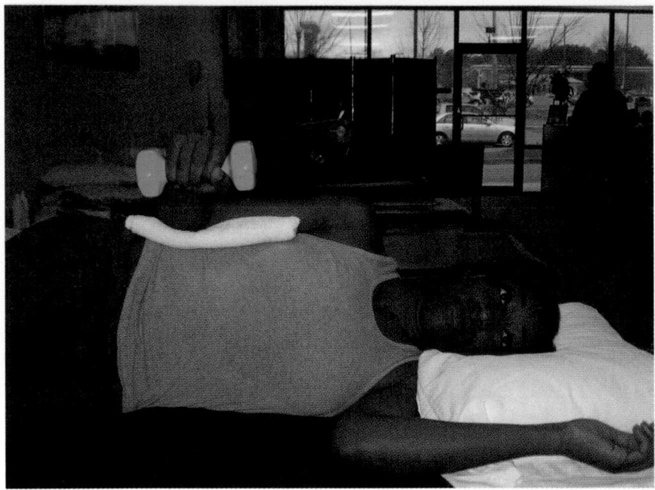

FIG 21-4 Side-lying external rotation.

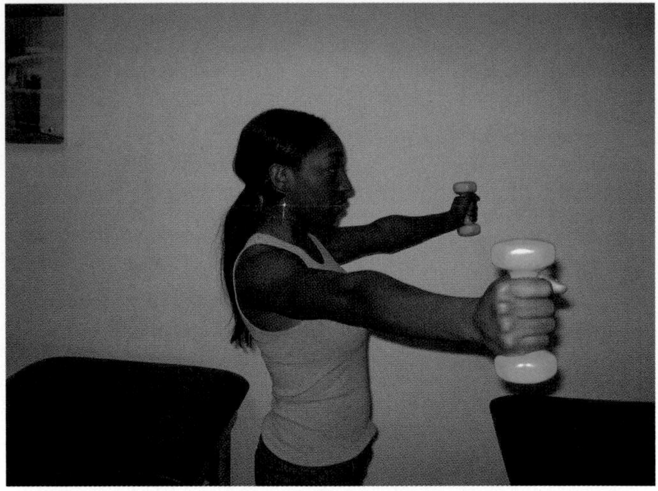

FIG 21-5 Scaption. Shoulder elevation in the plane of the scapula.

Initial strengthening activities that can begin during phase I generally include scapular stabilization exercises and light rotator cuff strengthening. Closed kinetic chain (CKC) loading, such as wall push-ups, can be an effective pain-free low-level muscle recruitment exercise. CKC exercise, which is known as distal fixed loading, provides cocontraction and triplane stabilization[45] with lower muscle contraction load than open kinetic chain (OKC) exercises.[6,9,47] When the patient demonstrates improved motion and ability to perform ADL without pain, a progression through a series of OKC muscle strengthening can begin. Shoulder rehabilitation exercises are often referred to as an OKC challenge.[44] Isotonic exercises that allow concentric and eccentric muscle contraction are more functional because they create free limb speed of motion. Eccentric exercises are considered by many authorities as the "missing link" in shoulder rehabilitation, and a special focus should be placed on isotonic eccentric exercises. This type of exercise is known to create a functional carryover of strengthening that leads to improved mobility. The PTA should instruct the patient to go slow with eccentric exercise because it can cause delayed-onset muscle soreness. Prone extension to the hip, side-lying external rotation, and scaption elevation without pain are some recommended exercises for rotator cuff recruitment toward strengthening (Fig. 21-4).[6,38] Specific rotator cuff strengthening exercises should focus on the supraspinatus muscle.[38] Studies demonstrate that the supraspinatus, infraspinatus, subscapularis, deltoid, latissimus dorsi, and pectoral muscles are effectively strengthened by arm elevation in the transverse plane, shoulder elevation with neutral rotation in the plane of the scapula (Fig. 21-5), prone horizontal shoulder abduction with external rotation (Fig. 21-6), and seated press-ups.[32]

Important Concepts

Eccentric exercises are considered by many authorities as the "missing link" in shoulder rehabilitation, and a special focus should be placed on isotonic eccentric exercises. This type of exercise is known to create a functional carryover of strengthening that leads to improved mobility.

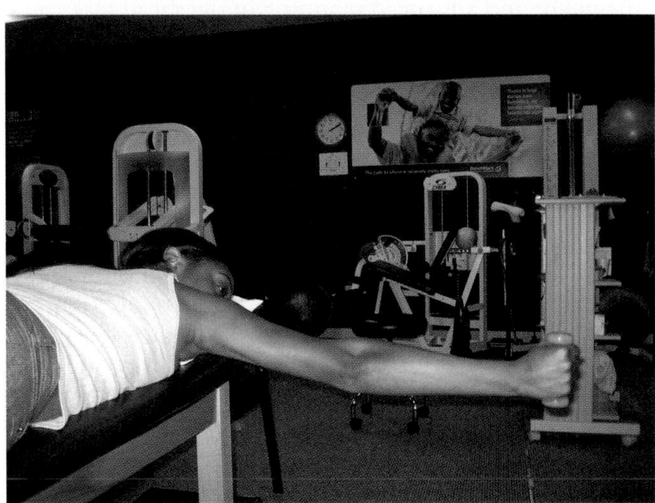

FIG 21-6 Prone horizontal shoulder abduction with external rotation.

Phase II, return to function, progresses with advanced scapular stabilization exercises that are encouraged as part of a comprehensive glenohumeral and scapulothoracic strengthening program. This phase employs progressive resistive strengthening via increased resistance while using OKC exercises. Electromyography studies[6,34] identified four basic scapular stabilization exercises that strengthen the upper, middle, and lower trapezius; the levator scapulae; the rhomboid major; the pectoralis minor; and the middle and lower serratus anterior muscles.[8,12] These exercises are rowing, scapular plane elevation (scaption), press-ups, and push-ups followed by scapular protraction. Exercises such as supine ceiling punch, also known as press-up with a plus, are performed to activate the serratus anterior to promote protraction. The function of protraction is to prepare the scapula to clear the subacromial space to allow elevation greater than 90°. As strength improves and when motion increases, a gradual return to normal function signifies the beginning of phase III, return to activity.[43]

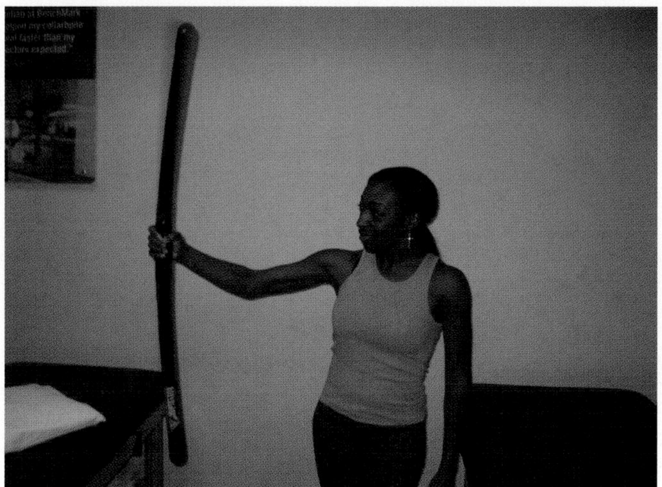

FIG 21-7 Oscillatory training (Bodyblade; Hymanson, Inc, Playa del Rey, CA) for deltoid.

Important Concepts

The function of protraction is to prepare the scapula to clear the subacromial space to allow elevation greater than 90°.

Functional recovery is slow and must proceed cautiously; overhead activities are introduced incrementally as the patient is able to demonstrate pain-free motion and the ability to perform strengthening activities. Some advanced return to activity phase exercises include oscillatory training (Bodyblade) using triplane positioning (Fig. 21-7).[40]

SURGICAL MANAGEMENT OF SHOULDER IMPINGEMENT AND ROTATOR CUFF TEARS

When physical therapy interventions fail to provide long-lasting relief and in cases of rotator cuff tears (Neer's stage III impingement, tendon degeneration, and cuff tears), various surgical procedures can be used to correct the underlying pathologic condition. With subacromial impingement not involving a specific rotator cuff tear, subacromial decompression (SAD) can be used to eliminate or diminish the abnormality causing the impingement between the humeral head and the undersurface of the acromion, allowing increased movement of the tendons without irritation. **Acromioplasty** includes beveling or reshaping of the acromion with detachment of the coracoacromial ligament. Distal clavicle excision may also be involved.[39] Acromioplasty may create complications such as deltoid weakness, excessive resection causing instability, and inadequate resection causing residual symptoms. If there is an associated rotator cuff tear (small tear <1 cm, medium tear <3 cm, large tear >5 cm), a SAD procedure is used in conjunction with direct repair of the rotator cuff defect. The SAD procedure can be performed as an open arthrotomy or as an arthroscopic procedure.[39]

Important Concepts

With subacromial impingement not involving a specific rotator cuff tear, subacromial decompression can be used to eliminate or diminish the abnormality causing the impingement between the humeral head and the undersurface of the acromion allowing increased movement of the tendons without irritation.

Rehabilitation after SAD or rotator cuff repair closely parallels nonoperative rehabilitation of rotator cuff impingement. However, time must be allowed for healing of the soft tissues and bone after surgery. Some clearly identified differences exist between rehabilitation procedures used for decompression and small cuff tears (<1 cm) and repairs of medium (<2 to 3 cm) and large (>4 to 5 cm) cuff tears with SAD.[39] With a small cuff tear repaired in conjunction with a decompression procedure, active motion and pain-free exercise can begin as soon as the patient can tolerate these activities.[39,43,44] However, if the rotator cuff tear is between 2 cm and 5 cm, tissue protection must be longer to allow for extensive soft tissue healing. If full active ROM is allowed too early, healing of the rotator cuff may be compromised because of the stresses placed on the repaired tissues. The type of surgical procedure used, mini-open procedure or arthroscopic approach, and the healing constraints must be considered for proper beginning of successful rehabilitation. Large cuff tears may require longer periods of time for recovery to achieve improved healing.[43]

Generally, recovery after SAD with or without rotator cuff repair follows a prescribed three-phase rehabilitation program.[44] Phase I, the prefunctional phase, lasts approximately 3 to 4 weeks[39,43,44] and focuses on control of pain and swelling with NSAIDs, oral analgesics, ice packs, ultrasound, phonophoresis (if needed), infrared laser therapy, and various degrees and durations of manual ROM, depending on the extent of tissue injury. The concept of early protected manual motion applies depending on the precise nature of the injury and which surgical procedure is used. The prefunctional phase should include increasing ROM, scapula stabilization beginning with retraction, and adding protraction when the patient has pain-free arm control.

With small rotator cuff repairs (<1 cm), isometric submaximal muscle sets of the shoulder extensors, flexors, abductors, external rotators, and internal rotators can begin as early as pain allows. Active assisted range of motion (AAROM) activities beginning with manual exercise must be performed pain-free. Active biceps and triceps exercises are performed in the neutral humerus position beginning with isometrics and progressing to light resistive exercises. ROM and strength gradually increase as pain and swelling are controlled.

At the end of this phase, the use of an upper body ergometer (UBE) may be introduced. The early use of CKC activity with double-arm wall push-ups may be helpful for low level recruitment of shoulder muscles.[43,45,47] With increased arm control strength and motion, phase II, the return to function phase, can begin. It generally lasts from

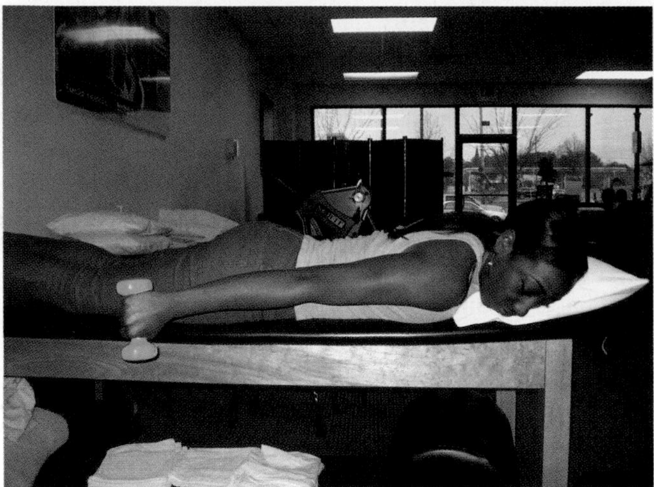

FIG 21-8 Prone extension to hip.

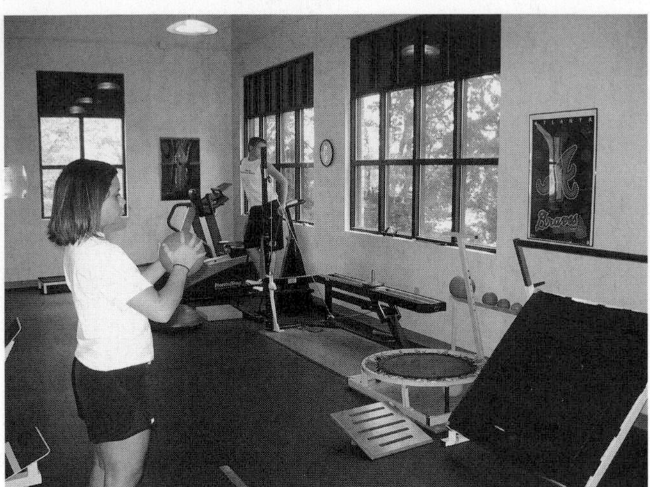

FIG 21-9 Plyometric activity with plyotoss exercise.

weeks 5 through 12 after surgery. During this phase, progressive motion can be used, although with caution for repetitive shoulder abduction and forward elevation above 90°. The use of band strengthening of the rotator cuff should be performed in a short-arc pattern of motion, normally in the standing position.[1,21,43] In addition, dumbbell isotonic concentric and eccentric exercises for recruitment of the humeral head decompression (rotator cuff) may begin using short-arc pain-free ROM. Short-arc movement patterns are designed to promote glenohumeral strengthening in the early phase of rehabilitation while limiting scapular involvement. This program is known as *positional recruitment* for the purpose of low-level strengthening and progresses according to the tolerance of the patient and demonstration of arm control.[43] During phase II, progressive strengthening exercises for elevation in scaption are performed allowing for what is known as shoulder hike. Prone positional exercise, such as prone extension to hip (Fig. 21-8) and short-arc prone scaption at 100°, and eccentric training of scaption have been very useful in treating shoulder hike.[6,32,38,43] Eccentric scaption is described as placement eccentric exercise to regain muscle control that is caused by rotator cuff weakness and is referred to as shoulder elevation hike dysfunction. This is a manual placement exercise into a scaption angle of the shoulder. Passive elevation is placing the shoulder 10° above the concentric angle in which the shoulder hike occurs. The PTA holds the shoulder at this angle and asks the patient to perform an isometric contraction and maintains control of this by manual assistance to secure the shoulder at this angle. After the patient has gained isometric control of this position, the PTA places his or her hand down at the start angle of the lift and allows the patient to lower the arm into the PTA's hand by a slow eccentric lowering of the elevated arm creating an eccentric placement. This exercise should be performed slowly with limited repetitions. Progressive resistive exercises (PREs) are a major part of the return to function phase. With some patients, based on good pain-free response to all rotator cuff exercise, advanced scapular stabilization and oscillatory training with the use of a Bodyblade may begin (see Fig. 21-7).

Important Concepts

Dumbbell isotonic concentric and eccentric exercises for recruitment of the humeral head decompression (rotator cuff) may begin using short-arc pain-free ROM. Short-arc movement patterns are designed to promote glenohumeral strengthening in the early phase of rehabilitation while limiting scapular involvement.

Phase III, the return to activity phase, can begin when the patient can demonstrate normal motion without symptoms and with improved strength. This phase lasts approximately from week 12 on. Return to activity always includes the continuation of PREs. This aspect of rehabilitation is for the long haul.[43] Advanced CKC exercises such as single-arm wall push-ups on an uneven surface may be introduced.[45] An advanced patient would be one at a higher level. Progressed further, stronger, and able to tolerate increased stresses (Fig. 21-9).

During the return to activity phase, core rotator cuff strengthening exercises of forward elevation, scaption, prone horizontal abduction with external rotation, and press-ups as well as scapular stabilization exercises of seated rows, prone scaption at 120° (Fig. 21-10), scaption, and press-ups for scapular protraction (push-ups with a plus)[23,34,38,43] form the foundation of improving strength that eventually leads to full functional recovery.

The prefunctional phases and periods of passive or manual control motion are extensive for rehabilitation after surgical repair of massive rotator cuff tears. Generally, no active shoulder motion or active concentric or eccentric strengthening is allowed for 2 to 3 months after surgery.[15] Extensive soft tissue healing must proceed unabated to foster the recovery of functional motion and strength.

The patient is initially placed in an abduction pillow or shoulder immobilization after surgery to allow the repaired tissues of the rotator cuff and deltoid to be placed in a shortened position. Early active muscle strengthening and active motion are avoided to allow for appropriate healing. Generally, manual control passive ROM with full motion restriction is allowed during the first several weeks of

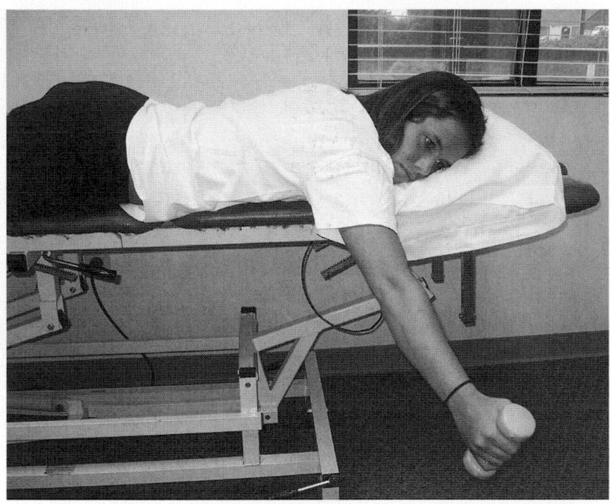

FIG 21-10 Prone scaption at 120°.

recovery. AAROM activities can begin 2 months after surgery.[15]

Submaximal isometrics and scapular stabilization exercises must be added cautiously 4 to 12 weeks after surgery.[15,43] Specific rotator cuff strengthening exercises[15] performed isotonically with dumbbells, TheraBand, and similar devices are reserved until 3 months after surgery to accommodate the healing constraints of the tendons and muscles of the rotator cuff and deltoid. Full functional recovery of motion and strength may take 10 to 12 months after repair of massive rotator cuff tears.[15,43]

GLENOHUMERAL JOINT INSTABILITY AND DISLOCATION

Dislocations and subluxations (partial dislocation) of the glenohumeral joint (the articulation between the humeral head and glenoid fossa of the scapula) frequently occur after indirect trauma with the arm abducted, elevated, and internally rotated (posterior dislocation).[18] The shoulder is the most commonly dislocated joint in the body,[18] and dislocation occurs in men more often than in women. Anterior dislocations occur more frequently than posterior dislocations.[18] Also, rotator cuff tears of various dimensions (small, <1 cm; medium, <3 cm; and large, >5 cm) occur with relative frequency. Rotator cuff tears can occur with acute anterior dislocations in patients older than 40 years.

Two associated injuries may occur as a result of acute glenohumeral dislocation and instability. Because the shoulder is the most mobile joint in the body, bony restrictions do not provide substantial restraint. The fibrocartilaginous glenoid labrum deepens the articulation between the humeral head and the bony glenoid fossa. Injury to the labrum can occur if forces are great enough to dislocate the humerus from its confines within the glenoid. This injury is referred to as a **Bankart lesion**[5,43] and is defined as "an avulsion of the capsule and glenoid labrum off of the anterior rim of the glenoid resulting from traumatic anterior dislocation of the shoulder."[24]

Important Concepts

The fibrocartilaginous glenoid labrum deepens the articulation between the humeral head and the bony glenoid fossa. Injury to the labrum can occur if forces are great enough to dislocate the humerus from its confines within the glenoid.

The head of the humerus is subject to injury as a result of anterior shoulder instability. A **Hill-Sachs lesion** is a compression or "impaction fracture" of the posterolateral aspect of the humeral head as a result of anterior shoulder instability.[11] This lesion results from instability and is not the essential cause of glenohumeral instability.[46]

As stated, anterior dislocations are more prevalent than posterior dislocations. However, shoulder instability can be defined as multidirectional, wherein the humeral head may sublux or dislocate anteriorly, inferiorly, and posteriorly.

NONOPERATIVE MANAGEMENT

The initial management of acute shoulder dislocations (anterior and posterior) calls for a period of protection lasting 4 to 6 weeks.[18] All positions that may reproduce the mechanism of dislocation are avoided. In some cases, immobilization is needed to promote healing.

Management of pain and swelling is addressed with physician-prescribed NSAIDs, analgesics, ice packs, electrical stimulation, or other physical agents such as ultrasound and infrared laser. During the protection period, the hand, wrist, and elbow of the affected shoulder must receive active motion and strengthening exercises that do not compromise the shoulder. Also, a general conditioning program of strength, flexibility, and endurance activities can begin. With an anterior shoulder subluxation (spontaneous reduction of the humeral head) or dislocation, the patient must avoid shoulder abduction and external rotation to allow proper capsular scarring and soft tissue healing to occur. Patients older than age 40 years who are not at significant risk of recurrent dislocation because of a relatively sedentary lifestyle may need only minimal protection for a couple of weeks before rehabilitation can begin and motion can be regained.[18]

The prefunctional phase of rehabilitation begins with manual control ROM, active assistive stretching for elevation, and assisted ROM exercises to help the patient regain lost motion if a relatively lengthy period of protection was warranted. Initial strengthening begins with submaximal isometric exercises that can be safely started while the patient's shoulder is placed in the neutral humeral position. Isometric shoulder adduction and abduction, internal and external rotation, and elevation and extension can be performed at a pain-free level. When the patient can demonstrate an increase from submaximal isometric contractions to near-maximal contractions, progressive internal and external rotation can begin with the affected shoulder in a minimal degree of abduction. When the symptoms of pain are reduced and the intensity and quality of muscle contractions are improved, the patient may increase ROM activities to forward elevation, extension, scapular mobility, and internal and external rotation and abduction. As the patient progresses to the return to function phase, combined shoulder abduction and external rotation are avoided. Some authorities recommend avoiding extremes of shoulder abduction and external rotation for 3 months after removal of the sling.[18] The hallmark of the return to function phase of recovery after anterior shoulder dislocation or subluxation is progressive strengthening of the rotator cuff, anterior shoulder muscles, and scapular stabilizers, with particular attention given to eccentric strengthening of the posterior rotator cuff (infraspinatus and teres minor).[43] Band and hand-held dumbbell weights are effective because of the wide variety of motions that can be addressed and can carry over to home exercises. The reader is referred to the previous section on rotator cuff exercises for a recommended home program.

Important Concepts

The hallmark of the return to function phase of recovery after anterior shoulder dislocation or subluxation is progressive strengthening of the rotator cuff, anterior shoulder muscles, and scapular stabilizers, with particular attention given to eccentric strengthening of the posterior rotator cuff (infraspinatus and teres minor).

Synchronous shoulder motion, or scapulohumeral rhythm, must be addressed before and throughout recovery from a shoulder dislocation. The 2:1 ratio of motion between the scapula and glenohumeral joint (meaning that for every 2° of glenohumeral flexion or abduction after the first 30° of shoulder motion, the scapula must rotate upwardly 1°) must be addressed early to prevent the facilitation of abnormal motions between the scapula and glenohumeral joint during strengthening activities. This can be accomplished adequately by focusing on normalized scapular motion and stabilization exercises during the return to function phase as long as symptoms of pain and harmful glenohumeral joint positions are avoided.

Throughout each phase of recovery, various tissues that contain the humeral head in the glenoid fossa (glenoid labrum, capsule, and ligaments; superior, middle, and inferior glenohumeral ligaments; and musculotendinous rotator cuff) can be stressed or torn. By definition, glenohumeral instability identifies ligamentous and capsular restraints as being "attenuated"[30,31]; the appropriate progressive application of strengthening activities for the rotator cuff and scapulothoracic muscles becomes central to the recovery of motion and function.

One way the PTA can address functional motions and stimulate the afferent neural input system is through CKC activities. CKC activities can enhance proprioception and promote dynamic joint stability.[18,31] Rhythmic stabilization through manual exercises and progression to other oscillation training such as the Bodyblade may be helpful.

Isotonic resistance exercises are challenging and stressful to the glenohumeral joint; consequently, many appropriate exercises must be modified to accommodate limitations of motion, pain, and the provocative positions of abduction and external rotation. The seated or supine chest press is an example of isotonic exercise that promotes anterior shoulder strength. However, this particular exercise can place the shoulder in a horizontally abducted position that stresses the anterior shoulder capsule, causing the head of the humerus to translate forward within the glenoid (Fig. 21-11). Progressive positional recruitment for strengthening using the PRE method is always continued throughout this phase of recovery.

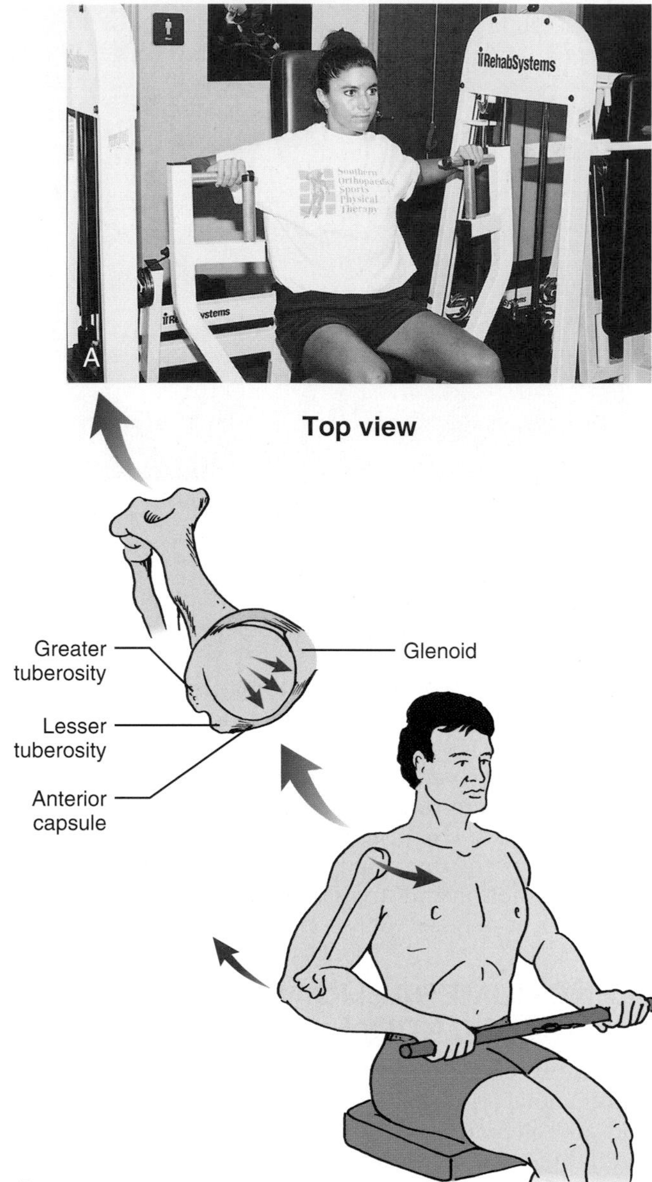

FIG 21-11 **A,** Seated chest press. This initial position can place stress on the anterior shoulder capsule. **B,** In this figure, notice how the head of the humerus can rock forward within the glenoid, causing stress to the anterior shoulder capsule.

Local muscle endurance activities are done using a UBE and CKC exercise with the use of hands on the stair stepper (Fig. 21-12, *A*). Weight-bearing CKC exercises, such as wall push-ups (Fig. 21-12, *B*) for triplane strengthening, can be introduced. These exercises provide proprioceptive stimulation to the mechanoreceptor system. Gradually, more challenging weight-bearing activities that demand progressive control of the glenohumeral joint in multiplane and diagonal motions are added (Fig. 21-13,

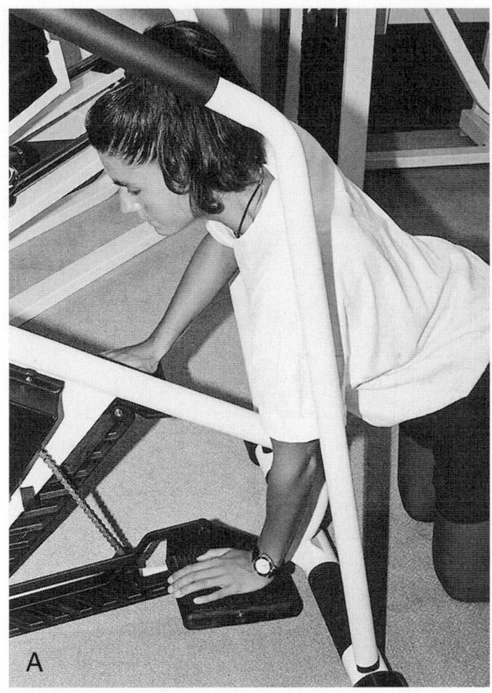

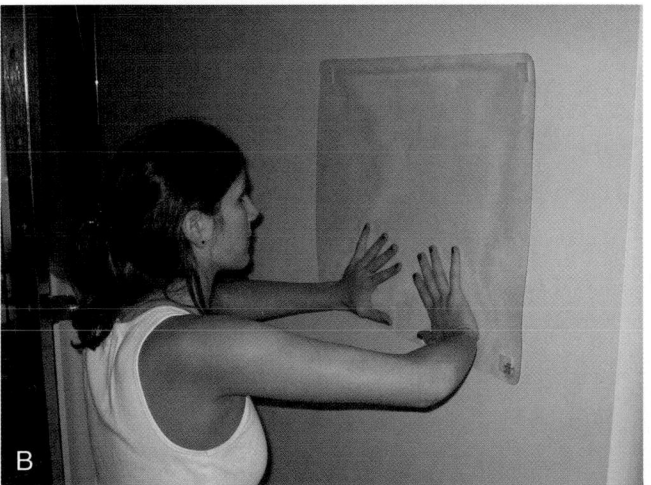

FIG 21-12 Closed kinetic chain exercises. **A,** Stair stepper activity. **B,** Wall push-up.

A-C). A balance board also can help train the shoulder muscles to respond and fire quickly for sufficient stabilization (Fig. 21-13, *D-E*).

Cable systems offer various exercises and positions that duplicate functional activities. Cable systems are particularly useful in athletic patients because sport-specific tasks can be reproduced with this equipment. In addition, a plyotoss (plyometric) exercise for stabilization is part of the return to activity phase. Plyometric ball toss against a rebounder is an excellent exercise for advanced patterns (Fig. 21-14).[7] Similar to advanced patients: advanced patterns would be patterns that are harder to perform, increased stress.

The process of recovery after shoulder dislocation matches the degree of injury. Full functional recovery is not always possible. In some cases after acute traumatic dislocation, minor stress causes the shoulder to dislocate again. With repeated episodes of shoulder dislocation or subluxation, recurrent anterior instability can result.[16,18] If patients fail to respond to an aggressive physical therapy program, the physician may choose one of several operative procedures to correct the instability. Patients with recurrent dislocations may undergo an anterior capsulolabral reconstruction.[11] Patients with multidirectional instability may require a procedure termed *capsular shift*.[26]

OPERATIVE MANAGEMENT AND REHABILITATION

Because posterior shoulder dislocations account for only 2% to 4% of all shoulder dislocations, this discussion focuses on repairs and rehabilitation procedures to enhance joint stability and promote function in patients with anterior glenohumeral instability. Surgical procedures for shoulder instability can be classified as open or arthroscopic techniques.[11,26]

The anterior capsulolabral reconstruction procedure essentially reattaches the capsule to the glenoid. Sometimes this is referred to as corrective surgery for capsular redundancy. All labral lesions are also repaired. A superior labrum anterior to posterior repair, which is the repair of the superior labral lesion, may also be needed.

Patients with anterior shoulder instability corrected via arthroscopy normally experience less postoperative pain and reduced soft tissue damage.[43] Rehabilitation after open or arthroscopic stabilization for anterior glenohumeral instability requires a prefunctional phase of rehabilitation that emphasizes protected ROM. Slow and protective external rotation is performed for up to 12 weeks postoperatively to ensure healing of all soft tissue. A recommended external rotation range of motion progressive increase is as follows:

- 0° to 30° for 3 weeks
- 30° to 45° for 6 weeks
- 45° to 75° for 9 weeks
- 75° to 90° for 12 weeks

Important Concepts

Slow and protective external rotation is performed for up to 12 weeks postoperatively to ensure healing of all soft tissue.

Initial postoperative care begins with a period of immobilization in a shoulder immobilizer to allow for appropriate soft tissue healing.[11] During this period, medications for pain and swelling may be prescribed by the physician. Frequently, ice packs are applied to the shoulder for 20 minutes three to five times daily as part of the home program to control postoperative pain and swelling. The patient also can actively perform finger, hand, wrist, and elbow mobility exercises. In addition, submaximal pain-free isometric exercises can be initiated while the arm is still in the immobilizer.

The degree and direction of shoulder motion allowed are specific to the surgical procedure, the wishes of the physician, and the direction of the PT. Generally, scapular protraction and retraction, manual control ROM, and assisted ROM exercises are performed to increase motion. The initiation of motion exercises is important because

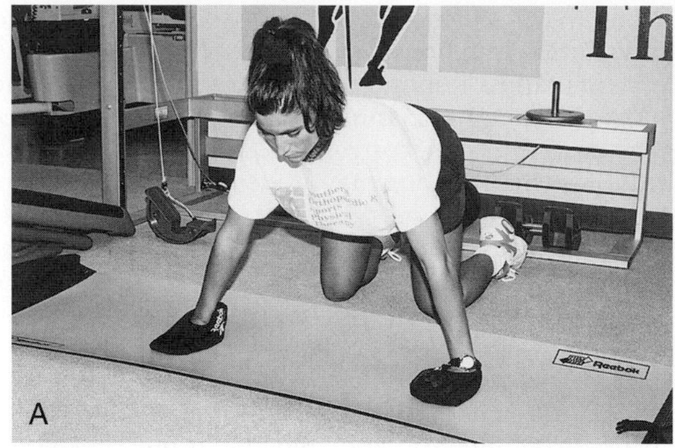

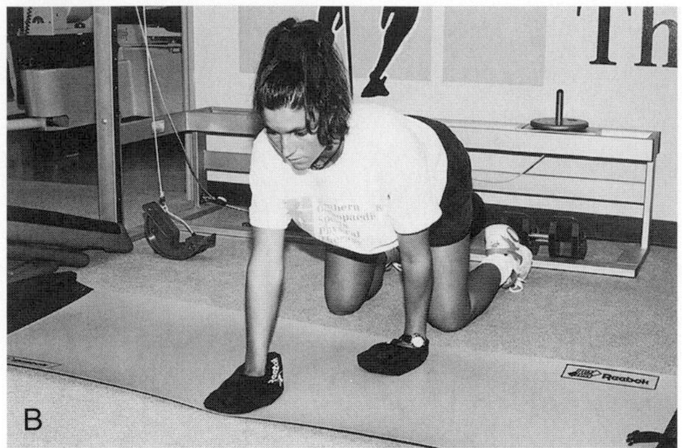

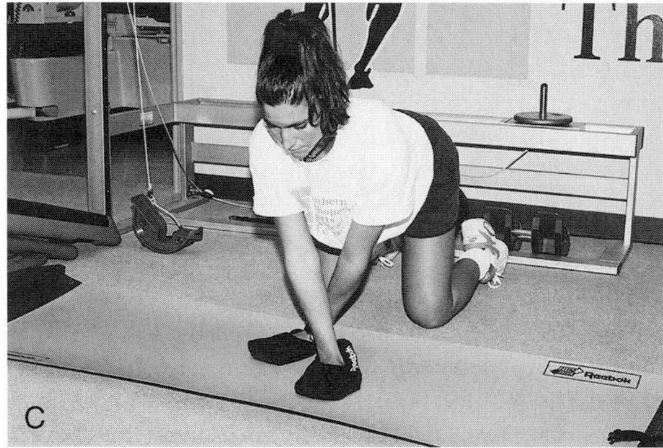

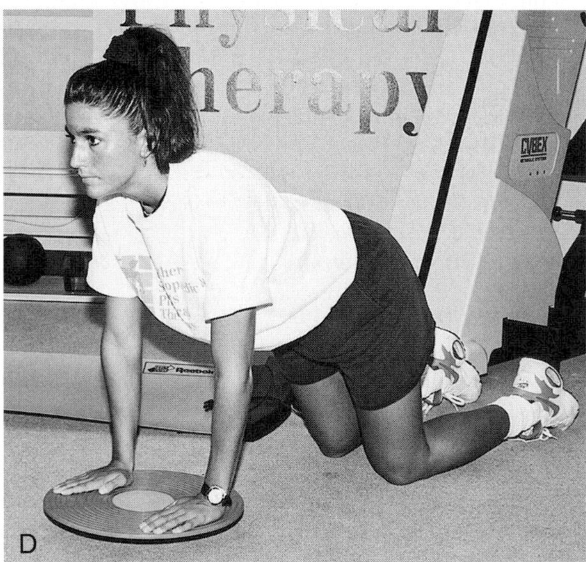

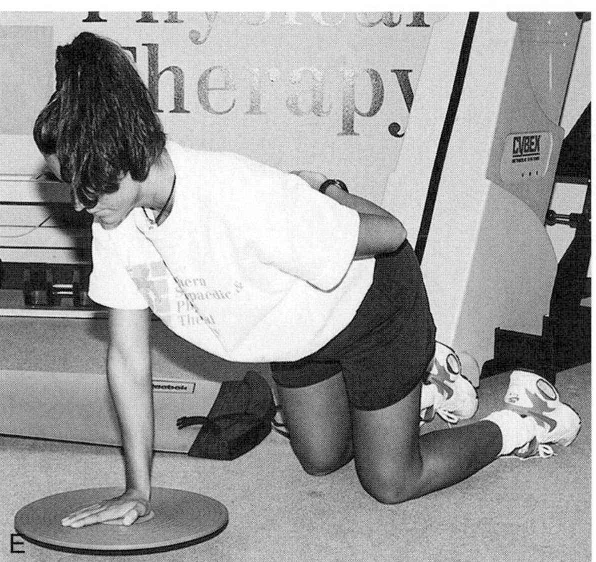

FIG 21-13 Multiplane and diagonal closed chain weight-bearing activities. **A,** Shoulder abduction and adduction on a slide board in a kneeling position. Extreme caution must be taken to ensure that a limited range of abduction be allowed when initiating this activity. **B,** Shoulder flexion and extension in a kneeling position. When beginning all slide board activities, the patient must be able to eccentrically and concentrically control the affected shoulder globally. **C,** Diagonal patterns on the slide board. **D,** Closed kinetic chain wobble board activity for stimulating shoulder stability. Both arms are used when introducing this exercise. **E,** When strength, control, and confidence improve, the patient can progress to one arm.

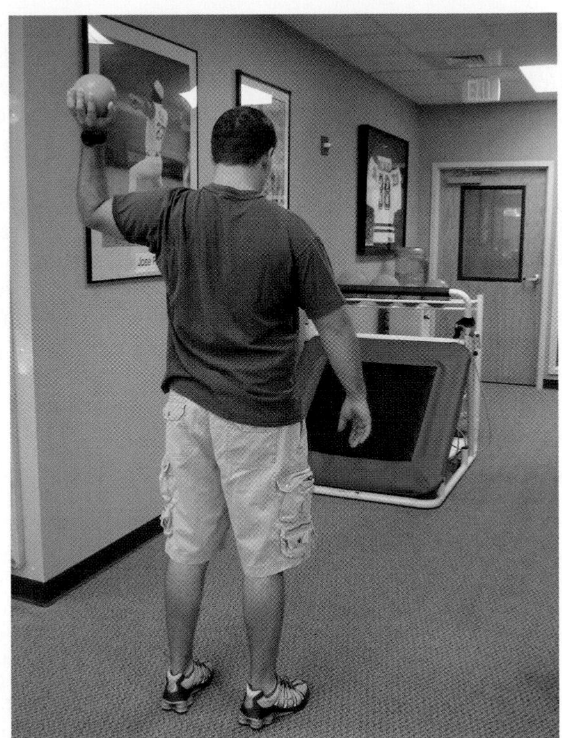

FIG 21-14 Plyometric drill: one-hand standing ball toss. *(From Johnson D, Mair S, Hosey R, et al:* Clinical sports medicine, *Philadelphia, 2006, Mosby.)*

faulty scapulothoracic and glenohumeral mobility can be affected early. Care must be taken to encourage scapular motion and glenohumeral mobility and to identify any limitations affecting normal scapulohumeral rhythm. Progressive elevation and scapular control is recommended early in this phase of rehabilitation. Elevation is normally progressed to 135° to tolerance after 6 weeks postoperatively. Slow progression of abduction is recommended. The PTA must be aware of the exact rationale behind limiting early active or passive shoulder abduction and external rotation.[43]

Progressive motion and strengthening exercises are allowed as the patient progresses to the return to function phase. Progressive shoulder strengthening must address both the glenohumeral and the scapulothoracic joints. To recover functional mobility of the shoulder, a program of positional recruitment is suggested. Because the scapula forms the base of support for glenohumeral motion, stabilization exercises must be advanced. As the patient demonstrates improved mobility without complaints of pain, the quality of muscle contraction (from submaximal to maximal) must be encouraged gradually. PREs using a TheraBand, dumbbells, or both within an active, pain-free ROM can begin, along with more challenging flexibility exercises, between 6 and 8 weeks after surgery.[1,11]

The eccentric contraction phase of each exercise must be encouraged. Applying this concept during the return to function phase involves emphasizing the eccentric loading phase of all internal rotation, abduction, external rotation, adduction, and shoulder elevation exercises.[7] Local muscle endurance also must be considered when the patient has achieved improved motion and strength. Usually an UBE or some other form of low-intensity, high-repetition, shoulder-specific activity is appropriate. Functional activities, proprioception, and CKC exercises are necessary for functional recovery.

Important Concepts

The eccentric contraction phase of each exercise must be encouraged. Applying this concept during the return to function phase involves emphasizing the eccentric loading phase of all internal rotation, abduction, external rotation, adduction, and shoulder elevation exercises.

During the return to activity phase of recovery, to stimulate the mechanoreceptor system, a complete program of advanced CKC exercises, plyotoss (plyometrics), and sport-specific training is designed. Generally, the length of rehabilitation after surgical stabilization of the glenohumeral joint ranges from 3 to 5 months.[7]

ADHESIVE CAPSULITIS

Adhesive capsulitis, which is also referred to as *frozen shoulder,* is characterized by decreased shoulder ROM, pain, inflammation, fibrous synovial adhesions, and reduction of the joint cavity.[1,3,6] Adhesive capsulitis occurs more commonly in female patients and affects patients between 40 and 60 years old.[6] The two distinct classifications of frozen shoulder are primary and secondary adhesive capsulitis. Primary idiopathic frozen shoulder is the most common lesion and occurs spontaneously from unknown causes. Secondary adhesive capsulitis generally occurs after trauma or immobilization.[6]

Important Concepts

Adhesive capsulitis occurs more commonly in women and affects patients 40 to 60 years old.

Secondary adhesive capsulitis can develop in older patients because of limited immobilization for as little as 1 or 2 days.[10] In the early stages of this disabling condition, pain occurs at rest and during activity.[10] However, as the condition progresses, pain gradually subsides and then spontaneously disappears. Severely restricted motion and profound loss of function remain.[10] During the acute painful phase, treatment is focused on controlling inflammation and symptoms of pain. Physician-prescribed analgesics, NSAIDs, and intraarticular steroid injections can provide some pain relief.[10]

Physical therapy interventions during this acute painful stage include the judicious use of ice, heat, ultrasound, phonophoresis, and infrared laser. Also central to this initial management phase is the stimulation of pain-free motion and relaxation of muscle guarding of the glenohumeral joint, cervical area, and scapulothoracic muscles.[22] Passive, active, and active assisted ROM exercise must occur within a pain-free ROM to stimulate removal of metabolic waste, increase local blood flow, and assist in the reduction of edema in the local tissues. Both wand and rope and pulley systems can be used early if they are performed in a slow, controlled, pain-free ROM. For severely restricted glenohumeral motion, the PT may prescribe the application of specific joint mobilization techniques to help modulate pain and reduce muscle guarding.[2,5,22,43] As addressed, grades I and II low-amplitude physiologic and accessory oscillations can help encourage relaxation while reducing pain.[22,43]

If the scapula is not stable and free from restriction while the patient attempts to regain shoulder motion and function, normal scapulohumeral rhythm cannot be obtained. Early scapular stabilization exercises[5,37,43] can be employed as long as pain does not inhibit the correct performance of the exercise. Normalized motion must precede specific strengthening activities to avoid developing faulty shoulder mechanics.

The complete restoration of glenohumeral joint mobility is the goal of treatment for the late stage of adhesive capsulitis. The PT must identify the appropriate application of increased joint mobilization techniques to address specific capsular restrictions and initiate more challenging progressive resistance exercises.[49] When the patient demonstrates improved glenohumeral motion and appropriate scapulohumeral rhythm, strengthening exercises can begin for the deltoid, scapular muscles, rotator cuff, and upper arm muscles.[13,43]

Although control of pain and inflammation is the primary feature of early physical therapy management, submaximal isometric exercise can be used to initiate strengthening if pain is not increased with exercise. Progression from submaximal isometrics to maximal isometrics usually precedes the use of a TheraBand or dumbbells for concentric and eccentric exercises. A comprehensive series of rotator cuff exercises[38,42] and scapular stabilization exercises[5] can be encouraged as early as pain and motion allow. To address normalized function, the patient does CKC resistance exercises and overhead loading along with proprioception exercises (e.g., balance board, slide board, and Plyoball) in a sequential, orderly fashion when sufficient strength, improved motion, and scapulohumeral rhythm have been established. Local muscle endurance activities focus on purposeful, functional movements that duplicate ADL. Pain control, restoration of motion, and improved function must be reinforced continually to encourage compliance with a home exercise program and the avoidance of positions that may exacerbate pain and muscle guarding.

ACROMIOCLAVICULAR SPRAINS AND DISLOCATIONS

Ligamentous sprains of the AC joint usually result from a fall on the acromion (direct force) or when force is transmitted from a fall on an outstretched arm proximally to the AC joint (indirect force). AC joint sprains and dislocations are graded according to the degree of injury to specific ligamentous structures (AC and coracoclavicular ligaments) as well as the position of the clavicle in complete rupture of the AC and the coracoclavicular ligaments, as follows:

- First-degree, grade I AC joint sprain: Characterized by partial tearing of the AC ligaments, with resultant joint tenderness over the AC joint, no joint instability or laxity of the ligament, and minimal loss of function.[33]
- Second-degree, grade II AC joint sprain: Complete rupture of the AC ligaments with partial tearing of the coracoacromial ligaments.[33] The patient has moderate pain, some dysfunction (reduction in shoulder abduction and adduction), and a palpable gap between the acromion and the clavicle.[2,32,33]
- Third-degree, grade III AC ligament injury: Dislocation between the acromion and clavicle where both the AC and the coracoclavicular ligaments are ruptured and the distal clavicle becomes displaced superiorly. Patients exhibit marked pain and severe limitation of shoulder motion. Three additional classifications have been proposed that describe the degree of vertical, posterior, and inferior separation of the clavicle in grade III AC dislocation.[33]

Important Concepts

AC joints and dislocations are graded according to the degree of injury to specific ligamentous structures (AC and coracoclavicular ligaments) and the position of the clavicle in complete rupture of the AC and the coracoclavicular ligaments.

Rehabilitation and management of grade I AC sprains focus on symptomatic relief. Typically, pain is controlled with the use of ice packs, NSAIDs, analgesics, and rest. Because the AC ligaments have been partially torn, the AC joint must be protected from further direct or indirect forces that may stress the AC ligaments. The patient may be allowed to resume activities within 2 weeks and usually does not require a rehabilitation program of significant duration.[2,33]

Grade II AC sprains require more direct attention to approximate the torn AC ligaments and allow for secure ligament healing. Usually this injury is managed nonoperatively using a shoulder immobilizer as needed for the short-term, and early ROM and stabilization exercises are begun.[33] Modalities of choice may be used as needed.

There is usually a palpable step-off between the acromion process and distal clavicle with grade II AC sprains. This deformity represents a permanent loss of joint continuity because of lost ligamentous support between acromion and clavicle.[33]

The rehabilitation program continues with the prefunctional phase for a grade II AC sprain; AAROM to active ROM exercises are allowed through pain-free ROM. Submaximal isometrics can be performed for all muscles of the shoulder girdle. However, care must be taken to avoid contractions that stress the AC joint; isometric strengthening may be progressed for return to function. During this phase of rehabilitation, inappropriate stress to the ligament should be avoided around the AC joint.

The return to function phase continues, using OKC and CKC advanced strengthening of the entire shoulder complex. Scapular stabilization continues to be vital for overall control of the upper extremity. PREs continue in the return to activity phase, including advanced scapular-cuff strengthening. Deltoid strengthening is advanced as tolerated. TheraBand and dumbbells are effective and versatile tools for compliance and carryover to a prescribed home exercise program. The performance of scapular and humerus elevation exercises helps approximate the torn ligaments and provides dynamic muscular support to the torn structures. It is recommended that eccentric training progress slowly, whereas plyometric with plyotoss exercises and advanced rhythmic stabilization exercises are helpful for more athletic patients. Rotator cuff strengthening is recommended throughout all the advanced phases of rehabilitation. In addition, a general conditioning program is warranted to improve or maintain aerobic fitness, strength, and flexibility.

The treatment of grade III AC sprains (dislocation of the distal clavicle and acromion process) may include surgical intervention. Although many surgeons advocate open surgical repair, others favor closed reduction, immobilization, and progressive rehabilitation. Nonoperative treatment of grade III AC sprains is centered on reducing the dislocation and maintaining the reduction.[33] The goal of the initial course of treatment in physical therapy is to minimize pain and swelling, with the modalities of choice including physician-prescribed NSAIDs, analgesics, and protection of the AC joint from unwanted stress. To ensure proper healing of the ligaments, the rehabilitation team must continuously reinforce compliance using the immobilizer for the recommended period prescribed by the treating physician.

While the patient is immobilized, submaximal isometric exercises can be initiated for the shoulder and scapula if no stress is applied to the healing ligaments. As with grade II AC sprains, the hand, wrist, and elbow of the affected arm can be safely and effectively strengthened during immobilization. Generally, nonoperative treatment of grade III sprains parallels the treatment plan for grade II sprains. The primary differences are the longer duration of immobilization and the more cautious and delayed application of motion and resistance exercises so as not to affect ligament healing adversely. In some cases, nonoperative treatment is ineffective, and surgical correction is indicated.

The surgeon may elect to perform open reduction with internal fixation (ORIF) of the AC joint to stabilize and approximate the joint. Another procedure calls for the surgeon to perform a modified reconstruction known as coracoacromial ligament transfer and clavicular reduction. An autogenous tendon graft material has been used more recently to reconstruct the AC joint.

Active motion and light resistance exercises for the hand, wrist, and elbow of the affected limb are encouraged in the early prefunction phase, normally lasting 4 to 6 weeks. Isometric exercises focus on the shoulder and scapular muscles when the AC joint is stabilized and protected from unwanted forces. Progressive active and active-assisted shoulder motion is allowed as pain resolves and soft tissue healing progresses. After this period of protection to support the surgical reconstruction, the return to function phase begins with progressive strengthening. Return to function closely follows the patient's level of motion and strength. As stated, heavy, intense resistance exercises must be based on the patient's tolerance. Advanced strengthening of the scapula, rotator cuff, and deltoids are included in the return to activity phase.

SCAPULAR FRACTURES

Most scapular fractures result from direct, severe trauma. There is a high incidence of significant associated injuries, including other fractures, glenohumeral dislocations, pneumothorax, and neurovascular injuries. Fractures of the scapular body are the most common and demonstrate the highest incidence of associated injuries. However, the treatment of fractures to the scapular body is conservative if associated injuries have not occurred, using ice and shoulder immobilization for 2 to 3 weeks. During the immobilization period, hand, wrist, and elbow exercises can be initiated for the affected arm along with a general conditioning program. Early manual control ROM exercises for the shoulder begin as the pain and swelling subside.

Isometric exercises performed submaximally also can be initiated early if the patient remains pain-free. As pain and swelling subside, strengthening exercises can be added within a pain-free ROM. Nonunion and malunion of this fracture are rare and usually are not associated with a loss of function or clinical symptoms.

The second most common scapular fracture occurs to the glenoid neck. If the fracture is extraarticular, healing can occur at 6 weeks, and management involves conservative symptomatic care. Glenoid fractures also can be intraarticular, where the fracture extends through the glenoid fossa. The treatment of these fractures depends on whether there is associated glenohumeral instability. If no instability is present, these fractures are treated with shoulder immobilization and a return to motion and strength. However, if there is glenohumeral instability associated with an intraarticular glenoid fracture, surgical repair is needed to stabilize the fragments. Usually an internal fixation device is inserted into the fracture fragments; immobilization is needed to minimize stress at the fracture site. Manual control exercises can be initiated soon after surgery to minimize postoperative joint stiffness. Although gentle manual control shoulder elevation and external rotation are initiated 2 to 3 weeks postoperatively, active stretching and resistance exercises must be deferred for 6 to 8 weeks to allow for secure bone healing.

CLAVICLE FRACTURES

Fractures of the clavicle occur as a result of direct or indirect trauma. These injuries are common and primarily affect men younger than 25 years of age. Care is focused on achieving reduction of the fracture fragments, maintaining the reduction, and minimizing the immobilization of the glenohumeral joint of the affected arm. Usually the patient is placed in a commercially available figure-of-eight bandage to maintain proper alignment of the area. The duration of immobilization varies, but authorities suggest that healing takes 4 to 6 weeks or longer.

During the initial period of immobilization with the figure-of-eight bandage, the hand, wrist, and elbow of the affected arm are exercised with active motion and resistance exercises. Unwanted stress to the fracture site is avoided during this period. In addition, the patient may perform submaximal isometrics for the shoulder and scapula when pain has been controlled. Manual exercises to the scapula are recommended before beginning OKC strengthening.[44]

Active shoulder elevation must not be greater than 50° to 70° until after 4 weeks (although patients may be encouraged to perform gentle active shoulder motion no greater than 60° when pain-free).[17] As the healing process continues and when bone healing is confirmed radiographically (approximately 4 to 6 weeks), greater degrees of shoulder motion are allowed, with PREs added as tolerated.

If the fracture is located at the distal end of the clavicle, ORIF may be more appropriate because these fractures tend to be unstable and do not maintain proper alignment with a figure-of-eight bandage. The fragments of a displaced distal clavicle fracture usually are secured with an intramedullary fixation pin.

PROXIMAL HUMERUS FRACTURES

Proximal humerus fractures usually are classified according to a four-part classification. The four parts are the humeral head, lesser tuberosity, greater tuberosity, and humeral shaft.

Physical therapy management of humerus fractures depends on the severity and complexity of the fracture as well as the means used to secure fixation of the fracture site. Generally, with nondisplaced one-part fractures (the most common type), the affected arm is placed in an immobilizer for a period of time, and the patient is given analgesics and encouraged to apply ice liberally to minimize pain and swelling. Within the first 2 weeks, gentle active motion is allowed as well as active motion of the elbow, wrist, and hand of the affected arm. The patient may be allowed to remove the immobilizer for active motion exercises a few times each day.

Submaximal shoulder isometrics are initiated as early as pain allows. Perhaps the most salient aspect of physical therapy care in proximal humerus fracture is the functional restoration of glenohumeral motion and strength after protracted periods of immobility to allow for appropriate bone healing. Early scapular motion exercises minimize the restriction of scapular mobility. Submaximal scapular stabilization exercises[43] also can be encouraged early, as pain allows, to provide a stable base for glenohumeral motion exercises. Manual glides for mobility of the scapula may be helpful. Manual glides to the glenohumeral joint may be needed if hypomobility is a side effect of prolonged immobilization. Progressive motion and resistance exercises for the deltoid, rotator cuff, and upper arm muscles closely parallel bone healing and the patient's ability to demonstrate improved motion without pain.

Other, more complex fractures can require ORIF with screws and a plate and prolonged periods of immobilization. As with all fractures, during immobility the patient can participate in a total body conditioning program that does not compromise the healing of the fracture. In addition, the hand, wrist, and elbow of the affected limb must be exercised without stressing the fracture site.

The ultimate task after the healing of humerus fractures is regaining purposeful, functional strength and motion of the glenohumeral joint. The time necessary to heal significant fractures may cause serious glenohumeral and scapular restrictions. The long-term healing restraints of bone form the primary guide for the physician and PT in deciding when to employ progressive motion activities and when to initiate strengthening tasks without compromising the fracture site.

Avascular necrosis may be a risk with some significant fractures (displaced fractures of the anatomic neck). For example, in older patients with advancing osteoporosis who have four-part proximal humerus fracture, internal fixation may be poor because of the osteopenic bone. A prosthetic humeral head, termed *hemiarthroplasty,* may be appropriate in this case.

As the fracture begins to stabilize and under the direction and supervision of the PT, some patients begin CKC exercises to stimulate the mechanoreceptor system (afferent neural input system) of the elbow, shoulder, and wrist and to effect proper bone healing (Wolff's law) by providing submaximal intermittent stress to the healing bone.

The PTA participates in the rehabilitation process of proximal humerus fractures by following and supervising a comprehensive program of early protected limited ROM and submaximal isometrics for the scapular stabilizers, rotator cuff, and upper arm muscles and by providing continued protection for the injured site. As pain resolves and motion and bone healing progress, the PTA must carefully observe the scapulothoracic and glenohumeral motion. If scapulohumeral rhythm is adversely affected, specific attention must be given to regaining a stable scapula and proper glenohumeral mobilization. In many cases, if a restriction is noted, the PT may use scapular and glenohumeral mobilization techniques to modulate pain and encourage improved motion. However, the fracture site must be secure and stable, with radiographic confirmation of this, and the physician must order this protocol before mobilization can begin.

Functional shoulder activities and resistance exercises are added gradually as bone healing advances and the patient demonstrates greater confidence, motion, and strength without pain. Proprioception and CKC activities also may be added during the return to function phase of recovery in preparation for normalized purposeful motion and strength of the involved limb.

TOTAL SHOULDER ARTHROPLASTY

With severe four-part fractures of the proximal humerus, avascular necrosis of the humeral head, osteoporosis, rheumatoid arthritis, and advanced osteoarthritis, the proximal humerus may be replaced with a prosthesis, or a total shoulder arthroplasty may be indicated. The condition of the rotator cuff is a significant feature in patients receiving a hemiarthroplasty or total shoulder arthroplasty. If a rotator cuff tear is repaired in addition to the arthroplasty, postoperative immobilization may last 4 to 6 weeks, with the affected arm held in an abduction splint to allow for healing of the repaired cuff.[4,48] When a patient has a massive rotator cuff tear or has had a revision of failed arthroplasty with rotator cuff tear, a reverse prosthesis procedure may be needed. This procedure requires the surgeon to place the humeral component in the glenoid socket and the glenoid component into the proximal humerus. The rehabilitation objectives are usually the same as a regular arthroplasty,[6] but in some cases the progress is slower.[4,48]

A rotator cuff repair added to shoulder arthroplasty guides the course of rehabilitation and dictates the need for protective or limited motion, which leads to a longer program of rehabilitation.[5] In terms of restoration of shoulder motion, if the rotator cuff is not repaired, progressive ROM through goal setting of the PT is carefully guided to regain functional motion.[50]

The prefunctional phase of rehabilitation after shoulder arthroplasty usually allows for early manual control assisted ROM and isometric exercises. Slow return toward external rotation is used to protect the healing of the subscapularis.[43]

Important Concepts

Slow return toward external rotation is used to protect the healing of the subscapularis.

Isometric exercise may depend on soft tissue healing and patient tolerance. Usually during the first postoperative week, the patient is allowed active exercise of the wrist, hand, and elbow of the affected shoulder. The postoperative immobilizer also is frequently removed for hygiene and exercises. By the end of the first week, the immobilization device may be removed, and manual control exercises are initiated and AAROM exercises are continued. At the end of the second postoperative week, the patient is introduced to scapular motion and stabilization exercises, while the quantity and quality of isometric exercises and motion exercises are progressed. The PTA must encourage compliance with a comprehensive home exercise program of motion and strength. Wand-assisted exercises and pulley systems can be used as part of the home ROM program. Return to function phase includes light resistive strengthening. More advanced scapular stabilization TheraBand exercises are useful for the home exercise program; this usually begins between 4 and 6 weeks postoperatively. Because the subscapularis has been taken down as part of this procedure, precautions are taken to protect against a return of external rotation that is too rapid. In addition, early strengthening of the subscapularis is avoided to allow adequate heading of this muscle.[43]

Important Concepts

Early strengthening of the subscapularis is avoided to allow adequate heading of this muscle.

If the patient has received a rotator cuff repair or neural prosthesis, the sequence of care and initiation of resistance exercise and active shoulder motion may be delayed. Functional use of the affected arm can be expected around 4 months postoperatively. The patient should participate in an active home exercise program long after discharge of rehabilitation.

MOBILIZATION OF THE SHOULDER

The precise application of specific peripheral joint mobilization techniques is extremely effective for pain reduction and restoration of normalized joint motion. In addition to various soft tissue injuries and fractures, immobilization frequently causes limitations in scapulothoracic and glenohumeral mobility. For a normalized scapulohumeral rhythm to be restored, any limitations in motion must be identified early in the rehabilitation period.

Important Concepts

For a normalized scapulohumeral rhythm to be restored, any limitations in motion must be identified early in the rehabilitation period.

During the initial immobilization, the PT documents all limitations of specific joint motion. Each limitation is addressed as part of the rehabilitation program. However, if the PTA recognizes delayed restoration of motion, reduced motion, or increased pain during the rehabilitation program, he or she must communicate this immediately to the PT.

The following scapular and glenohumeral mobilization techniques represent only a few of the many techniques available. The PT decides which specific technique is to be used; when to apply the technique; in which direction; and with what amplitude, grade, or oscillation.

Before the PTA uses any mobilization technique, the position and comfort of the patient must be assessed. The use of oral physician-prescribed analgesics, thermal agents (e.g., heat, ultrasound, ice), and proper body limb positioning enhances relaxation and compliance during treatment.

MOBILIZATION OF THE SCAPULOTHORACIC JOINT

While the patient is in a side-lying position on the unaffected side, the scapula can be effectively mobilized in a superior and inferior direction as well as distracted from the thorax. To distract the scapula, the PTA should stand facing the patient. The PTA should firmly grasp the medial or vertebral border of the affected scapula and purposefully distract the scapula away from the thorax (Fig. 21-15). To glide the scapula superiorly and inferiorly, the PTA should assume the same position and support the inferior border of the scapula. The PTA should use the hand on the inferior border to direct a force to glide the scapula in a superior direction, then use the hand on the superior border to direct a force to glide the scapula in an inferior direction.[24,43] In the same position, the PTA can perform a lateral scapular glide. This technique is helpful to loosen subscapular soft tissue that may have become hypomobile during the postoperative or prefunctional phase of rehabilitation.

MOBILIZATION OF THE GLENOHUMERAL JOINT

Inferior and posterior glide of the glenohumeral joint can be accomplished with the patient supine. The PTA should

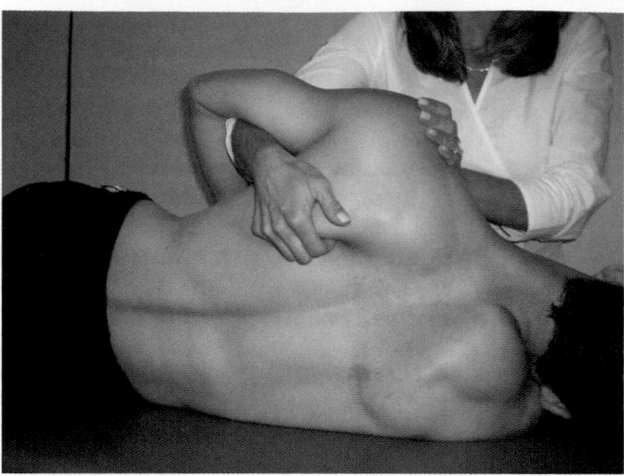

FIG 21-15 Vertebral border scapular lateral glide. *(From Skirven T, Osterman A, Fedorczyk J, et al:* Rehabilitation of the hand and upper extremity, *ed 6, Philadelphia, 2011, Mosby.)*

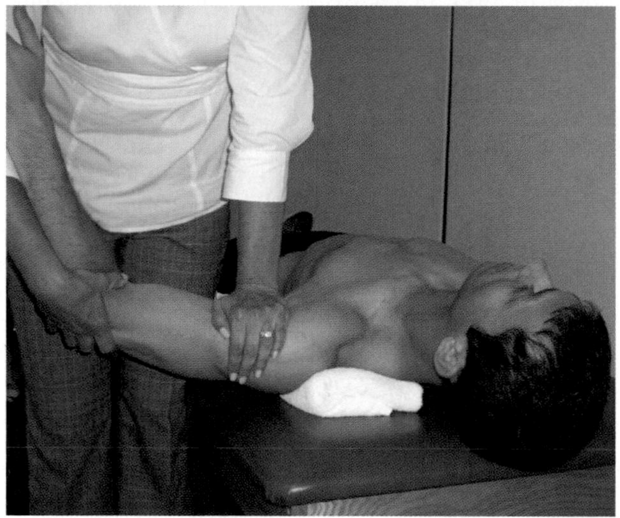

FIG 21-16 Inferior and posterior glide of the glenohumeral joint. *(From Skirven T, Osterman A, Fedorczyk J, et al:* Rehabilitation of the hand and upper extremity, *ed 6, Philadelphia, 2011, Mosby.)*

sit near the affected shoulder. The humeral head should be grasped firmly with one hand over the superior and anterior aspect of the humeral head and the other hand along the posterior aspect of the humerus. While applying distraction with the posterior distal hand, the PTA uses an inferior glide to the humeral head (Fig. 21-16). Mild inferior glides of the glenohumeral joint may be helpful in regaining motion owing to superior migration of the humeral head.[44]

Lateral distraction of the humeral head can also be achieved while the patient is supine. The PTA sits near the affected shoulder and abducts the shoulder to 45° with the arm supported by the PTA's hands. The PTA can use one or both hands to grasp the proximal humerus and direct a straight lateral force, effectively translating the humeral head from the glenoid (Fig. 21-17).

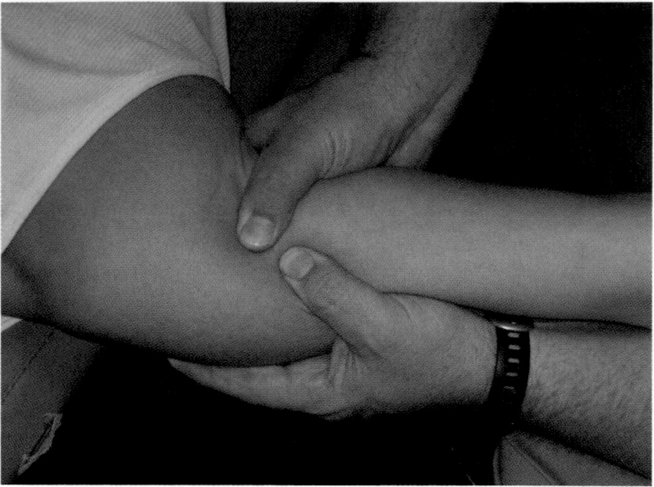

FIG 21-17 Lateral distraction of the humeral head.

GLOSSARY

Acromioplasty: Beveling or reshaping of the acromion with detachment of the coracoacromial ligament.

Bankart lesion: Dislocation of glenohumeral joint or repetitive subluxation may lead to fractures of the anteroinferior aspect of the glenoid rim.

Glenohumeral joint: Greatest range of motion and least stable of any joint. Center core of motion.

Hawkins-Kennedy test: Elevation of the shoulder to 90° in the scapular plane with internal rotation over pressure.

Hill-Sachs lesion: Glenohumeral joint dislocation or repetitive subluxation. May lead to bone defect on posterolateral aspect of humeral head. Hill-Sachs lesion is also called *impression fracture*.

Neer impingement test: Shoulder elevation with internal rotation, which compresses the rotator cuff against the coracoacromial arch.

Primary shoulder impingement: Refers to mechanical compression of the rotator cuff tendons, primarily the supraspinatus tendon, as they pass under the coracoacromial ligament between the acromion and coracoid process.

Scapular dyskinesis: Any alteration of normal position of the scapula that affects the pathology of the glenohumeral joint.

Secondary shoulder impingement: Relates to glenohumeral instability that creates a reduced subacromial space because the humeral head elevates and minimizes the area under the coracoacromial ligament.

REFERENCES

1. Anderson LL, Anderson CH, Mortenson OS, et al: Muscle activation and perceived loading during rehabilitation exercises: comparison of dumbbells and elastic resistance. *Phys Ther* 90:538–549, 2010.
2. Boissonnault WG, Janos SC: Dysfunction, evaluation and treatment of the shoulder. In Donatelli R, Wooden MJ, editors: *Orthopaedic physical therapy*, ed 3, St Louis, 2009, Churchill Livingstone.
3. Borstad JD, Dashottar A: Quantifying strain of posterior shoulder tissues during 5 simulated clinical tests: a cadaver study. *J Orthop Sports Phys Ther* 41(2):90–99, 2011.

4. Boudreau S, Boudreau E, Higgins L, et al: Rehabilitation following reverse total shoulder arthroplasty. *J Orthop Sports Phys Ther* 36(12):734–743, 2007.
5. Brudvig TJ, Kukkarni H, Shah S: The effect of therapeutic exercise and mobilization on patients with shoulder dysfunction: a systematic review with meta-analysis. *J Orthop Sports Phys Ther* 41(10):734–748, 2011.
6. Cricchio M, Frazer C: Scapulothoracic and scapulohumeral exercises: a narrative review of electromyographic studies. *J Hand Ther* 24:322–334, 2011.
7. Davies GJ, Krauschar DR, Brinks KF, et al: Neuromuscular static and dynamic stability of the shoulder: the key to functional performance. In Manske RC, editor: *Postsurgical orthopedic sports rehabilitation: knee & shoulder*, St Louis, 2006, Saunders.
8. De Mey K, Cagnie B, Van DeVelde A, et al: Trapezius muscle timing during selected shoulder rehabilitation exercises. *J Orthop Sports Phys Ther* 39(10):743–752, 2009.
9. Dillman C, Murray T, Hintermeister R: Biomechanical differences of open and closed chain exercises with respect to the shoulder. *J Sport Rehabil* 3:228–238, 1994.
10. Duralde XA, Pollock RG, Flatow EL, et al: Frozen shoulder: prevention, diagnosis and management. *J Musculoskel Med* 10(9):64–72, 1993.
11. Durall CJ, Giangarra C, Humphrey CS: Anterior capsulolabral reconstruction. In Manske R, editor: *Postsurgical orthopedic sports rehabilitation: knee & shoulder*, St Louis, 2006, Mosby.
12. Ekstrom RA, BiFulco KM, Lopau CJ, et al: Comparing the function of the upper and lower parts of the serratus anterior muscle using surface electromyography. *J Orthop Sports Ther* 34(5):235–243, 2004.
13. Ellen MI, Rogers DP, Gilhool JJ: Practitioner flexibility strengthens shoulder rehabilitation protocol. *Biomechanics* January:45–52, 2000.
14. Ellenbecker TS: *Clinical examination of the shoulder*, St Louis, 2004, Saunders.
15. Ellenbecker TS, Baile DS, Kibler WB: Rehabilitation after mini-open and arthroscopic repair of the rotator cuff. In Manske RC, editor: *Postsurgical orthopedic sports rehabilitation: knee & shoulder*, St Louis, 2006, Mosby.
16. Ghodadra NS, Provencher MT, Verma NN, et al: Open, mini-open and all-arthroscopic rotator cuff repair surgery: indications and implications for rehabilitation. *J Orthop Sports Phys Ther* 39(2):81–89, 2009.
17. Harris KD, Deyle GD, Gill NW, Howes RR: Manual physical therapy for injection-confirmed non acute acromioclavicular joint pain. *J Orthop Sports Phys Ther* 42(2):66–80, 2012.
18. Hayes K, Callanan M, Walton J, et al: Shoulder instability: management and rehabilitation. *J Orthop Sports Phys Ther* 32:497–509, 2002.
19. Heyworth BE, Williams RJ: Internal impingement of the shoulder. *Am J Sports Med* 37:1024–1047, 2009.
20. Hill Z, Sibilia K, Stone J, et al: Secondary impingement of the shoulder: examination and treatment used by physical therapist. *Orthop Phys Ther Pract* 20:14–20, 2008.
21. Hughes CJ, McBride A: The use of surface electromyography to determine muscle activation during isotonic and elastic resistance exercises from shoulder rehabilitation. *Orthop Phys Ther Pract* 2:18–23, 2005.
22. Jewell DV, Riddle DL, Thacker LR: Interventions associated with an increased or decreased likelihood of pain reduction and improved function in patients with adhesive capsulitis: a retrospective cohort study. *Phys Ther* 89:419–429, 2009.
23. Kamkar A, Irrgang J, Whitney SL: Nonoperative management of secondary shoulder impingement syndrome. *J Orthop Sports Phys Ther* 17:212–224, 1993.
24. Kolstad K, Tyler T, Nicholas S: Rehabilitation of the shoulder. In Kumbhare DA, Basmajian JV, editors: *Decision making and outcomes in sports rehabilitation*, Philadelphia, 2000, Churchill Livingstone.
25. Laudner KG, Sipes RC, Wilson JT: The acute effects of sleeper stretches on shoulder range of motion. *J Athl Train* 43(4):359–363, 2008.
26. Levinson M, Altchek D: Capsular shift procedures: Neer and multidirectional instabilities. In Manske R, editor: *Postsurgical orthopedic sports rehabilitation: knee & shoulder*, St Louis, 2006, Mosby.
27. Lunden JE, Muffenber M, Givens MR, et al: Reliability of shoulder internal rotation passive range of motion measurements in supine versus side-lying position. *J Orthop Sports Phys Ther* 30(9):589–594, 2010.
28. McClure P, Balacuis J, Heilland D, et al: A randomized controlled comparison to stretching procedures for posterior shoulder tightness. *J Orthop Sports Phys Ther* 37(3):108–114, 2007.
29. McClure PW, Bialker J, Neff N, et al: Shoulder function and 3-dimensional kinematics in people with shoulder impingement syndrome before and after a 6-week exercise program. *Phys Ther* 84:832–848, 2004.
30. McClure PW, Michener LA, Karduna AR: Shoulder function and 3-dimensional scapular kinematics in people with and without shoulder impingement syndrome. *Phys Ther* 86:1075–1090, 2006.
31. McCluskey GM, Getz BA: Pathophysiology of anterior shoulder instability. *J Athl Train* 35(3):268–272, 2000.
32. Macrina L, Reinhold M: Arm forces. *Train Conditioning* 18:48–51, 2008.
33. Matheson JW, Price CR: Rehabilitation after conservative and operative treatment of acromioclavicular joint injuries. In Manske R, editor: *Postsurgical orthopedic sports rehabilitation: knee & shoulder*, St Louis, 2006, Mosby.
34. Mosely JB, Jr, Jobe FW, Pink M, et al: EMG analysis of the scapular muscles during a shoulder rehabilitation program. *Am J Sports Med* 20(2):128–134, 1992.
35. Myers JB, Laudner KG, Pasquale MR, et al: Glenohumeral range of motion deficits and posterior shoulder tightness in throwers with pathologic internal impingement. *Am J Sports Med* 34:385–391, 2006.
36. Neer CS: Impingement lesions. *Clin Orthop Relat Res* 173:70–77, 1983.
37. Porterfield JA, DeRosa C: *Mechanical shoulder disorders: perspectives in functional anatomy*, vol 1, Philadelphia, 2004, Saunders, pp 129–159.
38. Reinold MM, Macrina LC, Wilk KE, et al: Electromyographic analysis of the supraspinatus and deltoid muscles during 3 command rehabilitation exercises. *J Athl Train* 43(4):464–469, 2007.
39. Schultz RA, Leetun DT, Warner CD: Subacromial impingement, acromioplasty and subacromial decompression. In Manske RC, editor: *Postsurgical orthopedic sports rehabilitation: knee & shoulder*, St Louis, 2006, Mosby.
40. Schultz RA, Warner C: Oscillatory devices accelerate proprioception training. *Biomechanics* May:85–90, 2001.
41. Tate AR, McClure PW, Young IA, Salvatori R, Michener LA: Comprehensive impairment-based exercise and manual therapy intervention for patients with subacromial impingement syndrome: a case series. *J Orthop Sports Phys Ther* 40(8):474–493, 2010.
42. Townsend H, Jobe FW, Pink M, Perry J: Electromyographic analysis of the glenohumeral muscles during a baseball rehabilitation program. *Am J Sports Med* 19:264–272, 1991.
43. Trundle TL: Orthopedic management of the shoulder. In Shankman GA, Manske RC, editors: *Fundamental orthopedic management for the physical therapist assistant*, ed 3, St Louis, 2011, Saunders.
44. Trundle TL: *Rotator cuff syndrome: from impingement to post operative rehab*, Brentwood, TN, 2012, Course Notes.
45. Tucci HT, Ciol MA, DeAraujo RC, et al: Activation of selected shoulder muscles during unilateral wall and bench press tasks under submaximal isometric effort. *J Orthop Sports Ther* 41(7):520–525, 2011.
46. Tyler TF, Nicholas SS, Seneviratne AN: The Bankart lesion. In Manske RC, editor: *Postsurgical orthopedic sports rehabilitation: knee & shoulder*, St Louis, 2006, Mosby.
47. Uhl TL, Carver TJ, Mattacola CG, et al: Shoulder musculature activation during upper extremity weight-bearing exercise. *J Orthop Sports Phys Ther* 33:109–117, 2003.
48. Unverzagt C, Omar L, Hughes C: Case report: rehabilitation outcomes for a patient following and implant of Reverse Delta III shoulder prosthesis. *Orthop Pract* 18(2):32–37, 2006.
49. Vermeulen HM, Rozing PM, Obermann WR, et al: Comparison of high-grade and low-grade mobilization techniques in the management of adhesive capsulitis of the shoulder: randomized controlled trial. *Phys Ther* 86:355–368, 2006.

50. Wilcox R, Arslanian L, Millett P: Rehabilitation following total shoulder arthroplasty. *J Orthop Sports Phys Ther* 35:821–836, 2005.

REVIEW QUESTIONS

Multiple Choice

1. Signs and symptoms of rotator cuff dysfunction may include:
   a. Compressive forces against the acromion.
   b. Deltoid weakness with scapular instability.
   c. Subacromial bursa fibrosis with or without bone spurs.
   d. a and b
   e. a and c
2. True functional type of exercise includes:
   a. Isometric and passive ROM.
   b. Static contraction.
   c. Isotonic concentric and eccentric mode of contraction.
   d. b and c
   e. All of the above
3. CKC loading includes:
   a. Distal fixed loading of the extremities.
   b. Movable body parts in space with free motion.
   c. Promotion of cocontraction.
   d. a and c
   e. b and c
4. Activation of the serratus anterior is vital to:
   a. Promote strengthening for arm abduction.
   b. Stabilize the glenohumeral joint.
   c. Prepare the scapula to clear the subacromial space to allow elevation greater than 90°.
   d. All of the above
5. A short-arc movement pattern of horizontal abduction with external rotation promotes muscle activation of:
   a. Scapular stabilization for advanced strengthening.
   b. Glenohumeral strengthening in early phase of rehabilitation.
   c. Rotator cuff strengthening without scapular involvement.
   d. All of the above
6. Primary impingement syndrome may involve:
   a. Weak rotator cuff muscles.
   b. Posterior and anterior capsular tightness.
   c. Spurs of degenerative joint disease changes.
   d. a and c
7. Nonoperative treatment for primary impingement may involve:
   a. Scapular stabilization.
   b. Rotator cuff strengthening.
   c. Capsular mobility and stretching.
   d. All of the above
   e. a and b
8. Acromioplasty is the operative approach to subacromion decompression and may have which of the following complications?
   a. Deltoid weakness secondary to surgical lesion
   b. Inadequate resection causing instability
   c. Excessive resection causing residual symptoms
   d. All the above
9. What should postoperative treatment progression for acromioplasty during the first phase include?
   a. Deltoid strengthening
   b. Inferior and posterior glides
   c. Rotator cuff isometric strengthening
   d. b and c
   e. a and c
10. The return to function phase of rehabilitation should include which of the following?
    a. Advanced rotator cuff strengthening
    b. Training of the deltoids
    c. High-level strengthening of scapular stabilization
    d. All of the above
    e. a and c
11. The return to function phase ("longest phase of rehab") should include:
    a. Isotonic strengthening.
    b. Elevation control and advanced scapular stabilization.
    c. Placement eccentric exercise for shoulder hike.
    d. a and c
    e. All of the above
12. Eccentric exercises are considered by many authorities as the "missing link" in rotator cuff rehabilitation. The published literature supports which of the following statements?
    a. Isotonic eccentric activity is more likely to create functional carryover.
    b. Eccentric muscle lengthening leads to controlled mobility.
    c. Eccentric overtraining would not cause soreness.
    d. a and b
    e. All of the above
13. Which stage of rotator cuff impingement occurs in patients younger than 25 years of age?
    a. Type 1
    b. Type 2
    c. Type 3
    d. Type 4
14. Which of the following is a benefit of closed kinetic chain exercises for the upper extremity?
    a. Isolates the rotator cuff musculature
    b. Single plane joint stabilization
    c. Encourages muscular cocontraction
    d. Higher muscle EMG than open kinetic chain
15. An injury to the anterior inferior labrum is considered which injury?
    a. Rotator cuff tear
    b. Bankart tear
    c. Hill-Sacks lesion
    d. None of the above

Short Answer

16. Explain the difference in primary and secondary shoulder impingement.
17. Describe the three most common static scapular positions that lead to the assessment of scapular dyskinesis.
18. Why are patients instructed to do posterior shoulder capsular stretching?

19. List the most common scapular stabilization exercises based on electromyographic studies for retraction and protraction.
20. Explain how the PTA would use manually placed eccentric exercises for the correction of shoulder hike dysfunction.

Fill in the Blank

21. Stage III rotator cuff impingement normally affects patients more than _______ years of age.
22. Capsular mobility has been shown to be helpful in ____________ motion to prepare the surrounding muscle to assist in shoulder _____________.
23. A reduction in available space in the shoulder is known as _________________.
24. A frozen shoulder is referred to as _______________.
25. CKC exercises provide _________________ and _________________ with lower muscle contraction load.

True/False

26. Age-related arthritic changes and bony osteophyte formation have no effect on subacromial impingement of the shoulder.
27. Posterior shoulder dislocations occur more often than anterior dislocations.
28. It is common for rotator cuff tears to occur with shoulder dislocation.
29. Scapular fractures occur from indirect and insignificant trauma.
30. Active muscle contractions of the deltoid are contraindicated during the prefunctional phase after rotator cuff repair.

Chapter 22

Orthopedic Management of the Elbow

Leonard C. Macrina

CHAPTER OUTLINE

LEARNING OBJECTIVES

1. Identify and describe the principles for common overuse soft tissue injuries of the elbow.
2. Discuss common methods of management and rehabilitation of overuse soft tissue injuries of the elbow.
3. Identify and describe intercondylar fractures, radial head fractures, olecranon fractures, and fracture-dislocations of the elbow.
4. Describe methods of management and rehabilitation of various fractures and fracture-dislocations of the elbow.
5. Describe techniques to improve range of motion of a stiff elbow including common joint mobilization techniques.

KEY TERMS

Epicondylitis
Lateral epicondylitis
Medial epicondylitis
Medial valgus stress overload
Ulnar collateral ligament (UCL)

Epicondylitis is any inflammatory condition of either the lateral or medial epicondyle of the distal humerus. This chapter introduces the physical therapist assistant (PTA) to common soft tissue injuries and fractures of the distal humerus and elbow. Specific attention is directed toward identifying treatment programs used to control pain and swelling and improve motion, strength, and function of the elbow after injury, surgery, or immobilization.

SOFT TISSUE INJURIES OF THE ELBOW

LATERAL EPICONDYLITIS

Commonly referred to as tennis elbow, lateral epicondylitis affects the common wrist extensor origin of the extensor carpi radialis longus, extensor carpi radialis brevis, extensor digitorum, and extensor digiti minimi.[13,56] The repetitive overuse of this area leads to tendinitis of the origin of the extensor carpi radialis brevis tendon (Fig. 22-1).[14,56] Lateral epicondylitis can affect anyone involved with repetitive activities of the wrist extensors.[55] Individuals who use hand tools (e.g., hammer, screwdriver, or pliers) and who participate in various activities involving wrist rotation, pulling, extending, and hand grasping can be affected by lateral epicondylitis.[55]

Generally, a patient with lateral epicondylitis has pain with palpation of the lateral epicondyle, with active or resisted wrist extension and occasionally with grasping of the affected hand.[13,46,55] Because this is a chronic overuse tendinitis, the intense inflammatory response in the affected area of the lateral epicondyle is "an attempt to increase the rate of tissue production to compensate for the increased rate of tissue microdamage."[55]

Important Concepts

It is critical that the PTA understand the different treatment strategies and presentations of an acute versus chronic lateral epicondylitis.

Initial acute management focuses on resolving pain and swelling with the judicious use of ice massage directly over the affected area, phonophoresis or iontophoresis, physician-prescribed analgesics and nonsteroidal

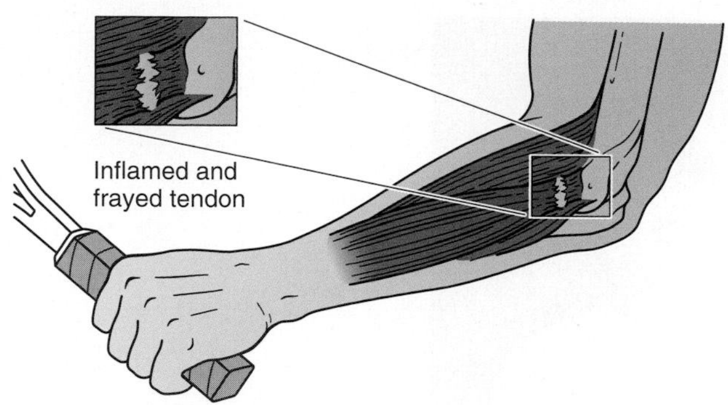

FIG 22-1 Lateral epicondylitis, or tennis elbow, affects the common wrist-extensor origin. *(From Salvo SG:* Mosby's pathology for massage therapists, *ed 3, St Louis, 2014, Mosby.)*

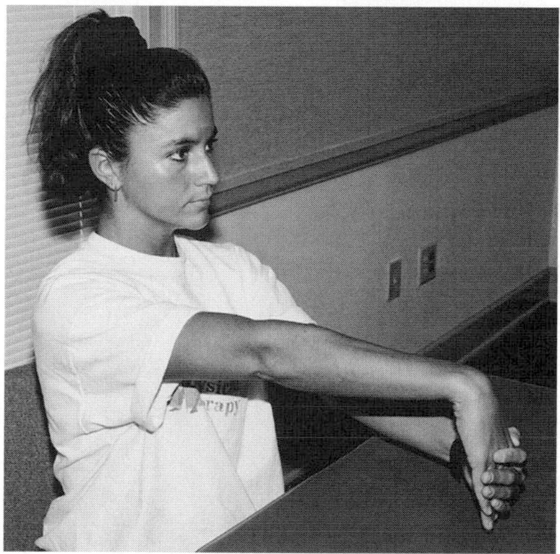

FIG 22-2 Stretching of the wrist extensors.

antiinflammatory drugs (NSAIDs), rest, and protection of the area from unwanted stress to allow for healing.[13,46,55] "Relative rest" rather than strict immobilization is used. A wrist cock-up splint can be used in severe cases to minimize stress on the inflamed wrist extensor tendons. The patient is allowed to remove the splint as needed to participate in controlled motion exercises that do not produce pain. Long-term, rigid immobilization is not indicated because the goal of treatment is not only to reduce pain and swelling but also to encourage proper collagen alignment and scar tissue maturation.[46] Without early protected motion, excessive tissue scarring and random collagen fiber alignment would severely limit normalized motion and function of the elbow and wrist.

During the initial healing stage, the PTA must encourage the patient to avoid any and all motions that may adversely affect healing. Short-term modifications in activities of daily living (ADL), sports, and job-related activities must be addressed to provide a pain-free environment for healing. When this initial program fails to bring significant relief of symptoms, some physicians elect to inject the area with a steroid to reduce the inflammation.[38,46] In addition, active gentle static stretching is advised for the wrist extensors to produce normalized, pain-free wrist flexion and extension (Fig. 22-2). Although specifically addressing treatment for the elbow, active motion and resistance exercises for the elbow and shoulder can be initiated if no wrist motion occurs to increase symptoms.

The PTA can enhance the effectiveness of low-load, long duration static stretching by applying moist heat packs (provided that the acute inflammatory process has ended) or ultrasound to the lateral epicondyle. These modalities help to stimulate local circulation and relieve congestion caused by metabolic waste products and relax soft tissues in preparation for stretching.

Resistance exercise can begin as pain is reduced with active motion exercises. Generally, submaximal isometrics are used for wrist extension, flexion, forearm pronation and supination, and radial and ulnar deviation. The PTA must carefully instruct the patient to perform all exercises within a pain-free range of motion (ROM). Throughout all phases of recovery, the patient must avoid stressful, pain-producing activities to prevent exacerbation of the inflammatory condition. Progressive motion exercises and increased resistance exercise is the foundation for a return to functional activities. Concentric and eccentric muscle contractions are added when the patient can demonstrate increased quality of multiple-angle isometric contractions. Care must be taken when initiating concentric and eccentric resistance exercises because frequently these contractions produce symptoms. Light resistance is advocated when having patients perform these exercises for the first time.

An important component for all resistance exercises used with lateral epicondylitis is the performance of slow, controlled eccentric contractions. Eccentric muscle contractions produce greater tension than either concentric or isometric exercise. In addition, energy use involving adenosine triphosphate (ATP) is less for eccentric exercise than for either concentric or isometric exercise. Eccentric muscle contractions are advocated by Curwin and Stanish[13] for the treatment of tennis elbow. The rationale for the performance of eccentric exercise is described by Reid and Kushner[49] as follows: "Exercising the muscle eccentrically allows it to withstand greater resistance and prevent injury, which occurs by eccentrically loading an inflexible muscle."[49,58]

Resistance exercises emphasizing the eccentric phase are shown in Fig. 22-3, *A* and *B*. A hammer is an effective strengthening tool for the treatment of lateral epicondylitis. However, when instructing the patient to perform pronation and supination of the forearm for the first time, the PTA should have the patient hold the hammer close to its head (Fig. 22-3, *C*). As the patient gains strength and can control the resistance of the hammer eccentrically, the patient should gradually hold the hammer at the midshaft. As strength improves, the patient should be allowed to hold the hammer at the end of the shaft, which requires greater eccentric muscle control, strength, and torque. In the same manner, strength can be gained for radial and ulnar deviation through use of the hammer. With a gradual return to functional activities, some physicians and therapists advocate the use of a counterforce brace to help dissipate the "overload forces" on the common origin of the wrist extensors (Fig. 22-3, *D*).[13,38,55]

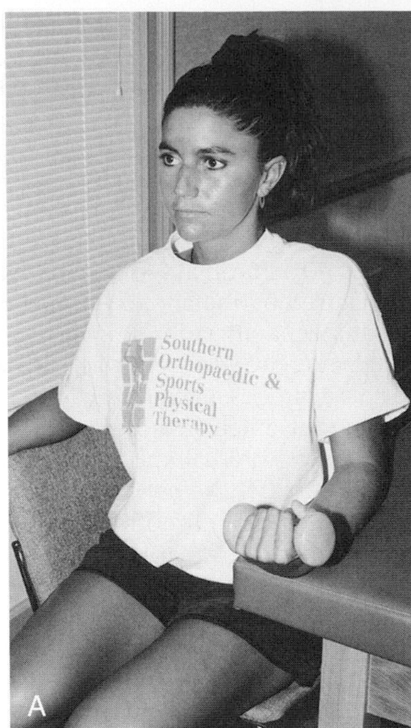

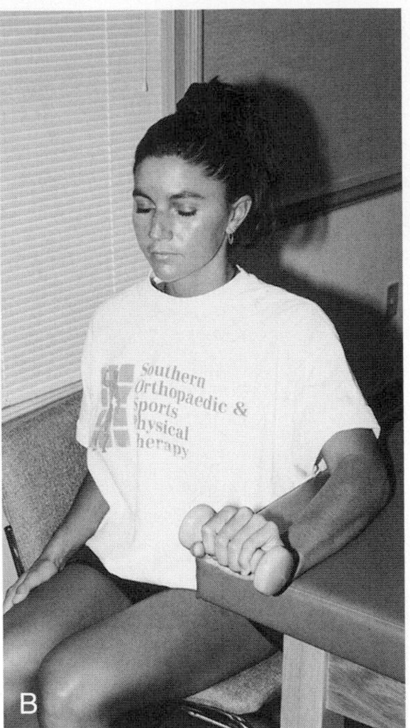

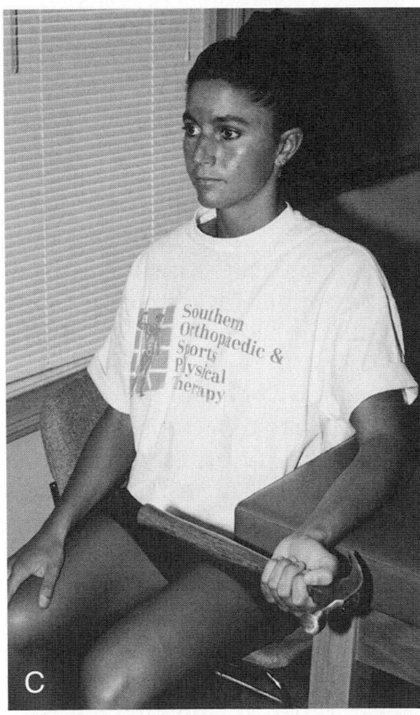

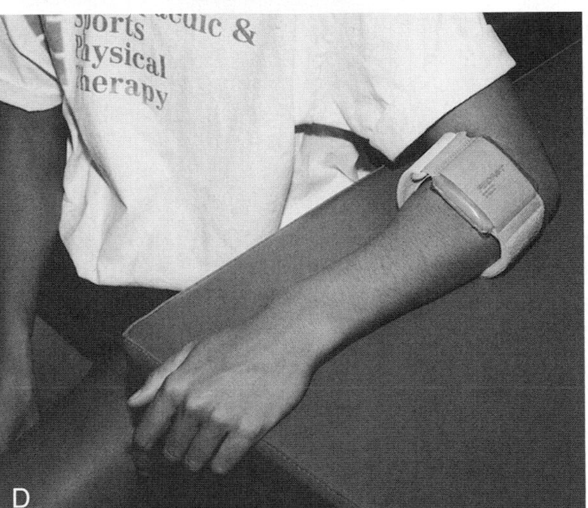

FIG 22-3 Common wrist and forearm strengthening exercises. **A,** Wrist flexion. **B,** Wrist extension. Encourage slow, controlled, nonballistic concentric and eccentric contractions. **C,** Pronation exercise with a hammer. The grip is held close to the head of the hammer when first introducing this exercise. **D,** A counterforce brace may help spread or dissipate overload force on the common wrist extensor origin.

Important Concepts

Eccentric strength training is the only exercise modality proven to improve chronic tendinitis, but it was proven in patients with Achilles tendinopathy.

Surgery is rarely necessary for this condition because physical therapy management frequently is effective. In rare instances when conservative means fail to reduce pain and improve function, the surgeon may elect to excise the "angiofibroblastic tissue at the origin of the extensor carpi radialis brevis muscle."[56]

MEDIAL EPICONDYLITIS

Medial epicondylitis is an overuse condition that affects the origin of the pronator teres, flexor carpi radialis, flexor digitorum sublimis, and flexor carpi ulnaris at the medial epicondyle of the elbow.[46] Although it occurs less

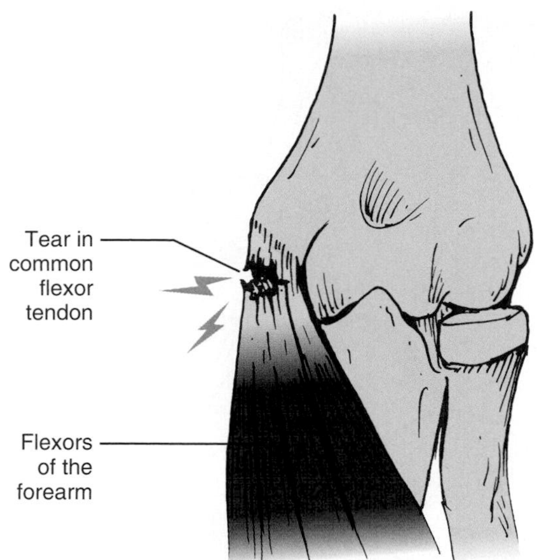

FIG 22-4 Medial epicondylitis, or golfer's elbow. Repetitive overuse injury.

often than lateral epicondylitis (the lateral epicondylitis-to-medial epicondylitis ratio is 7 : 1),[55] it is no less incapacitating to the patient. The dominant feature is pain with palpation over the medial epicondyle, with active motion, and particularly with resisted wrist flexion and full passive wrist extension (Fig. 22-4).[46,49]

The acute management phase of this inflammatory overuse condition, also referred to as golfer's elbow, concentrates on management of pain and swelling. Usually the physician prescribes NSAIDs and common modalities that may include massage, cold laser therapy, iontophoresis (Hybresis; DJO Global, Vista, CA), ultrasound, nitric oxide, and extracorporeal shock wave therapy. When used in combination with exercise or with other modalities, studies have shown improved tissue quality and outcomes.[1,9,16-18,21-23,26,30,40,43,45,47,48,54,59-61]

Conversely, the treatment for chronic tendinopathy, also known as tendinosis,[28,41,42] focuses on increasing circulation to promote collagen synthesis and collagen organization. The treatment includes heat, stretching, eccentrics, laser therapy, transverse massage, and soft tissue mobilization. All of these modalities are performed to increase circulation and promote tissue healing. Some authors have advocated dry needling for this pathology to promote tendon healing.[24,57]

Tendon loading by eccentric exercise and strength training has been shown to improve results in this patient population by increasing collagen synthesis[31] and realigning fiber orientation.[2,11,53] Other modalities such as laser therapy[9,16,30,54] and extracorporeal shock wave therapy[26,59,60] have shown promising results as well.

Important Concepts

Eccentric strength training in combination with manual therapy and relevant modalities should be the mainstay in treatment strategies.

Relative active rest (not immobilization), protection, and gentle active motion exercises are also encouraged in a pain-free ROM. The criteria-based treatment plan parallels treatment for lateral epicondylitis, although the focus is on the wrist flexors. Static low-load, long duration stretching[6,7] can proceed as pain allows. The PTA must encourage the patient to avoid repetitive flexion of the wrist and pronation of the forearm if these motions produce pain. Modifications in lifting, twisting, pulling, or turning of the wrist and forearm must accompany each phase of recovery to avoid stress on the medial structures. Moist heat and ultrasound can be applied to the medial epicondyle before stretching when motion has improved without pain. Resistance training can begin with submaximal isometrics, progressing to higher quality isometric multiple-angle contractions and ultimately to concentric and eccentric isotonic and isokinetic resistance exercises. The patient is instructed to use the shoulder of the affected limb actively and is strongly encouraged to follow a conditioning program to maintain or enhance cardiovascular fitness, strength, and flexibility throughout the rehabilitation process.

Although the resolution of pain and swelling is paramount for active use of the wrist and forearm, regaining lost motion caused by pain and muscular dysfunction is critical for function and a return to normal daily activities. The normal elbow ROM is 0° to approximately 145° of flexion.[56] However, most daily activities can be carried out within a functional ROM of 30° to 130° of flexion.[49,56] In addition, normal pronation of 75° and supination of 85° exceeds the functional arc of motion of 50° needed to carry out most ADLs. The PTA must encourage pain-free early protected motion to facilitate the collagen fiber alignment needed for functional scar maturation and purposeful motion to perform ADLs.

MEDIAL VALGUS STRESS OVERLOAD

Injuries to the elbow often occur in overhead athletes. The repetitive overhead motion involved in throwing is responsible for unique and sport-specific patterns of injuries to the elbow. These injuries are caused by chronic stress overload or repetitive microtraumatic stress observed during the overhead pitching motion as the elbow extends at greater than 2300°/sec, producing a medial shear force of 300 N and lateral compressive force of 900 N.[20,64] In addition, the valgus stress applied to the elbow during the acceleration phase of throwing is 64 N-m,[20,64] which exceeds the ultimate tensile strength of the **ulnar collateral ligament (UCL)**.[15] The medial aspect of the elbow undergoes tremendous tensile (distraction) forces, and the lateral aspect is forcefully compressed during the throwing motion.

Medial valgus stress overload, also known as valgus extension overload, occurs commonly among patients who participate in repetitive throwing and racquet sports such as javelin throwing, baseball, racquetball, and tennis.[14,39,46] Overhead athletes are susceptible to these specific elbow injuries. Numerous forces act on the elbow during the act of throwing,[20,64] including valgus stress with tension across the medial aspect of the elbow. These forces are maximal during the acceleration phase of throwing.

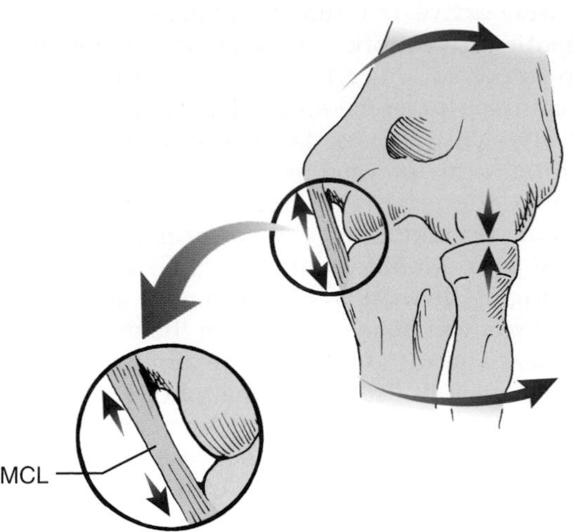

FIG 22-5 Medial valgus stress overload. Repetitive valgus stress to the elbow may stress the capsuloligamentous structures of the elbow. *MCL,* medial collateral ligament.

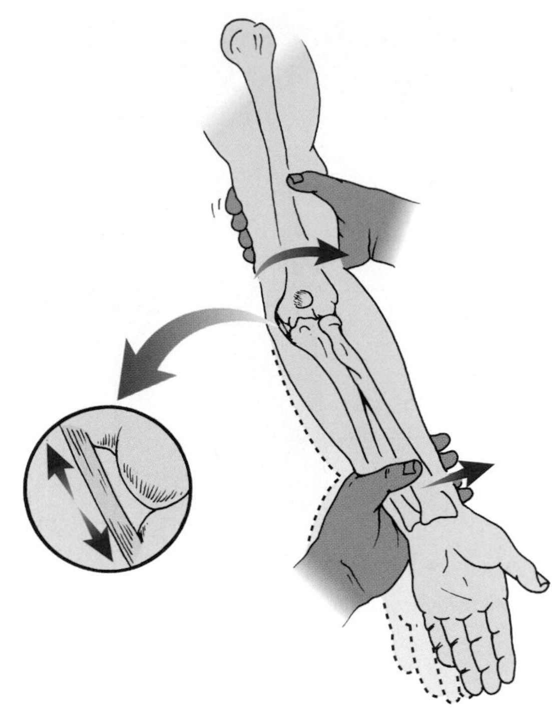

FIG 22-6 Clinical valgus stress examination to test the stability of the medial (ulnar) collateral ligament.

Compression forces are also applied to the lateral aspect of the elbow during the throwing motion. The posterior compartment is subject to tensile, compressive, and torsional forces during acceleration and deceleration phases. These forces may result in valgus extension overload within the posterior compartment leading to osteophyte formation, stress fractures of the olecranon, or physeal injury.[4,67] These stresses approach the ultimate failure load of the ligament with each throw. The repetitive nature of overhead throwing activities such as baseball pitching, javelin throwing, and football passing further increases the susceptibility of medial elbow injuries, including UCL injuries, by exposing the ligament to repetitive microtraumatic forces. Clinical differences exist between medial valgus stress overload and medial epicondylitis. Although medial epicondylitis represents a chronic overuse syndrome affecting the soft tissue musculotendinous origin of the wrist flexors and pronators, medial valgus stress overload occurs to the capsuloligamentous structures (medial [ulnar] collateral ligament) as a result of repetitive valgus stress to the elbow (Fig. 22-5).[14,39,46]

Patients usually complain of pain over the medial aspect of the elbow and the posterior aspect of the olecranon.[39,46] During initial evaluation by the physical therapist (PT), the PTA may observe the performance of ligament stability tests to confirm the presence of UCL laxity. The affected arm is held in 20° to 30° of flexion, while the humerus is held in full external rotation to unlock the olecranon process from the olecranon fossa. A medial or valgus stress is applied to the elbow to assess the stability of the medial (ulnar) collateral ligament (Fig. 22-6).[39,46]

Management of valgus stress injuries must take into account the healing constraints of ligaments. The patient may receive physician-prescribed NSAIDs, analgesics, ice massage, phonophoresis, or iontophoresis to reduce pain and swelling. Rest and protection of the injured medial ligamentous structures, while avoiding valgus stress, are the hallmarks of management. Because most of these injuries occur to active sports enthusiasts, the patient must omit activities that produce medial valgus stress. To ensure compliance, it may be necessary to suggest short-term rest from the activity, during which the patient should participate in running, cycling, and strength training in addition to flexibility exercises as long as no valgus load is applied to the elbow joint. Additionally, the wrist, hand, and shoulder of the affected limb must be exercised during each phase of recovery. As symptoms subside and ROM normalizes, dynamic stabilization and strengthening exercises are initiated. Emphasis is placed on improving eccentric strength of the elbow flexors in an attempt to control the rapid extension that occurs at the elbow during athletics. Manual resistance exercises of concentric and eccentric elbow flexion are performed as well as elbow flexion with exercise tubing. The athlete's throwing mechanics should be carefully assessed to determine if mechanical faults are causing the valgus extension overload symptoms or if a UCL injury is present.

Important Concepts

The PTA must address shoulder ROM or strength deficits because this may be the underlying cause of the medial elbow pain.

The elbow is predisposed to flexion contractures because of the intimate congruency of the joint articulations, the tightness of the joint capsule, and the tendency of the anterior capsule to develop adhesions after injury.[65] The brachialis muscle also attaches to the capsule and crosses the elbow joint before becoming a tendinous structure. Injury to the elbow may cause excessive scar tissue formation of the brachialis muscle and functional

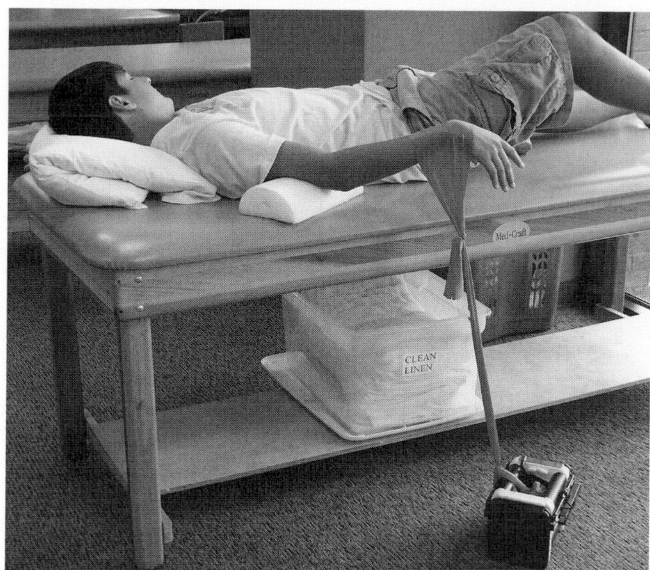

FIG 22-7 Low-load, long duration stretching technique to gain elbow extension range of motion.

splinting of the elbow.[65] Gentle low-load static stretching begins as soon as pain allows. The stretching regimen focuses on all wrist motions, forearm pronation and supination, and elbow flexion and extension as long as no pain occurs with these activities. If the patient continues to have difficulty achieving full extension using ROM and mobilization techniques, a low-load, long duration stretch may be performed to produce a deformation (creep) of the collagen tissue, resulting in tissue elongation.[27,52,62,63] This technique is extremely beneficial for regaining full elbow extension. The patient lies supine with a towel roll or foam placed under the distal brachium to act as a cushion and fulcrum. Light resistance exercise tubing is applied to the wrist of the patient and secured to the table or a dumbbell on the ground (Fig. 22-7). The patient is instructed to relax as much as possible for 10 to 15 minutes per treatment. The amount of resistance applied should be of low magnitude to enable the patient to perform the stretch for the entire duration without pain or muscle spasm. This technique should impart a low load over a prolonged period of time to achieve maximal benefits. Patients are instructed to perform this stretch technique several times per day, equaling 60 minutes of total end range time. Patients may perform a 15-minute stretch four times per day.[34] This program has been extremely beneficial for patients with a stiff elbow.

ULNAR NEUROPATHY (CUBITAL TUNNEL SYNDROME)

Numerous theories exist regarding the cause of ulnar neuropathy of the elbow in throwing athletes. Ulnar nerve changes can result from tensile forces, compressive forces, or nerve instability. Any one or a combination of these mechanisms may be responsible for ulnar nerve symptoms.

A leading mechanism for tensile force on the ulnar nerve is valgus stress. This valgus stress may be coupled with an external rotation-supination stress overload mechanism. The traction forces are magnified further when underlying valgus instability from UCL injuries is present. Ulnar neuropathy is often a secondary pathology of UCL insufficiency. Compression of the ulnar nerve is often due to hypertrophy of the surrounding soft tissues or the presence of scar tissue. The nerve may also be trapped between the two heads of the flexor carpi ulnaris. Repetitive flexion and extension of the elbow with an unstable nerve can irritate or inflame the nerve. The nerve may sublux or rest on the medial epicondyle rendering it vulnerable to direct trauma.

There are three stages of ulnar neuropathy.[3] The first stage includes an acute onset of radicular symptoms. The second stage includes a recurrence of symptoms as the athlete attempts to return to competition. The third stage comprises persistent motor weakness and sensory changes. When the athlete presents in the third stage of injury, conservative management may not be effective.

The nonoperative treatment of ulnar neuropathy focuses on diminishing ulnar nerve irritation, enhancing dynamic medial joint stability, and gradually returning the athlete to competition. NSAIDs are often prescribed, and rehabilitation includes iontophoresis and cryotherapy. After the diagnosis of ulnar neuropathy, throwing athletes are instructed to discontinue throwing activities for at least 4 weeks, depending on the severity and chronicity of symptoms. The use of a night splint with the elbow flexed to 45° may be beneficial to rest and decrease nerve irritation. The athlete progresses through the immediate motion and intermediate phases over the course of 4 to 6 weeks with emphasis placed on eccentric and dynamic stabilization drills. Plyometric exercises are used to facilitate further dynamic stabilization of the medial elbow. The athlete is allowed to begin an interval throwing program when full pain-free ROM and muscle performance is exhibited without neurologic symptoms. The athlete may gradually return to play if progression through the interval throwing program[50] does not unveil neurologic symptoms.

ULNAR COLLATERAL LIGAMENT SPRAIN

Injuries to the UCL are becoming increasingly more common in overhead throwing athletes, although the higher incidence of injury may be due to increased ability to diagnose these injuries. The elbow experiences a tremendous amount of valgus stress during overhead throwing.[19,64] The repetitive nature of overhead throwing activities such as baseball pitching, javelin throwing, and football passing further increase the susceptibility to UCL injury by exposing the ligament to repetitive microtraumatic forces.

Conservative treatment is attempted with partial tears and sprains of the UCL, although surgical reconstruction may be warranted for complete tears or if nonoperative treatment is unsuccessful. A brace may be used to restrict motion and prevent valgus loading. It may be beneficial to rest the UCL immediately after the initial painful episode of throwing to prevent additionally deleterious stresses on the ligament. Isometric exercises are performed for the shoulder, elbow, and wrist to prevent muscular atrophy. Ice and antiinflammatory medications are prescribed to control pain and inflammation.

Important Concepts

An active rest period of 6 to 8 weeks is typically recommended before the player attempts a throwing program.

ROM of flexion and extension is gradually increased by 5° to 10° per week during the second phase of treatment or as tolerated. Full pain-free ROM should be achieved by at least 3 to 4 weeks. Elbow flexion/extension motion is encouraged to promote collagen formation and alignment. An attempt to control valgus loading onto the elbow joint minimizes stress on the UCL.

The strengthening component of recovery must be modified to prevent any valgus stress or pain at end-range extension. This modification ensures that the healing ligament is not receiving any additional tensile forces that may affect the healing capacity. Full ROM (flexion/extension) concentric and eccentric resistance exercise is allowed with light weights as motion and pain dictate. Wrist and hand exercises are encouraged early and pose no threat to the healing ligament. In addition, forearm pronation and supination with use of a hammer (as outlined) is employed as the patient is able to demonstrate improved motion without pain. With time, the PT reassesses the stability of the UCLs. If these structures demonstrate improved stability without pain, a gradual return to throwing can commence.

Surgery is considered if conservative treatment fails to restore function and eliminate pain. Degenerative changes, which are usually present in adult patients, must be addressed surgically.[39,49] In general, an osteotomy is performed to remove osteophytes (bone spurs) and fibrotic, degenerated tissue.[39,49]

Acute rupture (grade III ligament rupture) of the UCL can occur in skeletally mature adults if valgus stress is applied suddenly with sufficient force (Fig. 22-8). First, these patients are managed conservatively with ice, NSAIDs, analgesics, and, most important, rest and protection. The progression from the acute, maximum protection phase to return-to-normal function parallels treatment outlined for valgus stress injuries. However, because the ligament has been ruptured, a longer period of recovery is needed as well as rest and joint protection from valgus stress. Normal elbow motion, including flexion, extension, pronation, and supination, should be encouraged as pain allows.

If early active protected joint motion and progressive resistance exercise have been used, authorities suggest that the injured patient can resume throwing activities approximately 3 to 4 months after injury.[39] However, surgery may be necessary to stabilize the joint if the patient does not demonstrate improved valgus stability and continues to have dysfunction.

Generally, if the UCL is ruptured midsubstance, a direct repair is carried out and a reconstructive procedure is performed. Typically, the palmaris longus or gracilis graft source is harvested and passed in a figure-of-eight pattern through drill holes in the sublime tubercle of the ulna and the medial epicondyle.[5] A subcutaneous ulnar nerve transposition is performed at the time of reconstruction. Some surgeons are presently performing UCL reconstruction using the docking procedure, as described by Rohrbough and colleagues.[51]

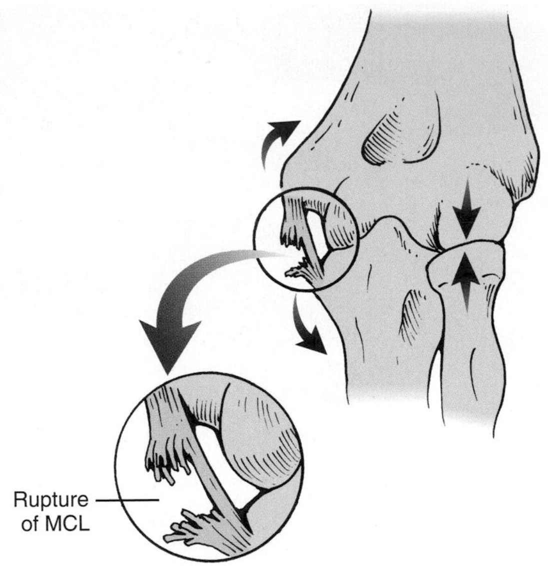

FIG 22-8 Sudden valgus force applied to a skeletally mature adult may result in rupture of the medial collateral ligament (*MCL*).

Postoperative rehabilitation begins immediately, with the patient's affected limb immobilized in a brace to protect against valgus stress. Instructions are given to perform hand, wrist, and shoulder exercises to maintain motion. Usually by the third week postoperatively, ROM should approach at least 20° of extension, while slowly progressing to 110° of elbow flexion.[14] The continuous use of ice and therapeutic agents (e.g., ultrasound, transcutaneous electrical nerve stimulation, galvanic stimulation)[49] are prescribed as necessary. Progressive resistance concentric and eccentric contractions are used for the wrist of the involved limb, whereas submaximal isometrics can begin for elbow flexion and extension.

Shoulder strengthening and flexibility exercises also can begin during the third week of recovery.[14] However, care must be taken to avoid external shoulder rotation exercises because this motion produces valgus stress on the elbow.[14]

Usually by 4 to 6 weeks after surgery, ROM should be 0° to 130°.[14] In addition, concentric and eccentric resistance exercises for elbow flexion and extension are added progressively as tolerated. Gentle forearm pronation and supination exercises can be made more challenging during this time frame. Functional training can begin 2 to 4 months after surgery with an emphasis on shoulder, elbow, and wrist strengthening; motion exercises; and plyometrics. Plyometric drills can be an extremely beneficial form of functional exercise for training the elbow in overhead athletes.[65,66] Plyometric exercises are performed using a weighted medicine ball during the latter stages of this phase to train the shoulder and elbow to develop and withstand high levels of stress (Fig. 22-9). Plyometric exercises are initially done with two hands performing a chest

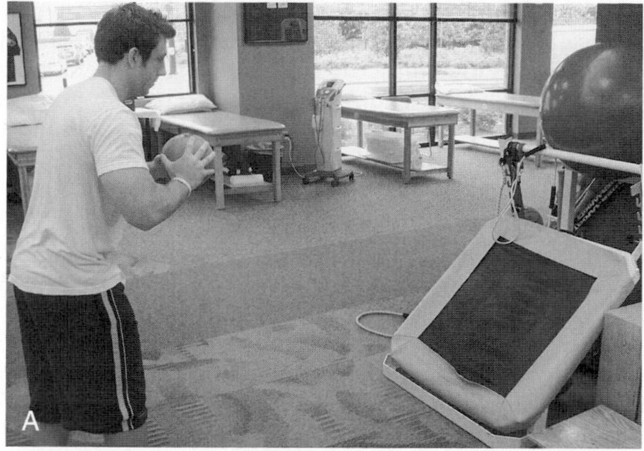

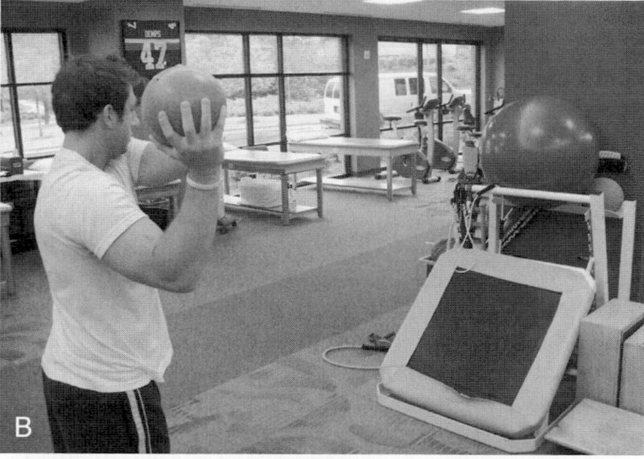

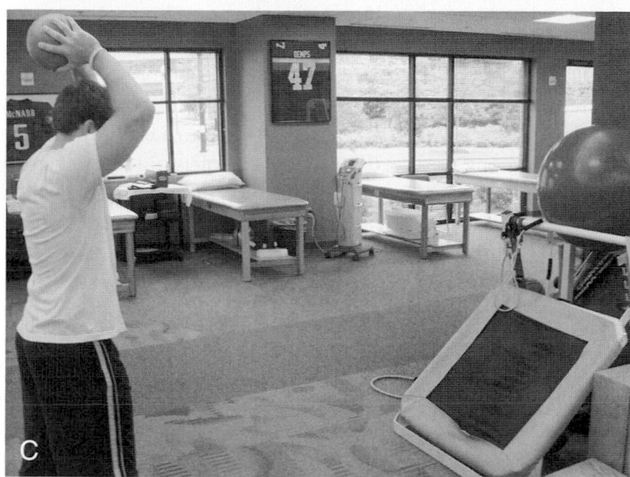

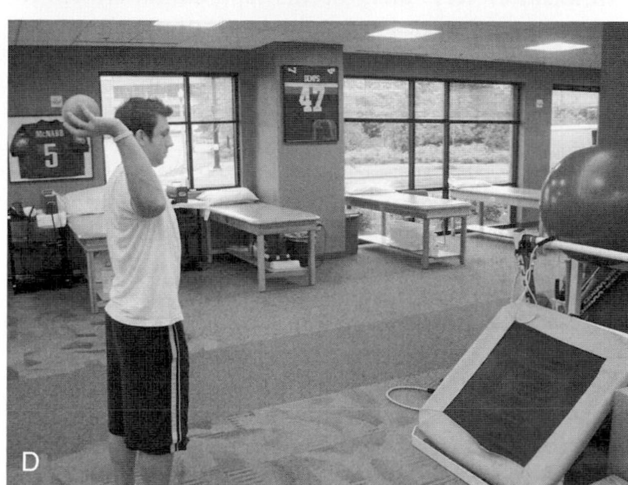

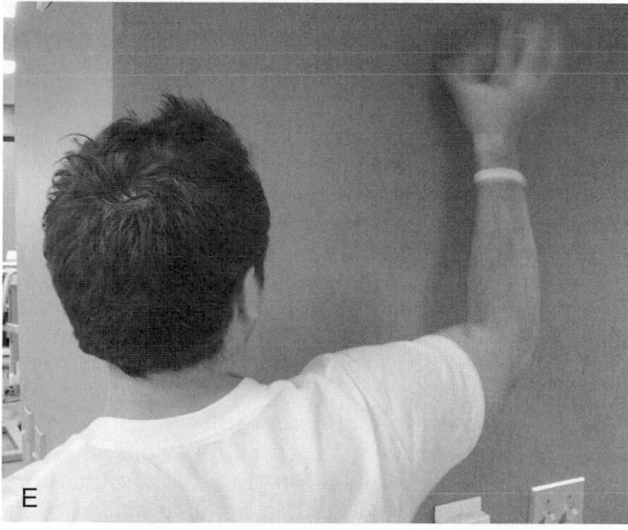

FIG 22-9 **A,** Two hands performing a chest pass. **B,** Side-to-side throw. **C,** Overhead soccer throw. **D,** 90/90 throws. **E,** Wall dribbles.

pass, side-to-side throw, and overhead soccer throw. These may be progressed to include one-hand activities such as 90/90 throws, external and internal rotation throws at 0° of abduction, and wall dribbles. On medical clearance, the athlete may initiate the formal interval sport program as described by Reinold and co-workers.[50] Patients returning to sports that involve the upper extremity, such as golf, tennis, javelin, baseball, and softball, are placed on an interval sport program.[50] Ultimately, it takes 10 to 12 months after elbow reconstruction and rehabilitation for valgus instability before a functional return to overhead, competitive sports is allowed.[39]

LATERAL COLLATERAL LIGAMENT INJURY

Stability of the elbow occurs mainly through the osseous configuration but secondarily through the medial and lateral collateral ligaments. In particular, the lateral ligament complex prevents rotational instability between the distal humerus and the proximal radius and ulna. However, disrupting the soft tissue constraints through a traumatic onset often results in subluxation or dislocation. The elbow is the second most commonly dislocated large joint after the shoulder.[32,33] Elbow dislocations are the most commonly dislocated joint in children younger than 10 years old.

Two main mechanisms of dislocation have been suggested. Elbow dislocations are thought to result from hyperextension, in which the olecranon process is forced into the olecranon fossa, and the trochlea is then levered over the coronoid process. Most elbow dislocations occur in a directly posterior or posterolateral direction. An anterior dislocation very rarely occurs (approximately 1% to 2%). A second proposed mechanism of injury is posterolateral rotation, in which combined forces of axial compression, elbow flexion, valgus stress, and forearm supination create a rotational displacement of the ulna on the distal humerus.

Nonoperative rehabilitation should begin immediately after the traumatic event. The focus of rehabilitation is to restore ROM within the limits of elbow stability, while slowly applying progressive stresses to the healing structures. Modalities to control pain and swelling, such as cryotherapy and a compressive sleeve, may be used. Additionally, a hinged elbow brace with the forearm in a neutral or slightly pronated position is used to protect against excessive valgus and varus forces. The brace should restrict ROM to approximately 30° to 90° initially with ROM progressively increased until full, pain-free ROM is achieved. A slow ROM progression for forearm supination and elbow extension protects the healing lateral collateral ligament structures.

Important Concepts

ROM progression should be based on the pain and end-feel during passive range of motion (PROM). The PTA should speed up or slow down the process based on progress of tissue healing.

Strengthening activities may be initiated early on to prevent atrophy resulting from immobilization. Multiple-angle isometrics may begin during the initial phase of 1 to 10 days postinjury. Progressive resistance exercises for the elbow are initiated during the intermediate phase (days 10 to 14 postinjury). During the advanced phase, weeks 2 through 8 postinjury, functional progressions and sport-specific activities are initiated. The athlete may be allowed to return to sports participation when sufficient strength, power, and endurance are obtained. A brace may be used during competition to prevent hyperextension and varus/valgus stresses.

Lateral Collateral Ligament Reconstruction

The reconstruction technique is intended to recreate the ulnar aspect of the lateral collateral ligament complex. O'Driscoll[44] recommended first repairing the avulsed origin of the lateral ligament complex to its isometric origin on the lateral epicondyle if possible. This repair is typically followed by augmentation of the repair with graft choices including the palmaris longus, lateral triceps tendon, and semitendinosus allograft or autograft and even a plantaris allograft. Physician preference often dictates which graft is used during the reconstruction.

The rehabilitation program is designed to protect the healing structures based on healing constraints, degree of soft tissue involvement, and the ultimate functional goal of the patient. The rehabilitation program for this specific surgical procedure is briefly described next.

The rehabilitation program is initiated immediately after the surgical procedure to ensure adequate healing and protection. The postoperative protocol has been broken down into three distinct phases to maximize functional outcomes: immediate postoperative phase, intermediate phase, and advanced phase. The rehabilitation specialist should make every attempt to use these guidelines; however, the progression rate may differ among patients depending on the exact surgical procedure, physician preference, and the patient's individual characteristics.

During the immediate postoperative phase (0 to 3 weeks), the patient is placed in a 90° posterior elbow splint with full forearm pronation. This splint is used for the first 3 weeks to allow adequate soft tissue healing of the graft within the bone tunnels. Gentle elbow ROM activities are permitted during this time, particularly supination, which is generally limited for the first 4 weeks. Wrist and shoulder PROM and active range of motion (AROM) activities may be performed as long as there are no pain symptoms along the lateral elbow. The PTA can be more aggressive with ROM at 6 weeks; full elbow ROM may take 10 to 12 weeks.

The patient may also begin gentle gripping exercises for the hand and isometric activities for the shoulder. Shoulder rotation (internal and external) isometric exercises may not be performed during this phase because of the varus and valgus moments at the elbow joint that may stress the healing soft tissue structures. By the end of the third postoperative week, the patient may initiate AROM activities for the shoulder musculature, including the full can exercise, lateral raises, and internal/external rotation with tubing.

During the intermediate phase (4 to 7 weeks), the patient may gradually increase elbow PROM and progress strengthening activities. The elbow joint is protected by a hinged brace set from 30° to 100°. This brace allows a moderate amount of motion but still prevents any deleterious end-range stresses. The patient may unlock the brace by 10° per week and may discontinue using the brace by the end of the sixth week. The rehabilitation specialist may begin elbow PROM with the forearm in neutral or slight pronation. Care should be taken not to push the elbow into end-range flexion or extension at this time. Full PROM may be expected by 8 to 10 weeks postoperatively. If full ROM has not been achieved, the low-load, long duration guidelines mentioned earlier in this chapter may assist in obtaining the remaining ROM.

During the intermediate phase, the strengthening activities should focus on dynamic stability of the medial and lateral musculature. The patient may begin light isotonic strengthening for the wrist, forearm, and elbow muscles. Also, the progressive strengthening program should emphasize the rotator cuff and scapula stabilizers. By week 6, the patient may advance to the Thrower's Ten program to enhance dynamic stability further. The Thrower's Ten program is a series or group of exercises that are intended to strength the entire upper extremity kinetic chain, including not only the shoulder, but also the elbow, forearm, and hand.

Important Concepts

Typical ligamentous healing takes 8 to 12 weeks, so the PTA must be careful in progressing the patient too quickly.

By week 8, the patient may progress to the advanced strengthening phase. The goals of this phase are to increase strength, power, and endurance while maintaining full elbow ROM. Aggressive strengthening exercises involving eccentric and plyometric contractions are also included, usually at 10 weeks postoperatively. These sport-specific activities are progressed through increasing the number of repetitions, increasing the weight of the medicine ball, or increasing the timed bouts of the activity to improve endurance. Beyond week 16, the patient is reassessed to determine strength levels before progressing to an interval sports program. Sufficient strength, generally within 15% of the contralateral side, and full ROM indicate the patient is ready to begin an interval program.[50]

FRACTURES OF THE ELBOW

FRACTURES OF THE DISTAL HUMERUS (SUPRACONDYLAR FRACTURES)

By definition, a supracondylar fracture is a transverse fracture of the distal third of the humerus.[35] These frequent injuries usually occur in children.[35,39,55] Supracondylar fractures generally are classified into two different types.[12,35,56] Type I is the most common and refers to an injury that occurs as a result of a fall on an extended, outstretched arm in which the distal humerus fragment is displaced posteriorly and is maintained in that position because of the strong pull of the triceps (Fig. 22-10, *A*).[12,56] Type II is considered a flexion injury and occurs after direct trauma to the posterior aspect of the elbow in which the distal humeral fragment lies anterior to the humerus (Fig. 22-10, *B*).[12,56]

The most common treatment of these fractures is by closed reduction and immobilization for 4 to 6 weeks. The affected arm is held in a flexed position to allow the triceps to help maintain the fracture in a stable position.[35,56] As with all other fractures, the initial phase of recovery focuses on motion and strengthening exercises for the contralateral limb; general body conditioning; and active motion of the hand, wrist, and shoulder of the injured limb, as long as no undue stress is directed at the fracture site.

Physical therapy treatment after immobilization focuses on gentle active motion exercises, which can be preceded by the use of moist heat or a warm whirlpool to encourage relaxation, remove wastes, and improve local circulation.

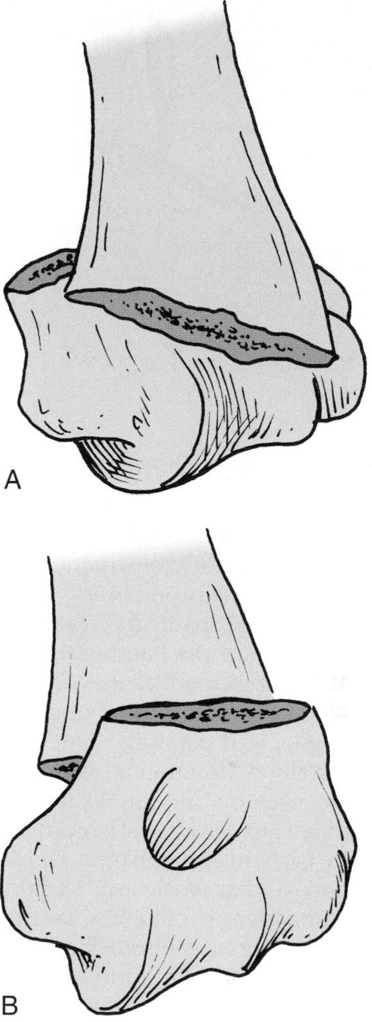

FIG 22-10 **A,** Supracondylar fracture type I, or extension-type fracture in which the distal humeral fragment is displaced posteriorly. **B,** Supracondylar fracture type II, or flexion-type fracture in which the distal humeral fragment is displaced anteriorly.

In most cases, progressive active motion of the elbow and resistance exercises proceed when radiographic evidence confirms solid union, a minimum of 6 weeks has elapsed since surgery (consistent with the healing constraints of bone tissue), and the patient demonstrates improved motion without pain.

Complications arising from supracondylar fractures[36] include nonunion, malunion, and joint contracture. Perhaps the most disastrous complication results from vascular compromise.[12,35,36,56] As the fracture fragments are displaced, hemorrhage beneath the deep fascia produces an ischemic injury that creates an arterial and venous obstruction (usually affecting the brachial artery), leading to Volkmann's ischemic contracture (Fig. 22-11).[12,36,55] Most importantly, the clinical signs and symptoms of ischemic obstruction may not be noticed until the end of immobilization.[12] The symptoms of Volkmann's ischemic contracture can occur throughout each phase of recovery after a supracondylar fracture.

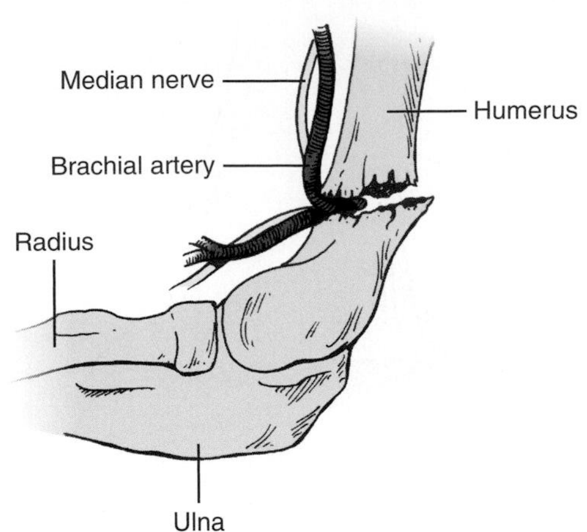

FIG 22-11 Volkmann ischemic contracture.

Stralka and Brasel[55] outlined six symptoms authorities defined as indicating vascular obstruction:

1. Severe pain in the forearm muscles
2. Limited and extremely painful finger movement
3. Purple discoloration of the hand with prominent veins
4. Initial paresthesia followed by loss of sensation
5. Loss of radial pulse and later loss of capillary return
6. Pallor, anesthesia, and paralysis

Restoration of elbow function after supracondylar fractures initially focuses on motion exercises that do not stress the fracture site. Passive stretching is contraindicated during the early healing phase.[35] Gentle active exercises for the upper arm, wrist, and shoulder should be performed to the patient's tolerance. Resistance exercises consisting of submaximal isometrics progressing to concentric and eccentric muscle contractions are allowed, pending confirmation of secure union of the fracture fragments.

INTERCONDYLAR T OR Y FRACTURES

In addition to nondisplaced or displaced transverse supracondylar fractures, potentially more significant fracture patterns can occur with falls or direct trauma to the elbow. Intercondylar fractures describe injuries that extend between the condyles of the distal humerus and involve the articular surfaces of the elbow joint.[12,35,36,56] According to Strege[56] and Miller,[36] there are four classifications of intercondylar fractures that display a T or Y configuration:[12,35,39]

- Type I: A nondisplaced fracture that extends between the two condyles (Fig. 22-12, *A*)
- Type II: A displaced fracture without rotation of the fracture fragments (Fig. 22-12, *B*)
- Type III: A displaced fracture with a rotational deformity (Fig. 22-12, *C*)
- Type IV: A severely comminuted fracture with significant separation between the two condyles (Fig. 22-12, *D*)

The type of fracture dictates a course of treatment that parallels the significance of the injury. With a type I nondisplaced fracture, treatment can be immobilization for approximately 3 weeks, followed by progressive, gentle AROM. Resistance exercises are deferred until secure bone union has been confirmed radiographically. With types II and III displaced fractures, the treatment is open reduction with internal fixation (ORIF) with the use of Kirschner wires, side plates, and lag screws to secure and stabilize the displaced fracture fragments (Fig. 22-13).[35,36,56] Type IV comminuted intercondylar fractures are treated differently for adults and elderly patients with poor bone quality (i.e., osteoporosis).[36,56] Adult patients are usually treated with an ORIF procedure to stabilize the fragments. However, in elderly patients with generally poor bone quality (osteopenic bone), a treatment procedure referred to as the "bag of bones technique" is used.[35,36,56] This technique calls for the use of a "collar and cuff" sling, with the affected elbow flexed as far as the limits of swelling and circulatory compromise allow.[56] With the elbow flexed and able to hang freely within the sling, gravity is used to help obtain possible reduction of the fracture fragments (Fig. 22-14).[36,56]

With intercondylar fractures of the elbow, the patient is instructed in a general conditioning program during immobilization while close attention is paid to avoid all stress to the affected arm. In addition, the wrist, hand, and shoulder of the affected limb may be exercised with active motion if prescribed by the physician and PT. With intercondylar fractures, the anatomic relationship of the elbow (being extremely compact, with significant bony stability) dictates that the restoration of purposeful, functional motion becomes paramount during recovery. Soft tissue scarring and bone callus formation can lead to early joint stiffness, arthrosis, and contractures.

During the early postimmobilization period, no passive manipulation or passive stretching can be performed.[56] Strege[56] reported an appreciable risk of joint ankylosis when passive stretching and manipulation are performed during early postinjury elbow rehabilitation.

Once wound closure has occurred after an ORIF procedure, the use of a whirlpool bath may aid local circulation, removal of waste, reduction in soft tissue congestion, and enhancement of soft tissue relaxation in preparation for protected AROM. Elbow flexion and extension and forearm pronation and supination are encouraged as prescribed by the physician and directed by the PT. Stable union of the fracture signifies more active involvement with progressive motion exercises and the initiation of resistance exercise training to regain strength. If the patient demonstrates loss of motion, the physician and PT may decide to perform specific joint mobilization techniques when bone union is secure; this does not conflict with the mentioned contraindication for passive manipulation and stretching immediately after immobilization. Some patients ultimately may have residual loss of motion. However, functional activities can be performed with flexion and extension of 30° to 130° and pronation and supination of 50°.[56]

RADIAL HEAD FRACTURES

A radial head fracture is another common fracture that occurs as a result of a fall on an outstretched arm. These fractures represent approximately one third of all elbow fractures and nearly 20% of all elbow trauma.[29]

The definition of the "carrying angle" of the elbow and the difference noted between men and women are

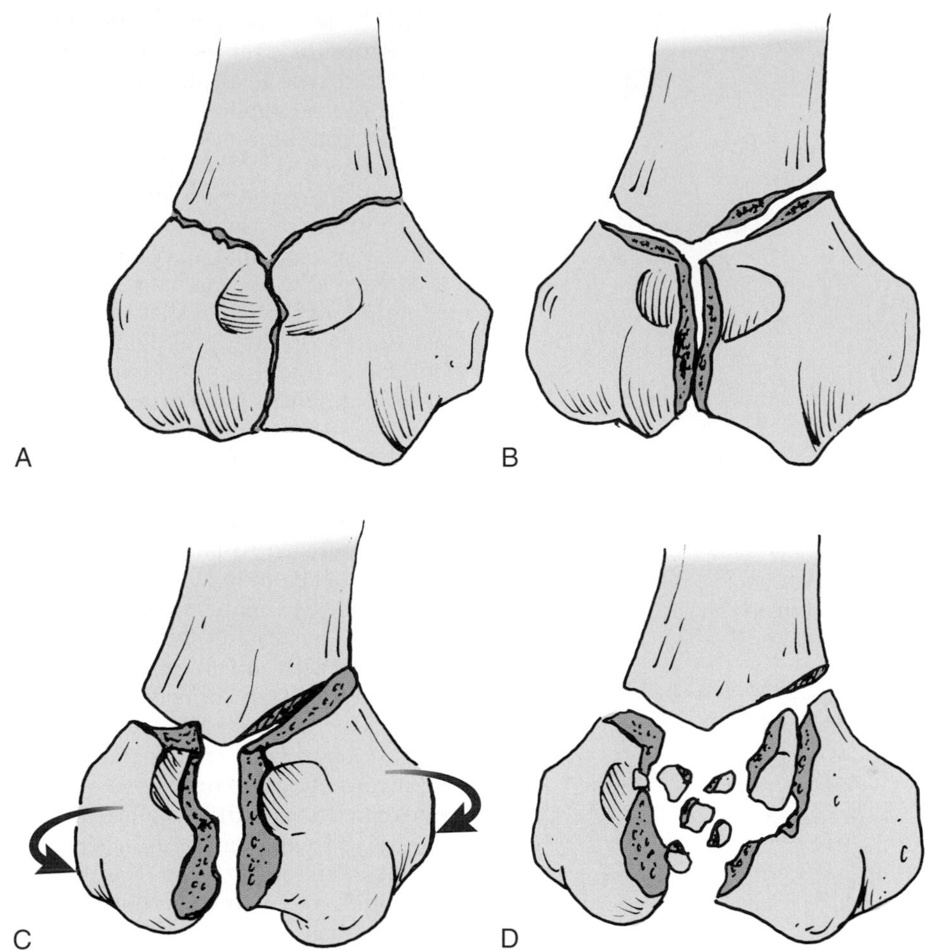

FIG 22-12 **A,** Type I intercondylar fracture, nondisplaced. **B,** Type II intercondylar fracture, displaced without rotation. **C,** Type III intercondylar fracture, displaced with rotation of fragments. **D,** Severely comminuted type IV intercondylar fracture with significant displacement.

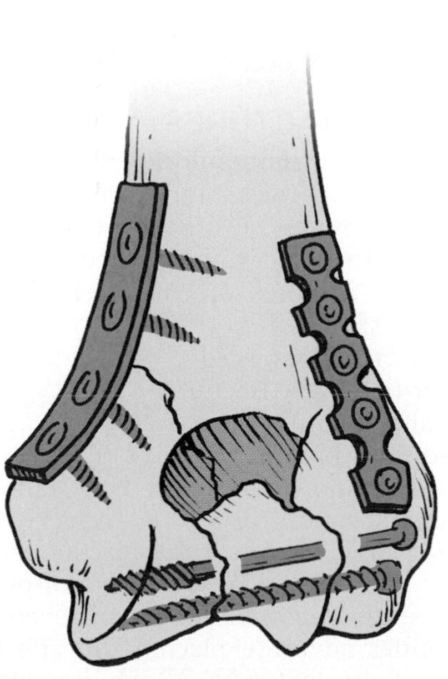

FIG 22-13 Displaced intercondylar fracture open reduction with internal fixation.

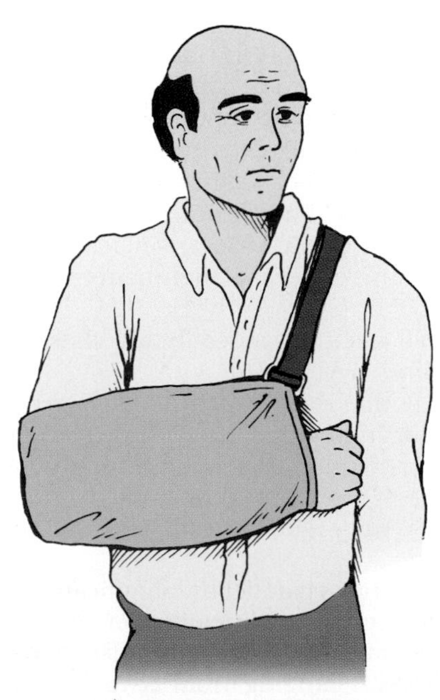

FIG 22-14 In cases in which elderly patients with osteoporosis sustain a severely comminuted intercondylar fracture, a treatment referred to as the bag of bones technique is used.

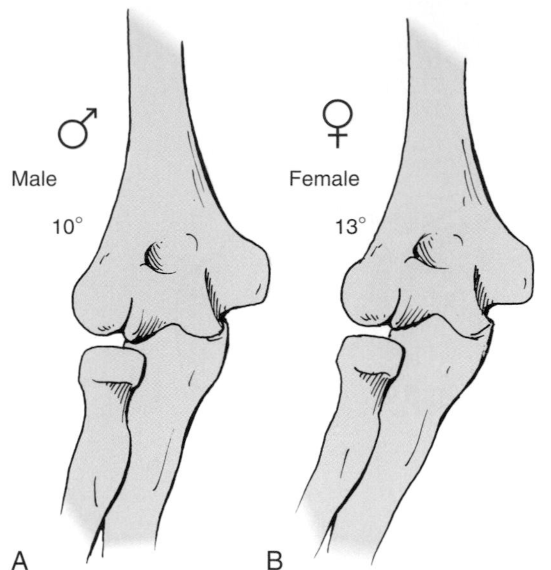

FIG 22-15 Elbow carrying angles.

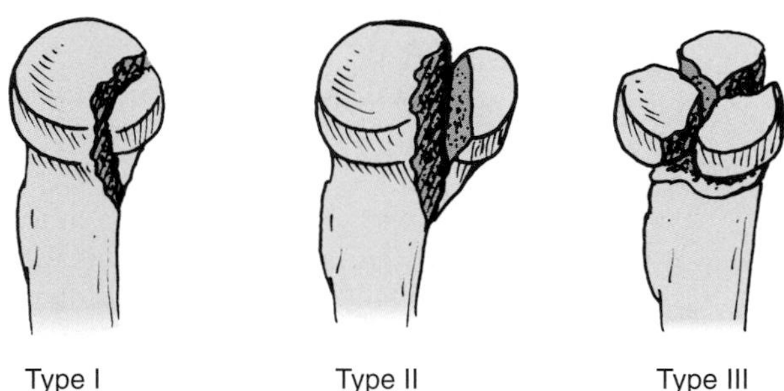

FIG 22-16 Radial head fractures. Type I, nondisplaced; type II, displaced; and type III, comminuted.

important in understanding radial head fractures. The carrying angle is formed between the intersection of the long axis of the humerus and the axis of the ulna, with the elbow joint in full extension.[56] A normal carrying angle for men is 10° of valgus; in women, it is 13° of valgus (Fig. 22-15).[56] The clinical relevance is that a fractured radial head can lead to an increased valgus deformity and the varus elbow malalignment called a "gunstock deformity."[29]

Radial head fractures generally are classified into four types, as follows (Fig. 22-16):

- Type I: A nondisplaced fracture
- Type II: A marginal fracture with displacement
- Type III: A comminuted fracture of the entire radial head
- Type IV: Any radial head fracture with elbow dislocation[56]

Treatment options parallel the significance of the injury and dictate the course of rehabilitation. Patients with type I nondisplaced radial head fractures usually need a period of immobilization ranging from 5 to 7 days to 3 to 4 weeks.[35,56] Usually, early active motion is allowed as soon as pain subsides. Because these fractures generally are stable (nondisplaced), healing occurs with very good results.[35] Terminal elbow extension may be recovered many months after type I radial head fractures.[35]

With a type II displaced fracture, the radial head can be excised or stabilized with an ORIF procedure. With a type III comminuted radial head fracture, the fractured area is excised.[29,35,36,56] Rehabilitation after an ORIF or radial head excision usually calls for immobilization in a hinged splint to protect the healing bone and surrounding soft tissues. As noted, excision of the radial head can lead to increased varus or valgus deformity. In either case, migration of the radial shaft may occur after excision and place stress on the distal ligamentous radioulnar articulation.[29,35,36] Any discomfort expressed by the patient at the distal radioulnar joint after excision of the radial head usually results from added stress on this area created by the disrupted proximal radial segment.[29,35,36] When the patient is immobilized, the hand, wrist, and shoulder of the affected limb are exercised as tolerated. The patient is also encouraged to participate in a general conditioning program of aerobic exercise, strength training, and flexibility exercises. Pain and swelling are typically managed satisfactorily by placing ice packs directly over the painful area. Early active ROM exercises are advocated 3 to 5 days postoperatively by some authorities or deferred for up to 3 weeks by others.[29,56] Restoration of motion is the cornerstone for recovery after radial head fractures. As noted, joint restrictions secondary to arthrofibrosis and contractures can occur, with pronation and supination most commonly affected after radial head fractures.

The PT may elect to perform specific joint mobilization techniques to enhance pronation and supination if secure fixation has occurred after an ORIF procedure. Once wound closure has occurred, a whirlpool bath can be an effective adjunct preceding motion exercises. After excision of the radial head, resistance exercises of elbow flexion and extension and forearm pronation and supination can begin as soon as pain and motion allow. These exercises may be deferred for longer periods if an ORIF procedure was performed so that stable bone union and soft tissue healing can occur.

OLECRANON FRACTURES

Olecranon fractures commonly result after a fall on the point of the elbow (olecranon process) or indirectly from forceful contraction of the triceps.[35] Generally, they are classified as either nondisplaced or displaced fractures. Displaced fractures of the olecranon have four subclassifications:[36]

- Avulsion fracture, displaced
- Oblique or transverse fracture
- Comminuted fracture
- Fracture-dislocation

The treatment for nondisplaced olecranon fractures requires immobilization for 6 to 8 weeks,[12,35] although 3 weeks or less is used in some cases (particularly in elderly patients).[36,56] The position in which nondisplaced olecranon fractures are immobilized is controversial, in that some authorities advocate placing the affected arm in extension or slight flexion,[8,12,29,35] whereas others recommend placing the affected arm in 45° to 90° of flexion.[36,56] The rationale for placing the elbow in 45° of flexion is the likelihood of the loss of flexion after immobilization.[56] In addition, Strege[56] suggested that immobilization should not exceed 45° because of the risk of displacing fracture fragments.

Usually, nondisplaced olecranon fractures are allowed gentle AROM exercises after 3 weeks of immobilization. Flexion of the affected arm should not exceed 90° for the first 6 to 8 weeks after injury so that fracture fragments can heal.[29,56] Displaced or comminuted fractures of the olecranon can be treated with an ORIF procedure to secure the fragments. With severely comminuted fractures, excision of 80% of the olecranon can occur without loss of joint stability.[36,56]

Physical therapy can begin during the initial stages of immobilization. Active motion of the hand, wrist, forearm (pronation and supination), and shoulder can commence when acute pain has subsided. A general physical conditioning program is allowed as soon as tolerated by the patient. Active elbow flexion must not exceed 90° for the first 2 months after injury. Active resistance exercises for elbow extension must be minimized because the forceful contraction of the triceps can displace the fracture fragments before secure bone healing at 8 weeks. Resistance exercises for elbow flexion can begin earlier if motion is limited and the muscle contractions are submaximal. Submaximal isometric triceps extensions can proceed when bony union has been verified. Progressive concentric and eccentric loading is added as motion increases and secure fixation of the fragments has occurred.

Progressive flexion and extension movements must proceed cautiously and slowly to prevent displacement of the fragments. In addition, the patient must be carefully instructed to perform resistance exercises initially well within the limits of pain and motion restrictions to allow for proper bone healing. The strong contractions of the biceps during flexion and the triceps during extension activities are effective to overcome gradually most motion limitations observed early after injury or surgery. Full recovery after olecranon fractures may take 6 months to 1 year.[29]

FRACTURE-DISLOCATIONS

A fall on an extended outreaching arm causes isolated elbow dislocations and combined fracture-dislocations (Fig. 22-17).[14,35,37,49,55] Conwell[12] reported that "with the exception of the shoulder, the elbow is the most frequently dislocated joint in the body." This injury occurs most often in men, with the nondominant arm representing about 60% of these injuries.[37]

Posterior elbow dislocations are the most common, whereas anterior dislocations represent 1% to 2% of all elbow dislocations.[37] Associated fractures of the radial head occur in approximately 10% of elbow dislocations.[37,55] In addition, associated neurovascular injuries can occur with either isolated elbow dislocations or fracture-dislocations.[35,37,55,56] Injuries involve the median, radial, and ulnar nerves and the brachial artery with elbow dislocations.[37,56]

Isolated posterior elbow dislocations are managed with closed reduction and immobilization.[12,14,35-37,55] The elbow is placed in 90° of flexion in a splint for approximately 3

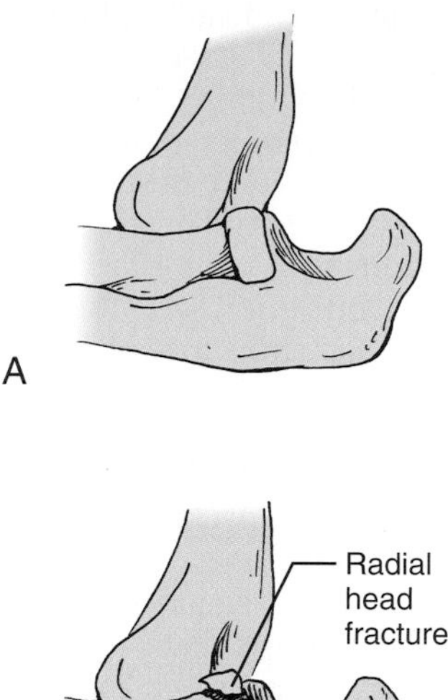

FIG 22-17 **A,** Posterior elbow dislocation without radial head fracture. **B,** Posterior elbow dislocation with radial head fracture.

weeks.[12,35,56] During this period, hand and shoulder motion is allowed if no offensive stress is applied to the elbow. PROM may be incorporated to help with pain control and early collagen alignment. Early AROM exercises can begin during the first week after reduction.[56] Active motion is not believed to cause this condition.[55] Gentle active flexion and extension exercises are added as pain, swelling, and soft tissue healing dictate. Because this injury represents a hyperextension trauma that significantly affects the joint capsule, muscle, tendon, and frequently ligamentous restraints, extensive soft tissue healing is necessary for a stable, functional joint. The joint capsule of the elbow may require 8 to 10 weeks to heal satisfactorily.[14] Restoration of elbow extension must proceed cautiously because the mechanism of injury is usually elbow hyperextension. Resistance exercises can begin as soft tissue healing progresses. Eccentric and concentric resistance exercises for the biceps can be emphasized to reduce hyperextension forces.[14] Resistance-type exercises are deferred for at least 3 weeks to allow for acute symptoms to subside. However, aggressive elbow extension must be prevented until 8 weeks have elapsed.[14,37]

The most common complication after elbow dislocation is loss of extension.[37,55,56] A 30° flexion contracture is common 10 weeks after dislocation, and a 10° flexion contracture is typically observed 2 years after injury.[37] However unacceptable this loss of motion may be, it does not represent an "overwhelming functional deficit."[56] Every effort should be made to regain full elbow extension because long-term deficits may affect the function of the patient.

The treatment of fracture-dislocations centers on the appropriate management of the fracture (most commonly the radial head) and reduction of the elbow. In most cases, radial head excision is performed to minimize the development of myositis ossificans.[55] With radial head excision, proximal migration of the radius can result in stress and pain to the distal radioulnar ligamentous articulation.[35,36,56]

Rehabilitation after fracture-dislocation of the elbow gains focus on early protected active motion. Passive stretching is strictly avoided during the early recovery phases of healing. With radial head excision, a loss of 25° to 30° of pronation and supination can be expected if postoperative immobilization lasts longer than 4 weeks.[55] As with isolated dislocation, loss of full elbow extension is common.

LITTLE LEAGUER'S ELBOW

Little leaguer's elbow is a spectrum of medial epicondylar apophyseal injury that ranges from microtrauma to the physis to fracture and displacement of the medial epicondyle through the apophysis. Pain of the medial elbow is common in adolescent throwers. The medial epicondyle physis is subject to repetitive tensile and valgus forces during the arm-cocking and acceleration phases of throwing. These forces may result in microtraumatic injury to the physis with potential fragmentation, hypertrophy, separation of the epiphysis, or avulsion of the medial epicondyle. Treatment varies based on the extent of injury.

Important Concepts

An active rest period of at least 8 weeks is recommended to allow the growth plate to heal and to prevent future issues. No throwing should be done during this time.

In the absence of an avulsion, a rehabilitation program similar to the nonoperative UCL program is initiated. Emphasis is placed initially on the reduction of pain and inflammation and the restoration of motion and strength. Strengthening exercises are performed in a gradual fashion. Isometrics are performed first before initiating light isotonic strengthening exercises. In young throwing athletes, we emphasize core, legs, and shoulder strengthening. Often these individuals exhibit poor core and scapula control along with weakness of the shoulder musculature. In addition, stretching exercises are performed to normalize shoulder ROM, especially into internal rotation and horizontal adduction. No heavy lifting, particularly where a valgus stress is placed on the elbow, is permitted for 12 to 14 weeks. An interval throwing program is initiated as tolerated when symptoms subside, typically after a rest period of 8 to 12 weeks.

In the presence of a nondisplaced or minimally displaced avulsion, a brief period of immobilization for approximately 7 to 14 days is encouraged, followed by a gradual progression of ROM, flexibility, and strength. An interval throwing program is usually allowed at 8 to 12 weeks. If the avulsion is displaced, an ORIF procedure may be required. See Box 22-1 for information on other elbow-related injuries and terms.

MOBILIZATION OF THE ELBOW

The rationale for specific joint mobilization is to avoid joint restrictions or hypomobility, which can limit the normal joint arthrokinematics.[10] In many instances, arthrofibrosis occurs as a result of immobilization and internal fixation methods used to stabilize fracture fragments.

The PT determines if mobilization is indicated after injury, surgery, or immobilization based on tissue healing constraints, the nature of the joint restriction (hypomobility of noncontractile tissue or articular surface dysfunction),[10] and whether passive motion is indicated for the treatment of joint limitations. The PT must clearly define the specific indications for mobilization with reference to the exact technique to be employed, rate of movement, amplitude of force, and direction of the force applied to the elbow. To obtain relaxation, the PTA must place the patient in a comfortable position, with specific attention paid to the support and stability of the shoulder, elbow, and arm of the patient. Before joint mobilization is applied, thermal agents are employed to reduce tissue congestion, aid in the removal of wastes, improve tissue extensibility, and enhance relaxation of the patient and the affected joint.

Injuries to the elbow that require mobilization should increase in flexion, extension, or both. Wooden[68] outlined three techniques used to enhance general motion, flexion, and extension of the elbow. To enhance general mobility of the elbow, the patient should be supine with the affected elbow flexed to 90°. The shoulder of the affected limb is held at the patient's side or in an abducted position. The PTA places both hands at the proximal aspect of the forearm and directs a straight lateral distraction force that directs the forearm away from the humerus (Fig. 22-18).

BOX 22-1 Elbow-Related Terms

Galeazzi's fracture: Radial shaft fracture at the distal metaphysis-diaphysis with radioulnar dislocation.

Ligament stability: Anterior band of the medial ulnar collateral ligament is the main ligamentous stabilizer.

Mobile WAD of Henry—descriptive eponym of common origin of wrist extensors: Brachioradialis, extensor carpi radialis brevis, and extensor carpi radialis longus.

Monteggia's fracture: Ulnar shaft—proximal aspect with radial head dislocation.

Pronator syndrome: Median nerve compression at the pronator teres muscle, bicipital aponeurosis (lacertus fibrosus), flexor digitorum superficialis, or other sites in the forearm.

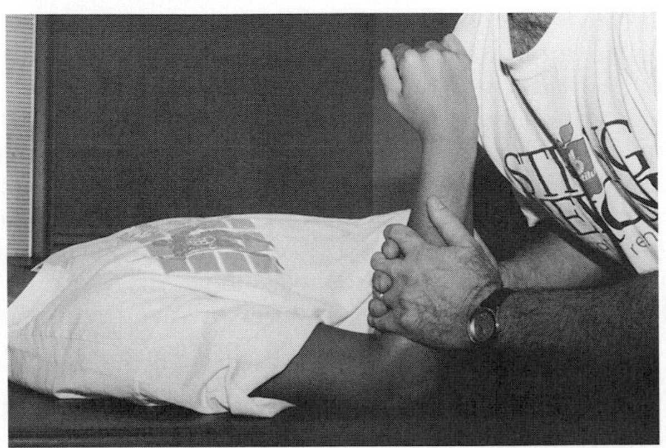

FIG 22-18 Elbow distraction.

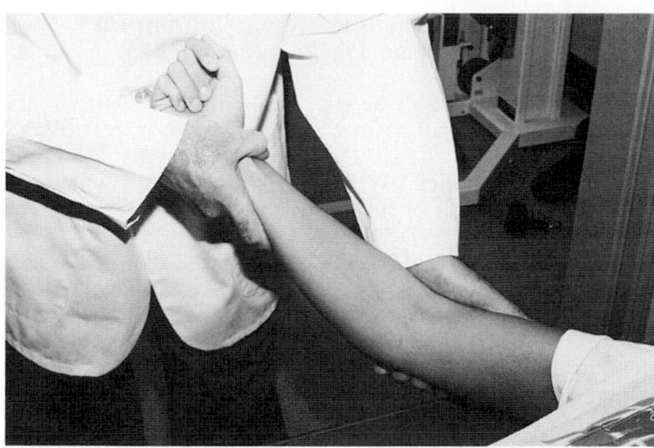

FIG 22-19 Valgus or humeral-ulna abduction.

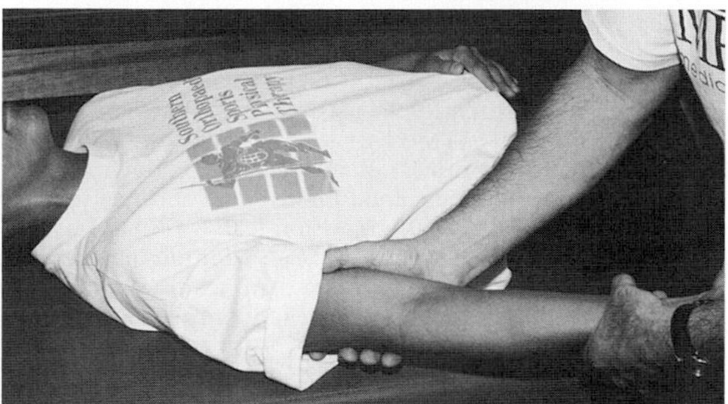

FIG 22-20 Varus or humeral-ulna adduction.

Humeral-ulnar abduction is employed to promote elbow extension.[68] The patient should be supine with the affected arm abducted and the elbow slightly flexed. The PT sits to the patient's affected side with one hand stabilizing the distal lateral humerus and the other hand firmly grasping the ulnar aspect of the distal forearm. In this position, the PT directs a valgus or abduction force to the elbow (Fig. 22-19).[68]

An adduction technique is applied to increase elbow flexion.[68] The patient remains supine with the affected arm abducted. The PT sits to the patient's affected side and stabilizes the distal humerus on the medial aspect with one hand, while placing the opposite hand on the distal radial aspect of the forearm. In this position, the PT directs a varus or adduction force to the elbow (Fig. 22-20).

These few techniques are representative of more common motions requiring mobilization. Other positions and techniques can be used to enhance elbow motion.[25]

GLOSSARY

Epicondylitis: An inflammatory condition of the epicondyle of the medial or lateral elbow.

Lateral epicondylitis: A form of tendinitis commonly referred to as *tennis elbow*.

Ligament stability: Anterior band of the medial ulnar collateral ligament is the main ligamentous stabilizer.

Medial epicondylitis: An overuse condition also known as *golfer's elbow*.

Medial valgus stress overload: A condition that occurs commonly among patients who participate in repetitive throwing and racquet sports; it is also known as *valgus extension overload*.

Ulnar collateral ligament (UCL): A thick triangular band at the medial aspect of the elbow uniting the distal aspect of the humerus to the proximal aspect of the ulna.

REFERENCES

1. Alfredson H: Chronic midportion Achilles tendinopathy: an update on research and treatment. *Clin Sports Med* 22:727–741, 2003.
2. Alfredson H, Pietila T, Jonsson P, et al: Heavy-load eccentric calf muscle training for the treatment of chronic Achilles tendinosis. *Am J Sports Med* 26:360–366, 1998.
3. Alley RM, Pappas AM: Acute and performance related injuries of the elbow. In Pappas AM, editor: *Upper Extremity Injuries in the Athlete*, New York, 1995, Churchill Livingstone, pp 339–364.
4. Andrews JR, Craven WM: Lesions of the posterior compartment of the elbow. *Clin Sports Med* 10:637–652, 1991.
5. Andrews JR, Jelsma RD, Joyse ME, et al: Open surgical procedures for injuries of the elbow in throwers. *Op Tech Sports Med* 4:109–113, 1996.
6. Bandy WD, Irion JM: The effect of time on static stretch on the flexibility of the hamstring muscles. *Phys Ther* 74:845–850, discussion 850–852, 1994.
7. Bandy WD, Irion JM: Briggler M. The effect of static stretch and dynamic range of motion training on the flexibility of the hamstring muscles. *J Orthop Sports Phys Ther* 27:295–300, 1998.
8. Bennett JB, Tullos HS: Acute injuries to the elbow. In Nicholas JA, Hershman EB, editors: *The Upper Extremity in Sports Medicine*, St Louis, 1990, Mosby.
9. Bjordal JM, Lopes-Martins RA, Iversen VV: A randomised, placebo controlled trial of low level laser therapy for activated Achilles tendinitis with microdialysis measurement of peritendinous prostaglandin E2 concentrations. *Br J Sports Med* 40:76–80, discussion 76–80, 2006.
10. Bowling RW, Rockar PA: The elbow complex. In Gould JA, editor: *Orthopaedics and Sports Physical Therapy*, ed 2, St Louis, 1990, Mosby.
11. Clement DB, Taunton JE, Smart GW: Achilles tendinitis and peritendinitis: etiology and treatment. *Am J Sports Med* 12:179–184, 1984.
12. Conwell HE: Injuries to the elbow. *Clin Symp* 21:35–62, 1969.
13. Curwin S, Stanish WD: *Tendinitis: Its Etiology and Treatment*, Lexington, MA, 1984, DC Heath.
14. Dickoff-Hoffman S, Foster D: Rehabilitation of elbow injuries. In Prentice WE, editor: *Rehabilitation Techniques in Sports Medicine*, St. Louis, 1994, Mosby.
15. Dillman CJ, Smutz P, Werner S: Valgus extension overload in baseball pitching. *Med Sci Sports Exerc* 23:S135, 1991.
16. England S, Farrell AJ, Coppock JS, et al: Low power laser therapy of shoulder tendonitis. *Scand J Rheumatol* 18:427–431, 1989.
17. Enwemeka CS: The effects of therapeutic ultrasound on tendon healing. A biomechanical study. *Am J Phys Med Rehabil* 68:283–287, 1989.
18. Enwemeka CS: Inflammation, cellularity, and fibrillogenesis in regenerating tendon: implications for tendon rehabilitation. *Phys Ther* 69:816–825, 1989.
19. Fleisig GS, Barrentine SW, Escamilla RF, et al: Biomechanics of overhand throwing with implications for injuries. *Sports Med* 21:421–437, 1996.
20. Fleisig GS, Escamilla RF: Biomechanics of the elbow in the throwing athlete. *Op Tech Sports Med* 4:62–68, 1996.
21. Gum SL, Reddy GK, Stehno-Bittel L, et al: Combined ultrasound, electrical stimulation, and laser promote collagen synthesis with moderate changes in tendon biomechanics. *Am J Phys Med Rehabil* 76:288–296, 1997.
22. Harvey W, Dyson M, Pond JB, et al: The stimulation of protein synthesis in human fibroblasts by therapeutic ultrasound. *Rheumatol Rehabil* 14:237, 1975.
23. Jackson BA, Schwane JA, Starcher BC: Effect of ultrasound therapy on the repair of Achilles tendon injuries in rats. *Med Sci Sports Exerc* 23:171–176, 1991.

24. James SL, Ali K, Pocock C, et al: Ultrasound guided dry needling and autologous blood injection for patellar tendinosis. *Br J Sports Med* 41:518–521, discussion 522, 2007.
25. Kisner C, Colby LA: *Therapeutic Exercise: Foundations and Techniques*, ed 6, Philadelphia, 2012, Davis.
26. Ko JY, Chen HS, Chen LM: Treatment of lateral epicondylitis of the elbow with shock waves. *Clin Orthop Relat Res* 387:60–67, 2001.
27. Kottke FJ, Pauley DL, Ptak RA: The rationale for prolonged stretching for correction of shortening of connective tissue. *Arch Phys Med Rehabil* 47:345–352, 1966.
28. Kraushaar BS, Nirschl RP: Tendinosis of the elbow (tennis elbow). Clinical features and findings of histological, immunohistochemical, and electron microscopy studies. *J Bone Joint Surg Am* 81:259–278, 1999.
29. LaCroix E: Treatment of common problems of the elbow, forearm and wrist joints. In Goldsteain GS, editor: *Geriatric Orthopaedics: Rehabilitative Management of Common Problems*, Gaithersburg, MD, 1991, Aspen Publishers.
30. Lam LK, Cheing GL: Effects of 904-nm low-level laser therapy in the management of lateral epicondylitis: a randomized controlled trial. *Photomed Laser Surg* 25:65–71, 2007.
31. Langberg H, Ellingsgaard H, Madsen T, et al: Eccentric rehabilitation exercise increases peritendinous type I collagen synthesis in humans with Achilles tendinosis. *Scand J Med Sci Sports* 17:61–66, 2007.
32. Linscheid RL, O'Driscoll SW: Elbow dislocation. In Morrey BF, editor: *The Elbow and Its Disorders*, ed 2, Philadelphia, 1993, Saunders, pp 441–452.
33. Linscheid RL, Wheeler DK: Elbow dislocations. *JAMA* 194:1171–1176, 1965.
34. McClure PW, Blackburn LG, Dusold C: The use of splints in the treatment of joint stiffness: biologic rationale and an algorithm for making clinical decisions. *Phys Ther* 74:1101–1107, 1994.
35. McRae R: Practical fracture treatment. In McRae R, editor: *Injuries about the Elbow*, New York, 1994, Churchill Livingstone.
36. Miller MD: *Review of Orthopaedics*, Philadelphia, 1992, Saunders.
37. Morrey BF: Elbow dislocation in the athlete. In DeLee JC, Drez D, editors: *Orthopaedic Sports Medicine: Principles and Practices*, vol 1, Philadelphia, 1994, Saunders.
38. Morrey BF, Regan WD: Tendinopathies about the elbow. In DeLee JC, Drez D, editors: *Orthopaedic Sports Medicine: Principles and Practice*, vol 1, Philadelphia, 1994, Saunders.
39. Morrey BF, Regan WD: Throwing injuries. In DeLee JC, Drez D, editors: *Orthopaedic Sports Medicine: Principles and Practice*, vol 1, Philadelphia, 1994, Saunders.
40. Murrell GA, Szabo C, Hannafin JA, et al: Modulation of tendon healing by nitric oxide. *Inflamm Res* 46:19–27, 1997.
41. Nirschl RP: Medial tennis elbow: surgical treatment. *Orthop Trans.* 7:298, 1983.
42. Nirschl RP, Ashman ES: Tennis elbow tendinosis (epicondylitis). *Instr Course Lect* 53:587–598, 2004.
43. Nowicki KD, Hummer CD, 3rd, Heidt RS, Jr, et al: Effects of iontophoretic versus injection administration of dexamethasone. *Med Sci Sports Exerc* 34:1294–1301, 2002.
44. O'Driscoll SW: Reconstruction of the lateral collateral ligament. In Yamaguchi K, King G, O'Driscoll SW, editors: *Advanced Reconstruction. Elbow*, Rosemont, IL, 2007, American Academy of Orthopaedic Surgeons, pp 159–165.
45. Paoloni JA, Appleyard RC, Nelson J, et al: Topical nitric oxide application in the treatment of chronic extensor tendinosis at the elbow: a randomized, double-blinded, placebo-controlled clinical trial. *Am J Sports Med* 31:915–920, 2003.
46. Parks JC: Overuse injuries of the elbow. In Nicholas JA, Hershman EB, editors: *The Upper Extremity in Sports Medicine*, St Louis, 1990, Mosby.
47. Reddy GK, Gum S, Stehno-Bittel L, et al: Biochemistry and biomechanics of healing tendon: Part II. Effects of combined laser therapy and electrical stimulation. *Med Sci Sports Exerc* 30:794–800, 1998.
48. Reddy GK, Stehno-Bittel L, Enwemeka CS: Laser photostimulation of collagen production in healing rabbit Achilles tendons. *Lasers Surg Med* 22:281–287, 1998.
49. Reid DC, Kushner S: The elbow region. In Donatelli R, Wooden MJ, editors: *Orthopaedic Physical Therapy*, New York, 1989, Churchill Livingstone.
50. Reinold MM, Wilk KE, Reed J, et al: Interval sport programs: guidelines for baseball, tennis, and golf. *J Orthop Sports Phys Ther* 32:293–298, 2002.
51. Rohrbough JT, Altchek DW, Hyman J, et al: Medial collateral ligament reconstruction of the elbow using the docking technique. *Am J Sports Med* 30:541–548, 2002.
52. Sapega AA, Quedenfeld TC, Moyer RA, et al: Biophysical factors in range-of-motion exercise. *Phys Sports Med* 9:57–65, 1981.
53. Shalabi A, Kristoffersen-Wilberg M, Svensson L, et al: Eccentric training of the gastrocnemius-soleus complex in chronic Achilles tendinopathy results in decreased tendon volume and intratendinous signal as evaluated by MRI. *Am J Sports Med* 32:1286–1296, 2004.
54. Stergioulas A, Stergioula M, Aarskog R, et al: Effects of low-level laser therapy and eccentric exercises in the treatment of recreational athletes with chronic Achilles tendinopathy. *Am J Sports Med* 36:881–887, 2008.
55. Stralka SW, Brasel JG: Elbow. In Richardson JK, Iglarsh ZA, editors: *Clinical Orthopaedic Physical Therapy*, Philadelphia, 1994, Saunders.
56. Strege D: Upper Extremity. In Loth TS, editor: *Orthopaedic Boards Review*, St, Louis, 1993, Mosby.
57. Suresh SP, Ali KE, Jones H, et al: Medial epicondylitis: is ultrasound guided autologous blood injection an effective treatment? *Br J Sports Med* 40:935–939, discussion 939, 2006.
58. Tyler TF, Thomas GC, Nicholas SJ, et al: Addition of isolated wrist extensor eccentric exercise to standard treatment for chronic lateral epicondylosis: a prospective randomized trial. *J Shoulder Elbow Surg* 19:917–922, 2010.
59. Wang CJ, Chen HS: Shock wave therapy for patients with lateral epicondylitis of the elbow: a one- to two-year follow-up study. *Am J Sports Med* 30:422–425, 2002.
60. Wang CJ, Ko JY, Chen HS: Treatment of calcifying tendinitis of the shoulder with shock wave therapy. *Clin Orthop Relat Res* 387:83–89, 2001.
61. Wang L, Qin L, Lu HB, et al: Extracorporeal shock wave therapy in treatment of delayed bone-tendon healing. *Am J Sports Med* 36:340–347, 2008.
62. Warren CG, Lehmann JF, Koblanski JN: Elongation of rat tail tendon: effect of load and temperature. *Arch Phys Med Rehabil* 52:465–474, 1971.
63. Warren CG, Lehmann JF, Koblanski JN: Heat and stretch procedures: an evaluation using rat tail tendon. *Arch Phys Med Rehabil* 57:122–126, 1976.
64. Werner SL, Fleisig GS, Dillman CJ, et al: Biomechanics of the elbow during baseball pitching. *J Orthop Sports Phys Ther* 17:274–278, 1993.
65. Wilk KE, Arrigo C, Andrews JR: Rehabilitation of the elbow in the throwing athlete. *J Orthop Sports Phys Ther* 17:305–317, 1993.
66. Wilk KE, Voight ML, Keirns MA, et al: Stretch-shortening drills for the upper extremities: theory and clinical application. *J Orthop Sports Phys Ther* 17:225–239, 1993.
67. Wilson FD, Andrews JR, Blackburn TA, et al: Valgus extension overload in the pitching elbow. *Am J Sports Med* 11:83–88, 1983.
68. Wooden MJ: Mobilization of the upper extremity. In Donatelli R, Wooden MJ, editors: *Orthopaedic Physical Therapy*, New York, 1989, Churchill Livingstone.

REVIEW QUESTIONS

Multiple Choice

1. Lateral epicondylitis is caused by which of the following?
   a. Acute direct trauma
   b. Concentric contraction of wrist flexors
   c. Overuse, repetitive motion disorder, cumulative trauma
   d. Eccentric loading of the biceps
   e. All of the above

2. Which of the following describe the muscles of the common wrist extensor origin? (Circle all that apply.)
   a. Biceps brachii
   b. Extensor carpi radialis longus
   c. Extensor carpi radialis brevis
   d. Extensor digitorum
   e. Brachioradialis
3. Which of the following is not advocated during the early recovery phase of rehabilitation for lateral epicondylitis?
   a. Ice
   b. Phonophoresis
   c. Functional activities
   d. Nonsteroidal antiinflammatory drugs (NSAIDs)
4. Which muscles make up the common flexor tendon of the medial epicondyle? (Circle all that apply.)
   a. Pronator teres
   b. Flexor carpi radialis
   c. Brachioradialis
   d. Flexor carpi ulnaris
   e. Biceps brachii
5. Which of the following is a type of supracondylar fracture?
   a. Type II
   b. Extension type
   c. Type I
   d. Flexion type
   e. All of the above
6. What is the most common treatment for supracondylar fractures?
   a. ORIF
   b. Rigid cast immobilization for 8 to 10 weeks
   c. Closed reduction and immobilization for 4 to 6 weeks
   d. Early active motion
7. Which of the following is considered the most significant complication after supracondylar fracture?
   a. Joint contracture
   b. Malunion
   c. Vascular compromise
   d. Nonunion
8. Because of general bone quality (osteoporosis), which of the following can be used for treatment in an elderly patient with a type IV intercondylar fracture?
   a. ORIF
   b. "Bag of bones" procedure
   c. Early active motion
   d. Fusion
9. Radial head fractures are generally classified into four types. Type I is defined as which of the following?
   a. Any radial head fracture with elbow dislocation
   b. A comminuted fracture
   c. A nondisplaced fracture
   d. A marginal fracture with displacement
10. Treatment of type I radial head fractures involves which of the following?
    a. ORIF procedure
    b. Immobilization for up to 4 weeks
    c. Excision
    d. Active motion
11. Type II radial head fractures always are treated with which of the following? (Circle all that apply.)
    a. ORIF
    b. Immobilization
    c. Excision
    d. Fusion
    e. Closed kinetic chain resistance
12. Which motion is most commonly affected (restricted) after radial head fractures? (Circle all that apply.)
    a. Flexion of the elbow
    b. Extension of the elbow
    c. Supination
    d. Pronation
    e. Radial deviation
13. What percentage of elbow dislocations are anterior?
    a. 10%
    b. 15%
    c. 1% to 2%
    d. 7%
14. What is the most common complication after elbow dislocation?
    a. Myositis ossificans
    b. Volkmann's ischemic contracture
    c. Loss of elbow extension
    d. Neurovascular compromise
15. Which of the following is the most common fracture that occurs with elbow dislocation?
    a. Supracondylar fractures
    b. Radial head fractures
    c. Radius fractures
    d. Ulnar fractures

Short Answer

16. Identify and describe common overuse soft tissue injuries of the elbow.
17. Discuss common methods of management and rehabilitation of overuse soft tissue injuries of the elbow.
18. Identify and describe intercondylar fractures, radial head fractures, olecranon fractures, and fracture-dislocations of the elbow.
19. Describe methods of management and rehabilitation of various fractures and fracture-dislocations of the elbow.
20. Describe common mobilization techniques for the elbow.

Fill in the Blank

21. The lateral epicondylitis-to-medial epicondylitis ratio is ______________.
22. The most common treatment of supracondylar fractures is by ______________and ______________for 4 to 6 weeks.
23. The normal elbow ROM is ______________ degrees to approximately ______________degrees of flexion.
24. Management of valgus stress injuries must take into account the ______________of ligaments.
25. A type ______________fracture is defined as a comminuted fracture of the entire radial head.

True/False

26. In severe cases of tennis elbow, the use of a wrist cock-up splint is advocated for the management of inflamed wrist extensor tendons.
27. During the subacute recovery phase of rehabilitation for lateral epicondylitis, initial instruction for patients to perform forearm pronation and supination must include the use of a hammer while holding the end of the shaft away from the head of the hammer.
28. Passive stretching is advocated during the early recovery phase of healing after supracondylar fractures.
29. A type IV intercondylar fracture, which is severely comminuted with significant separation, always is treated with an ORIF procedure.
30. Displaced or comminuted fractures of the olecranon can be treated with an ORIF procedure or, in cases of severely comminuted fractures, excision of up to 80% of the olecranon.

Chapter 23

Orthopedic Management of the Wrist and Hand

Marsha Lawrence

CHAPTER OUTLINE

LEARNING OBJECTIVES

1. Describe the extrinsic and intrinsic muscle systems in the hand and their roles in hand movement.
2. Identify and describe common metacarpal and phalanx fractures and methods of management and rehabilitation.
3. Identify methods of management and rehabilitation for common fractures of the wrist.
4. Describe and discuss methods of management and rehabilitation of ligament injuries of the wrist.
5. Discuss methods of management and rehabilitation of compression neuropathy of the wrist.
6. Describe common tendon disorders of the hand and their management.
7. Define Dupuytren's disease and options for surgical management.
8. Describe rehabilitation precautions after surgery for Dupuytren's disease.
9. Identify tendon lacerations and their management.
10. Identify methods of management and rehabilitation for complex regional pain syndrome.

KEY TERMS

Bennett fracture
Boxer's fracture
Carpal tunnel syndrome
Colles fracture
Complex regional pain syndrome (CRPS)
Compression neuropathy
de Quervain's disease
Dinner fork deformity
Dupuytren's disease
Extrinsic muscle system
Intrinsic muscle system
Mallet finger
Nerve entrapment
Smith fracture
Tendinitis
Tendinosis
Tendovaginitis
Trigger finger
Triangular fibrocartilage complex (TFCC)

The hand is our primary interface with our environment. We gather information from it and manipulate the world around us with it. We use our hands for communication and creativity, and any injury to either hand has a profound impact on our daily lives. This chapter reviews the anatomy and kinesiology of the hand and wrist and describes common orthopedic injuries and conditions and their treatment. The initial focus for all hand injuries is on interventions to control pain and swelling; protection of healing tissue and repaired structures; and progression to strategies for safely improving range of motion (ROM), strength, and functional use of the wrist and hand. The proximal joints place the hand in space, and they often are immobilized or unused as a consequence of the injured hand. The physical therapist assistant (PTA) must consider the upper quarter as a whole for successful treatment of the hand and wrist. The ultimate goal is to optimize the conditions for healing and maximize functional return.

Important Concept

Injuries to the hand require evaluation and often treatment of the entire upper extremity.

ANATOMY OF THE WRIST AND HAND

SKELETAL ANATOMY

The hand and wrist comprise 27 bones: 8 wrist bones, 5 metacarpals that compose the palm, and 14 phalanges that compose the fingers and thumb (Fig. 23-1). The shape and configuration of the bones form two transverse arches—the proximal arch along the carpals and the distal along the metacarpal heads—and one longitudinal arch from the midcarpals along the index and middle digits. These arches contribute to a mobile concavity of the palm allowing firm grasp of objects of varying size and shape (Fig. 23-2).[35]

CIRCULATION

Blood supply to the hand and wrist is from the radial and ulnar arteries (Fig. 23-3). They form the superficial and deep arches with the ulnar artery being the primary contributor to the superficial arch and radial artery being the primary source of the deep arch.[37] Three palmar digital arteries arise from the superficial arch, each splitting to supply the radial and ulnar digital arteries to the middle, ring, and small fingers and the ulnar index finger. The digital arteries to the thumb and radial index finger are from the deep arch.[37]

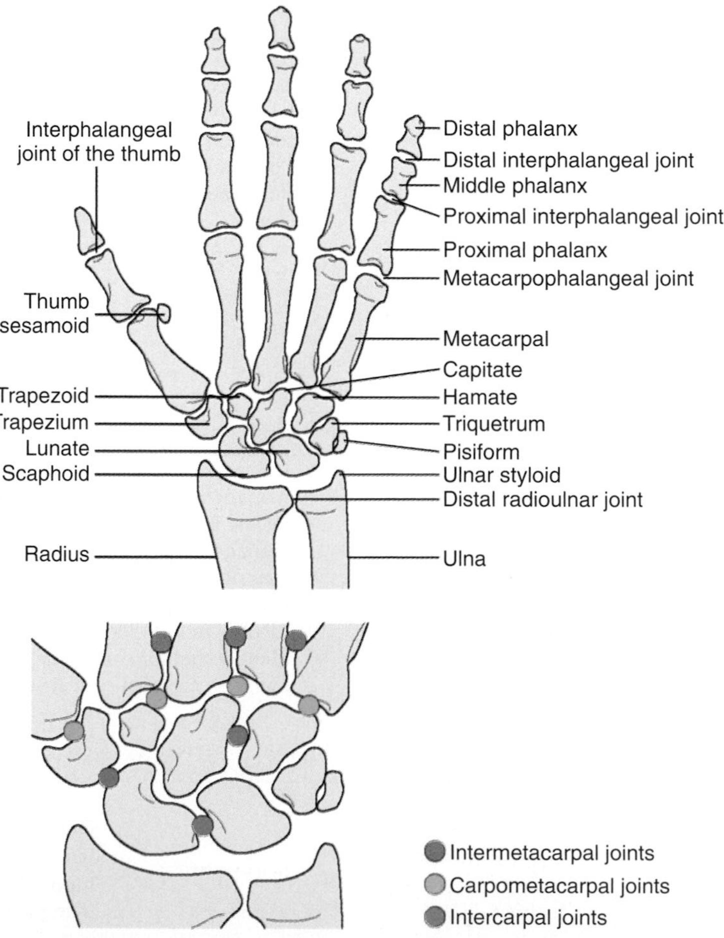

FIG 23-1 Skeletal anatomy of the hand and wrist. *(From Fam A, Lawry G, Kreder H:* Musculoskeletal examination and joint injection techniques, *Philadelphia, 2006, Mosby.)*

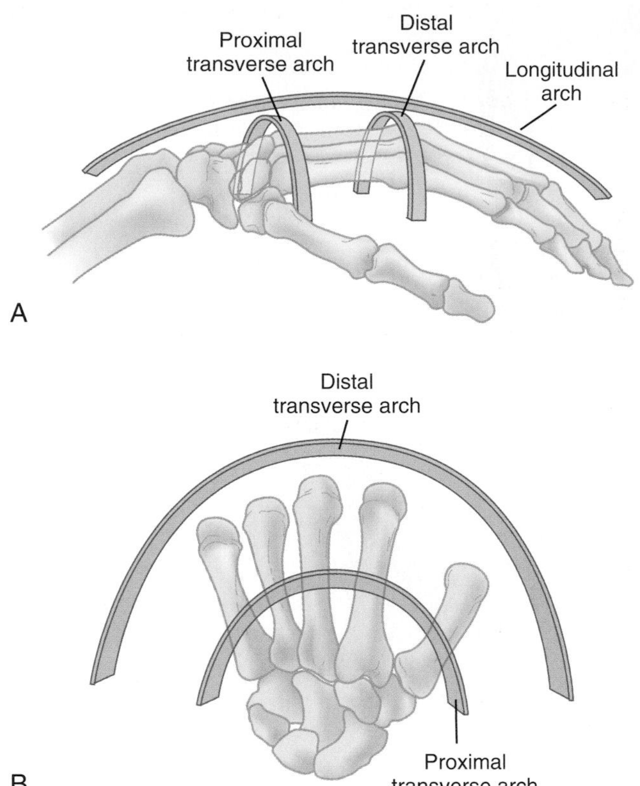

FIG 23-2 **A** and **B,** The transverse and longitudinal arches of the hand. *(From American Society for Surgery of the Hand:* Regional review course in hand surgery syllabus, *ed 10, Aurora, CO, 1990, ASSH.)*

MUSCULAR SYSTEM

The hand is powered by two muscular systems, the **intrinsic muscle system**, which comprises muscles that originate and insert within the hand, and the **extrinsic muscle system**, which comprises muscles that originate proximal to the hand and wrist and insert in the hand.

Intrinsic Muscle System

The intrinsic system can be divided into the thumb group, the digit group, and the small finger group (Fig. 23-4). There are four thumb intrinsic muscles. The abductor pollicis brevis, flexor pollicis brevis, and opponens pollicis make up the thenar eminence, and all are innervated by the median nerve; the adductor pollicis arises from the second and third metacarpals and inserts on the proximal phalanx of the thumb and is innervated by the ulnar nerve. These muscles function to position and stabilize the thumb carpometacarpal (CMC) joint and can contribute to thumb metacarpophalangeal (MP) joint motion.[35]

The hypothenar muscles are the abductor digiti minimi, flexor digiti minimi, and opponens digiti minimi. The palmaris brevis attaches the ulnar palmar aponeurosis to the skin of the medial palm.[37] These muscles are innervated by the ulnar nerve.

The digital intrinsic muscles are the volar and dorsal interossei and the lumbricales. The four lumbricales originate on the tendons of the flexor digitorum profundus and insert on the extensor mechanism of each finger. They have a dual innervation with the lateral two innervated by the median nerve and the medial two innervated by the ulnar nerve. They flex the MP joints and contribute to extension of the interphalangeal (IP) joints.

The interosseous muscles include three palmar interossei and four dorsal interossei. These muscles adduct and abduct the MP joints, respectively. They also contribute to flexion of the MP joints and extension of the IP joints. They are innervated by the ulnar nerve.

Extrinsic Muscle System

The extrinsic muscle system consists of the extensor/abductor muscles and the flexors of the wrist and digits. The extensor extrinsic muscle system is separated into six compartments at the dorsal wrist (Fig. 23-5). Compartments 1 and 3 contain tendons acting on the thumb, compartments 2 and 6 contain tendons acting at the wrist, and compartments 4 and 5 contain extensors of the digits. The radial nerve innervates all extrinsic extensors.

The extrinsic flexor system consists of the flexor carpi radialis and ulnaris and palmaris longus primarily acting on the wrist (Fig. 23-6), flexor pollicis longus acting on the thumb, and flexor digitorum superficialis and profundus acting primarily on the digits (Fig. 23-7). All are innervated by the median nerve except for the flexor carpi ulnaris and the flexor digitorum profundus to the ring and small digits, which are innervated by the ulnar nerve. The tendons for the digital flexors enter the hand through the carpal tunnel and enter digital sheaths at the MP joints of each respective digit. These sheaths play a critical role in the successful rehabilitation of flexor tendon lacerations occurring within the sheath.

> **Important Concept**
>
> Movement of the digits relies on extrinsic and intrinsic muscles to balance flexion and extension.

SENSORY SYSTEM

The median nerve provides most of the functional sensation for the hand innervating the palm and palmar surface of the radial three digits and the radial half of the fourth digit, with the ulnar nerve providing sensation to the fifth and ulnar half of the fourth as well as the ulnar palm and dorsum. The radial nerve provides sensation over the dorsal surface of the radial side of the hand (Fig. 23-8).

KINESIOLOGY OF THE WRIST AND HAND

The functional use of the hand never occurs in isolation. The mobility and stability of the proximal joints, the elbow, the forearm, and especially the wrist affect the efficiency of motion at the digits.

> **Important Concept**
>
> Complete functional restoration of the hand requires a balance of mobility and stability of the wrist, forearm, and elbow.

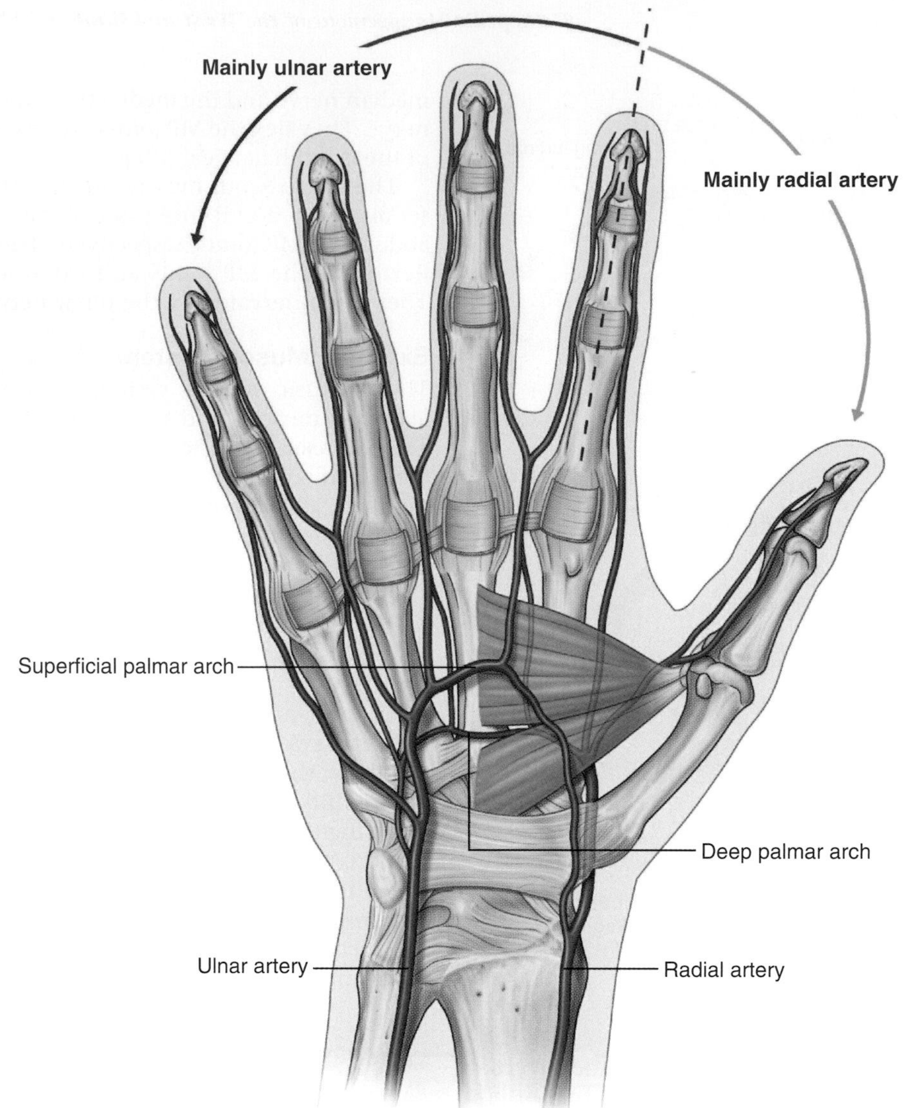

FIG 23-3 Circulation of the hand and wrist. *(From Drake RL, Vogl AW, Mitchell AWM:* Gray's anatomy for students, *ed 2, Philadelphia, 2010, Churchill Livingstone.)*

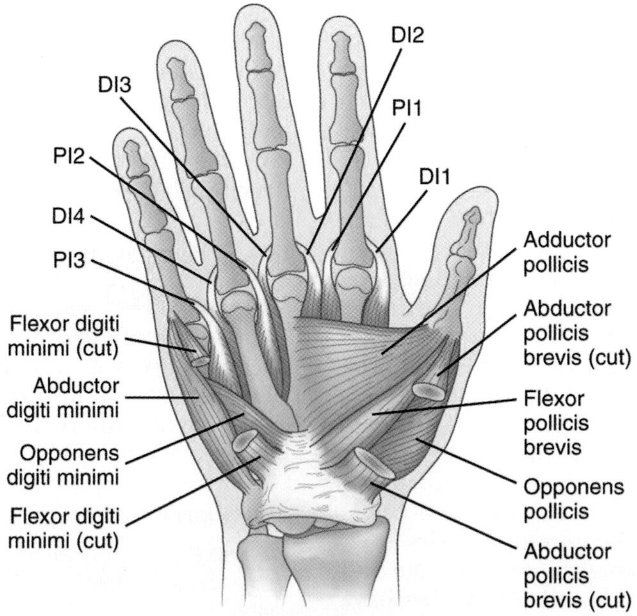

FIG 23-4 The intrinsic muscles of the hand have their origins and insertions within the wrist and hand. *(From Skirven T, Osterman A, Fedorczyk J, et al:* Rehabilitation of the hand and upper extremity, *ed 6, Philadelphia, 2011, Mosby.)*

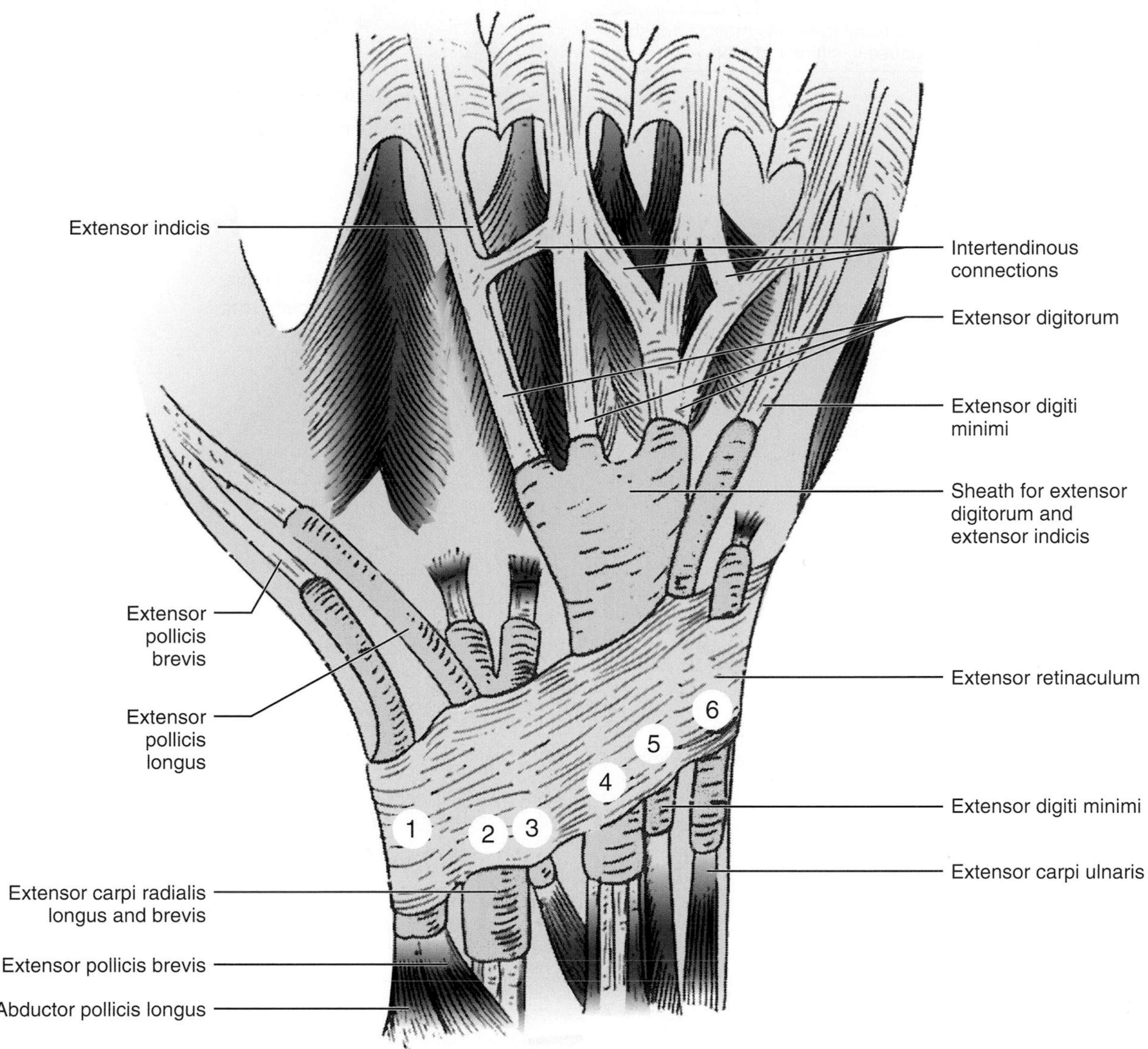

FIG 23-5 The extrinsic extensors originate proximal to the hand and insert in the hand. They are divided into compartments as they enter at the wrist. *(Modified from Miller M, Sekiya J:* Core knowledge in orthopaedics: sports medicine, *Philadelphia, 2006, Mosby.)*

KINESIOLOGY OF THE WRIST

The wrist consists of the radial carpal joint; the midcarpal joint, which divides the carpals into proximal and distal rows of four bones each; and the intercarpal joints. Flexion, extension, and radial and ulnar deviation are available at these joints. A functional diagonal movement from radial deviation and extension to ulnar deviation and flexion has been described as the "dart thrower's motion."[6] Extension and flexion of the wrist and radial and ulnar deviation occur at the radiocarpal and midcarpal joints, both being convex on concave.[35]

The wrist muscles work in force couples to move or stabilize the wrist. The extrinsic digit muscles can also move the wrist; however, their effectiveness in moving the digits is compromised if the wrist muscles are too weak to stabilize the wrist and allow the digit muscles to move the wrist.

KINESIOLOGY OF THE HAND

The CMC joints connect the hand to the wrist. The index and middle CMC joints are immobile, but a small amount of flexion is available at the ring and small CMC joints, allowing the hand to cup. The first CMC joint is positioned with the metacarpal medially rotated 90° in anatomic position. The thumb CMC joint is unique, and the base of the first metacarpal and the distal surface of the trapezium are saddle-shaped. In flexion and extension (movement medially and radially when the hand is in anatomic position), the joint is concave on convex; for abduction and adduction (movement anteriorly and posteriorly), the joint is convex on concave. Opposition at the first CMC joint occurs as a rotation.[35]

The MP joints are biconcave on biconvex and allow flexion and extension and abduction and adduction. Abduction is freer with the MP joints in extension, owing

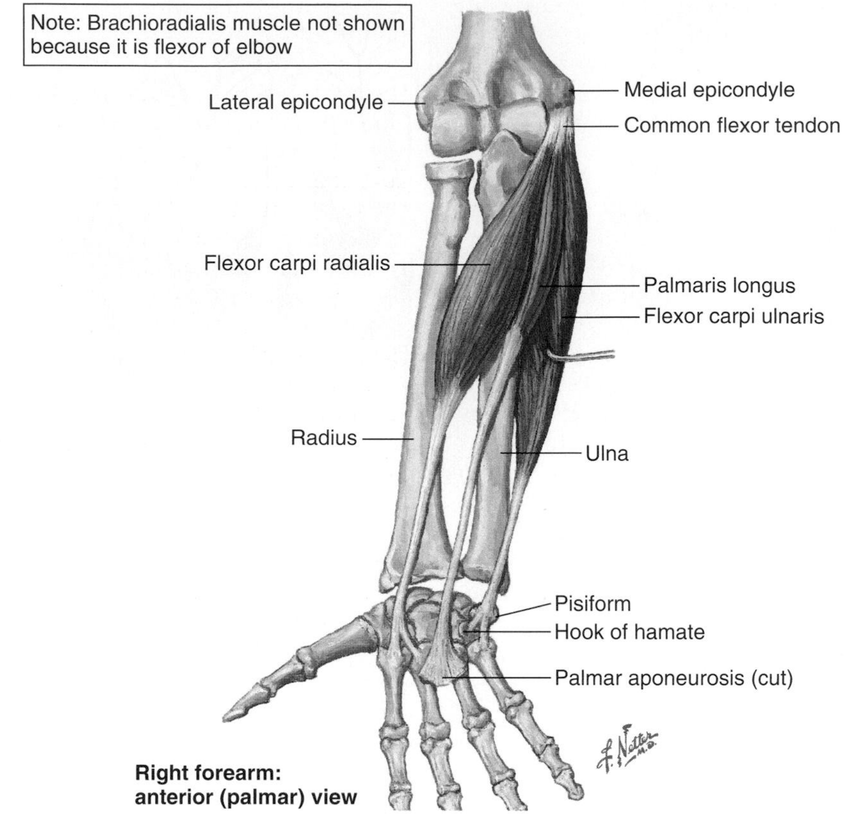

FIG 23-6 The extrinsic flexors of the wrist. *(From Cleland J, Koppenhave S, Su J:* Netter's orthopaedic clinical examination: an evidence-based approach, *ed 2, Philadelphia, 2011, Saunders.)*

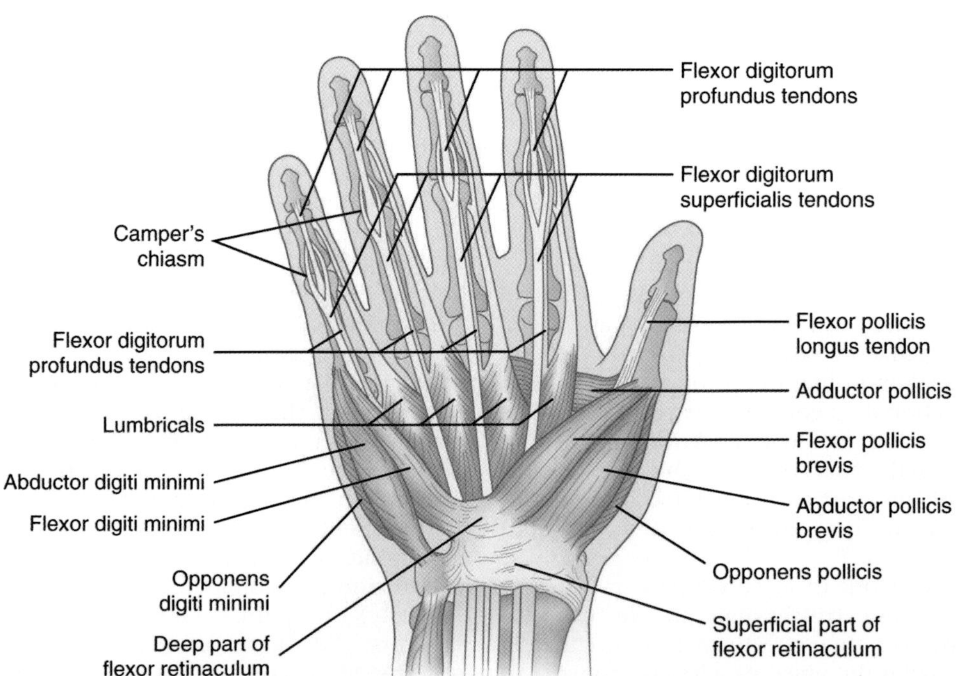

FIG 23-7 The extrinsic flexors of the digits. *(From Skirven T, Osterman A, Fedorczyk J, et al:* Rehabilitation of the hand and upper extremity, *ed 6, Philadelphia, 2011, Mosby.)*

to their shape and ligament structure. There are two sets of IP joints in each finger: the proximal interphalangeal (PIP) and distal interphalangeal (DIP). The thumb does not have a PIP joint. These joints are concave on convex and allow only flexion and extension.

EXAMINATION OF THE WRIST AND HAND

The examination should begin with the patient describing the onset of symptoms, the location, and the factors that exacerbate the symptoms or bring relative relief. The patient should be asked about the functional impact of the condition in activities at work, at home, and at recreation. Standardized, self-report functional measures can provide task-specific information and can be used to demonstrate functional improvement when administered periodically through the course of treatment. Any treatment already received and the result of that treatment should be noted. The patient's medical history, especially the presence of systemic diseases such as rheumatoid arthritis or diabetes, can influence the course of the condition. Social habits such as tobacco use also influence tissue healing.

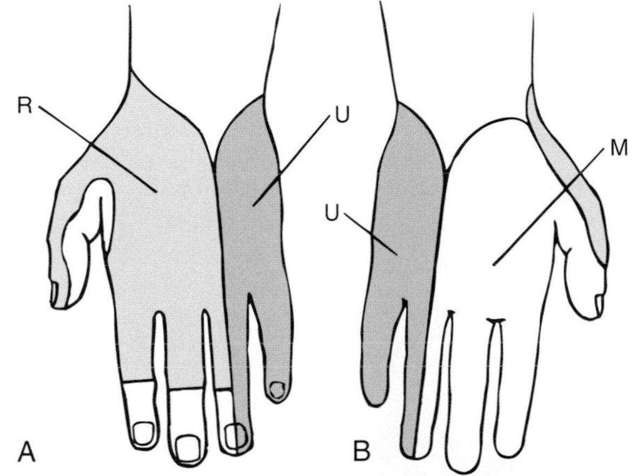

FIG 23-8 **A** and **B,** Sensation of the hand. *(From Mercier L:* Practical orthopedics, *ed 6, Philadelphia, 2008, Mosby.)*

The physical examination begins by comparing the hands side by side. Differences in skin color, the presence or absence of wrinkles over the dorsal joint surfaces, and the moistness of the fingertips should be observed. Bruises, abrasions, cuts, or wounds should be documented. Differences in hair density and nail growth may correlate with autonomic nerve dysfunction and should be noted. When the wrist is in neutral, the fingers should rest in a position of flexion increasing from radial to ulnar (Fig. 23-9). The patient's prehension patterns during use of the affected hand should be documented.

Objective tests and measures used to evaluate the hand, especially postoperatively, depend on the diagnosis. It is mandatory to understand what structures were repaired, the strength of the repairs, and the use of any internal fixation. The PTA must understand which measures can be used and which would be contraindicated. Use of active or passive wrist and finger extension with a newly repaired flexor tendon could rupture the repair. Edema can be recorded by measuring the circumference of the digits, wrist, and MP joints and comparing these measurements with the uninvolved side. The figure-of-eight method has also been shown to be a reliable way to assess hand and wrist volume (Fig. 23-10).[29] Sensation can be measured using static two-point discrimination or touch threshold with quantified, graded Semmes-Weinstein monofilaments.

Digit range of motion (ROM) (in the absence of any contraindications) is usually measured by having the patient make a fist and measuring each joint's position with the wrist in neutral; this is described as composite flexion. Composite extension should also be measured. The available motion at individual finger joints can be measured by holding the proximal joints in neutral and measuring the adjacent joint motion; this is noted as isolated joint motion. A quick measurement of improvement can be made by determining total active motion. Total active motion is measured by adding the flexion measurements of the MP, PIP, and DIP joints and subtracting the extension lag measurements to determine a final score. Extension past 0° is not included in determining total

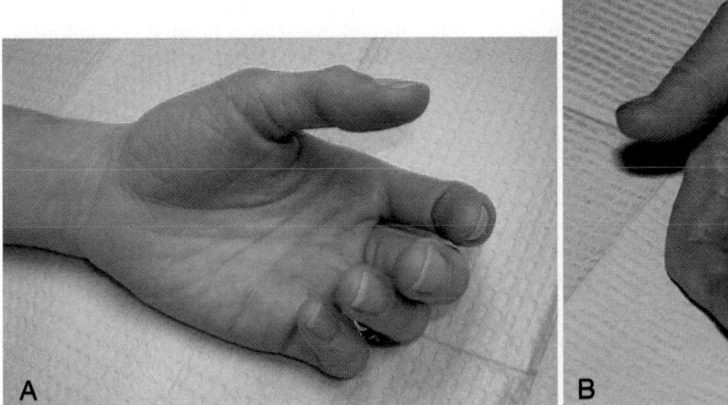

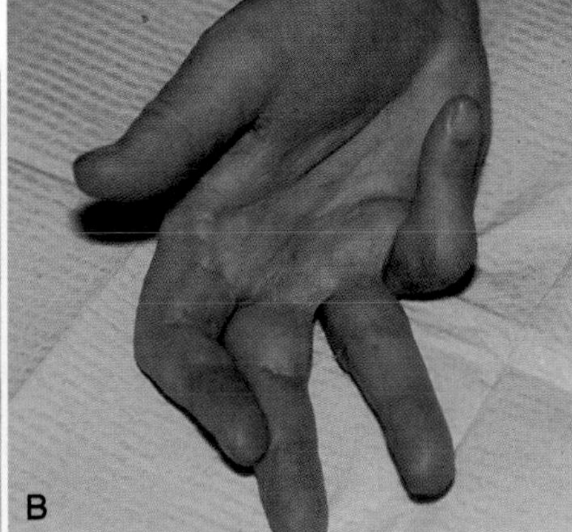

FIG 23-9 **A,** The natural flexion cascade from radial to ulnar. **B,** Dupuytren's effect on flexion cascade. *(From Skirven T, Osterman A, Fedorczyk J, et al:* Rehabilitation of the hand and upper extremity, *ed 6, Philadelphia, 2011, Mosby.)*

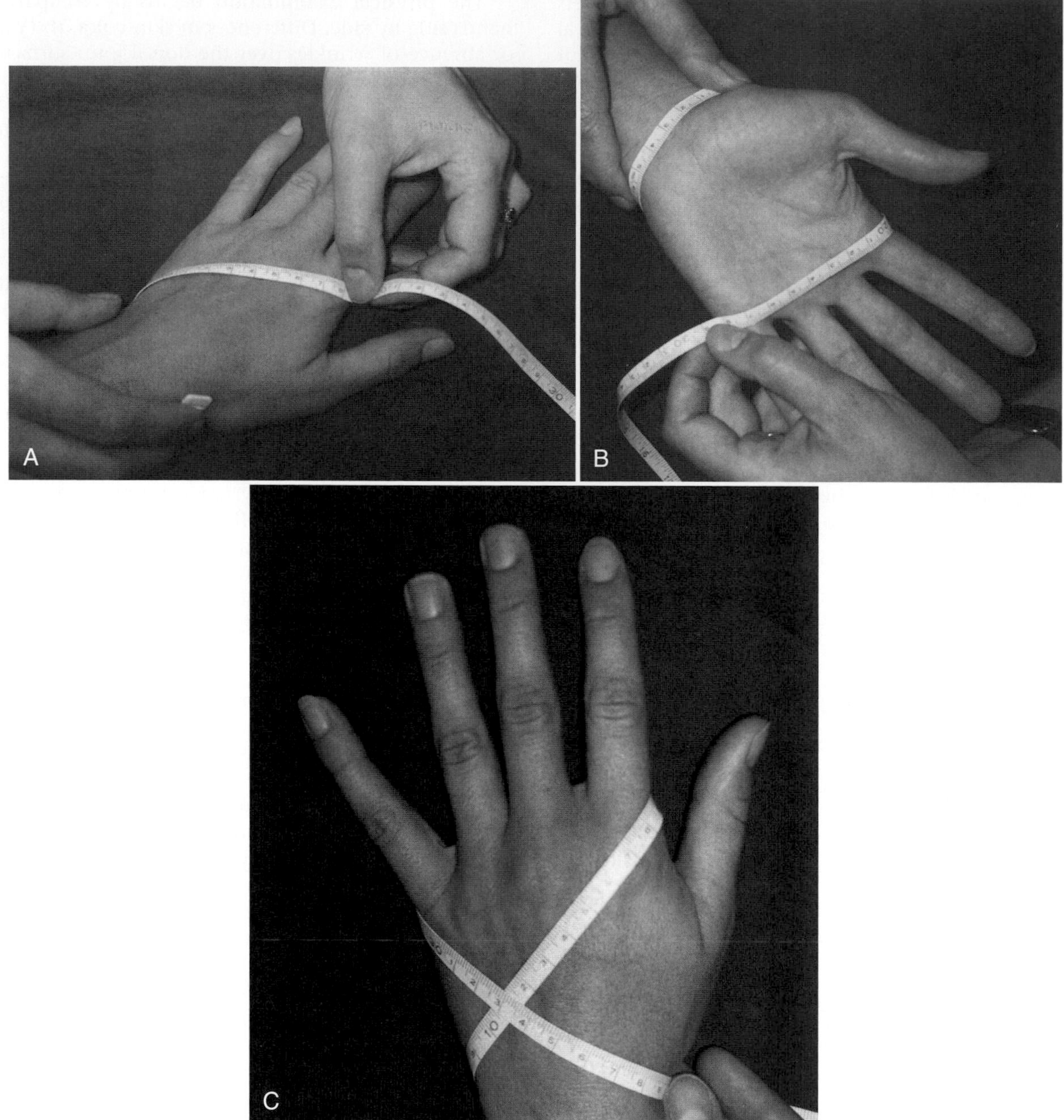

FIG 23-10 Volume measurement of the hand. **A,** Beginning at the radial styloid, extend measuring tape across the volar wrist crease. Continue around to the dorsum of the hand and angle up to the second metacarpal head. **B,** Continue ulnarly across the metacarpal heads on the palmar surface of the hand. **C,** Continue around the fifth metacarpal head to the dorsal surface of the hand and diagonally back to the radial styloid. *(From Maihafer GC, Llewellyn MA, Pillar WJ Jr, et al: A comparison of the figure-of-eight method and water volumetry in measurement of hand and wrist size,* J Hand Ther *16:305–310, 2003.)*

active motion (Table 23-1). As noted earlier, the extrinsic muscles work over multiple joints, so the proximal joints should be in neutral position when measuring ROM. If this position cannot be achieved comfortably, the position of the proximal joints should be recorded. Measurements are typically recorded as extension/flexion. Hyperextension can be recorded with a "+"sign before or an "H" after the numerical value. Normal values are variable depending on the digit and the thickness of the fingers with the ulnar digits having slightly more flexion at all the joints.[35]

TABLE 23-1 Active Range of Motion Values*

Joint	Extension	Flexion
MP	−30°	90°-115°
PIP	0°	100°-120°
DIP	0°	70°-90°
TAM	0°	260°-325°

DIP, distal interphalangeal; *MP,* metacarpophalangeal; *PIP,* proximal interphalangeal; *TAM,* total active motion.

*Active flexion increases from radial to ulnar digits. Comparing the TAM of the uninvolved side and sequentially in the same digit is a quick way to document range of motion progress.

Important Concept

The extrinsic and some intrinsic hand muscles exert force at multiple joints. The position of the proximal joints influences the available ROM of the distal joints.

For the thumb, the MP and IP joints can be measured in composite flexion and extension and isolated flexion and extension. Measurement of CMC abduction is variable, but the recommendation of the American Society of Hand Therapists is to use a ruler to measure the distance from the distal palmar crease directly over the third MP joint to the tip of the thumb.[3] Opposition can be recorded by the Kapandji method, noting which digit the thumb tip reaches (Fig. 23-11).[23] If strength measurements are not contraindicated, manual muscle testing and grip and pinch strength should be measured and compared with the uninvolved side.

PHASES OF HEALING

The complex structure of the hand requires careful attention to the phases of healing and the tissue response to treatment. Tissue healing occurs in three phases: inflammatory, fibroplastic, and maturation or remodeling.[27] The length of each phase is determined by the extent of the injury and the properties of the specific tissues involved.

Important Concept

The precise anatomy of the hand requires attention to detail. The practitioner must have full knowledge about which structures were damaged and how they were repaired before evaluating the patient's motion or strength.

The signs of inflammation are heat, redness, swelling, and pain. Although inflammation is a necessary step in healing, aggressive handling can prolong this stage and contribute to chronic inflammation and healing delays. Inflammation should begin to subside in 4 to 5 days with the onset of the fibroplastic stage, when new blood vessels enter the wound and collagen synthesis begins. This stage lasts until 3 weeks after the injury. Care should be taken during exercise to avoid placing too much tension on the wound or incision because this can lead to wound disruption, decreased healing strength, and wider scarring.[41] The primary goals are to reduce edema and pain and maintain active motion in the adjacent joints and begin gentle motion in the affected tissues, depending on the nature of the repairs. The maturation stage can continue from 3 weeks to many months as the wound gradually gains strength.[27] Therapy can progress to more aggressive motion and scar management depending on the diagnosis. These timelines are based on normal wound healing and should be adjusted for patients with additional considerations, such as diabetes or infection.

Important Concept

Successful treatment of hand injuries requires recognition of the phases of healing. Aggressive rehabilitation in the initial phases can prolong inflammation and delay recovery of functional use. The response to treatment should be closely monitored and the program advanced accordingly.

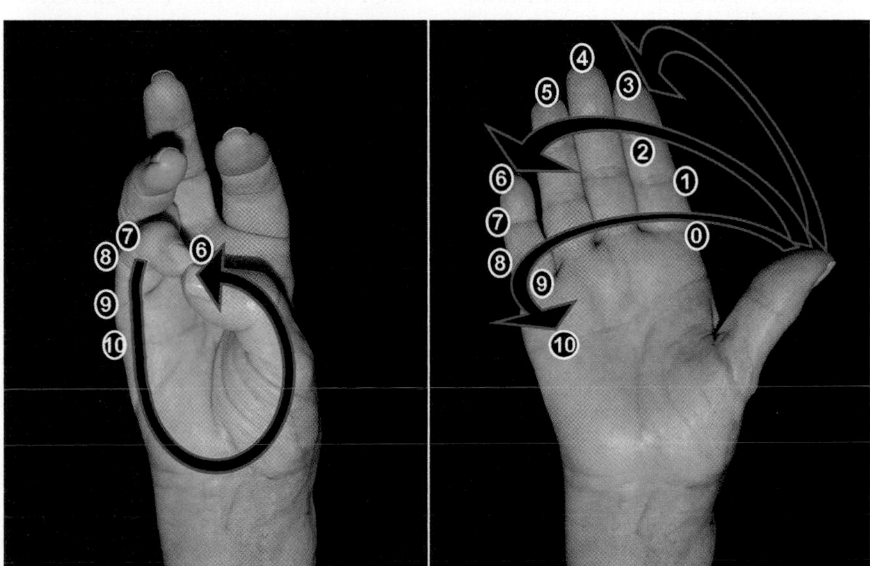

FIG 23-11 The Kapandje scale for recording thumb opposition. Opposition can be determined by assigning a numerical value to the segments of the hand as shown. Thumb opposition to the index finger tip would be a "3," and the distal palmar crease at the base of the small finger would be "10." *(From Ataker Y, Gudemez E, Ece SC, et al: Rehabilitation protocol after suspension arthroplasty of thumb carpometacarpal joint osteoarthritis,* J Hand Ther *25:374–383, 2012.)*

BONY INJURIES OF THE WRIST AND HAND

Fractures to the forearm, wrist, and digits are common. In general, their treatment and the timing of rehabilitation depend on the following:

1. The number of fragments in the fracture
2. The fragment orientation (displaced or in alignment)
3. The approach used to restore anatomic alignment (closed reduction or open reduction)
4. The method used to maintain the reduction (external fixation, involving casts or splints; internal fixation, involving pins, screws, or plates; or percutaneous fixation, involving pins that protrude through the skin into the bone)
5. Involvement of the articular surfaces

Before beginning any exercise program with patients with fractures, it is important to know how stable the reduction is. Exercise can begin earlier and more aggressively with strong and stable fixation. It is also important to review any two-joint muscles that may cross involved and uninvolved joints because exercise to the proximal, uninvolved joint may jeopardize the fixation at the distal joint.

Important Concept

In treating hand and wrist fractures, the stability of the reduction determines the timing and progression of the exercise program. The stability of the reduction also determines when movement of the proximal joints can begin, due to muscles spanning multiple joints.

DISTAL FOREARM FRACTURES

Radius

The most common distal radius fractures are **Colles fractures**.[19] Colles fracture is defined as a radius fracture within 2.5 cm of the wrist in which the distal fragment is displaced in a dorsal direction.[19] This injury is also known as a **dinner fork deformity** because of the resemblance resulting from the shape of the wrist and hand after this fracture (Fig. 23-12). This injury is usually the result of a fall on the palm of an outstretched hand. Treatment of these common fractures is controversial, and more than 85% require reduction.[19]

A **Smith fracture** is also referred to as a *reverse Colles fracture*.[19] The fracture usually occurs from a fall on the dorsum of the hand, with the resultant distal radial fragment displaced in a palmar direction (Fig. 23-13). The course of treatment is similar to the course of treatment for Colles fracture, and the rehabilitation is the same.

Rehabilitation starts as soon as stable immobilization has been achieved. The goals are to reduce edema through positioning and retrograde massage and to maintain digit ROM through exercise. The distal edge of the cast or splint must be proximal to the distal palmar crease to allow full flexion of the MP joints. "Six-pack" exercises are taught and performed hourly while awake (Fig. 23-14).[15] These exercises maintain MP and IP ligament length and encourage differential gliding of the finger and wrist tendons. Passive assistance may be needed to achieve full range. Light gripping and pinching and light use of the fingers are encouraged as long as there is no pain at the fracture site. Active forearm rotation within the limit of the cast should also be started. Shoulder pain should be evaluated by the supervising physical therapist (PT) because proximal injuries can be overlooked in light of the distal radius fracture.

Some distal radius fractures require immobilization of the elbow to prevent forearm rotation for the first 3 weeks.[40] When the cast is modified to free the elbow, active and passive exercise to the elbow can begin. The PT should be consulted before beginning resisted elbow flexion because of the attachment of the brachioradialis on the radial styloid. Strong contractions of this muscle may cause a loss of the fracture reduction.[40] Complications following distal radial fractures include loss of reduction of the fracture fragments, nonunion (the break does not heal), malunion (partial healing or poor alignment), tendon adhesions, median nerve compression, instability, Volkmann's ischemic contracture, and **complex regional pain syndrome (CRPS)**.[19] The patient's pain, circulation, and sensation should be monitored during each session, and the exercises should be adjusted accordingly.

When the cast is discontinued, the patient may be placed in a soft splint between exercise sessions until the wrist muscles are stronger. Active and active assisted ROM to the wrist and forearm are initiated, making sure combinations of motion, such as flexion and ulnar deviation, are performed. Patients should be taught to isolate the wrist muscles from the finger muscles because they will have a tendency to lead wrist motion with the finger muscles. Encouraging the patient to hold a paper towel

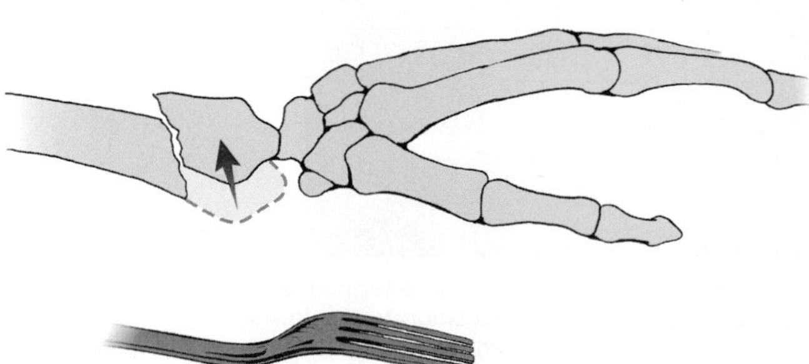

FIG 23-12 Colles fracture with resultant dinner fork deformity.

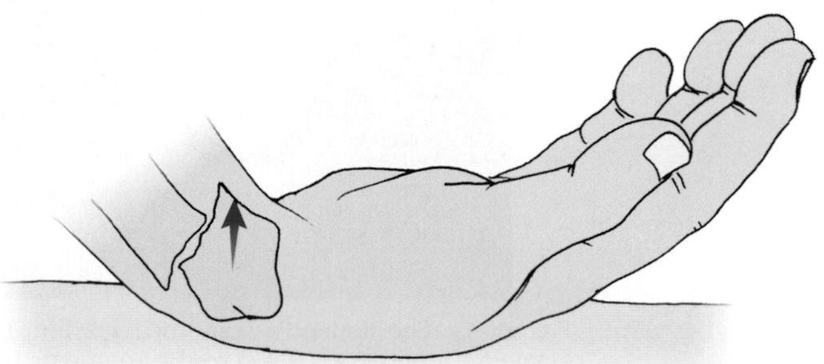

FIG 23-13 Smith fracture, also referred to as *reverse Colles fracture*. The mechanism of injury is usually a fall on the dorsum of the hand.

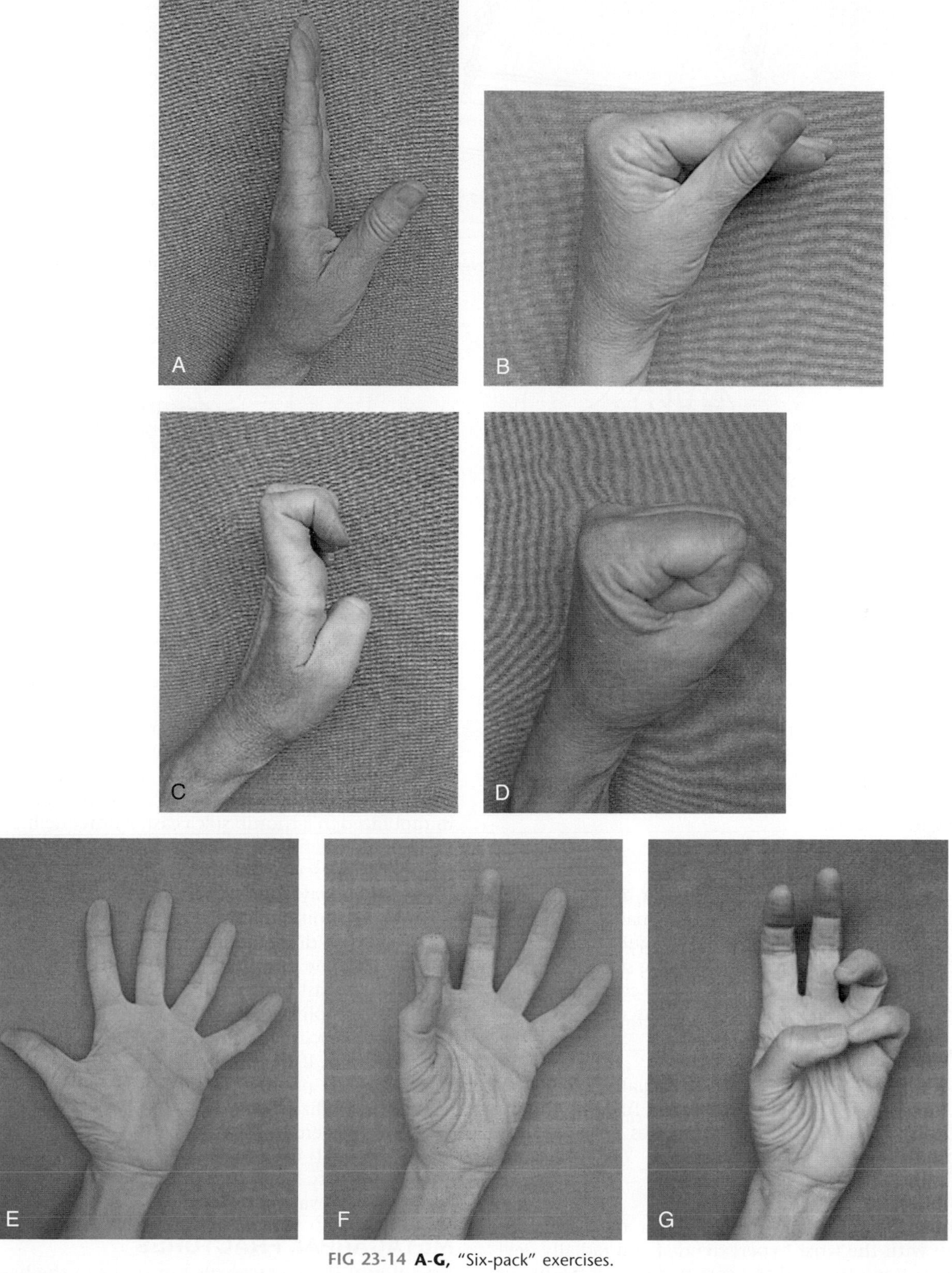

FIG 23-14 **A-G,** "Six-pack" exercises.

core while moving the wrist helps the patient to isolate the wrist muscles without adding resistance. Submaximal isometric exercises at various positions in the range are also started. Modalities to increase tissue extensibility or relieve pain are initiated as long as edema remains controlled. Strengthening is usually started 4 to 5 weeks after cast removal. The physician orders this only if the fracture site is no longer tender to palpation and evidence of bony union is seen. Closed chain weight bearing is also gradually started at this time. Joint mobilization can be

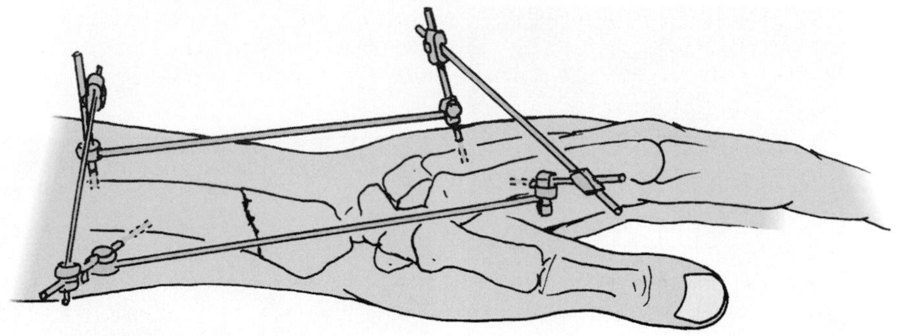

FIG 23-15 External fixator for stabilization of severely displaced, unstable comminuted fractures.

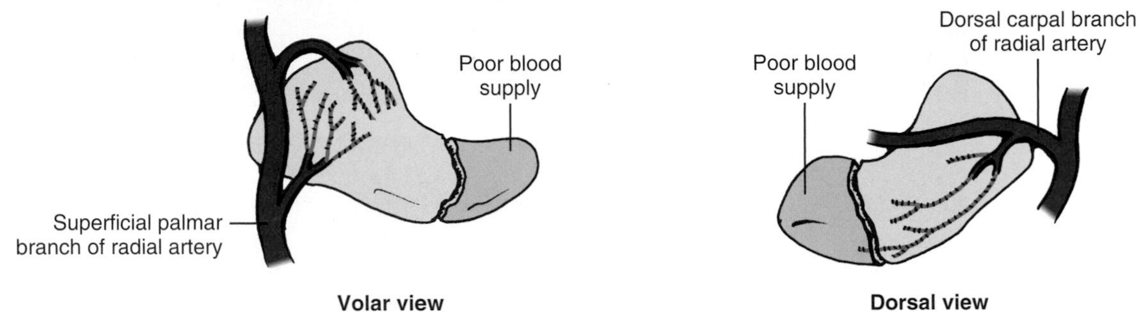

FIG 23-16 Vascular anatomy of the scaphoid. The proximal pole of the scaphoid has a poor blood supply. If fracture occurs in the proximal pole, there is the likelihood of avascular necrosis and resultant nonunion.

helpful in regaining full ROM. Patients generally return to work without restrictions about 10 weeks after cast removal.[40]

Patients with percutaneous fixation (sometimes called *external fixators*) can often follow the same exercise program outlined earlier (Fig. 23-15). The fixator stays in place until radiographs reveal evidence of bony healing, generally in 6 weeks.[15]

Ulna

Fractures of the distal ulna usually occur in combination with distal radius fractures.[32] Medical management and rehabilitation follow the above-outlined guidelines. Persistent pain with rotation or weight bearing suggests further evaluation of the triangular fibrocartilage complex (TFCC) is necessary to rule out tears (see later discussion).

CARPAL FRACTURES

Fractures of the carpal bones are also usually caused by a fall on the outstretched hand. Scaphoid fractures are the most common, and trapezoid fractures are the least common.[1]

Scaphoid Fractures

A scaphoid fracture is often the result of a minor fall on the palm with the wrist hyperextended and radially deviated.[1] It is often dismissed as a sprain, delaying treatment. Pain and swelling in the area of the anatomic snuffbox that do not resolve over a few weeks, pain with wrist extension, and decreased grip strength are signs indicating further evaluation is needed.

The location of the fracture within the scaphoid determines the method of treatment. The blood supply to this bone enters distally, leaving the proximal portion without direct circulation when it is separated by a fracture (Fig. 23-16). Fractures in the proximal third of the bone have a high incidence of nonunion, and fractures that do heal take much longer—12 to 24 weeks of immobilization compared with 5 to 6 weeks for the distal portion.[7,29,35] Fractures that are not displaced or can be reduced easily are immobilized in a thumb spica cast. Nonreducible fractures require internal fixation with rigid immobilization. If nonunion and avascular necrosis occur, bone grafts from the distal radius may be necessary.[1,7]

Rehabilitation should begin during immobilization as described for distal radial fractures. Edema reduction and ROM of the uninvolved distal joints are the primary focus. After cast removal, the patient usually wears a thumb spica splint between exercise sessions. Wrist exercises should focus on differential gliding of the wrist and finger muscles. If the patient is having difficulty regaining motion, static progressive splinting, dynamic splinting, and joint mobilization can help restore full ROM. Strengthening with exercise putty, sustained grip activities, and gradual closed chain activities progress to tolerance. Patients usually return to full activity within 12 weeks after cast removal.[7]

METACARPAL FRACTURES

Fractures of the metacarpals can occur in the base, shaft, neck, or head. These injuries are due to falls, jammed fingers, or direct blows.[44] Fractures that are nondisplaced or minimally displaced are placed in a cast or splint for 3 to 4 weeks, usually including the joint above and the joint below the fracture.[45] The MP joint is placed in 45° to 60° of flexion to prevent collateral ligament shortening.

Displaced fractures require surgical intervention and fixation by open or percutaneous techniques.

Fractures of the neck of the fourth or fifth metacarpal are called **boxer's fractures** (Fig. 23-17). These injuries occur when an individual strikes a hard object with a clenched fist. Ironically, these injuries are rarely seen in professional boxers.[45] Patients are immobilized with the wrist in slight extension and the MP joint flexed for 3 to 4 weeks.[44,45] The PIP joints are free to flex and extend often within 24 hours. Edema control sometimes requires the use of an Isotoner glove as well as massage and elevation.

Active ROM should emphasize isolated extensor digitorum communis motion, MP joint flexion, and composite flexion. Tendon adhesions to the fracture site or, in the case of open procedures, the skin, often limit gliding of the extensor tendons. A splint should be worn in between exercise sessions for an additional 2 weeks. At 6 weeks, passive ROM and resistance can be started emphasizing interossei strengthening to achieve full IP joint extension.[31] If the fixation is less stable, ROM may be delayed until 3 to 4 weeks and then follow the course outlined previously. When the incision has healed, scar mobilization techniques should be started.

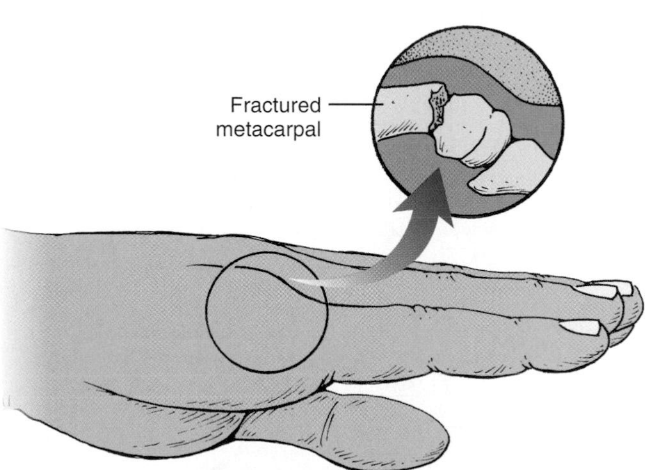

FIG 23-17 Boxer's fracture, or fighter's fracture.

Bennett Fracture

A **Bennett fracture** is a fracture of the palmar base of the first metacarpal.[45] The ligaments hold the fragment in place, but the remainder of the base is pulled radially and dorsally, resulting in a fracture-dislocation.[45] As with a boxer's fracture, treatment can be with closed reduction and rigid cast immobilization or with an open reduction with internal fixation (ORIF) procedure, depending on the severity of the fracture. There must be a solid union at the fracture site before active motion can begin. If closed reduction is used, immobilization lasts 6 weeks to promote stable union.[45] If an ORIF procedure is used, immobilization is slightly shorter because of the rigid internal fixation. Rehabilitation closely parallels the treatment for a boxer's fracture with emphasis on regaining the thumb web space, opposition, and composite flexion and extension. Resistance exercise, pinch, grip, and weight bearing on the palm with the thumb abducted can progress when stable fracture healing has occurred.

PHALANX FRACTURES

Phalanx fractures can occur at the neck, shaft, or base of the phalanx. Stable, closed, nondisplaced fractures are treated by buddy taping (Fig. 23-18, *A*) or with simple splints and immediate active ROM. More complex closed proximal and middle phalanx fractures should be placed in a hand-based splint for 3 to 4 weeks.[36] This splint should hold the MP joints in 50° to 70° flexion and the IP joints in 10° to 15° of flexion.[36] When radiographic evidence of healing is confirmed, ROM can progress. The most common complication is loss of PIP joint extension.[18] Blocking exercises can help prevent the tendons from adhering to the fracture site (Fig. 23-18, *B* and *C*).

The distal phalanx is the most frequently fractured bone in the hand.[33] These fractures are usually splinted in extension using a small aluminum splint leaving the PIP

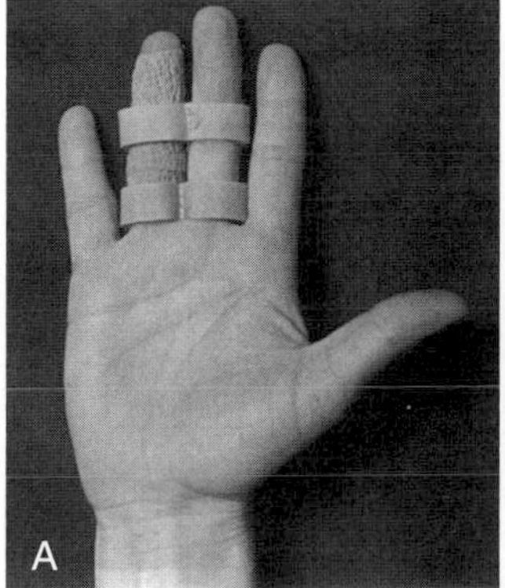

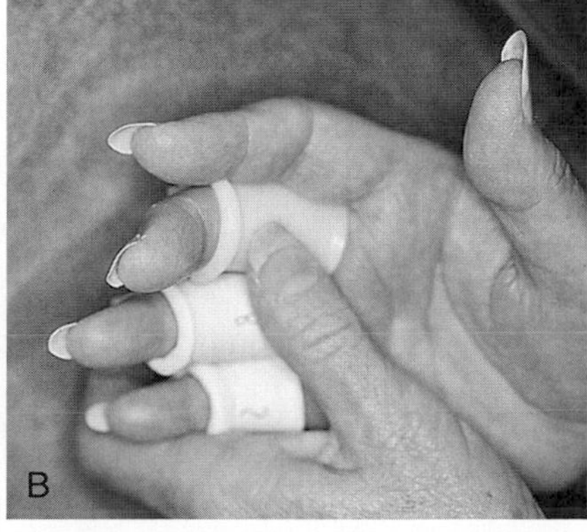

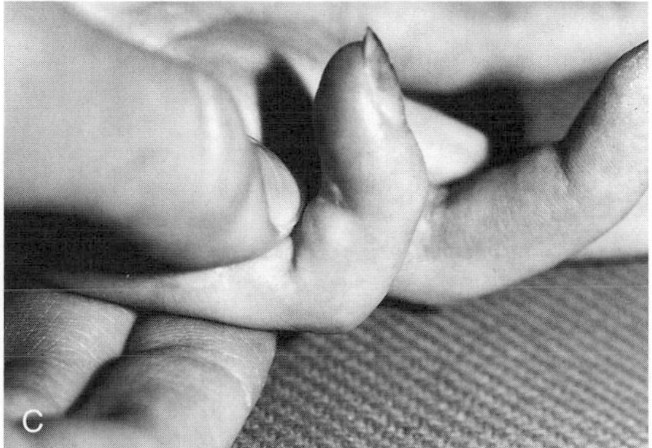

FIG 23-18 **A,** Buddy taping. **B,** Distal interphalangeal blocking exercises with the metacarpophalangeal in various positions. **C,** Manual blocking of the metacarpophalangeal during active flexion of the proximal interphalangeal joint. *(**A,** From Burke SL, Higgins JP, McClinton MA, et al:* Hand and upper extremity rehabilitation: a practical guide, *ed 3, St Louis, 2006, Churchill Livingstone; **B,** from Cooper C:* Fundamentals of hand therapy: clinical reasoning and treatment guidelines for common diagnoses of the upper extremity, *St Louis, 2007, Mosby; **C,** from Early MB:* Physical dysfunction practice skills for the occupational therapy assistant, *ed 2, St Louis, 2007, Mosby.)*

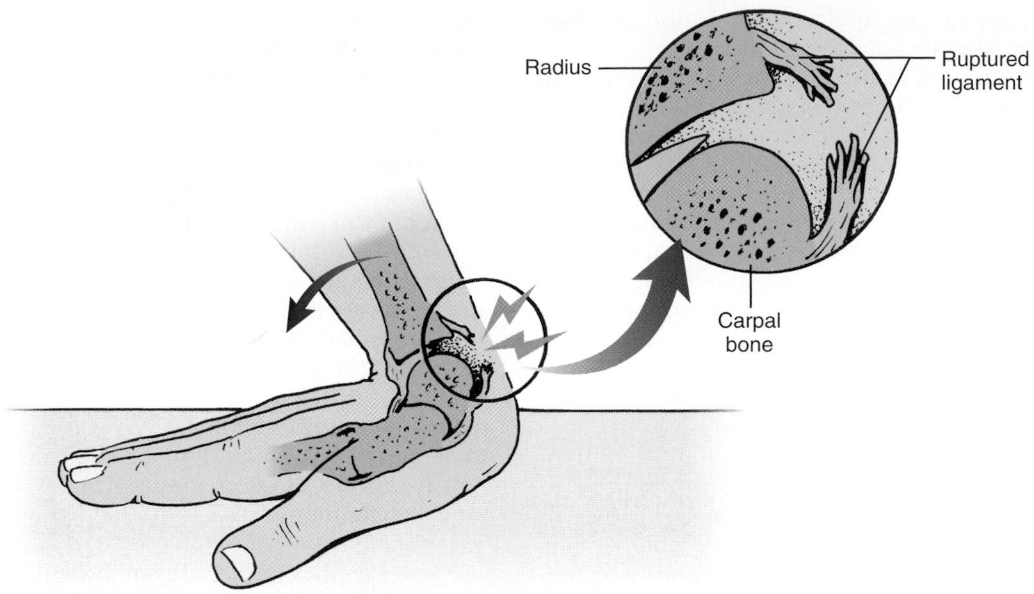

FIG 23-19 Hyperextension ligament sprain of the wrist.

joint free. Isolated PIP joint motion and MP joint motion can be started immediately. Resisted DIP joint flexion of the adjacent finger should be avoided because of the close connection of these tendons, especially in the ulnar three digits. When movement can begin at the DIP joint, (usually at 3 weeks), the emphasis is on composite digit flexion and coordinated use of the digits. Patients often bypass the injured digit in functional activities, so this is addressed in therapy with buddy taping and light grasping and pinching exercises that isolate the thumb and the involved finger. If the terminal extensor tendon is disrupted (see section on mallet finger later), the DIP joint is splinted for 6 to 8 weeks. Aggressive passive flexion should be avoided because it may lead to a loss of extension.[33] Often the nail bed is injured when the distal phalanx is fractured, leaving the finger hypersensitive and stiff. The nail may have been removed and then replaced to serve as a guide for the emerging nail. These patients are started on a program of desensitization, using touching, tapping, fluidotherapy, and vibration to overcome the hypersensitivity.

SOFT TISSUE INJURIES OF THE WRIST AND HAND

LIGAMENT INJURIES OF THE WRIST

Stability of the wrist depends primarily on intracapsular ligaments and not on intrinsic dynamic support from musculotendinous tissue.[50] Ligament sprains with varying degrees of carpal instability usually result from a fall with the wrist hyperextended (Fig. 23-19).[50]

Partial ligament injuries without carpal instability are immobilized in a short-arm cast or splint for 3 to 4 weeks. Severe ligament injuries lead to carpal instability, and reduction and maintenance of the alignment are more difficult. Options include rigid cast immobilization, closed reduction with percutaneous pinning, and ORIF (Fig. 23-20).[50] If cast immobilization is used to stabilize the joint, the patient is placed in the cast for 6 to 12 weeks, depending on the severity of the injury.[50] If closed reduction and internal fixation is required, the wrist is immobilized for about 2 months. The pins are removed after 2 months, and the arm is placed in a cast for an additional 4 weeks.[50] With an ORIF procedure, the ligaments are directly repaired, and the unstable carpal articulations are stabilized with wires or pins. The duration of immobilization is similar to that for closed reduction with percutaneous pinning.[50]

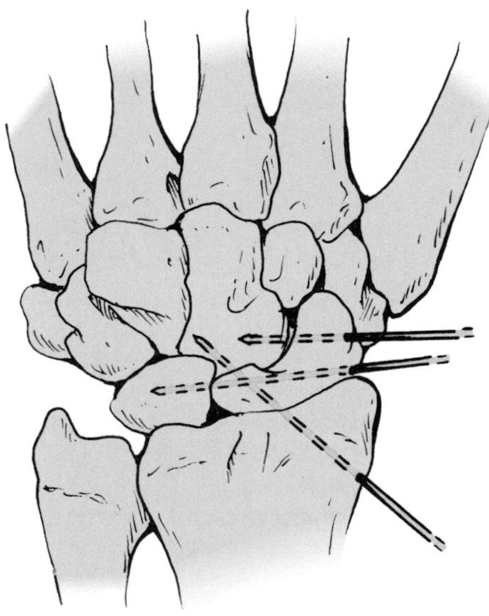

FIG 23-20 Insertion of pins for stabilization after ligament sprain with carpal instability.

Regardless of the severity of the injury, the principles for rehabilitation are the same.[19] The initial goals are to control pain and inflammation through the use of cold and electrical stimulation and to prevent edema through elevation, massage, light external compression wraps, and frequent digit active ROM within the limits of the immobilization. When the immobilization is removed, gentle, active, pain-free motion can begin in all planes. It is important to include forearm rotation and differential tendon glides between the wrist and fingers. As motion improves and pain subsides, submaximal isometric contractions can be used, progressing to resistance exercises and gradual closed chain exercises. The last step is to increase the speed of movement gradually. Exercising with a metronome is helpful. Sustained gripping and concentric and eccentric exercises improve wrist strength. Protection of the wrist continues well into the final recovery stages of rehabilitation, and the use of a wrist splint is encouraged in between exercise sessions.

Triangular Fibrocartilage Complex

Pain in the ulnar side of the wrist may indicate an injury to the **triangular fibrocartilage complex (TFCC)**. The TFCC is formed by ligaments and an articular disk between the ulna and the ulnar carpal bones.[26] Injury to the TFCC can occur from an axial force applied to the ulnar side of the wrist during weight bearing and gripping (as in gymnastics) or a fall on the palm with the forearm pronated. The ulna is longer compared with the radius when the forearm is pronated[26]; this can lead to an ulnocarpal impaction syndrome that results in a torn articular disk and damage to the ulnar head and lunate. Distal radial fractures resulting in a loss of radial length can also leave the ulna longer than the radius. The central disk of the complex has a poor blood supply, so healing tears in it is difficult.[54] Treatment initially involves rest and splinting of the wrist and elbow to prevent forearm rotation for 4 to 6 weeks followed by a gradual program of ROM exercises and progressive strengthening.[54] Exercises should begin in supination and progress to neutral, with pronated gripping and weight bearing being the final stage.[26] If symptoms are not relieved by conservative methods, arthroscopic débridement or ulnar shortening is considered.[54]

Skier's Thumb

Skier's thumb is an acute sprain of the ulnar collateral ligament of the thumb. The mechanism of injury is a sudden valgus stress and hyperextension of the thumb, which results in either a partial ligament tear or a complete rupture (Fig. 23-21).[51]

Partially torn ligaments can be treated nonsurgically with a thumb spica cast or rigid immobilization. The thumb CMC joint is abducted to 30°, and the IP joint is left free for exercise. The splint is worn continuously for 3 to 4 weeks.[20,54] Edema reduction techniques are used as needed. At 3 to 4 weeks, the splint can be removed for active thumb MP and composite CMC, MP, and IP joint motion. Progressive strengthening can begin at 5 to 6 weeks, and the protective splint is decreased except for heavy activities. Unrestricted use is delayed until 3 months postinjury.

Complete injuries may require surgery because they can be associated with a fracture of the proximal phalanx, or

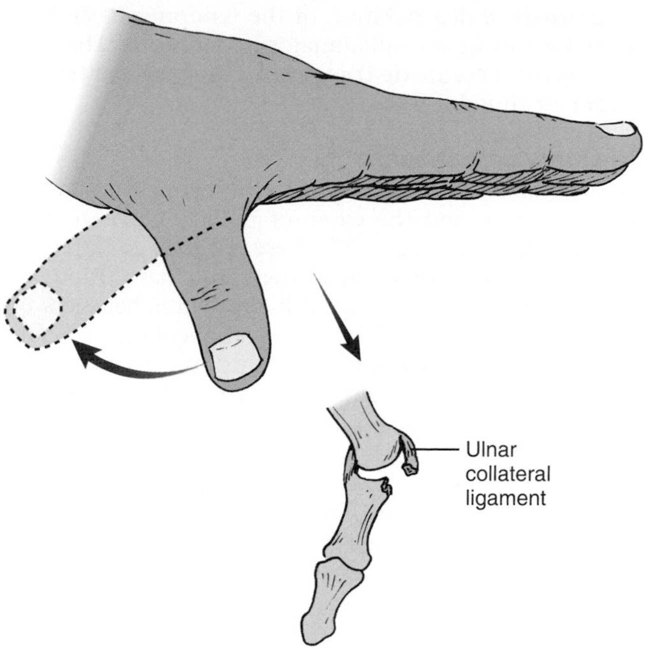

FIG 23-21 Skier's thumb, also referred to as *gamekeeper's thumb.* Sudden valgus stress and hyperextension can result in partial or complete rupture of the ulnar collateral ligament of the thumb.

the distal end of the ligament may be displaced by the adductor muscle insertion preventing healing (Stener's lesion).[20,54] A short-arm thumb spica cast is applied for approximately 4 weeks.[51] The IP joint is left free, and active flexion/extension is started immediately to prevent adherence of the extrinsic tendons. At 4 weeks, the cast is replaced by a splint, and the program progresses as discussed earlier except for strengthening, which should be cleared by the surgeon—usually at about 6 weeks. Scar massage and nightly application of silicon to the scar should help flexibility. The goal is a pain-free, stable thumb with pinch and grip values comparable to the uninjured hand. Unrestricted use is permitted around 3 months after surgery.[1]

TENDINOPATHIES

Tendons from the extrinsic muscles pass through fibro-osseous tunnels or under retinacula that serve as pulleys to hold the tendons in place, close to the bone, keeping them from "bowstringing" and improving their mechanical efficiency.[8] The tendons are subject to compressive stress, especially at the proximal edge of these pulleys, which can lead to thickening of the pulley and the tendon.

In some cases, the tendon develops a nodule that has difficulty gliding under the pulley. Some authors have suggested that people who use their hands in repetitive and forceful tasks have a higher incidence of nodules.[28,52]

Tendinopathies have been described by various names including **tendinitis,** referring to an inflammation of the tendon, or **tenosynovitis,** referring to inflammation of the synovial sheath of the tendon. **Tendovaginitis,** referring to inflammation of the tendon sheath, may be the most accurate description.[52] Some authors have suggested that the process is more accurately described as a

tendinosis, a degeneration of the tendon cells and collagen instead of an inflammatory condition.[4] The most common of these are **de Quervain's disease** and **trigger finger** or thumb.

De Quervain's Disease

De Quervain's disease is a condition affecting the abductor pollicis longus and the extensor pollicis brevis tendons and sheaths (Fig. 23-22).[28,52] These tendons comprise the first dorsal extensor compartment and pass through a fibro-osseous tunnel lined with synovium between the distal radius and the extensor retinaculum. Forceful, repeated thumb abduction and extension with medial and lateral deviation of the wrist creates friction that can lead to swelling and thickening of the connective tissue and narrowing of the tunnel.[20,52] The disease manifests as pain on the radial side of the wrist that is aggravated by use of the thumb. Swelling and, in some cases, nodules may be palpable. Pain is increased by ulnar deviation of the wrist when the thumb is clasped in the palm (Finkelstein test).[20,52] Traditional conservative management includes activity analysis and modification aimed at avoiding the provocative motions or wrist and thumb immobilization. In addition, ice and high-voltage, pulsed, galvanic electrical stimulation may improve symptoms. Iontophoresis is frequently ordered, but its effectiveness has not been established.[4] Passive motion in the pain-free range of the wrist and thumb should be performed daily, and progression to active motion can begin as tolerated. Strengthening can be initiated when active ROM is pain-free and should emphasize eccentric and concentric motions of the wrist and thumb. All muscles of both thumbs should be strengthened because they have been shown to be weak compared with normal individuals.[17] The speed of ROM should gradually be increased as the final step in rehabilitation. Patients should be prepared for a recovery time of months rather than weeks.[4]

If conservative care fails to relieve symptoms, the physician may inject the first dorsal compartment with a corticosteroid to reduce pain and inflammation. Chronic cases of de Quervain's disease require surgical release of the compartment. The affected wrist is immobilized for approximately 1 week with a compression bandage. The surgeon indicates when exercises can begin as directed by the PT, with specific attention directed to tendon gliding, pain, and scar management when the sutures are removed. Resistance can progress as outlined under the conservative program.

Trigger Finger

Trigger finger describes catching or sticking of a finger or thumb during flexion and extension. The patient reports resistance, usually to extension, that is overcome with increased effort. The condition can be associated with pain and progress to the digit being stuck in a bent position, requiring use of the other hand to straighten it. This catching is due to stress at the edge of the flexor tunnel, specifically the A1 pulley (Fig. 23-23).[28,52] The tendon and the pulley have been shown to thicken, limiting the ability of the tendon to glide.[28,52]

Therapy is targeted at preventing stress on the tendon and pulley by immobilization of the involved digit or digits and exercises that avoid simultaneous flexion of all three joints. Success rates of 73% to 87% have been reported with isolated PIP joint splinting in the digit and IP joint splinting in the thumb for individual digits[48] or isolated MP joint splinting in full extension[13] or isolated MP joint splinting in 10° to 15° flexion for multiple digits.

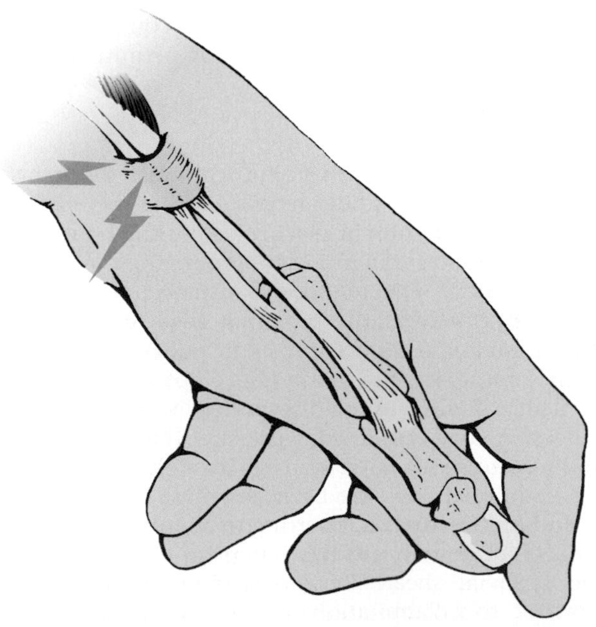

FIG 23-22 De Quervain's tenosynovitis. *(From Salvo S:* Mosby's pathology for massage therapists, *ed 3, St Louis, 2014, Mosby.)*

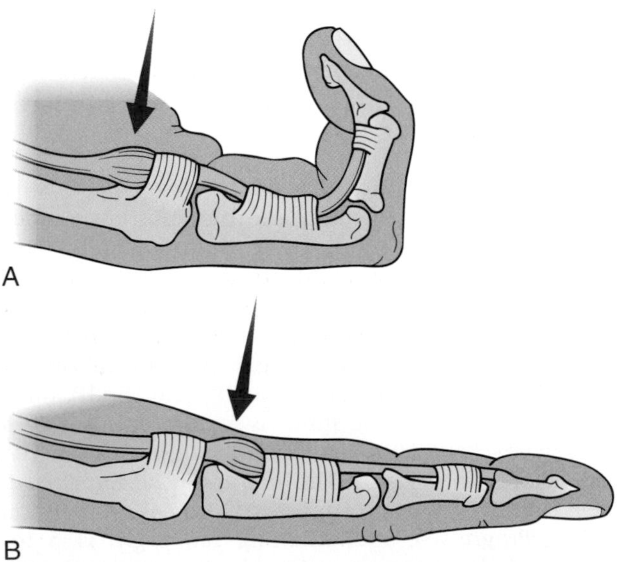

FIG 23-23 Trigger finger. **A,** With flexion, the swollen tendon "pops" through the A1 pulley. **B,** With extension, it must slide back through. The digit usually gets stuck in flexion, and the patient has to use the other hand to force the digit straight. *(Modified from Mercier L:* Practical orthopedics, *ed 6, Philadelphia, 2008, Mosby.)*

The splints are worn at all times for 3 to 10 weeks except for exercises. There is some disagreement about the best exercise approach, with passive isolated PIP joint flexion, passive composite flexion/extension, and active hook fisting (flexion of the DIP and PIP joints with the MP joints extended) recommended at varying intervals during the day. Active full excursion flexion/extension is avoided in the affected digits. Massage has also been recommended.[13]

Patients whose symptoms do not improve with conservative treatment may undergo corticosteroid injection.[52] In some cases, the injections do not relieve the triggering, and patients may require surgical release of the A1 pulley. This can also be done percutaneously in the surgeon's office. Therapy after pulley release includes edema and wound management and passive and active ROM as outlined earlier under conservative care. Isometric strengthening can begin at 3 weeks, but forceful, repetitive fisting or strong, sustained grasp should be minimized, especially in patients with a history of involvement of multiple digits.[28] Any catching reported by the patient or noted by the PTA is an indication that the program is progressing too quickly.

TENDON INJURIES

Tendon injuries are classified into zones according to the location of injury. There are different zones for extensor tendons compared with flexor tendons. The management of tendon injuries is precise and is determined by the level of injury, the type of repair, and any associated injuries.

Important Concept

Injuries to flexor tendons require precise rehabilitation based on the level of injury, the type of repair, and any associated injuries.

Extensor Tendon Injuries

Injuries to the extensor tendons are often treated as trivial, but they require careful management to maintain the dynamic balance of the fingers and wrist. Extensor muscles are weaker than the flexors, so restoration of strength is important. On the back of the hand, these tendons are superficial and have a large surface area that makes them susceptible to injury and adhesions.[42] An in-depth discussion of all levels of injury and methods of repair is beyond the scope of this text, but two of the more common injuries are discussed next. The PTA should follow the instructions of the PT precisely when working with a patient with an extensor tendon repair.

Mallet Finger. Interruption of the extensor tendon mechanism over the DIP joint (zones 1 and 2) is referred to as a **mallet finger.** These injuries can involve tendon only or can include a fracture of the distal phalanx (Fig. 23-24). The imbalance that is created by the unopposed force of the flexor digitorum profundus muscle positions the DIP joint in flexion and, with time, may lead to hyperextension of the PIP, resulting in a swan neck deformity.[42] The treatment is the same with either tendon rupture or

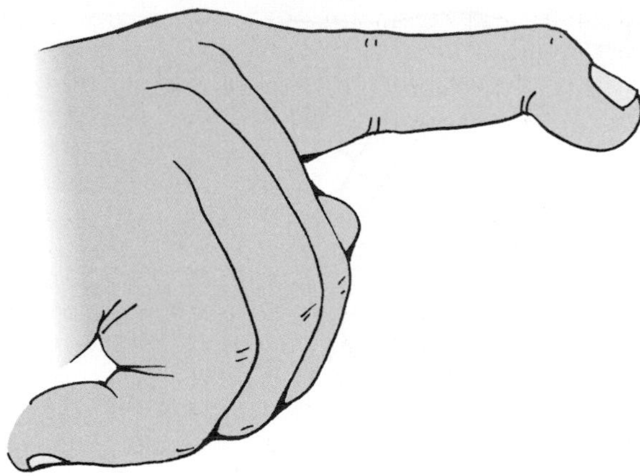

FIG 23-24 Mallet finger. Avulsion fracture or tendon rupture results in distal interphalangeal joint flexion contracture.

avulsion fracture. The recommended treatment of a closed injury is continuous, uninterrupted splinting of the DIP joint for 6 weeks in mild hyperextension that does not cause the skin to blanche.[13,42] The PIP joint is left free. The splint may require modification as swelling subsides, but care should be taken not to allow the DIP joint to change position during the adjustment. Active flexion/extension of the PIP joint begins immediately, but the adjacent finger DIP joints are not actively exercised. At 6 weeks, active flexion of the DIP joints begins. Initially, only 20° of flexion is allowed. The flexion angle is increased each week as long as full extension is maintained. Full active flexion is delayed until at least 3 months postinjury. The patient is advised against using a strong muscle effort, and passive flexion is contraindicated. The extension splint is reapplied at night for 4 more weeks. If an extension lag develops, full-time splinting is resumed.[10,42]

The patient should be informed that full motion may take 6 months. If the patient is noncompliant with the initial splinting, a Kirschner wire may be inserted to maintain the extended position. The wire is removed at 6 weeks, and the program progresses as discussed earlier.

Boutonnière Deformity. Interruption of the central tendon and triangular ligament at the PIP joint (zone 3) allows the head of the proximal phalanx to herniate dorsally resulting in a boutonnière deformity (Fig. 23-25).[42] This displacement leads to imbalance between the intrinsic and extrinsic muscles of the finger. The resultant position of the finger is flexion of the PIP joint and hyperextension of the DIP joint. If the deformity can be corrected passively, the finger is held in full PIP joint extension for 6 weeks with the MP and DIP joints free. The goal is to approximate the ends of the tendon so that they can heal together. The PTA should alert the PT if swelling decreases and the splint or cast is loose, requiring remolding. Active and passive DIP joint flexion is encouraged. After 6 weeks, active motion of the PIP joint is initiated, but the digit is splinted in between sessions for 2 to 4 weeks. Just as with a mallet finger, the patient gradually increases active flexion of the PIP joint. The splint is

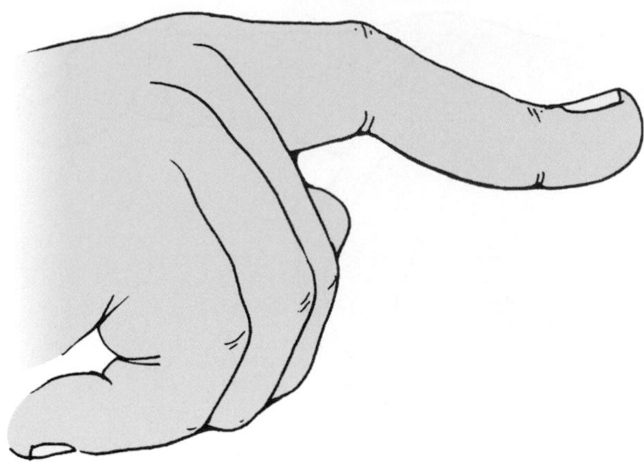

FIG 23-25 Boutonnière deformity. Proximal interphalangeal flexion with distal interphalangeal extension.

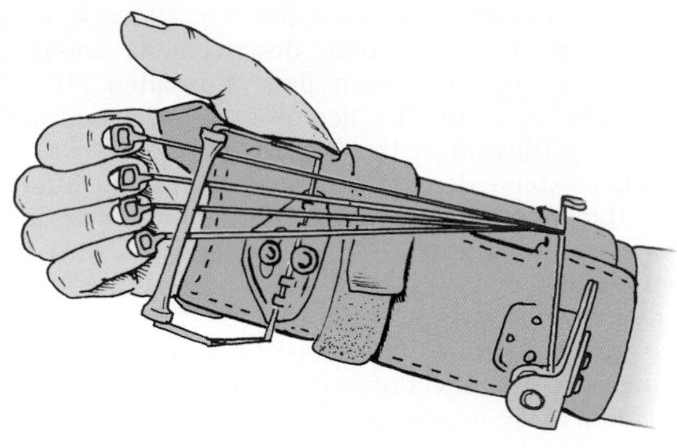

FIG 23-26 Postoperative protective splint with rubber band traction after flexor tendon repair.

gradually decreased as long as full PIP joint extension is maintained. The patient should be warned that treatment may be required for 6 to 9 months.[42]

If the deformity cannot be passively reduced or is associated with a fracture or other injury, surgical intervention is indicated. The postoperative course depends on the structures repaired and the specific procedure performed.

Important Concept

There are no trivial joint injuries in the hand. Extensor tendon injuries at the finger level resulting in mallet or boutonnière deformities require carefully balancing immobilization and movement and may take months to fully heal.

Flexor Tendon Injuries

The restoration of function after a flexor tendon injury requires careful balance between protecting the repair and gliding the tendon. The goal of surgery and therapy is a strong repair that glides freely. The flexor sheath and the pulley system in the digits provide a smooth gliding surface that is mechanically efficient. The level of the repair, the timing, the suture pattern and strength, and any associated nerve or blood vessel injury all affect the timing of therapy. Even the most carefully applied program can result in stretching or gapping of the repair or rupture. Failure to glide the tendon results in scarring within the pulley system and loss of active flexion. Ideally, these cases should be managed by a certified hand therapist (either a PT or an occupational therapist with advanced training in hand rehabilitation) who is in close communication with the hand surgeon.

As with extensor tendons, the flexor tendons are classified into zones. The most difficult is zone 2, which extends from the level of the MP joints to the insertion of the flexor digitorum superficialis just distal to the PIP joint. Injuries in this zone may involve both the flexor digitorum superficialis and the flexor digitorum profundus tendons.[46]

There is extensive literature on flexor tendon rehabilitation, but most programs fall into one of the following three categories, and the choice depends on the factors listed earlier and the patient's ability to comply.[46] In all of the methods, the flexor tendon is held on slack with varying degrees of wrist flexion or MP joint flexion, or both, with the IP joints in extension.

1. Immobilization: After repair, the wrist and hand are casted or splinted for 3 to 4 weeks before beginning active and passive exercise. Immobilization is generally reserved for children or adults who are unable to cooperate in their care.
2. Early passive mobilization: Passive flexion and active extension are allowed within the limits of the splint. Rubber band traction is sometimes used to pull the fingers passively into flexion (Fig. 23-26).
3. Early active mobilization: The tendon is moved actively within 48 hours of repair and within carefully outlined limits set by the surgeon. These programs are recommended only for the most compliant patient who can attend therapy frequently.

The splint is worn for about 4 weeks. After the initial 4 weeks, the splint may be modified to move the wrist into neutral, and active motion is progressed. Specific progression to isolated joint motion or passive extension should be discussed in detail with the PT and surgeon.

Strengthening is initiated at about 8 weeks, and the patient is generally informed that return to full, unrestricted use will take 3 months at a minimum.[46] If the tendon becomes adherent and cannot glide, surgery is considered to free the tendon from the scar.

CONNECTIVE TISSUE DISORDERS

Dupuytren's Disease

Dupuytren's disease in the hand is first observed with the formation of pits and firm nodules that lie just below the skin of the palm (Fig. 23-27).[30] The nodules can be composed of overactive fibroblasts producing collagen or can be from "bunching" of the skin in response to a longitudinal contraction of the underlying fascia.[30] This tissue is not random but appears along longitudinal tension lines in the palm or digits. The tissue undergoes

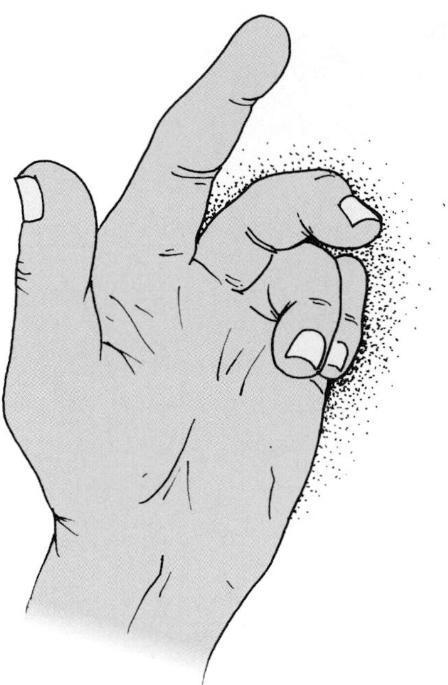

FIG 23-27 Dupuytren's contracture most commonly affects the ulnar digits, with flexion contracture of the ulnar metacarpophalangeal joint.

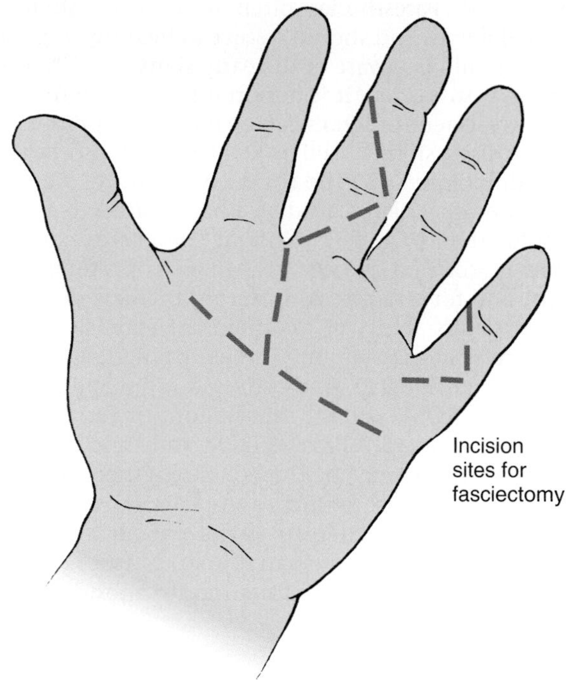

FIG 23-28 Fasciectomy for Dupuytren's contracture. The *dotted lines* represent the surgical incision, which is usually left open and not sutured together.

contraction and maturation resembling that of normal wound healing. There is no known "trigger," but the tissue can become thicker and eventually form cords that become firm and tendonlike causing the affected digits and thumb to lose extension. The progression is variable and is limited to nodules in some patients or progresses to full flexion of the affected digits in others. Patients may report some tenderness with pressure on the nodules, but pain is not a primary complaint. The greatest incidence is in white men of northern European descent, although it has been reported in all races and both sexes.[43] Initially, treatment is centered on patient reassurance and education. Reported conservative treatment includes injection of steroids that may soften the nodules or collagenases, which are chemicals known to break down collagen.[5]

When the disease interferes with function, a surgeon should be consulted. Physical therapy intervention preoperatively in the form of serial casting or serial static splinting may help in cases in which there are PIP joint contractures,[9] but it is not a substitute for surgery. There is disagreement regarding the best surgical approach for treatment, but there are four main techniques currently in the literature, as follows:[21]

1. Fasciotomy—dividing the cords by inserting a small blade or needle through the skin.
2. Regional or limited fasciectomy—removal of only the diseased fascia (Fig. 23-28).
3. Extensive fasciectomy—removal of the diseased tissue and any tissue with the potential of becoming diseased.
4. Dermofasciectomy—removal of the skin overlying the diseased tissue as well as the diseased tissue. The skin is replaced by a full-thickness skin graft, or the wound is left open in some cases to allow granulation. The goals for surgical intervention are correction of the deformity and control of the disease.[9]

The goals of physical therapy postoperatively are to optimize the conditions for wound repair; minimize wound tension, edema, and pain; minimize scarring; and optimize tendon gliding to restore ROM around the affected joints. Careful handling of the tissue is critical because aggressive stretching and splinting may be counterproductive, prolonging the inflammatory period and aggravating the disease.[9,12] Tissue affected by Dupuytren's disease has a lower tolerance to mechanical stress than normal tissue.[9]

After surgical release, the patient may be fitted with a dorsal blocking splint that allows active flexion but limits full extension at the MP joints.[9,12] This splint is used for the first 2 to 3 weeks to avoid tension and vascular compromise in the healing incisions, flaps, or grafts. The PTA should check the fit at each visit and alert the certified hand therapist when volume changes or improvements in the ROM necessitate splint adjustment. Wound care may include use of the whirlpool to loosen devitalized tissue, but care should be taken to avoid a completely dependent position because of edema concerns. Elevation, retrograde massage, and light external compression can assist with edema reduction. If a skin graft was used, the donor site should also be monitored. Active ROM emphasizing composite joint flexion and extension, abduction and adduction of the MP joints, and opposition of the thumb should begin immediately postoperatively, but care should be taken to avoid tension across the suture lines or pain. Sensation should be monitored, and protective techniques should be taught to patients whose sensibility is compromised. Paresthesias often result from stretching the digital nerves and should resolve as healing progresses. The PTA should be aware of the early signs of CRPS. If this condition is suspected, it is important to inform the PT so that the treatment program can be modified appropriately (see later discussion).[39] Active ROM should also begin at the proximal joints. By the third postoperative week, the dorsal splint may be replaced by a hand-based volar splint that holds the MP and IP joints in composite extension. A splint is worn an average of 3 months postoperatively at night and for short periods during the day, depending on the patient's ability to maintain the extension during wound and scar maturation. The use of night splinting is widespread, although a study showed night splinting did not improve ROM, patient satisfaction, or function in a 12-month follow-up.[22] Passive ROM and functional electrical stimulation may be added. Strengthening should begin with light isometrics and functional exercises. Aggressive grip strengthening is not encouraged. Closed chain weight bearing can begin as soon as wound healing permits and as the patient's function requires.

NERVE INJURIES

A **compression neuropathy** occurs when adjacent structures constrict a peripheral nerve, limiting its blood supply and resulting in impaired nerve conduction. Specific sites have been associated with compression of the radial, ulnar, and median nerves. If the adjacent tissue restricts gliding of the nerve, the nerve is subjected to stretch that can also result in paresthesias and pain. This is referred to as a **nerve entrapment.** The most common compression neuropathy in the upper extremity is that of the median nerve at the wrist.[47]

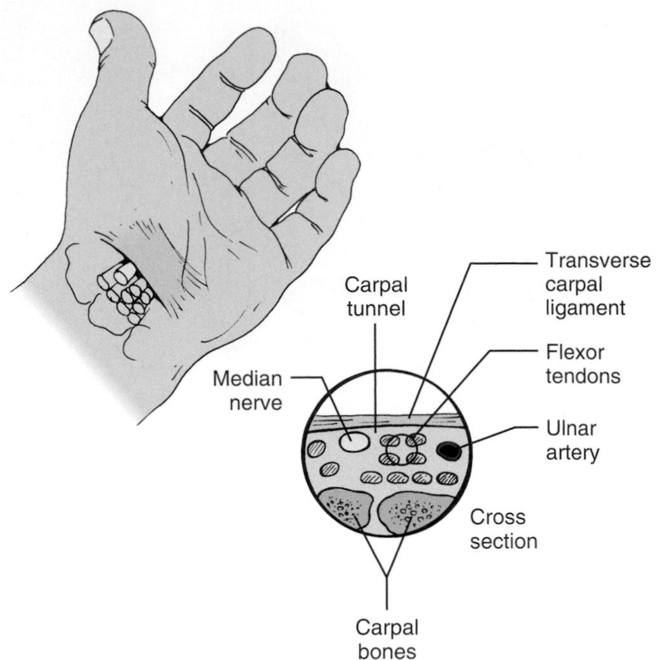

FIG 23-29 Carpal tunnel syndrome. Compression neuropathy of the median nerve.

Carpal Tunnel Syndrome

Carpal tunnel syndrome (CTS) refers to symptoms that occur when the median nerve is compressed or entrapped at the wrist. The carpal tunnel is formed by the carpal bones and the transverse carpal ligament and contains the median nerve and nine flexor tendons (Fig. 23-29). Increased friction and pressure within the tunnel constrict the nerve and produce sensory symptoms such as decreased sensation, pain, and tingling and motor problems, including loss of the thenar intrinsic muscles and loss of the first two lumbrical muscles.

There are many possible causes for CTS, including anatomic changes from arthritis, fractures, or cysts; systemic conditions such as diabetes, hypothyroidism, aging, pregnancy, or alcohol abuse; environmental factors such as solvent exposure or decreased temperatures; and occupational factors such as tasks requiring forceful, repeated motions in extreme postures (cumulative trauma) or vibration.[47] The clinical symptoms of CTS include numbness of the thumb and radial digits, tingling, pain that is often worse at night, clumsiness in hand activity, weakness of grip and pinch, atrophy of the thenar muscles, and swelling in the hand and forearm.[11,34]

Conservative physical therapy management of CTS focuses on identifying and altering the factors that compress and impair circulation to the nerve. These factors include wrist position, tendon load, and external force. Extreme flexion or extension of the wrist compresses the contents of the tunnel, so patient education should be directed to avoiding these positions. Anything that constricts the wrist, such as tight sleeves, watchbands, and bracelets, or applies pressure over the median nerve when the pronated arm is resting against a desk can contribute to the problem. Custom splints that hold the wrist in neutral should be worn at night[34] for several weeks to keep the carpal tunnel open. Deep (1-MHz) pulsed ultrasound, nerve gliding exercises, carpal bone mobilization, and yoga all have been suggested as being helpful in reducing the symptoms.[34] The evidence supporting these interventions is limited and in some cases conflicting.

Medical management may include nonsteroidal antiinflammatory drugs, or the physician may elect to inject the area with a corticosteroid to reduce pain and swelling.[11] Failure of nonoperative treatment and the presence of thenar intrinsic muscle atrophy are indications for surgical intervention. In surgery, the transverse carpal ligament is divided, and any inflammatory tissue is removed. The wrist is immobilized for 1 to 2 weeks, but digit ROM can begin immediately. The patient is taught to avoid simultaneous wrist and finger flexion to avoid bowstringing of the flexor tendons. Nerve gliding and differential tendon gliding exercises (Fig. 23-30) are emphasized to avoid adhesions.

When healing permits, scar massage is initiated, and silicon can be used. Gradual, controlled weight bearing on the palm is also helpful. The patient should be informed that full weight bearing may be painful for 6 months. Strengthening is started after suture removal and progressed as tolerated. Return to work should include patient education to avoid possible contributing factors as described earlier.

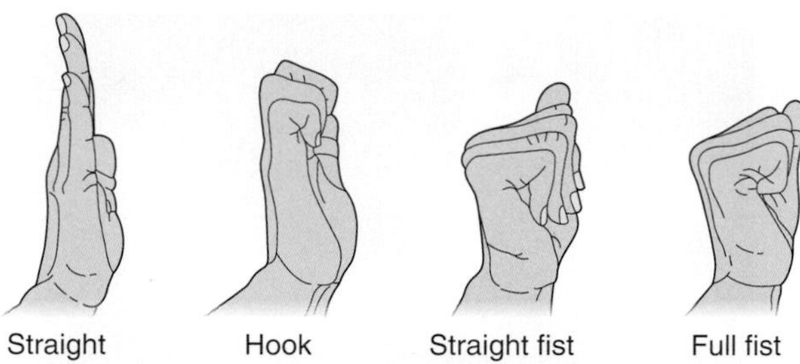

FIG 23-30 Nerve gliding and differential tendon gliding exercises. *(From Hayes EP, Carney K, Wolf J, et al: Carpal tunnel syndrome. In Skirven T, Osterman A, Fedorczyk J, et al:* Rehabilitation of the hand and upper extremity, *ed 6, St Louis, 2011, Mosby.)*

COMPLEX REGIONAL PAIN SYNDROME

One of the most difficult problems in hand rehabilitation is the treatment of CRPS. This term is used for clinical conditions in which the pain resulting from an injury is abnormally severe or prolonged compared with a normal postinjury response. CRPS includes the conditions reflex sympathetic dystrophy and causalgia, and these terms are no longer used.[24,55] CRPS is subdivided into type 1, without a nerve injury, and type 2, with a nerve injury. Both of these categories are further subdivided based on the presence or absence of sympathetic nerve involvement.[24]

Signs and Symptoms

The presentation of CRPS is variable, but there are four primary characteristics:

- Pain: This can range from localized pain to a delayed, abnormally painful reaction to light touch that extends beyond the actual location of the stimulus.[24,55] Patients often cannot tolerate any spontaneous touch; even air blowing on the extremity can produce extreme pain.
- Trophic changes: Atrophy results in differences in hair and nail growth; shiny, tight skin; loss of fat pads in the fingertips; and osteopenia.[24,25,55]
- Autonomic disturbances: The autonomic system controls microvascular perfusion and sweat gland activity. The patient may present with the affected fingers being warm or cool compared with the other side. There may be profuse sweating or extreme dryness of the skin. Edema usually is present. There may be dramatic color changes from pale and cyanotic to mottled to red and warm, all within the same treatment session. Increased sympathetic nerve activity may also lead to increased pilomotor activity (goose bumps).[24,25,55]
- Functional impairment: The patient is reluctant to use the hand or entire extremity because of pain. Fine and gross coordination are disturbed. A typical, imbalanced hand posture is assumed with the MP joints in extension and PIP joints in either flexion or extension. The patient may have difficulty localizing tactile stimuli and may have an altered perception of his or her own hand, regarding it as foreign.[16]

Incidence

CRPS is seen in both sexes but is most prevalent in 30- to 55-year-old women. There is a higher incidence in smokers. The most common injury associated with CRPS is fracture of the distal radius and ulna.[24] Patients often report a tight cast as their first sign of discomfort. Other surgeries complicated by postoperative CRPS include carpal tunnel release, first extensor compartment release, distal ulna surgery, and dermofasciectomy for Dupuytren's disease.[24]

Diagnosis

The diagnosis is made based on clinical criteria; early recognition and treatment are the best predictors of pain relief and functional recovery.[24] Bone scans, radiographs, cold stress tests, and microvascular perfusion tests contribute to confirmation of the diagnosis.[24,55] Evaluations of pain threshold, fine and gross coordination, grip strength, and ROM by the PT provide additional information.[24,25,55] The use of agents that interrupt the sympathetic nervous system differentiate types of CRPS, and these agents are used as part of the treatment when the sympathetic system is implicated.[24,25,54]

Treatment

A multidisciplinary approach including a surgeon, internist, pain specialist, PT, PTA, and psychologist or psychiatrist is recommended.[24,25,55] Pharmacologic management falls into two categories: (1) analgesics to relieve pain and (2) drugs that affect the sympathetic nerves, such as antidepressants and corticosteroids.[24,25] Surgery may be considered to correct the underlying source of pain if it is identified; this can be a nerve entrapment, neuroma, or joint derangement.[24]

The PTA is in the optimal position to observe and report the patient's response to treatment and may be the first clinician to notice the onset of symptoms. Care should be taken to avoid increasing the symptoms. Pain control must be implemented before therapy can progress. Pain control may be helped by the use of heat or cold modalities, contrast baths in which extremes of temperature are avoided, transcutaneous electrical nerve stimulation, continuous passive motion, and hydrotherapy. Desensitization programs and sensory reeducation techniques can help. Graded motor imagery, a program designed to improve cortical organization through the use of laterality training, imagined hand movements, and mirror visual feedback, has shown promise as an intervention (Fig. 23-31).[38] Edema should be treated through positioning, compression garments, and intermittent compression pumps because the patient may not tolerate retrograde massage.

The entire limb should be treated with special attention to the shoulder because adhesive capsulitis is frequently present.[54] Maintenance of motion is a primary goal. Splints are used between exercise sessions to help prevent contractures and reduce pain. Active ROM with special attention to the MP and PIP joints, isometrics, and gentle pain-free passive ROM can be used. Light bimanual activities can help integrate the involved extremity and restore movement patterns. Aerobic activities to increase cardiac output may help stabilize the vasomotor system and assist the patient to feel some physical accomplishment. Joint mobilization is not indicated and can be detrimental. Positive results have been reported for stress loading programs. These programs use active distraction and compression of

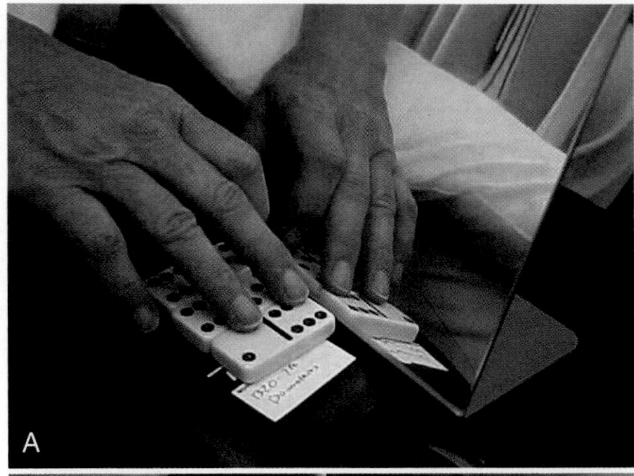

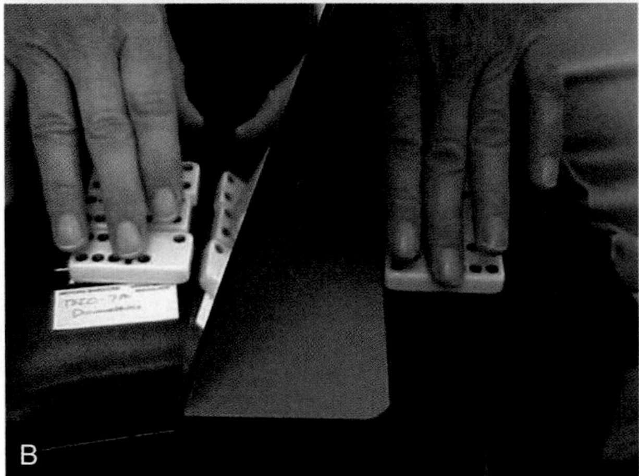

FIG 23-31 Mirror imagery. **A,** The unaffected hand is placed in front of the mirror. In the mirror, the right hand looks like the left affected hand. **B,** The patient watches the mirror image and receives positive visual feedback that the affected hand is moving normally. *(From Skirven T, Osterman A, Fedorczyk J, et al:* Rehabilitation of the hand and upper extremity, *ed 6, Philadelphia, 2011, Mosby.)*

the extremity during which the patient alternates weight-bearing scrubbing with weighted carrying. This approach provides proprioceptive input to the extremity without joint motion.[49]

The treatment of patients with CRPS requires patience and creativity on the part of the PTA. Recovery is usually gradual and is dependent on the full, active participation of the patient.

MOBILIZATION OF THE WRIST AND HAND

The term *joint mobilization* is used to describe skilled passive movements of the joints applied by a PT at varying speeds and amplitudes to reduce pain and improve motion.[2] These techniques use arthrokinematic motions or "joint play" motions that cannot be isolated by the patient actively but are necessary to achieve the physiologic motions at joints. The specific applications of these techniques are determined by the PT; however, evidence-based guidelines have not been established.[14]

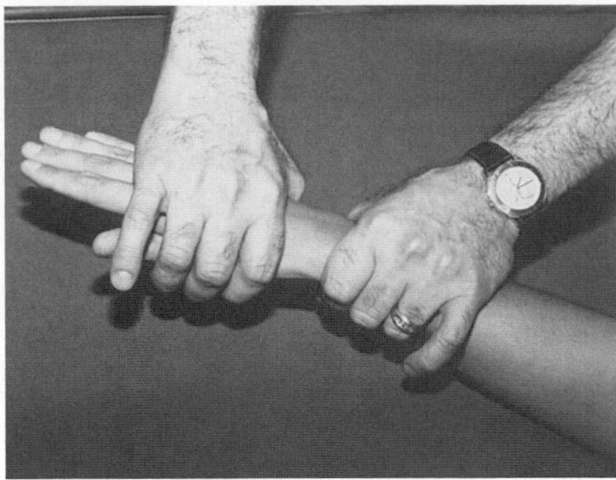

FIG 23-32 Anterior-posterior, medial, and lateral glides of the wrist.

Heat modalities, electrical stimulation, and gentle active exercise can be used immediately before mobilization to encourage soft tissue relaxation and evacuation of waste from the injured area. The position of the patient is a critical feature of effective mobilization. The injured extremity must be positioned to provide comfort, relaxation, and support, while affording the clinician access to the extremity.

As with other joints, many different techniques are used. This discussion introduces only a few of the more common and easily performed techniques. The intricate and complex nature of the wrist and hand demands mastery of anatomy, kinesiology, pathomechanics of injury, and arthrokinematics for effective performance of the more difficult techniques described in orthopedic texts.

MOBILIZATION OF THE WRIST

There are two primary joints at the wrist, the radiocarpal and the midcarpal. Both of these joints are convex on concave (distal on proximal). The intercarpal joints have a smaller contribution to overall wrist motion.[35] Anterior, posterior, medial, and lateral glides of the wrist are performed with the patient either sitting with the affected arm supported or supine. The PT uses one hand to stabilize the proximal bones while moving the distal row of carpal bones with the other hand (Fig. 23-32).[53] The movements are graded by amplitude and by the amount of available motion they use. A grade 1 movement is a small-amplitude movement in the beginning of the available range, and a grade 5 movement is a small-amplitude movement at the end of the available range of movement.[14]

Distraction of the wrist can be done with the patient either sitting or supine. The hand position is exactly the same as described for performing glides, but the direction of force is distal or longitudinal to the radius and ulna. This direction of force moves the carpal bones away from the stabilized radius and ulna (Fig. 23-33).[53]

MOBILIZATION OF THE HAND

Anterior, posterior, medial, and lateral glides of the MP joint can be performed with the patient supine or sitting. The PT uses one hand to stabilize the shaft of the affected

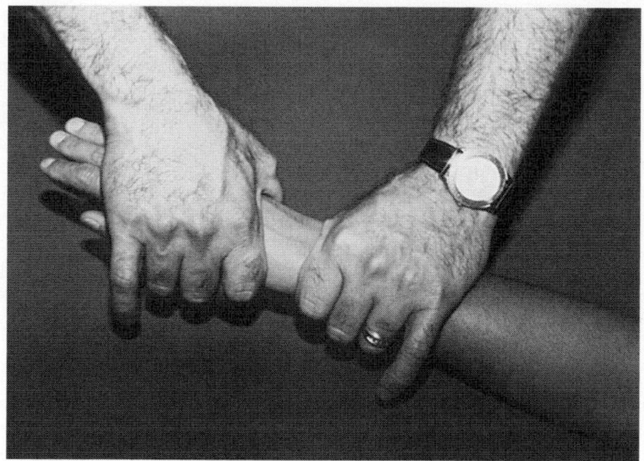

FIG 23-33 Long-axis or longitudinal distraction of the wrist.

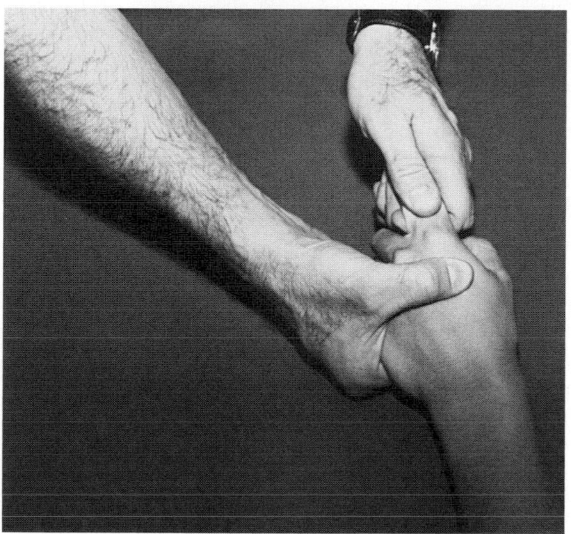

FIG 23-34 Anterior-posterior, medial, and lateral glides of the metacarpophalangeal joint.

metacarpal while firmly grasping the proximal phalanx with the other hand. With the metacarpal firmly stabilized, the hand contacting the phalanx can direct an anterior, posterior, or medial and lateral force that glides the MP joint (Fig. 23-34).[53]

Distraction of the MP joint is performed with the patient supine or sitting. With the hand placement the same as for glides, the direction of force is applied to distract the phalanx from the stabilized metacarpal (Fig. 23-35).[53] Anterior and posterior glides of the IP joint can be performed with the joint in slight flexion. Active or passive physiologic movement of the joint usually follows the mobilization.

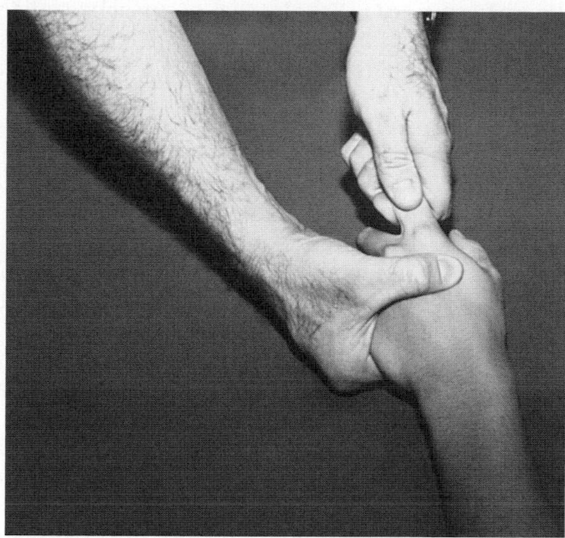

FIG 23-35 Long-axis or longitudinal distraction of the metacarpophalangeal joint.

GLOSSARY

Bennett fracture: Fracture of the palmar base of the proximal first metacarpal.

Boxer's fracture: Fracture of the neck of the fourth or fifth metacarpal caused by a strike to a hard object with a clenched fist.

Carpal tunnel syndrome: A group of symptoms that occur when the median nerve is compressed or entrapped at the wrist.

Colles fracture: A radius fracture within 2.5 cm of the wrist in which the distal fragment is displaced in a dorsal direction.

Complex regional pain syndrome (CRPS): A condition in which pain after an injury or surgery is disproportionate or prolonged beyond that of a typical response.

Compression neuropathy: Disorder that occurs when adjacent structures constrict a peripheral nerve, limiting its blood supply and resulting in impaired nerve conduction.

De Quervain's disease: Tenosynovitis or tendinosis of the abductor pollicis longus and extensor pollicis brevis tendons and sheaths near the radial styloid characterized by pain in the radial side of the wrist and thumb, especially with use.

Dinner fork deformity: A deformity seen after Colles fracture with the position of the wrist and forearm resembling a dinner fork.

Dupuytren's disease: A disease process in which the balance of collagen formation and breakdown is disrupted leading to excess collagen that is seen in the palm as thickening, pits, and nodules; this can lead to Dupuytren's contracture, a flexion contracture of one or more digits that is due to the collagen deposited and the action of myofibroblasts.

Extrinsic muscle system: Muscles acting on the joints of the wrist and hand that originate in the arm and insert in the hand.

Intrinsic muscle system: Muscles acting on the joints of the hand and wrist that originate and insert within the hand and wrist.

Mallet finger: Interruption of the extensor tendon mechanism over the distal interphalangeal joint.

Nerve entrapment: Disorder that occurs when adjacent tissue restricts gliding of the nerve. The nerve is subjected to stretch that can result in paresthesias and pain.

Smith fracture: A type of fracture also known as a *reverse Colles fracture* that occurs from a fall on the dorsum of the hand, with the resultant distal radial fragment displaced in a palmar direction.

Tendinitis: Inflammation of a tendon.

Tendinosis: A degeneration of tendon cells without inflammation; this is usually a chronic process that leads to decreased tendon strength.

Tendovaginitis: Inflammation of the tendon sheath.

Trigger finger: Resistance to motion in a finger as a result of narrowing of the pulley system and enlargement of the tendon. The finger can become stuck in a bent position and requires additional force to extend it.

Triangular fibrocartilage complex (TFCC): A structure between the ulna and the ulnar carpal bones composed of an articular disk and ligaments that helps stabilize the distal radial ulnar joint and protects the ulnar carpal bones, especially during compressive loading.

REFERENCES

1. Amadio PC, Taleisnik J: Fractures of the carpal bones. In Green DP, Hotchkiss RN, Pederson WC, editors: *Green's operative hand surgery*, Philadelphia, 1999, Churchill Livingstone.
2. American Physical Therapy Association: Guide to Physical Therapist Practice. Second Edition. American Physical Therapy Association. *Phys Ther* 81:9–746, 2001.
3. American Society of Hand Therapists: *Clinical Assessment and Recommendations*, Chicago, 1992, American Society of Hand Therapists.
4. Ashe MC, McCauley T, Khan KM: Tendinopathies in the upper extremity: a paradigm shift. *J Hand Ther* 17:329–334, 2004.
5. Badalamente MA, Hurst LC: Efficacy and safety of injectable mixed collagenase subtypes in the treatment of Dupyutren's contracture. *J Hand Surg [Am]* 32:767–774, 2007.
6. Berger RA: Anatomy and kinesiology of the wrist. In Skirven TM, Osterman AL, Fedorczyk JM, et al, editors: *Rehabilitation of the hand and upper extremity*, Philadelphia, 2011, Mosby.
7. Brach P, Goitz R: An update on the management of carpal fractures. *J Hand Ther* 16:152–160, 2003.
8. Brand PW, Hollister AM, Agee JM: Transmission. In Brand PW, Hollister AM, editors: *Clinical mechanics of the hand*, St Louis, 1999, Mosby.
9. Davis P, Eaton C: Hand therapy for Dupuytren's contracture. In Eaton C, Seegenschmiedt MH, Bayat A, et al, editors: *Dupuytren's disease and related hyperproliferative disorders*, Berlin, 2012, Springer-Verlag.
10. Evans RB: Clinical management of extensor tendon injuries: the therapist's perspective. In Skirven TM, Osterman AL, Fedorczyk JM, et al, editors: *Rehabilitation of the hand and upper extremity*, Philadelphia, 2011, Mosby.
11. Evans RB: Therapist's management of carpal tunnel syndrome: a practical approach. In Skirven TM, Osterman AL, Fedorczyk JM, et al, editors: *Rehabilitation of the hand and upper extremity*, Philadelphia, 2011, Mosby.
12. Evans RB, Dell PC, Fioldowski P: A clinical report of the effect of mechanical stress on functional results after fasciectomy for Dupuytren's contracture. *J Hand Ther* 15:331–339, 2002.
13. Evans RB, Hunter JM, Burkhalter WE: Conservative management of trigger finger: a new approach. *J Hand Ther* 2:59–68, 1988.
14. Fedorczyk F: Manual therapy in the management of upper extremity musculoskeletal disorders. In Skirven TM, Osterman AL, Fedorczyk JM, et al, editors: *Rehabilitation of the hand and upper extremity*, Philadelphia, 2011, Mosby.
15. Fernandez DL, Palmer AK: Fractures of the distal radius. In Green DP, Hotchkiss RN, Pederson WC, editors: *Green's operative hand surgery*, Philadelphia, 1999, Churchill Livingstone.
16. Forderreuther S, Sailer U, Straube A: Impaired self-perception of the hand in complex regional pain syndrome. *Pain* 110:756–761, 2004.
17. Forget N, Piotte F, Bourbonnais D, et al: Thumb strength and mobility in de Quervain's disease. *J Hand Ther* 19:441–442, 2006.
18. Freedland AE, Hardy MA, Singletary S: Rehabilitation for proximal phalangeal fractures. *J Hand Ther* 16:129–142, 2003.
19. Frykman GK, Kropp WE: Fractures and traumatic conditions of the wrist. In Hunter JM, Mackin EJ, Callahan AD, editors: *Rehabilitation of the hand: surgery and therapy*, St Louis, 1995, Mosby.
20. Glickel SZ, Barron OA, Eaton RG: Dislocations and ligament injuries in the digits. In Green DP, Hotchkiss RN, Pederson WC, editors: *Green's operative hand surgery*, Philadelphia, 1999, Churchill Livingstone.
21. Hurst L: Dupuytren's disease: surgical management. In Skirven TM, Osterman AL, Fedorczyk JM, et al, editors: *Rehabilitation of the hand and upper extremity*, Philadelphia, 2011, Mosby.
22. Jerosch-Herold C, Shepstone L, Chojnowski AJ, et al: Night-time splinting after fasciectomy or dermofasciectomy for Dupuytren's contracture: a pragmatic, multi-centre, randomized controlled trial. In Eaton C, Seegenschmiedt MH, Bayat A, et al, editors: *Dupuytren's disease and related hyperproliferative disorders*, Berlin, 2012, Springer-Verlag.
23. Kapandji AI: Clinical evaluation of the thumb's opposition. *J Hand Ther* 5:102–106, 1992.
24. Koman AL, Poehling GG, Smith TL: Complex regional pain syndrome: reflex sympathetic dystrophy and causalgia. In Green DP, Hotchkiss RN, Pederson WC, editors: *Green's operative hand surgery*, Philadelphia, 1999, Churchill Livingstone.
25. Lankford LL: Reflex sympathetic dystrophy. In Hunter JM, Mackin EJ, Callahan AD, editors: *Rehabilitation of the hand: surgery and therapy*, St Louis, 1995, Mosby.
26. La Stayo PC, Lee MJ: The forearm complex: anatomy, biomechanics and clinical considerations. *J Hand Ther* 19:137–145, 2006.
27. Lawrence WT: Physiology of the acute wound. *Clin Plast Surg* 25:321–340, 1998.
28. Lee MP, Biafora SJ, Zelouf DS: Management of hand and wrist tendinopathies. In Skirven TM, Osterman AL, Fedorczyk JM, et al, editors: *Rehabilitation of the hand and upper extremity*, Philadelphia, 2011, Mosby.
29. Maihafer GC, Llewellyn MA, Pillar WJ, et al: A Comparison of the figure-of-eight method and water volumetry in measurement of hand and wrist size. *J Hand Ther* 16:305–310, 2003.
30. McGrouther DA: Dupuytren's contracture. In Green DP, Hotchkiss RN, Pederson WC, editors: *Green's operative hand surgery*, Philadelphia, 1999, Churchill Livingstone.
31. McNemar TB, Howell JW, Chang E: Management of metacarpal fractures. *J Hand Ther* 16:143–151, 2003.
32. Melone CP: Fractures of the wrist. In Nicholas JA, Hershman EB, editors: *The upper extremity in sports medicine*, St Louis, 1990, Mosby.
33. Meyer FM, Wilson RL: Management of non-articular fractures of the hand. In Hunter JM, Mackin EJ, Callahan AD, editors: *Rehabilitation of the hand: surgery and therapy*, St Louis, 1995, Mosby.
34. Muller M, Tsui D, Schnurr R, et al: Effectiveness of hand therapy interventions in primary management of carpal tunnel syndrome: a systematic review. *J Hand Ther* 17:210–228, 2004.
35. Neumann DA: *Kinesiology of the musculoskeletal system*, St Louis, 2010, Mosby.
36. Page S, Stern PJ: Complications and range of motion following plate fixation of metacarpal and phalangeal fractures. *J Hand Surg [Am]* 23:827–832, 1998.
37. Pratt NE: Anatomy and kinesiology of the hand. In Skirven TM, Osterman AL, Fedorczyk JM, et al, editors: *Rehabilitation of the hand and upper extremity*, Philadelphia, 2011, Mosby.

38. Priganc VW, Stralka SW: Graded motor imagery. *J Hand Ther* 24:164–169, 2011.
39. Prosser R, Conolly WB: Complications following surgical treatment for Dupuytren's contracture. *J Hand Ther* 9:344–348, 1996.
40. Reiss B: Therapists' management of distal radial fractures. In Hunter JM, Mackin EJ, Callahan AD, editors: *Rehabilitation of the hand: surgery and therapy*, St Louis, 1995, Mosby.
41. Rohrich RJ: The biology of wound healing. Techniques of wound closure, abnormal scars, evenomation, Select Readings in Plastic Surgery 5:1, 1988.
42. Rosenthal EA, Elhassan BT: The extensor tendons: evaluation and surgical management. In Skirven TM, Osterman AL, Fedorczyk JM, et al, editors: *Rehabilitation of the hand and upper extremity*, Philadelphia, 2011, Mosby.
43. Ross DC: Epidemiology of Dupuytren's disease. *Hand Clin* 15:53–62, 1999.
44. Singletary S, Freeland AE, Jarrett CA: Metacarpal fractures in athletes: treatment, rehabilitation and safe early return to play. *J Hand Ther* 16:171–179, 2003.
45. Stern PJ: Fractures of the metacarpals and phalanges. In Green DP, Hotchkiss RN, Pederson WC, editors: *Green's operative hand surgery*, Philadelphia, 1999, Churchill Livingstone.
46. Stewart KM, Van Strien G: Postoperative management of flexor tendon injuries. In Hunter JM, Mackin EJ, Callahan AD, editors: *Rehabilitation of the hand: surgery and therapy*, St Louis, 1995, Mosby.
47. Szabo RM: Entrapment and compression neuropathies. In Green DP, Hotchkiss RN, Pederson WC, editors: *Green's operative hand surgery*, Philadelphia, 1999, Churchill Livingstone.
48. Valdes K: A retrospective review to determine the long-term efficacy of orthotic devices for trigger finger. *J Hand Ther* 25:89–96, 2012.
49. Watson HK, Carlson L: Treatment of reflex sympathetic dystrophy of the hand with an active "stress loading" program. *J Hand Surg [Am]* 12:779–785, 1987.
50. Wilgis EFS, Yates AY: Wrist pain. In Nicholas JA, Hershman EB, editors: *The Upper Extremity in Sports Medicine*, St Louis, 1990, Mosby.
51. Wilson RL, Hazen J: Management of joint injuries and intraarticular fractures of the hand. In Hunter JM, Mackin EJ, Callahan AD, editors: *Rehabilitation of the hand: surgery and therapy*, St Louis, 1995, Mosby.
52. Wolfe SW: Tenosynovitis. In Green DP, Hotchkiss RN, Pederson WC, editors: *Green's operative hand surgery*, Philadelphia, 1999, Churchill Livingstone.
53. Wooden MJ: Mobilization of the upper extremity. In Donatelli RA, Wooden MJ, editors: *Orthopaedic Physical Therapy*, New York, 1989, Churchill Livingstone.
54. Wright HH, Rettig AC: Management of common sports injuries. In Hunter JM, Mackin EJ, Callahan AD, editors: *Rehabilitation of the hand: surgery and therapy*, St Louis, 1995, Mosby.
55. Zhongyu L, Smith BP, Smith TL, et al: Diagnosis and management of complex regional pain syndrome complicating upper extremity recovery. *J Hand Ther* 18:270–276, 2005.

REVIEW QUESTIONS

Multiple Choice

1. Immediate postoperative rehabilitation after dermofasciectomy for Dupuytren's disease should include which of the following?
   a. Wound care
   b. Active ROM
   c. Stretching
   d. All of the above
   e. a and b
2. Therapy for a 3-week-old mallet injury on the ring finger should include:
   a. Isolated active ROM of the adjacent finger joints.
   b. Isolated active ROM of the ring finger PIP joint.
   c. Splinting of the ring finger DIP at night only.
   d. Splinting of the ring finger DIP and PIP at all times for 6 weeks.
3. A Bennett fracture is a fracture of the:
   a. Volar base of the first metacarpal.
   b. Head of the fourth or fifth metacarpals.
   c. Distal phalanx of the thumb.
   d. Scaphoid.
4. A patient's index finger active ROM measured with the wrist in neutral is as follows: MP, 0°/75°, PIP, −25°/90°, DIP, −10°/45°. What is the total active motion?
   a. 210°
   b. 245°
   c. 175°
   d. 185°
5. A patient complains that she is unable to abduct her fifth finger. Which of the following injuries is consistent with this presentation?
   a. Laceration of the flexor digitorum profundus to the fifth digit
   b. Bennett fracture
   c. Laceration of the extensor digiti minimi
   d. Laceration of the ulnar nerve at the wrist
6. Which of the following lesions would be the most limiting for patient function?
   a. Radial nerve laceration at the wrist
   b. Ulnar digital nerve laceration at the middle finger PIP joint
   c. Median nerve laceration at the wrist
   d. Radial digital nerve laceration at the index finger proximal phalanx
7. The signs of inflammation are:
   a. Pain, warmth, redness, and swelling.
   b. Bleeding, swelling, perspiration, and loss of sensation.
   c. Blisters, swelling, pale skin, and stiffness.
   d. Pus, swelling, pain, and increased perspiration.
8. Which of the following statements bests describes Colles fracture?
   a. One or more of the carpal bones is broken.
   b. The distal ulna is fractured and displaced ulnarly.
   c. The distal radius is fractured and displaced radially.
   d. The distal radius is fractured, and the distal fragment is displaced dorsally.
9. Which of the following statements about skier's thumb is not true?
   a. The thumb IP joint can begin active ROM immediately.
   b. Surgery is always required to treat these injuries.
   c. The injury occurs from hyperextension and abduction of the thumb MP joint.
   d. The patient is placed in a thumb spica splint or cast for 3 to 4 weeks.
10. Which of the following terms describes de Quervain's disease?
   a. Fibroplasia
   b. Neuritis
   c. Tinnitus
   d. Tendovaginitis

11. Which of the following is not a typical approach to the treatment of flexor tendon lacerations in zone 2?
    a. Immobilization for 3 to 4 weeks followed by active and passive exercises
    b. Early active mobilization in a specific, specified range
    c. Early active strengthening within the splint
    d. Early passive mobilization with the splint
12. Which of the following muscles is not affected by CTS?
    a. Adductor pollicis
    b. Opponens pollicis
    c. Flexor pollicis brevis
    d. Abductor pollicis brevis
13. CRPS:
    a. Always involves an injury to a peripheral sensory nerve.
    b. Produces pain proportional to the extent of the tissue injury.
    c. Is more prevalent in left-handed men.
    d. Is most commonly seen after distal radius and ulnar fractures.
14. Which one of the following is not a sign or symptom of CRPS?
    a. Inflammation
    b. Trophic changes
    c. Loss of hand function
    d. Profuse sweating of the fingers
15. Nonsurgical treatment of a boxer's fracture includes:
    a. Splinting the wrist and MP and IP joints of the affected digit.
    b. Edema control.
    c. Immediate active ROM of the IP joints of the affected digits.
    d. Immobilization of the wrist and MP joint of the affected digit.
    e. b, c, and d
    f. a and b

Short Answer

16. Name the most common compression neuropathy of the wrist and describe symptoms associated with it.
17. Demonstrate the "six-pack" exercises.
18. Identify the injuries or deformities in the following figures.

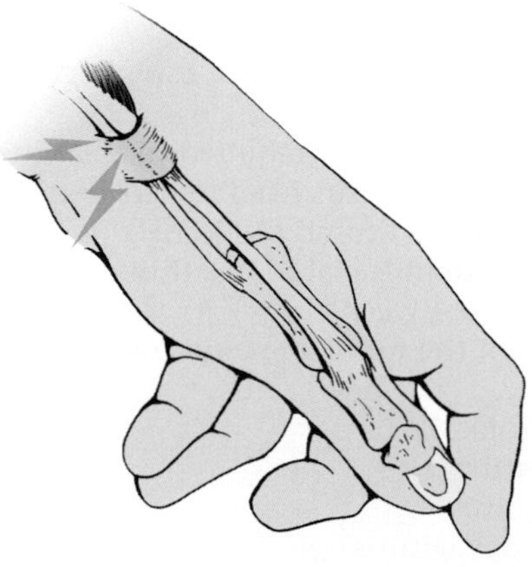

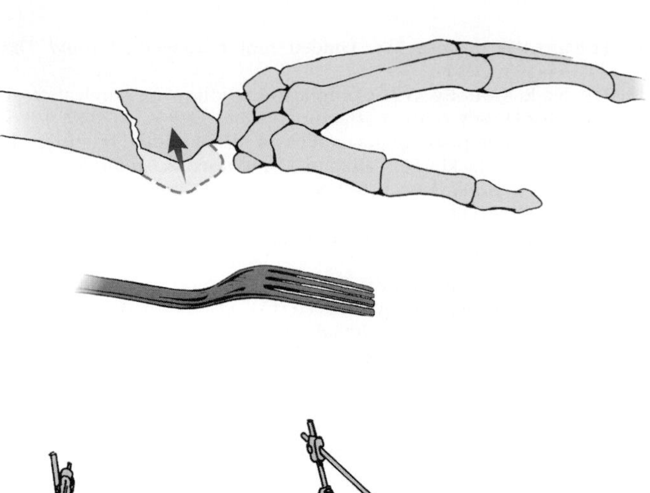

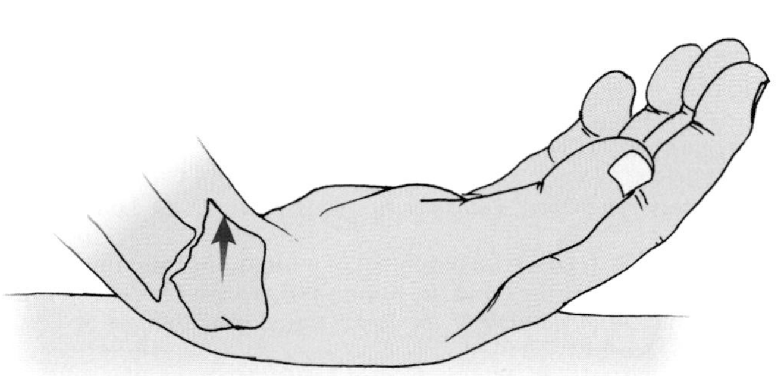

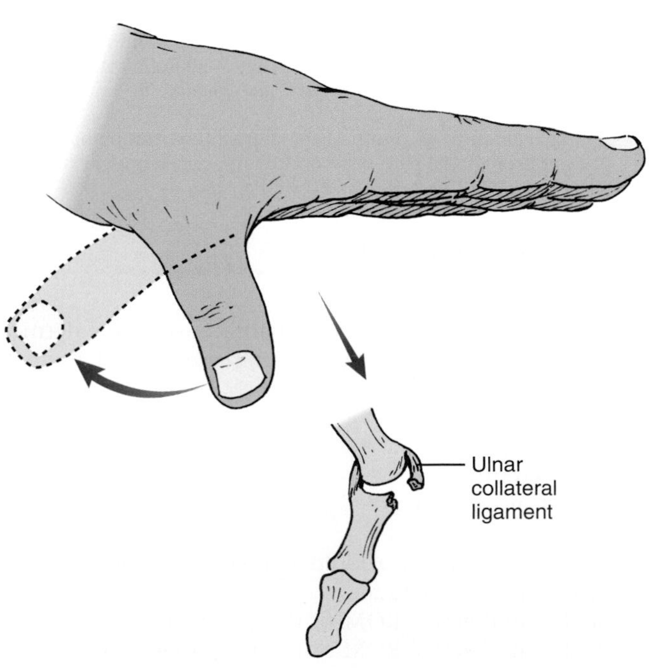

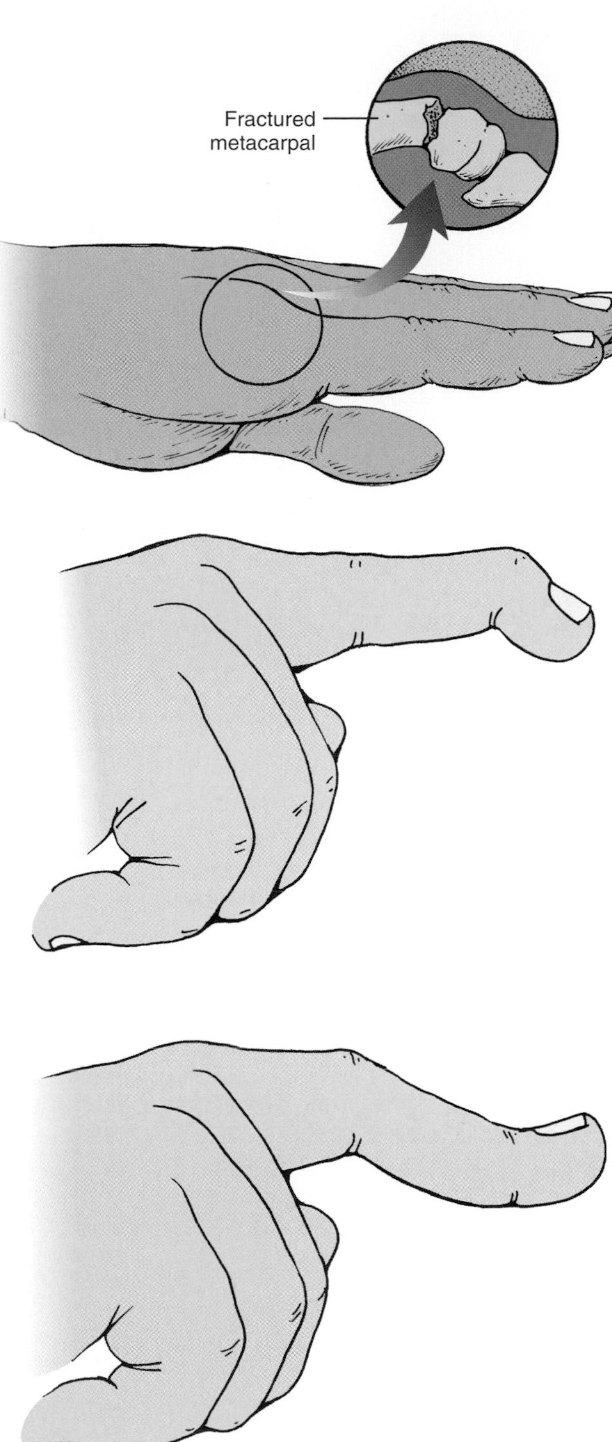

19. Describe the conservative approach to treating trigger finger.
20. Name five intrinsic muscles of the hand.

Fill in the Blank

21. The intrinsic muscles of the hand are innervated by the _________ and the ________ nerves.
22. A fall on the palm with the forearm pronated can result in a tear of the _________.
23. Working on finger active ROM by strapping two fingers together is called __________.
24. A rupture or avulsion fracture of the extensor tendon that results in a DIP joint flexion contracture is called ______________.
25. A rupture or stretch of the central extensor tendon at the PIP joint that creates PIP flexion with DIP extension is called a ________________.

True/False

26. Generally, motions that produce repetitive ulnar deviations can create tenosynovitis at the first dorsal compartment of the wrist.
27. The stability of the carpals depends primarily on musculotendinous support and intracapsular ligaments.
28. Active ROM of the fingers in a patient with Colles fracture should start when the cast is removed.
29. Although occasionally tender nodules are present, Dupuytren's disease is commonly not painful.
30. There is usually a direct relationship between the severity of injury and the degree of pain experienced by people with CRPS.

Part V

Management of Orthopedic Patients by Condition

In this section, the physical therapist assistant (PTA) is introduced to essential, common, and foundational principles of rheumatic diseases; pain management; and components of bracing, orthotics, and prosthetics. New to the fourth edition is a chapter on "Orthopedic Management Concepts Specific to Women." Within the daily provision of physical therapy practice, spanning most settings, the PTA will be exposed to and responsible for the delivery of services related to rheumatic disease and pain; the application of bracing, orthotics, and prosthetics; and treatment of pelvic floor dysfunctions in female patients. The management of these critical conditions and provision of physical therapy services require knowledge of sound scientific principles of anatomy, physiology, and pathomechanics. However, most important is the sober and responsible application of treatment strategies delivered under the direction of the supervising physical therapist, which is addressed in this section.

Consistent with the body of information in this text, the PTA is presented information related to foundations of disease processes and pathology of rheumatic diseases as well as neuroanatomy and pathophysiology of pain management. The PTA is introduced to the materials, components, use, and application of various braces, orthotics and prosthetics. In Chapter 27, the PTA is introduced to treatment concepts specific to women and the pelvic floor. Foremost in this section is the relevant clinical application of therapeutic interventions in light of the basic science motif established and endorsed throughout the text.

In the study of this section, students and clinicians are strongly encouraged to review Part II ("Review of Tissue Healing," Chapters 8 through 13), Part III ("Basis for Movement," Chapters 14 through 16), and Part IV ("Management of Orthopedic Patients by Region," Chapters 17 through 23) carefully and thoroughly. Each of these sections provides the essential material on which to ground practical, functional, and purposeful interventions using established basic science knowledge of tissue healing, biomechanics, and orthopedic pathologic conditions.

Chapter 24

Orthopedic Management of Rheumatic Disorders

Steven Elliott

CHAPTER OUTLINE

LEARNING OBJECTIVES

1. Discuss different types of arthritis.
2. Discuss similarities and differences of osteoarthritis and rheumatoid arthritis.
3. Discuss the effects and benefits and limitations of exercise for patients with arthritis.
4. Discuss common methods of medical management and rehabilitation of arthritic conditions.
5. Discuss principles of joint protection.
6. Discuss pathophysiology of rheumatic disorders.

KEY TERMS

Atrophy
Closed chain exercises
Connective tissue
Infection
Inflammation
Malaise
Open chain exercises
Proteoglycan

Arthritis affects the lives of 50 million Americans, and it is the leading cause of disability in American adults.[13] The U.S. Centers for Disease Control and Prevention estimated that by 2020 nearly 60 million people would be affected by rheumatic disease, which is a blanket term covering more than 100 different conditions that may cause pain, stiffness, and sometimes swelling in or around joints.[2,22] Individuals with arthritis can experience pain, joint stiffness, swelling, and overall decrease in functional ability.[34] The causes of arthritis are not fully understood. The prevalence of arthritis increases with age, and it is more commonly found in women than in men.[22,34]

ARTHRITIS

OSTEOARTHRITIS

Osteoarthritis (OA) is the most common form of arthritis[6,10,14] and is considered to be a painful and disabling joint disorder.[2,22,27,38] There is no single cause of OA; a combination of biomechanical, metabolic, and genetic

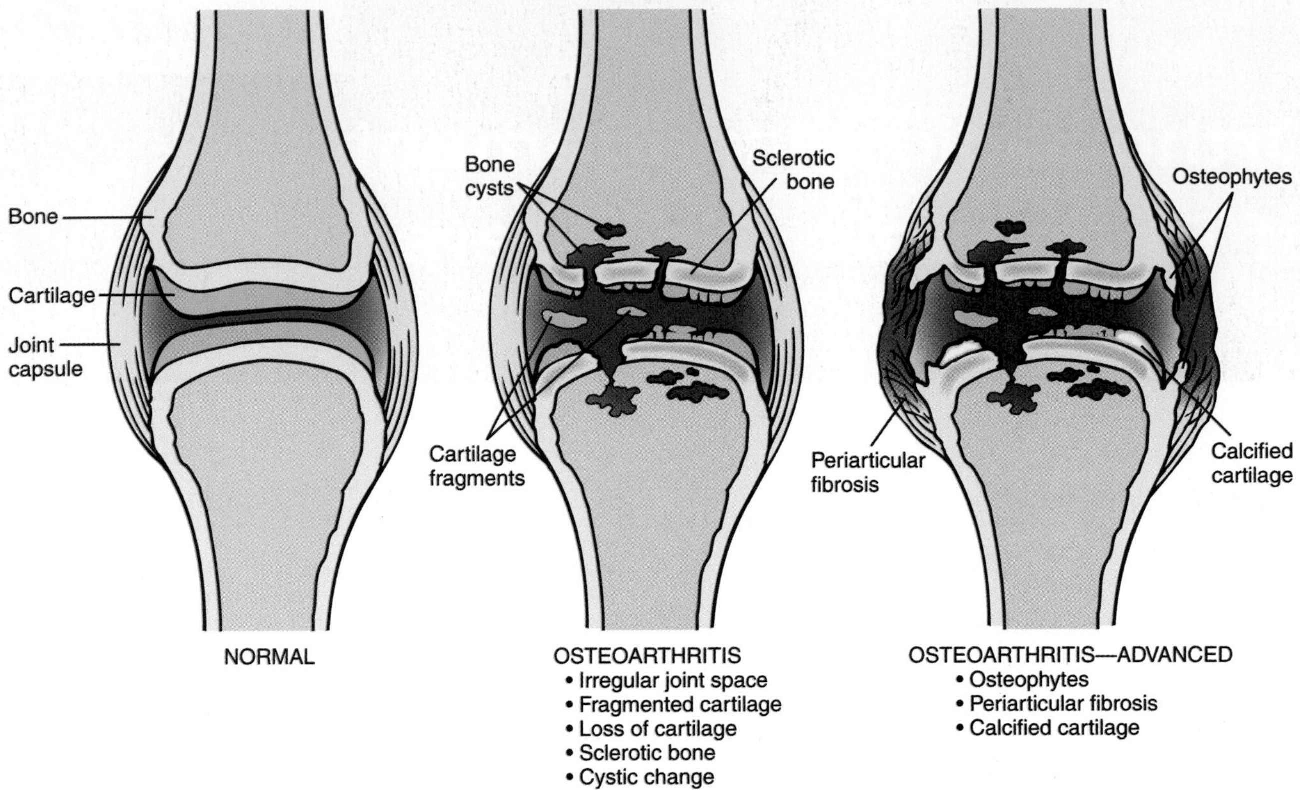

FIG 24-1 Schematic presentation of the pathologic changes in osteoarthritis. Fragmentation and loss of cartilage denude the subchondral bone, which undergoes sclerosis and cystic change. Osteophytes form on the lateral side and protrude into the adjacent soft tissues, causing irritation, inflammation, and fibrosis. *(From Damjanov I:* Pathology for the health professions, *ed 4, St Louis, 2012, Saunders.)*

factors may be causative.[6,10,14,36,38] The prevalence of OA has been shown to increase with age, and OA is more common in women older than 45 years of age.[55] Risk factors associated with OA include obesity, trauma, **infection,** and repeated joint overuse.[2,22,27,38,55]

OA primarily affects the articular cartilage (which is composed of type II collagen, chondrocytes, and proteoglycans) that surrounds the subchondral bone secondary to chemical and mechanical factors (Fig. 24-1).[2,6,10,14,36] Patients with OA have decreased synthesis and increased catabolism of the cartilage matrix. OA initially damages the cartilage, causing it to become thinner and decreasing **proteoglycan** synthesis. Initially, chondrocytes can maintain the cartilaginous matrix (which consists of proteoglycans and collagen), but over time focal **inflammation** of the synovial membrane develops, releasing cytokines, which increase the release of metalloproteinases.[2,6,10,14] Metalloproteinase further breaks down cartilage collagen and proteoglycans.[2,6,10,14,22]

OA most commonly affects weight-bearing joints, such as the knee, hip, or spine.[2,22,34,36,55] Joints in the hands can also be affected; the first carpometacarpal joint, distal and proximal interphalangeal (DIP and PIP) joints, and the first metatarsophalangeal joint are other common sites for OA.[6,10,36] In patients with OA of the hands, Bouchard's and Heberden's nodes, bony overgrowths at the PIP and DIP joints, are often present (Fig. 24-2).[14,27,36,39] Pain associated with OA usually occurs with activity and is relieved with rest.[27,36] Other signs of OA include morning stiffness lasting 20 to 30 minutes, joint locking, a gel sensation in the joint, a bony appearance of the joint, crepitus, and effusion.[18,23] Radiographic imaging can show a progression of subchondral bone sclerosis and cysts, osteophytes, and joint space narrowing.[19,36] Carpal tunnel syndrome can be present in conjunction with OA and rheumatoid arthritis (RA).[39]

Important Concept

Osteoarthritis is a disease that primarily affects the articular cartilage which surrounds the subchondral bone. OA affects many joints but most commonly those that are weight bearing. OA pain usually occurs with activity and is relieved with rest.

Management of Osteoarthritis

Although there is no cure for OA, preventive measures can be taken in hopes of slowing down the progression of the disease and assisting in symptom management. Obesity places extra stress on joints and is a key risk factor that can be prevented or remedied with proper diet and exercise.[10,27,36] Research has shown that every pound of body weight increases the forces in the knee by 2 to 3 pounds during single-leg stance.[52] The addition of vitamin D and calcium to a patient's diet can also reduce the occurrence and progression of OA.[27] Muscle weakness, repetitive motions, or trauma contribute to the onset of OA.[36,55] Studies also have shown that immobilizing the joint for longer than 30 days can increase the risk of cartilage damage.[4] Given the positive and negative effects of

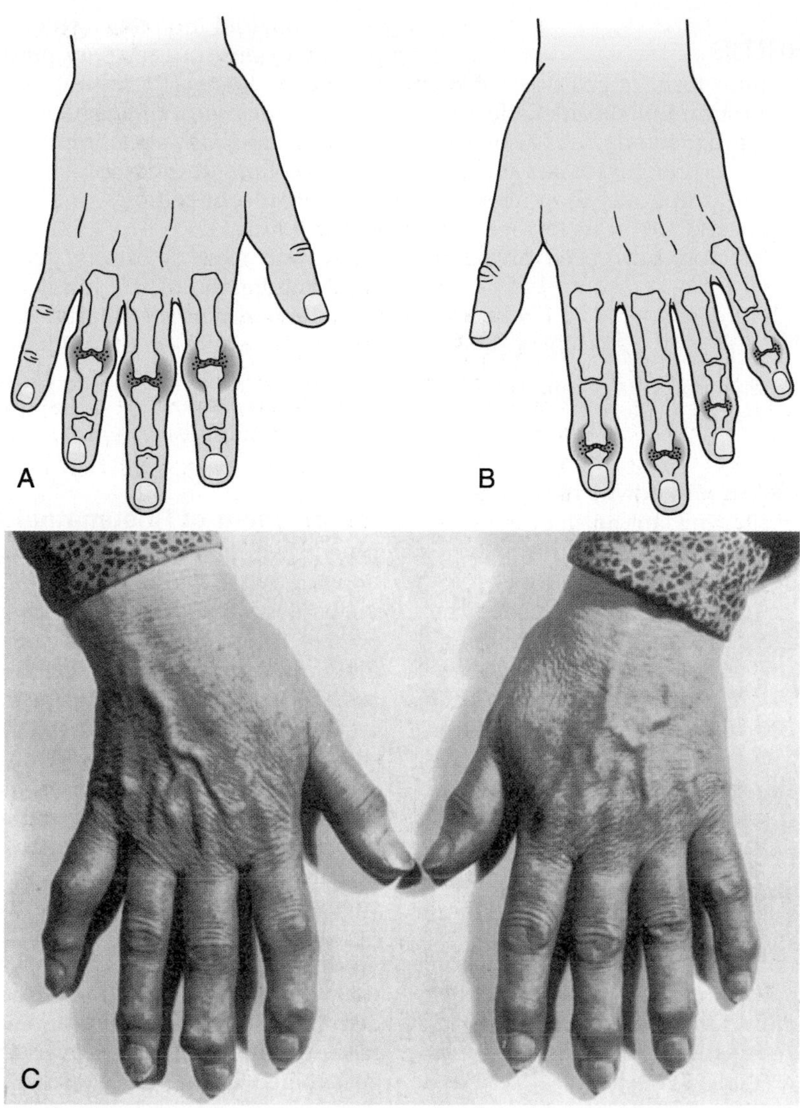

FIG 24-2 Degenerative joint disease (osteoarthritis) of both hands. **A,** Bouchard's nodes. **B,** Heberden's nodes. **C,** Osteoarthritic enlargement of the distal interphalangeal joints (Heberden's nodes) and the proximal interphalangeal joints (Bouchard's nodes) is present. The metacarpophalangeal joints are not affected. *(**A** and **B**, From Magee DJ:* Orthopedic physical assessment, *ed 6, St Louis, 2014, Saunders;* ***C**, from Polley HF, Hunder GG:* Rheumatologic interviewing and physical examination of the joints, *Philadelphia, 1978, Saunders.)*

changes in behavior, it is imperative to educate patients about joint protection, health behavior changes, and the importance of gentle pain-free exercise in the management of arthritis. Patients should be educated about the progression of the disease and the potential benefit of pain management with supportive devices. Joint protection and modalities can also be helpful in the management of symptoms. Exercise should be low impact as opposed to high impact to avoid joint damage and pain.[60]

As mentioned, research has shown that every 1 pound of body weight increases the forces in the knee by 2 to 3 pounds during single-leg stance.[52] Exercise, specifically flexibility and strength training, has been shown to decrease pain and improve function in individuals with OA.[36] Maintaining flexibility is an important first step because it helps decrease stiffness and allows for more comfortable movement.[2] Slow progression of the exercise program is important to avoid exacerbation of symptoms. Patients should be progressed to 15 minutes of stretching without an increase in symptoms before initiating strength training.[2,36] Strength training improves the ability to absorb shock, support joints, and protect from injury.[2,38] When choosing an appropriate exercise, it is important to keep in mind how much stress is being placed on the joint. **Closed chain** weight-bearing **exercises** can create shear and compressive forces across the lower extremity joints and may be a contraindication depending on the severity of OA. **Open chain exercises** are encouraged in patients with OA.

Important Concept

Exercise, specifically flexibility, and strength training have been shown to decrease pain and improve function in those with OA.

RHEUMATOID ARTHRITIS

RA is the second most common form of arthritis.[35] RA is an inflammatory, systemic autoimmune disorder affecting the synovial tissue.[18,50,65] The progression of RA also leads to difficulty with activities of daily living (ADL) and disability. RA affects women more commonly than men and occurs in adults between 20 and 40 years of age.[2,20,27] Genetic and environmental factors have been linked as causes of RA.[1,4,27,63]

Important Concept

Rheumatoid arthritis is an inflammatory, systemic autoimmune disorder affecting the synovial tissue.

The exact etiology of RA is unknown; it is believed to involve a trigger contributing to an autoimmune response.[2,20,50] The immune response causes the body to attack its own tissue, leading to breakdown of joints.[2,20,65] RA affects the synovial lining, which expands, damaging the extracellular matrix, cartilage, and bone.[2,20,38,59] This autoimmune response also activates T cells, which secrete cytokines, causing expansion of the synovial layer. Cytokines increase activation of fibroblastlike cells and macrophages leading to breakdown of cartilage and bone (Fig. 24-3).[2,20,63]

Early signs and symptoms associated with RA include fatigue, weight loss, fever, and musculoskeletal pain. Later signs or symptoms include pain, tenderness, swelling, redness, and stiffness in specific joints.[2,9,20,27,63] In contrast to OA, RA morning stiffness can last hours or all day. Fatigue associated with RA may cause patients to need to rest through the day.[2,63] Extraarticular manifestations can affect the lungs, heart, blood vessels, eyes, skin, and other organs.[2,9,27,65] It is important for the physical therapist assistant (PTA) to be able to distinguish the main differences between OA and RA (Table 24-1).

Rheumatoid nodules, which occur on bony prominences, extensor surfaces, or pressure points, are a unique feature of RA.[2,27,50,65] Several common joint deformities occur at the digits and toes, as follows[49,63]:

- Metacarpophalangeal joints
  - Swelling of the joint
  - Volar subluxation
- PIP joints
  - Swan neck deformity (hyperextension of PIP joint and flexion of DIP joint)
  - Boutonnière deformity (flexion of PIP joint with hyperextension of DIP joint)
- Toes
  - Hallux valgus
  - Hammer toes

Management of Rheumatoid Arthritis

When treating a patient with RA, education and prevention are vital. Some important objectives of physical therapy and occupational therapy have a common theme of prevention: prevent pain; deformities; loss of normal function; and loss of normal social, physical, and work capabilities. An exercise routine should start with range of motion (ROM) exercises in pain-free ranges,[2,20] and patients with RA should be informed not to overstretch an inflamed tissue to avoid any tears. To prevent contractures and muscular **atrophy,** it is crucial to maintain full ROM of joints through a graded exercise routine.[20] Muscle conditioning is also a key component of management, and strength can be increased through gentle isometric and dynamic exercise. Application of heat before exercise can result in better performance.[27] During an acute exacerbation, submaximal pain-free isometric exercises are recommended. During subacute and chronic phases, patients can implement dynamic exercise. Vigorous activity should be avoided during an exacerbation of symptoms. Any

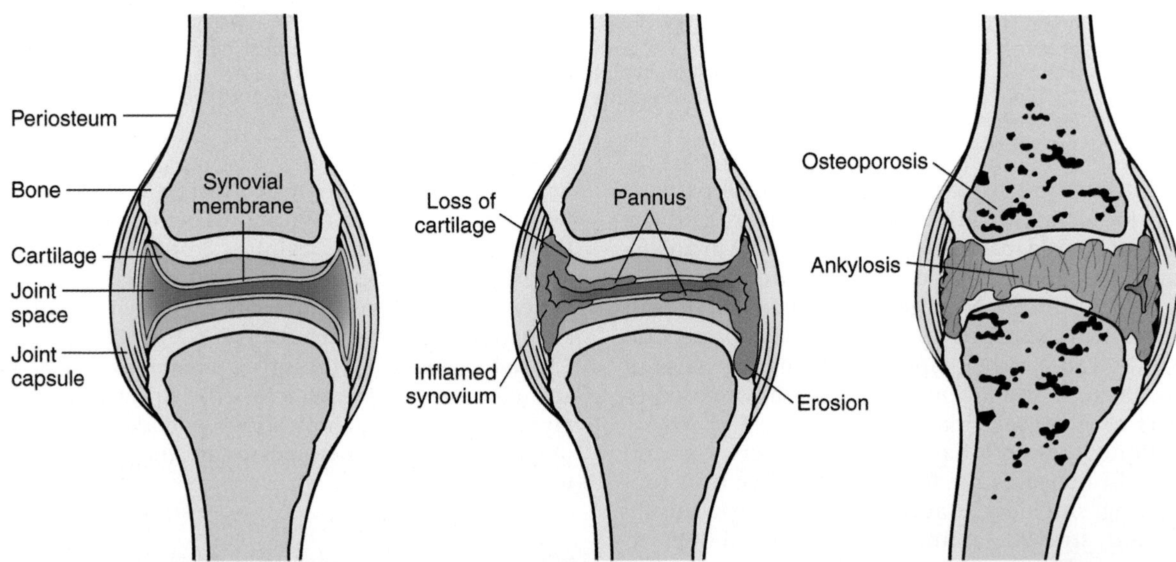

FIG 24-3 Schematic presentation of the pathologic changes in rheumatoid arthritis. Inflammation (synovitis) leads to pannus formation, obliteration of the articular space, and ankylosis. The periarticular bone shows disuse atrophy in the form of osteoporosis. *(From Damjanov I:* Pathology for the health professions, *ed 4, St Louis, 2012, Saunders.)*

TABLE 24-1 Differential Diagnosis between Rheumatoid Arthritis and Osteoarthritis

Characteristic	RA	OA
Joints affected	Any joint but more frequently wrists, hands, elbows, shoulders, knees, ankles	DIP > PIP CMC Spine Hip Knee
Age	Any age; most common ages 20-60 years	More common >40 years
Gender	More common in women	More common in men <45 years and women >45 years
Relative severity	More than OA	Less than RA
Disease pathogenesis	Autoimmune: immune system attacks body	Condition of wear and tear with aging or injury and chemical factors
Joint involvement	Symmetric	Asymmetric
Joint destruction	From inflammation	From biomechanical stress
Deformities	Swan neck MP joint ulnar deviation Wrist subluxation Boutonnière deformity	Heberden's nodes Bouchard's nodes CMC joint instability
Erythrocyte sedimentation rate	Markedly increased	Mild increase
Connective tissue flexibility	Increased	Decreased
Morning stiffness	>1 hour	<30 minutes
Rheumatoid factor	Positive in 70%	Negative
Imaging	Juxtaarticular osteoporosis, erosions	Osteophytes Eburnation Reduced joint space
Management	Physical therapy/occupational therapy NSAIDs Gold Penicillamine Many new biologics	Acetaminophen Weight loss Joint replacement Exercise
NSAID response	Usually some relief	Variable relief

CMC, carpometacarpal; *DIP,* distal interphalangeal; *MP,* metacarpophalangeal; *NSAID,* nonsteroidal antiinflammatory drug; *OA,* osteoarthritis; *PIP,* proximal interphalangeal; RA, rheumatoid arthritis.

exercise that causes pain longer than 1 hour after exercise should be eliminated.[27]

The current management approach with medication is to start early with disease-modifying antirheumatic drugs (DMARDs) because they have been shown to slow RA progression. Nonsteroidal antiinflammatory drugs (NSAIDs) are the most commonly used drugs to decrease pain and swelling and increase ROM. Corticosteroids are also used for swelling, pain, and fatigue and tend to decrease symptoms faster. Biologic response modifiers block cytokines decreasing the breakdown of cartilage and bone.[20,21,33] The pathophysiology of these drugs will be explained in greater detail later.

Important Concept

For those with RA, it is very important to use management based on the phase of exacerbation that the patient is presently in.

REACTIVE ARTHRITIS

Reactive arthritis, or Reiter's syndrome, most commonly manifests as an abrupt onset of arthritis in young men who present with the triad of conjunctivitis, urethritis, and oligoarticular arthritis.[9,25,27] Conjunctivitis, also known as *pinkeye,* is inflammation of the conjunctiva (outermost layer of eye and inner surface of eyelid). Urethritis is inflammation of the urethra and manifests as painful urination. Oligoarthritis is a form of arthritis with inflammation in two to four joints. Reiter's syndrome usually manifests within days or weeks of a dysenteric or sexually transmitted infection.[25,27] The arthritis is usually asymmetric and initially involves the weight-bearing joints, such as the toes, ankles, and knees, then ascends to the axial skeleton and upper extremities.[9,25,27] Other symptoms that occur with Reiter's syndrome are oral ulcers, penile lesions, keratoderma blennorrhagicum, and plantar heel pain.[9,27] Approximately 80% of individuals with Reiter's syndrome are positive for human leukocyte antigen B27 (HLA-B27).[9,27] The HLA system is the name of the major histocompatibility complex in humans. The major HLA antigens are essential elements in immune function. Sacroiliitis is observed in about 60% of patients with chronic Reiter's syndrome. Management of Reiter's syndrome includes NSAIDs and physical therapy.

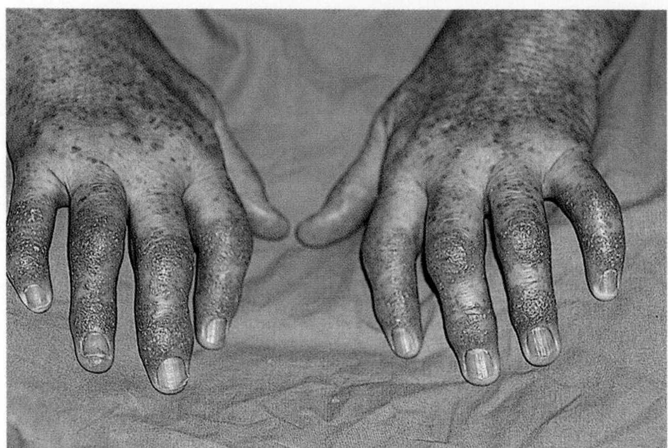

FIG 24-4 Deforming arthritis of the hands in a person with psoriatic arthritis. *(From Callen JP, Greer K, Paller A, et al:* Color atlas of dermatology, *ed 2, Philadelphia, 2000, Saunders.)*

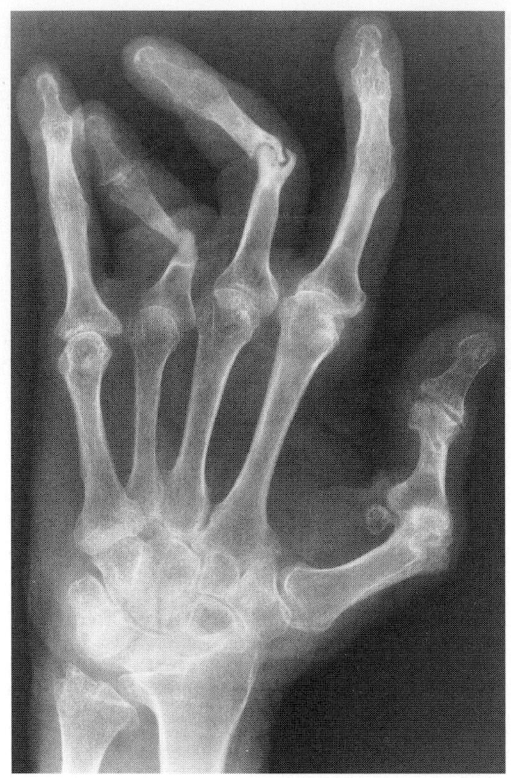

FIG 24-5 Pencil-in-cup deformity in the third proximal interphalangeal joint and bony ankylosis involving the wrist and phalanges of the second and fifth digits. *(From Eisenberg RL:* Comprehensive radiographic pathology, *ed 4, St Louis, 2008, Mosby.)*

PSORIATIC ARTHRITIS

Psoriatic arthritis is a seronegative inflammatory joint disease that affects a small percentage of people with psoriasis.[19,27] Psoriasis is an inherited chronic inflammatory skin disease that is characterized by silvery scales on a bright red plaque (Fig. 24-4).[7,19] In most cases, the skin disease precedes arthritis symptoms by several months to years.[15] Psoriatic arthritis closely resembles RA but has differences such as DIP joint involvement, psoriasis or family history of psoriasis, nail pitting, and "sausage" appearance of digits.[9,20,27] Gender does not appear to predispose one to psoriatic arthritis. It generally begins between ages 30 and 50 years.[15,19,25] Psoriatic arthritis is usually asymmetric and involves the small joints of the hands and feet.[9,19,44] However, larger axial joints, such as the sacroiliac joint, can be affected in later phases of the disease. Sacroiliitis usually occurs unilaterally, whereas ankylosing spondylitis is bilateral.[19,25] Imaging reveals a "pencil-in-cup" deformity caused by erosion and destruction of the phalanx bones that makes them look like a sharpened pencil at the end of the bone (Fig. 24-5).[7,9,44] Psoriatic arthritis also can cause fingernail thickening, pitting, and separation from the nail bed.[15] Finally, periosteal reactions (formation of new bone) can be seen on x-rays.

Management of psoriatic arthritis is similar to management of RA.[9,25,44] Although there is no cure for psoriatic arthritis, NSAIDs can be used to treat inflammatory symptoms.[7,19] Most of the time the disease is mild and not destructive, and treatment consists of symptom management.[7,19]

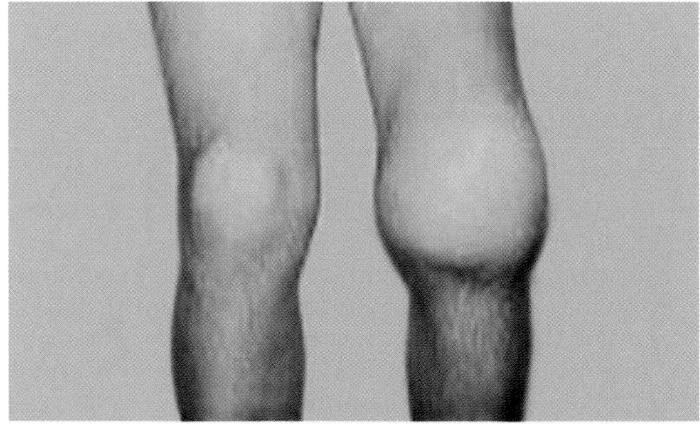

FIG 24-6 An affected knee in a patient with pauciarticular juvenile rheumatoid arthritis. *(From Kliegman RM:* Nelson essentials of pediatrics, *ed 5, St Louis, 2006, Saunders.)*

JUVENILE RHEUMATOID ARTHRITIS

Many acute and chronic rheumatic diseases exist in children with juvenile rheumatoid arthritis (JRA) being one of the most common.[62] JRA, a chronic inflammatory disease, actually covers three types of childhood arthritis: pauciarticular, polyarticular, and systemic.[9,19,44,62] The etiology of JRA is unknown, but it is thought to be triggered by environmental factors or infection in children with a genetic predisposition.[19,62] "JRA is similar to adult RA in the fact that the immune system mistakenly attacks the joints and organs, causing inflammation, destruction, fatigue, and other local and systemic effects."[19] JRA occurs before age 16 years and affects girls more commonly.[9,19,62] To confirm diagnosis, the child must have arthritis for at least 6 consecutive weeks.[62] Other symptoms of JRA are fever, rash, fatigue, anemia, loss of appetite, stiffness, irritability, altered mobility, and change in ADL.[62]

Pauciarticular JRA is characterized by asymmetric synovitis of four or fewer joints.[9,19,62] There are usually no systemic features, and it most commonly affects the knee, elbow, and ankle (Fig. 24-6).[19,62] Two subtypes of pauciarticular JRA exist: early onset and late onset.[9,19,62] Early-onset pauciarticular JRA occurs before age 5 years and usually affects girls. When left untreated, early-onset pauciarticular JRA can result in iridocyclitis, which can lead to visual impairments.[9,19,62] The second subtype, late-onset pauciarticular JRA, occurs between ages 10 and 12 years and is more common in boys. This subtype affects large weight-bearing joints and entheses (insertion point of tendon into bone).[62] These children often have spinal involvement that may develop into a spondyloarthropathy.[19,62]

Polyarticular JRA is synovitis in more than four joints and is more common in girls.[9,19,62] It usually manifests with symmetric involvement of the small joints of the hands or feet, wrists, elbows, shoulders, knees, hips, ankles, cervical spine, and temporomandibular joints.[19,62] Bursitis and tendinitis can occur because tendons and bursae also are lined with synovial tissue. In contrast to pauciarticular JRA, polyarticular JRA can have systemic features, including low-grade fever, anemia, leukocytosis, mild hepatosplenomegaly, and lymphadenopathy.[62]

The last type of JRA is systemic JRA (Still's disease), which can occur at any age and does not favor girls or boys.[19,62] Systemic JRA is characterized by a rash, synovitis in one or more joints, and an intermittent high-grade fever.[9,19,62] The fever usually occurs in the afternoon and evening and abates when the child feels better.[19,62] Because fever can precede all other symptoms, these children are often initially evaluated for fever of unknown origin.[62] The rash usually appears with the fever and is salmon pink, is 2 to 5 mm in diameter, and has an erythematous perimeter.[62] Other signs and symptoms of systemic JRA include **malaise,** irritability, anemia, hepatitis, peptic ulcer disease, leukocytosis, thrombocytosis, lymphadenopathy, hepatomegaly, splenomegaly, pericarditis, and pleuritis.[19,62]

Management of Juvenile Rheumatoid Arthritis

Management for children with JRA involves a combination of medication, physical therapy, and occupational therapy. The main objectives of therapy should be to control pain and inflammation, promote mobility, and improve function.[19,62] Control of pain and inflammation is usually obtained with NSAIDs, which have been shown to decrease stiffness, pain, and swelling in children with JRA. Other medications used with JRA are corticosteroids, DMARDs, infliximab, and immunosuppressants.[19,62] ROM is the strongest indicator of functional disability in children with systemic JRA.[19] All joints should be gently put through the full ROM twice a day to maintain good mobility.[62] Heat can be used before stretching to help warm the muscles and decrease pain before stretching. Gentle splinting can also be used to help maintain ROM.[62] Aquatic therapy is an appropriate management for JRA because the heat can help relax the muscles and decrease pain.[62] Although patients with JRA are children, education in joint protection and energy conservation is still important. The therapist should always try to make the exercise program fun, interesting, and interactive to keep the child involved.[62]

SEPTIC ARTHRITIS

Septic arthritis is the invasion of a joint by an infectious agent causing arthritis. Septic arthritis usually occurs from a bacterial infection, but the infection can be viral, mycobacterial, or fungal. Bacteria are introduced into the joint by the bloodstream from an infection elsewhere or from direct penetration after a wound, surgery, or local infection.[58] Two common types of septic arthritis are gonococcal and nongonococcal.[27,58]

Gonococcal Arthritis

Gonococcal arthritis usually occurs in healthy individuals and is two to three times more common in women.[27,58] Initially, the patient experiences 1 to 4 days of noninflammatory joint pain in the wrist, ankle, knee, and elbow. Chronic arthritis and tendinitis are common symptoms preceding gonococcal arthritis.[58] Patients tend to have characteristic asymptomatic skin lesions with 2 to 10 small necrotic pustules over the extremities, especially the palms and soles.[27]

Management of Gonococcal Arthritis. Gonococcal arthritis usually responds well to drug therapy in 24 to 48 hours and is not as destructive as nongonococcal bacterial infections.[27,58]

Nongonococcal Arthritis

Nongonococcal bacterial infections are primarily monarticular and occur in large weight-bearing joints and wrists.[27,58] Individuals with previous joint damage from a disease such as RA and intravenous drug users have an increased risk of infection.[27,58] *Staphylococcus aureus* is the most common cause of nongonococcal septic arthritis.[27,58] Nongonococcal septic arthritis is marked by a sudden onset of acute arthritis with pain, swelling, and heat in one joint.[27] The hip, wrist, shoulder, and ankle all can be affected, but the knee is most commonly affected. Chills and fever often accompany the symptoms of nongonococcal septic arthritis.[27]

Management of Nongonococcal Arthritis. Management should be initiated quickly with systemic antibiotics addressing the causative organism. If the specific organism cannot be determined, bacterial antibiotics are recommended.[27] Aspiration of the affected joint keeps the joint free of destructive exudates.[27,58] Early intervention is important because ankylosis and articular damage can occur if management is delayed. Immobilization and heat can help decrease joint pain.[27] Rest, elevation, and immobilization are used during the acute phase of the disease.

As stated previously, early diagnosis and management are important because of the potential for harm if septic arthritis is untreated.[58] Risk factors to keep in mind are infection elsewhere in the body, very old or young age, presence of other systemic diseases, recent joint aspiration or surgery, prosthetic joints, immunosuppression, and intravenous drug abuse.[19,58] An infected joint is painful and tender and has limited motion but may not have redness, heat, and swelling, especially if treatment includes immunosuppressants.[58] Gentle passive and active ROM can be started when the patient tolerates to prevent contractures and loss of strength.

ARTHRITIC CONDITIONS OF THE SPINE

Arthritic conditions of the spine, termed *spondyloarthropathies,* mainly affect the axial skeleton. Clinically, the patient has low back pain that increases with rest and improves with activity. Spondyloarthropathies have the following characteristics:

- They run in families.
- They are more common in men.
- Onset is before age 40 years.
- Patients generally have inflammatory arthritis of the spine or the large peripheral joints.
- Patients lack autoantibodies in the serum.
- They are associated with the presence of HLA-B27.[27]

Ankylosing Spondylitis

Ankylosing spondylitis is a type of inflammation that affects the synovium of the spinal arthrodial joints and all the joint ligaments of the spine at their insertion points into the bone (enthesitis). It begins in the sacroiliac joints in nearly all patients and spreads superiorly up the spine.[25] As the disease progresses, the spine becomes more rigid (ankylosed) and develops flexion deformities.[25] The disease also leads to formation of bony bridges called *syndesmophytes* between the vertebrae. Structurally, patients lose the lumbar curve, have reduced chest expansion, and have an increase in thoracic kyphosis.[25,32] Other changes noted in radiographic imaging are squaring of vertebrae and destruction of the sacroiliac joints (Fig. 24-7).[44]

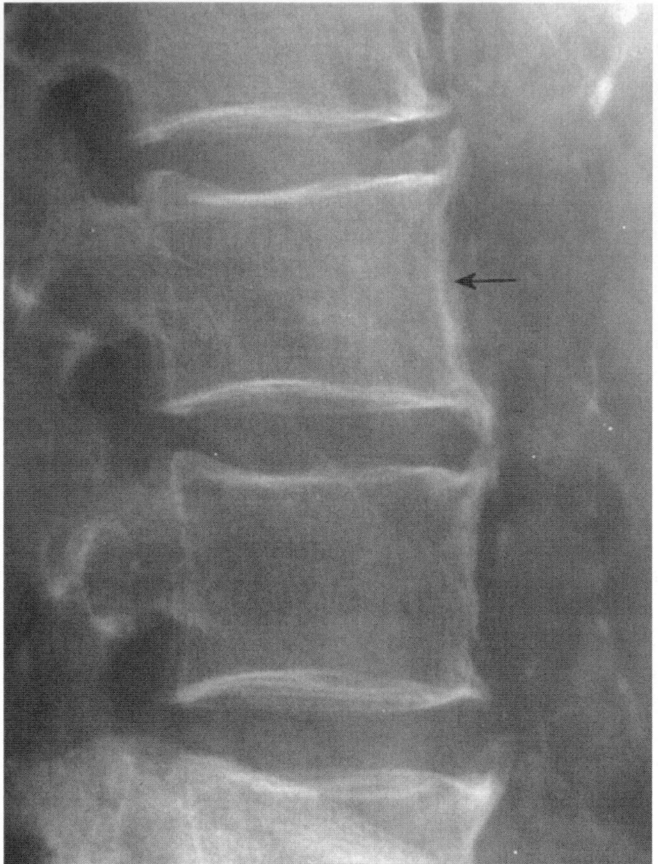

FIG 24-7 Ankylosing spondylitis of the spine. There is vertebral body squaring resulting from mineralization of the anterior longitudinal ligament, which fills in the normal anterior concavity of the vertebral body *(arrow). (From Adam A, Dixon AK, Grainger RG, et al, editors:* Grainger & Allison's diagnostic radiology: a textbook of medical imaging, *ed 5, Philadelphia, 2008, Churchill Livingstone.)*

Ankylosing spondylitis has a greater incidence in men, and the age of onset is usually in the late teens to early 20s.[25] Hypomobility is likely to be seen in men between ages 40 and 50 years and in women older than 50 years.[39] Patients with ankylosing spondylitis usually complain of alternating buttock pain that radiates down the thigh and that increases with rest but decreases with activity, a hot bath, or a shower.[25] Patients may show signs of peripheral arthritis, such as swelling, redness, and tenderness. Constitutional symptoms include fever, fatigue, weight loss, and elevated erythrocyte sedimentation rate.[25] Ankylosing spondylitis often is confused with sacroiliac arthritis; however, there are several differences between these two diseases (Table 24-2).

Management of Ankylosing Spondylitis. Management of ankylosing spondylitis includes physical therapy and drug therapy. It is suggested that early rehabilitation of ankylosing spondylitis improves functional mobility and posture reducing the impact of disability.[25,26,28] Therapeutic exercise along with antiinflammatory drug therapy is important in managing ankylosing spondylitis. Benefits of exercise include improved mobility, posture, and function.[26,28] Education is key to starting management of patients with ankylosing spondylitis. Patients should try to exercise when pain level is low and they are least tired. Starting an exercise session with heat application and light motion exercises can help loosen the joints and decrease pain for exercise.[25] Before starting the patient on a strengthening regimen, the therapist should always try to improve mobility of the spine, which can reduce pain and stiffness in the patient.[25] Physical therapy should focus on stretching the anterior flexor muscles and strengthening the extensors. Specifically, therapy should focus on strengthening the postural muscles, back and neck extensors, shoulder retractors, and hip extensors and abductors.[25] A prone program is a good management option to stretch the anterior muscles.[25] Postural exercises are also beneficial, including standing against a wall with heels, buttocks, and shoulders touching the wall. Also, patients should try to sleep with as much extension as tolerable and lay prone at least 15 minutes a day.[25] Aquatic therapy is another management option that can help reduce discomfort and provide an avenue for relaxation, maintaining assisted ROM, and gentle strengthening.[25] Finally, breathing exercises are important because of the decreased chest expansion that occurs with ankylosing spondylitis.

Pharmacologic intervention usually includes NSAIDs to help decrease pain and stiffness, allowing for normal ADL and exercise. Indomethacin is the most effective NSAID used with ankylosing spondylitis for decreasing night pain and morning stiffness.[25,27] Sulfasalazine, which reduces levels of acute phase reactants, may act as a "disease-modifying" agent. Sulfasalazine can decrease the

TABLE 24-2 Differential Diagnosis between Ankylosing Spondylitis and Sacroiliac Arthritis

Characteristic	Ankylosing Spondylitis	Sacroiliac Arthritis
History	Bilateral sacroiliac pain that may refer to posterior thigh Morning stiffness Male predominance	Bilateral sacroiliac pain referring to gluteal area (S1-S2 dermatomes) Morning stiffness (prolonged) Coughing painful
Observation	Stiff, controlled movement of pelvis	Controlled movement of pelvis
Active movement	Decreased	Side flexion and extension full Slight limitation of flexion
Passive movement	Decreased	Normal
Resisted isometric movement	Pain and weakness, especially if sacroiliac joints are stressed	Pain, especially if sacroiliac joints are stressed
Special tests	Sacral stress tests probably positive	Sacral stress tests probably positive
Sensation and reflexes	Normal	Normal
Palpation	Tender over sacroiliac joints	Tender over sacroiliac joints
Diagnostic imaging	X-rays diagnostic	X-rays diagnostic
Laboratory tests	Erythrocyte sedimentation rate increased HLA-B27 human leukocyte antigen present in 80%	Normal

From Magee DJ: *Orthopedic physical assessment,* ed 5, St Louis, 2008, Saunders.

peripheral symptoms associated with ankylosing spondylitis. It is reasonable to prescribe immunosuppressant drugs for severely affected patients who cannot participate in physical therapy.[25,27]

NONARTHRITIC RHEUMATIC DISEASES

GOUT

Gout is a metabolic disorder characterized by deposition of monosodium urate crystals in the joints, soft tissue, kidneys, and other connective tissue (Fig. 24-8).[9,19,27,58] When urate crystals are present, they can cause acute or chronic inflammation by stimulating inflammatory mediators.[9,19,27,44,58] The deposition of monosodium urate crystals is the outcome of hyperuricemia, which is the presence of high levels of uric acid in the blood. Hyperuricemia is due to the overproduction or underexcretion (or both) of uric acid.[9,19,27,44,58] Overproduction of uric acid is more common in individuals with a history of lymphoma, leukemia, or psoriasis.[19,27] Overproduction can also be due to enzyme abnormalities, hematologic malignancies, or other causes of rapid cell turnover.[58] Underexcretion of uric acid is more common with obesity, fasting, medication (e.g., diuretics, cyclosporine), renal insufficiency, hypertension, hypothyroidism, hyperparathyroidism, and acidosis.[19,27,58] Alcoholism increases risk of gout by increasing production and decreasing renal excretion of uric acid.[19,27,58]

Gout most commonly affects men older than 30 years; occasional cases occur in postmenopausal women.[9,19,27,58] Gout is characterized by acute monarticular onset of inflammatory arthritis that is worse at night. Although the metatarsophalangeal joint of the great toe is the most common site of pain, the ankle, knee, wrist, elbow, and fingers all can be affected.[19,27,58] The involved joints usually become tender, swollen, warm, and red.[19,27,58] A fever often occurs along with the joint complaints.[19,27] The early initial episodes last 3 to 10 days, and then a patient can go months to years with no symptoms.[19,27,58] Severe gouty attacks suddenly return with more frequency affecting more joints and lasting longer.[19,27,58] The gout can become chronic with multiple-joint damage leading to loss of function and disability.[19,27] Tophi, visible deposits of crystallized monosodium urate, usually occur several years after the first episode of gout.

Management of Gout

Management of acute gout focuses on the arthritis first and then addresses the hyperuricemia.[19,27] NSAIDs are most commonly used for pharmacologic management of acute gout and decrease inflammation and pain.[19,27,58] Corticosteroids are also used, but mainly when a patient has a contraindication for NSAIDs.[27] Another management option is to prescribe drugs to inhibit tubular reabsorption of uric acid to promote urinary excretion.[53] Rest, elevation, and joint protection are important during attacks of acute gout to promote decreased inflammation further.[19,58] Hyperuricemia is addressed between or after the acute attacks to help prevent future episodes.[19,27,58] Management during symptom-free periods includes changes in diet, avoidance of hyperuricemic medications, colchicine, and reduction of serum uric acid. Dietary changes that can decrease the risk of gout are weight loss, moderation of alcohol, and avoidance of high-purine foods.[19,27] Controlling hyperuricemia is important to prevent gout from becoming chronic.[19]

Important Concept

Gout is a nonarthritic rheumatic disease that is characterized by deposition of monosodium urate crystals in the joints, soft tissue, kidneys and other connective tissue. Management of gout focuses on arthritis and also addresses the hyperuriemia via medications.

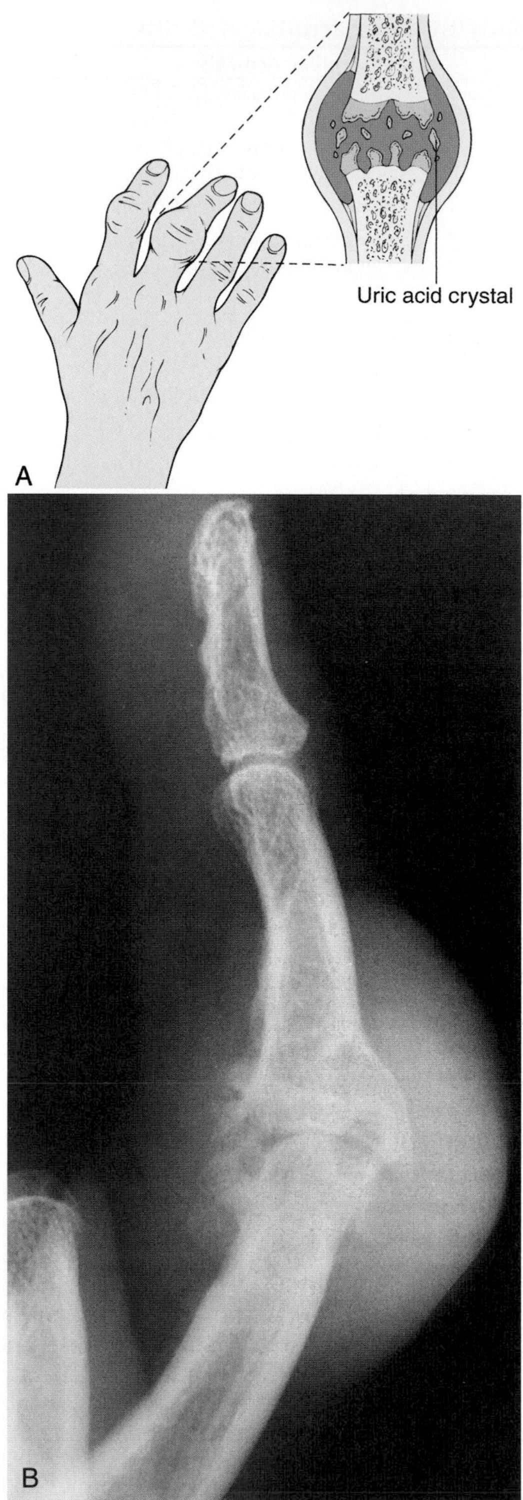

FIG 24-8 Gout. **A,** Deposits of uric acid crystals in the connective tissue have a chemotactic effect and cause exudation of leukocytes into the joint. **B,** Severe joint effusion and periarticular swelling of the proximal interphalangeal joint of the finger. *(**A,** From Frazier MS, Drzymkowski JW:* Essentials of human diseases and conditions, *ed 2, Philadelphia, 2000, Saunders; **B,** From Eisenberg RL:* Comprehensive radiographic pathology, *ed 4, St Louis, 2008, Mosby.)*

FIBROMYALGIA

Fibromyalgia is a chronic widespread muscle pain syndrome.[12,19,27,31] Fibromyalgia is defined as widespread pain lasting at least 3 months with physical findings of 11 to 18 tender points (Fig. 24-9).[12,19,31] Common characteristics of fibromyalgia are chronic widespread pain, aching, fatigue, and stiffness. Patients may also complain of headaches, sleep disorders, mood disorders, irritable bowel syndrome, and paresthesias.[40] Fibromyalgia is most common in women between the ages of 20 and 50 years.[12,19,27] The exact etiology and pathogenesis of fibromyalgia are not fully understood, but disturbances in different systems of the body are thought to be involved. One common thought is that pain results from abnormalities of central sensory processing.[12] More recent research characterizes fibromyalgia as a biologic disorder associated with neurohormonal dysfunction of the autonomic nervous system because of the objective biochemical, endocrine, and physiologic abnormalities.[19] Abnormalities in the hypothalamic-pituitary-adrenal axis, reproductive hormone axis, autonomic nervous system, and immune system have been found in patients with fibromyalgia.[19] The onset of fibromyalgia may be due to prolonged stress or anxiety, trauma, rapid steroid withdrawal, hypothyroidism, and viral and nonviral infections.[12,19] Fibromyalgia may start as localized pain and after months or years become widespread.[12] The pain associated with fibromyalgia is often described as burning or aching and sometimes tender, stiff, throbbing, and sore.[12,19] Although fibromyalgia pain is widespread, patients have one or two locations that are the worst, which are usually the neck, shoulders, and back.[12,27,31] Sleep disturbance is another, more common symptom in fibromyalgia.[12,19,27] Patients complain of exhaustion even after a night of sleep, which is because of the disordered non–rapid eye movement sleep.[48] Also, patients with fibromyalgia have increased motor activity and restlessness during sleep, which accounts for increased fatigue.[48] Other common symptoms are fatigue, subjective numbness, chronic headaches, dizziness, Raynaud's phenomenon, and irritable bowel and bladder.[12,19,27,31] Symptoms tend to be exacerbated with noise, stress, tiredness, weather changes, trauma, noxious smells, and too much or too little exercise.[12,19,40]

Management of Fibromyalgia

The first step in treating patients with fibromyalgia is to ensure the patients understand they have a diagnosed syndrome that is a legitimate disorder with real symptoms and there is an effective management.[12,27] The management for fibromyalgia needs to be multidisciplinary and address education, stress management, nutrition, lifestyle training, medication, muscle pain, and exercise.[19] Pharmacologic management focuses on managing the pain and sleep disturbances.[12] Antidepressants are commonly used for fibromyalgia because of their positive effects on pain, sleep, and fatigue.[12,31] Antidepressants work well with some patients because the chemicals in the body that control pain and sleep also control mood.[31] Other drugs used to treat fibromyalgia are muscle relaxants, antianxiety medications, and sleep aids.[15]

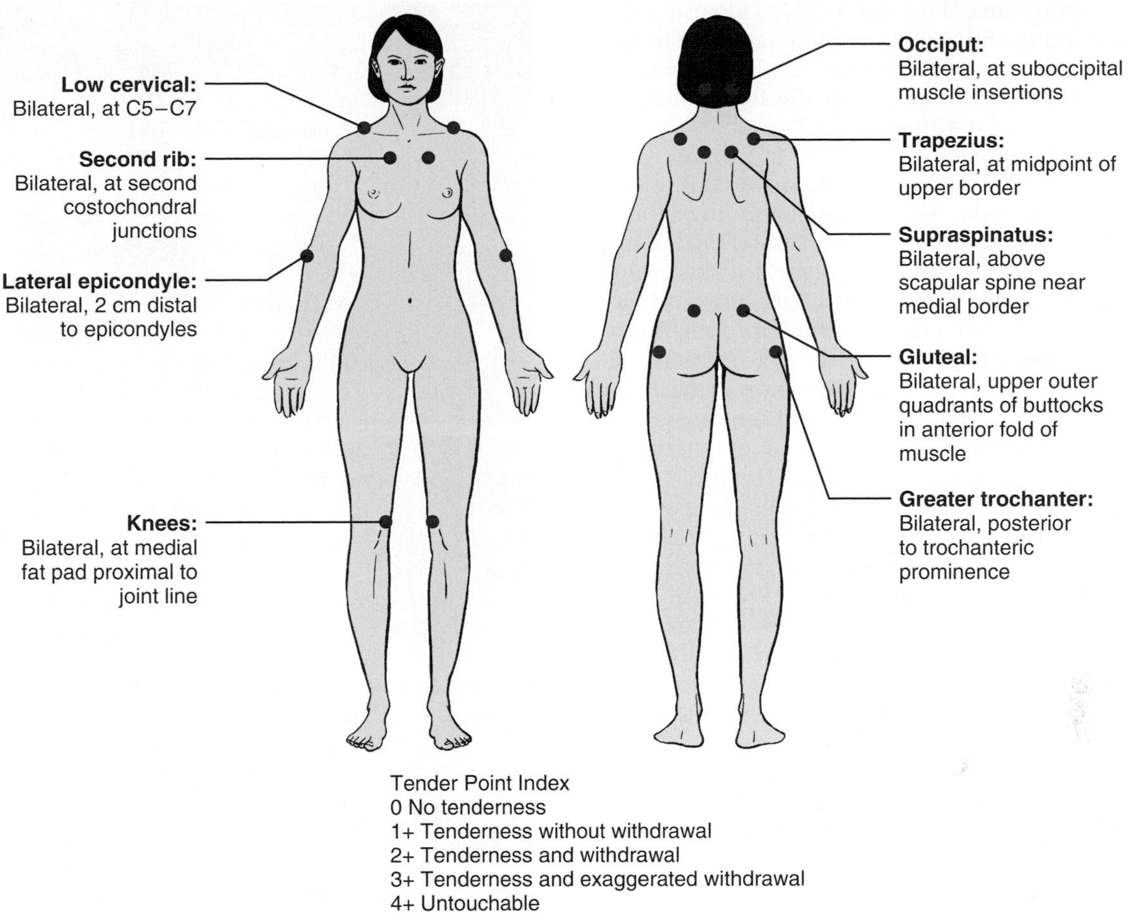

FIG 24-9 Anatomic locations of tender points associated with fibromyalgia. *(From Goodman CC, Snyder T:* Differential diagnosis for physical therapists: screening for referral, *ed 4, Philadelphia, 2007, Saunders.)*

Exercise is an important aspect of fibromyalgia management and is shown to have numerous benefits.[12,19,27,31] The exercise program should not be progressed too fast, and it is suggested to have patients start below a level they believe they can accomplish.[12] Modalities are useful in decreasing acute pain allowing patients to start an exercise program.[19,31] Stretching can help improve flexibility and decrease pain. Stretching should be done in a pain-free range and can start with 10- to 15-second holds and progress up to 1 minute. It is important to perform stretches at least once a day. Heat alone can help with muscle pain, but it is also beneficial to use heat before stretching.[12,31] Aerobic exercise has been shown to decrease pain and improve function in patients with fibromyalgia.[12,31] The exercise routine can be broken into several shorter bouts throughout the day or one longer 30-minute session. Depending on fitness level, some patients may need to start with 5 minutes of exercise daily and work up to 30 minutes slowly. It is very important that the patient avoid overexertion because this can lead to increased symptoms.[12] Strengthening can help reduce the risk of muscle damage, but the patient should attempt to reduce eccentric muscle work.[12] Patients should pause for about 4 seconds between repetitions to allow for complete muscle relaxation. Lifting above the head and shoulders should be avoided to reduce risk of shoulder girdle injury or overuse. Water therapy or aerobics is a good alternative because the warmth and decreased pressures can lead to better relaxation.[12]

SYSTEMIC LUPUS ERYTHEMATOSUS

Systemic lupus erythematosus (SLE) is a chronic inflammatory autoimmune disorder that may affect multiple organ systems.[9,19,27,51] SLE is most common in women during their childbearing years and is rarely found in older individuals.[9,19,27,51] In SLE, the body produces antibodies against itself.[19] The antigen-antibody complexes in tissues suppress the body's immunity and damage tissues. The etiology of SLE is unknown, but environmental and genetic factors are believed to be the most related with evidence also supporting interrelated immunologic and hormonal factors.[19] Many risk factors exist for SLE with hereditary factors at the forefront, along with physical and mental stress, streptococcal or viral infections, exposure to sunlight or ultraviolet light, and abnormal estrogen metabolism.[19] Physical therapy diagnosis for SLE is not difficult if the patient presents with common symptoms associated with SLE. The diagnostic criteria of the American Rheumatism Association for SLE require the patient to show 4 or more of the 11 symptoms. If the patient shows fewer symptoms, the diagnosis is made using clinical judgment along with supportive laboratory testing.[27,51]

The clinical symptoms of patients with SLE are variable. The severity of SLE can vary drastically from a treatable rash or fatigue to a life-threatening illness.[27,51] The skin, joints, lungs, kidneys, blood, and other organs and tissues can be affected.[19,27,44,51] General signs of SLE include fever, fatigue, anorexia, weight loss, and myalgias.[27,51] Joint involvement is an early symptom and occurs in more than 90% of patients.[27] Symmetric polyarthritis is common in any joint but is usually found in small joints of hands, wrists, and knees.[19,51] SLE manifests similar to RA, but it is not usually destructive or deforming.[19,27,44,51] When SLE is present, deformities such as ulnar deviation or swan neck deformity can occur. Tenosynovitis and tendon ruptures also can occur.[19,51] Recurrent inflammation of tendons and other supportive structures of the joints can lead to ulnar deviation of the second to fifth fingers and subluxation of the metacarpophalangeal joints, which is referred to as *Jaccoud's arthropathy*.[51,64] Jaccoud's arthropathy may be correctable with no radiographic signs of erosion.[51] Also, patients should be observed for signs of osteonecrosis or septic arthritis, which manifest as persistent monarthritis primarily in the shoulders, hips, or knees.[51]

Another common symptom in SLE is skin rashes over areas exposed to sunlight. Butterfly rash is an acute inflammatory rash over the nose and checks.[19,27,44,51] Discoid lupus is characterized by raised, red, scaly, and scarring rashes that can develop around the face, scalp, ears, and upper extremities (Fig. 24-10).[19,27,51] Other cutaneous manifestations include alopecia, oral ulcers, fingertip lesions, periungual erythema, nail-fold infarcts, splinter hemorrhages, livedo reticularis, urticaria, panniculitis, and Raynaud's phenomenon.[19,27,51] Other clinical findings in SLE are associated with the renal, hematologic, cardiopulmonary, immune, and central nervous systems.[19,27,51]

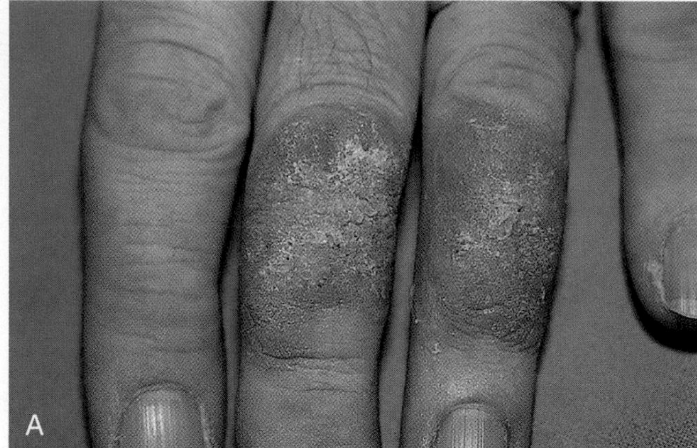

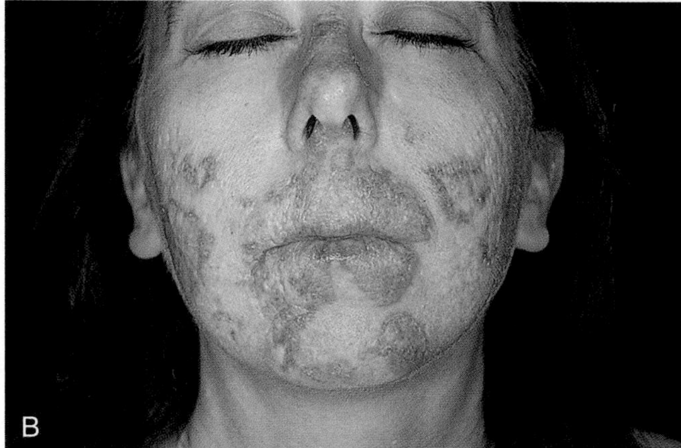

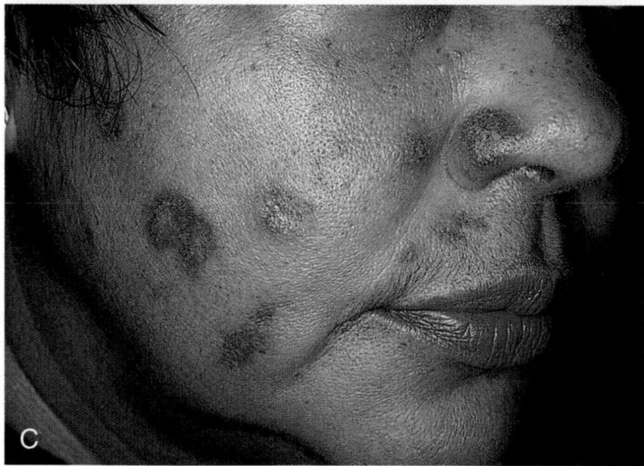

FIG 24-10 Discoid lupus erythematosus. Patients with skin changes associated with discoid lupus erythematosus can present with a variety of signs. **A,** Hypertrophic discoid lupus erythematosus with prominent adherent scale. **B,** Round or oval cutaneous lesions can occur on the face or other parts of the body. **C,** Round or oval cutaneous lesions as they appear on a dark-skinned individual. *(From Callen JP, Greer K, Paller A, et al:* Color atlas of dermatology, *ed 2, Philadelphia, 2000, Saunders.)*

Management of Systemic Lupus Erythematosus

SLE is marked by remissions and relapses, and management is focused on addressing symptoms quickly during an exacerbation.[27,51] Patient education is important for successful management of SLE. Relapses are less likely if activities are controlled and sometimes limited.[19] Also, after an exacerbation, return to activity should be slow and pain-free.[19] Medical management of joint pain is similar to RA, with NSAIDs as the primary medication for minor symptoms.[27,51] Patients should be cautioned against prolonged sun exposure and should use sunscreen regularly. Topical corticosteroids are often used for rashes or skin lesions.[27,51] Because of the use of corticosteroids, patients have a higher risk of osteoporosis, and weight-bearing exercises should be incorporated into the management plan.

OSTEOPOROSIS

Osteoporosis is a disease characterized by low bone mass and microarchitectural deterioration of bone tissue, which leads to enhanced bone fragility and a consequent increase in fracture risk (Fig. 24-11).[41] The decrease in bone mass is due to decreased osteoblast activity, which builds bone, or increased osteoclast activity, which reabsorbs bone, or both.[61] Remodeling of bone, which maintains bone mass, is performed by osteoblasts and osteoclasts and occurs about every 120 days. However, between the ages of 30 and 40 years, bone resorption starts to exceed bone formation, and density decreases.[37] The bone becomes weaker

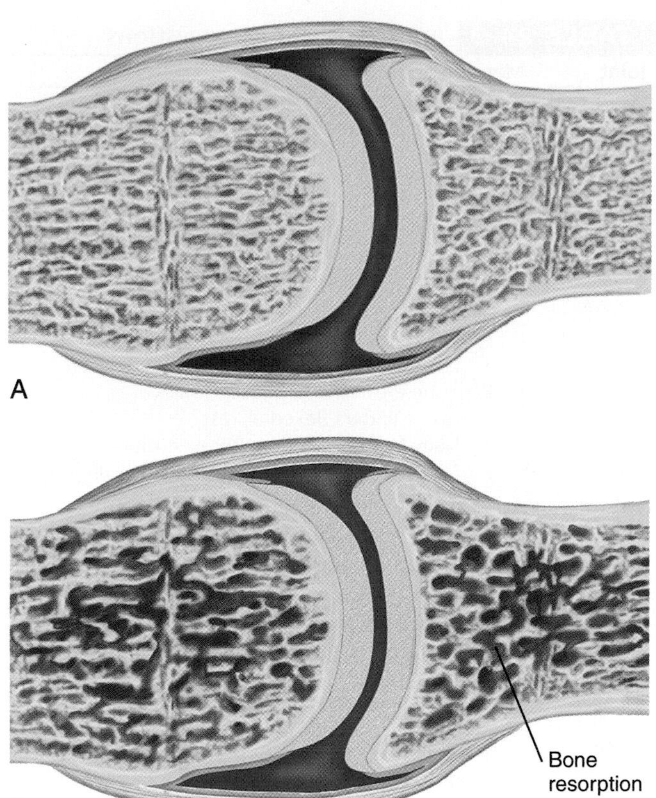

FIG 24-11 Osteoporosis. **A,** Normal bone and joint. **B,** Osteoporotic changes shown with bone resorption greater than bone formation resulting in weakened trabeculae and increasing risk for fracture. *(From Jarvis C:* Physical examination and health assessment, *ed 3, Philadelphia, 2000, Saunders.)*

because of the decreased quantity of bone; however, the quality of bone remaining has not been altered.[9,44]

Many risk factors are associated with osteoporosis, including a sedentary lifestyle, white or Asian race, thin body frame, smoking, excessive alcohol intake, immobilization, early menopause, low calcium and vitamin D intake, and corticosteroid treatment.[37,44] Osteoporosis is more common in women and is directly associated with age. Peak bone mass is usually reached by age 20 to 25 years and then slowly declines, especially after menopause. In men, the peak bone mass is generally higher, and the decline in bone mass is less rapid.[41]

Clinical features associated with osteoporosis are kyphosis, vertebral compression fractures, hip fracture, and distal radius fractures.[41] However, a definitive diagnosis is made by measuring bone mineral density. The most popular method to measure bone mineral density is dual-energy x-ray absorptiometry.

Measures to prevent osteoporosis include a proper diet with adequate calcium and vitamin D, weight-bearing exercises, and an estrogen therapy evaluation at menopause.[44] Prevention or management of osteoporosis needs to include weight-bearing activities and strength along with endurance exercise.[53] Management of osteoporosis should include a combination of medication (bisphosphonates, teriparatide, strontium ranelate), nutrition (calcium and vitamin D), and exercise (aerobic, weight-bearing, and resistance exercise). Getting the correct amount of vitamin D and calcium is important for healthy bones. Calcium alone does not lead to strong bones because vitamin D is needed to transport the calcium into the bone.[15] Strength training exercises are important for postmenopausal women with osteoporosis because they can increase or stabilize bone density of the hip and spine, while improving muscle mass, strength, and balance.[38] Increasing the strength of the back extensors can help decrease symptoms of osteoporosis.[38]

TREATMENT IN RHEUMATIC DISEASE

The primary goal of treatment is to improve function of the patient allowing for a better quality of life. Secondary goals include the following:

- Decrease pain
- Maintain or increase ROM
- Maintain or increase strength
- Increase joint stability in an attempt to prevent deformities
- Decrease biomechanical stress on joints with joint protection techniques
- Improve efficiency and safety of gait
- Promote independence with ADL
- Educate about joint protection, energy conservation techniques, functional abilities, and limitations

These goals can be achieved with an eclectic management program including modalities, gentle pain-free assisted ROM, non–weight-bearing aerobic training, and education.[30] A systematic review by Hurkmans found exercise to be beneficial in decreasing a patient's signs and symptoms of arthritis.[30]

REHABILITATIVE MANAGEMENT OF RHEUMATIC DISORDERS

Modalities

Modalities are not a cure for disease, but there is research to support that they can help decrease symptoms and allow for better function.

Cold. During an acute exacerbation of symptoms, patients should use cold to decrease inflammation, pain, and swelling.[15,24] Cold has been shown to have beneficial effects on pain, function, and stiffness.[24] Cold should be avoided in patients with inadequate thermoregulatory response.[24] Cold decreases pain by slowing or blocking nerve conduction, decreasing activity of the muscle spindle, and releasing endorphins. Veins in the tissues contract because of the coldness and decrease blood flow and capillary pressure decreasing swelling.[24] Histamine release is blocked by cold, which also decreases inflammation. Treatment of patients with RA with ice has not been reported to have any significant effects in the literature.[67]

Heat. During subacute or chronic phases of rheumatic diseases, heat is more appropriate to decrease pain and increase ROM.[24] Heat should be avoided during an acute phase of inflammatory arthritis and in people who have decreased thermoregulatory response. Other

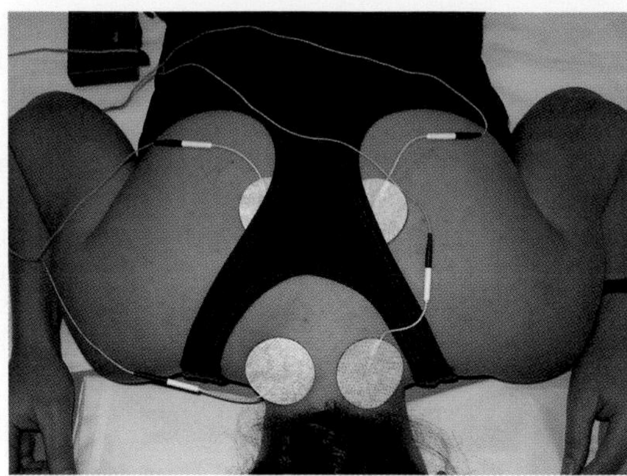

FIG 24-12 Treatment of upper back and neck pain with electrical stimulation. *(From Cameron MH:* Physical agents in rehabilitation: from research to practice, *ed 3, St Louis, 2009, Saunders.)*

contraindications include swelling, fever, infection, hemorrhage, or malignancy.[24] Heat can increase the pain threshold, increase blood flow, wash out pain-producing metabolites, and decrease muscle guarding.[15,24] Heat increases the extensibility of **connective tissue** and should be combined with a low-stress prolonged stretch to increase flexibility.[24] In patients with RA, improved ROM, improved grip and pinch strength, and reduced pain and stiffness were found with paraffin wax baths.[67]

Electrical Stimulation. Transcutaneous electrical nerve stimulation (TENS) is effective in decreasing pain (Fig. 24-12).[24] A TENS unit should never be placed close to the heart in a patient with a pacemaker.[16] TENS uses the gate theory to block pain by stimulating larger sensory fibers, which then block the smaller pain C fibers. C fibers innervate the synovium and joint capsule, so blocking pain perception in these fibers is beneficial to decreasing pain in patients with arthritis. A systematic review by Brosseau and colleagues[11] found TENS to help decrease pain in RA.

Range of Motion

ROM and gentle stretching are an important component of exercise in arthritis because they can relieve stiffness, increase joint mobility, and increase muscle length.[47] Intensity, duration, and frequency of ROM and stretching should take into consideration the phase of arthritis (Table 24-3).

In the acute phase, patients should decrease activity and rest the inflamed joint.[47] Splinting also helps to reduce pain and inflammation by immobilizing or supporting the joint.[23] Reduced stress on the joint capsule and synovial lining through splinting reduces pain and inflammation.[23] Rest is needed during the acute phase, but gentle ROM to maintain joint motion is still important. The goal of ROM and gentle stretching in the acute phase is not to gain flexibility but to maintain it, so the tissues should not be overstretched. Tensile strength is decreased in inflamed tissues, and tears are more likely to occur. ROM exercise should be performed at least once a day to maintain proper flexibility.[47]

TABLE 24-3 Joint Protection Suggestions

Joint	Management Suggestion

Hand	AROM without pain including digit flexion, wrist flexion and extension, wrist ulnar deviation (with RA)
	Maintain thumb web space
	MP
	• Avoid power grasp, lateral pinch
	• Use palm over fingers to open jars
	• Two hands instead of one
	• Swan neck
	  • Avoid intrinsic plus
	  • Encourage PIP flexion with MP extension
	• Boutonnière
	  • Avoid fingers flexed at rest
	  • Daily DIP flexion with PIP extension ROM
	  • Stress MTP extension with PIP and DIP flexion

Wrist	Avoid stirring with utensil diagonal in palm Avoid heavy lifting (hook grasp for bag)
Elbow	Avoid flexion contractures by positioning in gentle extension at rest Gentle supination/pronation to maintain AROM
Shoulders	Avoid decreased ROM all planes Tenderness inferior and lateral coracoids Be careful of GH subluxation
Spine	Core stabilization
Hip	Avoid sitting with legs crossed Avoid asymmetric weight bearing Open seat ankle Avoid loss of abduction and rotation Avoid flexion contracture
Knees	Stand up with knees apart to prevent valgus Avoid hyperextension
Feet	Arch supports Hallux valgus Sit to stand with COG forward

AROM, assisted range of motion; *COG,* center of gravity; *DIP,* distal interphalangeal; *GH,* glenohumeral; *MP,* metacarpophalangeal; *MTP,* metatarsophalangeal; *PIP,* proximal interphalangeal; *RA,* rheumatoid arthritis; *ROM,* range of motion.

During the subacute or chronic phase of arthritis, a goal may be to increase flexibility, so a gentle stretch at the end of joint ROM should be maintained. Intensity of the stretch should be gentle during subacute arthritis and aggressive during the chronic phase. Stretching should be performed two to three times a day with two to five repetitions performed on each joint.[47] If symptoms are subacute, five warmups with two to five more aggressive stretches can help improve motion. When joint symptoms are chronic, three to five warmups with one to two maximum tolerated stretches are recommended. Each stretch should be held 10 to 30 seconds depending on the pain involved.[47] Pain should never last longer than 1 to 2 hours after exercise; if pain persists longer than 2 hours, the intensity of exercise needs to be decreased.

Strengthening

Therapeutic exercise programs for individuals with RA and OA must take into account the arthritic process, including the amount of inflammation, joint stability, and muscle atrophy.[5] Muscle balance and conditioning are important aspects of physical activity because they provide joint stabilization and help the patient remain functional and independent with ADL.[37] In OA, regular exercise has been shown to decrease joint pain and disability.[57] Exercise in patients with RA increases muscle strength and functional capacity.[46] Gentle resistive training can improve muscle disability, physical performance, and pain. Strong muscles can help absorb shock through a joint, whereas weak muscles cannot provide stability or control.[47] Strengthening is important but is more effective when using the correct resistance for the phase of disease. During an acute phase, resistive exercises need to be gentle with little pressure on the joints so that symptoms are not increased. Isometric exercises—exercises during which muscles are contracted without joint movement—are recommended because of the minimal increase in joint pressure. Increased strength can also occur with isometric contractions held 6 seconds at 70% maximum effort and repeated 5 to 10 times a day.[47] Placing the joint at midrange during contractions allows for safer exercise. If symptoms increase, intensity should be decreased to avoid joint irritation; if pain does not subside 1 to 2 hours after exercise, the exercises should be stopped until the patient is past the acute phase of an arthritis flare.

When a patient reaches the subacute phase, isotonic exercises—exercises during which the muscle contracts against a constant load resulting in joint movement—should be implemented.[47] The exercises should be performed through a pain-free ROM; the American College of Sports Medicine states that three sets of 8 to 10 repetitions should be performed for each exercise.[1] If the patient is older than 50 years, 10 to 15 repetitions are recommended.[47] The appropriate amount of resistance is determined when the patient is able to perform all repetitions with no increase in symptoms but a minor feeling of fatigue at the end of each set. When a patient can perform all repetitions easily, resistance should be increased slightly (1 to 2 pounds).[37] When working with larger muscle groups, such as the chest, back, or leg, an increase of 5 pounds should not aggravate symptoms. Although the joint is not in an acute flare, precautions should be taken to avoid exacerbation of symptoms. Open chain exercises are less stressful on the joint because the weight of the body is not sustained by the joint. All major muscle groups should be addressed during exercise, but focus should be placed on muscles crossing the joint or joints affected by arthritis.

Patients in the chronic phase of arthritis should be able to perform more progressive activity without increasing joint symptoms. During this phase, physical therapy should challenge the patient with increased intensity and repetitions. Exercises should be performed through the full available ROM of each joint; incorporating proprioceptive neuromuscular facilitation patterns allows for more muscles to be recruited for each motion and helps prepare the patient for more functional movements. Balance activities should also be performed to decrease risk of falls and train the body further functionally. Strength training should be performed two to three times a week and not repeated 2 days in a row to allow for proper recovery. When performing any exercises, the patient should always be positioned for optimal joint protection.

Aerobic Exercise

Aerobic activities are beneficial to all individuals for overall health and to decrease the risk of disease. Patients with arthritis often believe that rest is the only answer to decrease joint pain, but inactivity may exacerbate arthritic symptoms.[37] RA has many extraarticular manifestations, so aerobic exercise is an especially important part of management. Aerobic activity should be performed three to five times a week for 20 to 30 minutes continuously.[1] If the patient cannot tolerate 30 minutes of continuous exercise, the patient should be encouraged to perform several shorter activities throughout the day that add up to 30 minutes. As the patient's cardiovascular endurance improves, the amount of time spent in continuous exercise may increase. The intensity of exercise should be 70% to 85% of the patient's maximum heart rate (calculated as 220 minus age). The therapist should also explain to the patient that any hobby or activity that increases the heart rate can be considered exercise.

Aquatic Therapy

Water is an excellent medium to allow for an increase in pain-free movement, while decreasing the stress on the joints. Aquatic exercise is unique because it can support, resist, or assist with exercises depending on the motion. Decreased joint compression, muscle relaxation, and sensory input from the pressure and temperature in the water help to decrease pain,[47] so aquatic therapy programs can increase strength, flexibility, and aerobic fitness in patients with knee or hip OA.[66] The resistance of water provides a means to strengthen muscles: The faster a patient moves through the water, the more resistance the patient experiences. Fins or water weights can be used to provide more resistance and progress strengthening. The buoyancy of the water helps unload the body's weight-bearing joints, which can decrease stress and pain. As the patient's pain decreases and strength and endurance improve, the water level can be decreased to allow for more weight bearing. Recommendations from Minor[45] are as follows:

- Select a pool with a water temperature of 84°F to 92°F (29°C to 33°C).
- Exercise in sufficiently deep water to minimize joint compression (midchest to shoulder level).
- Use nonslip, padded footwear to reduce foot discomfort.
- Perform aquatic exercise programs specifically designed for people with arthritis.
- Receive instruction in proper technique before starting a swimming or deep water running program.

Important Concept

The management of rheumatic disease will include the trial of many forms of modalities that may include but not be limited to heat, cold, or electrical modalities. Range of motion and strengthening will also be used as indicated based on the degree and or acuteness of pathology.

MEDICAL MANAGEMENT OF RHEUMATIC DISORDERS

Drugs play an important role in rheumatic disorders by delaying the progression of the diseases and controlling the symptoms. Although the drugs are helpful in their own way to the specific diseases, there are side effects and risks, so the risk-to-benefit ratio needs to be carefully considered when deciding about drug use. As a PTA, it is important to know the effects of the different drugs to explain those effects to patients. It is important to educate patients about complying with their medication schedule because many drugs take months to start working and need to be taken regularly to get an appropriate amount in the bloodstream. There are numerous drugs to help rheumatic disorders, and they fall into the following categories: analgesics, NSAIDs, corticosteroids, biologic response modifiers, and DMARDs.

Analgesics

The role of medication in the treatment of arthritis is dictated by the referring physician or via prescription of a physician. The descriptions presented in this chapter are for educational purposes only and not intended to take the place of physician consultation.

The main role of an analgesic is to decrease pain, which is prevalent in patients with rheumatic disorders. Analgesics are primarily used with OA or in the early phases of RA, where inflammation is not as prevalent.[43] Several analgesics are available for patients with rheumatic disorders, most notably acetaminophen, oxycodone, propoxyphene, and tramadol. Acetaminophen is one of the safest and most cost-effective drugs available. Other pain reducers, such as propoxyphene, oxycodone, and tramadol, are often used but have more side effects and higher risk of dependence. Tramadol is the least likely to cause dependence and is often used first; however, tramadol contains opioids, which decrease the sensation of pain through the central nervous system. Opioids can cause sleepiness, dizziness, and constipation.[43] Education about side effects is important so patients can report any side effects.

Nonsteroidal Antiinflammatory Drugs

NSAIDs have analgesic and antiinflammatory effects but have no effect on arthritis progression.[19] There are many NSAIDs, including ibuprofen (Motrin), aspirin, naproxen, indomethacin, meloxicam (Mobic), choline, and magnesium salicylates.[15,43] NSAIDs inhibit cyclooxygenase (COX), which is an enzyme that converts arachidonic acid to prostaglandin, a molecule that has many roles including the promotion of inflammation and pain. COX has two different isomers: COX-1 and COX-2. COX-1 may be the main contributor in the adverse side effect of gastric bleeding and ulcers. COX-2 is mainly involved in inflammation of tissues; COX-2 inhibition may be the key factor in the use of NSAIDs.[27,43]

NSAIDs given at a lower dosage act more as an analgesic, and NSAIDs given at a higher dosage have more of an antiinflammatory effect. Low doses of NSAIDs may be more appropriate with OA and early-phase RA.[8] Late-phase or severe RA may require a higher dosage. Educating the patient about the importance of regularly taking their NSAID to get proper dosage is important. Symptoms should decrease in the first 2 to 3 weeks of NSAID use; however, some patients respond better to different medications, so a different NSAID should be tried if the patient does not feel any improvement after 3 weeks.[27] Side effects to watch for include gastrointestinal bleeding and ulcers, dizziness, headaches, and drowsiness. Nausea and abdominal irritation are common and can be reduced by taking medication with food.[43]

Corticosteroids

Patients with inflammation as a primary symptom and patients who do not respond to NSAIDs are good candidates for corticosteroids.[8] Several corticosteroids are available, including prednisone, dexamethasone, hydrocortisone, and betamethasone.[27,43] Corticosteroids are primarily used on a short-term basis to decrease symptoms and allow for other management methods to be used, such as physical therapy. Although corticosteroids usually provide the fastest and most effective antiinflammatory response, long-term use has been shown to increase the risk of osteoporosis. Patients using corticosteroids should take precautions to ensure they get adequate calcium and vitamin D. Corticosteroids given by intraarticular injection should not be repeated more than three to four times in a year because of increased loss of blood supply to the bones. Oral and intravenous options are also available for administering corticosteroids. Most patients experience a decrease in symptoms within 24 hours of receiving a dose. Corticosteroids are often given along with NSAIDs or DMARDs.[19]

Disease-Modifying Antirheumatic Drugs

DMARDs are generally started as soon as a definite diagnosis of rheumatoid disease is made because they work in the early phases of the inflammatory process, can decrease arthritic symptoms, and possibly decrease the rate of damage to bone and cartilage.[19,27,43] DMARDs decrease this damage by suppressing the immune system, but they generally take several weeks to months to produce effects.[15] DMARDs are primarily used in patients with RA and SLE, but they may also be used in patients with psoriatic arthritis and ankylosing spondylitis.[15,43]

There are several types of DMARDs, including methotrexate, oral gold, penicillamine, sulfasalazine, and antimalarial drugs. Methotrexate is generally the first option for severe RA because of its long-term efficiency and its antiinflammatory and immunosuppressant effects.[15,27,43] Methotrexate tends to produce results within 2 to 6 weeks, as opposed to other DMARDs, which can take 6 months.[27,43] As stated earlier, it is important for the PTA to be cognitive of side effects for each drug. Side effects of methotrexate include nausea, vomiting, diarrhea, mouth ulcers, decreased white blood cell count, megaloblastic anemia, and liver fibrosis or cirrhosis.[43]

Oral gold was one of the first DMARDs that demonstrated improved symptoms in most patients, but it has several side effects that have a negative impact on the risk-to-benefit ratio. Penicillamine was another DMARD used; it has many adverse side effects with about the same amount of beneficial results as oral gold. Sulfasalazine has been shown to be effective in treating spondyloarthropathies and JRA.[15,43] Sulfasalazine has antibacterial, antiinflammatory, and immunomodulatory properties and has been shown to inhibit tumor necrosis factor (TNF) α, which coordinates the autoimmune process.[43,56]

Biologic Response Modifiers

The main purpose of biologic agents is to inhibit the chemicals that are key factors in the inflammation and autoimmune processes. In contrast to DMARDs, biologic response modifiers target specific components of the immune system, avoiding its widespread suppression.[15] Two chemicals that current RA drugs address are TNF and interleukin-1. TNF is a cytokine that activates lymphocytes and leukocytes, two inflammatory cell types that destroy the synovium of joints.[27,43] TNF inhibitors can be more effective than methotrexate in early phases of RA, but the two have been used in combination with favorable results.[27] Side effects are minimal with TNF inhibitors but can include fever, chills, dyspnea, hypotension, and possibly higher chances of infection.[44] Interleukin-1 receptor antagonist is designed to slow the rate of joint damage; this is done by blocking interleukin-1 α and β, which play a role in immune and inflammatory responses in the body.

Supplements

Over-the-counter glucosamine and chondroitin sulfate are two safe supplements widely used for pain with arthritis.[43] Glucosamine is a natural substance that is a precursor in the synthesis of glycosaminoglycans, which are present in cartilage. Glucosamine helps the body build and repair cartilage.[29] Chondroitin sulfate is a glycosaminoglycan and is thought to draw fluid into the cartilage, allowing for better joint function and protection from destructive enzymes.[29,43] No serious side effects have been documented with either of these supplements, and they are readily available.[29,43,54] According to Richy and colleagues,[54] patients taking glucosamine and chondroitin reported improved scores on a visual analog scale for pain and mobility. These two supplements have an excellent safety record and have been shown to be effective in managing the symptoms of arthritis in the knee and hip.[42]

SURGICAL MANAGEMENT OF RHEUMATIC DISORDERS

Surgery should be considered only after conservative management, such as rehabilitation, has been shown to be ineffective in relieving symptoms or improving function. There are always risks when undergoing surgery, and the PTA should encourage the patient to ask his or her physician questions about the surgery being recommended. There are numerous surgical options, including the following:

- Synovectomy
- Osteotomy
- Resection
- Arthrodesis
- Arthroscopy
- Arthroplasty

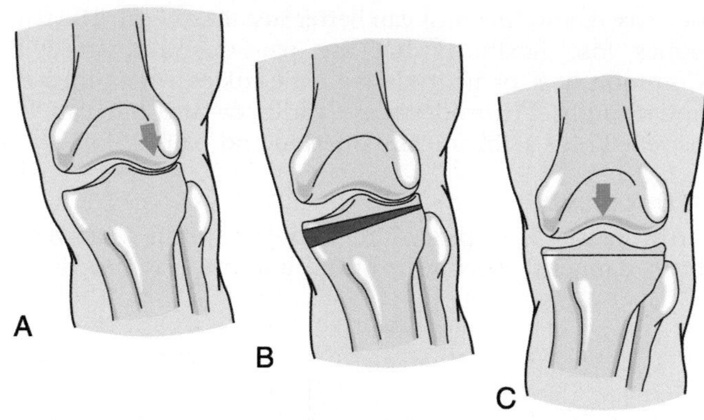

FIG 24-13 Osteotomy of tibia for genu valgum (valgus deformity); anterior view of left knee. **A,** Weight-bearing force is concentrated on one compartment of the knee. **B,** Wedge of bone is removed from tibia. The amount of bone removed is determined by how much correction in angulation is necessary. **C,** Distal portion of tibia is swung to proximal portion. Correction of angulation obtained allows weight-bearing forces to be more evenly distributed through both compartments of the knee. *(From Monahan FD:* Phipps' medical-surgical nursing: health and illness perspectives, *ed 8, St Louis, 2007, Mosby.)*

Synovectomy

Synovectomy is the removal of synovium infected with inflammation. Removing the inflamed synovium can decrease symptoms and prevent or slow destruction of a joint.[15] Synovium does grow back, so the long-term benefits of a synovectomy are unknown.[27]

Osteotomy

An osteotomy is a procedure in which bone is cut to change the alignment of the joint to a better position (Fig. 24-13). Osteotomy can improve the weight-bearing position of the lower extremities to aid in ambulation and is commonly used to correct coxa vara, genu valgum, and genu varum.[15] Osteotomy is one option that can be used to delay the need for a total joint replacement. During the rehabilitation of a patient after osteotomy, the therapist needs to be careful not to cause trauma or torque on the extremity until the bone heals. ROM and exercise should be done in a gentle manner, and increased discomfort in these activities should last no longer than 1 hour. Osteotomy may be used for a patient with a spondyloarthropathy disease who has severe deformities of the lumbar spine.[25]

RESECTION

In resection, part or all of a bone is removed from a stiff or immobile joint, creating a space between the bones (Fig. 24-14). The empty space fills with scar tissue, which can be more flexible.[15] Patients with severe arthritis of the foot can have bone resection in the foot to improve walking and pain. Other common sites for resections are the wrist, thumb, and elbow. The main goal of the surgery is to improve function and decrease pain.

Arthrodesis

Arthrodesis is the artificial ossification between two bones or a bone fusion (Fig. 24-15). By fusing, the joint pain is decreased, and the joint can better sustain weight. The two bones lose flexibility but are pain-free and sturdy.[15] Common sites for arthrodesis are the ankles, wrists, fingers, and thumbs. Arthrodesis use varies by site but can be beneficial for a chronically infected and painful joint.[27]

Arthroplasty

Arthroplasty is a procedure to repair joints that have been damaged, become painful, and are less functional (see Fig. 18-8). Total joint replacement is a very successful method for decreasing pain and improving functional ability. The arthritic joint is replaced with metal, ceramic, and plastic parts. The two most common joint replacements are knee and hip, but shoulder, elbow, ankle, and knuckles also can be replaced.[27] In general, patients are expected to return to functional levels of strength, mobility, and ROM after 6 months.[3] Hip and knee arthroplasties are common surgical interventions in patients with OA[36]; total hip arthroplasty is the most common procedure in patients with ankylosing spondylitis.[25]

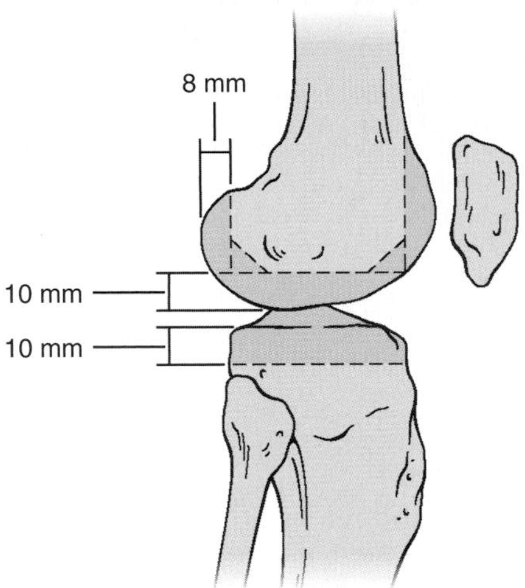

FIG 24-14 In the measured resection technique, as much bone or cartilage (or both) is removed as will be replaced by the thickness of the arthroplasty components. This method attempts to restore the anatomic joint line level. *(From Magee DJ:* Pathology and intervention in musculoskeletal rehabilitation, *St Louis, 2009, Mosby.)*

Arthroscopy

Arthroscopy is not a procedure but rather a means of performing a procedure. An arthroscope is a thin tube with a light at the end connected to a screen. Arthroscopic surgery allows for exploration of a joint to determine what is wrong and to determine how extensive the damage is. Biopsies, cutting loose tissue, repairing cartilage, and smoothing rough surfaces all can be done arthroscopically. Arthroscopic surgery can have a faster recovery time than more invasive procedures because only small incisions are required, and minimal anesthesia is used. Surgeries commonly performed arthroscopically include meniscus repairs, rotator cuff repairs, cartilage damage repairs, and labral tear repair.

GLOSSARY

Atrophy: A wasting away; a decrease in size of an organ or tissue.

Closed chain exercises: Distal end of extremity is fixed to the ground or to a device; for example, keeping your feet on the ground while bending the knees.

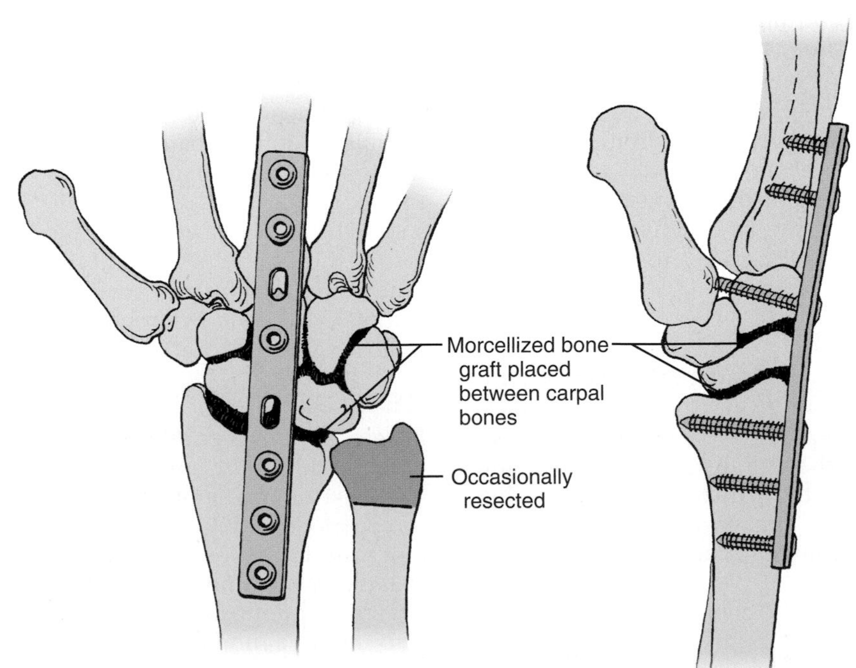

FIG 24-15 Total wrist arthrodesis. *(From Burke SL:* Hand and upper extremity rehabilitation: a practical guide, *ed 3, St Louis, 2006, Churchill Livingstone.)*

Connective tissue: Tissue that supports and connects other tissues and parts of the body. Connective tissue has comparatively few cells. Its bulk consists of intercellular substance or matrix, the nature of which gives each connective tissue its particular properties.

Infection: The presence and growth of a microorganism that produces tissue damage.

Inflammation: Nonspecific response that occurs in reaction to any type of bodily injury. Symptoms include rubor (redness), calor (heat), tumor (swelling), and dolor (pain).

Malaise: Discomfort, uneasiness, or indisposition, often indicative of infection.

Open chain exercises: Distal end of extremity is not fixed and can move freely; for example, if you raise one foot off the ground, you can move the leg in any direction.

Proteoglycan: A glycoprotein that retains water providing more absorptive properties to the cartilage.[2]

REFERENCES

1. American College of Sports Medicine: *ACSM's guidelines for exercise testing and prescription*, ed 6, Philadelphia, 2000, Lippincott Williams & Wilkins.
2. American Pain Society: *Guideline on the management of pain in osteoarthritis, rheumatoid arthritis, and juvenile chronic arthritis*, ed 2, Glenview, IL, 2002, American Pain Society.
3. American Physical Therapy Association: *Guide to physical therapist practice*, Alexandria, VA, 2003, American Physical Therapy Association.
4. Andrews JR, Harrelson GL, Wilk KE: *Physical rehabilitation of the injured athlete*, ed 3, Philadelphia, 2004, Saunders.
5. Beardmore TD: Rehabilitation of patients with rheumatic diseases. In Klippel JH, editor: *Primer on the rheumatic diseases*, ed 13, New York, 2008, Springer, pp 599–608.
6. Berenbaum F: Osteoarthritis: B. Pathology and pathogenesis. In Klippel JH, editor: *Primer on the rheumatic diseases*, ed 13, New York, 2008, Springer, pp 229–234.
7. Berger TG: Skin, hair, and nails. In Tierney LM, McPhee SJ, Papadakis MA, editors: *Current medical diagnosis and treatment*, New York, 2006, Lange.
8. Bolten WW: Differential analgesic treatment in arthrosis and arthritis. *MMW Fortschr Med* 146:40–42, 2004.
9. Brinker MR, Miller MD: *Fundamentals of orthopaedics*, Philadelphia, 1999, Saunders.
10. Brinker MR, O'Conner DP: Basic sciences. In Miller MD, Brinker MR, editors: *Review of orthopedics*, ed 3, Philadelphia, 2008, Saunders.
11. Brosseau L, Yonge KA, Welch V, et al: Transcutaneous electrical nerve stimulation (TENS) for the treatment of rheumatoid arthritis in the hand. *Cochrane Database Syst Rev* (2):CD004377, 2003.
12. Burckhardt CS: Fibromyalgia. In Robbins L, Burckhardt CS, Hannan MT, et al, editors: *Clinical care in the rheumatic diseases*, Atlanta, 2001, Association of Rheumatology Health Professionals.
13. Cheng YJ, Hootman JM, Murphy LB, et al: Prevalence of doctor-diagnosed arthritis and arthritis-attributable activity limitation—United States, 2007–2009. *MMWR Morb Mortal Wkly Rep* 59:1261–1265, 2010.
14. Dieppe P: Osteoarthritis: A. Clinical features. In Klippel JH, editor: *Primer on the rheumatic diseases*, ed 13, New York, 2008, Springer, pp 224–228.
15. Dunkin MA: *The Arthritis Foundation's guide to managing your arthritis*, Atlanta, 2001, Arthritis Foundation.
16. Foley RA: Transcutaneous electrical nerve stimulation. In Hayes KW, editor: *Manual for physical agents*, Saddle River, NJ, 2000, Prentice Hall.
17. Fumagalli M, Sarzi-Puttini P, Atzeni F: Hand osteoarthritis. *Semin Arthritis Rheum* 34(Suppl 2):47–52, 2005.
18. Gabriel SE, Crowson CS, O'Fallon WM: Comorbidity in arthritis. *J Rheumatol* 26:2475–2479, 1999.
19. Goodman CC: *Pathology: implications for the physical therapist*, ed 2, St Louis, 2009, Saunders.
20. Gornisiewicz M, Moreland LW: Rheumatoid arthritis. In Robbins L, Burckhardt CS, Hannan MT, et al, editors: *Clinical care in the rheumatic diseases*, Atlanta, 2001, Association of Rheumatology Health Professionals.
21. Hafstrom I, Albertsson K, Boonen A, et al: Remission achieved after 2 years treatment with low-dose prednisone in addition to disease-modifying anti-rheumatic drugs in early rheumatoid arthritis is associated with reduced joint destruction still present after 4 years: an open 2-year continuation study. *Ann Rheum Dis* 68:508–513, 2009.
22. Hannan MT: Epidemiology of rheumatic diseases. In Robbins L, Burckhardt CS, Hannan MT, et al, editors: *Clinical care in the rheumatic diseases*, Atlanta, 2001, Association of Rheumatology Health Professionals.
23. Harrell PB: Splinting of the hand. In Robbins L, Burckhardt CS, Hannan MT, et al, editors: *Clinical care in the rheumatic diseases*, Atlanta, 2001, Association of Rheumatology Health Professionals.
24. Hayes KW: Physical modalities. In Robbins L, Burckhardt CS, Hannan MT, et al, editors: *Clinical care in the rheumatic diseases*, Atlanta, 2001, Association of Rheumatology Health Professionals.
25. Helewa A, Stokes B: Spondylarthropathies. In Robbins L, Burckhardt CS, Hannan MT, et al, editors: *Clinical care in the rheumatic diseases*, Atlanta, 2001, Association of Rheumatology Health Professionals.
26. Helliwell PS, Abbott Chamberlain MS: A randomized trial of three different physiotherapy regimes in ankylosing spondylitis. *Physiotherapy* 82:85–90, 1996.
27. Hellmann DB, Stone JH: Arthritis and musculoskeletal disorders. In Tierney LM, McPhee SJ, Papadakis MA, editors: *Current medical diagnosis and treatment*, New York, 2006, Lange.
28. Hidding A, Van der Linden S, De Witte L: Therapeutic effect of individual physical therapy in ankylosing spondylitis related to disease duration. *Clin Rheumatol* 12:334–340, 1993.
29. Horstman J: *Arthritis Foundation's guide to alternative therapies*, Atlanta, 1999, Arthritis Foundation.
30. Hurkmans E, van der Giesen FJ, VlietVlieland TP, et al: Dynamic exercise programs (aerobic capacity and/or muscle strength training) in patients with rheumatoid arthritis. *Cochrane Database Syst Rev* (4):CD006853, 2009.
31. Kelly J, Devonshire R: *Taking charge of fibromyalgia: a self-management program for your fibromyalgia syndrome*, Wayzata, MN, 2001, Fibromyalgia Educational Systems.
32. Kishiyama JL, Adelman DC: Allergic and immunologic disorders. In Tierney LM, McPhee SJ, Papadakis MA, editors: *Current medical diagnosis and treatment*, New York, 2006, Lange.
33. Klareskog L, Catrina AI, Paget S: Rheumatoid arthritis. *Lancet* 373:659–672, 2009.
34. Koopman WJ: *Arthritis and allied conditions: a textbook of rheumatology*, Philadelphia, 2001, Lippincott Williams & Wilkins.
35. Lawrence RC, Felson DT, Helmick CG, et al: Estimates of the prevalence of arthritis and other rheumatic conditions in the United States. Part II. *Arthritis Rheum* 58:26–35, 2008.
36. Lozada CJ, Altman RD: Osteoarthritis. In Robbins L, Burckhardt CS, Hannan MT, et al, editors: *Clinical care in the rheumatic diseases*, Atlanta, 2001, Association of Rheumatology Health Professionals.
37. Luggen AS, Meiner SE: *Care of arthritis in the older adult*, New York, 2002, Springer.
38. Lundon K: *Orthopedic rehabilitation science: principles for clinical management of bone*, Boston, 2000, Butterworth-Heinemann.
39. Magee DJ: *Orthopedic physical assessment*, ed 5, St Louis, 2009, Saunders.
40. Mannerkorpi K, Iverson MD: The use of exercise and rehabilitation regimens. In Wallace DJ, Clauw DJ, editors: *Fibromyalgia and other central pain syndromes*, Philadelphia, 2005, Lippincott Williams & Wilkins.
41. Maricic MJ: Osteoporosis. In Robbins L, Burckhardt CS, Hannan MT, et al, editors: *Clinical care in the rheumatic diseases*, Atlanta, 2001, Association of Rheumatology Health Professionals.
42. McAlindon TE, Lavalley MP, Gulin JP, et al: Glucosamine and chondroitin for treatment of osteoarthritis: a systematic quality assessment and analysis. *JAMA* 283:1469–1475, 2000.

43. Miller DR: Pharmacologic interventions in the 21st century. In Robbins L, Burckhardt CS, Hannan MT, et al, editors: *Clinical care in the rheumatic diseases*, Atlanta, 2001, Association of Rheumatology Health Professionals.
44. Miller MD: *Review of orthopaedics*, ed 3, Philadelphia, 2000, Saunders.
45. Minor MA: Exercise in the treatment of osteoarthritis. *Rheum Dis Clin North Am* 25:387–415, 1999.
46. Minor MA, Hewitt JE, Webel RR, et al: Efficacy of physical conditioning exercise in patients with rheumatoid arthritis and osteoarthritis. *Arthritis Rheum* 32:1396–1405, 1989.
47. Minor MA, Westby MD: Rest and exercise. In Robbins L, Burckhardt CS, Hannan MT, et al, editors: *Clinical care in the rheumatic diseases*, Atlanta, 2001, Association of Rheumatology Health Professionals.
48. Moldofsky H, MacFarlane JG: Sleep and its potential role in chronic pain and fatigue. In Wallace DJ, Clauw DJ, editors: *Fibromyalgia and other central pain syndromes*, Philadelphia, 2005, Lippincott Williams & Wilkins.
49. Nichols LA: History and physical assessment. In Robbins L, Burckhardt CS, Hannan MT, et al, editors: *Clinical care in the rheumatic diseases*, Atlanta, 2001, Association of Rheumatology Health Professionals.
50. Oegema TR, Lewis JL, Mikecz K, et al: Osteoarthritis and rheumatoid arthritis. In Einhorn TA, O'Keefe RJ, Buckwalter JA, editors: *Orthopaedic basic science*, ed 3, Rosemont, IL, 2007, American Academy of Orthopaedic Surgeons, pp 395–413.
51. Ramsey-Goldman R: Connective tissue diseases. In Robbins L, Burckhardt CS, Hannan MT, et al, editors: *Clinical care in the rheumatic diseases*, Atlanta, 2001, Association of Rheumatology Health Professionals.
52. Rayman M, Callaghan A: *Nutrition and arthritis*, Danvers, Mass, 2006, Blackwell.
53. Rhoades RA, Tanner GA: *Medical physiology*, Baltimore, 2003, Lippincott Williams & Wilkins.
54. Richy F, Bruyere O, Ethgen O, et al: Structural and symptomatic efficacy of glucosamine and chondroitin in knee osteoarthritis. *Arch Intern Med* 163:1514–1522, 2003.
55. Roach HI, Tilley S: The pathogenesis of osteoarthritis. In Bronner F, Farach-Carson MC, editors: *Bone and osteoarthritis: Topics in bone biology*, London, 2008, Springer-Verlag.
56. Rodenburg RJ, Ganga A, vanLent PL, et al: The antiinflammatory drug sulfasalazine inhibits tumor necrosis factor alpha expression in macrophages by inducing apoptosis. *Arthritis Rheum* 43:1941–1950, 2000.
57. Rogers MW, Wilder FV: The effects of strength training among persons with hand osteoarthritis: a two-year follow up study. *J Hand Ther* 20:244–250, 2007.
58. Schumacher RH, Gall EP: *Rheumatoid arthritis: an illustrated guide to pathology, diagnosis, and management*, Philadelphia, 1988, Lippincott.
59. Scott DL, Kingsley GH: *Inflammatory arthritis in clinical practice*, London, 2008, Springer-Verlag.
60. Semble EL, Loeser RF, Wise CM: Therapeutic exercise for rheumatoid arthritis and osteoarthritis. *Semin Arthritis Rheum* 20:32–40, 1990.
61. Sherwood L: *Human physiology from cells to systems*, ed 2, Independence, KY, 2010, Brooks Cole.
62. Taylor J, Erlandson D: Pediatric rheumatic disorders. In Robbins L, Burckhardt CS, Hannan MT, et al, editors: *Clinical care in the rheumatic diseases*, Atlanta, 2001, Association of Rheumatology Health Professionals.
63. Tehlirian CV, Bathon JM: Rheumatoid arthritis: A. clinical and laboratory manifestations. In Klippel JH, editor: *Primer on the rheumatic diseases*, ed 13, New York, 2008, Springer, pp 114–121.
64. Van Vugt RM, Derksen RH, Kater J, et al: Deforming arthropathy or lupus and rhupus hands in systemic lupus erythematosus. *Ann Rheum Dis* 57:540–544, 1998.
65. Waldburger JM, Firestein GS: Rheumatoid arthritis: B. epidemiology, pathology, and pathogenesis. In Klippel JH, editor: *Primer on the rheumatic diseases*, ed 13, New York, 2008, Springer, pp 122–132.
66. Wang TJ, Belza B, Thompson EF, et al: Effects of aquatic exercise on flexibility, strength, and aerobic fitness in adults with osteoarthritis of the hip or knee. *J Adv Nurs* 57:141–152, 2007.
67. Welch V, Brosseau L, Casimiro L, et al: Thermotherapy for treating rheumatoid arthritis. *Cochrane Database Syst Rev* (2):CD002826, 2002.

REVIEW QUESTIONS

Multiple Choice

1. Which of the following is not found in articular cartilage?
   A. Type I collagen
   B. Type II collagen
   C. Chondrocytes
   D. Proteoglycans
2. What is the role of metalloproteinase in OA?
   A. Increases type II collagen production
   B. Decreases type I collagen production
   C. Increases proteoglycan production
   D. Breaks down cartilage collagen and proteoglycans
3. Which of the following joints is least likely to be affected by OA?
   A. Knee
   B. Shoulder
   C. Spine
   D. Hip
4. Addition of which of the following can reduce the progression of OA?
   A. Vitamin B and potassium
   B. Vitamin D and potassium
   C. Vitamin B and calcium
   D. Vitamin D and calcium
5. Patients with OA should begin a strengthening program after they have progressed to what amount of stretching without an increase in symptoms?
   A. 5 minutes
   B. 10 minutes
   C. 15 minutes
   D. 30 minutes
6. Which of the following types of exercise are contraindicated in advanced OA?
   A. Open chain
   B. Isotonic
   C. Closed chain
   D. Isometric
7. Which of the following is an early sign of RA?
   A. Swelling
   B. Weight loss
   C. Redness
   D. Stiffness in specific joints
8. Which of the following is a swan neck deformity in the finger?
   A. Hyperextension of PIP and flexion of DIP
   B. Flexion of PIP with hyperextension of DIP
   C. Hyperflexion of PIP with extension of DIP
   D. Hyperextension of DIP and flexion of PIP
9. At what phase of RA are pain-free isomtreic exercises recommended?
   A. Acute
   B. Subacute
   C. Chronic
   D. Prolonged chronic

10. In what type of arthritis is it common to see a "pencil-in-cup" deformity on imaging studies?
    A. Reiter's syndrome
    B. Psoriatic arthritis
    C. OA
    D. RA
11. In order to confirm the diagnosis of JRA, how long must children have symptoms of arthritis?
    A. 2 consecutive weeks
    B. 4 consecutive weeks
    C. 6 consecutive weeks
    D. 8 consecutive weeks
12. What is the strongest indicator of functional disability in children with systemic JRA?
    A. Pain
    B. Strength
    C. ROM
    D. Emotional status
13. Where does the rash associated with SLE occur?
    A. On the backs of the hands
    B. Over the nose and cheeks
    C. On the dorsum of the feet
    D. Over the shoulders
14. Which of the following is not a risk factor for osteoporosis?
    A. Sedentary lifestyle
    B. Smoking
    C. Small body frame
    D. African-American race
15. During what phase of arthritis should splinting be used?
    A. Acute
    B. Subacute
    C. Chronic
    D. Prolonged chronic

Short Answer

16. Name at least five characteristics that can predispose someone to arthritis.
17. Discuss at least seven differences between OA and RA.
18. List two examples from each of these types of drugs: analgesics, NSAIDs, corticosteroids, DMARDs, and biologic response modifiers.
19. List the three types of JRA and how many joints are affected by each disease.
20. List four diagnosis criteria for SLE.

Fill in the Blank

21. Pain associated with OA usually _______ with activity and is ______ with rest.
22. _______increase activation of fibroblast-like cells and macrophages leading to breakdown of cartilage and bone in patients with RA.
23. Approximately 80% of individuals with _________ are positive for HLA-B27.
24. Recurrent inflammation of tendons and other supportive structures of the joints can lead to ulnar deviation of the second to fifth fingers and subluxation of the metacarpophalangeal joints, which is referred to as __________.
25. Patients with inflammation as a primary symptom or who do not respond to NSAIDs are good candidates for __________.

True/False

26. Arthritis is more common in women.
27. During the acute phase of arthritis, patients should rest and not stretch or exercise.
28. The intensity of exercise should be 50% of the patient's maximum heart rate.
29. A prone program is recommended for a patient with ankylosing spondylitis.
30. Patients with SLE should be cautioned against prolonged sun exposure.

Chapter 25

Orthopedic Management of Pain and Pain Syndromes

Adriaan Louw, Terry Cox

CHAPTER OUTLINE

LEARNING OBJECTIVES

1. Describe how pain can be a burden to the patient and society.
2. Detail a brief history of how pain has been treated in the past.
3. Describe a biopsychosocial model for treating pain.
4. Describe how pain is a multisystem output.
5. Describe a neuromatrix and how it relates to a person's neural signature.
6. Describe how the medical terminology used can influence a patient's level of fear and anxiety.
7. Describe how multiple body systems can be influenced by a persistent pain state.
8. Describe the bidirectional approach for treatment of patients with a persistent pain state.
9. Identify the 12 treatment principles for treating patients that present with a persistent pain state.
10. Apply knowledge of the 12 treatment principles in the context of therapeutic neuroscience education for patients with persistent pain.

KEY TERMS

Adrenaline
Biopsychosocial model
Cartesian model of pain
Chronic pain
Cortisol
Ion channels
Nerve sensitization
Neuromatrix theory
Nociception
Pain
Pain neurotag
"Red flags"
Pain gate
Therapeutic neuroscience education (TNE)

THE PATIENT WITH CHRONIC PAIN

A middle-aged woman enters physical therapy seeking help for low-back pain (LBP). After a thorough examination, gentle exercises, education, and provision of a home exercise program (HEP), the patient is sent home, asked to walk, perform her HEP, and return for follow-up care. Feeling she was not understood, the patient created a drawing of her pain to make the physical therapist (PT) and assistant physical therapist (PTA) have a better realization of her LBP (Fig. 25-1). This patient's drawing is a small window affording a view of a problem affecting more Americans than any other disease state: chronic pain.

Pain is a normal, human experience. Without the ability to experience pain, humans would not survive. However, living in pain is not normal. As pain rates increase, physical therapy practitioners will encounter, on an ever-increasing scale, the complexities and challenges associated with treating patients experiencing pain, especially chronic pain. **Chronic pain** is pain that persists beyond normal tissue healing time, which is generally thought to be between 3 and 6 months.[106,167] In the United States, it is estimated that approximately 116 million Americans have persistent pain.[72] Chronic pain rates have been steadily increasing with epidemiologic data from the early 1990s showing one in seven people experiencing persistent pain and more recent data indicating that closer to one in four people are currently affected.[106,167]

What treatments can we offer patients with chronic pain? Traditional treatments such as electrical stimulation,

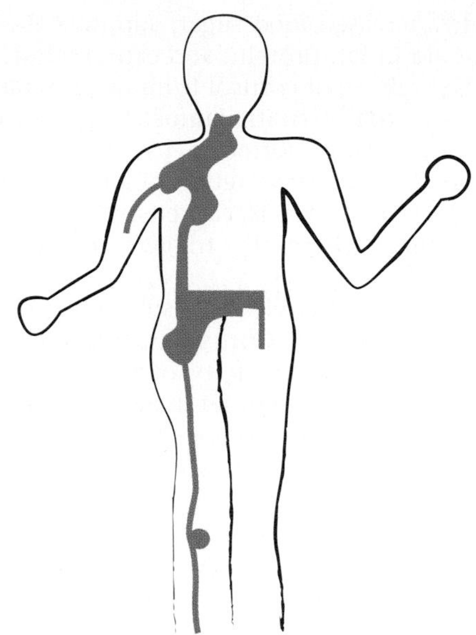

FIG 25-1 A patient's drawing of her low-back pain.

transcutaneous electrical neuromuscular stimulation (TENS), and therapeutic ultrasound are of little value because the pain is spread over various body parts. The good news is that there is "gold level" evidence at the present time for certain treatment strategies aimed at treating these very challenging patients. A Cochrane review highlighted two commonly used therapeutic approaches to help patients with chronic pain: aerobic exercise and cognitive behavioral therapy (specialized education).[14] A cynical physical therapy practitioner will likely read this comment and state, "Sure, they need to exercise, but they hurt all the time!" Education can be used, but a practitioner who uses a tissue model to educate people about pain will likely struggle treating these patients.[83,128,156] The goal of this chapter is to update physical therapy practitioners on the latest neuroscience view of pain and how such a viewpoint allows practitioners not only to understand why approaches such as education and exercise can help patients with chronic pain but also to provide real-life clinical strategies to help these patients.

THE LION METAPHOR

An easy way to reconceptualize pain, or more specifically chronic pain, is the basic threat response.[93,146] The basic threat response, often assigned to the sympathetic nervous system, is the fight-and-flight response. However, the stress response during an immediate threat is significantly more complex and involves various other bodily systems. An example the authors like to use in patient education about the stress response is the scenario of a big roaring African lion entering the room.

To deal with this immediate threat, the body reacts with various systems:

- Adrenaline: **Adrenaline** is a centrally acting neurotransmitter and a hormone affecting almost all body tissues, but it is best known to regulate heart rate, blood vessel and air passage diameters, and metabolic shifts.[146] The action varies, depending on the tissues and adrenergic receptors; for example, high levels of adrenaline cause smooth muscle relaxation in the airways but cause contraction of the smooth muscle that lines most arterioles. Adrenaline works via the sympathetic nervous system. In response to a perceived threat, the heart rate increases rapidly to pump blood through the body to areas needing blood and oxygen. Adrenaline causes hypervigilance. If a lion enters the room, it is not time for a nap.[140]
- Muscles: In an immediate threat response, large muscles able to evade the threat or face the threat are needed. Big, strong leg muscles activate to run away. Arm muscles activate to "punch the lion." Smaller muscles are not needed, such as postural muscles or even stabilizing muscles.[66,82,112] Deactivating these muscles for the immediate threat seems like a good strategy, and they should be switched back on when the threat has been removed.
- Language: When startled with a threat such as the lion, you will likely say a few choice words in a loud, sharp, and abrasive voice.[154]
- Breathing: With the impending threat, breathing becomes faster and shallower.
- Gastrointestinal system: Digestion of food is slowed down and even put on hold, allowing for all possible energy and blood flow to be allocated to the immediate, much needed systems.
- Other: Other responses can involve reproduction, pain, motivation, and memory.

When the lion is captured by a gamekeeper or animal control officer, the stress response dissipates, and homeostasis allows the systems to normalize and prepare for the next stress response.[146] This process occurs daily as people are faced with differing stressors. However, the system is designed to elevate and then calm down; it is not designed to continue to run at elevated levels for prolonged periods. How does this pertain to a patient with chronic pain? Living in pain is not normal and becomes a stressor, similar to a lion. Apart from the pain, various psychosocial issues have been correlated to a chronic pain experience.[79,168] These psychosocial issues increase threat and ultimately the pain experience. The most common psychosocial issues identified to perpetuate pain include various explanations for pain, failed treatments, fear, anxiety, family issues, and job and money issues. Put together, the lion is a metaphorical description of these psychosocial issues that occur along with the daily pain (Fig. 25-2).

During this acute stress response, adrenaline levels are increased. It is thought that adrenosensitive **ion channels** (nerve sensors) open, allowing for an easier firing of the nervous system and the resultant pain response. Clinically, the patient may experience pain secondary to stress, anxiety, or fear and not just injured or damaged tissues. This pain response may explain increased pain experiences reported during high-stress scenarios, such as spinal surgery, litigation, or whiplash injuries. In chronic pain, the stress response is protracted. If the stressors and biopsychosocial factors (lion) remain in place for months or years, the resultant chemical activation will have significant repercussions for the nervous system, tissues, and brain. The stress biology analogy would be the lion following a patient for months. The stress response is primarily executed by adrenaline initially, followed by cortisol changes in the body.

Adrenaline is a fast-acting neurotransmitter and likely very effective in the immediate stress response, which should last no longer than several minutes. **Cortisol** is a more potent and longer lasting chemical, similar in effect to adrenaline but produced to deal with longer lasting threats.[146] Cortisol is a glucocorticoid steroid hormone produced by the adrenal gland and is more formally known as hydrocortisone.[146] The primary function of cortisol is to increase blood sugar; suppress the immune system; and aid in fat, protein, and carbohydrate metabolism.[139,149] The release of cortisol from the adrenal gland is controlled by the hypothalamus. The secretion of corticotropin-releasing hormone by the hypothalamus triggers anterior pituitary secretion of adrenocorticotropic hormone (ACTH). ACTH is carried by the cells to the vascular cortex, where it triggers blood secretion (Fig. 25-3).[50,93,162]

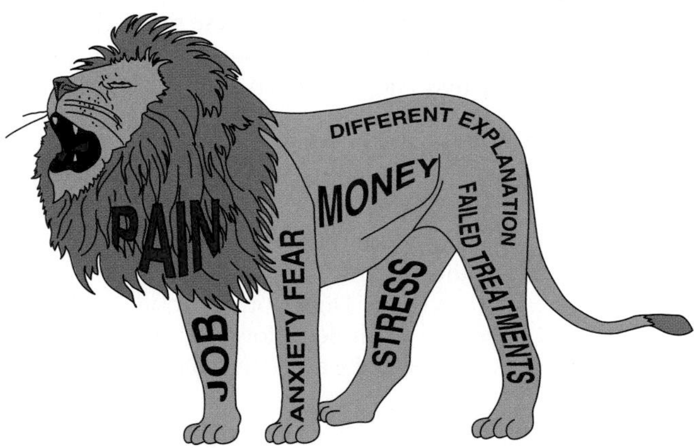

FIG 25-2 A lion as a metaphor for stressors associated with a persistent pain state. *(From Louw A:* Why do I hurt? A neuroscience approach to pain, *Minneapolis, 2013, OPTP.)*

Cortisol prevents the release of substances in the body that cause inflammation. Cortisol is used to treat conditions resulting from overactivity of the B cell–mediated antibody response, such as inflammatory and rheumatoid diseases and allergies. Low-potency hydrocortisone is used to treat skin conditions such as rashes and eczema. Elevated levels of cortisol, if prolonged, can lead to proteolysis and muscle wasting. Cortisol has a daily pattern, typically peaking around 8 A.M. with the lowest level between midnight and 4 A.M., or 3 to 5 hours after sleep initiation.[22,34]

Cortisol levels are affected by changes in ACTH; depression; psychological stress; and physiologic stressors such as illness, surgery, fear, injury, and pain. Changes in cortisol levels have been linked to a reduction in bone formation and thought to be responsible for the mechanism behind stress dwarfism.[161] Cortisol works along with adrenaline to create short-term memories. Long-term exposure to cortisol damages hippocampus cells, limiting learning and altering memory.[108] Cortisol dysregulation increases blood pressure; shuts down the reproductive system; and is associated with weight gain, appetite changes, and obesity.

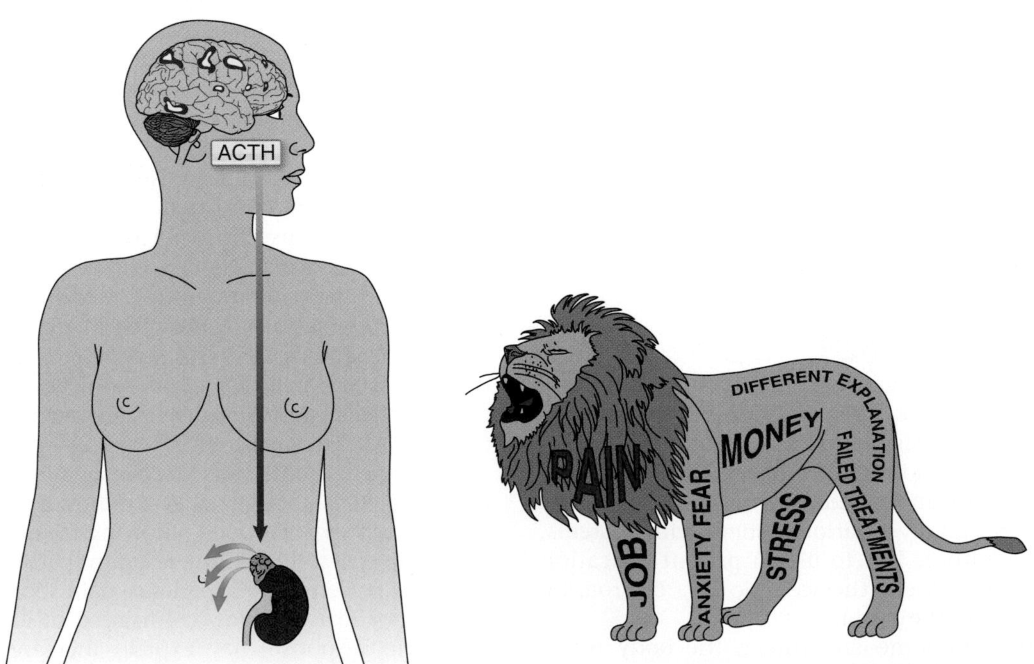

FIG 25-3 Release of cortisol from the adrenal gland in response to threat is controlled by the hypothalamus via corticotropin-releasing hormone, which triggers secretion of adrenocorticotropic hormone (ACTH) from the anterior pituitary gland. ACTH triggers release of cortisol into the bloodstream. *(From Louw A, Puentedura EJ:* Therapeutic neuroscience education, *Minneapolis, 2013, OPTP.)*

A more significant effect of cortisol change is its effect on the immune system, specifically proinflammatory cytokines. Cytokines are immune molecules, and they affect tissue healing significantly.[29] During infections or trauma, cytokines such as interleukin-6 increase 1000-fold, allowing for more ion channels specific to cytokines to open up, potentially resulting in increased sensitivity. This process occurs during a bout of the flu. A major stimulus for the production of cytokines is cortisol. With increased cytokines, there is the further possibility of increased inflammatory processes all over the body, including keeping tissues inflamed.

Pain is complex. Modern understanding of pain has been updated to include a neuroscience approach to pain from a therapeutic perspective.[91,104,111,115] This detailed discussion on the stress response should allow physical therapy practitioners to appreciate how various chemicals contribute to a pain experience and how pain is a multiple-system response to threat (Fig. 25-4).[93] An integral part of the pain experience in a patient is now believed to be mainly due to complex biologic and physiologic processes in the nervous system, brain, endocrine system, and immune system, which are often included under the term *neuroscience* (see Fig. 25-4). In the past 20 years, physical therapy has attained a greater understanding of the neuroscience of pain, resulting in a neuroscience approach to pain. This neuroscience approach is gaining popularity and becoming a part of physical therapy curricula, continuing education classes, and clinical practice.

This elaborate neuroscience description of pain provides physical therapy practitioners a rationale and treatment model to understand why aerobic exercise and education have gained "gold level" evidence for treating people with pain.[14] It is proposed that if a PTA is to provide optimal assistance to a PT treating a patient with pain, he

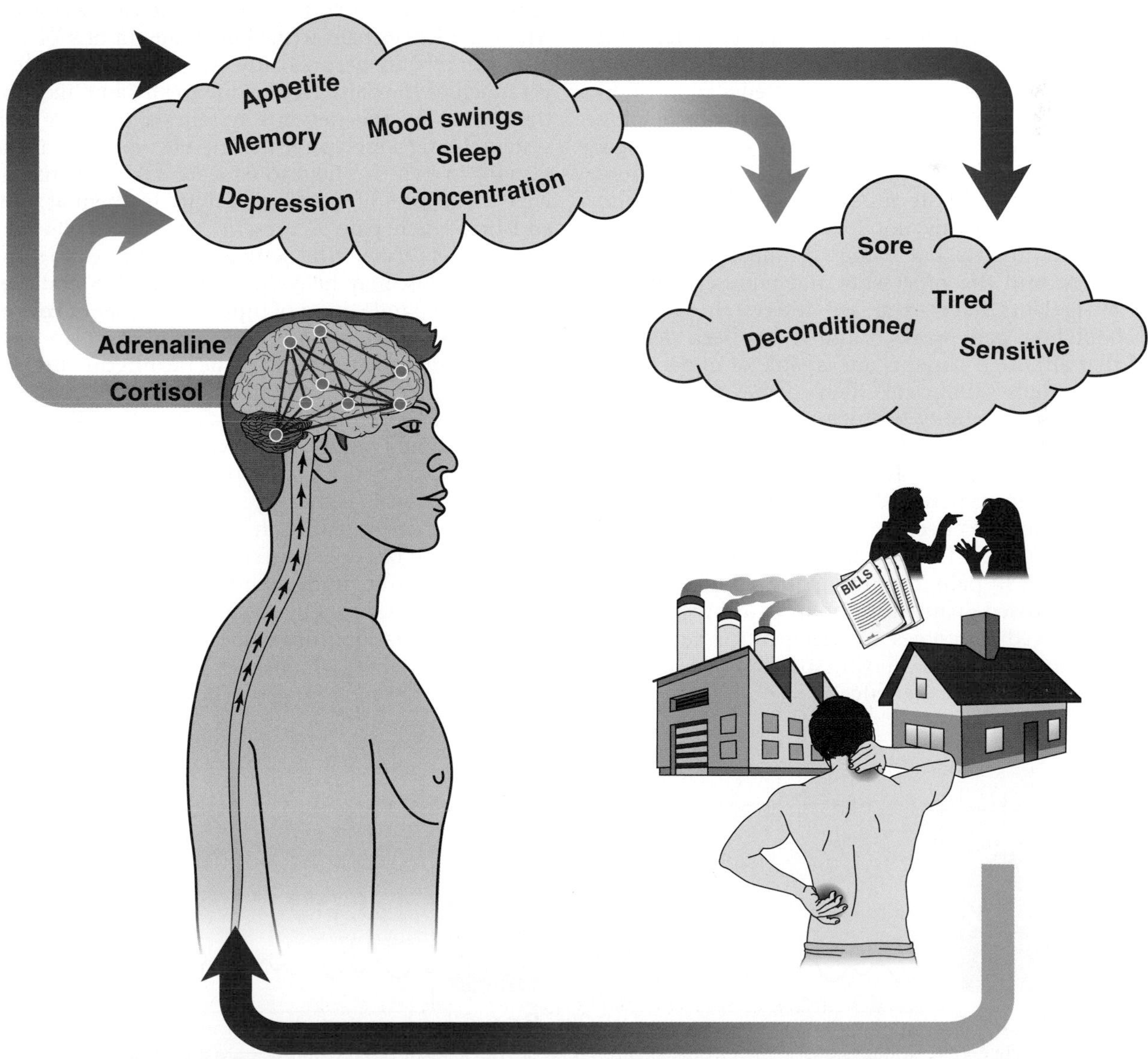

FIG 25-4 The pain mechanism model based on the mature organism model by Gifford.[51] *(From Louw A, Puentedura EJ:* Therapeutic neuroscience education, *Minneapolis, 2013, OPTP.)*

or she also needs to have an updated neuroscience view of pain. This chapter aims to update the PTA on the neuroscience of pain, with the goal being to incorporate this knowledge into clinical treatments such as patient education, exercise, and movement.

COGNITIVE THERAPY

PATIENT EDUCATION

Most education programs used for orthopedic patient populations, such as the patient with LBP described earlier, employ anatomic and biomechanical models for addressing pain, which not only have been shown to have limited efficacy[11] but also may lead to an increase in fear, anxiety, and stress in patients, negatively affecting outcomes.[97,132] Several educational strategies are advocated for patients with LBP, including biomechanical/back school type of education, evidence-based guideline education (i.e., the Back Book[13]), cognitive behavioral therapy,[74] and most recently **therapeutic neuroscience education (TNE)**.[112,122,123]

Research in educational strategies for patients with chronic LBP finds an increased advocacy of TNE.[112,122] Neuroscience education is a cognitive-based education intervention that aims to reduce pain and disability by helping patients gain an increased understanding of the biologic process underpinning their pain state.[142] TNE differs from traditional education strategies such as back school and biomechanical models by not focusing on anatomic or biomechanical models but rather on neurophysiology, neurobiology, and the processing and representation of pain.[102,142] Patients have expressed interest in knowing more about how pain works,[92] and it has been demonstrated that although patients are capable of understanding the neurophysiology of their pain, professionals underestimate their ability to understand the "complex" issues related to pain.[124]

Studies that use TNE have shown that it decreases patients' fear, changes patients' perception of their pain,[110] and has an immediate effect on improvements in patients' attitudes about pain.[15] TNE has also been shown to result in improvements in pain, cognition, and physical performance[112]; increased pain thresholds during physical tasks[122]; improved outcomes of therapeutic exercises[123]; and significant reduction in widespread brain activity characteristic of a pain experience.[113]

It is strongly recommended that the PTA develop a greater understanding of the new neuroscience view of pain (as described in this chapter) and develop an ability to use it in clinical practice. In an ideal practice setting, the primary PT would initiate the TNE, and the PTA would continue supporting and teaching the same updated view of pain, providing a true team approach. Apart from one-on-one "sit-down" education sessions, it is imperative for the PTA to realize that most education/cognitive restructuring is done while performing traditional movement-based therapies such as exercise, mobilization, soft tissue treatment, and other therapeutic approaches.[91] Part of this TNE approach involves developing a new "pain language" using metaphors and examples to explain to patients how pain really works and what pain may mean.[49,91] An easy example is nerve sensitivity, and this applies to the patient with LBP who described widespread pain discussed at the beginning of this chapter (see Fig 25-1). It is now believed that most of the pain a patient experiences is due not only to an injury or disease state such as arthritis but also to a heightened sensitivity of the nervous system. In such a case, the patient who experiences pain while performing a task or exercise may think the tissues are badly injured because of the pain, yet much of the pain may be due to an "amplification" of the signals by the nervous system—a sensitive nervous system. Using a metaphor that nerves work like an "alarm system," a PTA can help to educate a patient that nerves have some level of electrical activity in them at all times and that when pain is present, the nerves elevate their resting levels of electrical activity to become extra sensitive. This metaphor may help the patient understand that the pain is not an indication of injury but rather of **increased nerve sensitization** (Fig. 25-5, *A* and *B*).[88-90] In this case, treatment may focus around tissue healing and therapeutic strategies to help calm the nervous system down, such as education and aerobic exercise.[88] Additionally, this new language should purge old, provocative terminology, such as *torn, ripped,* and *rupture,* to avoid increased fear and anxiety. Education is therapy.

This reconceptualization of pain (sensitive nerves versus injured back or tissues) is a key element of TNE and warrants a greater understanding of "how pain works." Pain is 100% produced by the brain. The processing of the brain of information from tissues, environment, thoughts, beliefs, experiences, memories, and various senses is referred to as the neuromatrix. The **neuromatrix theory**

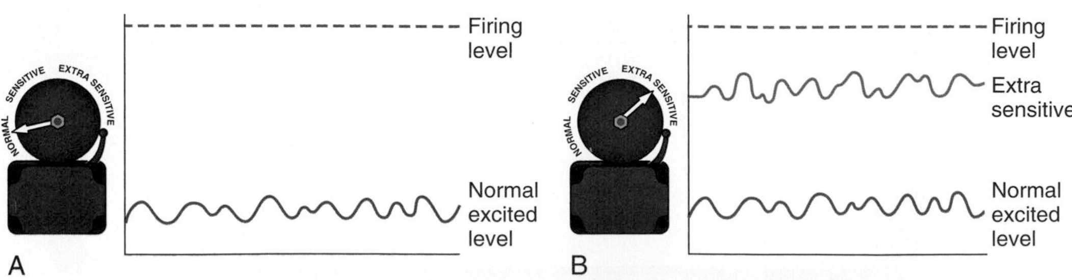

FIG 25-5 Graphic representation of nerve sensitization. **A,** The nervous system depicts normal, resting levels of electrical activity. **B,** An extra sensitive nervous system is shown, indicating low tolerance for activity and exercise. *(From Louw A:* Your nerves are having back surgery, *Minneapolis, 2012, OPTP.)*

was introduced in 1996 by Melzack.[103,111] To understand the processing of the brain of this nociceptive information and ultimately a pain experience, we need to dispel the belief that there is a specific "pain area" within the brain, such that when you hit your thumb with a hammer, this area activates so that you experience pain.[105] This single "pain area" notion was dispelled by observations of patients after cerebral lobotomy and cerebral hemispherectomy.[5,75] Multiple studies involving functional brain scanning have shown that during a painful experience many different brain areas are active, and these areas have been more comprehensively described.[43,44,105,111] The pain neuromatrix is best defined as a collection of brain areas activated during a pain experience (Fig. 25-6).[134]

For years, scientists were aware that certain areas of the brain (i.e., anterior cingulate cortex, thalamus, and sensory cortex) were activated during a pain experience. The neuromatrix theory conceptualized that these activated neuronal areas communicate with each other as a network as a means to protect—hence the name *pain neuromatrix,* or pain neural signature or map. The neuromatrix allows us to update our view of pain, based on the definition of pain by Moseley:[111] "Pain is a multiple system output, activated by an individual's specific pain neuromatrix. The pain neuromatrix is activated when the body tissues are in danger and action is required."

The key to this definition for those new to this updated pain model is to recognize that pain is an output or decision of the brain. To understand the modern neuroscience definition of pain, a few key issues need to be discussed briefly.

Output

It is commonly thought that C and A-delta nerve fibers conduct pain. With an injury, such as an ankle sprain, A-delta fibers activate instantly followed by C fibers, and pain signals are sent to the spinal cord and ultimately the brain, "telling" the person he or she is in pain.[89] In the metaphorical lion description, this teaching has a devastating effect. If a lion jumps into a room and a person steps on a thumbtack with his or her bare foot while running to escape the lion, surely the thumbtack (pain) is not felt. In this case, the brain analyzes the threats (lion versus thumbtack) via the neuromatrix and chooses not to produce pain. All of the signals that the ankle can send to the brain via complex electrochemical communication

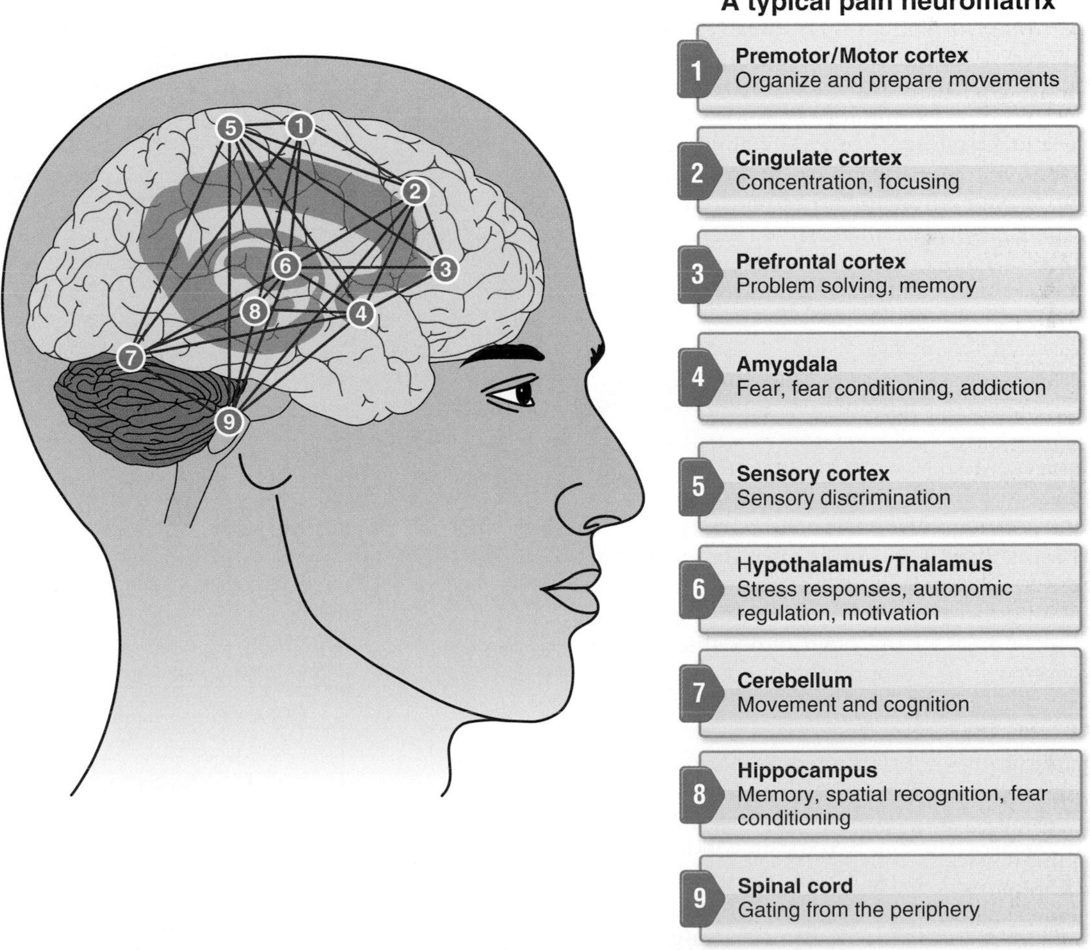

FIG 25-6 A typical pain neurotag involves activity from many brain areas. *(From Puentedura EJ, Louw A: A neuroscience approach to managing athletes with low back pain,* Phys Ther Sport *13[3]:123-133, 2012.)*

are **nociception**, or danger signals. If the ankle sent "pain messages," the pain could grab the attention of the fleeing person, which may slow the person down or even stop him or her resulting in a bigger threat—being eaten by the lion. Pain as an output allows physical therapy practitioners to see the value of treatments such as TNE. If pain is based on a perception of threat, a well-meaning, neuroscience-influenced practitioner may help reconstruct a threat such as a "bulging disk" and influence how much pain is produced by the brain.

Important Concepts

Pain Is an Output

Critical to understanding an updated, modern concept of pain is the realization that pain is an output. It is a construct of the brain based on information that the brain has available to it and the brain's perception of threat. Such information can include nociceptive input coming in from the body, past experiences stored in the brain, the current environment including if the body is in danger, health of the entire human organism, and cultural and social biases.

Individual Neuromatrix

Every person is different. Every pain experience is different and is unique to the individual. It is already established that various areas of the brain activate during a pain experience and form part of a "typical" neuromatrix, or simply stated these areas are active in all people who experience pain. Multiple studies involving functional brain scanning have shown that many different brain areas are active during a painful experience, and these areas have been more comprehensively described (Table 25-1).[43,44,105,111] The end result of a pain experience is a neural signature or map within the brain, which is referred to as a *neurotag* or *neuromatrix* (see Fig. 25-6).[105,111,134]

Important Concepts

Pain Neurotag

Also called an "individual pain neuromatrix" or a "pain neurosignature," the concept of a **pain neurotag** is foundational to understanding the neuromatrix theory of pain. A pain neurotag is the network of areas of the brain that communicate when an individual has a pain experience. It is important for understanding that pain is an experience that uses multiple areas of the brain rather than a pain area of the brain, which was previously thought.

Further examination of a typical pain neurotag reveals two key clinical issues for physical therapy practitioners treating patients with chronic pain. First, if during a painful experience, an area of the brain typically designated to perform another task (e.g., motor control in transversus abdominis contraction) in the therapeutic application of spinal stabilization exercises, the pain processing is likely to influence the motor control. Several studies have shown that cognitions such as fear and catastrophizing can have a significant impact on motor control.[112,117,118] Second, each person's map is different and individualized[111]; this underscores the clinical notion that treatment should be individualized for the patient and may be a reason why one-on-one education produces superior results to group education.[91,124] The individual nature of a person's pain experience is due to the complexity of neuronal activation, synaptic activity, and neurotransmitters and modulators. The primary "pain map" can also be influenced by neighboring neural circuits, which will likely influence the pain experience (Fig. 25-7).[134]

Important Concepts

Neurons That Fire Together, Wire Together

Based on the Hebbian theory, this concept is important for understanding how the neuromatrix affects people experiencing persistent pain. As a presynaptic cell repeatedly excites a postsynaptic cell, the efficiency of the connection is enhanced. This is the basic mechanism for the concept of synaptic plasticity.

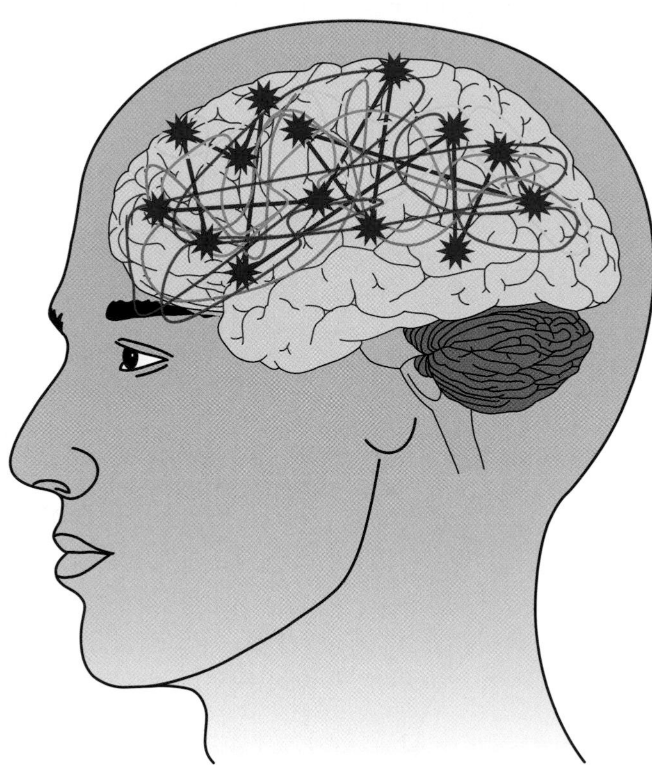

KEY

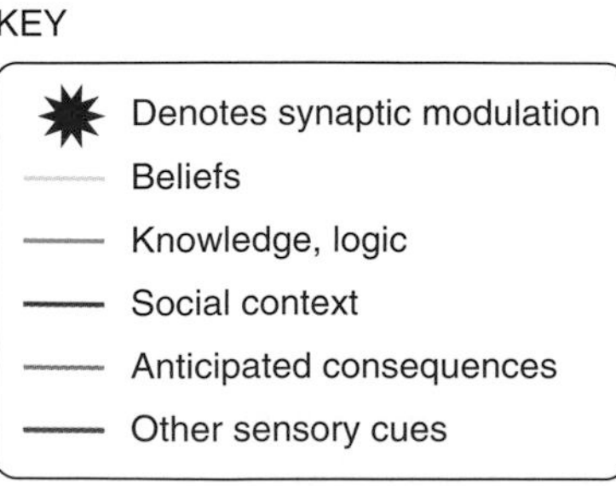

FIG 25-7 The primary "pain map" also can be influenced by neighboring neural circuits. *(From Puentedura EJ, Louw A: A neuroscience approach to managing athletes with low back pain,* Phys Ther Sport *13[3]:123-133, 2012.)*

TABLE 25-1 Areas of the Brain Involved in Processing a Painful Experience

Area	Functions	Location

1. Amygdala	• Almond-shaped group of nuclei located deep within the medial temporal lobes of the brain
	• Part of the limbic system
	• Processing and memory of emotional reactions
	  • Fear
	  • Addictions
	• One of the most active areas during a pain experience
		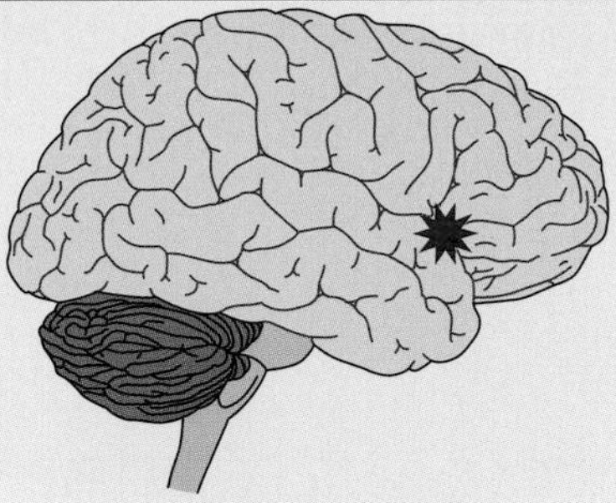

2. Primary somatosensory cortex	• Somatic sensation • Visual stimuli • Movement planning	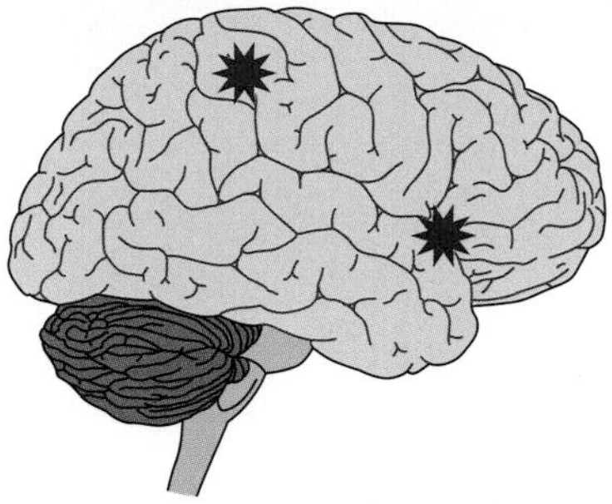
3. Hippocampus	• Part of the limbic system • Consolidation of information from short-term to long-term memory • Spatial navigation	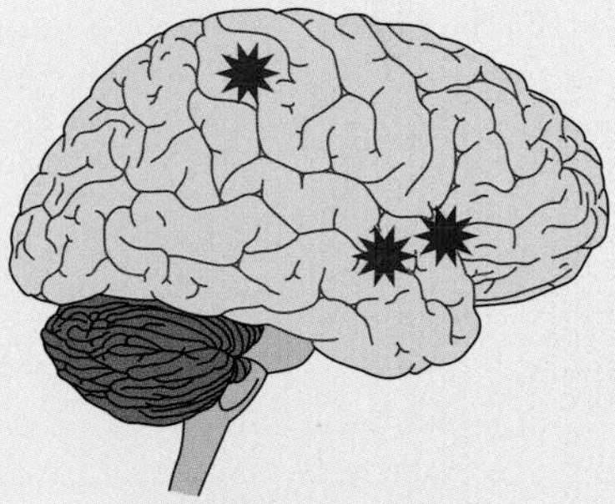

4. Anterior cingulate cortex	• Plays a role in various autonomic functions
	  • Blood pressure regulation
	  • Heart rate regulation
	• Plays a role in rational cognitive functions
	  • Reward anticipation
	  • Decision making
	  • Empathy
	  • Emotion
	• Concentration
	• Focus
		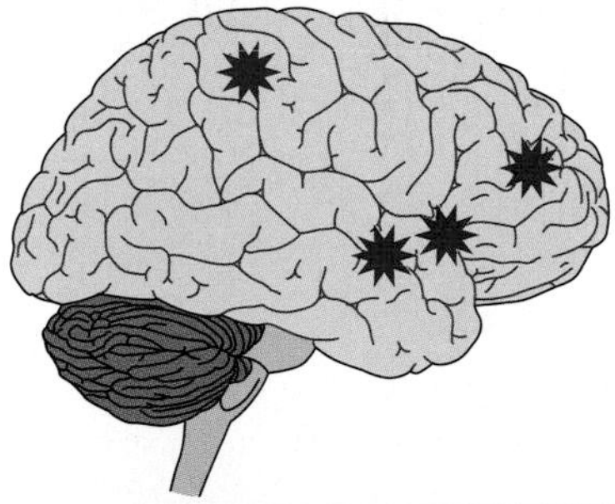

5. Primary motor cortex	• Works in association with other motor areas, including premotor cortex, supplementary motor area, posterior parietal cortex, and several subcortical brain regions, to plan and execute movements	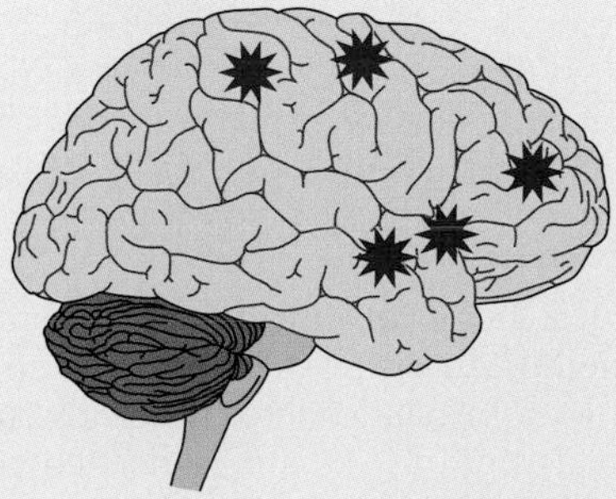

Continued

TABLE 25-1 Areas of the Brain Involved in Processing a Painful Experience—cont'd

Area	Functions	Location

6. Hypothalamus	• Below the thalamus and above the brainstem
	• Links to the nervous system via the endocrine system via the pituitary gland
	• Autonomic nervous system
	• Controls various functions
	  • Body temperature
	  • Hunger and thirst
	  • Fatigue and sleep
		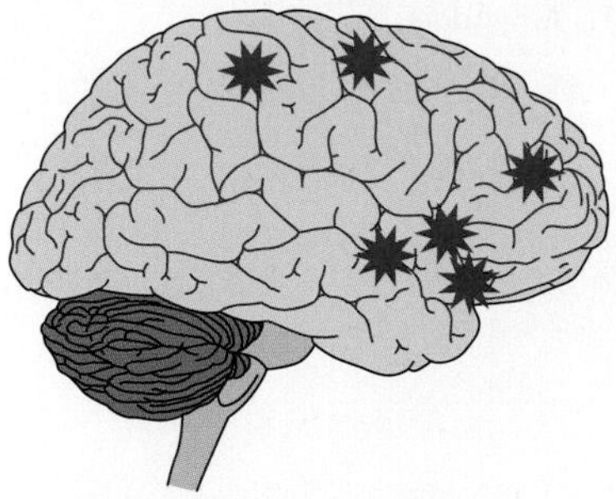

7. Thalamus	• Relaying sensory and motor signals to the cerebral cortex • Consciousness • Sleep • Alertness	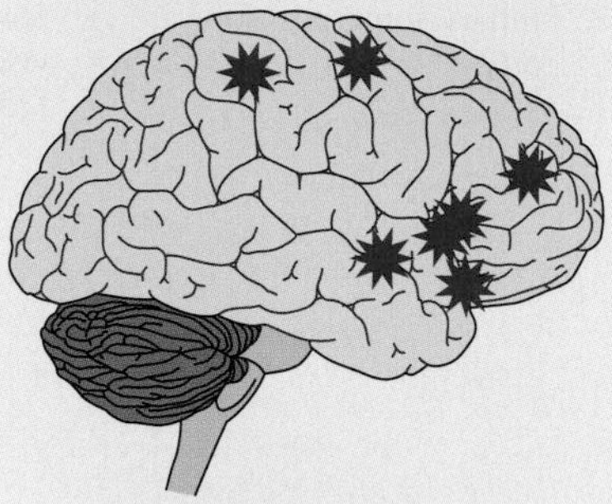
8. Prefrontal cortex	• Planning complex cognitive behavior • Personality expression • Decision making • Moderating social behavior	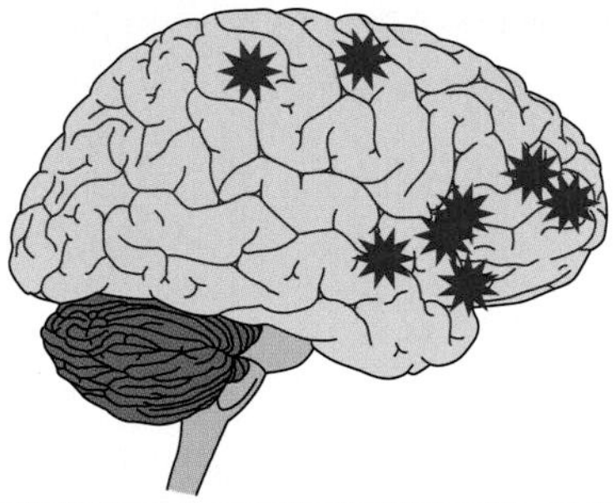
9. Cerebellum	• Movement • Balance, proprioception • Fear • Coordination	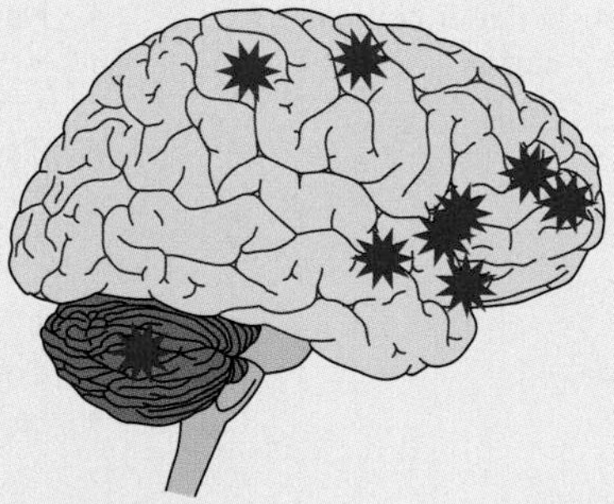

Perceptions

On receipt of information from tissues, environment, memories, and other sensory input via the neuromatrix, the brain has to determine how much danger the person is facing and if pain is needed to protect. Pain is again individualized based on many variables, and one person's pain experience is not the same as another. *Threat* can be defined as an expression of intent to inflict injury or damage. As it pertains to pain, it could be argued that people may have different threats, based on various factors. For example, in a whiplash study comparing illness and care-seeking behaviors for whiplash-associated disorders by physicians with personnel with no medical training, a significant difference was observed.[164] Both groups sustained similar injuries; however, the perception of the injury and recovery was seen as a major difference in the ensuing care-seeking behaviors between the groups. Pain is based on perception of threat because perceptions include the individualistic nature of pain.[115] The decision that there is danger increases activity along facilitative pathways in the central nervous system to send additional information to the brain (Fig. 25-8, *A*).[172] If the end result of the neuronal circuitry is that there is no real threat, pain will not be produced to protect, and descending pathways will modulate the threat messages (Fig. 25-8, *B*).[111,115]

This refinement of the definition of pain (perception of threat) is a key point in the treatment of pain. It is believed that educating patients more about their pain directly (TNE) targets the perception of threat, and the cortical reorganization of the perception of threat is likely a significant contributor to the effectiveness of pain education.[91,122]

> **Important Concepts**
>
> **Perception of Threat**
>
> Based on the brain's most basic function, survival, the brain processes information from nociceptors and puts that information into context, weighs the information, and decides if there is danger. If the conclusion is that there is a threat of danger and action is required, pain is produced to protect the organism. If the conclusion is that there is no real threat, descending pathways are used to modulate the danger messages, and the result is no pain.

Multiple Systems

The section describing the lion metaphor illustrates numerous biologic systems that are involved in a pain experience. These biologic system changes explain various issues in patients with chronic pain, such as fatigue, difficulty sleeping, a sensitive gastrointestinal system, and widespread sensitivity.

> **Important Concepts**
>
> **Pain Is a Multiple System Output**
>
> Pain involves the nervous system, but it does not stop there. There is strong scientific and anecdotal evidence that nearly every system of the body is influenced by a pain experience. When we understand that these multiple systems are involved in the pain experience, it becomes easier to understand a patient's multiple complaints that relate to the various systems involved.

AEROBIC EXERCISE

The second "gold level" approach to chronic pain is aerobic exercise. An understanding of the vast biologic changes, driven by various stress chemicals (Fig. 25-4), should provide an initial understanding of why aerobic exercise can help patients with chronic pain. The overall health benefits of aerobic exercise cannot be overstated. In terms of neuroscience, aerobic exercise should be seen as a very powerful tool in helping a patient who is experiencing pain.[8,9,14,18,53,54,141,151] Aerobic exercise in and of itself has been shown to help decrease pain by causing an immediate postexercise hypalgesia.[12,21,67-70,80,150] There is also ample evidence that aerobic exercise improves sleep,[20,136,158,175] motor function,[135] memory,[107,133,159] and cortisol levels[169]; aids the immune system[4,7,19,56,155,171]; decreases chronic inflammation[56]; decreases anxiety[126]; decreases depression symptoms[6,28,126,130]; improves mood[67,131,148]; decreases nerve sensitivity[125]; and is just as effective as antidepressants in patients with chronic pain.[6]

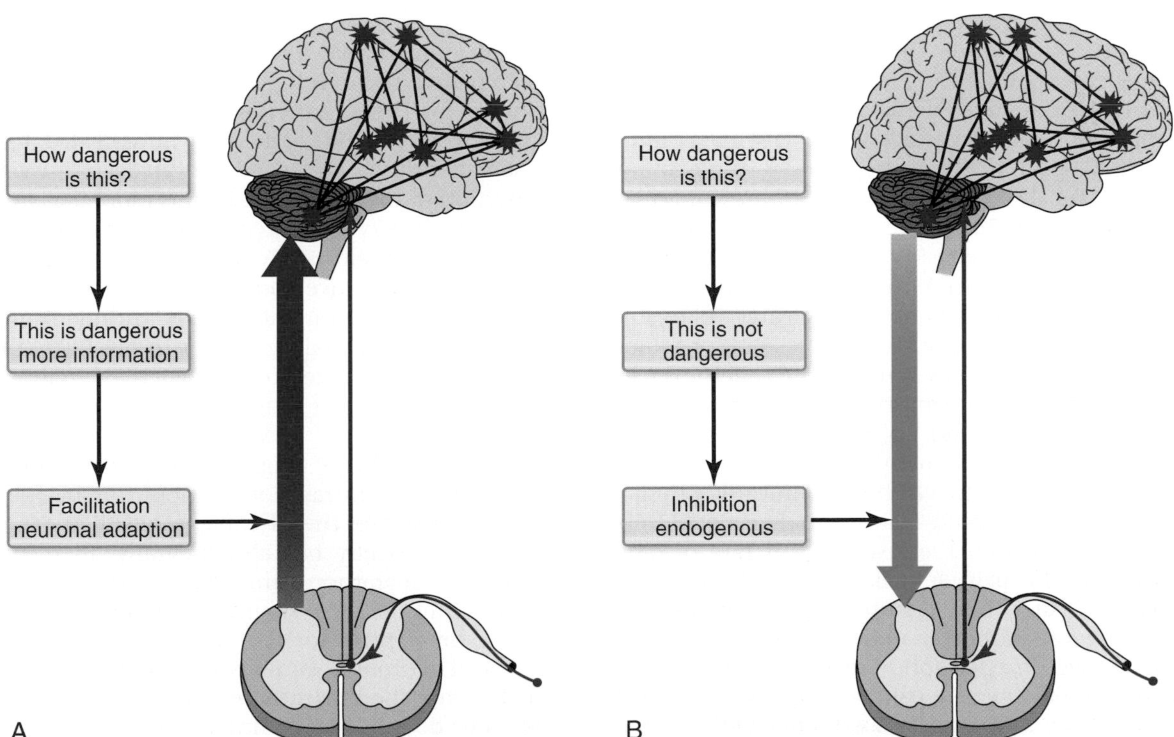

FIG 25-8 Danger messages from the body are received by the brain, and if the brain concludes that danger is real, facilitation is unregulated to provide more information about the threat (**A**). If the brain concludes that there is no danger, inhibitory activity modulates the danger messages (**B**). *(From Louw A:* Why do I hurt? A neuroscience approach to pain, *Minneapolis, 2013, OPTP.)*

Physical therapy practitioners must have the necessary skills to highlight effectively the importance and benefit of an aerobic exercise program to their patients. Patients experiencing chronic pain are often reluctant to engage in exercise because they experience pain with activity and movements, and they may believe the pain signals harm to their tissues. TNE aims to help patients reconceptualize their pain.[115] Once TNE has helped a patient reconceptualize his or her pain, the patient needs to be introduced to the benefits of aerobic exercise from a neuroscience perspective. Benefits include changes in adrenaline, decreased activation of the ion channels (nerve sensors), decreased firing of the nervous system, decreased upregulation of the central nervous system, improved respiration, improved sleep, decreased pain, improved immunity, regulation of cortisol, improved oxygenation of the brain, improved mood, improved cognitions, improved memory, improved appetite, decreased depression, oxygenation and energizing of tissues, decreased sensitivity of tissues, and improved blood flow throughout the body.[93]

After TNE, physical therapy practitioners may consider various strategies to help patients remain compliant with their HEP. Strategies include using an exercise log book,[25,71,98,114,174] providing no more than five exercises for the HEP,[31,101] educating the patient more about the importance of exercise,[46,47,100,101,109] making the exercises personal to the patient rather than using a generic approach,[2,147] treating pain before and during the exercise program,[30,33,101] keeping instructions simple,[1,96] constantly motivating patients,[1,147] and using low-cost equipment when possible.[1]

Two important considerations in aerobic exercise are dosage and frequency. Aerobic exercise is working out at an intensity of 60% to 70% of one's age-predicted maximum heart rate (HR). Commonly, age-predicted maximum HR is calculated as 220 minus a person's age. For example, a 40-year-old patient would have a maximum HR of 180 (220 – 40). In this example, 60% of maximum HR would be 108 (180 × 0.6), and 70% of maximum HR would be 126 (180 × 0.7); this would mean that a 40-year-old patient should be exercising at a target HR of 108 to 126 beats per minute (bpm). With reference to pain, it has been shown that aerobic exercise at greater than 50% maximum oxygen consumption ($\dot{V}O_2max$) and for a duration greater than 10 minutes is required to elicit exercise analgesia.[68] Without discussing the complexities of individualized maximum HR and $\dot{V}O_2max$, it is suggested that most patients with chronic pain should aim to increase their exercise HR to 100 to 110 bpm. Clinically, physical therapy practitioners should realize this is probably not that much elevated from the resting heart rate of most patients with chronic pain. A brisk walk may be all that is needed. Patients are often fearful that aerobic exercise means running a marathon or enduring boot camp–style vigorous exercises. This perception may cause undue stress and fear, which may increase pain. Therapists should seek to calm any fears and anxiety associated with aerobic exercise by reviewing this information with the patient. A good example of this approach is a study on patients with chronic fatigue syndrome.[48] Patients with chronic fatigue syndrome started with 5 to 15 minutes of walking 5 days per week and tolerated it well. By adding 1 to 2 minutes per day, the patients worked their way up to 30 minutes. They had the choice to substitute walking with bicycling or swimming. After the 12-week study, more than half of the patients reported feeling substantially better. After 1 year, 63% of the participants were still doing very well. In a second group of patients, who were given stretches and relaxation exercises, only 25% reported improvement at the same follow-up point.

Important Concepts

Treatment for Patients with Persistent Pain

Best evidence indicates that a combination of a bottom-up and top-down approach is the best method for treating patients with chronic pain. Using a traditional model of treatment that includes physical therapy modalities, therapeutic exercise, and manual therapy may lead to minimal improvement in pain and function and further frustration for the patient and the physical therapy practitioner. A multimodal approach that includes therapeutic neuroscience education at its core along with well-timed traditional treatments is the approach most well supported from an evidence-based approach. The education component must be reinforced throughout the entire episode of care.

Exercising with a Sensitive Alarm System

The evidence for exercise is compelling—but the patient is in pain! The biggest issue physical therapy practitioners will face is the patient's pain. Patients know that exercise is good for them; they know it may even help; but you (the clinician) do not understand—they hurt, and the more they exercise, the more they hurt. It cannot be stressed enough that exercise should be discussed only after a patient has developed a better understanding of his or her pain. The key message of TNE is that tissues and injuries heal over time. After they have healed, tissues can be sore, sensitive, and deconditioned, and a significant proportion of the continued pain is more likely due to an oversensitive nervous system. The "alarm system" is too sensitive in a patient with chronic pain. It takes only a few pulls on the resistance band for the alarm to go off. The important message for the patient to understand is that the alarm is not signaling further injury but rather "sensitivity." It may be helpful to review or draw the extra sensitive nerves for a patient as he or she embarks on exercise (Fig. 25-9).[89]

Patients can also be taught mantras or self-talk. Athletes frequently use mantras. For example, a marathon runner trying to qualify for the Olympic team will prepare himself not only physically but also mentally. In this case, an experienced marathon runner knows the real race starts 20 miles into the race. He may mentally prepare through self-talk or mantras for that time of the race when the going will get tough. Patients in pain are really no different. Patients should learn two mantras—"sore but safe" and "hurt does not equal harm."

Conversely, other mantras are more likely to be detrimental to a patient with chronic pain. Two in particular are "no pain; no gain" (Fig. 25-10) and "if it hurts, don't do it" (Fig. 25-11).

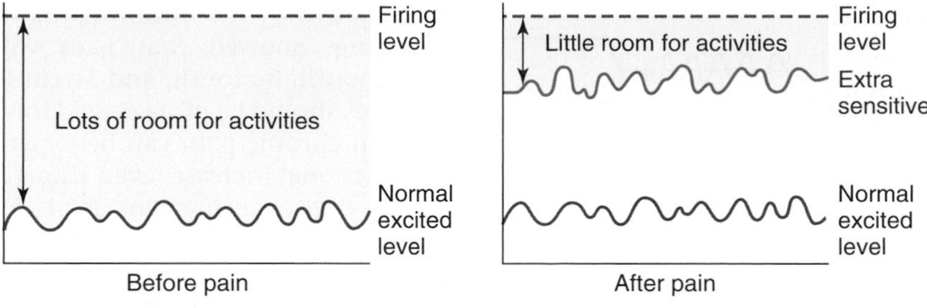

FIG 25-9 The nervous system may be "extra sensitive," and that is why activity increases pain. *(From Louw A:* Your nerves are having back surgery, *Minneapolis, 2012, OPTP.)*

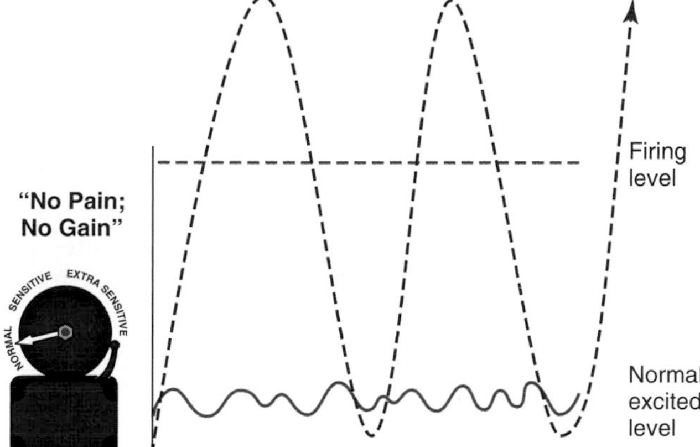

FIG 25-10 The detrimental consequences of following a "no pain, no gain" mantra when a patient has chronic pain. *(From Louw A, Puentedura EJ:* Therapeutic neuroscience education, *Minneapolis, 2013, OPTP.)*

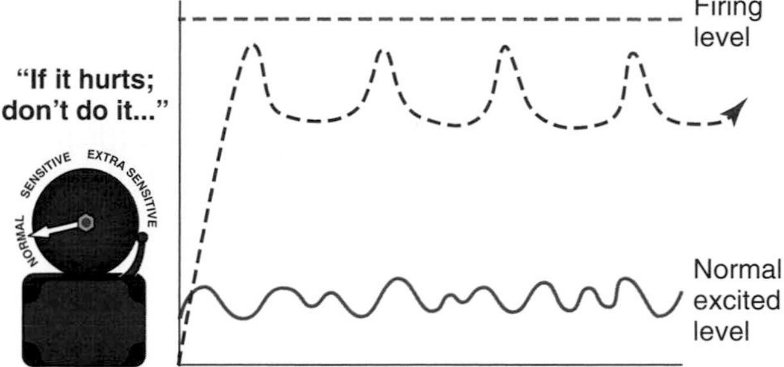

FIG 25-11 The detrimental consequences of following a "if it hurts, don't do it" mantra when a patient has chronic pain. *(From Louw A, Puentedura EJ:* Therapeutic neuroscience education, *Minneapolis, 2013, OPTP.)*

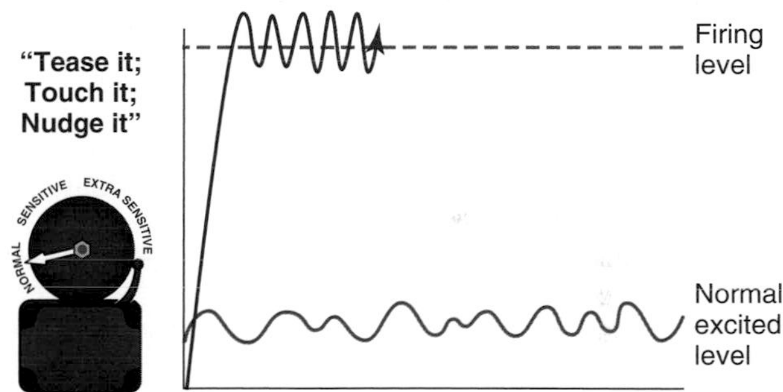

FIG 25-12 The concept of exercising and performing activities to the point of onset of discomfort, or "tease it; touch it; nudge it," where "it" is pain. *(From Louw A, Puentedura EJ:* Therapeutic neuroscience education, *Minneapolis, 2013, OPTP.)*

In the "no pain; no gain" approach, patients may work themselves hard, disregard the pain barrier, and push right through it. Pain protects, and so the patient will crash. He or she may valiantly try again, and the same will happen. This is the classic "boom-bust" cycle, which will overwhelm the patient and they will learn that it does not help to push hard into pain. With failure, resentment, depression, and fear, pain is likely to be increased, and the pain will be produced earlier over time to protect and will get worse.

In an acute injury (e.g., an athlete rehabilitating from an ankle sprain), this model of "no pain; no gain" may pose no problems, but it is not likely to work in a patient with chronic pain. However, it is worth noting that an athlete that fights his or her way through "no pain; no gain" likely understands the pain. The athlete knows what the pain means and does not fear it. Knowledge is important in reducing fear. Pain that is understood does not induce fear and anxiety.

The second mantra, "if it hurts, don't do it" is probably much more common in patients with chronic pain. This approach is associated with fear, anxiety, and uncertainty. It could also be argued that an approach such as this awakens the alarm system by making patients focus on the exact moment they experience pain. Given the sensitivity of the nervous system, a patient's ability to execute meaningful, progressive tasks and exercise becomes considerably diminished, and no progress is made. Given that fear and anxiety increase nerve sensitivity, the tolerances decrease over time limiting exercise and movement more and more; this is the classic fear avoidance model.

Because both of the previous approaches present significant limitations, physical therapy practitioners may be left questioning what they can or should do. An alternative approach of "tease it; touch it; nudge it" (Fig. 25-12) appears to lead to better outcomes over time for this patient population. In such an approach, patients are instructed to exercise or perform a task until some slight discomfort is experienced but not to crash through the discomfort into pain or to stop short of pain.

Armed with improved knowledge about the neurobiology of pain, mantras, and coaching from physical therapy practitioners, the patient will succeed. Over time, as patients reap the benefits of exercising, the "pain

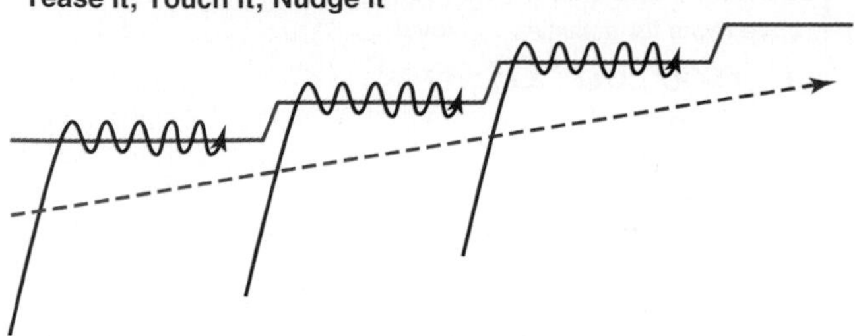

FIG 25-13 Over time, the patient will be able to perform more repetitions, longer sets, and over a longer time period as the pain threshold increases and allows the patient to do more without experiencing pain. *(From Louw A, Puentedura EJ:* Therapeutic neuroscience education, *Minneapolis, 2013, OPTP.)*

threshold" increases, allowing them to push a little further with the exercise. Over time, the numbers, distance, and time increase: 5 minutes of walking becomes 6, followed by 7, and so forth (Fig. 25-13).

Important Concepts

Dealing with a Sensitive Alarm System

It is important that patients understand that there are neurobiologic reasons for why they are more sensitive to activities. As the alarm system "wakes up" and remains awakened, it becomes easier for a threat or danger message to be sent to the brain for processing. As patients gain understanding of this concept, it more easily explains why they are able to perform less activity and why some activities that should not provoke pain now do so. This understanding is a first step in reducing the heightened sensitivity of the alarm system and providing some strategies for guidelines to increase activities, movements, and exercises.

Additional Treatment Ideas

Evidence-based medicine is the application of the best available treatment for the individual patient.[143] A review of the current best evidence for treating patients with chronic pain, including spinal disorders, provides the PTA with some guidelines that can be added to the aforementioned TNE and aerobic exercise.

- Identify patients with **"red flags."** The first rule of medicine is "do no harm." Although the PTA does not perform the initial evaluation, he or she should constantly be an extension of the primary PT. This includes being vigilant and observant to any signs and symptoms that may cause concern. Patients with "red flags" should be referred for additional testing and medical treatment.
- Provide prognostication. This may be one of the most difficult aspects of treatment. However, it is imperative for the physical therapy practitioner to provide the patient with clear timelines regarding expected outcomes. In acute or subacute pain states, timelines may be easier to develop. However, care should be taken not to focus only on pain in the patient with chronic pain. In patients with chronic pain, outcome studies on pain ratings showed that pain will decrease at typical 3-month, 6-month, and 1-year follow-ups,[110,123] yet the focus should be more geared toward function. A patient with chronic pain can be expected to have significant functional increase, even though there is pain.[94] This is one of the mechanisms of "de-focusing" the patient on his or her pain.[170] The clinician should clearly explain to the patient his or her expectations regarding pain and function. An important aspect is the issue that tissues heal. Tissues have predicted stages of healing that are well known by physical therapy practitioners.[152] In contrast to tissue healing, pain can persist well beyond the normal stages of healing, and neuroscience education should allow a patient to understand pain is not a sign of injury or slow healing but of sensitivity, as described in the previous section.
- Promote self-care. A powerful treatment approach for patients with pain is to teach patients strategies to help themselves. This approach fosters greater independence and helps with the development of coping strategies—teaching the patient that he or she is able to help treat his or her own pain[73,141]; this also creates less dependence on the physical therapy practitioner. Self-help includes the development of an aerobic exercise program; systematic application of stretches; and use of modalities such as ice/heat, meditation, relaxation, breathing exercises, problem solving, and time management. An important "neuroscience" aspect of self-care is to have the patient apply treatments such as heat, cold, or a TENS unit specific to a task or time of day and not pain. By focusing on applying treatments "when it hurts," it could be argued that the pain neural signature will be activated more easily and be limited in its effect. For example, a housewife may know that she develops a lot of pain after 30 minutes of standing and cooking dinner every night, and instead of waiting until she feels the pain (and likely be overly focused on "when it hurts"), she can be instructed to plan on applying the TENS unit before starting dinner and on completion to remove the TENS unit.
- Get patients active and moving as early as possible and appropriately after injury. There are many reasons to get patients to move soon after injury or surgery. Reasons from a biologic perspective include blood flow and removal of irritant substances and from a psychological aspect include coping strategies and empowerment. However, the mounting body of evidence regarding neuroplastic changes in the brain underscores the importance of early movement after surgery or injury. Studies using functional magnetic resonance imaging showed that after an injury or immobilization of a body part (i.e., fingers), the representation of that body part in the brain is altered in 30 minutes.[153] What is important about this finding is that when a body part is distorted (i.e., low back), it is linked to persistent pain.[43,45] Studies using functional magnetic resonance imaging further demonstrated that movement or exercise of the affected area changes the map of the affected body part to a more normal representation in the brain, which is associated with decreased pain and functional

improvement.[157] The neurobiology of this process is best described as a process whereby an injured area that loses its normal movement develops a "poorer" map in the brain—it becomes "smudged." By moving the body part, the map of that part is "retrained," and the brain develops a healthy view of the injured area; this correlates to improvement. Movement after injury can be seen as homuncular refreshment—keeping the maps well defined and healthy after injury.

- Decrease unnecessary fear related to movement, leisure activities, and work activities. Several factors are associated with the development and maintenance of pain. For example, epidemiologic data indicate that 6% of patients with LBP account for almost 50% of expenditures associated with the treatment of LBP.[86,87] With countries spending more and more money to treat LBP, scientists started investigating the factors associated with the development of chronic LBP. The list is exhaustive; however, a lot of studies have focused on fear. Several authors believe that the fear of pain, fear of injury, or fear of reinjury may be the most potent factor in the development of chronic LBP. This belief led to the development of questionnaires to examine the level of fear a patient may have, such as the Fear Avoidance Beliefs Questionnaire.[23,55,132,165] From a treatment perspective, physical therapy practitioners should aim to decrease fear; this is the essence of neuroscience education. It is believed that decreased fear in essence "calms" the brain down, making the threat less.[113] The PT and the PTA should aim to develop a greater understanding (after the evaluation) as to what the patient is afraid of and address these issues. The patient may have an unrealistic expectation that a particular movement or exercise will injure tissue, which may lead to an increase in fear. Several studies using neuroscience education that addresses a patient's fears have shown improvement in movements such as straight leg raise and forward flexion following this education.[94,112,122]
- Help the patient experience success. A big focus of the evaluation is to determine "what a patient cannot do," and then treatment is aimed at restoring the functional deficit. It is recommended that clinicians also point out positive features—such as a nice movement or muscle contraction. This also applies to the treatments. Encouragement is important. Patients with chronic pain typically have numerous psychological comorbidities, such as depression, poor body image, and lack of self-confidence.
- Make any treatment strategy closely linked to evidence of the biologic nature of the problem rather than a syndrome or the geography of the pain. Physical therapy practitioners are encouraged to get away from a syndrome and areas of pain. LBP refers only to the fact that the area of pain is not in the front and is below the shoulder blades. The geography (where the pain is) does not tell the patient anything about the underlying pathology or explain why treatments may be beneficial. Likewise, syndromes are uninformative. Failed back surgery syndrome informs the patient only that he or she had spinal surgery that did not provide the desired results. There is growing evidence that the more patients understand the biology behind their pain, the better their understanding of the pathology and the proposed treatment plan.[91] This is another cornerstone of neuroscience education—"biologizing" a patient's pain. Physical therapy practitioners should explain to patients what happens on a biologic level that causes the pain and what can be done about it. An example is a patient who states he or she experiences arm pain when he or she becomes stressed. A neuroscience educational session would aim to explain to the patient that nerves have receptors or sensors and research has shown that some sensors are very sensitive to "stress chemicals" such as adrenaline.[89] When the patient gets stressed and these stress chemical levels increase, the nerves increase their level of excitement ("buzz" higher) and are more likely to "fire" and send danger messages, which could be interpreted by the brain as pain. This explanation may be followed by a biologic description of strategies to decrease stress and calm the nervous system.
- Use any measures possible to reduce pain. With all the knowledge available on the development of central sensitization, it seems imperative to decrease the constant barrage of danger messages to the central nervous system as soon as possible.[172,173] With persistent input from the periphery, the central nervous system upregulates, which may lead to long-lasting changes. Physical therapy practitioners should use all means to decrease pain; this includes the use of medication, modalities, education, and hands-on treatment. Although it is proposed that clinicians move "beyond" the gate control theory of pain,[104] treatments such as manual therapy and skillful delivery of modalities or even a well-placed orthosis or taping technique can alter nociception and ultimately the pain experience.

GATE CONTROL

Apart from the **Cartesian model of pain**, it could be argued that the gate control theory, more commonly referred to as the **pain gate**, is the predominant mechanism physical therapy practitioners use to understand pain and develop treatments to modulate a patient's pain experience. Since the early 1900s, scientists focused their attention on various nerve fibers, ultimately leading to a widely accepted classification of nerve fibers based on size and speed of conduction—A, B, and C fibers.[3,27] These nerve fibers are also typically categorized as being responsible for things such a pain, light touch, or pressure.[17]

- Type A fibers are the thickest and fastest conducting; they are myelinated; they have a diameter of 1.5 to 20 μm; and their speed of conduction ranges from 4 to 120 m/sec, which shows that they can conduct impulses quickly. Examples of type A fibers are skeleton muscle fibers and afferent fibers to the skin.
- Type B fibers are medium in size (i.e., they are smaller than type A fibers but larger than type C); they are myelinated; they have a diameter of 1.5 to 3.5 μm; and their speed of conduction is 3 to 15 m/sec, which shows that they conduct impulses more slowly than type A fibers. Examples of type B fibers are preganglionic autonomic efferents.

- Type C fibers are the smallest and thinnest. They are nonmyelinated; they have a diameter of 0.1 to 2 μm; and their speed of conduction is 0.5 to 4 m/sec, which shows that they have the slowest conduction of impulses. Examples of type C fibers are postganglionic autonomic efferents and afferent fibers to skin. Many PTs are taught that C fibers are "pain fibers" and responsible, along with A-delta fibers, for "conducting pain."

Based on the specialized activity of nerves, Melzack and Wall developed the gate control theory. According to this theory, information is sent to the dorsal horn of the spinal cord and ultimately to the brain from various nerve fibers, including thin "pain" fibers and larger diameter fibers dealing with touch, pressure, and vibration. Along the way, the information can be modulated or altered by various interactions, including inhibition by the substantia gelatinosa. Many physical treatments, such as large-amplitude passive range of motion, TENS, massage, and electrical stimulation, are thought to control pain partly by activating low-threshold, large-diameter, nonnociceptive sensory nerve fibers dealing with touch, pressure, and vibration, which inhibit pain transmission by closing the gate to pain transmission at the spinal cord level (Fig. 25-14). Anecdotally, this activation of sensory nerve fibers explains why people rub an injury site or even "walk it off," stimulating nerve fibers that in essence override the "pain signals."

Although the gate control theory explains many observations regarding pain and modulation, it has various shortcomings in light of updated research in regard to pain.[104,105,111] Gate control cannot account for phantom limb pain in patients with amputations or pain in quadriplegics; it also cannot account for the complex immune and inflammatory processes that have been shown to be key components in pain. The pain gate does not take into consideration emotions or descending inhibitory pathways of the brain. Melzack, one of the original authors of the pain gate, has urged clinicians to recognize the shortcomings of the pain gate and embrace the current, more updated view of pain, the brain, and neuromatrix.[103-105]

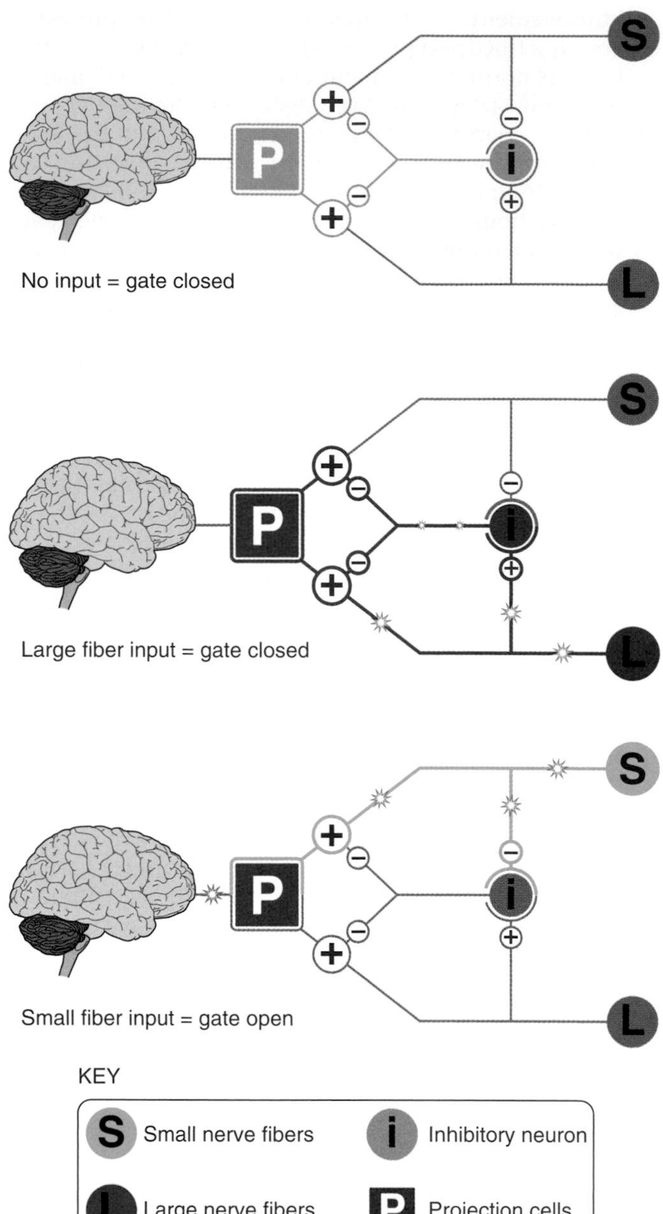

FIG 25-14 Gate control. *(From Melzack R, Wall PD: Pain mechanisms: a new theory,* Science *150:971-979, 1965.)*

Minimize Number of Treatments and Contacts with Medical Personnel

The ideal scenario is for a patient with pain to develop a greater understanding of his or her pain and for a treatment plan to be created focused on development of independence and the ability of the patient to help himself or herself. Physical therapy practitioners should aim to develop this independence through encouragement, HEP, and education. Many patients most likely receive many unnecessary treatments by physical therapy practitioners that have, perhaps unknowingly, fostered a dependence on the physical therapy practitioners rather than independence. Treating pain is challenging. Even if a physical therapy practitioner anticipates a long process, it is advised that the practitioner consider a series of treatments. After the first treatments, the patient would continue with home exercises and treatment strategies (i.e., breathing, meditation) and then return again a few weeks (or months) later for reassessment and to work toward the next level of goals and strategies followed by a short-term reprieve from therapy. This approach is more advisable than having a patient attend therapy indefinitely. For example, a patient may attend therapy for eight visits and be sent home with a HEP, walking program, and work on short-term goals, to be set up to return to therapy in 6 to 8 weeks for a few sessions of reassessment and adjustment of the exercises and goals and then again embark on a period of working on these at home.

Consider Multidisciplinary Management

No single treatment is a cure. The reality of chronic pain is that these patients may have many comorbidities, long-lasting physical and emotional changes, and medication needs. Patients may benefit from several health care providers, including a physical therapist, psychologist, pain management physician, and dietitian.

Assess and Assist Recovery of General Physical Fitness

Aerobic exercise has already been discussed in detail.

Strengthening. In contrast to all the available research on aerobic exercise and pain, less is known about strengthening. Additionally, there does not appear to be any compelling evidence that patients experiencing chronic pain will have become significantly weakened. Bed rest, limited movement, and generally decreased functioning may take a toll, but most of these patients will have become deconditioned, rather than exhibiting true muscle weakness. The available evidence for strengthening in patients with chronic pain suggests the use of lighter weight and resistance exercise along with higher repetitions.[10,160] Clinically, lighter weight, higher repetition exercises can be thought of as toning exercises and another way to bring about increased heart rate, blood flow, and oxygenation of tissues.

It should also be recognized that educating a patient that he or she is in need of strengthening exercises may imply to the patient weakness, which may produce fear and anxiety. Resistance exercises should be considered conditioning exercises. As with aerobic exercise, conditioning exercises should be preceded by TNE and a reminder to patients of the extra sensitivity of their nervous system. Patients should understand that receiving signals from the body part being exercised is normal and likely does not signal true tissue damage. Finally, conditioning exercises should not focus on pain. Patients should be encouraged to focus on a certain number of repetitions, duration, or distance. Not only will this help to de-focus pain, but also it should reinforce the message that pain is not important in this case.

Spinal Stabilization. The amount of research on spinal stabilization for LBP over the past 2 decades has been impressive.[137,138] Much of that research has focused on muscle properties, fine-wire needle electromyography findings in healthy volunteers and volunteers with pain, muscle contractile properties, pain inhibition, effect of fear and catastrophization on motor control, imaging studies, and physical tests associated with motor control.[57-61,63-65,119,121] More recently, similar research related to the cervical spine focusing on deep cervical spine flexors for cervical spine stabilization was published.[78] This research again focused on muscle and contractile properties in symptomatic individuals and subsequently in patient groups with neck pain, headache, and traumatic injuries to the cervical spine.[35-41,76,77] The purpose of this section is not to review spinal stabilization theory but to discuss the clinical application of spinal stabilization in patients with chronic pain.

Spinal stabilization has been proposed as a treatment for patients with chronic LBP.[16,26,52,62] Despite the popularity of spinal stabilization, controversy has surrounded an approach whereby therapists teach patients a very specific approach focusing on specific muscles (i.e., transversus abdominis), a definite sequence of retraining those muscles, and use of equipment such as biofeedback units and diagnostic ultrasound.[16,24,81] This approach is often referred to as "specific" spinal stabilization and was summarized by Richardson and Hodges as "firing the right muscles at the right time, in the right sequence for the right amount of time and then disengaging at the appropriate time."[137] This approach is attributed to researchers from Queensland University, including Richardson, Hodges, Jull, and Hides.[137,138]

In contrast to the "specific" approach, it has also been postulated that stabilization can be performed as a more generalized approach—not overly concerned about specific muscles, sequences of contraction, or careful monitoring or quantification of contractions. This more generalized approach has been promoted mainly by McGill.[42,144,163] From the clinical perspective, therapists are likely to be using one approach or the other (Fig. 25-15).

The major contention surrounding the differing spinal stabilization approaches is the paucity of evidence for either approach. Current evidence, focusing on systematic reviews and high-quality randomized controlled trials, has failed to show that spinal stabilization exercises are superior to other forms of exercise and therapy for patients with LBP.[16,26,81,99,127,129]

It is not our aim to describe spinal stabilization in detail but to offer useful strategies for patients with chronic LBP.

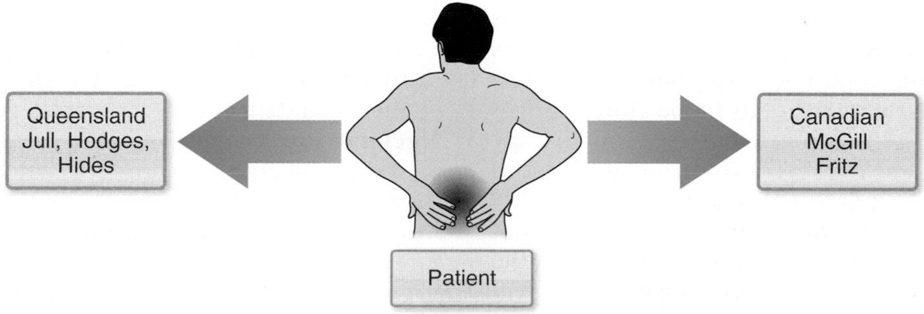

FIG 25-15 Spinal stabilization for low-back pain can be approached from two different points of view: a "specific" motor control approach promoted by researchers from Queensland versus a more "general" strengthening approach advocated by researchers from Canada (McGill) and the United States (Fritz). *(From Louw A, Puentedura EJ:* Therapeutic neuroscience education, *Minneapolis, 2013, OPTP.)*

Although it may be appropriate to focus on a "specific" motor control approach with some patients, we believe there is a stronger argument for a more "generalized" approach for patients with chronic LBP. This belief is based on the realization that patients with persistent pain struggle to perform small, well-coordinated tasks, such as the tasks required during the "specific" spinal stabilization approach. Various factors may contribute to this struggle, including the motor cortex being used in the pain neuromatrix,[134] decreased importance in fine motor control when facing threat,[145] altered cortical representation of the low back (i.e., smudging),[43,116] psychological issues affecting motor control,[120] and problems with pelvic position sense.[95] The "generalized" approach we advocate for such patients would mean teaching patients a simple bracing exercise and then shifting focus quickly to more functional movements and tasks.

When considering spinal stabilization concepts from a neuroscience perspective, care should be given to the language used when educating patients about their need for stabilization. Patients may assume stabilization means "instability" or weakness, which may induce fear. Additionally, if a physical therapy practitioner decides to opt for the "specific" spinal stabilization approach with its stronger focus and emphasis on specific muscles and sequences of motor control retraining, it may ultimately end in frustration on the part of the patient because they will be unable to perform a simple abdominal drawing in maneuver.

> **Important Concepts**
>
> **Spinal Stabilization for Patients with Persistent Pain**
> Although a popular way to train patients with LBP, segmental, specific stabilization training may not be the correct choice for patients experiencing persistent pain. The motor areas in the brain are likely occupied too much with the pain experience as part of the individual's neuromatrix to be efficient or effective at the fine control required for segmental stabilization training. A more general broad approach to stabilization is likely a better choice.

Posture Exercises. If we recall the cascade of events that are likely to occur in the stress response such as when a lion enters the room, we understand how postural changes can occur, especially over a long period of time. Patients are likely to report pain associated with postural demands, but this may also be due in part to blood flow changes (i.e., ischemia).[166] It is important that physical therapy practitioners understand that even if posture is perceived to be poor, it may not correlate to pain and pathology.[32,84,85] A critical point to be made with respect to posture is that as long as there is the perception of threat (i.e., lion in the room), there will be little chance for posture to be restored. Given the neuroscience premise of postural changes, therapists are clinically challenged to teach patients self-correcting exercises, develop reminder strategies, and focus on aerobic exercise to help oxygenate the sensitive postural muscles.[82]

CONCLUSION

Pain is complex. Many patients experience long-lasting pain, and PTs and PTAs are increasingly called on to help these patients, such as the woman described at the beginning of the chapter who brought in her pain drawing. Emerging pain science research validates the notion that a movement-based profession such as physical therapy is ideal to "take on pain" by virtue of its biologic background, movement focus, hands-on nature, psychology background, and use of exercise as well as the sheer numbers of PTs and PTAs. However, a major shortcoming is knowledge of pain. Physical therapy practitioners are well versed in biologic models (anatomy, biomechanics, and pathoanatomy) but not models associated with pain. In addition to individual physical therapy practitioners familiarizing themselves with pain science research, it is recommended that pain science research become a cornerstone of education in physical therapy. Physical therapy practitioners can then take their rightful place as the neuromusculoskeletal specialists they are and help patients experiencing chronic pain who are desperately in need of their help.

GLOSSARY

Adrenaline: A neurotransmitter and hormone that affects nearly all body tissues.

Biopsychosocial model: A model of treatment that encompasses not only biologic factors but also psychological and social factors.

Cartesian model of pain: An overly simplistic view of pain originating from Rene Descartes in 1664 that explained pain as being transmitted via nerve pathways or wires from a nociceptive source to the brain.

Chronic pain: Pain that persists past normal tissue healing time.

Cortisol: A potent and long-lasting chemical produced in the adrenal gland that is similar to adrenaline but deals with more long-lasting threats.

Ion channels: Nerve sensors that are normally located along the body of an axon where myelin is absent. These sensors can open and close based on a stimulus specific for the type of ion channel.

Nerve sensitization: Occurs when a nerve becomes more easily excitable for various reasons.

Neuromatrix theory: A theory introduced by Melzack in 1996 that focuses more on the brain and theorizes that pain is produced by the brain when it perceives there is a danger and action is required.

Nociception: Danger messages produced by the nervous system; fibers that carry this information are termed *nociceptors*.

Pain: According to the International Association for the Study of Pain, pain is an unpleasant sensory and emotional experience that follows actual or potential tissue damage or is described in terms of such damage.

Pain neurotag: Also known as *pain neurosignature* or *pain map,* a pain neurotag is the network of areas within the brain that communicate with each other as a means to protect and result in a perception of pain.

"Red flags": Signs, symptoms, or subjective information that may indicate a more sinister source of a patient's pain.

Pain gate: Based on the gate control theory by Melzack and Wall in 1965, in which pain is controlled via stimulation of low-threshold, large-diameter sensory nerve fibers to close the gate to pain transmission at the spinal cord level.

Therapeutic neuroscience education (TNE): An important component of a comprehensive plan of care for patients with persistent pain to improve a patient's understanding of the latest science regarding the source and management of a pain experience.

REFERENCES

1. Ainsworth KD, Hagino CC: A survey of Ontario chiropractors: their views on maximizing patient compliance to prescribed home exercise. *J Can Chiropr Assoc* 50(2):140–155, 2006.
2. Asenlof P, Denison E, et al: Individually tailored treatment targeting motor behavior, cognition, and disability: 2 experimental single-case studies of patients with recurrent and persistent musculoskeletal pain in primary health care. *Phys Ther* 85(10):1061–1077, 2005.
3. Barker RA, Barasi S: *Neuroscience at a Glance*, Oxford, 1999, Blackwell.
4. Bauer T, Weisser B: [Effect of aerobic endurance exercise on immune function in elderly athletes]. *Praxis (Bern 1994)* 91(5):153–158, 2002.
5. Bear MF, Connors BW, Paradiso MA: *Neuroscience. Exploring the Brain*, Baltimore, 1996, Williams & Wilkins.
6. Blumenthal JA, Babyak MA, et al: Exercise and pharmacotherapy in the treatment of major depressive disorder. *Psychosom Med* 69(7):587–596, 2007.
7. Boas SR, Danduran MJ, et al: Immune modulation following aerobic exercise in children with cystic fibrosis. *Int J Sports Med* 21(4):294–301, 2000.
8. Bonifazi M, Suman AL, et al: Changes in salivary cortisol and corticosteroid receptor-alpha mRNA expression following a 3-week multidisciplinary treatment program in patients with fibromyalgia. *Psychoneuroendocrinology* 31(9):1076–1086, 2006.
9. Brosseau L, Wells GA, et al: Ottawa Panel evidence-based clinical practice guidelines for aerobic fitness exercises in the management of fibromyalgia: part 1. *Phys Ther* 88(7):857–871, 2008.
10. Brosseau L, Wells GA, et al: Ottawa Panel evidence-based clinical practice guidelines for strengthening exercises in the management of fibromyalgia: part 2. *Phys Ther* 88(7):873–886, 2008.
11. Brox JI, Storheim K, et al: Systematic review of back schools, brief education, and fear-avoidance training for chronic low back pain. *Spine J* 8(6):948–958, 2008.
12. Bruce B, Fries JF, et al: Aerobic exercise and its impact on musculoskeletal pain in older adults: a 14 year prospective, longitudinal study. *Arthritis Res Ther* 7(6):R1263–R1270, 2005.
13. Burton AK, Waddell G, et al: Information and advice to patients with back pain can have a positive effect. A randomized controlled trial of a novel educational booklet in primary care. *Spine* 24(23):2484–2491, 1999.
14. Busch AJ, Barber KA, et al: Exercise for treating fibromyalgia syndrome. *Cochrane Database Syst Rev* (4):CD003786, 2007.
15. Butler D, Moseley G: *Explain Pain*, Adelaide, 2003, Noigroup.
16. Cairns MC, Foster NE, et al: Randomized controlled trial of specific spinal stabilization exercises and conventional physiotherapy for recurrent low back pain. *Spine* 31(19):E670–E681, 2006.
17. Carter R: *The Human Brain Book*, New York, 2009, Dorling Kindersley Limited.
18. Carville SF, Arendt-Nielsen S, et al: EULAR evidence-based recommendations for the management of fibromyalgia syndrome. *Ann Rheum Dis* 67(4):536–541, 2008.
19. Castellano V, White LJ: Serum brain-derived neurotrophic factor response to aerobic exercise in multiple sclerosis. *J Neurol Sci* 269(1–2):85–91, 2008.
20. Catai AM, Chacon-Mikahil MP, et al: Effects of aerobic exercise training on heart rate variability during wakefulness and sleep and cardiorespiratory responses of young and middle-aged healthy men. *Braz J Med Biol Res* 35(6):741–752, 2002.
21. Chatzitheodorou D, Kabitsis C, et al: A pilot study of the effects of high-intensity aerobic exercise versus passive interventions on pain, disability, psychological strain, and serum cortisol concentrations in people with chronic low back pain. *Phys Ther* 87(3):304–312, 2007.
22. Chervin RD, Teodorescu M, et al: Objective measures of disordered sleep in fibromyalgia. *J Rheumatol* 36(9):2009–2016, 2009.
23. Cleland JA, Fritz JM, et al: Psychometric properties of the Fear-Avoidance Beliefs Questionnaire and Tampa Scale of Kinesiophobia in patients with neck pain. *Am J Phys Med Rehabil* 87(2):109–117, 2008.
24. Cleland JA, Whitman JM, et al: Manual physical therapy, cervical traction, and strengthening exercises in patients with cervical radiculopathy: a case series. *J Orthop Sports Phys Ther* 35(12):802–811, 2005.
25. Cox KL, Burke V, et al: Controlled comparison of retention and adherence in home- vs center-initiated exercise interventions in women ages 40-65 years: The S.W.E.A.T. Study (Sedentary Women Exercise Adherence Trial). *Prev Med* 36(1):17–29, 2003.
26. Critchley DJ, Ratcliffe J, et al: Effectiveness and cost-effectiveness of three types of physiotherapy used to reduce chronic low back pain disability: a pragmatic randomized trial with economic evaluation. *Spine* 32(14):1474–1481, 2007.
27. Delcomyn F: *Foundations of Neurobiology*, New York, 1998, W.H. Freeman.
28. Dimeo F, Bauer M, et al: Benefits from aerobic exercise in patients with major depression: a pilot study. *Br J Sports Med* 35(2):114–117, 2001.
29. Dinarello CA: Overview of cytokines and their role in pain. In Watkins LR, Maier SF, editors: *Cytokines and Pain*, Basel, 1999, Birkhauser.
30. Dobkin PL, Sita A, et al: Predictors of adherence to treatment in women with fibromyalgia. *Clin J Pain* 22(3):286–294, 2006.
31. Duncan KA, Pozehl B: Staying on course: the effects of an adherence facilitation intervention on home exercise participation. *Prog Cardiovasc Nurs* 17(2):59–65, 2002.
32. Edmondston SJ, Chan HY, et al: Postural neck pain: an investigation of habitual sitting posture, perception of "good" posture and cervicothoracic kinaesthesia. *Man Ther* 12(4):363–371, 2007.
33. Engstrom LO, Oberg B: Patient adherence in an individualized rehabilitation programme: a clinical follow-up. *Scand J Public Health* 33(1):11–18, 2005.
34. Fabian LA, McGuire L, et al: The association of the cortisol awakening response with experimental pain ratings. *Psychoneuroendocrinology* 34(8):1247–1251, 2009.
35. Falla D, Bilenkij G, et al: Patients with chronic neck pain demonstrate altered patterns of muscle activation during performance of a functional upper limb task. *Spine* 29(13):1436–1440, 2004.
36. Falla D, Jull G, et al: Feedforward activity of the cervical flexor muscles during voluntary arm movements is delayed in chronic neck pain. *Exp Brain Res* 157(1):43–48, 2004.
37. Falla D, Jull G, et al: Neck flexor muscle fatigue is side specific in patients with unilateral neck pain. *Eur J Pain* 8(1):71–77, 2004.
38. Falla D, Jull G, et al: An endurance-strength training regime is effective in reducing myoelectric manifestations of cervical flexor muscle fatigue in females with chronic neck pain. *Clin Neurophysiol* 117(4):828–837, 2006.
39. Falla D, Jull G, et al: Further evaluation of an EMG technique for assessment of the deep cervical flexor muscles. *J Electromyogr Kinesiol* 16(6):621–628, 2006.
40. Falla D, Jull G, et al: Effect of neck exercise on sitting posture in patients with chronic neck pain. *Phys Ther* 87(4):408–417, 2007.
41. Falla D, O'Leary S, et al: Recruitment of the deep cervical flexor muscles during a postural-correction exercise performed in sitting. *Man Ther* 12(2):139–143, 2007.
42. Fenwick CM, Brown SH, et al: Comparison of different rowing exercises: trunk muscle activation and lumbar spine motion, load, and stiffness. *J Strength Cond Res* 23(5):1408–1417, 2009.

43. Flor H: The functional organization of the brain in chronic pain. *Prog Brain Res* 129:313–322, 2000.
44. Flor H: *The image of pain*, Glasgow, 2003, Scotland.
45. Flor H, Braun C, et al: Extensive reorganisation of primary somatosensory cortex in chronic back pain patients. *Neurosci Lett* 244:5–8, 1997.
46. Friedrich M, Gittler G, et al: Combined exercise and motivation program: effect on the compliance and level of disability of patients with chronic low back pain: a randomized controlled trial. *Arch Phys Med Rehabil* 79(5):475–487, 1998.
47. Friedrich M, Gittler G, et al: Long-term effect of a combined exercise and motivational program on the level of disability of patients with chronic low back pain. *Spine (Phila Pa 1976)* 30(9):995–1000, 2005.
48. Fulcher KY, White PD: Randomised controlled trial of graded exercise in patients with the chronic fatigue syndrome. *BMJ* 314(7095):1647–1652, 1997.
49. Gallagher L, McAuley J, et al: A randomized-controlled trial of using a book of metaphors to reconceptualize pain and decrease catastrophizing in people with chronic pain. *Clin J Pain* 29(1):20–25, 2013.
50. Geiss A, Rohleder N, et al: Predicting the failure of disc surgery by a hypofunctional HPA axis: evidence from a prospective study on patients undergoing disc surgery. *Pain* 114(1–2):104–117, 2005.
51. Gifford LS: Pain, the tissues and the nervous system. *Physiotherapy* 84:27–33, 1998.
52. Goldby LJ, Moore AP, et al: A randomized controlled trial investigating the efficiency of musculoskeletal physiotherapy on chronic low back disorder. *Spine* 31(10):1083–1093, 2006.
53. Goldenberg DL, Burckhardt C, et al: Management of fibromyalgia syndrome. *JAMA* 292(19):2388–2395, 2004.
54. Gowans SE, deHueck A, et al: Effect of a randomized, controlled trial of exercise on mood and physical function in individuals with fibromyalgia. *Arthritis Rheum* 45(6):519–529, 2001.
55. Grotle M, Vollestad NK, et al: Clinical course and impact of fear-avoidance beliefs in low back pain: prospective cohort study of acute and chronic low back pain: II. *Spine (Phila Pa 1976)* 31(9):1038–1046, 2006.
56. Haaland DA, Sabljic TF, et al: Is regular exercise a friend or foe of the aging immune system? A systematic review. *Clin J Sport Med* 18(6):539–548, 2008.
57. Hides JA, Belavy DL, et al: Magnetic resonance imaging assessment of trunk muscles during prolonged bed rest. *Spine (Phila Pa 1976)* 32(15):1687–1692, 2007.
58. Hides JA, Richardson CA, et al: Magnetic resonance imaging and ultrasonography of the lumbar multifidus muscle. Comparison of two different modalities. *Spine (Phila Pa 1976)* 20(1):54–58, 1995.
59. Hides JA, Richardson CA, et al: Multifidus muscle recovery is not automatic after resolution of acute, first-episode low back pain. *Spine (Phila Pa 1976)* 21(23):2763–2769, 1996.
60. Hodges P, Cresswell A, et al: Preparatory trunk motion accompanies rapid upper limb movement. *Exp Brain Res* 124(1):69–79, 1999.
61. Hodges PW: Changes in motor planning of feedforward postural responses of the trunk muscles in low back pain. *Exp Brain Res* 141(2):261–266, 2001.
62. Hodges PW: Core stability exercise in chronic low back pain. *Orthop Clin North Am* 34(2):245–254, 2003.
63. Hodges PW, Cresswell AG, et al: Perturbed upper limb movements cause short-latency postural responses in trunk muscles. *Exp Brain Res* 138(2):243–250, 2001.
64. Hodges PW, Moseley GL, et al: Experimental muscle pain changes feedforward postural responses of the trunk muscles. *Exp Brain Res* 151(2):262–271, 2003.
65. Hodges PW, Richardson CA: Relationship between limb movement speed and associated contraction of the trunk muscles. *Ergonomics* 40(11):1220–1230, 1997.
66. Hodges PW, Richardson CA: Delayed postural contraction of transversus abdominis in low back pain associated with movement of the lower limb. *J Spinal Disord* 11(1):46–56, 1998.
67. Hoffman MD, Hoffman DR: Does aerobic exercise improve pain perception and mood? A review of the evidence related to healthy and chronic pain subjects. *Curr Pain Headache Rep* 11(2):93–97, 2007.
68. Hoffman MD, Shepanski MA, et al: Intensity and duration threshold for aerobic exercise-induced analgesia to pressure pain. *Arch Phys Med Rehabil* 85(7):1183–1187, 2004.
69. Hoffman MD, Shepanski MA, et al: Experimentally induced pain perception is acutely reduced by aerobic exercise in people with chronic low back pain. *J Rehabil Res Dev* 42(2):183–190, 2005.
70. Hurkmans E, van der Giesen FJ, et al: Dynamic exercise programs (aerobic capacity and/or muscle strength training) in patients with rheumatoid arthritis. *Cochrane Database Syst Rev* (4): CD006853, 2009.
71. Hurling R, Catt M, et al: Using internet and mobile phone technology to deliver an automated physical activity program: randomized controlled trial. *J Med Internet Res* 9(2):e7, 2007.
72. Institute of Medicine: Relieving Pain in America: A Blueprint for Transforming Prevention, Care, Education and Research. 2011. Available at http://iom.edu/~/media/Files/Report%20Files/2011/Relieving-Pain-in-America-A-Blueprint-for-Transforming-Prevention-Care-Education-Research/Pain%20Research%202011%20Report%20Brief.pdf.
73. Iversen MD, Hammond A, et al: Self-management of rheumatic diseases: state of the art and future perspectives. *Ann Rheum Dis* 69(6):955–963, 2010.
74. Johnson RE, Jones GT, et al: Active exercise, education, and cognitive behavioral therapy for persistent disabling low back pain: a randomized controlled trial. *Spine (Phila Pa 1976)* 32(15):1578–1585, 2007.
75. Juan S: *The Odd Brain: Mysteries of Our Weird & Wonderful Brains Explained*, New York, 2006, MJF Books.
76. Jull G, Barrett C, et al: Further clinical clarification of the muscle dysfunction in cervical headache. *Cephalalgia* 19(3):179–185, 1999.
77. Jull G, Kristjansson E, et al: Impairment in the cervical flexors: a comparison of whiplash and insidious onset neck pain patients. *Man Ther* 9(2):89–94, 2004.
78. Jull G, Sterling M, et al: *Whiplash, Headache, and Neck Pain: Research-Based Directions for Physical Therapies*, Philadelphia, 2008, Churchill Livingstone.
79. Kendall N, Watson P: Identifying psychosocial yellow flags and modifying management. In Topical Issues. In Gifford LS, editor: *Pain 2*, Falmouth, 2000, CNS Press.
80. Koltyn KF, Garvin AW, et al: Perception of pain following aerobic exercise. *Med Sci Sports Exerc* 28(11):1418–1421, 1996.
81. Koumantakis GA, Watson PJ, et al: Trunk muscle stabilization training plus general exercise versus general exercise only: randomized controlled trial of patients with recurrent low back pain. *Phys Ther* 85(3):209–225, 2005.
82. Larsson SE, Cai H, et al: Microcirculation in the upper trapezius muscle during sustained shoulder load in healthy women—an endurance study using percutaneous laser-Doppler flowmetry and surface electromyography. *Eur J Appl Physiol Occup Physiol* 70(5):451–456, 1995.
83. Latimer J, Maher C, et al: The attitudes and beliefs of physiotherapy students to chronic back pain. *Clin J Pain* 20(1):45–50, 2004.
84. Lewis JS, Green A, et al: Subacromial impingement syndrome: the role of posture and muscle imbalance. *J Shoulder Elbow Surg* 14(4):385–392, 2005.
85. Lewis JS, Wright C, et al: Subacromial impingement syndrome: the effect of changing posture on shoulder range of movement. *J Orthop Sports Phys Ther* 35(2):72–87, 2005.
86. Linton SJ: The socioeconomic impact of chronic back pain: is anyone benefiting? *Pain* 75(2–3):163–168, 1998.
87. Linton SJ: A review of psychological risk factors in back and neck pain. *Spine (Phila Pa 1976)* 25:1148–1156, 2000.
88. Louw A: *Your Nerves Are Having Back Surgery*, Minneapolis, 2012, OPTP.
89. Louw A: *Why Do I Hurt? A Neuroscience Approach to Pain*, Minneapolis, 2013, OPTP.
90. Louw A, Butler DS, et al: Development of a preoperative neuroscience educational program for patients with lumbar radiculopathy. *Am J Phys Med Rehabil* 92(5):446–452, 2013.

91. Louw A, Diener I, et al: The effect of neuroscience education on pain, disability, anxiety, and stress in chronic musculoskeletal pain. *Arch Phys Med Rehabil* 92(12):2041–2056, 2011.
92. Louw A, Louw Q, et al: Preoperative education for lumbar surgery for radiculopathy. *S Afr J Physiother* 65(2):3–8, 2009.
93. Louw A, Puentedura EJ: *Therapeutic Neuroscience Education*, Minneapolis, 2013, OPTP.
94. Louw A, Puentedura EL, et al: Use of an abbreviated neuroscience education approach in the treatment of chronic low back pain: A case report. *Physiother Theory Pract* 28(1):50–62, 2012.
95. Luomajoki H, Moseley GL: Tactile acuity and lumbopelvic motor control in patients with back pain and healthy controls. *Br J Sports Med* 45(5):437–440, 2011.
96. Lysack C, Dama M, et al: A compliance and satisfaction with home exercise: a comparison of computer-assisted video instruction and routine rehabilitation practice. *J Allied Health* 34(2):76–82, 2005.
97. Maier-Riehle B, Harter M: The effects of back schools—a meta-analysis. *Int J Rehabil Res* 24(3):199–206, 2001.
98. Mailloux J, Finno M, et al: Long-term exercise adherence in the elderly with chronic low back pain. *Am J Phys Med Rehabil* 85(2):120–126, 2006.
99. Mannion AF, Caporaso F, et al: Spine stabilisation exercises in the treatment of chronic low back pain: a good clinical outcome is not associated with improved abdominal muscle function. *Eur Spine J* 21(7):1301–1310, 2012.
100. Mayoux-Benhamou A, Giraudet-Le Quintrec JS, et al: Influence of patient education on exercise compliance in rheumatoid arthritis: a prospective 12-month randomized controlled trial. *J Rheumatol* 35(2):216–223, 2008.
101. Medina-Mirapeix F, Escolar-Reina P, et al: Predictive factors of adherence to frequency and duration components in home exercise programs for neck and low back pain: an observational study. *BMC Musculoskelet Disord* 10:155, 2009.
102. Meeus M, Nijs J, et al: Pain physiology education improves pain beliefs in patients with chronic fatigue syndrome compared with pacing and self-management education: a double-blind randomized controlled trial. *Arch Phys Med Rehabil* 91(8):1153–1159, 2010.
103. Melzack R: Gate control theory: on the evolution of pain. *Pain Forum* 5:128–138, 1996.
104. Melzack R: From the gate to the neuromatrix. *Pain Suppl* 6:S121–S126, 1999.
105. Melzack R: Pain and the neuromatrix in the brain. *J Dent Educ* 65:1378–1382, 2001.
106. Merskey H, Bogduk N: *Classification of Chronic Pain*, Seattle, 1994, IASP Press.
107. Miles C, Hardman E: State-dependent memory produced by aerobic exercise. *Ergonomics* 41(1):20–28, 1998.
108. Mohs R, Mease P, et al: The effect of duloxetine treatment on cognition in patients with fibromyalgia. *Psychosom Med* 74(6): 628–634, 2012.
109. Mori DL, Sogg S, et al: Predictors of exercise compliance in individuals with Gulf War veterans illnesses: Department of Veterans Affairs Cooperative Study 470. *Mil Med* 171(9):917–923, 2006.
110. Moseley GL: Joining forces—combining cognition-targeted motor control training with group or individual pain physiology education: a successful treatment for chronic low back pain. *J Man Manip Therap* 11(2):88–94, 2003.
111. Moseley GL: A pain neuromatrix approach to patients with chronic pain. *Man Ther* 8(3):130–140, 2003.
112. Moseley GL: Evidence for a direct relationship between cognitive and physical change during an education intervention in people with chronic low back pain. *Eur J Pain* 8(1):39–45, 2004.
113. Moseley GL: Widespread brain activity during an abdominal task markedly reduced after pain physiology education: fMRI evaluation of a single patient with chronic low back pain. *Aust J Physiother* 51(1):49–52, 2005.
114. Moseley GL: Do training diaries affect and reflect adherence to home programs? *Arthritis Rheum* 55(4):662–664, 2006.
115. Moseley GL: Reconceptualising pain according to modern pain sciences. *Phys Ther Rev* 12:169–178, 2007.
116. Moseley GL: I can't find it! Distorted body image and tactile dysfunction in patients with chronic back pain. *Pain* 140(1):239–243, 2008.
117. Moseley GL, Brhyn L, et al: The threat of predictable and unpredictable pain: differential effects on central nervous system processing? *Aust J Physiother* 49(4):263–267, 2003.
118. Moseley GL, Hodges PW: Chronic pain and motor control. In Jull G, Boyling J, editors: *Grieves Modern Manual Therapy of the Vertebral column*, Edinburgh, 2002, Churchill-Livingstone.
119. Moseley GL, Hodges PW: Are the changes in postural control associated with low back pain caused by pain interference? *Clin J Pain* 21(4):323–329, 2005.
120. Moseley GL, Hodges PW: Reduced variability of postural strategy prevents normalization of motor changes induced by back pain: a risk factor for chronic trouble? *Behav Neurosci* 120(2):474–476, 2006.
121. Moseley GL, Nicholas MK, et al: Does anticipation of back pain predispose to back trouble? *Brain* 127(Pt 10):2339–2347, 2004.
122. Moseley GL, Nicholas MK, et al: A randomized controlled trial of intensive neurophysiology education in chronic low back pain. *Clin J Pain* 20(5):324–330, 2004.
123. Moseley L: Combined physiotherapy and education is efficacious for chronic low back pain. *Aust J Physiother* 48(4):297–302, 2002.
124. Moseley L: Unraveling the barriers to reconceptualization of the problem in chronic pain: the actual and perceived ability of patients and health professionals to understand the neurophysiology. *J Pain* 4(4):184–189, 2003.
125. Nathan PA, Wilcox A, et al: Effects of an aerobic exercise program on median nerve conduction and symptoms associated with carpal tunnel syndrome. *J Occup Environ Med* 43(10):840–843, 2001.
126. Newman CL, Motta RW: The effects of aerobic exercise on childhood PTSD, anxiety, and depression. *Int J Emerg Ment Health* 9(2):133–158, 2007.
127. Niemisto L, Rissanen P, et al: Cost-effectiveness of combined manipulation, stabilizing exercises, and physician consultation compared to physician consultation alone for chronic low back pain: a prospective randomized trial with 2-year follow-up. *Spine (Phila Pa 1976)* 30(10):1109–1115, 2005.
128. Nijs J, Roussel N, et al: Thinking beyond muscles and joints: therapists' and patients' attitudes and beliefs regarding chronic musculoskeletal pain are key to applying effective treatment. *Man Ther* 18(2):96–102, 2013.
129. Nilsson-Wikmar L, Holm K, et al: Effect of three different physical therapy treatments on pain and activity in pregnant women with pelvic girdle pain: a randomized clinical trial with 3, 6, and 12 months follow-up postpartum. *Spine (Phila Pa 1976)* 30(8):850–856, 2005.
130. Oman RF, Oman KK: A case-control study of psychosocial and aerobic exercise factors in women with symptoms of depression. *J Psychol* 137(4):338–350, 2003.
131. Petruzzello SJ, Tate AK: Brain activation, affect, and aerobic exercise: an examination of both state-independent and state-dependent relationships. *Psychophysiology* 34(5):527–533, 1997.
132. Poiraudeau S, Rannou F, et al: Fear-avoidance beliefs about back pain in patients with subacute low back pain. *Pain* 124(3):305–311, 2006.
133. Pontifex MB, Hillman CH, et al: The effect of acute aerobic and resistance exercise on working memory. *Med Sci Sports Exerc* 41(4):927–934, 2009.
134. Puentedura EJ, Louw A: A neuroscience approach to managing athletes with low back pain. *Phys Ther Sport* 13(3):123–133, 2012.
135. Quaney BM, Boyd LA, et al: Aerobic exercise improves cognition and motor function poststroke. *Neurorehabil Neural Repair* 23(9):879–885, 2009.
136. Reid KJ, Baron KG, et al: Aerobic exercise improves self-reported sleep and quality of life in older adults with insomnia. *Sleep Med* 11(9):934–940, 2010.
137. Richardson C, Hodges P, et al: *Therapeutic Exercise for Lumbopelvic Stabilization*, London, 2004, Churchill Livingstone.
138. Richardson C, Jull GA, et al: *Therapeutic Exercise for Spinal Segmental Stabilization in Low Back Pain*, London, 1999, Churchill Livingstone.
139. Riva R, Mork PJ, et al: Comparison of the cortisol awakening response in women with shoulder and neck pain and women with fibromyalgia. *Psychoneuroendocrinology* 37(2):299–306, 2012.
140. Riva R, Mork PJ, et al: Catecholamines and heart rate in female fibromyalgia patients. *J Psychosom Res* 72(1):51–57, 2012.

141. Rooks DS, Gautam S, et al: Group exercise, education, and combination self-management in women with fibromyalgia: a randomized trial. *Arch Intern Med* 167(20):2192–2200, 2007.
142. Ryan CG, Gray HG, et al: Pain biology education and exercise classes compared to pain biology education alone for individuals with chronic low back pain: a pilot randomised controlled trial. *Man Ther* 15(4):382–387, 2010.
143. Sackett DL: Evidence-based medicine. *Spine (Phila Pa 1976)* 23(10):1085–1086, 1998.
144. Sanchez-Zuriaga D, Vera-Garcia FJ, et al: Trunk muscle activation patterns and spine kinematics when using an oscillating blade: influence of different postures and blade orientations. *Arch Phys Med Rehabil* 90(6):1055–1060, 2009.
145. Sapolsky R: *Why Zebras Don't Get Ulcers*, New York, 1994, W.H. Freeman & Co.
146. Sapolsky RM: *Why Zebras Don't Get Ulcers: An Updated Guide to Stress, Stress-Related Diseases, and Coping*, New York, 1998, W.H. Freeman & Co.
147. Scales R, Miller JH: Motivational techniques for improving compliance with an exercise program: skills for primary care clinicians. *Curr Sports Med Rep* 2(3):166–172, 2003.
148. Sculco AD, Paup DC, et al: Effects of aerobic exercise on low back pain patients in treatment. *Spine J* 1(2):95–101, 2001.
149. Segal TY, Hindmarsh PC, et al: Disturbed adrenal function in adolescents with chronic fatigue syndrome. *J Pediatr Endocrinol Metab* 18(3):295–301, 2005.
150. Sharma NK, Ryals JM, et al: Aerobic exercise alters analgesia and neurotrophin-3 synthesis in an animal model of chronic widespread pain. *Phys Ther* 90(5):714–725, 2010.
151. Sim J, Adams N: Systematic review of randomized controlled trials of nonpharmacological interventions for fibromyalgia. *Clin J Pain* 18(5):324–336, 2002.
152. Smart KM, Blake C, et al: Mechanisms-based classifications of musculoskeletal pain: part 3 of 3: symptoms and signs of nociceptive pain in patients with low back (+/–leg) pain. *Man Ther* 17(4):352–357, 2012.
153. Stavrinou ML, Della Penna S, et al: Temporal dynamics of plastic changes in human primary somatosensory cortex after finger webbing. *Cereb Cortex* 17(9):2134–2142, 2007.
154. Stephens R, Atkins J, et al: Swearing as a response to pain. *Neuroreport* 20(12):1056–1060, 2009.
155. Stringer WW, Berezovskaya M, et al: The effect of exercise training on aerobic fitness, immune indices, and quality of life in HIV+ patients. *Med Sci Sports Exerc* 30(1):11–16, 1998.
156. Timm KE: A randomized-control study of active and passive treatments for chronic low back pain following L5 laminectomy. *J Orthop Sports Phys Ther* 20(6):276–286, 1994.
157. Tsao H, Galea MP, et al: Reorganization of the motor cortex is associated with postural control deficits in recurrent low back pain. *Brain* 131(Pt 8):2161–2171, 2008.
158. Ucok K, Aycicek A, et al: Aerobic and anaerobic exercise capacities in obstructive sleep apnea and associations with subcutaneous fat distributions. *Lung* 187(1):29–36, 2009.
159. Uysal N, Tugyan K, et al: The effects of regular aerobic exercise in adolescent period on hippocampal neuron density, apoptosis and spatial memory. *Neurosci Lett* 383(3):241–245, 2005.
160. Valkeinen H, Hakkinen K, et al: Muscle hypertrophy, strength development, and serum hormones during strength training in elderly women with fibromyalgia. *Scand J Rheumatol* 34(4):309–314, 2005.
161. van de Ven M, Andressoo JO, et al: Adaptive stress response in segmental progeria resembles long-lived dwarfism and calorie restriction in mice. *PLoS Genet* 2(12):e192, 2006.
162. Van Houdenhove B, Van Den Eede F, et al: Does hypothalamic-pituitary-adrenal axis hypofunction in chronic fatigue syndrome reflect a "crash" in the stress system? *Med Hypotheses* 72(6):701–705, 2009.
163. Vera-Garcia FJ, Brown SH, et al: Effects of different levels of torso coactivation on trunk muscular and kinematic responses to posteriorly applied sudden loads. *Clin Biomech (Bristol, Avon)* 21(5):443–455, 2006.
164. Virani SN, Ferrari R, et al: Physician resistance to the late whiplash syndrome. *J Rheumatol* 28(9):2096–2099, 2001.
165. Waddell G, Newton M, et al: A fear-avoidance beliefs questionnaire (FABQ) and the role of fear avoidance beliefs in chronic low back pain and disability. *Pain* 52:157–168, 1993.
166. Wakefield E, Holtermann A, et al: The effect of delayed onset of muscle soreness on habitual trapezius activity. *Eur J Pain* 15(6):577–583, 2011.
167. Wall PD, Melzack R: *Textbook of Pain*, London, 2005, Elsevier.
168. Watson P, Kendall N: Assessing psychosocial yellow flags. In Gifford LS, editor: *Topical Issues in Pain 2*, Falmouth, 2000, CNS Press.
169. Wedekind D, Sprute A, et al: Nocturnal urinary cortisol excretion over a randomized controlled trial with paroxetine vs. placebo combined with relaxation training or aerobic exercise in panic disorder. *Curr Pharm Des* 14(33):3518–3524, 2008.
170. Wilson D, Williams M, et al: Language and the pain experience. *Physiother Res Int* 14(1):56–65, 2009.
171. Woods JA, Ceddia MA, et al: Effects of 6 months of moderate aerobic exercise training on immune function in the elderly. *Mech Ageing Dev* 109(1):1–19, 1999.
172. Woolf CJ: Central sensitization: uncovering the relation between pain and plasticity. *Anesthesiology* 106(4):864–867, 2007.
173. Woolf CJ, Shortland P, et al: Sensitization of high mechanothreshold superficial dorsal horn and flexor motor neurones following chemosensitive primary afferent activation. *Pain* 58(2):141–155, 1994.
174. Wu G, Keyes L, et al: Comparison of telecommunication, community, and home-based Tai Chi exercise programs on compliance and effectiveness in elders at risk for falls. *Arch Phys Med Rehabil* 91(6):849–856, 2010.
175. Yamamoto U, Mohri M, et al: Six-month aerobic exercise training ameliorates central sleep apnea in patients with chronic heart failure. *J Card Fail* 13(10):825–829, 2007.

REVIEW QUESTIONS

Multiple Choice

1. Which of the following theories might explain why an individual would rub his or her elbow after striking it on a doorframe?
   a. Cartesian theory
   b. Neuromatrix theory
   c. Gate control theory
   d. Hebbian theory
2. Which of the following statements is true?
   a. Pain is carried on A nerve fibers to the brain and spinal cord.
   b. Pain is carried on large C nerve fibers to the brain and spinal cord.
   c. Tissues contain nociceptors that can send a danger signal to the spinal cord and brain.
   d. Danger messages are sent to the spinal cord only where they are interpreted as pain.
3. Which of the following statements is true?
   a. The pain area of the brain can enlarge based on the degree of pain that a patient is experiencing.
   b. Because pain uses multiple areas of the brain, it may influence adjacent areas of the brain so that their normal function is made less efficient.
   c. Pain is controlled by the motor areas of the brain and can cause movement dysfunction.
   d. All of the above are true
4. Which of the following can influence the extent to which the brain will produce pain for protection?
   a. How a patient perceives the health of the tissues
   b. The amount of damage in the tissues
   c. Which specific tissues have been injured
   d. Whether or not the pain fibers are blocked

5. Which of the following systems is the main system involved during the fight-or-flight response?
   a. Endocrine system
   b. Parasympathetic system
   c. Immune system
   d. Sympathetic system
6. Which of the following hormones can affect almost all body tissues; can regulate heart rate, blood vessel and air passage diameter, and shifts in metabolic activity; and is very active during the fight-or-flight response?
   a. Adrenaline
   b. Cytokine
   c. Cortisol
   d. Interleukin-6
7. Which of the following substances is produced by the adrenal gland and prevents the release of substances that cause inflammation?
   a. Adrenaline
   b. Cytokines
   c. Interleukin-6
   d. Cortisol
8. Which approach for treatment of individuals in pain is generally associated with psychology, counseling, or psychotherapy?
   a. Bottom-up approach
   b. Top-down approach
   c. Bidirectional approach
   d. Inside-out approach
9. Which of the following models for educating a patient about his or her pain has been shown to increase a patient's fear and anxiety?
   a. Neuromatrix theory model
   b. Hebbian theory model
   c. Anatomic and biomechanical model
   d. All of the above
10. Which of the following statements regarding the education component of a comprehensive pain program is true?
    a. Education is best done all in one session, after which no further mention of education is made during the remainder of the patient's therapy.
    b. The PTA and PT should work as a team with the PTA reinforcing the education that the PT provides even during the traditional movement-based therapies.
    c. The education component is best done after all other therapies have been exhausted.
    d. The PTA has no role in the comprehensive pain program.
11. Which of the following concepts should be emphasized during neuroscience education?
    a. When there is pain, it is an indication that tissues are damaged and are not healing.
    b. When there is pain, there is something wrong with the damaged tissues.
    c. Pain that persists after tissues heal may be due to a sensitive nervous system.
    d. Patients should focus on their pain and adhere to "no pain, no gain."
12. Which of the following has been described as one of the most potent factors in the development of chronic LBP and is the essence of neuroscience education?
    a. Fear
    b. Continued use of poor lifting techniques
    c. Overuse of pain medications
    d. Poor sustained postures
13. Which of the following strategies is referred to as one of the cornerstones of neuroscience education and can help a patient to understand his or her pain better as well as the treatment plan?
    a. Using anatomic models
    b. Explaining the biology of a patient's pain
    c. Explaining how pain can be blocked with pain medication
    d. Having a patient ignore pain and continue with activities that may even cause the pain to flare up
14. Which of the following best describes the recommended format for neuroscience education for patients with persistent pain?
    a. Patients should be seen at least three times per week.
    b. Patients should be encouraged to depend on the physical therapy practitioner for treatments even if there is not much accomplished during an individual treatment session.
    c. Patients should be given a series of treatments as necessary followed by home exercises and treatment strategies and be seen a few weeks later for reassessment and advancement.
    d. Patients should be seen once and then discharged on a home program.
15. Which of the following "mantras" should not be used with a patient experiencing persistent pain?
    a. "Sore but safe"
    b. "Hurt does not equal harm"
    d. "Tease it, touch it, nudge it" (that is, the pain)
    c. "If it hurts, don't do it"

Short Answer

16. Describe the shortcomings of the Cartesian model of pain.
17. Based on the modern understanding of pain in this chapter, write your own definition of pain.
18. Describe the concept of pain being a multiple system output.
19. What is a normal biologic process that is aimed at protecting the body tissues and is the start of the healing and repair process?
20. Briefly describe what is meant by a bottom-up approach to the treatment of pain.

Fill in the Blank

21. The ________________ theory states that pain is involved in multiple brain areas rather than a single "pain area."
22. A pain ________________ is the networking of various brain areas that together make up an individual pain experience.

23. _______________ is the most recent educational strategy advocated by the authors for the treatment of patients experiencing chronic pain.
24. Studies have shown that after an injury or immobilization of a body part, the representation of the injured or immobilized body part is altered in the brain in _______________ minutes.
25. _______________ exercise has been shown to help decrease pain via a postexercise hyperalgesia, improve sleep and motor function, aid the immune system, improve mood and anxiety, and decrease nerve sensitivity.

True/False

26. An individual's pain level is reflective of the amount of tissue damage.
27. Pain can be thought of as input coming from the periphery and carried by pain nerve fibers to the brain.
28. Pain is a response by the brain based on threat.
29. Stress response is a normal response for all humans when in a stressful situation, and the changes should return to normal when the stressor is relieved.
30. According to the chapter, the authors believe that using an updated view of pain and the evidence for treatment based on a neuroscience approach is a treatment for pain rather than just managing pain.

Chapter 26

Orthopedic Management of Orthotics and Prosthetics

Leslie K. King

CHAPTER OUTLINE

LEARNING OBJECTIVES

1. Define the terms *orthotics* and *prosthetics.*
2. Obtain a basic understanding of materials.
3. Learn the nomenclature—the naming of orthoses and prostheses in relation to the joint they support or replace.
4. Describe the key differences when off-the-shelf orthoses can be chosen instead of custom fabricated orthoses.
5. Have a general understanding of orthotic options for supporting major joints in the body.
6. List levels of amputation sites and the reasons for amputation.
7. Develop an understanding of basic prosthetic componentry and how the selection of componentry relates to patient function and outcome.

KEY TERMS

Body powered prosthesis
Brace
Componentry
Doff
Don
Footdrop
Liner
Myoelectric prosthesis
Orthosis
Packing out
Prosthesis
Sock management
Socket
Splint

When selecting an appropriate **orthosis** or **prosthesis** for a patient, numerous options are available for either prefabricated or custom fabricated devices. The plethora of possible manufacturers makes it increasingly difficult to select the best device simply because of the number of optimal choices. The proper selection of each device is based on diagnosis, functional goals, and the patient's cognitive and physical abilities to **don** and **doff** and use these devices properly.

The process developed for naming orthoses and prostheses is simple. The International Standards Organization recognizes common descriptors for orthoses and prostheses based on the acronyms from the body joint or joints that are supported or replaced (Table 26-1). This method of nomenclature is effective and easily learned.

Important Concepts

Nomenclature is the system developed in which we name devices (e.g., below knee amputee = BK).

ORTHOTICS

An orthosis is a product or device that supports a body part or joint. These devices provide the patient with stability, support, positioning, and protection. Orthoses range

TABLE 26-1 International Standards Organization Naming Conventions for Orthoses and Prostheses

Device Type	Amputation Level		Nomenclature
Orthoses	Upper extremity	Finger orthosis	FO
		Hand orthosis	HO
		Wrist-hand orthosis	WHO
		Wrist orthosis	WO
		Elbow orthosis	EO
		Elbow-wrist-hand orthosis	EWHO
		Shoulder orthosis	SO
	Spinal	Cervicothoracolumbosacral orthosis	CTLSO
		Cervical orthosis	CO
		Thoracolumbosacral orthosis	TLSO
		Lumbosacral orthosis	LSO
		Sacroiliac orthosis	SIO
	Lower extremity	Foot orthosis	FO
		Knee orthosis	KO
		Ankle-foot orthosis	AFO
		Knee-ankle-foot orthosis	KAFO
		Hip-knee-ankle-foot orthosis	HKAFO
Prostheses	Upper extremity	Shoulder disarticulation	SD
		Transhumeral	TH
		Elbow disarticulation	ED
		Transradial	TR
		Wrist disarticulation	WD
	Lower extremity	Hip disarticulation	HD
		Transfemoral	TF
		Knee disarticulation	KD
		Transtibial	TT
		Ankle disarticulation	Symes
		Transmetatarsal amputation	TMA

From Shurr DG, Michael JW: *Prosthetics and orthotics,* ed 2, Upper Saddle River, NJ, 2002, Prentice Hall, p 16.

from a prefabricated wrist **splint** to a custom fabricated reciprocating gait orthosis. Orthoses are tools used to help a patient become more independent and functional with tasks such as activities of daily living and ambulation. Selecting the proper device is crucial in providing the patient with optimal support, results, care, and outcome results.

Important Concepts

An orthosis is a device that supports the body.

Two key terms are commonly used when discussing orthotics: splinting and bracing. *Splinting* is a term used today and most often refers to an orthosis that immobilizes a joint, such as a finger splint used to hold a broken phalange immobile or a hip spica splint fitted to a patient after hip repair or replacement that allows only a specific range of motion (ROM) as the rehabilitation protocol requires. *Bracing* is a term that is still used today by the lay population, but it is a dated term for clinicians. The term *orthotic* is derived from the Greek *ortho,* meaning to straighten. Today, orthotics relates to biomechanical and musculoskeletal support and correction of abnormalities within the human body.

PROSTHETICS

A prosthesis is any device that replaces a body part, including arms, legs, partial feet, hands, ears, and breasts. The goal for each prosthesis is to provide function, body balance, ease of use, and optimal cosmesis to restore self-image, quality of life, and independence (Table 26-2). Prostheses are custom fabricated and require adjustments and realignment on a regular basis.

TABLE 26-2 Specifications for the Ideal Prosthesis/Orthosis

Need	Definition
Function	Meets the user's needs, simple, easily learned, dependable
Comfort	Fits well, easy to don/doff, lightweight, adjustable
Cosmesis	Looks, smells, sounds "normal," cleans easily, stain-resistant
Fabrication	Fast, modular, readily and widely available
Economics	Affordable, worth cost of monetary investment

From Shurr DG, Michael JW: *Prosthetics and orthotics,* ed 2, Upper Saddle River, NJ, 2002, Prentice Hall, p 29.

Important Concepts

A prosthesis is a device that replaces a body part.

The amount of **componentry,** or parts of a prosthesis, depends on the involved level of amputation. For an upper extremity prosthesis, the components may include a **socket,** shoulder joint, pylon, elbow joint, wrist unit, and hand, depending on where the amputation site is located along the arm. For a lower extremity prosthesis, the components are similar to an upper extremity prosthesis, but the hands and wrists are replaced by feet, knees, and hip joints. Each of the components (for upper extremity and lower extremity prostheses) plays a specific role in whether the prosthesis is ultimately used successfully by the patient. For example, the socket is the custom fabricated portion created from a mold of the patient's residual limb. This mold is obtained by casting the patient or by computer-aided manufacturing, a process during which the residual limb is scanned using a computer-aided design program. Proper fit of the socket is crucial, and intimacy of the fit is directly related to the patient's end result for use and wear time. The rest of the prosthetic componentry is carefully selected from the vast list of products available from manufacturers. Hands, elbows, and shoulder joints are chosen by the prosthetist to assemble the most appropriate and functional prosthesis.

Prosthetic socks are applied on top of the **liners** as a means to fill up the volume inside the socket. Prosthetic socks are available in different thicknesses referred to as *ply.* As the amputee retains or loses fluid throughout the course of the day, adding or removing a sock is done to maintain the optimal fit of the socket. This process is referred to as **sock management.**

Important Concepts

Sock management is the technique of controlling the proper fit of the prosthetic socket by adding or removing prosthetic socks throughout the day.

Prostheses may also incorporate silicone liners for suspension and cushion. Liners are fabricated out of materials such as silicone, polyurethane, and gel elastomers. These materials are chosen because of their ease of use for donning or doffing, quality of hygiene, and durability. To obtain proper limb length, a pylon, which is an aluminum or stainless steel tube, is fitted between the foot and the socket or knee unit.

FITTING FOR ORTHOSES OR PROSTHESES

As each orthosis or prosthesis is being fabricated or fitted, the functional goals of each patient are key to making the most appropriate selection for componentry. The patient's weight, age, activity level, and potential to regain independence and agility are the factors used to determine which type of orthosis or type of material to choose.

When selecting orthotic or prosthetic components, it is important to consider how the patient will be using the device. Requirements vary per person and may be necessary for safety, ambulation, prevention of deformity, or transferring from one seated position to another.

Material Selection

When fabricating orthoses and prostheses, the material selection is the first consideration of the process. Multiple types of thermoplastics, metals, carbon fiber composites, and interface materials are available. Each type of material has certain desirable characteristics or properties that best suit each patient's needs. Body weight, activity level, amount of rigidity needed, flexibility of material, energy-storing properties, amount of cushioning required, and patient strength all are variables to consider when selecting fabrication materials (Table 26-3).

TABLE 26-3 Important Characteristics of Prosthetic and Orthotic Materials

Need	Definition
Strength	Maximum external load that can be withstood
Stiffness	Stress/strain or force-to-displacement ratio
Durability	Ability to withstand repeated loading
Density	Weight per unit volume
Corrosion resistance	Resistance to chemical degradation
Ease of fabrication	Equipment and techniques needed to shape it

From Shurr DG, Michael JW: *Prosthetics and orthotics,* ed 2, Upper Saddle River, NJ, 2002, Prentice Hall, p 29.

Plastic

Plastics used in orthoses and prostheses are copolymer, thermoplastic polyethylene, polypropylene, and acrylics. Plastics used for custom orthoses such as ankle-foot orthoses (AFOs), knee-ankle-foot orthoses (KAFOs), and upper extremity bracing are chosen for thermal properties and level of rigidity or flexibility and weight of material. When fabricating a lower extremity **brace**, a thicker, stronger plastic should be chosen over a thin plastic, which may be used for an upper extremity splint. The heaviness, strength, and rigidity necessary for supporting body weight would not be necessary for an upper extremity brace.

Metal

Metals most commonly used in orthoses are aluminum and steel alloys, titanium, copper, and bronze. These metals are used when designing and fabricating short leg braces or AFOs and KAFOs and for pylons in prostheses. They are strong, lightweight, and noncorrosive. Metals are also used in knee orthoses and casings for prosthetic knees and torsion units.

Carbon Fiber Composites

Carbon fiber composites are being used more commonly in custom and prefabricated orthoses. Floor reaction, anterior tibial shell AFOs, footplates, knee bracing, and KAFOs all use varying layers and pattern designs of carbon composites. The patterns create varying degrees of strength, flexibility, weight, and energy-storing properties. This advancement in the ability to provide a support that is lightweight and conserves energy has been beneficial to all users. Reduced energy output for ambulation during the day is a tangible benefit. The potential of wearing a less cumbersome device under clothing is a cosmetic advantage and provides a more optimal, intimate fit of the device. Lastly, the energy-storing property provides each patient with the ability to work and walk for longer periods of time, resulting in a more productive and happier individual. This same technology of layering carbon fiber in multiple, pattern-specific directions is used in the production of prosthetic feet to produce the same lightweight, yet strong, energy return benefit.

Interface Material

Interface material is used for cushioning an orthosis or prosthesis for comfort and fit and for fabricating custom arch supports. Varying durometers of firmness and multiple thicknesses and color options (which is a bonus when working with children) make obtaining the best option available possible. Plastazote, PPT, and pelite are some of the most commonly used interface materials. These product properties include vacuum molding, closed or open cell, and whether the material is subject to **packing out**, will resist packing out, or will not pack out. Packing out is what happens to the material over time and use, and the result is the material compresses and eventually collapses.

DEVICE SELECTION

According to information gathered from the patient and the prescription ordered by the physician, an assessment must be made by the physical therapist (PT) as to whether the patient may need to be fitted with an orthosis. Often this device can be ordered through an orthotic/prosthetic clinic. A prefabricated orthosis is designed with the size and measurements of a high percentage of the general population taken into account. The first option is to fit the patient with a prefabricated orthosis, as long as the patient's measurements are within the measurement guidelines provided by the manufacturer, and proper fit and function are not compromised. The prefabricated orthosis can be an appropriate and cost-saving selection. When the patient's size or skeletal deformities do not allow for proper fit of a prefabricated orthosis, the patient is casted, scanned, and measured as needed to custom fabricate the orthotic device. Custom fabricated orthoses include wrist splints, knee orthoses, and diabetic shoes.

The advancements made in prefabricated orthoses have created a wide range of readily available prefabricated products. A large percentage of the general population can be fitted with these new devices. However, adjustments and changes are necessary for a custom fit and optimal patient benefit. Certain indications, diseases, and deformities require custom fabricated splints, including progressive, dynamic, and static varieties. A progressive splint is one that can be modified as the patient's rehabilitation progresses so that it accommodates those changes and still provides the necessary support from a greater to lesser support and allows for increases in ROM. Dynamic splinting uses springs or tension rod joints to apply a constant resistance or assistance for flexion or extension. The amount of tension is adjustable and can be set to meet rehabilitation protocols. Lastly, static splinting holds the joint or joints in a specific position.

All prosthetic devices are fabricated by combining a custom-made socket designed from a mold or scanned file taken of the residual limb and selected componentry for the rest of the prosthesis that will be replacing the amputated body part. Depending on patient size, measurements, and deformity, items such as liners can be custom fabricated if a prefabricated item does not fit properly. Patients who exceed the recommended weight limit for prefabricated prosthetic feet and knee units can also be fitted with a custom fabricated component.

ORTHOSES

Upper Extremity

Fingers, Hand, and Wrist. A splint for the fingers and hand should support only the affected joint or joints and allow the unaffected joints free ROM. Single joint splints for the fingers are available, such as proximal interphalangeal and distal interphalangeal splints, which maintain or promote active ROM in the phalanges after sprains, fractures, or contractures. Some splints maintain or hold the joint in a fixed position, whereas dynamic splints that are spring-loaded allow the patient some movement of flexion or extension, while applying constant force in the desired direction (Fig. 26-1). One particular type of wrist-hand-finger orthosis (WHFO) is the Thomas suspension splint. The function of this splint is to apply tension to the wrist joint and thumb to dorsiflex the wrist for diagnoses such as radial palsy. The long opponens splint is often used for flexion contractures, nerve or tendon damage resulting from traumatic accidents, or rheumatoid arthritis. These splints offer dynamic finger extension and allow the patient to use flexors needed for gripping.

Another example of a functional custom fabricated WHFO is the tenodesis splint (also known as a *wrist action splint*) (Fig. 26-2). This splint is used to increase functional levels and independence mainly for quadriplegia. The design is ultra-lightweight and uses the available ability to flex the wrist to accentuate the natural movement of opposition for gripping objects by using the three-jaw chuck pinch position. The wrist-driven wrist-hand orthosis employs the flexor hinge principle. The fingers and thumb are stabilized in the position of function. A small amount of wrist extensor strength creates flexion motion in the metacarpophalangeal joints to produce adequate pinch for various daily activities. Because it is custom fabricated, this style of splint requires a cast of the hand and forearm and measurements for fabrication.

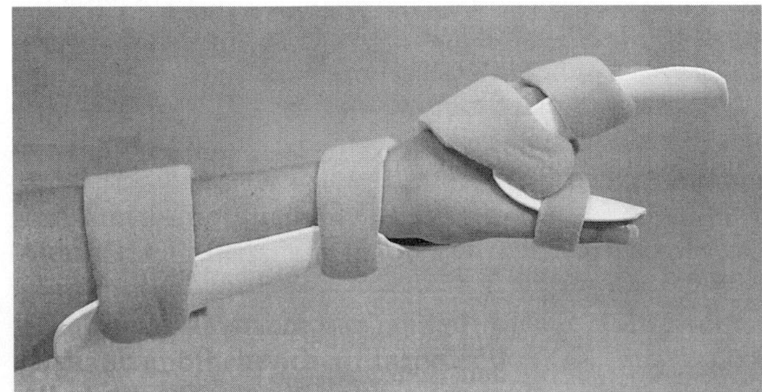

FIG 26-1 Static immobilization splint. This static splint immobilizes the thumb, fingers, and wrist. *(From Coppard BM, Lohman H: Introduction to orthotics: a clinical reasoning and problem-solving approach, ed 4, St Louis, 2015, Mosby.)*

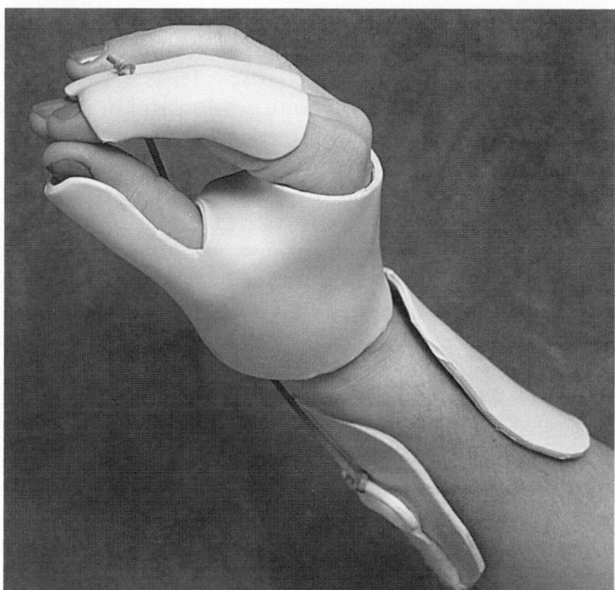

FIG 26-2 A tenodesis splint uses active wrist extension to aid passive finger flexion. *(From Coppard BM, Lohman H:* Introduction to orthotics: a clinical reasoning and problem-solving approach, *ed 4, St Louis, 2015, Mosby.)*

Multiple orthotic options are available for supporting the hand and wrist, depending on the diagnosis and desired limitations for movement. For diagnoses such as carpal tunnel syndrome, tendinitis, or a sprain, a cock-up wrist splint, which holds the wrist in a neutral position, is the most common choice (Fig. 26-3, *A*). This splint is a prefabricated brace that is readily available in various sizes. For diagnoses such as a contracture secondary to a cerebrovascular accident or rheumatoid arthritis, a prefabricated malleable WHFO will suffice. This orthosis is progressive in design because the wrist joint and finger platform is easily flexed or extended to accommodate gains made by stretching protocols in physical therapy sessions. These prefabricated, lightweight splints are called *platform* or *resting splints* and provide static positioning (Fig. 26-3, *B*). Some soft versions of these splints are more skin-friendly because they offer the option of a cover that can be removed and washed, which promotes good hygiene.

Elbow. Fitting choices for elbow orthoses can usually be prefabricated. A lateral epicondylitis splint (a band with a silicone or air pocket), is used to disperse the pressure placed on the tendon caused by use over a greater area, decreasing the point of high stress and pain (Fig. 26-4). ROM splints that limit active ROM or provide pressure to increase ROM can also be purchased as prefabricated orthoses. The Flex POP Elbow Orthosis by RCAI (St. Petersburg, FL) provides rehabilitation for joint stiffness and contractures, instabilities, strains, sprains, and ligament repairs. This ROM elbow orthosis offers flexion/extension stop sets at 5° increments, which allows changes to be made in therapy sessions as the patient progresses. Dynamic elbow splints can be used when the function desired is to gain ROM by applying a constant stretch to

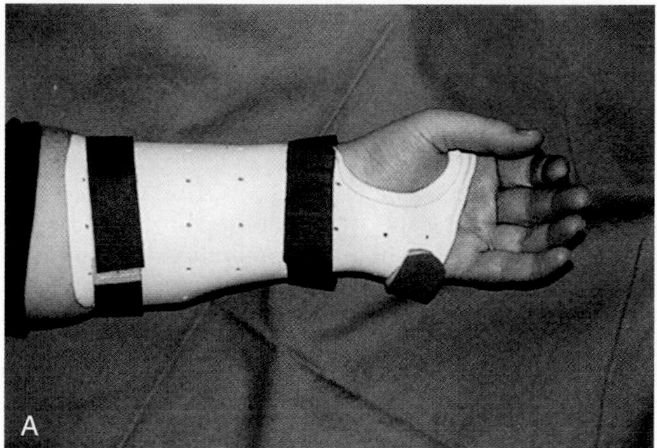

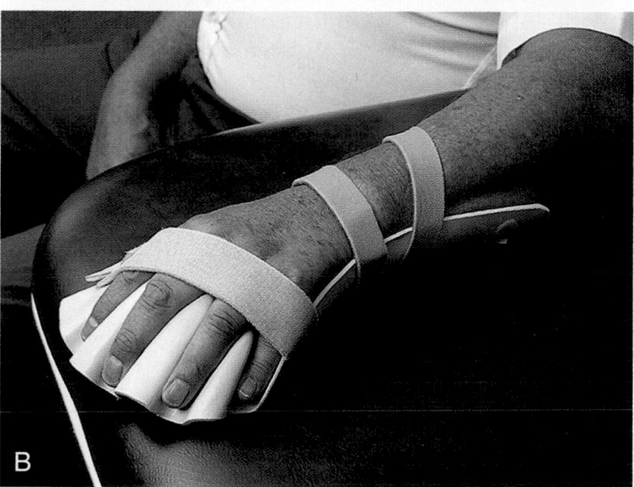

FIG 26-3 **A,** Completed radial bar cock-up splint. **B,** Positional resting splint. *(**A,** From Early MB:* Physical dysfunction practice skills for the occupational therapy assistant, *ed 2, St Louis, 2007, Mosby; **B,** from Pierson FM, Fairchild S:* Principles & techniques of patient care, *ed 4, St Louis, 2008, Saunders.)*

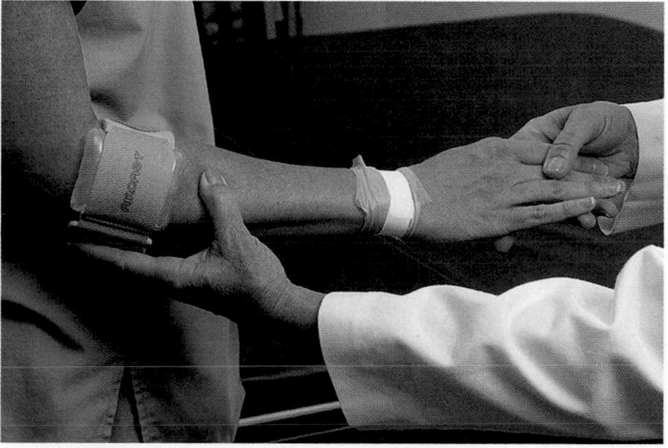

FIG 26-4 Tennis elbow strap applied. *(From Pierson FM, Fairchild S:* Principles & techniques of patient care, *ed 4, St Louis, 2008, Saunders.)*

the elbow joint tendons and muscles. Protocols are set for wear time and when the tension placed on the joint can be increased. Static splints can be set to a designated degree of flexion or extension and, depending on the style or brand, may or may not be adjustable. The physician's prescription, rehabilitation protocols, and the patient's level of compliance and tolerance all contribute to the decision-making process when fitting these types of elbow splints. Elbow contractures can be caused by various injuries or diseases, such as cerebral palsy and cerebrovascular accident.

Shoulder. Shoulder splinting for immobilization can use a sling and swath or a shoulder immobilizer that supports the shoulder joint. One common design uses a chest band, upper arm cuff, and forearm cuff that is adjustable and positions the arm securely against the body (Fig. 26-5). If the required position is abduction, an airplane splint can be fitted.

Specialized Orthoses for the Upper Extremity. Activities of daily living require a multitude of orthoses to promote independence for individuals who have experienced a stroke or debilitating injury. There are hand and wrist splints that are adapted to hold a fork when feeding oneself or other items such as a pen, hairbrush, and toothbrush (Fig. 26-6). Many types of foam are available to place around utensils and items with handles to increase their circumference, decreasing the grip strength and ROM needed to hold and use such items.

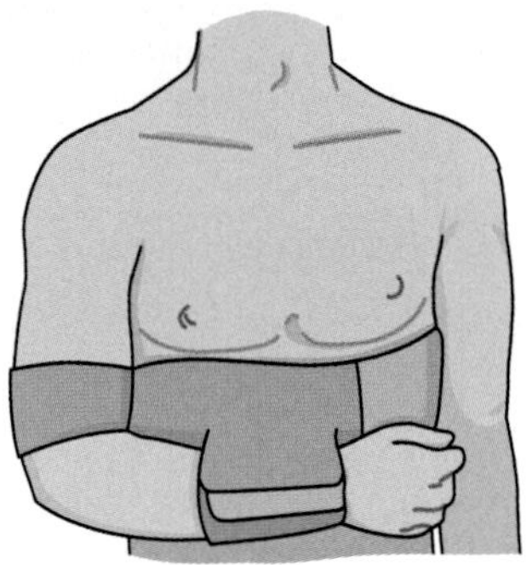

FIG 26-5 Shoulder immobilizer. *(Redrawn from Beare PG, Meyers JL:* Principles and practice of adult health nursing, *ed 3, 1998, Mosby; in Elkin MK:* Nursing interventions & clinical skills, *ed 4, St Louis, 2008, Mosby.)*

Fracture splinting uses a compression method for stabilization of the fracture site. The compression of fluid and soft tissue around the fracture site is key when providing a femoral, humeral, radial, or ulnar splint. These splints can be modified to a custom fit by heating or adding a soft interface material to provide added comfort. The fracture splint is a bivalve, two-piece orthosis and uses adjustable hook and loop strapping (Fig. 26-7). The splint allows movement of the unaffected joints, such as elbow and wrist for ulnar fracture. The technique and principles used in splinting for upper extremity fractures are the same for lower extremity fractures.

Spine and Trunk

Cervical Spine. Cervical orthoses are fitted for the purpose of supporting the cervical muscles; limiting rotation, flexion, and extension; or immobilization of the cervical spine. A soft cervical collar can be fitted for lesser injuries such as sprains and strains. The soft collar is a prefabricated orthosis made of foam with a cotton cover and has a hook and loop closure in the back (Fig. 26-8). They are available in different heights and lengths. A cervicothoracic orthosis is a semirigid, two-piece brace that can be fitted for whiplash, degenerative joint disease, arthritis, and presurgical or postsurgical repairs. These collars are adjustable in height, circumference, and rigidity, but, as with all bracing, the therapist must always check pressure points to ensure there is no skin breakdown.

Lumbosacral Spine. For spinal support, numerous custom and off-the-shelf products are available. The severity of the injury, pain, or disease determines the amount of support required for each individual. The more that the patient wears the orthosis, the more dependent he or she becomes on it because the abdominal muscles are not

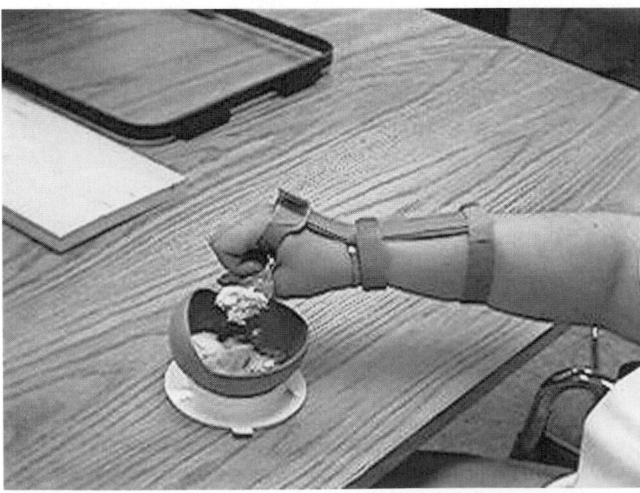

FIG 26-6 Eating using a special splint with a utensil holder fitted to the hand. *(From Early MB:* Physical dysfunction practice skills for the occupational therapy assistant, *ed 2, St Louis, 2007, Mosby.)*

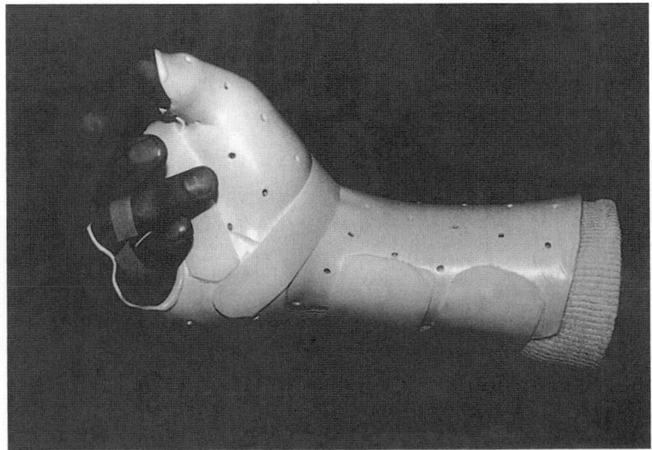

FIG 26-7 Designed to facilitate adjustments as edema diminishes, this two-piece metacarpal fracture splint has excellent contiguous fit. *(Courtesy Lin Beribak, OTR/L, CHT, Chicago, IL. In Fess EE, Gettle K, Philips C, et al:* Hand and upper extremity splinting: principles and methods, *ed 3, St Louis, 2005, Mosby.)*

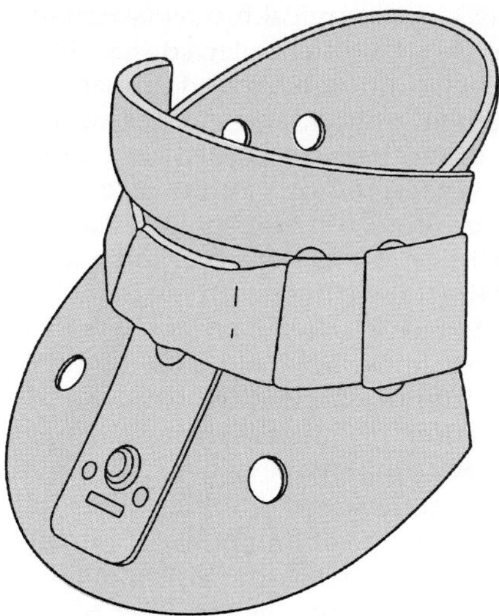

FIG 26-8 The Philadelphia collar, with an anterior opening for tracheostomy care. *(Modified from Shurr DG: Prosthetics, orthotics and orthopaedic rehabilitation. In Clark CR, Bonfiglio M, editors:* Orthopaedics: essentials of diagnosis and treatment, *New York, 1994, Churchill Livingstone.)*

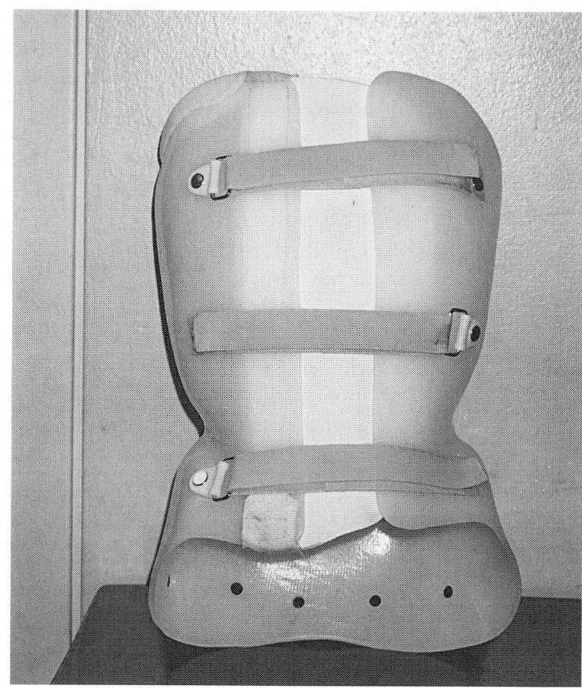

FIG 26-9 The Wilmington brace is a custom-molded, total-contact thoracolumbosacral orthosis. *(From Campbell S:* Physical therapy for children, *ed 3, St Louis, 2007, Saunders.)*

working to support the spine, as the device is doing the work of the muscles. With this concept in mind, the least amount of support necessary is always the best option.

Trunk support encompasses abdominal binders, rigid panel supports, hyperextension braces, and custom fabricated scoliosis orthoses. Each orthosis requires certain specific circumferential measurements, length measurements, and width measurements and, for custom bracing, casting or scan of the torso to create a mold. When making a custom spinal orthosis, material selection becomes very important. Selecting the necessary amount of rigidity with the least amount of weight is crucial.

The most flexible and the least rigid lumbosacral orthosis (LSO) is the abdominal binder. This orthosis is a stretchy surgical elastic binder that is available in varying widths and lengths to provide optimal fit to a wide range of sizes. The LSO provides support and compression to the abdominal muscles, which support the lower back. The abdominal binder is most often fitted for low-back pain.

Pregnancy supports are abdominal binders and are available for use during pregnancy. They provide relief to the lumbar spine and support and assistance with unloading the abdomen while compressing the hip complex.

There are numerous styles of rigid back panel LSOs. Depending on where the injury or disease is in the lumbar region, there are two choices for which orthosis style to fit. If the region lies between L1 and L5, there are supports that fit and support this narrow region. This type of orthosis limits motion in the sagittal plane. This support is created by intracavity pressure to reduce the intervertebral load on the disks. The Aspen QuickDraw RAP is an example of a prefabricated orthosis that falls into this category. This LSO is easy to don and doff, which contributes to the compliance of the patient in wearing the support. It is fabricated of a material that is made to be worn next to the skin. This decreases the occurrence of migration. The fabric is lightweight and breathable, which makes cleaning easier and prolongs the life of the orthosis and increases the patient's hygiene. The back panel has a pocket in which to insert the customizable rigid panel, and a hot or cold pack can be placed in the pocket for therapeutic benefit. This LSO uses effective compression and leverage to give strong support and immediate pain relief.[3]

An LSO can be transformed into a thoracolumbosacral orthosis (TLSO) by adding shoulder straps, chest panel, and torso straps. With the additional strapping and pads, the region of support now includes the posterior side from the sacrococcygeal junction to just inferior to the scapular spine. The anterior section of the TLSO extends from the symphysis pubis to the sternal notch, restricting motion in the transverse and sagittal planes and restricting gross trunk movement (Fig. 26-9). TLSOs also provide intracavity pressure to the lumbar and lower thoracic region. Typically, using the least software and hardware necessary makes it easier to don and doff the orthosis. A higher level of compliance by the wearer is required when adding more componentry (or pieces) to the orthosis.[2]

Hyperextension TLSOs are worn on the anterior side of the body. They operate and function by using a three-point pressure system to maintain full extension and allow for healing of stress fractures. Two pads are used on the anterior portion of the trunk: a sternal pad that sits below the sternal notch and a pubis pad that sits just superior to the symphysis pubis. A third pad is on the posterior side attached to the strap, and it applies pressure in the center of the spine. This orthosis is typically indicated for stress fractures resulting from osteoporosis, and it is commonly used by elderly women. Because the design of the TLSO is to hold the wearer in good posture, compliance is often an issue with wearing this support, as good posture often decreases with age.

To provide complete spinal support throughout the cervical to lumbar vertebrae, a cervicothoracolumbosacral orthosis (CTLSO) should be fitted. A CTLSO has a mandibular piece on which the chin rests (Fig. 26-10). A forehead strap is also incorporated to assist in controlling the rotation on the head. This type of orthosis is very rigid and immobilizing. These devices are usually fitted for degenerative diseases, for fractures, or after spinal surgeries.

Lower Extremity

Sprains, fractures, torn ligaments, arthritis, footdrop, and paralysis all require specific orthoses depending on the diagnosis. Similar to upper extremity orthoses, lower extremity orthoses have prefabricated and custom options. Necessary support, varying degrees of immobilization, and function all are required criteria to be met in each fitting.

Hip. The realm of splinting for the hip joint encompasses immobilization during injury, presurgical and postsurgical intervention, and limited ROM control to meet rehabilitation protocols. When splinting for hip dislocations, subluxations, or postsurgical hip replacement, a hip spica abduction orthosis is often selected (Fig. 26-11). The hip orthosis provides hip stability and proper hip alignment, limits unwanted motion, and reduces stress on the hip. The hip orthosis is prefabricated and offers hip joint options to provide the best orthosis to meet individual rehabilitation protocols. Hip joints have settings for flexion, extension, abduction, and adduction. The pelvic section and the thigh cuff section can be ordered individually for optimum fit. The interface is soft and can be removed for cleaning. Depending on the need, either one or two hip joint hinges and thigh cuffs can be attached to the pelvic section, making the orthosis adaptable for one or two leg spica supports.[11]

Certain neuromuscular disorders, especially cerebral palsy, are associated with pronounced instability and poor balance secondary to spastic hip adduction. This hip adduction creates a very narrow base of support when sitting and standing, causing crouched posture, genu valgum, foot pronation, and poor gait. One hip orthosis on the market today that may be helpful for these conditions is called the *S.W.A.S.H.* (Sitting Walking And Standing Hip orthosis), manufactured by Allard (Rockaway, NJ) (Fig. 26-12). This orthosis is designed for children with neuromuscular diagnoses, such as spastic hemiplegia, quadriplegia, low trunk tone, or cerebral palsy, or who have a risk of hip displacement. This orthosis should not be fitted to patients with chronic hip dislocation or fixed hip flexion contracture greater than 20°. The S.W.A.S.H. is designed to reduce hip adduction, promote hip abduction,

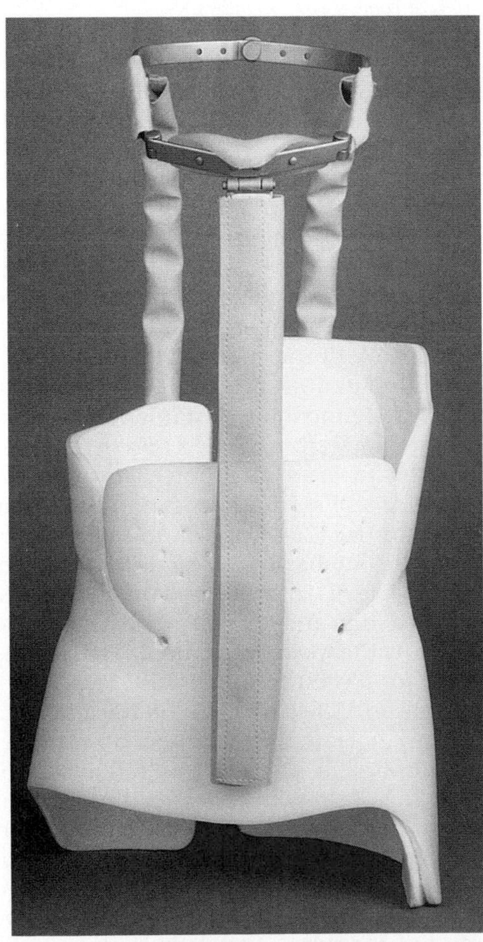

FIG 26-10 Milwaukee brace. Note the tightly fitting pelvic section and the superstructure with its ringlike chin and occipital supports. *(From Lusardi MM, Nielson CC:* Orthotics and prosthetics in rehabilitation, *ed 2, St Louis, 2007, Saunders.)*

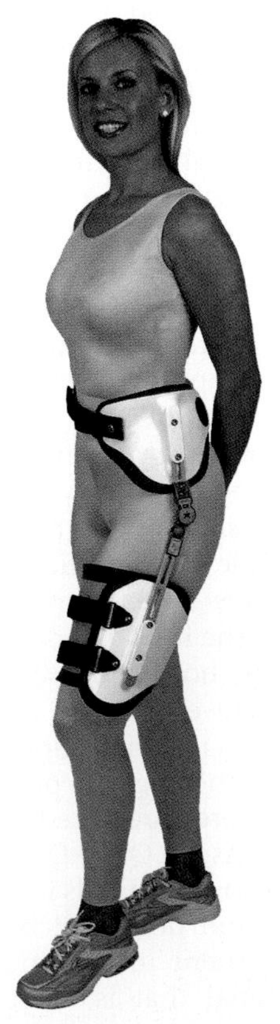

FIG 26-11 Hip abduction orthosis. *(Courtesy of Orthomerica Products, Inc. © 2015.)*

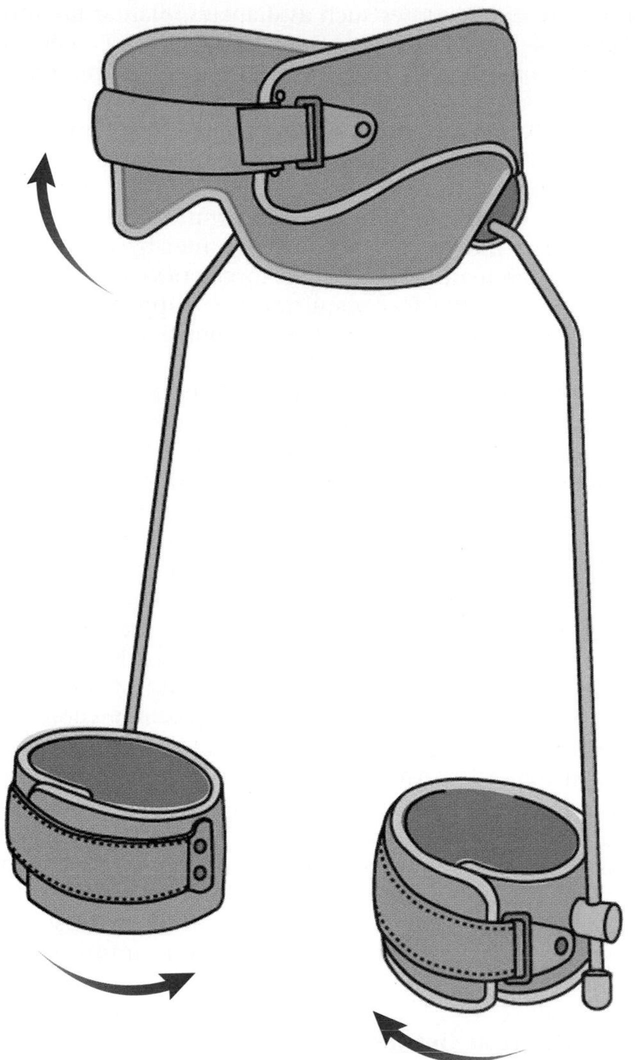

FIG 26-12 S.W.A.S.H. orthosis.

and allow for better control in gait and sitting. This orthosis has been shown to reduce hip adduction and tone, improve hip alignment and ambulation, and create greater independence for patients over time. Maximum success can be achieved with ongoing therapy while wearing this device. The S.W.A.S.H. also allows for greater interaction during play and rehabilitation because it frees the patient's hands.[1]

Knee. Knee orthoses range from a neoprene sleeve to a structured combined instability orthosis that has a rigid frame and is hinged at the knee joint. A knee sleeve can be selected when the knee instability is not significant. Reasons to select a knee sleeve may be that heat is desired to relieve pain in an arthritic joint or to provide proprioceptive cues. Diagnoses such as knee pain or mild osteoarthritis can be qualified for the fitting of the knee sleeve.

Patellar tracking knee orthoses are usually fitted for patients with patellofemoral syndrome, patellar tracking problems, or patellar dislocations. The main symptom for these conditions is knee pain in front of the knee exacerbated during squatting or climbing steps. Patellar tracking orthoses are usually a neoprene fabric with an additional strap that presses against the patella to promote normal tracking during ambulation and prevent further dislocations or injury. Increasing quadriceps strength is also beneficial.

A hinged knee orthosis may be indicated when more significant knee pain or mild instabilities are involved. A knee sprain or strain or possible meniscal tear is an indication for fitting of a hinged knee brace. By adding the hinges to the knee orthosis, medial and lateral stability is gained; the hinged splint provides more stability. A hinged knee orthosis may be neoprene with hinges, a single upright hinge with strapping for placement and support, or a more structured combined instability brace (Fig. 26-13). Combined instability orthoses are used for anterior

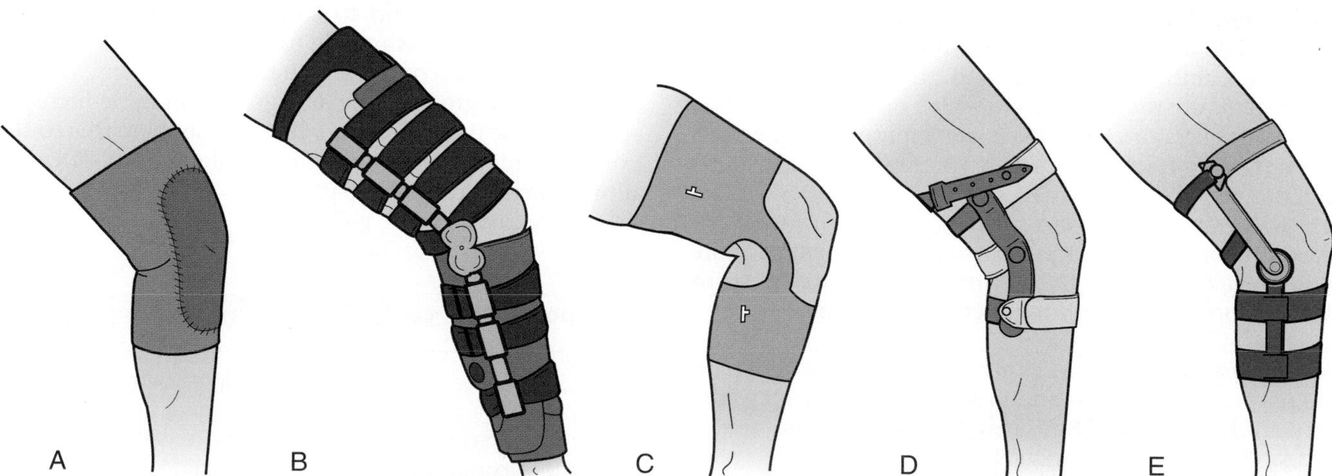

FIG 26-13 Knee orthoses. **A,** Soft neoprene knee sleeve. **B,** Postoperative knee orthosis controls flexion range of motion and extension range of motion with adjustable joints. **C,** Prophylactic knee orthosis with lateral joint. **D,** Rehabilitative design to control knee hyperextension. **E,** Custom knee orthosis to stabilize injured knee. *(Modified from Coppard BM, Lohman H:* Introduction to orthotics: a clinical reasoning & problem-solving approach, *ed 4, St Louis, 2015, Mosby.)*

cruciate ligament tears, posterior cruciate ligament tears, medial collateral ligament tears, or meniscal tears. These orthoses are also fitted for prophylactic needs for athletes to prevent ligament injuries or instabilities. Combined instability knee orthoses can be either prefabricated or custom-made depending on the size and deformity of the knee. These braces provide protection against hyperextension and medial and lateral shifting.

Specific osteoarthritis knee braces are available for the diagnosis of osteoarthritis with medial or lateral compartment failure involved. This particular style of knee orthosis is designed to assist with realigning the skeleton to unload the compressed side of the knee joint. By decreasing the load on the compressed compartment, pain is decreased, and degeneration in the joint is slowed. By providing proper support and correction to the compromised joint, the likelihood of increasing the patient's quality of life and mobility is the main goal to maintain a healthy lifestyle. These knee braces are available in prefabricated or custom sizes. Custom knee orthoses require casting and measuring.

Postoperative knee orthoses use a knee hinge with adjustable ROM settings that can be changed as rehabilitation protocols are met and changed. The knee brace can be set to hold a certain position or allow only desired ROM as prescribed by the physician or reassessed by the PT or the physical therapist assistant (PTA). This type of knee orthosis is generally not meant for long-term use, and the patient either graduates out of a knee orthosis altogether or moves into a knee orthosis that is less bulky, is more durable, and has a more specific design depending on the diagnosis.

Ankle. Two common choices are available when providing an orthosis for an ankle sprain. The stirrup splint allows free dorsiflexion and plantar flexion to occur, while providing limitations to inversion and eversion to prevent the sprain from recurring. This splint is often used for patients who experience frequent ankle sprains. The other type of orthosis is the ankle gauntlet. This splint provides more immobilization in all planes of motion and is easily worn inside a tennis shoe. Depending on the diagnosis, the physician's prescription, and the patient's history, assessments are made regarding which orthosis to provide.

Boot walkers or cam walkers are appropriate selections when treating fractures or severe sprains or for immobilizing the foot or ankle after surgery. These orthoses are removable for bathing and sleeping. The sole of the boot walker incorporates a rocker bottom to assimilate a more natural gait. The length of time the orthosis is worn depends on the patient's required healing time.

Foot. Custom foot orthoses are another means of obtaining proper foot position and protecting areas of increased pressure in the foot. The transverse arch and the medial and lateral longitudinal arches can be supported. By creating pocketed areas of relief for the plantar surface of the foot, degenerative processes can be slowed down, while correcting skeletal alignment of the foot. Prominent bony landmarks, such as the metatarsal heads, navicular, talus, and cuneiform bones, can be supported or relieved. Patients with diagnoses such as diabetes, plantar fasciitis, heel spurs, pronation, ulcerations, and collapsed arches all benefit from the use of custom-made arch supports to correct the position of the foot and assist with a better gait pattern. Numerous materials are available to meet the needs of each individual patient, including, but not limited to, carbon fiber, cork, pelite, Plastazote, and elastomer gel offering a wide range of firmness from rigidity to softness. Individual needs can be met by combining two or more materials to obtain forgiveness and cushion in portions of the foot requiring soft support and firm support to align the foot in the best position possible.

Shoe Wear. When treating a patient for foot problems, proper shoe wear is pertinent. The shoe becomes an integral part of the brace when the AFO or KAFO is a metal upright attached to the shoe as well as when the shoe is necessary to seat a plastic or carbon fiber AFO properly in it for stable ambulation. If the patient is not diabetic, a high-quality walking shoe or tennis shoe is recommended for use. If the patient is diabetic, insurance companies will cover the cost of the shoes, and there are numerous options for diabetic shoe brands and styles. Each manufacturer must meet set guidelines to qualify for diabetic shoes status. Diabetic shoes are as seamless as possible and have extra depth to accommodate custom arch supports and custom AFOs. Most brands also incorporate a hidden rocker bottom to decrease pressure on the metatarsal heads. For a patient who has such deformity that an off-the-shelf pair of shoes will not fit, custom shoes can be fabricated. Custom shoes are made from a cast or scanned file of the patient's feet. Numerous options exist, so any needed design is possible and the fit is intimate and protective.

Combination Orthoses

Ankle-Foot Orthoses. Diagnoses such as cerebrovascular accident, multiple sclerosis, spinal cord injury, and various neuropathies can cause a condition known as **footdrop.** This condition causes the patient to lose the ability to fire the peroneal nerve and to contract the anterior tibialis muscle. The patient is unable to pick the toe up by dorsiflexing the ankle complex. When this happens, the frequency of dragging the toe during the gait cycle increases and can cause the patient to fall. AFOs can help this condition by holding the ankle/foot complex at 90°. The AFO allows dorsiflexion as the patient rolls over the foot during the stance phase of the gait cycle.

> **Important Concepts**
>
> Footdrop is a common condition resulting from brain injury, cerebrovascular accident, multiple sclerosis, or cerebral palsy. The peroneal nerve is damaged, or the brain is not communicating properly to cause dorsiflexion of the ankle/foot complex.

Most AFOs limit inversion and eversion and place the foot in a subtalar neutral position if obtainable. A pelite liner can also be molded into a custom AFO as a soft interface, creating a more comfortable, padded support for the patient. Diabetic patients especially need custom AFOs to decrease the potential for developing sores or ulcers that may not heal because of rubbing or areas of high pressure. When a custom AFO is fabricated, areas of relief are built into the orthosis. These areas accommodate heavy callused areas and ulcerations and provide support and relief for collapsed arches that cannot be corrected. Plastic AFOs are in complete contact with the patient's foot and calf and are fitted inside a shoe, causing the shoe to be an integral part of the orthosis. Shoe wear is limited to mostly lace or hook and loop attachments because this feature of the shoes seats the heel of the AFO into the shoe. Slip-on shoes do not work as well because they allow the heel to slip in and out of the shoe too easily.

There are several types of AFOs, including leaf spring, solid ankle, free ankle, and dorsi-assist (Fig. 26-14). These orthoses fall into two categories, static and dynamic, with both types consisting of either prefabricated or custom fabricated devices. Static orthoses prohibit motion at the ankle, and dynamic orthoses permit ankle motion, primarily in the sagittal plane. The solid ankle AFO, the anterior floor reaction brace, and the patellar tendon–bearing AFO are examples of static AFOs. The dynamic group includes posterior leaf spring and hinged-ankle (articulating) AFO designs.[9] Dynamic AFOs are contraindicated in patients with severe edema, nonhealing diabetic ulcers, and severe foot deformity.

Important Concepts

AFOs fall into two categories, static (solid ankle AFOs) and dynamic (AFOs that allow dorsiflexion and plantar flexion).

The simplest and most cost-effective AFO is the leaf spring. The leaf spring AFO fits under the plantar surface of the foot and into the shoe. It extends up the posterior portion of the calf and has a single strap just distal to the fibula head. It is lightweight, streamlined, and effective, especially if no other instabilities or weaknesses are present. The leaf spring is available in a wide variety of sizes of foot length, foot width, and height of the upright portion.

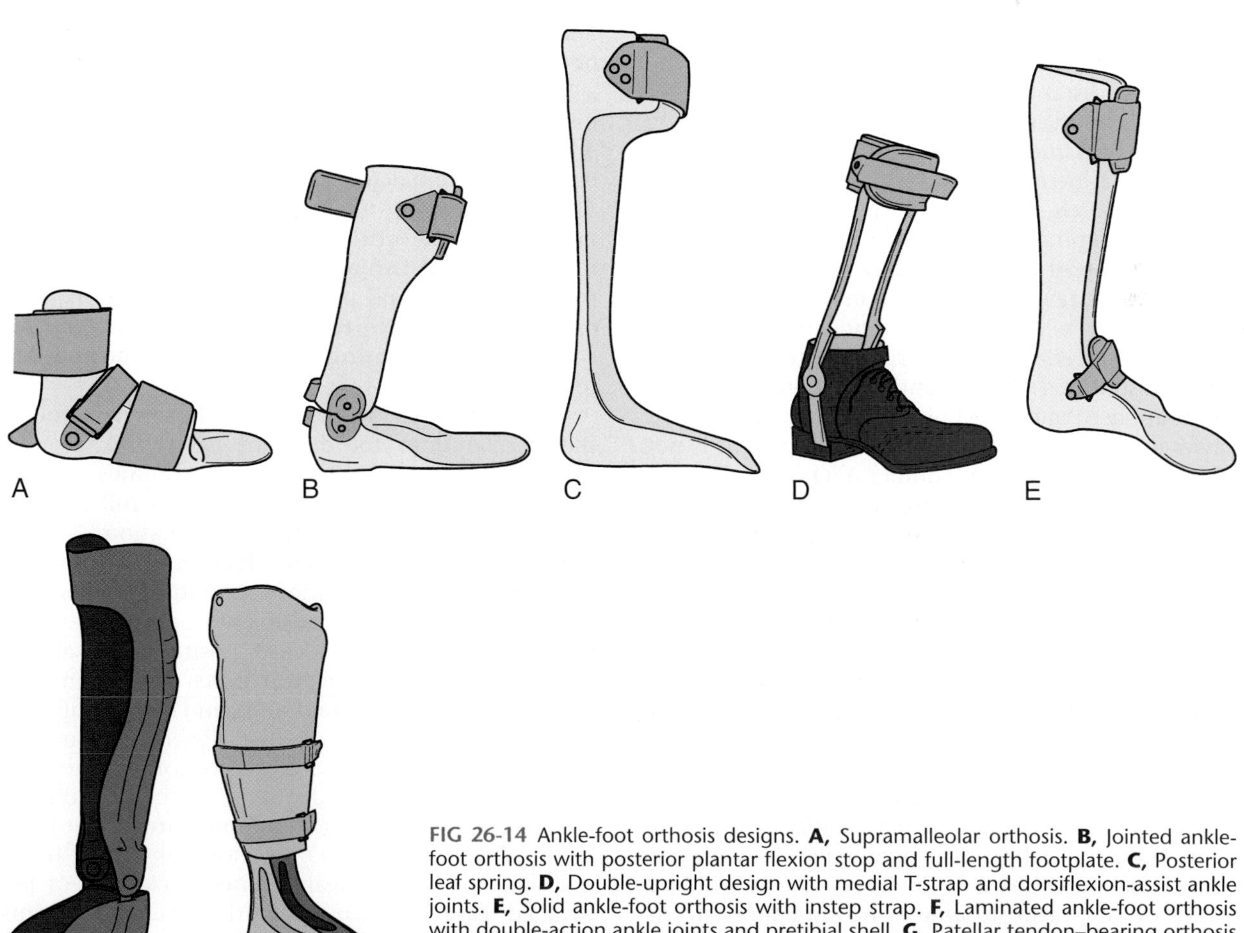

FIG 26-14 Ankle-foot orthosis designs. **A,** Supramalleolar orthosis. **B,** Jointed ankle-foot orthosis with posterior plantar flexion stop and full-length footplate. **C,** Posterior leaf spring. **D,** Double-upright design with medial T-strap and dorsiflexion-assist ankle joints. **E,** Solid ankle-foot orthosis with instep strap. **F,** Laminated ankle-foot orthosis with double-action ankle joints and pretibial shell. **G,** Patellar tendon–bearing orthosis for load-bearing relief of the foot and ankle complex with carbon fiber reinforcements at the ankle. *(Modified from Coppard BM, Lohman H:* Introduction to splinting: a clinical reasoning & problem-solving approach, *ed 3, St Louis, 2008, Mosby.)*

The solid ankle AFO provides the highest level of support and immobilization. The dorsi-assist ankle joint allows and assists dorsiflexion, whereas plantar flexion can be limited to stopping at 90° or free plantar flexion. A free ankle AFO allows free plantar flexion and dorsiflexion.

Prefabricated versus custom ankle-foot orthoses. If a prefabricated AFO does not fit properly under the foot or have proper contouring around the malleoli, a custom AFO can be made. Fabricating a custom AFO provides a more intimate fit and creates an orthosis that the patient can wear for longer periods of time, which increases compliance and quality of life. The custom AFO incorporates areas of relief for bony prominences such as malleoli; dropped or collapsed bones of the foot, such as the navicular or talus; and dropped, callused, or ulcerated metatarsal heads. When fabricating a custom AFO, the design of the orthosis depends on patient requirements and the practitioner's expertise in componentry selection. If minimal support is required, the trim lines can be very narrow, allowing more movement and flexibility, and it is less limiting. If the trim lines are wide and encompass the malleoli, the AFO is more rigid and immobilizing, providing increased levels of ankle stability and immobilization.

Plastic versus metal ankle-foot orthoses. The plastic AFO is total contact, and this feature is not an option for certain patient populations. For patients who present with edema in the lower extremities, the metal AFO is a good choice because it does not touch the patient except for the single strap just distal to the fibula head; this allows for edema accumulation during the day without rubbing along all of the trim lines that the plastic AFO has. Another reason to select a metal AFO is that it enables incorporation of a custom arch support into the shoe. There would not be enough depth in a shoe for a plastic AFO and a custom arch support. A metal AFO, more commonly known as a *short-leg brace,* consists of metal uprights contoured specifically to each patient and attached to the shoe using a metal stirrup that is riveted into the sole of the shoe. The options of solid ankle, limited motion, or dorsi-assist apply to metal and plastic bracing. Metal AFOs are heavier and less cosmetic, but when the patient is not a candidate for a plastic total contact AFO, a metal brace must be fabricated. Metal orthoses are most commonly fitted for patients with postpolio syndrome, cerebrovascular accidents, spinal cord injuries, cerebral palsy, and multiple sclerosis. Making the proper selection for metal type used for the uprights in a lower extremity brace is crucial for optimal patient outcome. For instance, if the patient is of small stature, experiencing weakness, or fairly inactive, choosing aluminum uprights for the patient's bracing allows the practitioner to provide a material with required strength and adequate support for ambulation without fabricating a brace that would be too heavy for the patient to use. The consideration of patient ability is a crucial factor in choosing fabrication materials. Providing a patient with an orthosis that is too heavy for use will lead to nonuse of the orthosis and noncompliance of the patient, increasing the likelihood of injury and further progression of the deformity. The shoe attached to the orthosis is considered to be a part of the orthosis. Shoe selection is limited to walking shoes and other closed heel and toe shoes. Refer to the previous section on shoe wear for more information about shoes.

Specialized ankle-foot orthoses. Certain conditions may not require custom-made AFOs and benefit from alternative styles of specialized orthoses. The ToeOFF, an orthosis to aid gait manufactured by Allard USA (Rockaway, NJ), is used for many different conditions, such as footdrop, partial foot amputation, posterior tibial tendon dysfunction, and Achilles tendinitis. The carbon fiber, anterior shell design aids in obtaining a more natural gait and can be worn for walking and running.

The Charcot restraint orthotic walker (CROW) is another type of specialized custom AFO. The CROW is one form of a custom fabricated boot using a clamshell two-piece design and a rocker bottom sole. The CROW provides a custom, intimate fit to eliminate friction, shear forces, and motion inside the boot to promote the healing process for nonhealing decubitus ulcers or fractures of the foot or Charcot deformities. Because it is removable, the boot helps to promote proper hygiene. Often patients who are fitted with a CROW are also receiving wound care treatment. The CROW has an anterior/posterior bivalve construction and is fabricated using a mold of the patient's lower leg. The closure for the CROW uses a butterfly chafe design with hook and loop for ease of don and doff.

Knee-Ankle-Foot Orthoses. When instability, deformity, or both are present in the knee as well as the foot and ankle, a KAFO can be fabricated. The KAFO extends from just distal of the femoral head to the foot. Often fitting both a knee orthosis and an AFO is tried but is not always successful or optimal for patient outcomes. Because of the difficulty in trying to fit a patient with the two components of a knee orthosis and an AFO, the fit is compromised where the two orthoses meet or overlap. Frequently, there is rubbing and pinching at this junction. The knee orthosis would have to extend down past the proximal edge of the AFO causing the purchase of the knee orthosis to be sacrificed.

Types of knee-ankle-foot orthoses. For the KAFO, there are options for different types of knee joints to accommodate various levels of instabilities (Fig. 26-15). Locked knee joints hold the patient in full extension to prevent knee buckling during ambulation. The patient must use hip hiking or circumduction to progress the limb forward during ambulation, providing supported and secure ambulation. The use of drop locks enables the patient to release the locked position and allow knee flexion for sitting. The drop locks can be unlocked by simply grasping with the hands and pulling up until the joint is cleared or by the use of a trigger release mechanism attached to the upper, lateral portion of the KAFO. If quadriceps strength is adequate, a free knee joint can be used to allow full ROM and a more natural gait for ambulation. This type of KAFO will not lock during heel strike and will not protect against knee buckling. For patients with a disease such as osteoarthritis or deformity, this type of orthosis provides adequate support for ambulation owing to the patient having adequate quadriceps strength, while still providing medial and lateral support.

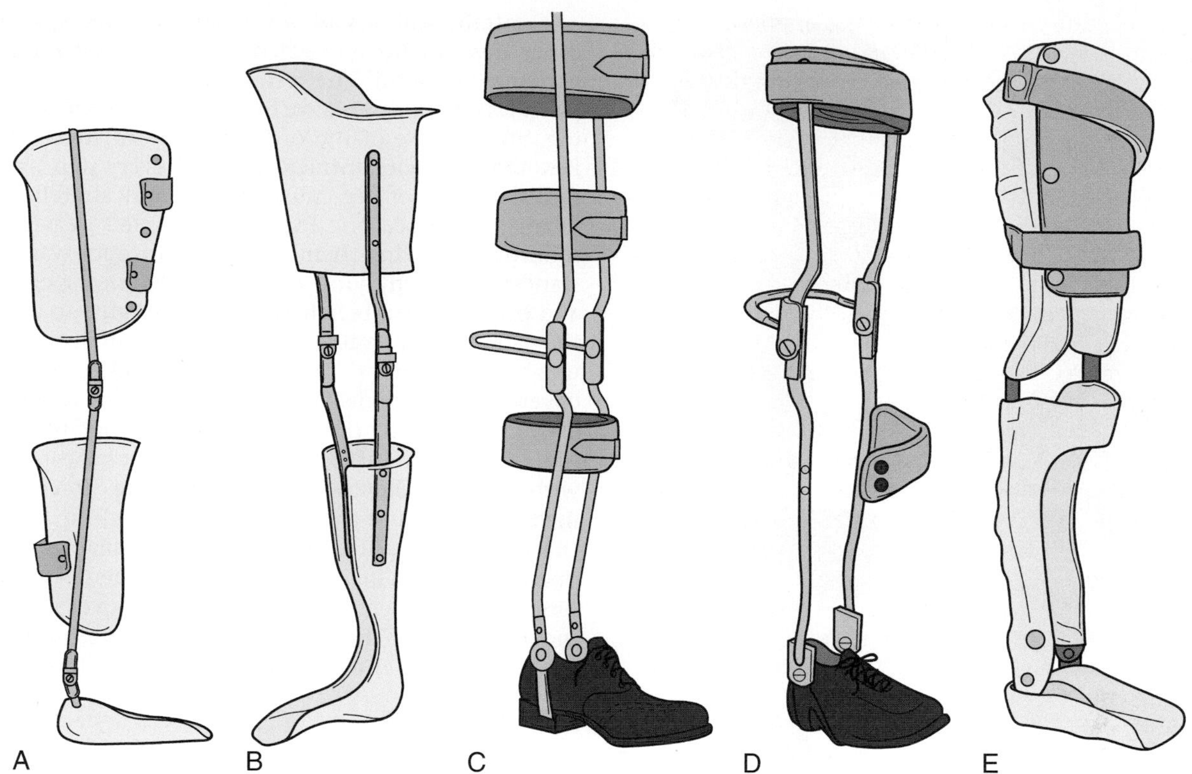

FIG 26-15 Various knee-ankle-foot orthoses. **A,** Thermoplastic orthosis with molded footplate, jointed ankle, long anterior tibial shell, drop locks, and circumferential thigh shell. **B,** Thermoplastic orthosis with molded footplate, solid ankle, drop locks, and quadrilateral thigh shell. **C,** Double-upright orthosis attached to shoe, with jointed ankle, posterior calf band, bail lock knee, and two posterior thigh bands. **D,** Scott-Craig orthosis with double-action ankle joints, pivot anterior tibial band, bail lock knee, and posterior thigh band. **E,** Laminated orthosis with molded footplate, double-action ankle, pretibial shell, free knee, and posterior thigh shell with long anterior tongue. *(Modified from Coppard BM, Lohman H:* Introduction to splinting: a clinical reasoning & problem-solving approach, *ed 3, St Louis, 2008, Mosby.)*

In recent years, the benefits of technologic advances have become substantial in the realm of KAFOs. New knee joint designs that allow a locked knee at heel strike or full knee extension and a free knee swing during the swing phase of the gait cycle are becoming more widely prescribed and fitted. The mechanism for locking and unlocking the knee unit is determined by the manufacturer, and each design has a slightly different patient population selection.

The Free Walk KAFO by Otto Bock (Minneapolis, MN)[14] helps achieve a more natural gait by locking during the stance phase and unlocking during the swing phase. The automatic lock is initiated by knee extension moment and is released to swing freely only when a knee extension moment and dorsiflexion occur simultaneously in terminal stance. The KAFO joint requires the simultaneous extension moment and 10° of dorsiflexion to release the lock, making it safe for descents and ascents. The Free Walk has an open frame design that uses only one upright instead of two (Fig. 26-16, *A*). The upright is on the lateral side of the leg. The locking mechanism control cable is contained in the tubular stainless steel sidebar. The Free Walk is a custom fabricated orthosis, but the patient must be able to obtain a knee extension moment and dorsiflexion of ankle and foot to operate this device.[7]

Fillauer (Chattanooga, TN) designed a dynamic KAFO called the Swing Phase Lock (SPL). The SPL KAFO uses a simple internal pendulum mechanism to lock and unlock the knee depending on the angle of the joint in the sagittal plane (Fig. 26-16, *B*). During the gait cycle, the knee joint locks just before heel strike for support during stance and unlocks the knee at heel off in preparation for swing phase. The SPL KAFO has three modes of operation controlled by a proximal remote push-button switch: automatic lock and unlock, manual unlock, and manual lock. These three modes allow the patient to select automatic lock for walking, unlock for sitting, or lock for standing. Candidates for this KAFO are patients with postpolio syndrome, spinal involvement, cerebrovascular accident, peripheral paresis or paralysis, nerve inflammations, neurologic failures, myopathies, and MS or similar diseases. Contraindications are knee flexion contractures greater than 10°, central paralysis, hip flexion contractures, hip musculature involvement, poor balance/coordination, and knee hyperextension greater than 10°.[7] Both KAFOs described here eliminate the need for circumduction or hip hiking as seen in the traditional KAFOs.

Hip-Knee-Ankle-Foot Orthoses. The HKAFO supports all of the joints that it crosses. Different styles, materials, and

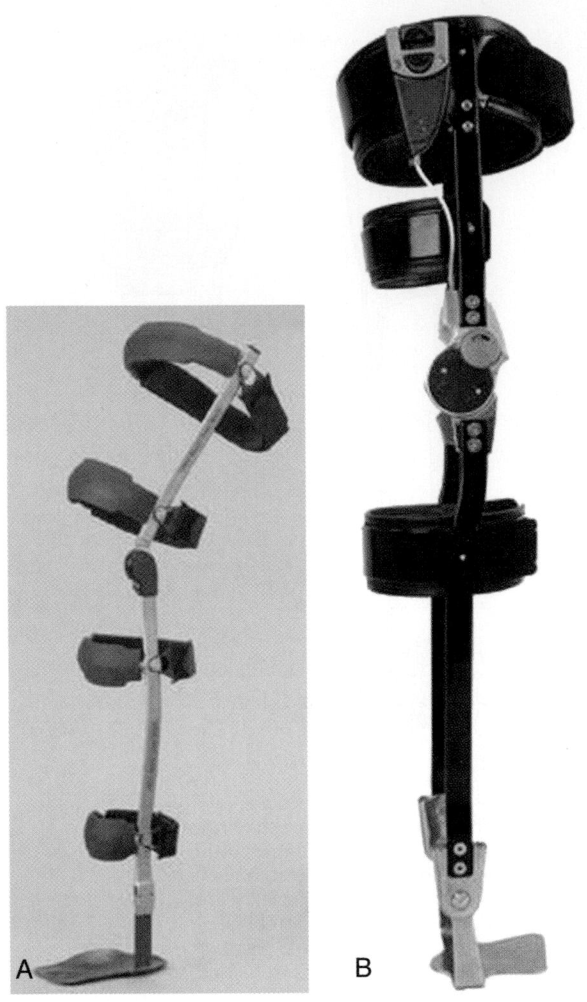

FIG 26-16 Joint designs for knee-ankle-foot orthoses. To view the most up-to-date models, please visit the manufacturer websites. **A,** FreeWalk open frame design. **B,** Swing Phase Lock knee-ankle-foot orthosis.

componentry are available to design every orthosis specifically to each individual's needs (Fig. 26-17). Some styles of HKAFO can be heavy and cumbersome simply because of the bulk of the orthosis and the number of anatomic joints that it crosses, creating a steep learning curve for the patient, PT, and PTA. Practicing the donning and doffing process and focusing rehabilitation sessions on upper body strength, ROM, and developing a successful gait pattern are a few of the hurdles that face the patient, PT, PTA, family members, and caregivers. In addition to the physical demands, the emotional stressors should be addressed by setting clear, concise, attainable goals and ensuring that each individual has the patience needed to fulfill the physical therapy sessions and protocols. Indications are spina bifida, traumatic paraplegia, muscular dystrophy, and osteogenesis imperfecta. The patient must have plantigrade feet, knees should not have flexion contractures greater than 5° to 10°, hips should be free of contractures and flexible (not rigid or spastic), upper extremity strength should be good, the patient should be well motivated and have a supportive family, and goals and expectations should be realistic.

Contraindications are severe contractures, spasticity or other involuntary movements, obesity, and poor upper extremity strength. The reciprocating gait orthosis (RGO) provides excellent walking function and hands-free standing, and the use of the orthosis helps to stretch the hip flexors to prevent contractures. With every step, as one leg flexes, the other leg must extend and stretch the hip flexors. The isocentric RGO can be fitted in patients 17 months old, giving them a better chance for walking and standing and enjoying earlier the physiologic, skeletal, and psychological benefits of being upright. To ambulate, the patient must be able to use forearm crutches to provide upper body support. A tripod gait is often used when covering a greater distance is required, such as when outdoors. When using the isocentric RGO inside the home or indoors, the patient can use a normal ambulation pattern with crutches. The RGO is a custom-made device in which measurements and a cast of the torso and hip portion of the patient is required. Two styles are available. One is an open design in which the wearer dons the device by slipping into the open posterior side. It fits over all clothing including shoes. The second style fits more intimately to the patient, and the ankle-foot portion fits into a shoe.[6]

PROSTHESES

As discussed at the beginning of the chapter, a prosthesis replaces a body part. The process for fabricating a custom prosthesis has several steps, as follows:

1. Evaluation to determine the type of prosthesis to be fabricated based on activity level, strength, amputation site, personal goals set, and insurance guidelines
2. Casting or scanning of the patient's affected body area and manufacture of a check socket to assess fit
3. Fabrication of the permanent socket and assembly of the prosthesis
4. Fitting of the prosthesis and delivery of all necessary componentry and accessories

The patient also has the option of a protective, cosmetic covering on the prosthesis. This covering is custom-made and matches the existing limb in color and shape as closely as possible. The patient returns as necessary for follow-up appointments.

Reasons for Amputations

Amputations are performed for numerous reasons, including traumatic injury, cancer, infections, and diabetes. Many amputees are born with congenital deformities in which the limb did not develop, or the limb deformity is so great that it must be amputated. The younger the amputee, the better the outcome in most cases because there is a longer period of time available to learn coping skills, compensation techniques, and ways to adapt physically to the environment. The younger the amputee, the greater the likelihood that the amputee will have higher levels of flexibility, strength, and balance and have marked improvements at a faster rate. Congenital amputees, whether upper or lower extremity, learn many ways to compensate for the absence of the limb, becoming very efficient in ambulation or tasks that require upper extremity involvement and dexterity. The psychological involvement can also be lessened for congenital or very young

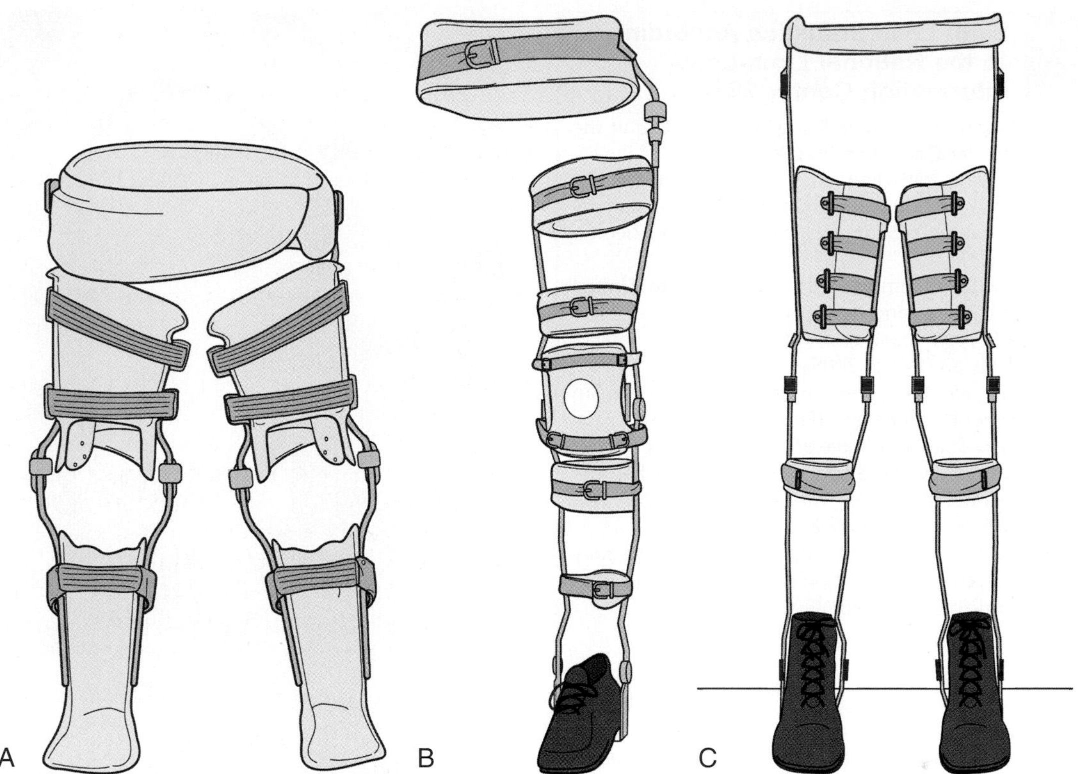

FIG 26-17 Hip-knee-ankle-foot orthoses. **A,** Bilateral thermoplastic hip-knee-ankle-foot orthosis. **B,** Unilateral double-upright hip-knee-ankle-foot orthosis. **C,** Bilateral double-upright hip-knee-ankle-foot orthosis. *(Modified from Coppard BM, Lohman H:* Introduction to orthotics: a clinical reasoning & problem-solving approach, *ed 4, St Louis, 2015, Mosby.)*

amputees for issues such as self-image if the family maintains a positive attitude. Experts in the pediatric prosthetics field believe that as long as the parents, extended family, and support team maintain a positive attitude toward the missing limb or deficiency, whether acquired or congenital, the child will also have a positive attitude and outlook on life. If the parents do not handle the limb deficiency well, it is likely that the child also will not cope well with the limb loss. When the patient or family begins to have difficulty coping with the limb loss, referral to a psychologist, a peer group, or both becomes essential. The earlier the intervention and support for the family and the child, the better the outcome.[4]

See Box 26-1 for statistics on limb loss. Table 26-4 lists the possible causes for amputation.

Suspension Methods

Suspension of a prosthesis refers to the manner in which the prosthesis is held onto the residual limb. Locking pins, suction valves, patella straps, harnesses, and simply the design of the socket all are means by which the prosthesis is suspended. Proper suspension of the prosthesis is a key factor in fit, function, and usability of the prosthesis.

Important Concepts

Suspension is the means by which a prosthesis is held on.

TABLE 26-4 Causes of Amputation

Cause	Rationale
Dysvascular-related amputations	Problems associated with the blood vessels: 38.30 per 100,000 in 1988 increased to 46.19 per 100,000 in 1996 Lower limb amputations: 97% In all age groups, the highest risks were for males and African-Americans
Trauma-related amputations	Upper extremity accounts for 68.6% Males were at slightly higher risk For males and females, risk of traumatic amputation increased steadily with age, reaching its highest level among people ≥85 years old
Cancer-related amputations	Most common occurrence in the lower limb accounting for 36% No notable differences found between sexes and races and lower occurrence rate found in African-Americans
Congenital-related incidences	Rates for newborns were 26 per 100,000 live births, relatively unchanged over the study period Upper limb accounted for 58.5%

From National Limb Loss Information Center. Amputation Statistics by Cause: Limb Loss in the United States. Published by the National Limb Loss Information Center. Available online: http://www.amputee-coalition.org/fact_sheets/limbloss_us.html. Accessed March 27, 2015.

BOX 26-1 Limb Loss Statistics According to the National Limb Loss Information Center 2012

- There are nearly 2 million people living with limb loss in the United States (Ziegler-Graham et al, 2008).
- Among people living with limb loss, the main causes are vascular disease (54%), including diabetes and peripheral arterial disease; trauma (45%); and cancer (<2%) (Ziegler-Graham et al, 2008).
- Approximately 185,000 amputations occur in the United States each year (Owings and Kozak, 1998).
- In 2009, hospital costs associated with amputation totaled more than $8.3 billion (HCUP, 2009).
- African-Americans are four times more likely to have an amputation than white Americans (Fisher et al, 2008).
- Nearly half of individuals who have an amputation as a result of vascular disease die within 5 years; this is higher than the 5-year mortality rates for breast cancer, colon cancer, and prostate cancer (Robbins et al, 2008).
- Of individuals with diabetes who have a lower extremity amputation, 55% require amputation of the second leg within 2 to 3 years (Pandian et al, 1998).

References

Fisher ES, Goodman DC, Chandra A: *Disparities in Health and Health Care among Medicare Beneficiaries: A Brief Report of the Dartmouth Atlas Project,* Robert Wood Johnson Foundation, 2008.

Healthcare Cost and Utilization Project (HCUP): *HCUP Nationwide Inpatient Sample (NIS),* Rockville, 2009, Agency for Healthcare Research and Quality.

Owings M, Kozak LJ: *National Center for Health Statistics: Ambulatory and Inpatient Procedures in the United States, 1996,* Hyattsville, MD, 1998, U.S. Department of Health and Human Services, Centers for Disease Control and Prevention, National Center for Health Statistics.

Pandian G, Hamid F, Hammond M: Rehabilitation of the patient with peripheral vascular disease and diabetic foot problems. In DeLisa JA, Gans BM, editors. *Rehabilitation medicine: principles and practice,* ed 3, Philadelphia: Lippincott-Raven; 1998.

Robbins JM, Strauss G, Aron D, et al: Mortality rates and diabetic foot ulcers. J Am Podiatr Med Assoc 98(6):489–493, 2008.

Ziegler-Graham K, MacKenzie EJ, Ephraim PL, et al: Estimating the prevalence of limb loss in the United States: 2005 to 2050. Arch Phys Med Rehabil 89(3):422–429, 2008.

From National Limb Loss Information Center: Amputation Statistics by Cause: Limb Loss in the United States. Published by the National Limb Loss Information Center. Available online: http://www.amputee-coalition.org/limb-loss-resource-center/resources-by-topic/limb-loss-statistics/limb-loss-statistics/. Accessed March 27, 2015.

Locking Pins. Many prostheses, whether upper or lower extremity, are suspended by the use of a liner with a locking pin. The pin is located on the distal end of the liner and slips into a locking mechanism that is housed within the distal end of the socket (Fig. 26-18). A liner is a means of interface that lies between the skin and the socket. Liners are made of silicone, polypropylene, elastomer gels, or urethane blends. The liners act as a cushion for shock absorbency, prevent abrasions, and protect against shearing forces and skin breakdown of the residual limb. This type of suspension provides a secure attachment, and because of the visual and audible cues made as the pin engages into the lock, this type of suspension provides a factor of emotional security that the prosthesis is donned correctly. There is a release button to press that disengages the lock and allows the prosthesis to be removed.

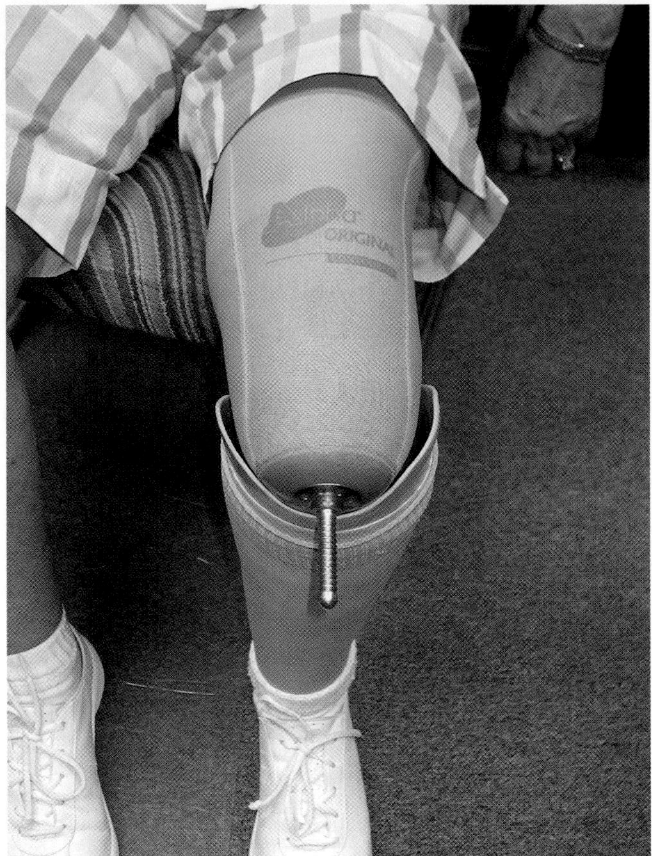

FIG 26-18 Alpha Locking Liner with pin. The pin engages the lock in the distal socket.

The Alpha Liner is composed of a unique, mineral oil–based, thermoplastic, elastomer gel with durable fabric covering that makes the liner last longer. The mineral oil within the liner seeps into the skin, creating a skin-friendly environment. This gel liner also conforms to the shape of the residual limb providing a custom fit. The Alpha Liner is available in prefabricated and custom-made variations for pediatric, transfemoral, transtibial, and upper extremity amputees. Liners are also available without the distal umbrella for pin attachment and provide an interface between the socket and the limb.[10]

Suction/Vacuum Suspension. Suction is also a viable and desirable way to suspend a prosthesis. Suction creates an airtight socket through the use of an expulsion valve. At the distal end of the prosthesis, there is a valve through which the wearer pulls a thin sock, which pulls the residual limb completely into the socket, and then the valve cap is placed back into the opening to create a closed environment (Fig. 26-19). The top cap of the valve uses an expulsion valve that the amputee can press to release air that may get trapped inside the socket to regain optimal fit.

The use of a vacuum system within the socket provides multiple benefits to the amputee. Fluid fluctuation

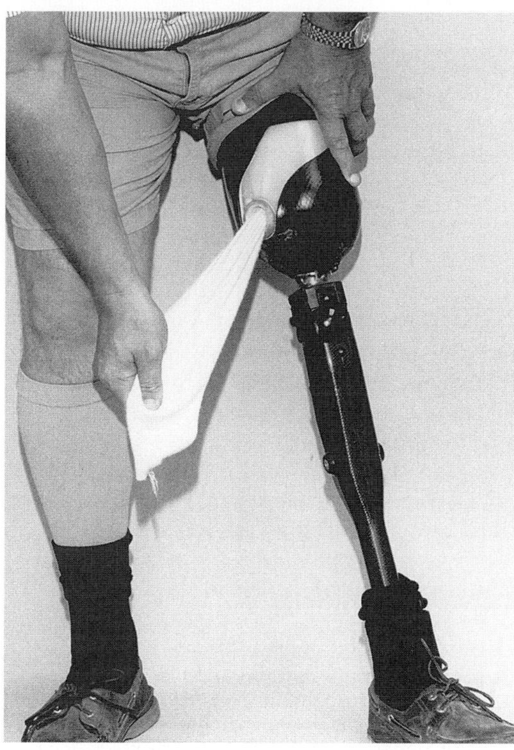

FIG 26-19 Patient donning a suction socket using a pull sock. The air expulsion valve has been removed so that the sock can be pulled completely out of the socket. *(From Lusardi MM, Nielsen CC, editors:* Orthotics and prosthetics in rehabilitation, *ed 2, St Louis, 2006, Butterworth-Heinemann.)*

throughout the course of the day is better managed, less pistoning occurs, and circulation is enhanced, contributing to a healthier residual limb. One of the main problems that amputees experience on a daily basis is the control of volume change within the socket during the length of the day. The more active the amputee, the more volume loss the individual experiences throughout the day. Traditionally, the way to control volume changes inside the socket is to add prosthetic socks as the residual limb volume decreases. If the amputee does not use sock management effectively, chaffing and pistoning become a problem and cause skin breakdown.

Important Concepts

By using a method of pulling air out of the socket, a more intimate fit is created, which offers multiple benefits.

Patella Straps. A patella strap can be added to a transtibial prosthesis to provide suspension above the femoral condyles, while still allowing full flexion and extension. This strap can be made out of leather or other strapping materials and secured with buckles or hook and loop closures.

Supracondylar suspension is obtained by the design of the socket. By creating a snug, intimate fit just superior to the femoral or humeral condyles, this design creates a suspension that is easy to use, maintains appropriate fit, and allows for full ROM.

BOX 26-2 Advantages and Disadvantages of Using a Harness

Advantages

- Harness generates enough power and excursion (length of movement) to open/close the terminal device
- Harness can be worn under clothing
- Ease of donning and doffing
- Easy to learn
- Patient gets immediate biofeedback when movement is elicited

Disadvantages

- Movements can be unnatural
- Harness may be cumbersome (may require a waist belt)
- Depending on level of amputation, a harness may not generate enough power and excursion. Nerve impingement syndrome can occur over time from the axilla pressure applied to the contralateral limb or both sides if the amputee is bilateral

Data from Uellendahl JE, Uellendahl EN: Body-powered upper-limb, prosthetic designs. In Carroll K, Edelstein JE, editors: *Prosthetics and patient management: a comprehensive clinical approach,* Thorofare, NJ, 2006, Slack.

Harnesses. For upper extremity prostheses, a harness is widely used for suspension. The harness not only suspends the prosthesis but also acts as a mechanism for control of the terminal device (TD) or hand for opening and closing the hand for grip (Fig. 26-20). The hand can be one of several types of hooks or a hand that has more cosmesis and looks like a real hand. By elevating or depressing the shoulder or scapular manipulations, the cables that connect to the hand are tightened, and this tension on the cable opens the hand. The harness also operates the elbow unit for transhumeral amputees. Separate cables, controls, and body movements are necessary to lock and unlock the elbow joint.

There are many designs for harnesses. The style desired is the most simple that will provide the amputee with the ability to control the TD. Harnessing uses the body's movements and transmits them to the cable portion of the harness and causes movement of the TD. The movements necessary for TD control are glenohumeral forward flexion, biscapular abduction, shoulder depression and elevation, and chest expansion. The correct harness can be chosen based on the level of amputation and the amputee's strength and ROM. Different motions can be used to control the TD or the elbow joint. Each movement must be mastered to use the prosthesis efficiently.[15] Advantages and disadvantages to using a harness are summarized in Box 26-2.

Important Concepts

Suspension of an upper extremity prosthesis can be a body harness or a suction or pin system.

Limb Design. One more technique used to suspend a prosthesis is a joint and corset. This type of suspension is usually reserved for transtibial amputees who also have knee conditions such as osteoarthritis, ligament or

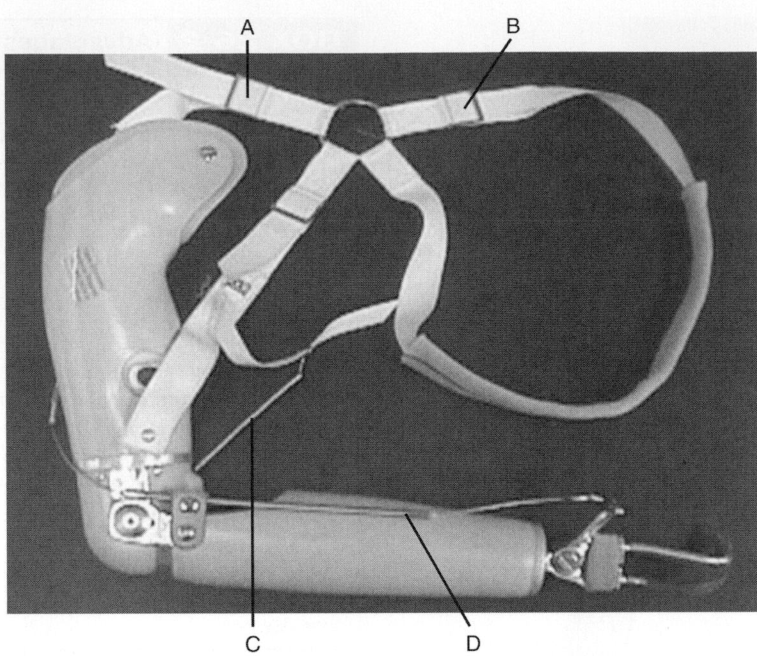

FIG 26-20 The figure-of-eight harness with posterior ring and cable control systems used in a conventional (body-powered) transhumeral prosthesis includes an anterior suspension loop *(A)*, the contralateral axillary loop *(B)*, a cable to control locking and unlocking of the elbow mechanism *(C)*, and a cable that will lift the forearm if the elbow unit is unlocked or operate the terminal device if the elbow unit is locked *(D)*. *(From Lusardi MM, Nielsen CC, editors:* Orthotics and prosthetics in rehabilitation, *ed 2, St Louis, 2006, Butterworth-Heinemann.)*

meniscal damage, or other instabilities on the amputated side. A pair of metal knee joints is incorporated into the socket, making sure to maintain the knee center alignment. The upper thigh portion, called the *corset,* is commonly fabricated from leather and is attached to the upper half of the knee joint encompassing the thigh. The corset portion is laced up because this technique provides suspension for the prosthesis as well as a functional knee brace. Another advantage of the corset is that it helps to unload the residual limb by transferring the weight of the prosthesis to the thigh portion of the limb, preventing further injury or degeneration of the involved knee.

Upper Extremity Prostheses

Body Powered Versus Myoelectric. The difference between an upper extremity **body powered prosthesis** and a **myoelectric prosthesis** is that the body powered prosthesis operates by the amputee moving a body part to elicit the movement of the TD. A myoelectric prosthesis is controlled by the ability to stimulate the antagonist and agonist muscle group. The electrodes seated within the socket wall directly receive the stimuli to produce movement. For example, if the amputee flexes the wrist extensor muscle group, that contraction will translate into opening the terminal device, or hand. This type of prosthesis does not require a harness for suspension or TD control. As with any device fitted to a patient, the patient must have the cognitive ability to use the device, the physical ability to operate the device, and clearly understood goals and limitations for use of the device.

The learning curve for using myoelectric components is greater than the learning curve for body powered components. Software packages are available that can be used during a physical therapy session to assist with learning control of the speed and the strength of the muscle contractions needed for different tasks, whether the desired motion is opening or closing the TD (hand) or rotating the wrist unit.

Prosthetic Shoulders. Shoulder joints do not have as many options as elbows and hands. Most shoulder components are friction controlled, allowing for movements of abduction, flexion, and extension of the humeral joint. The amount of friction can be changed depending on tasks and need. Some shoulder components also provide an extension stop with full humeral flexion.

Prosthetic Elbows. Body powered elbow components are controlled by friction or locking positions. The elbows with locking positions have 11 positions in which to place the elbow and can assist in lifting. The units that are friction controlled can be manually placed in desired flexion or extension. The elbows are available in adult or pediatric sizes (Fig. 26-21).

Myoelectric elbow units are also a consideration. One type is the DynamicArm, a myoelectric prosthetic elbow unit by Otto Bock. This unit lifts loads up to 13 pounds and offers a feature called Automated Forearm Balance (AFB). AFB stores energy when the arm is extended and reuses it for flexion, which results in a smooth, natural

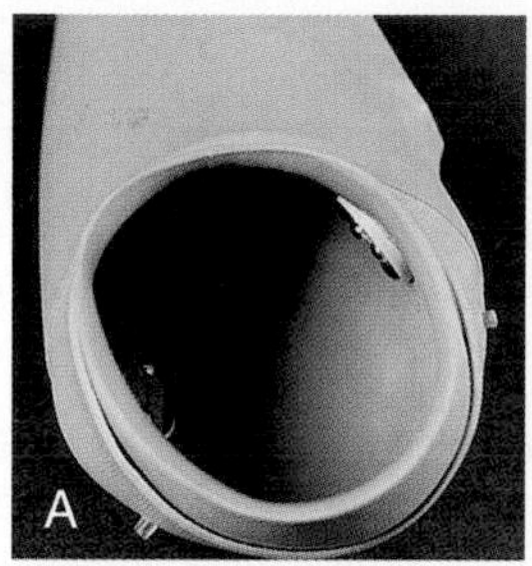
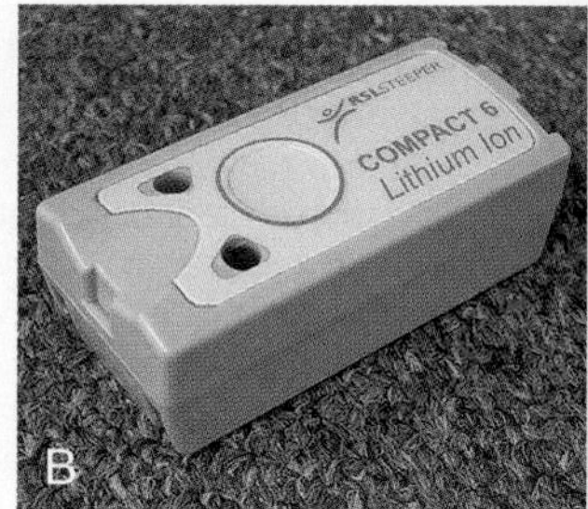

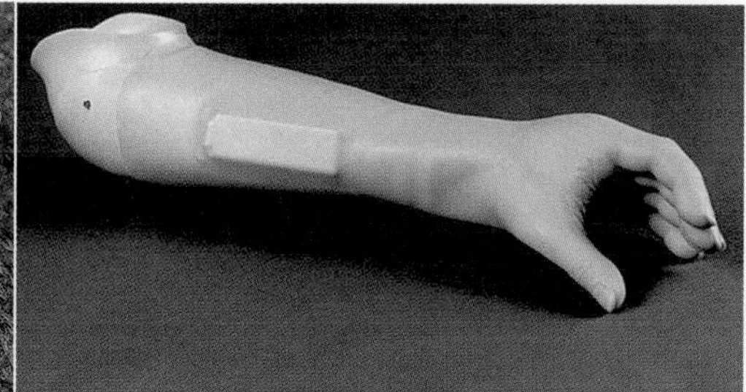
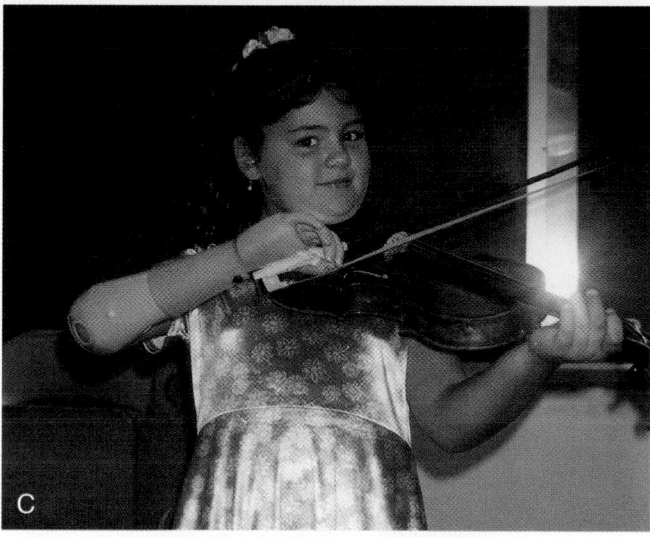

FIG 26-21 Myoelectric transradial prosthesis. **A,** Electrode placement within the socket. **B,** The battery pack is positioned in the forearm. **C,** Playing the violin with a myoelectric prosthesis. *(**A** and **B**, From Zenie J: Prosthetic options for persons with upper extremity amputation. In Lusardi MM, Nielsen CC, editors:* Orthotics and prosthetics in rehabilitation, *ed 2, St Louis, 2006, Butterworth-Heinemann; **C**, courtesy MH Mandelbaum Orthotic & Prosthetic Services.)*

swing during walking. The DynamicArm unlocks easily, even when under load. It can be positioned without having to send an unlocking signal, which enables the user to make fewer compensatory movements while providing a more natural appearance.[13]

Prosthetic Wrists. Wrist units provide a connection between the hand and the prosthetic forearm or socket. Some wrists can be manually twisted against a constant friction to allow for positioning of the hand. Other wrist units are myoelectric and a cocontraction of the agonist and antagonist muscle groups is required to control the wrist unit to achieve pronation or supination of the hand. Quick disconnect wrist units can be fabricated into the distal end of the socket for ease of changing out the prosthetic hand.

Prosthetic Hands. Prosthetic hands can be body powered or myoelectric. The hands can use a protective glove, which provides cosmesis. They are many sizes and designs. A passive hand has a gripping function that is opened by the sound hand and closes automatically. This type of hand is used by a wearer who possibly cannot cognitively understand how to operate a hand, is physically unable to operate a hand, or does not wish to learn how to use one and still has the need for body balance and symmetry. Voluntary opening and voluntary closing hands are controlled by a cable-activated prosthesis. The voluntary opening hand opens when the cable is pulled and closes under a spring tension. The voluntary closing hand uses the opposite technique.

There are two main types of TDs or hands offered: hooks and hands (Fig. 26-22). Both can be either body powered, where the hand is controlled by a cable system through a harness, or myoelectrically powered, where the hand is controlled by muscle stimulus received by sensors placed within the socket.

Hooks come in a variety of shapes and sizes to accommodate children and adults. The various shapes are offered to make different tasks easier to accomplish. Hooks can be body powered or myoelectric. The body powered hooks are opened by pulling the cable and closed automatically under spring or rubber band tension. Multiple rubber bands can be placed on the TD to increase the grip strength for different tasks. Hooks are also available for specific recreational tasks, such as designs for fishing, bowling, and wearing a baseball glove. Assistive TDs are also available that attach to the wrist unit. These TDs include saws, knives, gardening tools, spoons, and kitchen tools.

Mastectomy Products. Numerous options are available for patients after mastectomy. Prefabricated silicone breast

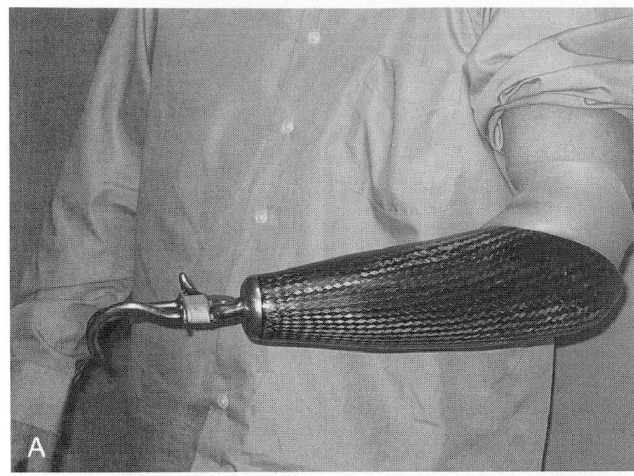

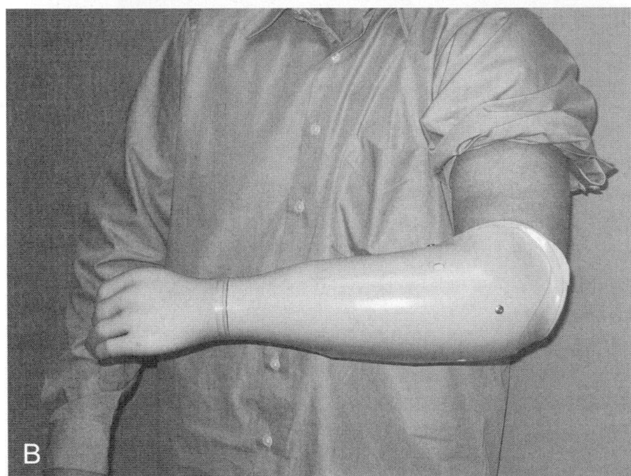

FIG 26-22 Two types of prosthetic hands. **A,** Hook. **B,** Hand.

forms range in size, shape, and color, and it is possible to fit most patients with a prefabricated breast form. When the heaviness of a silicone form is not desired, foam-filled forms are available, which are very lightweight but not as shapely. External garments or camisoles are also offered as an alternative to a bra, which is an especially nice offering for use during or after radiation because it fits loosely and does not rub against the already compromised skin tissue. Many mastectomy bras also are available in various sizes and colors. There are custom fabricated breast forms for patients who have difficulty with the prosthesis slipping inside the bra or chaffing the skin or who have more radical scar tissue or severe chest wall deformity. The chest wall must be casted or scanned for the fabrication of the form. The goal for mastectomy forms and products is to balance the body with weight distribution and cosmesis.

Lower Extremity Prostheses

Componentry Selection Guidelines. When selecting the appropriate foot or knee for each patient, there are set medical guidelines for levels of ambulation to direct the prosthetist's choice. Depending on the activity and ambulation abilities or potential of each amputee, the Medicare chart presented in Box 26-3 can be adhered to when selecting the foot or knee for each prosthesis. Careful consideration and evaluation for this potential to regain ambulatory ability is a crucial step in determining appropriate componentry. The PTA and the prosthetist can make optimal decisions as a team and create better outcomes for the patient.

BOX 26-3 Activity Guidelines K0 through K4

- K0 does not have the ability or potential to ambulate or transfer safely with or without assistance, and a prosthesis does not enhance quality of life or mobility.
- K1 has the ability or potential to use a prosthesis for transfers or ambulation on level surfaces at a fixed cadence. Typical of a limited household ambulatory individual.
- K2 has the ability or potential for ambulation with the ability to traverse low-level environmental barriers such as curbs, stairs, or uneven surfaces. Typical of a limited community ambulatory individual.
- K3 has the ability or potential for ambulation with variable cadence. Typical of a community ambulatory individual who has the ability to traverse most environmental barriers and may have vocational, therapeutic, or exercise activity that demands prosthetic use beyond simple locomotion.
- K4 has the ability or potential for prosthetic ambulation that exceeds basic ambulation skills, exhibiting high impact, stress, or energy levels, typical of the prosthetic demands of a child, active adult, or athlete.

From DMERC Medicare Advisory Bulletin. Columbia, SC, 1994, DMERC, pp 95–145.

An additional tool that can be used when evaluating the activity level of the amputee is the Amputee Mobility Predictor Questionnaire and the Amputee Mobility Predictor Testing Methodology.[8] These evaluation tools were developed by Robert Gailey, PhD, PT, and are widely used in the clinical setting to determine the functional level of each amputee. By gathering qualitative data, the PT, PTA, and prosthetist can have shared data to use while collaborating on treatment plans for patients.

Important Concepts

Amputee Mobility Predictor can be used to assess a patient's current and potential for ambulation.

Prosthetic Knees

Types of Knees. A prosthetic knee functions as a means of support and ambulation. Providing the proper combination of stability, shock absorption, and agility is the key to selecting and fitting the right knee to each patient.

Locking knee. A locking knee is inherently the most stable and safest knee. This knee has a manual switch or button that unlocks the knee and allows flexion for sitting. During ambulation, the knee remains locked throughout the gait cycle. This feature allows the amputee to ambulate and roll over the knee without fear of buckling, decreasing the percentage of falls. Because the knee does not bend during swing phase, hip hiking or circumduction may be used to propel the prosthesis.

Weight activated knee. A weight activated or stance control knee unit provides some limited locked knee moments and allows free swing during the swing phase of the gait. To lock the knee for a safe stance phase, the knee must reach full extension at heel strike. Most weight activated knees have a built-in angle of flexion of approximately 15° before breaking and releasing the knee for swing phase. As the amputee rolls over the foot and the knee begins to break, the knee releases the locked, safe position and flexes and then swings forward freely. This swing phase of the knee units is adjustable and can be set to meet each individual's cadence requirements. The use of hydraulics or pneumatics controls the rate of swing by increasing or decreasing the viscosity or pressure of fluids or air within the knee component.

Microprocessor knee. Today's technology provides control features that have not been offered until more recently. The use of computerized componentry to control swing and stance phase has provided transfemoral amputees with a new type of freedom. The C-Leg, Rheo Knee, Plié MPC Knee, and Smart Adaptive are examples of microprocessor knee components (Fig. 26-23). Each knee works on a slightly different mechanism of gait, but this freedom of cadence change without the fear of falling and less use of mental focus required by traditional knee units provides huge gains for transfemoral amputees.[12]

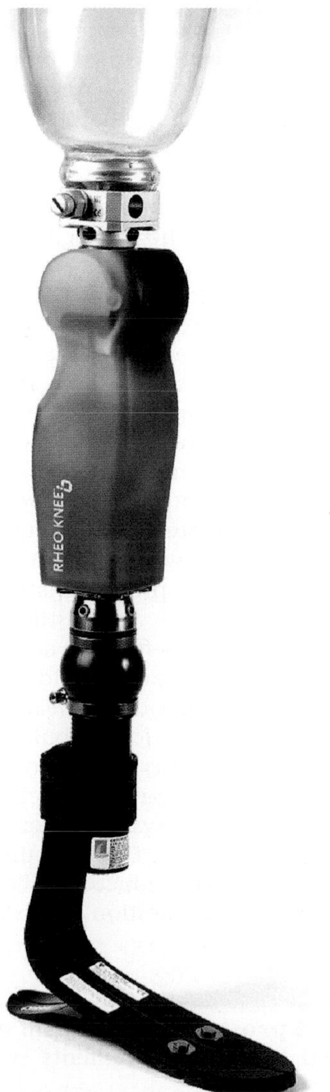

FIG 26-23 Microprocessor-controlled knee unit. *(Photo of Rheo Knee courtesy Össur, Aliso Viejo, CA.)*

Prosthetic Feet. Prosthetic feet types are best described by the function that each provides. There are three general types of prosthetic feet: solid ankle cushion heel (SACH), single-axis, and dynamic (Fig. 26-24).

The SACH foot does not allow any motion. This foot is most commonly used on a temporary prosthesis or for an amputee who will be using the prosthesis for transfers only. The SACH foot provides stability and shock absorption at heel strike.

The single-axis foot allows motion for dorsiflexion and plantar flexion. Single-axis feet use bumpers in the forefoot and hindfoot for shock absorption. These bumpers come in various durometers or stiffness to make the amount of cushion as customized as possible. Single-axis feet are fitted to transfemoral or transtibial amputees with low activity level who traverse uneven ground on a daily basis, traveling between their homes and their vehicles, but who are still relatively low-activity amputees.

The third type of prosthetic foot is the multiaxial, dynamic foot. This type of foot is most commonly selected because of the ability to mimic the complex ROM, rotation, stability, and shock absorption of the natural foot and ankle. Any lower extremity amputee can be fitted with this type of foot. It is usually selected for more active amputees, such as community ambulators and people who like to go hiking or walking for exercise or therapy. Dynamic feet allow motion in all directions and provide energy return to the amputee. As the heel of the foot strikes the ground and some form of compression is acquired at the heel and ankle portion of the foot, energy is retained in the material from which the foot keel is fabricated. As the amputee rolls over the midfoot and forefoot section, this stored energy is returned at toe off and acts springlike to help propel the amputee forward just as the sound limb foot and ankle complex functions. The goals for this type of foot are to restore normal ROM, function, and shock absorption. The Element Foot by Fillauer is a great example of a carbon, shock-absorbent, energy-returning foot (Fig. 26-25).

OTHER PROSTHETIC PRODUCTS

The replacement of body parts such as ears, noses, fingers, and toes falls within the realm of prosthetics. This process consists of making an impression of the existing ear or finger and duplicating it as closely as possible in size and color. These prostheses are functional and assist with tasks such as typing, hearing, and walking. The prosthesis can be suspended in a variety of manners depending on the available site for attachment. Adhesive glues and suction are often used for suspension. These prostheses are made of vinyl or silicone and are custom fabricated.

SUMMARY

This introduction to orthotics and prosthetics has provided a brief overview of products and indications for use of the orthotic or prosthetic componentry. There are many considerations involved with each patient, and

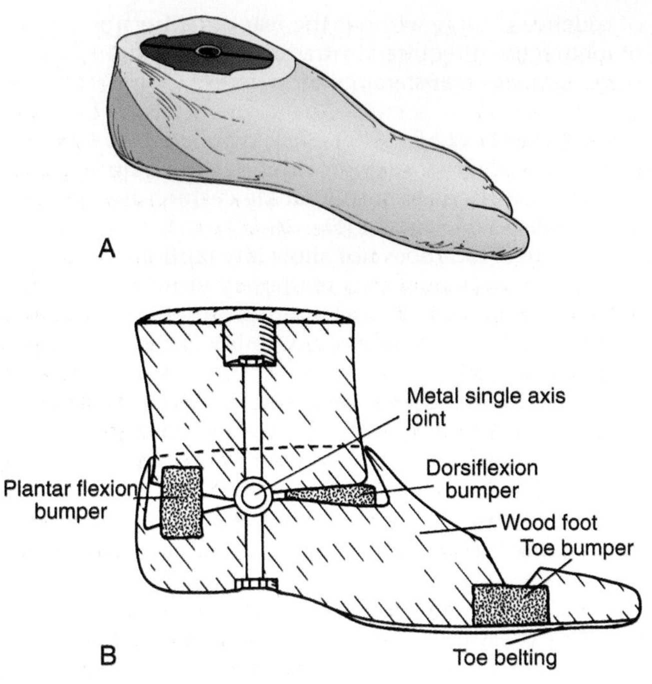

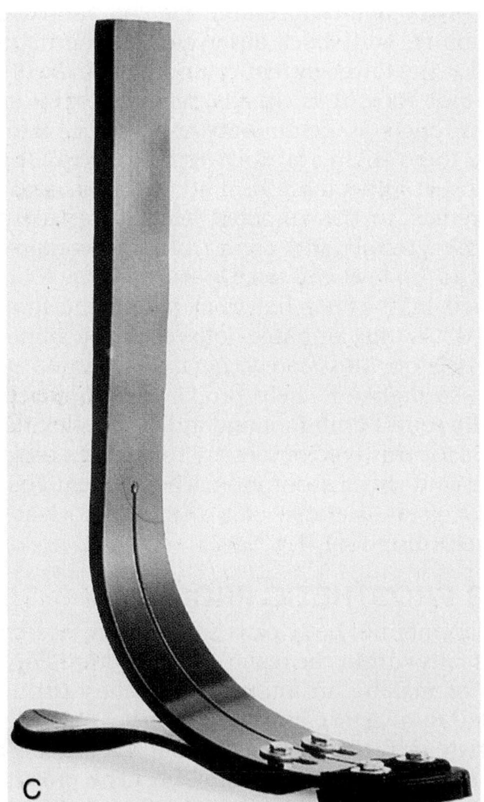

FIG 26-24 Types of prosthetic feet. **A,** Solid ankle cushion heel foot. **B,** Single-axis foot. **C,** Flex-foot. *(**A,** From Cameron MH, Monroe LG:* Physical rehabilitation: evidence-based examination, evaluation, and intervention, *St Louis, 2008, Saunders; **B,** from Fergason J: Prosthetic feet. In Lusardi MM, Nielsen CC, editors:* Orthotics and prosthetics in rehabilitation, *St Louis, 2000, Butterworth-Heinemann; **C,** photo courtesy Össur North America, Aliso Viejo, CA.)*

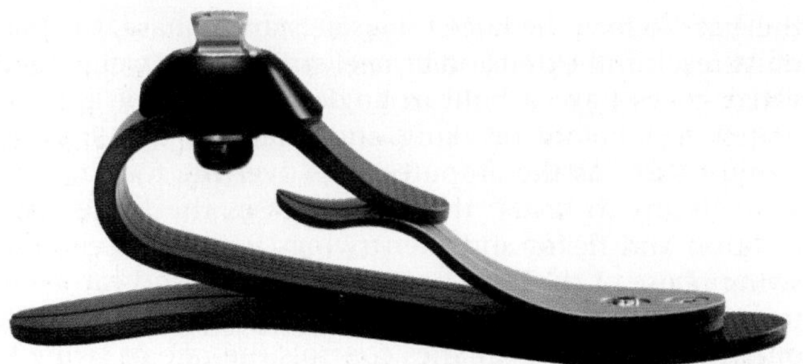

FIG 26-25 Fillauer Element foot. *(Courtesy of Fillauer© Companies, Inc., Chattanooga, TN.)*

familiarizing oneself can be time-consuming and ongoing throughout one's career. When fitting an orthosis, the main concerns are finding a proper fit, not compromising the patient's function, using as little orthotic support as required, and supporting only the joint or joints that are deficient in strength or ROM or have deformity. Prosthetic componentry for lower extremity amputees should be selected based on the patient's ability to ambulate using the Activity Guidelines chart to gauge the selection process (see Box 26-3). For upper extremity amputees, the choice can be decided based on ability to operate the TD and the patient's active ROM and strength. Physical therapy before receipt of a prosthesis is beginning to be discussed among professionals in the medical field. According to the American Geriatrics Society, which comprises more than 6800 health care professionals who are focused on the issues of the aging, more than 75% of all amputations are performed on persons older than 65 years. Approximately 90% of those amputations are lower limb, and approximately two thirds of lower limb amputations are transtibial. According to the Amputee Coalition of America, more than 65% of all amputations performed on people age 50 years and older are due to diabetes or peripheral vascular disease. What can help the patient to have a satisfying quality of life and achieve functional goals after amputation? "Approximately 75 percent of older adults can regain their ability to walk with or without assistive devices if they undergo the proper rehabilitation program before and after they receive … a prosthesis."[8] For optimal preparation of the patient before the amputation surgery, the physical therapy program should address strength, stamina, flexibility, and improved heart and lung function. Wearing a prosthesis for ambulation requires an increased level of energy consumption of about 60%. Providing a multidisciplinary team approach to each patient, including a PT, physician, physiatrist, counselor, and prosthetist, enables the patient to be better prepared mentally and physically and more educated about the process and the answer to the question of exactly what is a prosthesis.[5]

GLOSSARY

Body powered prosthesis: Movement of the prosthesis is controlled by body movements such as shoulder elevation or extension.

Brace: A term, now mostly used outside of a clinical setting, referring to a splint.

Componentry: The parts of a prosthesis or orthosis.

Doff: To remove a prosthesis or orthosis.

Don: To fasten a residual limb onto the body or apply an orthosis.

Footdrop: A condition in which the foot drops into a plantar flexed position as a result of nerve damage. This causes the leg to drag during gait secondary to a loss of function in the peroneal nerve. This loss of nerve function can be caused by conditions such as cerebrovascular accident, multiple sclerosis, spinal cord injury, or various neuropathies.

Liner: An interface that lies between the skin and the prosthetic socket. The liner acts as a cushion for shock absorbency and to protect against abrasions, shear forcing, and skin breakdown of the residual limb.

Myoelectric prosthesis: Small contractures of muscle stimulate electrodes placed inside the socket, and electrical impulses cause movement of the hand, wrist, or elbow.

Orthosis: A device that provides biomechanical and musculoskeletal support and correction of abnormalities within the human body.

Packing out: What happens to the material lining a prosthesis over time. Through general wear and tear during use of a device, the material compresses and eventually collapses.

Prosthesis: A device that replaces a body part, including arms, legs, partial feet, hands, ears, and breasts.

Sock management: The process of adding or removing a prosthetic sock to maintain the optimal fit of the socket as the amputee retains or loses fluid throughout the course of the day.

Socket: The custom fabricated portion of a prosthesis created from a mold of the patient's residual limb.

Splint: An orthosis that immobilizes a joint and allows only a specific range of motion as rehabilitation protocol requires.

REFERENCES

1. Allard USA: S.W.A.S.H. (website): www.allardusa.com. Accessed April 18, 2010.
2. Aspen Medical Products, Inc.: Aspen TLSO LumboSacral Bracing System (website): www.aspenmp.com. Accessed September 21, 2008.
3. Aspen Medical Products, Inc.: QuickDraw RAP LumboSacral Bracing (website): www.aspenmp.com. Accessed September 21, 2008.
4. Fairley M: Early prosthetic fitting—yes or no? *The O & P EDGE* 7(4):26–34, 2008.
5. Fairley M: Preprosthetic therapy: is it needed? Does it help? *The O & P EDGE* 7(10):34–40, 2008.
6. Fillauer Companies: Continuing the Climb, Chattanooga, TN, 2001, The Isocentric RGO (website): www.fillauer.com.
7. Fillauer Companies: Swing Phase Lock (SPL), Chattanooga, TN, 2004 (website): www.fillauer.com.
8. Gailey RS, Roach KE, Applegate EB, et al: The amputee mobility predictor: an instrument to assess determinants of the lower-limb amputee's ability to ambulate. *Arch Phys Med Rehabil* 83(5):613–627, 2002.
9. Lusardi MM: *Orthotics and prosthetics in rehabilitation*, ed 2, St Louis, 2008, Butterworth-Heinemann.
10. Ohio Willow Wood: Liners and suspension (online PDF): www.owwco.com/pdf/catalog/B/oww%20catalog%20sec%20B_006.pdf. Accessed April 18, 2010.
11. Otto Bock HealthCare: ABD LockSystem Hip Abduction Orthosis (website): www.ottobock.ca. Accessed September 21, 2008.
12. Otto Bock HealthCare: C-Leg Clinical and Technical Information (website): www.ottobockus.com. Accessed June 20, 2008.
13. Otto Bock HealthCare: DynamicArm 12K100 (website): www.ottobockus.com. Accessed October 26, 2008.
14. Otto Bock HealthCare: FreeWalk Stance Control System (website): www.ottobockus.com. Accessed May 13, 2008.
15. Uellendahl JE, Uellendahl EN: Body-powered upper-limb, prosthetic designs. In Carroll K, Edelstein JE, editors: *Prosthetics and patient management: a comprehensive clinical approach*, Thorofare, NJ, 2006, Slack.

REVIEW QUESTIONS

Multiple Choice

1. A device that replaces a body part is:
   a. A prosthesis.
   b. An orthosis.
   c. Both a and b
2. A device that supports a body part or joint is:
   a. A prosthesis.
   b. An orthosis.
   c. Both a and b
3. To properly stabilize a fracture the splint should be placed:
   a. Above the joint.
   b. Below the joint.
   c. Above and below the joint.
4. Spinal orthoses can be:
   a. Flexible.
   b. Rigid.
   c. A combination of both flexible and rigid materials.
5. Ankle foot orthoses can effectively treat:
   a. Sprains.
   b. Contractures.
   c. Both a and b
6. Materials for fabricating orthotics include:
   a. Polypropylene plastic.
   b. Pelite foam.
   c. Both a and b
7. A prosthetic knee can provide all of the following except:
   a. Knee extension.
   b. Shock absorption.
   c. Knee hyperextension.
8. Prosthetic components include all of the following except:
   a. Knee joints.
   b. Wrist splints.
   c. Feet.
9. Prosthetic hands have the ability to:
   a. Open.
   b. Close.
   c. Both a and b
10. A prosthetic wrist component can:
    a. Flex.
    b. Rotate.
    c. Both a and b
11. A WalkAide device will help achieve:
    a. Dorsiflexion.
    b. Plantar flexion.
    c. Both a and b

12. A carbon fiber anterior shell AFO can assist with:
    a. Energy return.
    b. Ankle stability.
    c. Both a and b
13. A reciprocating gait orthosis will benefit someone with:
    a. Paralysis.
    b. A fracture.
    c. Both a and b
14. A microprocessor knee will:
    a. Closely replicate normal gait pattern.
    b. Provide hypermobility of the knee joint.
    c. Be less stable.
15. Prosthetic feet are selected by taking into account a patient's:
    a. Activity level.
    b. Shoe size.
    c. Both a and b

Short Answer

16. Describe the difference between custom fitted and custom fabricated.
17. Describe how a SACH foot differs from a single axis foot.
18. Describe the differences in a body powered upper extremity prosthesis and a myoelectric prosthesis.
19. When splinting an injured joint, explain why you would or would not brace more than the injured joint.
20. List the different professions that should be involved in the multidisciplinary team approach for improved patient outcomes.

Fill in the Blank

21. A patient presents with weak quadriceps, knee buckling, and footdrop. The appropriate orthosis is a ________________.
22. A new amputee is being treated and is ready for a prosthesis. Appropriate team members include the physical therapist, prosthetist, counselor, physiatrist, and ________________.
23. A paraplegic patient expresses the desire to walk using orthotics. An appropriate selection to support hips, knees, ankles, and feet would be the ________________.
24. An ____________________ will support the ankle complex and the foot to properly assist with ambulation.
25. An ____________________________ orthosis is not custom-made.

True/False

26. Nomenclature for prostheses and orthoses is based on the person who invented the device.
27. Ears can be considered to be a prosthesis.
28. Custom arch supports should not be fitted unless there is a specific diagnosis of deformity.
29. Some KAFOs can provide free swing and a locked knee at full knee extension.
30. The younger the amputee, the less successful he or she will be.

Chapter 27

Musculoskeletal-Related Dysfunctions of the Pelvic Floor

Jennifer E. Celso

CHAPTER OUTLINE

LEARNING OBJECTIVES

1. Identify anatomic structures of the pelvis and pelvic floor, including bony structures that border the pelvic floor and ligamentous, muscular, and fascial components of the pelvic floor.
2. Describe the biomechanics of the pelvic floor.
3. Identify common pelvic floor dysfunctions.
4. Recognize reasons for medical referral for lumbopelvic pain or dysfunction.
5. Discuss clinical applications of physical therapy interventions for common pelvic floor dysfunctions.
6. Identify orthopedic conditions of the low back or hip in which pelvic floor dysfunction may be involved.

KEY TERMS

Abdominal pelvic dyssynergia
Anal incontinence
Anismus
Bladder sphincter dyssynergia
Chronic pelvic pain
Coccygodynia
Constipation
Cystocele
Cystourethrocele
Dyspareunia
Electromyographic biofeedback
Enterocele
Interstitial cystitis (IC)
Irritable bowel syndrome (IBS)
Kegel exercises
Levator ani syndrome
Nonrelaxing pelvic floor dysfunction
Nonrelaxing puborectalis
Pelvic floor dyssynergia
Piriformis syndrome
Proctalgia fugax
Pudendal neuralgia
Rectocele
Sacroiliac joint dysfunction
Sciatica
Urethral syndrome
Urethrocele
Urinary incontinence (UI)
Urinary retention
Uterovaginal/vaginal prolapse
Vaginismus
Vulvar vestibulitis
Vulvodynia

The pelvic floor commonly is forgotten when treating general orthopedic conditions. However, the pelvic floor is an integral part of the kinetic chain and system of movement. Whether the dysfunction is seen in the upper or lower extremities of a high-level athlete, the low back of a recently postpartum mother, or the hip of an inactive geriatric patient, the pelvic floor has an important stabilization function in performance of activities in all of these individuals. Without proper pelvic floor function, increased stress and strain are placed on other pieces of the kinetic chain, leading to possible overuse, injury, and pain. This chapter introduces the reader to normal pelvic floor function, pelvic floor dysfunctions, and pelvic floor strengthening exercises and emphasizes the importance of pelvic floor function in relationship to other orthopedic conditions of the spine, hip, sacrum, and pelvis. An anatomic review of the pelvic floor is provided to assist in understanding this relationship and in developing a specific home exercise program for patients exhibiting these dysfunctions.

ANATOMIC REVIEW

As shown in Figs. 27-1 through 27-5, the pelvic floor is bordered by the pubic symphysis and pubic rami anteriorly (Fig. 27-1), the ischial tuberosities (Fig. 27-2, *A*) and acetabulum laterally (Fig. 27-1), and the sacrum and coccyx posteriorly (Fig. 27-3). The bony pelvis is stabilized by ligamentous, muscular, and fascial support. The sacrum and pelvis are supported by the anterior longitudinal ligament (Fig. 27-1), iliolumbar ligament (Fig. 27-4), anterior sacroiliac ligament (Fig. 27-4, *A*), sacrotuberous ligaments (Figs. 27-1 and 27-5), sacrospinous ligaments (Figs. 27-3 and 27-5), anterior sacrococcygeal ligaments (Fig. 27-1), lateral sacrococcygeal ligaments (not shown), deep and superficial posterior sacrococcygeal ligaments (not shown), posterior sacroiliac ligaments (Fig. 27-3), and supraspinous ligaments (Fig. 27-1).

The pelvic floor consists of three layers of musculature commonly categorized into the urogenital triangle, deep urogenital triangle, and anal triangle as shown in Fig. 27-2, *B*. The urogenital triangle, the most superficial

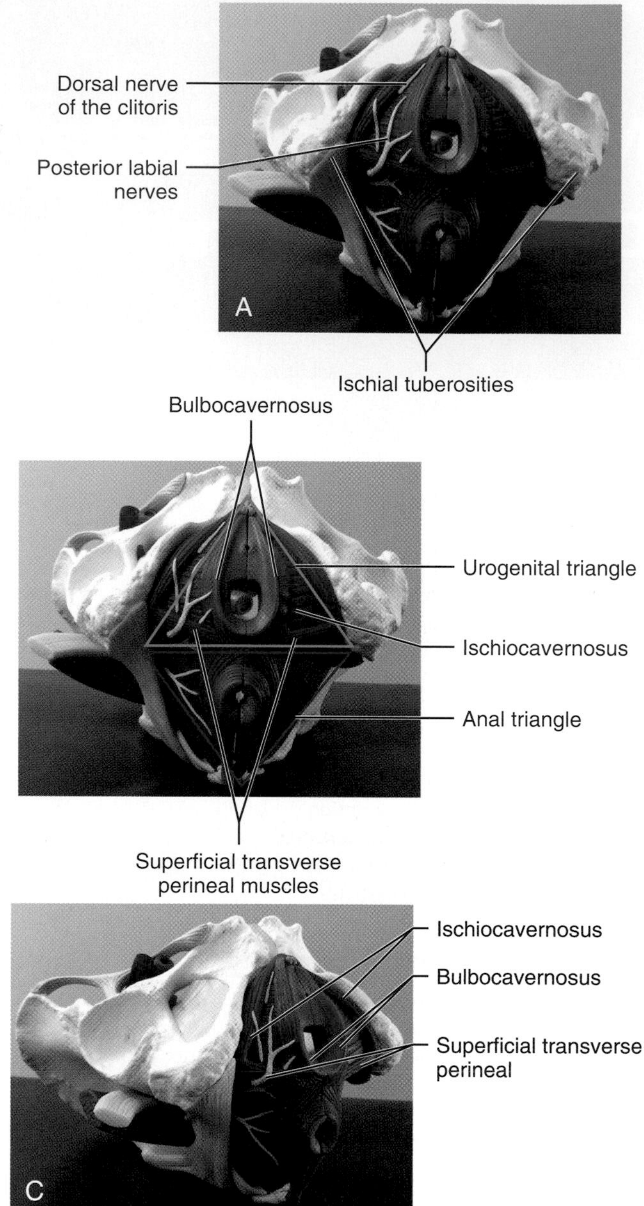

FIG 27-2 **A-C,** Inferior view of the pelvic floor.

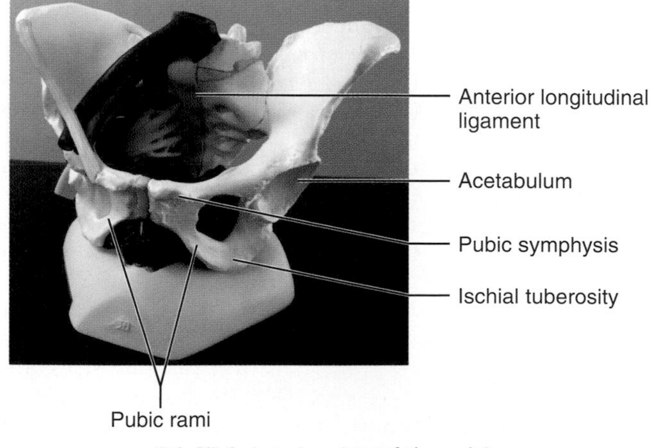

FIG 27-1 Anterior view of the pelvis.

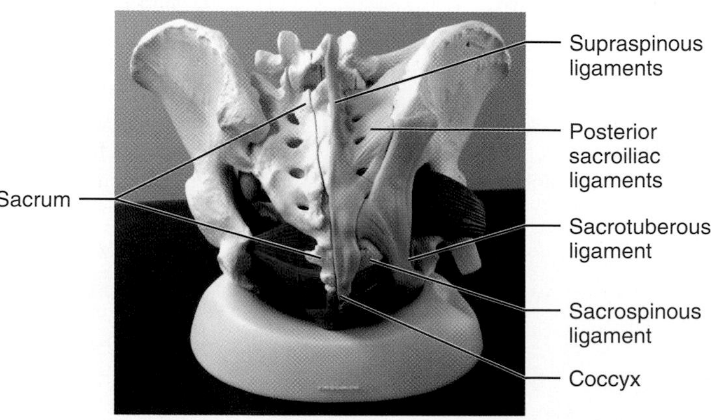

FIG 27-3 Posterior view of the pelvis and sacrum.

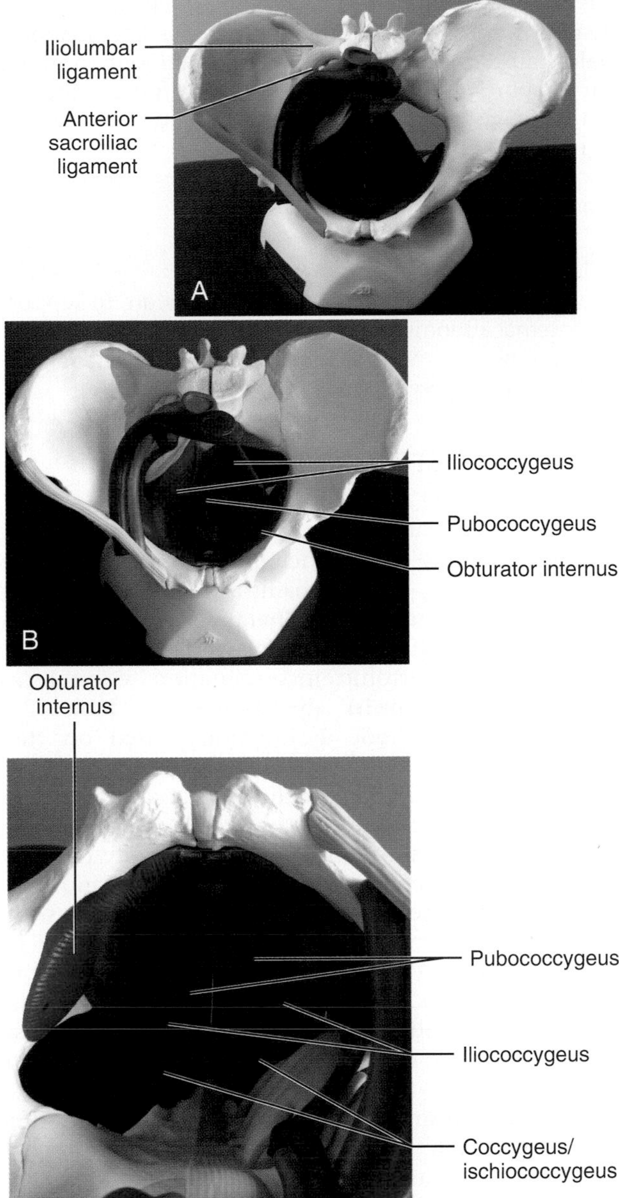

FIG 27-4 **A-C,** Superior view of the pelvic floor.

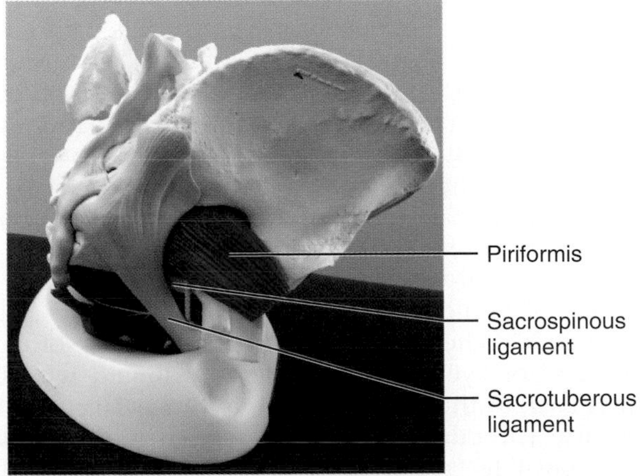

FIG 27-5 Lateral view of the sacral ligaments.

layer of musculature, consists of the bulbocavernosus (bulbospongiosus in males), ischiocavernosus, and superficial transverse perineal muscles (Fig. 27-2, *B* and *C*) as well as the superficial Colles' fascia, which is continuous with Scarpa's fascia of the abdomen. These muscles function together to maintain urinary continence and to aid in sexual appreciation. The deep urogenital triangle lies on the internal surface of the urogenital triangle and consists of the deep transverse perineal muscles, urethral sphincter, and inferior fascial layer. This layer of muscles accomplishes a sphincteric function for maintaining urinary continence. The deepest layer of muscles (the pelvic diaphragm) consists of the levator ani muscles (pubococcygeus and iliococcygeus), the coccygeus (also called the ischiococcygeus), and the piriformis and obturator internus muscles of the hip (Fig. 27-4, *B* and *C*). This muscle layer supports the bony pelvis and the abdominopelvic organs and provides stabilization for hip muscles.

Important Concept

The pelvic floor consists of three layers of muscle categorized into the urogenital triangle, the deep urogenital triangle, and the anal triangle. The urogenital triangle consists of the bulbocavernosus (bulobospongiosus in males), ischiocavernosus, and superficial transverse perineal muscles. The deep urogenital triangle consists of the deep transverse perineal muscles, urethral sphincter, and inferior fascial layer. The deepest layer of muscles (the pelvic diaphragm) consists of the levator ani muscles (pubococcygeus and iliococcygeus), the coccygeus (also called the ischiococcygeus), and the piriformis and obturator internus muscles of the hip.

The pelvic floor consists of two continuous layers of fascia (the parietal pelvic fascia and the visceral pelvic fascia, together referred to as the endopelvic fascia) that form the tendinous arch of the levator ani. The arcus tendineus attaches to the pubic bone ventrally and the ischial spine dorsally and serves as an attachment for portions of the levator ani muscles and the obturator internus muscle of each hip.[4]

Innervation of the pelvic floor is supplied by ventral sacral roots 2 through 5 via the levator ani and the pudendal nerves. The pudendal nerve originates from sacral roots 2 through 4, enters the pelvic floor anterior and inferior to the sacrospinous ligament just medial to the ischial spine, and courses through the gluteal region between the sacrospinous and sacrotuberous ligaments. The pudendal nerve travels along the obturator internus muscle as it enters the pudendal canal and splits into three branches: the inferior rectal nerve (Fig. 27-6), which supplies the external anal sphincter and perianal/gluteal skin; the perineal nerve (Fig. 27-6), which supplies the superficial transverse perineal bulbocavernosus in females or bulbospongiosus in males and ischiocavernosus muscles; and the dorsal nerve of the clitoris (Fig. 27-2, *A*) in females or the dorsal nerve of the penis in males.[73,74] The levator ani nerve originates from the ventral rami of sacral spinal

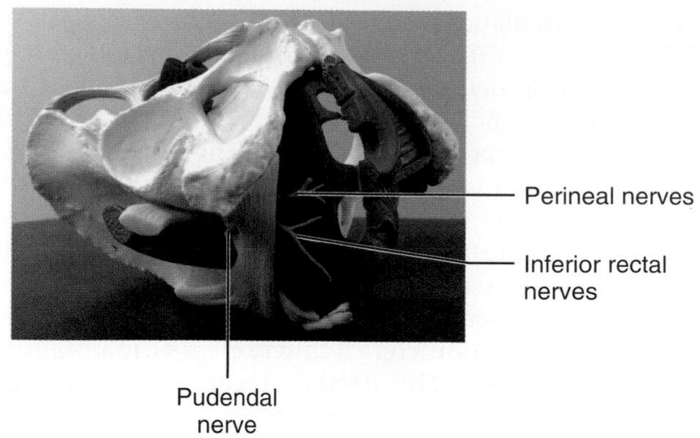

FIG 27-6 Inferolateral view of branches of the pudendal nerve.

roots 3 through 5 and supplies the iliococcygeus, pubococcygeus, and coccygeus muscles.[10]

Arterial supply to the pelvic floor originates from the common iliac arteries through the internal iliac artery via the umbilical, obturator, inferior vesical, middle rectal, vaginal, superior and inferior gluteal, iliolumbar, lateral sacral, and external and internal pudendal arteries as well as the internal pudendal and deep dorsal arteries of the penis or clitoris.[73] Venous drainage of the pelvis occurs through the internal iliac veins and their tributaries by combining with the external iliac vein, turning into the common iliac vein, which empties into the inferior vena cava.[73]

BIOMECHANICS OF THE PELVIC FLOOR

FUNCTIONS OF THE PELVIC FLOOR

The muscles, ligaments, and connective tissue of the pelvic floor create a three-dimensional arrangement.[4] The pelvic floor supports the internal abdominopelvic organs, maintains urinary and fecal continence, aids in sexual appreciation, and supports the bony pelvis. Structures such as the vaginal wall, the endopelvic fascia, the arcus tendineus fascia pelvis, and the levator ani muscles together provide most of the support to the abdominopelvic organs and especially the urethra.[4] Without such support, dysfunctions such as **urinary incontinence (UI)** and pelvic organ prolapse (POP) could occur. These and other dysfunctions are discussed later in this chapter. There is an intertwined relationship between the levator ani muscles and the endopelvic fascia. The endopelvic fascia may provide a source of stability and attachment for the levator ani; however, the levator ani muscles also protect the endopelvic fascia and pelvic ligaments from excessive loads.[5] In addition to support, the pelvic floor must allow flexibility for functions such as childbirth, urination, and defecation.[5] The levator ani has been shown to stretch up to 259% of its resting length to accommodate for vaginal delivery[62]; this equates to a 3.26 stretch ratio, whereas the maximum stretch ratio tolerated by striated muscle is only 1.5.[5]

A combination of phasic and tonic fibers makes up the pelvic floor musculature. Tonic slow-twitch fibers comprise approximately 70% of the muscle fibers, whereas 30% are made up of phasic fast-twitch fibers.[71] The constant strain put on the pelvic fascia and ligaments would cause these structures to stretch out, and lose their supportive effectiveness, if it were not for the constant tonic contractions of the levator ani.[76] The importance of this fibrous makeup also comes into play when prescribing pelvic floor exercises for strengthening purposes.

Important Concept

The four main functions of the pelvic floor are to support the internal abdominopelvic organs, maintain urinary and fecal continence, support the bony pelvis, and aid in sexual appreciation.

COMMON DYSFUNCTIONS OF THE PELVIC FLOOR

The pelvic floor musculature may become dysfunctional secondary to many causes, including, but not limited to, childbirth, surgery, trauma, pain, and skeletal malalignments. The American Physical Therapy Association Section on Women's Health categorizes pelvic floor dysfunctions as supportive, hypertonic, incoordination, visceral, and **chronic pelvic pain** dysfunctions.[101] Table 27-1 summarizes pelvic floor dysfunctions based on these categories.

Supportive dysfunctions include UI and anal incontinence, POP, pelvic muscle weakness, disuse atrophy, and neurologic dysfunctions; pelvic pain, dyspareunia, constipation, dysmenorrhea, voiding difficulty, and pelvic tension myalgia are categorized by hypertonic dysfunctions. Incoordination dysfunctions include urinary frequency and urgency and paradoxical pelvic floor. Chronic pelvic pain, or pain lasting longer than 6 months and not relieved by medication or other measures, can be caused by the above-mentioned dysfunctions. **Irritable bowel syndrome (IBS)**, fibroids, endometriosis, urinary tract infection, and dysmenorrhea represent visceral dysfunctions of the pelvic floor, but these are not addressed in detail in this chapter.

Screening for Medical Referral for Lumbopelvic Pain or Dysfunction

Medical screening should always be considered for pain that occurs in the lumbopelvic regions. This pain could be related to gynecologic, gastrointestinal, or urologic causes.[39] Although the physical therapist (PT) should screen for this during a patient's initial examination, the physical therapist assistant (PTA) must be aware of these potential medical causes of musculoskeletal pain/dysfunction and alert the PT of any noticed concerns during treatment sessions.

It is important when screening for medical referral to be aware of "yellow flags" (cautionary) and "red flags" (warning).[38,39] When a patient presents with three or more "red flags" or "yellow flags," the PTA should refer the patient back to the PT to determine if medical referral is necessary. The purpose of this section is to inform the PTA of possible "red flags" associated with pain in the sacral region that may or may not be related to the pelvic

TABLE 27-1 Categories of Pelvic Floor Dysfunction

Supportive Dysfunctions	Hypertonic Dysfunctions	Incoordination Dysfunctions	Visceral Dysfunctions	Chronic Pelvic Pain Syndromes
Incontinence (urinary/fecal)	Muscle dysfunctions (levator ani syndrome, vaginismus, anismus)	Abdominal pelvic dyssynergia	Urologic (detrusor instability, interstitial cystitis, urethral syndrome)	Urologic (interstitial cystitis)
Pelvic organ prolapse (cystocele, urethrocele, rectocele)	Joint dysfunctions (coccygodynia, pelvic asymmetry)	Habitual use of accessory muscles	Gynecologic (endometriosis, dysmenorrhea/ PMS, PID)	Gynecologic (endometriosis, PID, vulvar disorders such as vulvodynia, vulvar vestibulitis)
Musculoskeletal dysfunctions (ligamentous laxity, pelvic floor muscle weakness, disuse atrophy)	Connective tissue dysfunctions (scar adhesions, trigger points)	Bladder sphincter dyssynergia	Colorectal (IBS)	Colorectal (IBS, constipation)
Neurologic dysfunctions (MS, diabetes, Parkinson's disease, stroke)	Neurologic dysfunctions (upper motor neuron lesions)	Nonrelaxing puborectalis		

IBS, irritable bowel syndrome; *MS,* multiple sclerosis; *PID,* pelvic inflammatory disease; *PMS,* premenstrual syndrome.
From Wilder E (ed): The gynecological manual, ed 2, Alexandria, VA, 2002, APTA, Section on Women's Health, p. 67.

floor or be visceral in nature (Table 27-2). According to Goodman and Snyder,[39] the most typical systemic diseases that refer pain to the sacrum and sacroiliac joint include endocarditis, prostate or reproductive cancers, gynecologic disorders such as endometriosis or pelvic inflammatory disease, and disorders of the large intestine (e.g., ulcerative colitis, Crohn's disease, colon cancer, or IBS). If the PTA suspects a cluster of the above-mentioned "red flags" are present in a patient combined with a lack of expected progress in response to interventions provided, it is imperative to communicate these concerns to the supervising PT.

Supportive Dysfunctions

Urinary Incontinence and Anal Incontinence. UI, defined by the International Continence Society as any involuntary loss of urine, can be categorized further according to patient symptoms as urgency urinary incontinence (urge incontinence), stress urinary incontinence (SUI), mixed urinary incontinence, nocturnal enuresis, postmicturition dribble, and continuous urinary leakage.[1] **Anal incontinence** is defined by the International Continence Society as any involuntary loss of fecal material or flatus.[1] The prevalence of UI in the literature depends significantly on the type of UI studied and the age range of the study. A study of SUI of women 31 to 54 years old showed a prevalence of 39.4%.[103] Another study including women 20 years old and older showed a much lower prevalence of nearly 15%.[68] A review of 36 studies in the general population found that most studies reported a prevalence of any form of UI in the range of 25% to 45%.[72] Urinary continence is maintained when sphincteric pressure around the urethra exceeds that of the contracting detrusor muscle of the bladder and intraabdominal pressure. The pelvic floor muscles have a key role in maintaining that sphincteric pressure around the urethra. In the presence of pelvic floor dysfunction, continence can be compromised. Table 27-3 summarizes the various types of incontinence.

Pelvic Organ Prolapse. Chen and Ng[23] defined POP as an anatomic support deficit of the pelvic viscera that may result from a series of long-term failures of the supporting and suspension mechanisms of the uterus and vaginal wall. Although prevalence rates vary, POP has been shown to affect approximately 50% of women 20 to 60 years old.[7] The incidence of POP increases significantly with age, with 20% incidence seen in women 20 to 29 years old, 50% seen in women 30 to 39 years old, 77% seen in women 40 to 49 years old, and 75% seen in women 50 to 59 years old. POP also increases significantly with childbirth as follows: 3.6% in nulliparous, 6.5% in primiparous, 23% in secundiparous, 33% in tertiparous, and 47% in quadriparous women.[7] POP accounts for 17% to 20% of all major gynecologic surgical procedures.[7] Risk factors for POP include increased body mass index, history of fetal macrosomia or miscarriages, menopause, previous gynecologic surgical operations, and a history of metabolic disorders including diabetes mellitus.[7]

The American Urogynecologic Society developed the Pelvic Organ Prolapse Quantification classification system to determine the level of severity of POP through a staging method.[78] Table 27-4 defines the stages of POP severity. Persu and colleagues[78] also described the common classifications of POP as defined by the viscera involved or the anatomic structure affected. Table 27-5 describes POP as defined by the viscera involved compared with classifying POP by the anatomic vaginal wall affected by the prolapse. The latter system uses terms such as *anterior vaginal wall prolapse* to describe **cystoceles** and **urethroceles;** *apical vaginal wall prolapse* to describe **enteroceles,** uterine prolapse, or uterovaginal/vaginal vault prolapses; and *posterior vaginal wall prolapse* to describe **rectoceles.** This system is often preferred because of the uncertainty

TABLE 27-2 "Red Flags" and Differential Diagnosis

"Red Flags"	Associated with Back Pain of Systemic Origin	Associated with Sacroiliac/ Sacral Pain or Symptoms	Associated with Pelvic Pain or Symptoms
History	• <20 years old or >50 years old • Previous history of cancer • History of falls or trauma (screen for fracture, osteoporosis, domestic violence, alcohol use)	• Sacroiliac/sacral pain without history of trauma or overuse (rule out assault, anal intercourse) • Previous history of cancer • Previous history of gastrointestinal disease (ulcerative colitis, Crohn's disease, irritable bowel syndrome)	• History of reproductive, colon, or breast cancer • History of dysmenorrhea, ovarian cysts, pelvic inflammatory disease, sexually transmitted disease • Endometriosis • Chronic bladder or urinary tract infections • History of bladder or pelvic surgeries, especially hysterectomy • Recent abortion or miscarriage • History of assault, incest, or trauma • History of prolonged labor; use of forceps or vacuum extraction during delivery • History of multiple births • Chronic yeast/vaginal infections • History of varicose veins in lower extremities
Risk factors	• Recent urinary tract infection • History of injection drug use • Immunocompromised condition	• Osteoporosis • Sexually transmitted infection/disease • Long-term use of antibiotics (e.g., for colitis)	• Recent intrauterine contraceptive device (rejection) or long-term use, especially without medical follow-up (scar tissue) • Perimenopause, menopause (vaginitis) • Sexual activity without use of condom • Multiple sexual partners • Childbirth, recent abortion, multiple abortions
Clinical presentation	• Failure to improve with conservative care (>4-6 weeks) • Pain not relieved by rest or recumbency • Severe, constant nighttime pain • Back pain accompanied by abdominal, pelvic, or hip pain • Significant morning stiffness with limitation in spinal movement	• Lack of objective findings for sacroiliac/sacral pain • Anterior pelvic, suprapubic, or low abdominal pain at same level as the sacrum	• Poorly localized, diffuse; client unable to point to one spot • Aggravated by increased intraabdominal pressure • Pelvic pain is not affected by specific movements but gets worse toward end of day or after standing for prolonged period • May be temporarily relieved by position change (getting off feet, resting or elevating the legs) • Pelvic pain is not reduced or eliminated by scar or soft tissue mobilization or by trigger point release of myofascial structures in the pelvic cavity • Positive McBurney's, Blumberg's, or iliopsoas/obturator sign
Associated signs and symptoms	• Constitutional symptoms (fever, chills, unexplained weight loss) • Progressive, neurologic deficit; saddle anesthesia • Skin rash	• Pain relieved by passing gas or having a bowel movement • Presence of gastrointestinal, gynecologic, or urologic signs and symptoms	• Vaginal or penile discharge • Urologic signs or symptoms • Unreported abdominal pain • Dyspareunia • Constitutional symptoms • Missed menses or unexplained/ unexpected spotting of blood (possible ectopic pregnancy)—ask about shoulder pain • Headache, fatigue, irritability

From Goodman CC, Snyder TE: *Differential diagnosis for physical therapists: screening for referral*, ed 4, St Louis, 2007, Saunders.

TABLE 27-3 Types of Incontinence

Type	Definition
Urgency urinary incontinence	Involuntary leakage accompanied by or immediately preceded by urgency
Stress urinary incontinence	Involuntary leakage on effort or exertion or on sneezing or coughing
Mixed urinary incontinence	Involuntary leakage associated with urgency and with effort, exertion, sneezing, and coughing
Nocturnal enuresis	Any involuntary loss of urine occurring during sleep
Postmicturition dribble	Involuntary loss of urine immediately after passing urine, usually after leaving the toilet in men or after rising from the toilet in women
Continuous incontinence	Continuous leakage
Fecal incontinence	Any involuntary loss of fecal material
Flatus incontinence	Any involuntary loss of gas (flatus)

TABLE 27-4 Stages of Pelvic Organ Prolapse

Stage	Definition
0	No prolapse
1	Most distal portion of prolapse is >1 cm above the level of the hymen
2	Most distal portion of prolapse is ≤1 cm proximal or distal to the hymenal plane
3	Most distal portion of prolapse protrudes >1 cm below the hymen but no farther than 2 cm less than the total vaginal length
4	Vaginal eversion is essentially complete

Adapted from Persu C, Chapple CR, Chauni V, et al: Pelvic organ prolapse quantification system (POP-Q)—a new era in pelvic organ prolapse staging. *J Med Life* 4(1):75-81, 2011.

TABLE 27-5 Types of Pelvic Organ Prolapse

Type of Prolapse	Definition
Urethrocele	Prolapse of lower anterior vaginal wall involving the urethra only
Cystocele	Prolapse of upper anterior vaginal wall involving the bladder
Cystourethrocele	Prolapse of upper and lower anterior vaginal wall involving the urethra and bladder
Uterovaginal prolapse	Prolapse of uterus, cervix, and upper vagina
Enterocele	Prolapse of upper posterior wall of the vagina usually containing loops of small bowel
Rectocele	Prolapse of lower posterior wall of the vagina involving the rectum

Adapted from Persu C, Chapple CR, Chauni V, et al: Pelvic organ prolapse quantification system (POP-Q)—a new era in pelvic organ prolapse staging. *J Med Life* 4(1):75-81, 2011.

of what visceral structure is actually causing the specific prolapse to occur. Abrams and associates[1] described commonly reported symptoms of POP based on the International Continence Society as a feeling of a bulge at the vaginal opening, LBP, pelvic heaviness, a dragging sensation, or a need to replace the prolapse digitally to allow for defecation or urination.

Hypertonic Dysfunctions

Hypertonic dysfunctions occur when the pelvic floor muscles are in a state of increased tension or prolonged state of contraction with the inability to relax. When this condition occurs, the urethral meatus, the vaginal introitus, and the anus are forced closed and demonstrate difficulty relaxing for normal functional opening to allow for urination, intercourse, tampon or speculum insertion of the vagina, or defecation functions. Wallace describes in Wilder's manual,[101] common primary presentations of patients with hypertonus as a pain, pressure, or ache (that is usually poorly localized) in the perivaginal and perirectal regions, lower abdominal quadrants, and pelvis (suprapubic or coccyx or both) and sometimes down the posterior thigh. *The Gynecological Manual* published by the American Physical Therapy Association Section on Women's Health summarizes common terminology associated with hypertonic dysfunction of the pelvic floor.[101]

The term ***nonrelaxing pelvic floor dysfunction*** encompasses many of the hypertonic pelvic floor conditions that involve a specific muscle or specific dysfunction, including the following. **Levator ani syndrome** refers to a spasm of the levator ani muscles that can cause pain in the buttock, posterior thigh, coccyx, hip, or low back. **Nonrelaxing puborectalis** also may be referred to as *puborectalis syndrome* or *paradoxical puborectalis contraction* and causes bowel movement dysfunction or constipation or both. **Anismus** is a muscle spasm of the anal sphincter that causes rectal/anal pain that restricts the anal opening. **Proctalgia fugax** is a muscle spasm of the anal sphincter that causes sharp fleeting rectal pain that can last seconds to 20 to 30 minutes and can occur during the day but occurs frequently in the middle of the night.[53]

Hypertonic pelvic floor muscles can also cause pain and tenderness that is noticed usually in sitting but that does not increase with defecation in a condition known as **coccygodynia** (pain of the coccyx) as well as **urethral syndrome,** which can cause urinary urgency and frequency; suprapubic pelvic or perineal pressure; and urethral pain, burning, and sensitivity. This syndrome occurs in the absence of infection and causes pain after voiding.[54] If the hypertonic pelvic floor muscle entraps the pudendal nerve, a condition called ***pudendal neuralgia*** may develop, and the patient may complain of constant unprovoked localized burning, itching, or a sensation of dryness that can be unilateral.[44,45]

Other manifestations of hypertonicity in the pelvic floor muscles include voiding dysfunctions such as **urinary retention** (inability to void urine because of muscle spasms around the urethra) and **constipation.** Constipation is defined by the Rome Foundation Rome III Diagnostic Criteria for Functional Gastrointestinal Disorders[63] as having at least two of the following symptoms for at least 3 months with symptom onset at least 6 months before diagnosis:

1. Straining during at least 25% of defecations
2. Lumpy or hard stools in at least 25% of defecations
3. Sensation of incomplete evacuation for at least 25% of defecations
4. Sensation of anorectal obstruction/blockage for at least 25% of defecations
5. Manual maneuvers to facilitate at least 25% of defecations (e.g., digital evacuation, support of the pelvic floor)
6. Fewer than three defecations per week

Prevalence rates of constipation are between 2.6% and 26.9% of adults (≥15 years old) and between 3% and 5% of children (<15 years old).[22,29,88] Although constipation can occur because of poor fiber intake, medication side effects, or other pathologic disorders of the body, pelvic floor muscle hypertonus in the form of anismus can also cause constipation by resisting defecation at the anal sphincter.[98]

Dyspareunia is pain before, during, or after intercourse.[70] There are many causes for dyspareunia; however, most causes are directly or indirectly related to hypertonus of the pelvic floor. According to Steege and colleagues,[93] **vaginismus** is a common cause of dyspareunia secondary to the involuntary contraction and spasm of the bulbocavernosus muscle, making vaginal penetration difficult, painful, or impossible. Pain with vaginal penetration could also occur with the attempt to insert tampons during menses or insertion of a speculum for gynecologic examination. Dyspareunia can be described further as *deep dyspareunia,* which describes pain with deep vaginal penetration, and *entry dyspareunia,* which refers to pain with initial penetration of the vaginal introitus.[51] Dyspareunia can also occur secondary to chronic vulvar pain syndromes such as **vulvodynia** and **vulvar vestibulitis,** which are discussed later in the section on chronic pelvic pain. The World Health Organization looked at 54 studies in a systematic review of pelvic pain and determined that 31 of the studies showed the prevalence of dyspareunia in greater than 35,000 women to be 45.7%.[59]

Incoordination Dysfunctions

Another type of pelvic floor dysfunction involves the inability of the patient to coordinate the necessary muscles of the abdominal wall and the pelvic floor to urinate or defecate. This can be described as **abdominal pelvic dyssynergia**, **bladder sphincter dyssynergia** (also referred to as *detrusor sphincter dyssynergia*), or **pelvic floor dyssynergia**.[9,81,82] For example, during defecation, the abdominal wall muscles must contract while the pelvic floor muscles simultaneously relax. If the opposite action occurs, defecation cannot occur because of the closure around the anus. Similarly, urination occurs when the detrusor muscle contracts and the urethral sphincters and pelvic floor muscles relax; however, when there is incoordination of this reciprocal pattern, urination cannot occur.[79]

Chronic Pelvic Pain

Chronic pelvic pain is defined by the International Pain Society as pain in the lower abdomen, vvulva/vagina, perineum, anus, or coccyx that lasts longer than 6 months. Chronic pelvic pain disorders are considered to be as prevalent as asthma and back pain affecting approximately 39 per 1000 women who see primary care physicians for their discomfort.[106] It has also been reported that primary care physicians do not feel comfortable with the diagnoses and that there is an educational need for general practitioners regarding chronic pelvic pain syndromes.[67]

Conditions considered as chronic may also be categorized as viscerally related pelvic floor disorders because they may involve various abdominopelvic organs, such as the uterus, ovaries, colon, rectum, and bladder. Chronic pelvic pain conditions include, but are not limited to, the **interstitial cystitis (IC)**, vulvodynia, vulvar vestibulitis, and IBS.

IC (also referred to as *painful bladder syndrome*) is defined by the Interstitial Cystitis Association as a bladder condition that usually consists of multiple symptoms. Most patients with IC have recurring pelvic pain, pressure, or discomfort in the bladder and pelvic region and urinary frequency (up to 60 voiding episodes per day in severe cases) and urgency. IC is diagnosed based on the presence of pain related to the bladder that is usually accompanied by urinary urgency and frequency as long as other bladder conditions causing these symptoms have been ruled out. More difficult cases of IC may require a cystoscopy with hydrodistention for diagnosis. There are two types of IC, ulcerative (approximately 5% to 10% of patients) and nonulcerative (approximately 90% of patients).[50] Patients with nonulcerative IC exhibit pinpoint hemorrhages, also called glomerulations, in the wall of the bladder, whereas patients with ulcerative IC present with Hunner's ulcers (patches of red, bleeding areas on the bladder wall). In March 2011, the American Urological Association released clinical guidelines for the diagnosis and treatment of IC, including patient behavioral/dietary restrictions, medications, surgical options, and physical therapy to treat any related pelvic floor dysfunction.[50]

Vulvar pain syndromes such as vulvodynia and vulvar vestibulitis cause the patient significant irritation and discomfort in the vulva. Such discomforts may include itching, burning, and a rawlike sensation that can cause dyspareunia and other functional limitations related to the inability to wear tight-fitting clothing or discomfort with walking or exercise such as bicycling or horseback riding (activities in which there is direct contact or pressure on the perineum).

IBS is diagnosed based on the Rome III Diagnostic Criteria for Functional Gastrointestinal Disorders as follows: recurrent abdominal pain or discomfort at least 3 days/month in the last 3 months associated with two or more of the following:[63]

1. Improvement with defecation
2. Onset associated with a change in frequency of stool
3. Onset associated with a change in form (appearance) of stool

Worldwide prevalence of IBS ranges from 11% to 20%. IBS affects women more than men and is more common in individuals younger than age 50.[60]

Important Concept

The main categories of pelvic floor dysfunction are supportive, hypertonic, incoordination, visceral, and chronic pelvic pain.

INTERVENTIONS FOR PELVIC FLOOR DYSFUNCTION

Physical therapy for pelvic floor disorders has been proven effective for many years.[21,55,56,58] Conservative interventions for the above-mentioned dysfunctions consist of therapeutic exercises (pelvic floor exercises), biofeedback in its many forms, electrical stimulation, and forms of manual therapy. Although pelvic floor exercises have been shown to be the most effective conservative intervention for conditions such as UI, a combination of the above-mentioned interventions benefits many individuals with pelvic floor dysfunction.[17,20,31,34,46,58]

THERAPEUTIC EXERCISE PRESCRIPTION

To determine the appropriate therapeutic exercise prescription for a patient with pelvic floor dysfunction, the PTA should consider whether to up-train versus down-train the pelvic floor muscles. In supportive dysfunctions, up-training (strengthening) should be considered. Caution should be used with hypertonic dysfunctions, and down-training (teaching relaxation) of the pelvic floor muscles may be more appropriate.

It is well documented in several systematic reviews that pelvic floor exercises are beneficial for pelvic floor dysfunctions such as UI in women and men.[17,20,31] Kegel first studied pelvic floor exercises/contractions in 1948 and found benefits in patients with UI if the patients performed the pelvic floor contraction exercises (**Kegel exercises**) correctly and consistently. He originally recommended 300 to 500 repetitions per day for full benefit. However, in 1996, the Agency for Health Care Policy and Research assessed the research and found that between 30 and 80 repetitions per day for at least 8 weeks, but maybe indefinitely, is sufficient for pelvic floor strengthening to prevent UI.[33] However, it is important to determine the appropriate number and type of pelvic floor exercises to prescribe to patients because of the varied muscle fiber composition. Many patients initially report "I've tried those and they don't work!" In reality, the exercises would work if properly prescribed.

Practitioners specially trained in intravaginal/rectal manual muscle testing of the pelvic floor use Laycock's PERFECT Scale for pelvic floor assessment to determine an appropriate exercise prescription for each individual patient. *PERFECT* is an acronym for power (*P*), endurance (*E*), repetitions (*R*), fast contractions (*F*), and every contraction timed (*ECT*).[61] Table 27-6 describes each of the PERFECT measurements in detail.

The internal assessment consists of a digital palpation by inserting one gloved examination finger into the vagina or rectum (Fig. 27-7) and asking the patient to perform a maximal voluntary pelvic floor contraction and holding as long as the examiner continues to feel the contraction sustained at the original power/strength or no longer than 10 seconds. As soon as the patient starts to lose the contraction, the examiner asks the patient to rest for 4 seconds. The examiner repeats this until the patient is unable to contract at the same power/strength anymore or up to 10 repetitions. The patient is asked to rest for 1 minute and then to contract the pelvic floor with quick 1-second pelvic floor contractions with only 1 second of rest time between contractions, and the examiner counts how many contractions the patient can perform at the same strength (up to a maximum of 10 contractions). The examiner determines the power/strength of the patient's maximum voluntary contraction using the modified Oxford Scale of 0 to 5 (0 meaning no palpable movement of muscle fibers and 5 meaning a very strong, symmetric squeeze). Table 27-7 presents Laycock's proposed

TABLE 27-6 Laycock's Proposed Definitions of PERFECT Score for Pelvic Floor Strength Assessment

Perfect	Laycock's Proposed Definition
P = Power (strength)	MVC is measured on modified Oxford Scale of 0-5 (see Table 27-7 for scale definitions/equivalents)
E = Endurance	Number of seconds (up to 10) that MVC can be maintained by patient before strength is reduced by ≥35%
R = Repetitions	Number of repetitions (up to 10) of specific MVC (at above-noted endurance hold time) that patient can perform while allowing only 4 seconds rest between each contraction
F = Fast contractions	After a short rest (at least 1 minute), the number (up to 10) of 1-second MVCs is assessed
ECT = Every Contraction Timed	This reminds the examiner to time and record the above sequence of events

MVC, maximum voluntary contraction.
Adapted from Laycock J, Jerwood D: Pelvic floor muscle assessment: the PERFECT scheme. *Physiotherapy* 87(12):631-642, 2001.

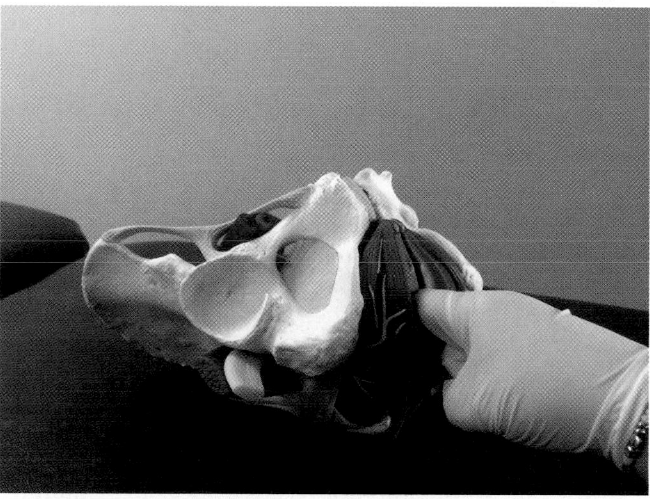

FIG 27-7 Internal examination of pelvic floor strength.

TABLE 27-7 Laycock's Proposed Definitions of Strength on Modified Oxford Scale

Oxford Scale	Laycock's Proposed Definition
0	No discernible muscle contraction
1	Flicker or pulsation is felt under examiner's finger
2	Increase in tension is detected, without any discernible lift
3	Muscle tension is further enhanced and characterized by lifting of muscle belly and elevation of posterior vaginal wall; stronger muscle contraction can be observed as a drawing in of the perineum and anus
4	Increased tension and good contraction are present, which are capable of elevating posterior vaginal wall against resistance (digital pressure applied to posterior vaginal wall)
5	Strong resistance can be applied to elevation of posterior vaginal wall; the examining finger is squeezed and drawn into the vagina (similar to a hungry baby sucking a finger).

Adapted from Laycock J, Jerwood D: Pelvic floor muscle assessment: the PERFECT scheme. *Physiotherapy* 87(12):631-642, 2001.

definitions of strength on this modified Oxford Scale.[61] The examiner also needs to count how many seconds the endurance contractions lasted and the number of fast contractions the patient was able to perform. The PERFECT score is documented as P/E/R//F. For example, if a patient is able to contract the pelvic floor symmetrically around the examination finger as well as provide a lift or elevation of the anus/posterior vaginal wall for four repetitions of 6-second endurance holds and then performs eight quick pelvic floor contractions at the same strength, the PERFECT score would be documented as 3/6/4//8. The PERFECT score is used by the examiner to determine the appropriate number of repetitions and the appropriate hold time (based on the principle of overload) to prescribe as a daily home exercise program as described subsequently.

If the practitioner has not received specialized training in internal assessment, an alternative assessment can be used to ensure proper isolation and contraction of the pelvic floor. This technique requires the patient to lie in the hook lying position while the examiner sits next to the patient with the arm resting on the table. Using a lumbrical hold around the ischial tuberosity with the examiner's fingertips resting medial to the ischial tuberosity/pubic rami, inferior to the pubic symphysis, and anterior to the coccyx, the examiner asks for a pelvic floor contraction and feels for an inward pull of the perineum (Fig. 27-8). Although the examiner cannot obtain an exact modified Oxford Scale score of strength, he or she can determine if there is any contraction of the muscle felt, if it is symmetric, and if there is an actual superior translation of the pelvic floor muscles. This information can assist in determining the strengthening therapeutic exercise prescription for this individual patient.

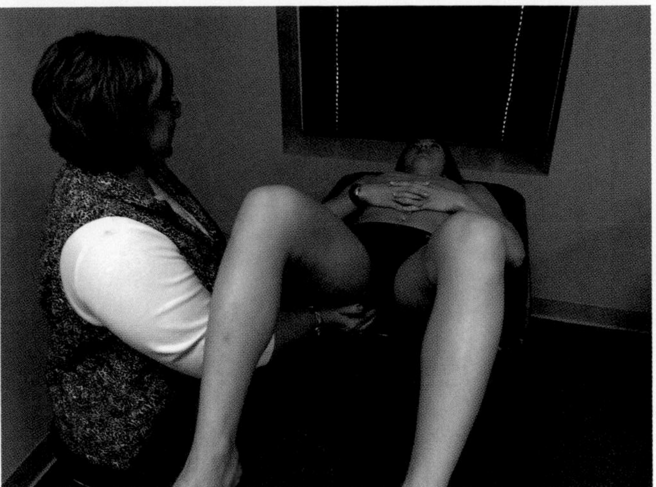

FIG 27-8 External examination of pelvic floor contractions.

Important Concept

Pelvic floor exercises have been shown to be the most effective conservative intervention for conditions such as UI.

Exercise Prescription for Strengthening

Before beginning a strengthening program for the pelvic floor, it is imperative that the PTA determine the patient's ability to perform a proper diaphragmatic breath. The respiratory diaphragm and pelvic floor have been shown to work together to control increased intraabdominal pressure.[66,105] Coordination of relaxing the pelvic floor with inhalation or depression of the respiratory diaphragm is very important to avoid increasing this intraabdominal pressure. The excursion (stretch) that occurs to the pelvic floor with proper diaphragmatic inhalation also provides a good quick stretch to facilitate proper contraction of the pelvic floor on exhalation.

Determining the Type of Pelvic Floor Exercise to Prescribe

As with strengthening any other muscle group, the PTA should determine whether to use endurance or quick as well as concentric or eccentric contractions for this patient. There are many types of pelvic floor contractions to choose from (Table 27-8).

Important Concept

It is imperative that the PTA determine the patient's ability to perform a proper diaphragmatic breath. The respiratory diaphragm and pelvic floor have been shown to work together to control increased intraabdominal pressure.

Selection of Exercise Position

If the patient's strength is measured at 0 to 2 on the modified Oxford Scale, the PTA should choose a training position that is either gravity assisted or gravity eliminated. A patient with a strength of 3 to 5 would need some form of

TABLE 27-8 Types of Pelvic Floor Exercises

Type of Pelvic Floor Exercise	Description	Purpose
Endurance Kegel	Patient pulls pelvic floor up and in on exhalation and holds Kegel (without holding breath) for 5-10 seconds up to 20 seconds.	Strengthen tonic muscle fibers for supportive and endurance functions
Quick Kegel	Patient quickly pulls pelvic floor up and in for 1-2 seconds.	Strengthen and train phasic muscle fibers for quick response
Combination Kegel	Patient pulls pelvic floor up and in on exhalation and holds Kegel (without holding breath), and when holding all the way in, patient does quick flick Kegels at the "top" of the endurance contraction	Advanced strengthening options to exercise tonic and phasic muscle fibers in combination with one another
Elevator Kegel	Patient gradually (in a steplike pattern) pulls pelvic floor up and in on exhalation to "first floor," "second floor," "third floor," and "fourth floor or top." Patient then releases contraction to "third floor," "second floor," and "first floor" and finally completely releases contraction.	Advanced strengthening of tonic muscle fibers eccentrically

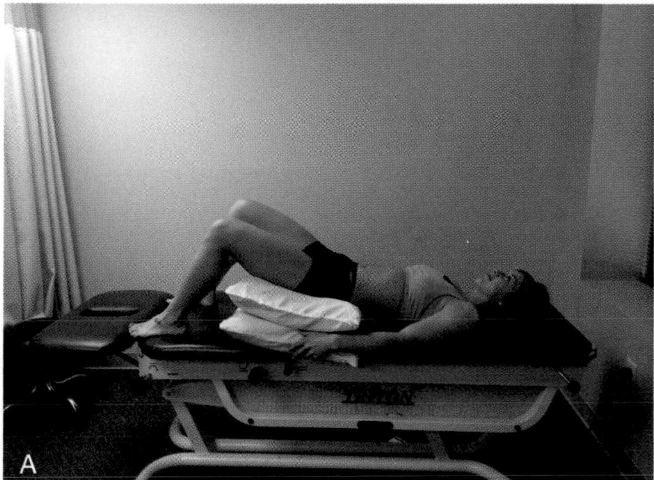

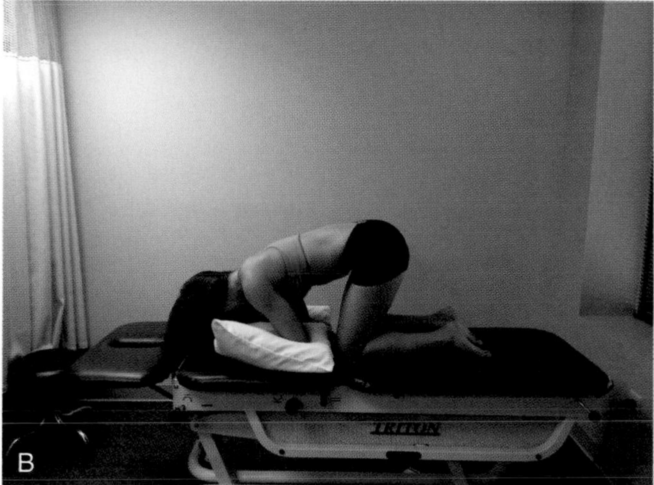

FIG 27-9 Gravity-assisted positioning. **A,** Inverted hook lying. **B,** Inverted quadruped position.

gravity resistance to continue to overload the muscle for strengthening, and a gravity-resisted position would be the ideal starting position for the patient to perform pelvic floor exercises. Refer to Figs. 27-9 through 27-12 for examples of gravity-assisted, gravity-eliminated, and gravity-resisted positions to have the patient perform pelvic floor exercises.

Weighted Vaginal Cones

For pelvic floor muscle strengths of grades 3 to 5, the PTA may choose to prescribe the use of vaginal weights or weighted vaginal cones. These cones are made to insert into the vagina and are of various weights to progress the amount of resistance being added to the pelvic floor contractions. A systematic review of randomized controlled trials demonstrated that the use of weighted vaginal cones may be beneficial to patients with UI.[43] There are various types and brands of vaginal weights with their own recommended instructional use. The PTA should refer to the instructions of each brand for exercise prescription specifics. Fig. 27-13 shows a few of the vaginal weight options that are available to patients.

Exercise Prescription for Relaxation of the Short Pelvic Floor

Caution should be used when determining the appropriate pelvic floor intervention. If the PTA chooses to strengthen a pelvic floor that is shortened or hypertonic and painful, the patient may experience increased symptoms. Hypertonic conditions may require down-training the pelvic floor muscles to improve function or eliminate pain.[35] Although biofeedback (which is discussed later in this chapter) is commonly used for down-training the pelvic floor, some therapeutic exercises have also been shown to be beneficial in relaxing the pelvic floor muscles.

Diaphragmatic breathing has been shown to decrease heart rate and relax respiratory muscles and neck and shoulder muscles.[11,80] This theory can also be applied to relaxation of abdominal and pelvic floor muscles when treating the short or hypertonic pelvic floor. It is important to teach the patient with pelvic floor dysfunction how to coordinate the pelvic diaphragm with the respiratory diaphragm; however, to accomplish this, the patient must be able to perform proper diaphragmatic breathing. As described earlier, when the respiratory diaphragm contracts with inhalation, it descends into the abdominal cavity; the pelvic diaphragm should relax and stretch on

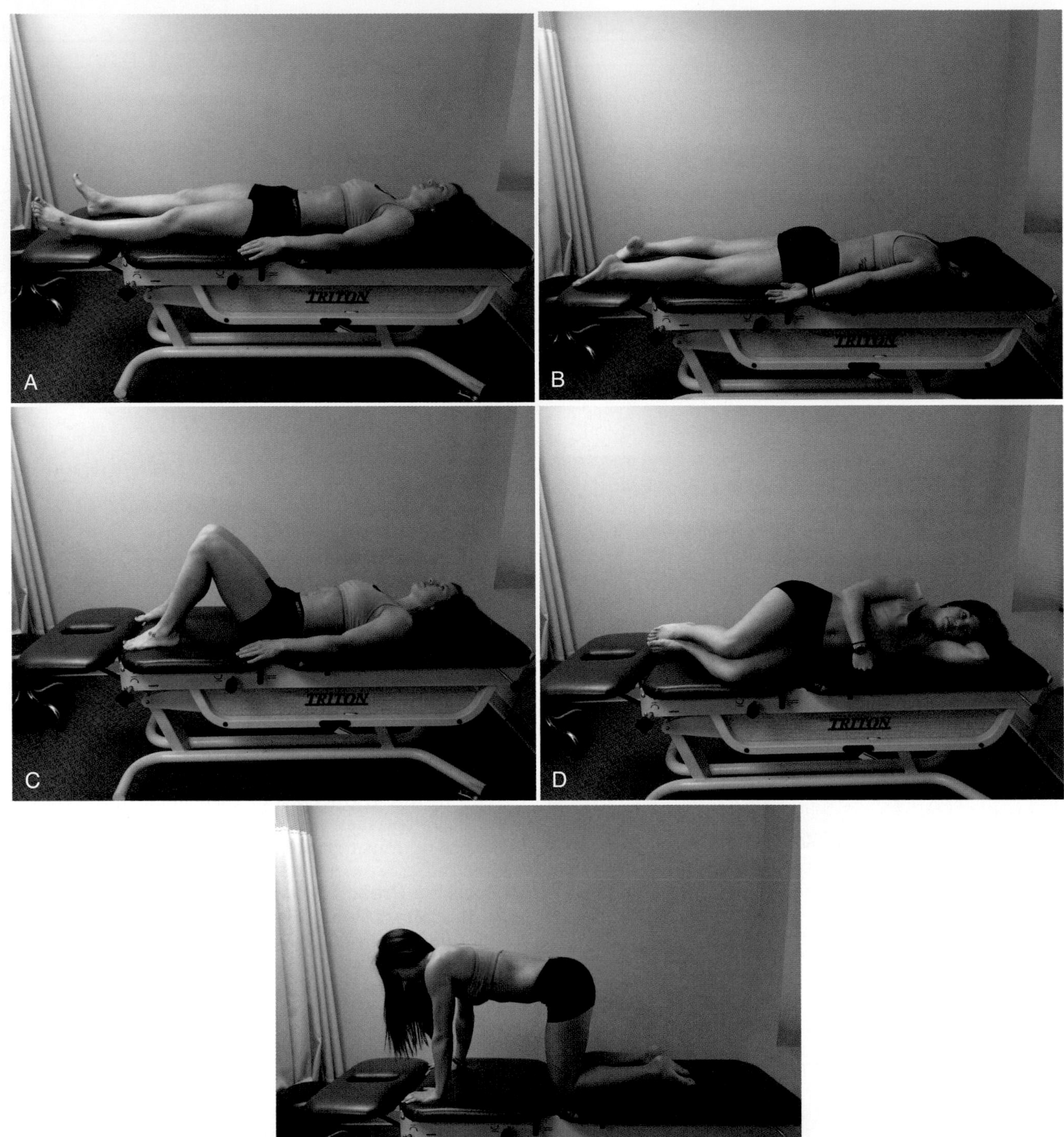

FIG 27-10 Gravity-eliminated positioning. **A,** Supine. **B,** Prone. **C,** Hook lying. **D,** Side-lying. **E,** Quadruped.

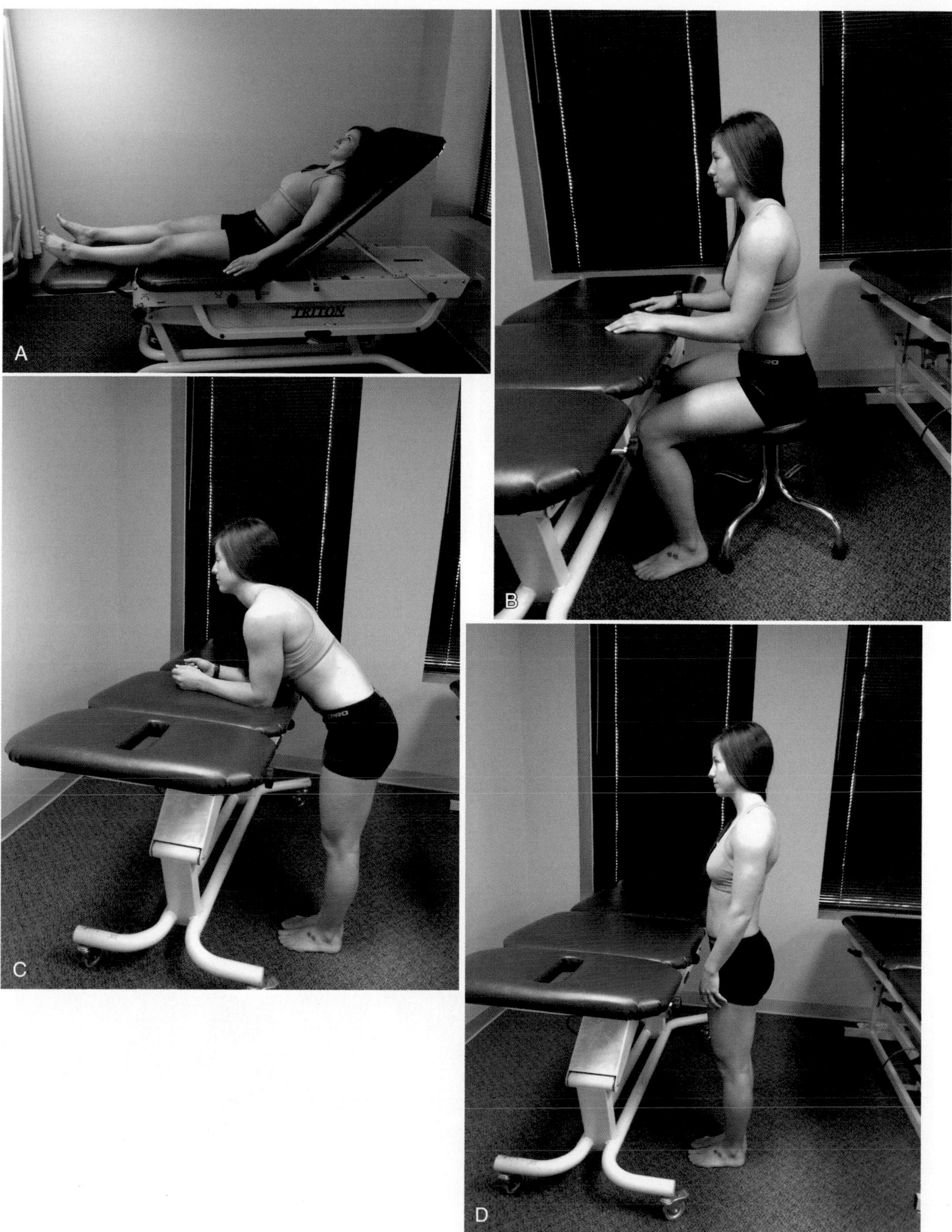

FIG 27-11 Gravity-resisted positioning. **A,** Reclined. **B,** Sitting. **C,** Modified standing. **D,** Standing.

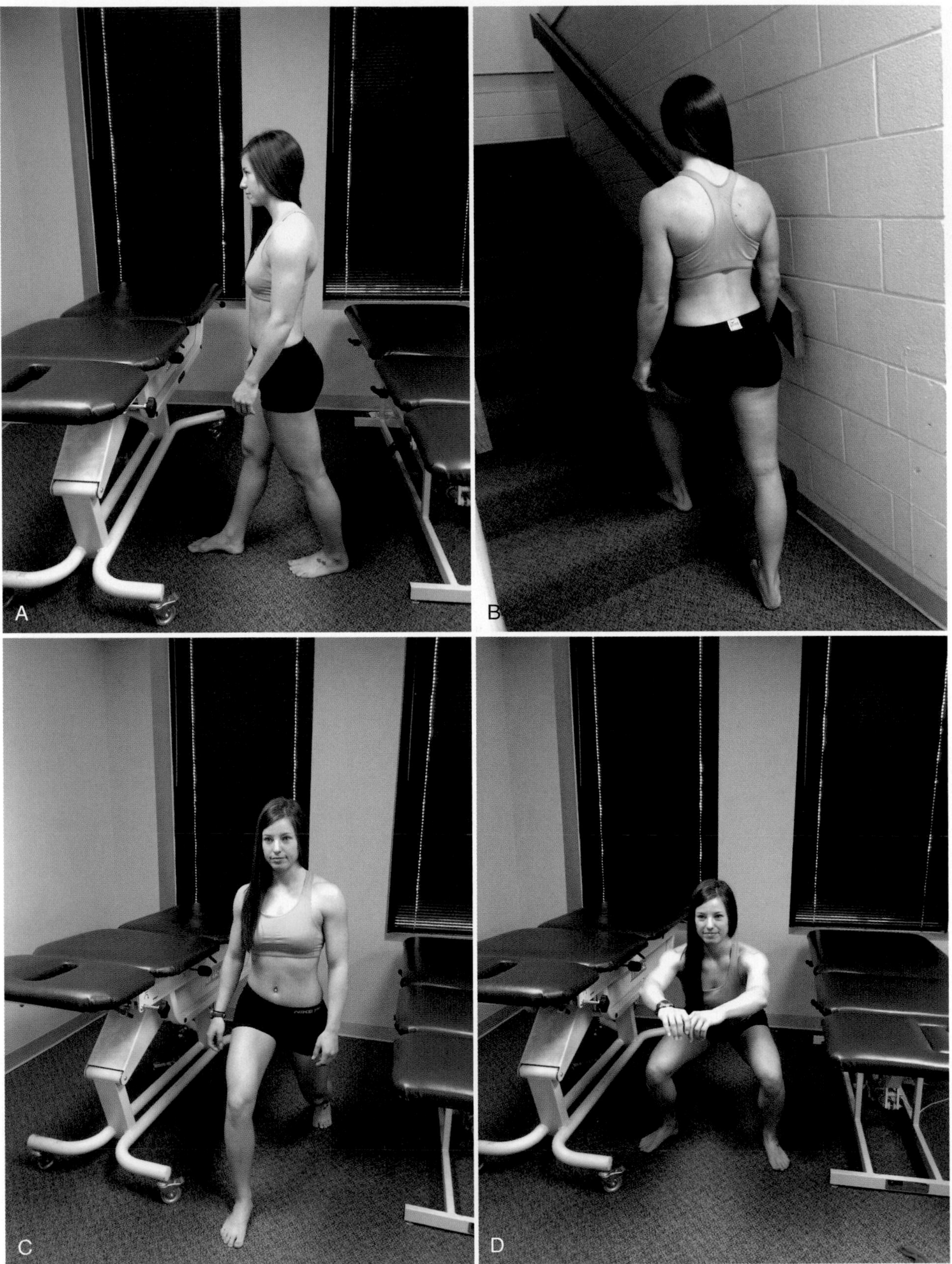

FIG 27-12 Gravity-resisted/functional advanced positioning. **A,** Staggered standing. **B,** Stairs. **C,** Lunges. **D,** Squats.

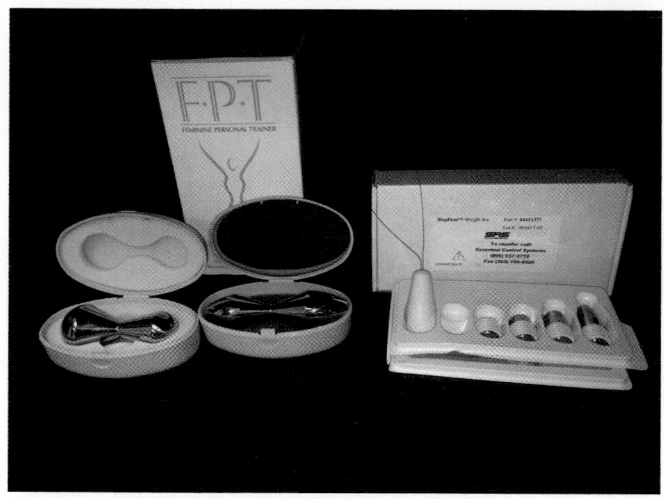

FIG 27-13 Vaginal weights and cones.

inhalation to avoid increasing intraabdominal pressure. During exhalation, the respiratory diaphragm ascends superiorly into the rib cage, allowing for increased space in the abdominal cavity accommodating the ascending pelvic diaphragm during the concentric contraction of a Kegel exercise. However, in hypertonic pelvic floor conditions, the emphasis should be placed on a slow inhalation with a slow stretch of the pelvic floor diaphragm using diaphragmatic breathing to inhibit pelvic floor contraction.

Important Concept

Caution should be used when determining the appropriate pelvic floor intervention. If the PTA chooses to strengthen a pelvic floor that is shortened or hypertonic and painful, the patient may experience increased symptoms.

Muscle energy techniques (METs), an intervention commonly used with patients who demonstrate pelvic floor dysfunctions secondary to malalignments of the lumbopelvic or sacral regions, involve the patient actively and isometrically contracting specific muscles to realign the bony segments of a joint. Although there is no current research on the direct effects of METs on pelvic floor dysfunction, numerous studies show that METs can reduce Oswestry Disability Index scores for low-back pain and reduce sacroiliac pain and malalignment.[13,27,28,90,102] Owing to the reduction of malalignments of the sacrum, the pelvic floor muscles are able to relax out of their hypertonic state with the use of METs.

Stretching the Pelvic Floor Muscles

The shortened pelvic floor muscles seen in hypertonic conditions need to be lengthened to allow for decreased pain and pressure in and around the vaginal and anal openings and on the musculoskeletal system around the pelvis. Manual stretching to the pelvic floor can be done directly with insertion of the patient's thumb into the posterior portion of the vaginal opening. The PTA instructs the patient to perform continuous U-shaped strokes from the anterior portion of the vaginal opening on one side, down toward the perineal body, and back up to the other side of the anterior portion of the vaginal opening. Circumferential stretching can be done with vaginal dilators as described subsequently.

Vaginal dilators (as shown in Fig. 27-14) have commonly been used in the prevention of vaginal stenosis after radiation therapy for cervical cancer and after pelvic reconstructive surgeries.[2,95] These dilators can also provide an effective tool to stretch the shortened hypertonic pelvic floor muscles gradually with progressive use of the increased diameter. The patient is taught to relax in a reclined position and perform a gentle contraction of the pelvic floor muscles and insert a small portion of the lubricated small dilator on relaxing the pelvic floor contraction and to proceed in the same manner until the dilator is inserted at least halfway. The patient can relax passively with the dilator placed vaginally or can apply an inferior pressure on the dilator, while inserted vaginally, to apply a mechanical stretch to the pelvic floor muscles. When the patient is able to insert the small dilator without pain or resistance from the vaginal opening, she should perform the same exercise described here using the next size dilator (increasing in dilator diameter until the patient can tolerate the dilator that relates to her functional need).

Lower extremity or spinal stretches of muscles that attach on the thoracic, lumbar, or sacral spines or the pelvis should also be considered for patients with pelvic floor dysfunctions. Such muscles include, but are not limited to, the abdominal muscles, quadratus lumborum, iliopsoas complex, thoracolumbar paraspinals, piriformis, gluteal muscles, hamstrings, iliotibial band, and adductors.

MANUAL SOFT TISSUE AND NEUROMUSCULAR INTERVENTIONS TO TREAT MYOFASCIAL PAIN ASSOCIATED WITH HYPERTONIC CONDITIONS OF THE PELVIC FLOOR

Many soft tissue techniques and neuromuscular interventions that are commonly used in other regions of the body, such as contract-relax, reciprocal inhibition, trigger point release, and strain counterstrain, are also used as interventions for myofascial pain associated with a hypertonic pelvic floor. It is not within the scope of this chapter to cover the theoretical or physiologic mechanisms of these interventions; however, they are mentioned as possible interventions to consider. The following internal versions of these techniques should be used only by someone who has been specifically trained in vaginal and rectal muscle examinations.

Proprioceptive neuromuscular facilitation techniques, such as contract-relax and reciprocal inhibition, have also been used as mechanisms to relax and stretch the hypertonic short pelvic floor without the use of vaginal dilators as described earlier. During the use of contract-relax, the PTA inserts one finger vaginally and asks for a voluntary

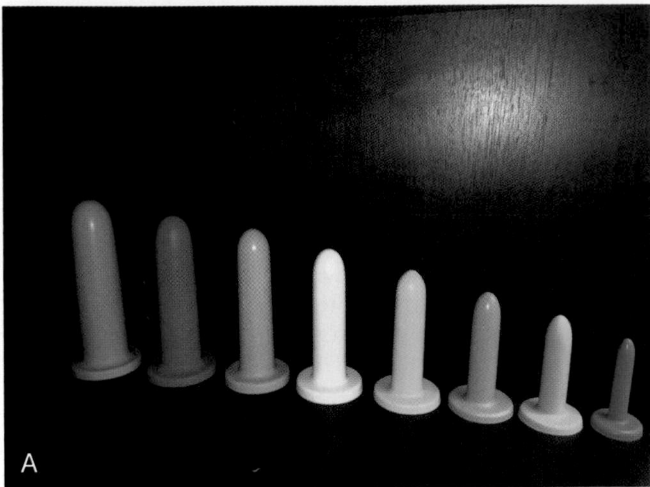

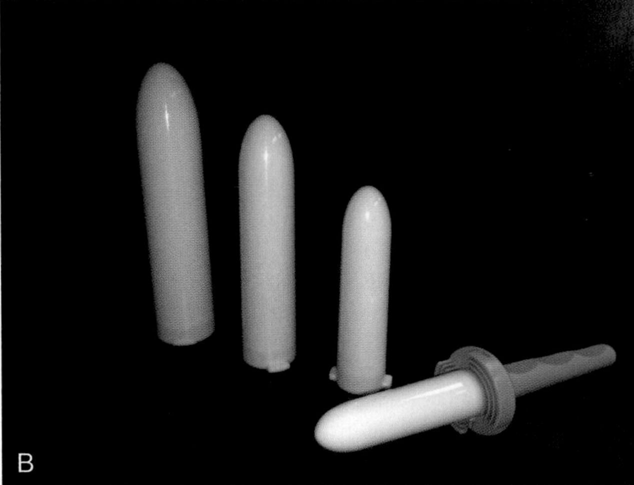

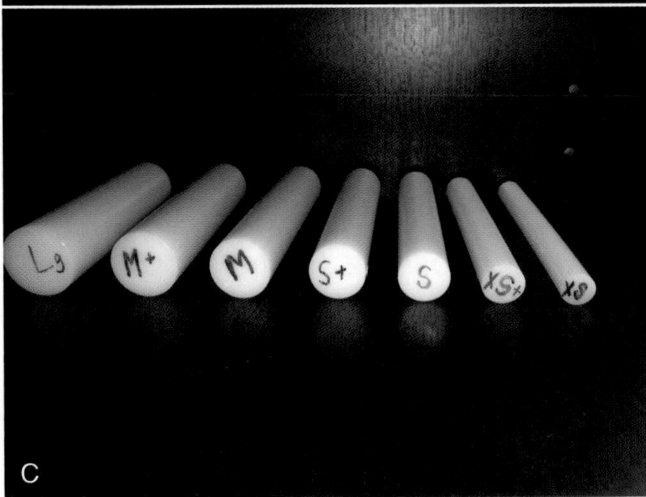

FIG 27-14 **A,** Vaginal dilators. **B,** Vaginismus vaginal dilators. **C,** Syracuse vaginal dilators.

contraction of the levator ani muscles and then applies a gentle posterior stretch on voluntary relaxation of the concentric contraction. Reciprocal inhibition using the abdominal muscles to create a Valsalva maneuver can also relax the pelvic floor muscles.[35]

Trigger point release, the use of ischemic pressure at the localized and painful nodule within the muscle that can refer pain to specific areas of the body, is another option to lengthen and relax hypertonic pelvic floor muscles. Trigger points can cause weakness, stiffness, and restricted range of motion in muscles.[64,100] Intravaginal and intrarectal and external trigger point releases all have been used in the treatment of pelvic floor trigger points.[77]

Strain counterstrain is a technique of passively positioning a muscle in a shortened position to allow the muscle spindle to reset and break the muscle contraction cycle. The research related to its effectiveness is conflicting. Somprasong and colleagues,[92] Dardzinski and co-workers,[26] Ibanez-Garcia and associates,[49] and Mesequer and colleagues[69] all reported success in pain reduction and improved range of motion when using strain counterstrain. However, Blanco and colleagues[14] reported an inability of strain counterstrain to improve range of motion in their 2006 study.[14,92] Most of the above-mentioned studies were done with the masseter muscle, and more research is needed on the effects of strain counterstrain on the pelvic floor muscles.

MODALITIES

The use of modalities such as electrical stimulation and biofeedback is common practice in women and men with UI and other pelvic floor dysfunctions. A combination of the two interventions was shown to improve male UI after radical prostatectomy much faster than pelvic floor muscle exercises alone.[94]

Biofeedback

Biofeedback, a method by which a patient is made aware of the physiologic state of targeted muscles, comes in many forms.[51] For example, visual, audible, and tactile feedback all can benefit pelvic floor muscle retraining. **Electromyographic biofeedback (EMG)**, a form of biofeedback that can be used to measure the electrical activity of muscles (Fig. 27-15, *A*) EMG has been shown to be another effective intervention for the treatment of pelvic floor disorders.[16] Although some studies showed no added benefit of electromyography (EMG) compared with pelvic floor exercises in the treatment of UI,[34,46] others showed benefit.[6,44] Fig. 27-15, *B,* demonstrates the external pelvic floor sensors used for pelvic floor biofeedback. The external sensors are used for surface EMG; the two active sensors are placed perianally parallel to the pubococcygeus muscle fibers, and the ground sensor is placed on the muscle belly of the gluteus medius.

Internal vaginal and rectal sensors also exist for use with EMG systems and are used when the PT also wants to elicit a proprioceptive (or tactile) response from the patient for a pelvic floor contraction. Internal sensors are more expensive and are not preferred by some practitioners. Biofeedback can be used to assist with up-training or down-training the pelvic floor muscles using visual and audible cues to facilitate pelvic floor contractions. However, EMG also picks up the electrical activity of surrounding muscles, so the PTA should visually examine the patient to ensure no substitution or use of accessory muscles when targeting an isolated pelvic floor contraction. Abdominal, gluteal, and adductor contractions represent common accessory/substitution patterns seen with pelvic floor contraction.

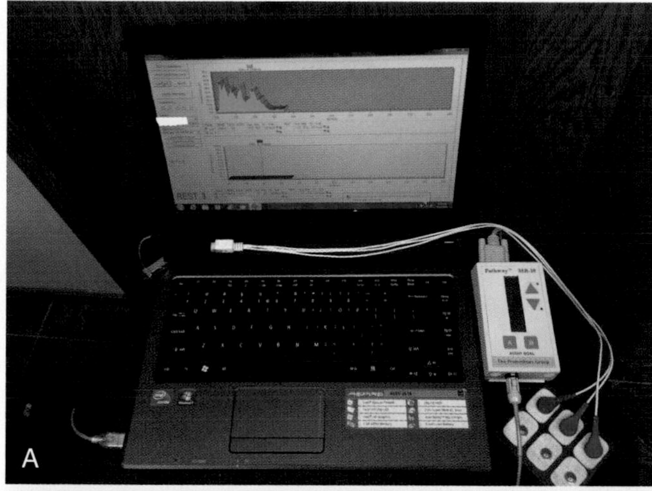

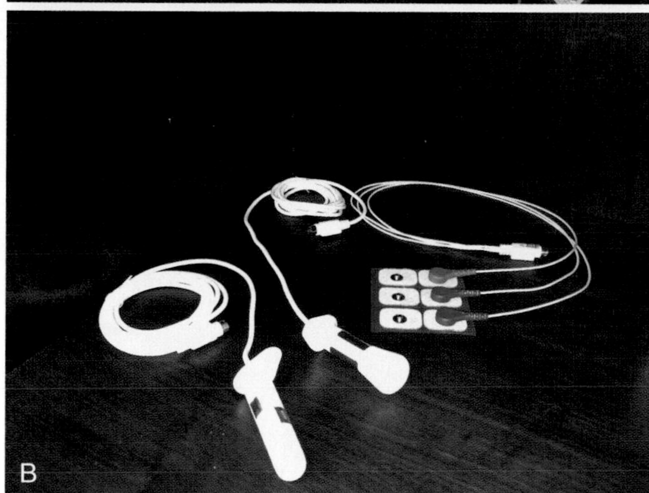

FIG 27-15 **A,** Surface EMG biofeedback with Synergy software. **B,** Surface EMG surface and internal electrodes.

Transabdominal ultrasound provides a visual form of biofeedback because the patient can visually see contraction of the muscle belly in the abdominal wall or a superior translation of the bladder that occurs when the pelvic floor muscles contract properly. Galea and associates[37] demonstrated effective use of transabdominal ultrasound for biofeedback of pelvic floor muscle function in a randomized controlled trial when teaching pelvic floor muscle contractions to older women with UI.

Electrical Stimulation

Electrical stimulation, also commonly used in the treatment of pelvic floor dysfunction, has been shown to be an effective treatment for strengthening the pelvic floor muscles to treat various types of UI, POP, and erectile dysfunction.[12] Contraindications for the use of electrical stimulation apply; Box 27-1 lists these contraindications.

Types and Parameters of Electrical Stimulation Used for Pelvic Floor Disorders. Intravaginal/intrarectal electrical stimulation uses a sensor that may be inserted into the vagina or rectum to deliver electrical stimulation internally. This intervention has been shown to be effective in the treatment of urge incontinence.[89]

BOX 27-1 Contraindications of Electrical Stimulation for Pelvic Floor Disorders

- Pregnancy
- Pacemaker
- Active vaginal or rectal infection
- Active vaginal or rectal bleeding
- Impaired sensation

Intravaginal electrical stimulation has also been referred to as transvaginal electrical stimulation and when used with biofeedback was shown to improve SUI in women.[97] Yamanishi and co-workers[104] and Mariotti and associates[65] determined that intrarectal electrical stimulation with pelvic floor exercises resulted in a faster resolution of post-prostatectomy UI compared with pelvic floor exercises alone. Sand and colleagues[86] also demonstrated positive results with intravaginal electrical stimulation in women with UI. Frequencies and duty cycles of 12.5 Hz continuous and 50 Hz with a 10-second on cycle and 20-second off cycle for 15 minutes three to five times per week are commonly used for treatment of urge incontinence and SUI, respectively.

Surface electrical stimulation is another option for treatment of UI. This method does not require the use of a personal intravaginal sensor and is more cost-effective and less invasive. Various authors have tested different pad placements and parameters for surface electrical stimulation and have reported promising results. Correia and colleagues[25] placed two suprapubic external pads and two external pads near the ischial tuberosities with a frequency of 50 Hz, pulse duration of 700 µsec, a duration of 20 minutes with a cycle of 4 seconds on and 8 seconds off with a 2-second rise and 2-second fall, two times per week for 6 weeks. Another option for pad placement was tested in male subjects with UI after prostatectomy and consisted of placement of all pads surrounding the T10-L2 spinal levels with a frequency of 4 Hz, pulse width of 1 µsec, for a duration of 20 minutes three times per week.[3]

Transcutaneous electrical nerve stimulation at S2-S3 with a 10-Hz frequency, pulse duration of 200 msec, and a biphasic waveform for 2 hours daily was shown to decrease urge UI in children.[41] Samhan and colleagues[85] found the use of suprapubic transcutaneous electrical nerve stimulation daily for 20 minutes, five times per week, with a mean frequency of 100 Hz and an intensity of 25 mA effective in the treatment of chronic pelvic pain syndrome in men.

CONSIDERING THE PELVIC FLOOR WHEN TREATING OTHER ORTHOPEDIC CONDITIONS

Low-back pain is one of the most common conditions treated by PTs.[52] The PTA should be aware of and screen for pelvic floor dysfunctions when treating low-back pain.[32] Simultaneous treatment of pelvic floor dysfunction may speed recovery time for low-back pain. Studies have shown associations between low-back pain and UI, likely secondary to the fact that the pelvic floor plays such a vital role in the stabilization of the lumbopelvic region as well as its role in continence of bladder and bowel.[19,32,57,91] Women with disorders of continence and respiration have a significantly higher prevalence of back pain than women who do not have these disorders, owing to the role of the pelvic floor and respiratory diaphragm in postural control and respiration.[91] In 1999, Gurel and Atar[40] also discovered a relationship between back pain, dyspareunia, and chronic pelvic pain. A synergistic response exists between the deep abdominal muscles and the pelvic floor.[87] The pelvic floor is an essential part of trunk and lumbopelvic stability.[83] Instability of the trunk can occur when the transverse abdominis, the pelvic floor muscles, and the respiratory diaphragm do not work together to control increases in intraabdominal pressure.[47,87] Other researchers looked at the association between UI and falls in the elderly population.[18,24,42,95,96] Additionally, the severity of UI significantly correlates with static balance ability.[57]

In addition to associations between the pelvic floor and the lumbopelvic region, the PTA should consider the pelvic floor as essential when treating hip dysfunctions or when rehabilitating after hip surgeries such as total hip replacements or hip fracture repairs. Baba and colleagues[8] looked at anterior and posterior approaches to perform hip arthroplasty and found differences in the posterior approach dissecting the short external rotators and the anterior approach not dissecting these muscles. There were different influences on the pelvic floor muscles that subsequently affected UI.

PIRIFORMIS SYNDROME AND SCIATICA AND THE RELATIONSHIP WITH PELVIC FLOOR DYSFUNCTION

Sciatica is a neuromusculoskeletal pain down the leg in the path of the dermatomatic distribution of the sciatic nerve.[48] Although the primary cause of sciatica is believed to be compression of the nerve root via a herniated intervertebral disk, Freighburg and Vinkle proposed and Robinson confirmed that compression of the nerve trunk from the piriformis muscle can also cause sciatica symptoms, and so the condition is termed ***piriformis syndrome***.[48]

As mentioned in the section on anatomic review, the pelvic diaphragm consists of the muscles of the levator ani and coccygeus muscles as well as the piriformis and obturator internus muscles of the hip. The pelvic floor shares an attachment with the obturator internus via the tendinous arch of the levator ani muscle in which the obturator internus attaches laterally and the levator ani attaches medially. Any excessive activity of the levator ani could cause increased tension on the obturator internus muscle. It has been shown that the sciatic nerve occasionally passes between the piriformis muscle and the obturator internus muscle and should be considered in differential diagnosis of piriformis syndrome.[75] The PTA should watch for poor results of sciatica symptom relief when treating for piriformis syndrome. An external technique to palpate the obturator internus can be performed with the patient in side-lying position with the top hip and knee flexed to 90° and fully supported by a bolster or pillows to keep it parallel to the treatment table. The PTA should sit behind the patient on a treatment stool with the elbow resting on the treatment table. The PTA can palpate the obturator internus by finding the patient's ischial tuberosity with the opposite thumb to guide the PTA's other hand inferior to the ischial tuberosity using a lumbrical grip and directing the examining fingers medially and superiorly past the ischial tuberosity. When the PTA passes the ischial tuberosity, he or she drops the examining elbow down toward the table to appreciate the obturator foramen with the examining fingers. The PTA asks the patient to externally rotate the hip, and the obturator internus muscle belly should swell on top of the PTA's fingers. The patient should be warned that it will feel like the PTA is going to palpate the anus; however, the exact location of the examining fingers is just lateral to the anus. This technique can be done through very loose, thin shorts or underwear but not through any thicker material to avoid improper placement. If there is significant pain or tension in the obturator internus, the PTA can perform trigger point release or contract relax techniques to release this muscle and decrease the compression being placed on the sciatic nerve. Fig. 27-16 demonstrates this technique. If the patient does not experience relief of pain and symptoms,

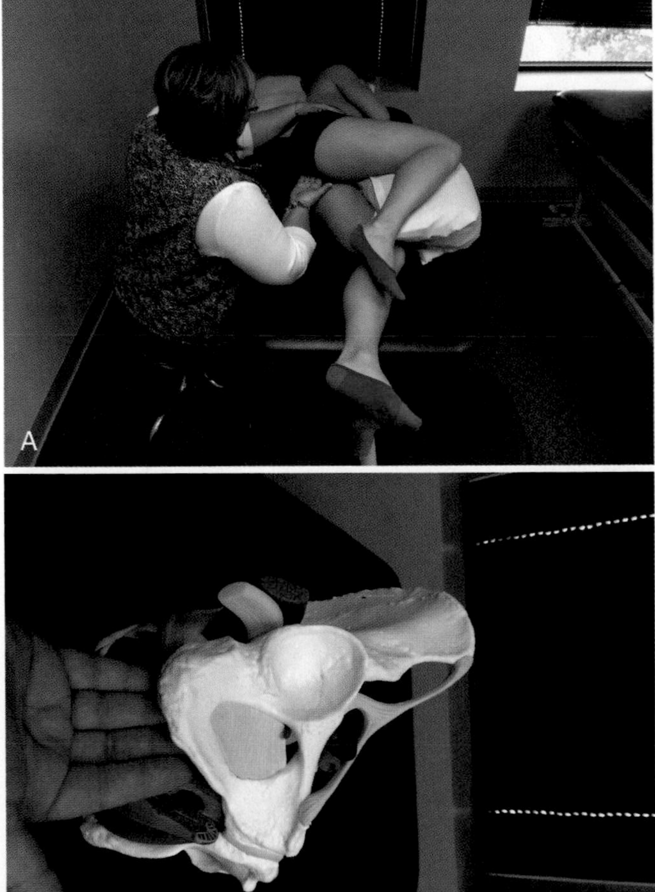

FIG 27-16 **A,** External technique for releasing obturator internus. **B,** External technique for releasing obturator internus (skeletal model view).

it is possible that dysfunction in the pelvic floor muscles may be the root of the problem. This anatomic connection the pelvic floor shares with muscles of the hip could also be the cause of other hip dysfunctions caused by muscular imbalances. Bo and Stein[15] revealed that several trunk and hip muscles are synergists of the pelvic floor musculature. According to Sahrmann,[84] muscular imbalances between synergistic muscles can cause microtrauma that leads to macrotrauma and finally results in musculoskeletal pain syndromes.

SACROILIAC JOINT DYSFUNCTION AND LONG DORSAL SACROILIAC AND SACROTUBEROUS LIGAMENTS IN RELATIONSHIP TO THE COCCYX

Sacroiliac joint dysfunction is described as pain in or around the region of the sacroiliac joint that is likely to be due to malalignment or abnormal movement of the sacroiliac joints.[30,36] Vlemming and colleagues[99] discussed the possible role of the long dorsal sacroiliac and sacrotuberous ligaments in women with posterior pelvic pain. The long dorsal sacroiliac ligament initiates just caudal to the posterior superior iliac spine down to the sacrococcygeal segment. The sacrotuberous ligament has connections with the gluteus maximus muscle, the long head of the biceps femoris muscle, the sacrospinous ligament, and the iliococcygeus muscle.[99] It stands to reason, based on the principles of force closure, that if there is too much tension on one long dorsal sacroiliac ligament, the sacroiliac joint may have too much pressure on it with resulting pain. Sacral nutations or counternutations or both can cause this imbalance of tension among these ligaments. However, another cause for the increased tension could come from coccygeal deviations. Because of the connections of the coccygeus and iliococcygeus muscles with the coccyx as well as the sacroiliac ligaments, the PTA not only should correct malalignments of the sacrum and coccyx but also should look for dysfunctions in the pelvic floor muscles possibly causing these malalignments.

Important Concept

The PTA should be aware of and screen for pelvic floor dysfunctions when treating LBP, piriformis syndrome, sacroiliac joint dysfunction, or any other lumbopelvic, sacral, or hip dysfunction.

SUMMARY

The PTA is encouraged to consider the pelvic floor and its function and possible dysfunction when treating general orthopedic conditions of the lumbopelvic, sacral, or hip area based on the above-mentioned anatomic relationships. Pelvic floor dysfunction may be resolved with interventions to coordinate, strengthen, or lengthen the pelvic floor muscles. Pelvic floor strengthening has repeatedly been shown to be the most effective intervention for supportive dysfunctions; however, other manual therapy techniques and modalities have also been shown to be beneficial. The PTA is encouraged to screen patients for pelvic floor dysfunctions to avoid missing an essential musculoskeletal component of functional movement or pain syndromes.

GLOSSARY

Abdominal pelvic dyssynergia: A condition in which the patient is unable to coordinate the necessary muscles of the abdominal wall and the pelvic floor to urinate or defecate. Also referred to as *bladder sphincter dyssynergia, detrusor sphincter dyssynergia,* and *pelvic floor dyssynergia.*

Anal incontinence: Any involuntary loss of fecal material or flatus.

Anismus: A muscle spasm of the anal sphincter that causes rectal/anal pain that restricts the anal opening.

Bladder sphincter dyssynergia: See *abdominal pelvic dyssynergia.*

Chronic pelvic pain: Pain in the lower abdomen, vulva/vagina, perineum, anus, or tailbone that lasts longer than 6 months.

Coccygodynia: Pain of the coccyx.

Constipation: A condition that is defined by having at least two of the following findings for at least 3 months with onset at least 6 months before diagnosis: (1) straining during at least 25% of defecations; (2) lumpy or hard stools in at least 25% of defecations; (3) sensation of incomplete evacuation for at least 25% of defecations; (4) sensation of anorectal obstruction or blockage for at least 25% of defecations; (5) manual maneuvers to facilitate at least 25% of defecations (e.g., digital evacuation, support of the pelvic floor); (6) fewer than three defecations per week.

Cystocele: A prolapse of the bladder.

Cystourethrocele: A prolapse of the urethra and the bladder.

Dyspareunia: Pain before, during, or after intercourse.

Electromyographic biofeedback: A form of biofeedback that can be used to measure the electrical activity of muscles.

Enterocele: A prolapse of the upper posterior wall of the vagina usually containing loops of small bowel.

Interstitial cystitis (IC): A bladder condition that usually consists of multiple symptoms. Most patients with IC have recurring pelvic pain, pressure, or discomfort in the bladder and pelvic region and urinary frequency (up to 60 voiding episodes per day in severe cases) and urgency. May also be referred to as *painful bladder syndrome.*

Irritable bowel syndrome (IBS): Recurrent abdominal pain or discomfort at least 3 days/month in the last 3 months associated with two or more of the following: (1) improvement with defecation; (2) onset associated with a change in frequency of stool; (3) onset associated with a change in form (appearance) of stool.

Kegel exercises: Voluntary muscle contractions of the pelvic floor. Also referred to as *pelvic floor contractions* or *exercises.*

Levator ani syndrome: A spasm of the levator ani muscles that can cause pain in the buttock, posterior thigh, coccyx, hip, or low back.

Nonrelaxing pelvic floor dysfunction: A term used to encompass many of the hypertonic pelvic floor conditions that involve a specific muscle or specific dysfunction, including levator ani syndrome, nonrelaxing puborectalis, anismus, and proctalgia fugax.

Nonrelaxing puborectalis: Causes bowel movement dysfunction or constipation. Also may be referred to as *puborectalis syndrome* or *paradoxical puborectalis contraction*.

Pelvic floor dyssynergia: See *abdominal pelvic dyssynergia*.

Piriformis syndrome: A compression of the nerve trunk of the sciatic nerve from the piriformis muscle that can also cause sciatica symptoms.

Proctalgia fugax: A muscle spasm of the anal sphincter that causes sharp fleeting rectal pain that can last seconds to 20 to 30 minutes and can occur during the day but occurs frequently in the middle of the night.

Pudendal neuralgia: An entrapment of the pudendal nerve that leads to complaints of constant unprovoked localized burning, itching, or a sensation of dryness that can be unilateral in the perineal area.

Rectocele: A prolapse of the lower posterior wall of the vagina involving the rectum.

Sacroiliac joint dysfunction: Pain in or around the region of the sacroiliac joint that is likely to be due to malalignment or abnormal movement of the sacroiliac joints.

Sciatica: A neuromusculoskeletal pain down the leg in the path of the dermatomatic distribution of the sciatic nerve.

Urethral syndrome: A condition that can cause urinary urgency and frequency; suprapubic pelvic or perineal pressure; and urethral pain, burning, and sensitivity. This syndrome occurs in the absence of infection and causes pain after voiding.

Urethrocele: A prolapse of the urethra.

Urinary incontinence (UI): The condition of any involuntary loss of urine, which can be categorized further according to patient symptoms as urgency urinary incontinence (urge incontinence), stress urinary incontinence, mixed urinary incontinence, nocturnal enuresis, postmicturition dribble, and continuous urinary leakage.

Urinary retention: The inability to void urine secondary to muscle spasms around the urethra.

Uterovaginal/vaginal prolapse: A prolapse of the uterus, cervix, and upper vagina. Also referred to as *uterine prolapse*.

Vaginismus: An involuntary contraction and spasm of the bulbocavernosus muscle, making vaginal penetration difficult, painful, or impossible.

Vulvar vestibulitis: Pain or inflammation of the vulvar vestibule.

Vulvodynia: Pain in the vulva.

REFERENCES

1. Abrams P, Cardozo L, Fall M, et al: The standardization of terminology of lower urinary tract function: report from the standardization sub-committee of the International Continence Society. *Neurourol Urodyn* 21:167–178, 2002.
2. Antosh D, Gutman R, Park A, et al: Vaginal dilators for prevention of dyspareunia after prolapse surgery. *Obstet Gynecol* 121(6):1273–1280, 2013.
3. Araujo de Sousa M, Dantas J, Alves T, et al: Surface electrical nerve stimulation in post-prostatectomy urinary incontinence: case reports. *Rev Terapia Man* 46:908–913, 2011.
4. Ashton-Miller J, DeLancey J: Functional anatomy of the female pelvic floor. *Ann N Y Acad Sci* 1101:266–296, 2007.
5. Ashton-Miller J, DeLancey J: On the biomechanics of vaginal birth and common sequelae. *Annu Rev Biomed Eng* 11:163–176, 2009.
6. Aukee P, Immonen P, et al: The effect of home biofeedback training on stress incontinence. *Acta Obstet Gynecol Scand* 83:973–977, 2004.
7. Awwad J, Sayegh R, Yeretzian J, et al: Prevalence, risk factors, and predictors of pelvic organ prolapse: a community-based study. *Menopause* 19(11):1235–1241, 2012.
8. Baba T, Homma Y, Takazawa N, et al: Is urinary incontinence the hidden secret complications after total hip arthroplasty? *Eur J Orthop Surg Traumatol* 24(8):1455–1460, 2014.
9. Bannister T: Physical therapy management of pelvic floor dyssynergia. *J Womens Health Phys Therap* 33(1):16–21, 2008.
10. Barber MD, Bremer RE, Thor KB, et al: Innervation of the female levator ani muscles. *Am J Obstet Gynecol* 187:64–71, 2002.
11. Bell J, Saltikov J: Mitchell's relaxation technique: is it effective? *Physiotherapy* 86(9):473–478, 2000.
12. Berghmans B, Hendriks E, Bernards A, et al: Electrical stimulation with non-implanted electrodes for urinary incontinence in men. *Cochrane Database Syst Rev* (6):CD001202, 2013.
13. Bindra S, Kumar M, Singh P, et al: A study on the efficacy of muscle energy techniques as compared to conventional therapy in chronic low back pain due to sacroiliac joint dysfunction. *Indian J Physiother Occup Ther* 6(1):200–203, 2012.
14. Blanco C, Fernandez-de-las-Penas C, Xumet J, et al: Changes in active mouth opening following a single treatment of latent myofascial trigger points in the masseter muscle involving post-isometric relaxation or strain counter-strain. *J Bodyw Mov Ther* 10:197–205, 2006.
15. Bo K, Sherburn M: Evaluation of female pelvic-floor muscle function and strength. *Phys Ther* 85(3):269–282, 2005.
16. Bo K, Stein R: Needle EMG registration of striated urethral wall and pelvic floor muscle activity patterns during cough, Valsalva, hip adductor, and gluteal muscle contractions in nulliparous healthy females. *Neurourol Urodyn* 13:35–41, 1994.
17. Boyle R, Hay-Smith EJ, Cody JD, et al: Pelvic floor muscle training for prevention and treatment of urinary and faecal incontinence in antenatal and postnatal women. *Cochrane Database Syst Rev* (10):CD007471, 2012.
18. Brown JS, Vittinghoff E, Wyman JF, et al: Urinary incontinence: does it increase risk for falls and fractures? Study of Osteoporotic Fractures Research Group. *J Am Geriatr Soc* 48:721–725, 2000.
19. Bush H, Pagorek S, Kuperstein J, et al: The association of chronic back pain and stress urinary incontinence: a cross-sectional study. *J Womens Health Phys Therap* 37(1):11–18, 2013.
20. Campbell SE, Glazener CM, Hunter KF, et al: Conservative management for postprostatectomy urinary incontinence. *Cochrane Database Syst Rev* (1):CD001843, 2012.
21. Castro RA, Arruda RM, Zanetti M, et al: Single blind, randomized, controlled trial of pelvic floor muscle training, electrical stimulation, vaginal cones, and no active treatment in the management of stress urinary incontinence. *Clinics* 64:465–472, 2008.
22. Chase J, Shields N: A systematic review of the efficacy of non-pharmacological, non-surgical and non-behavioural treatments of functional chronic constipation in children. *Aust N Z Cont J* 17(2):40–50, 2011.
23. Chen G-D, Ng S-C: Updated definition of female pelvic organ prolapse. *Incont Pelvic Floor Dysfunct* 1(4):121–124, 2007.
24. Chiarelli PE, Mackenzie LA, Osmotherly PG: Urinary incontinence is associated with an increase in falls: a systematic review. *Aust J Physiother* 55:89–95, 2009.
25. Correia G, Pereira V, Hirakawa H, et al: Effects of surface and intravaginal electrical stimulation in the treatment of women with stress urinary incontinence: randomized controlled trial. *Eur J Obstet Gynecol Reprod Biol* 173:113–118, 2014.

26. Dardzinski J, Ostrov B, Hamann L: Myofascial pain unresponsive to standard treatment successful use of strain counter-strain technique with physical therapy. *J Clin Rheumatol* 6:169–174, 2000.
27. Day J, Nitz A: The effect of muscle energy techniques on disability and pain scores in individuals with low back pain. *J Sport Rehabil* 21:194–198, 2012.
28. Dhinkaran M, Sareen A, Arora T: Comparative analysis of muscle energy technique and conventional physiotherapy in treatment of sacroiliac joint dysfunction. *Indian J Physiother Occup Ther* 5(4):127–130, 2011.
29. Diamanti A, Bracci F, Reale A, et al: Incidence, clinical presentation, and management of constipation in a pediatric ED. *Am J Emerg Med* 28(2):189–194, 2010.
30. Dreyfuss P, Dreyer S, Griffin J, et al: Positive sacroiliac screening tests in asymptomatic adults. *Spine (Phila Pa 1976)* 19:1138–1143, 1994.
31. Dumoulin C, Hay-Smith J: Pelvic floor muscle training versus no treatment, or inactive control treatments, for urinary incontinence in women. *Cochrane Database Syst Rev* (1):CD005654, 2010.
32. Eliasson K, Elfving B, Nordgren B, et al: Urinary incontinence in women with low back pain. *Man Ther* 13:206–212, 2008.
33. Fantel JA, Newman DK, Colling J: Urinary incontinence in adults: acute and chronic management: 1996 update AHCPR Clinical Practice Guidelines, No. 2. Department of Health and Human Services. Public Health Service, Agency for Health Care Policy and Research. AHCPR Publication No. 96-0682.
34. Fitz F, Magalhães Resende A, Stüpp L, et al: Biofeedback for the treatment of female pelvic floor muscle dysfunction: a systematic review and meta-analysis. *Int Urogynecol J* 23:1495–1516, 2012.
35. FitzGerald M, Kotarinos R: Rehabilitation of the short pelvic floor II: treatment of the patient with the short pelvic floor. *Int Urogynecol J* 14:269–275, 2003.
36. Fortin JD, Aprill DN, Ponthieux B, et al: Sacroiliac joint: pain referral maps upon applying a new injection/arthrography technique, part II: clinical evaluation. *Spine (Phila Pa 1976)* 19:1483–1489, 1994.
37. Galea M, Tisseverasinghe S, Sherburn M: A randomised controlled trial of transabdominal ultrasound biofeedback for pelvic floor muscle training in older women with urinary incontinence. *Aust N Z Cont J* 19(2):38–44, 2013.
38. Goodman CC, Boissonnault WG: *Pathology: Implications for the Physical Therapist*, Philadelphia, 1998, Saunders.
39. Goodman CC, Snyder TE: *Differential Diagnosis for Physical Therapists: Screening for Referral*, St Louis, 2007, Saunders.
40. Gurel H, Atar GS: Dyspareunia, back pain and chronic pelvic pain: the importance of this pain complex in gynecological practice and its relation with grandmultiparity and pelvic relaxation. *Gynecol Obstet Invest* 48:119–122, 1999.
41. Hagstroem S, Mahler B, Madsen B, et al: Transcutaneous electrical nerve stimulation for refractory daytime urinary urge incontinence. *J Urol* 182:2072–2078, 2009.
42. Hasegawa J, Kuzuya M, Iguchi A: Urinary incontinence and behavioral symptoms are independent risk factors for recurrent and injurious falls, respectively, among residents in long-term care facilities. *Arch Gerontol Geriatr* 50:77–81, 2010.
43. Herbison GP, Dean N: Weighted vaginal cones for urinary incontinence. *Cochrane Database Syst Rev* (7):CD002114, 2013.
44. Herderschee R, Hay-Smith EJ, Herbison GP, et al: Feedback or biofeedback to augment pelvic floor muscle training for urinary incontinence in women. *Cochrane Database Syst Rev* (7):CD009252, 2011.
45. Hibner M, Desai N, Robertson L, Nour M: Pudendal neuralgia. *J Minim Invasive Gynecol* 17(2):148–153, 2010.
46. Hirakawa T, Suzuki S, Kato K, et al: Randomized controlled trial of pelvic floor muscle training with or without biofeedback for urinary incontinence. *Int Urogynecol J* 24:1347–1354, 2013.
47. Hodges PW, Gandevia SC: Changes in intra-abdominal pressure during postural and respiratory activation of the human diaphragm. *J Appl Physiol (1985)* 89:967–976, 2000.
48. Hopayion K, Song F, Riera R, et al: The clinical features of the piriformis syndrome: a systematic review. *Eur Spine J* 19:2095–2109, 2010.
49. Ibanez-Garcia J, Alburquerque-Sendin F, Blanco C, et al: Changes in masseter muscle trigger points following strain counter-strain or neuromuscular technique. *J Bodyw Mov Ther* 13:2–10, 2009.
50. Interstitial Cystitis Association (web site). www.ichelp.org. Accessed December 12, 2013.
51. Irion J, Irion G: *Women's Health in Physical Therapy*, Baltimore, 2010, Lippincott Williams & Wilkins.
52. Jette AM, Smith K, Haley SM, et al: Physical therapy episodes of care for patients with low back pain. *Phys Ther* 74(2):101–110, 1994.
53. Jeyarajah S, Purkayastha S: Proctalgia fugax. *CMAJ* 185(5):417, 2013.
54. Kaur H, Arunkalaivanan A: Urethral pain syndrome and its management. *Obstet Gynecol Surv* 62(5):348–351, 2007.
55. Kegel A: Progressive resistance exercise in the functional restoration of muscles. *Am J Obstet Gynecol* 56:238–249, 1948.
56. Kegel AH: Stress incontinence and genital relaxation. *Ciba Clin Symp* 4(2):35–52, 1952.
57. Kim J, Kim S, Oh D, et al: Correlation between the severity of female urinary incontinence and concomitant morbidities: A multi-center cross-sectional clinical study. *Int Neurourol J* 14:220–226, 2010.
58. Knorst M, Resende T, Santos T, et al: The effect of outpatient physical therapy intervention on pelvic floor muscles in women with urinary incontinence. *Braz J Phys Ther* 17(5):442–449, 2013.
59. Latthe P, Latthe M, Say L, et al: WHO systematic review of prevalence of chronic pelvic pain: a neglected reproductive health morbidity. *BMC Public Health* 6:177, 2006.
60. Lavelle R, Ford A: Global prevalence of and risk factors for irritable bowel syndrome: a meta-analysis. *Clin Gastroenterol Hepatol* 10(7):712–721, 2012.
61. Laycock J, Jerwood D: Pelvic floor muscle assessment: The PERFECT scheme. *Physiotherapy* 87(12):631–642, 2001.
62. Lien KC, Mooney B, DeLancey JO, et al: Levator ani muscle stretch induced by simulated vaginal birth. *Obstet Gynecol* 103:31–40, 2004.
63. Longstreth G, Thompson G, Chey W, et al: Functional bowel disorders. *Gastroenterology* 130:1480–1491, 2006.
64. Lucus K: Latent myofascial trigger points: their effect on muscle activation and movement efficiency. *J Bodyw Mov Ther* 8(3):160–166, 2003.
65. Mariotti G, Sciarra A, Gentilucci A, et al: Early recovery of urinary continence after radical prostatectomy using early pelvic floor electrical stimulation and biofeedback associated treatment. *J Urol* 181:1788–1793, 2009.
66. Masatsune Y, Neumann P, Gill V: Pelvic floor and abdominal muscle interaction: EMG activity and intraabdominal pressure. *Int Urogynecol J* 13:125–132, 2002.
67. McGowin L, Escott D, Luker K, et al: Is chronic pelvic pain a comfortable diagnosis for primary care practitioners: a qualitative study. *BMC Fam Pract* 11:7, 2010.
68. Melville JL, Katon W, Delaney K, et al: Urinary incontinence in US women: a population-based study. *Arch Intern Med* 165:537–542, 2005.
69. Meseguer A, Fernandez-de-las-Penas C, Navarro-Poza J, et al: Immediate effects of the strain counter-strain technique in local pain evoked by tender points in the upper trapezius muscle. *Clin Chiropr* 9:112–118, 2006.
70. Messelink B, Benson T, Berghamans B, et al: Standardization of terminology of pelvic floor muscle function and dysfunction: report from the pelvic floor clinical assessment group of the International Continence Society. *Neurourol Urodyn* 24:374–380, 2005.
71. Miller J, Kasper C, Sampselle C: Review of muscle physiology with application to pelvic muscle exercise. *Urol Nurs* 14:92–97, 1994.
72. Milsom I, Altman D, Lapitan MC, et al: *Epidemiology of UI and faecal incontinence and pelvic organ prolapse. Proceedings of 4th International Consultation on Incontinence, July 5–8 2008*, vol 1, 2009, Health Publications Ltd, pp 37–111.
73. Moore K, Dalley A: *Clinically Oriented Anatomy*, ed 4, Philadelphia, 1999, Lippincott, Williams & Wilkins.
74. Montoya T, Calver L, Carrick KS, et al: Anatomic relationships of the pudendal nerve branches. *Am J Obstet Gynecol* 205:504–505, 2011.

75. Murata Y, Ogata S, Ikeda Y: An unusual cause of sciatic pain as a result of the dynamic motion of the obturator internus muscle. *Spine J* 9:16–18, 2009.
76. Parks AG, Porter NH, Melzak J: Experimental study of the reflex mechanism controlling muscles of floor. *Dis Colon Rectum* 5:407–414, 1962.
77. Pastore E, Katzman W: Recognizing myofascial pelvic pain in the female patient with chronic pelvic pain. *J Obstet Gynecol Neonatal Nurs* 41:680–691, 2012.
78. Persu C, Chapple CR, Cauni V, et al: Pelvic organ prolapse quantification system (POP-Q)—a new era in pelvic organ prolapse staging. *J Med Life* 4(1):75–81, 2011.
79. Pichon B, Bloch F: Management of detrusor sphincter dyssynergia. *Curr Bladder Dysfunct Rep* 8(2):114–122, 2013.
80. Prem V, Rao B, Gundmi A: Comparison of Jacobson's progressive muscle relaxation and diaphragmatic breathing on cardiorespiratory parameters in health adults—a randomized cross-over trial. *Indian J Physiother Occup Ther* 5(3):117–121, 2011.
81. Rao SS: Dyssynergic defecation. *Gastroenterol Clin North Am* 30:97–114, 2001.
82. Rao SS, Tuteja AK, Vellema T, et al: Dyssynergic defecation: demographics, symptoms, stool patterns, and quality of life. *J Clin Gasteroenterol* 38:680–685, 2004.
83. Richardson C, Jull G, Hodges P, et al: *Therapeutic Exercise for Spinal Segmental Stabilization in Low Back Pain*, Edinburgh, 1999, Churchill Livingstone.
84. Sahrmann SA: *Diagnosis and Treatment of Movement Impairment Syndromes*, St Louis, 2002, Mosby.
85. Samhan A, Abd-Elhalim N, Elnegmy E, et al: The effect of transcutaneous electrical nerve stimulation in the treatment of chronic pelvic pain syndrome: an evidence based electromyographic studies. *Indian J Physiother Occup Ther* 5(3):14–17, 2011.
86. Sand PK, Richardson DA, Staskin DR, et al: Pelvic floor electrical stimulation in the treatment of genuine stress incontinence: a multicenter, placebo-controlled trial. *Am J Obstet Gynecol* 173(1):26–35, 1995.
87. Sapsford RR, Hodges PW, Richardson CA, et al: Co-activation of the abdominal and pelvic floor muscles during voluntary exercises. *Neurourol Urodyn* 20:31–42, 2001.
88. Schmidt F, Santos V: Prevalence of constipation in the general adult population. *J Wound Ostomy Continence Nurs* 41(1):70–76, 2014.
89. Schreiner L, Guimarães dos Santos T, Anton de Souza A, et al: Electrical stimulation for urinary incontinence in women: a systematic review. *Int Braz J Urol* 39:454–464, 2013.
90. Selkow N, Grindstaff T, Cross K, et al: Short-term effect of muscle energy technique on pain in individuals with non-specific lumbopelvic pain: a pilot study. *J Man Manip Ther* 17(1):14–18, 2009.
91. Smith M, Russell A, Hodges P: Disorders of breathing and continence have a stronger association with back pain than obesity and physical activity. *Aust J Physiother* 52:11–16, 2006.
92. Somprasong S, Mekhora K, Vachalathiti R, et al: Effects of strain counter-strain and stretching techniques in active myofascial pain syndrome. *J Phys Ther Sci* 23:889–893, 2011.
93. Steege JE, Metzger DA, Levy BS: *Chronic Pelvic Pain: An Integrated Approach*, Philadelphia, 1998, Saunders.
94. Taher M, Hassan A, Amansour A: Effect of pelvic floor electrical stimulation and biofeedback on the recovery of urinary continence after radical prostatectomy. *Türk Fiz Tıp Rehab Derg* 58:170–176, 2012.
95. Tanner P, Lindsay J, Kerrison S, et al: Prevention of vaginal stenosis after treatment for gynecologic cancer. *Aust J Cancer Nurs* 12(1):21–27, 2011.
96. Teo JS, Briffa NK, Devine A, et al: Do sleep problems or urinary incontinence predict falls in elderly women? *Aust J Physiother* 52:19–24, 2006.
97. Terlikowski R, Dobrzycka B, Kinalski M, et al: Transvaginal electrical stimulation with surface-EMG biofeedback in managing stress urinary incontinence in women of premenopausal age: a double-blind, placebo-controlled, randomized clinical trial. *Int Urogynecol J* 24:1631–1638, 2013.
98. Toglia MR: Pathology of anorectal dysfunction. *Obstet Gynecol Clin North Am* 25(4):771–781, 1998.
99. Vlemming A, De Vries H, Mens J, et al: Possible role of the long dorsal sacroiliac ligament in women with peripartum pelvic pain. *Acta Obstet Gynecol Scand* 81:430–436, 2002.
100. Weissmann R: Considerations with regard to biomechanics related to myofascial trigger point therapy. *Physiotherapie* 35(10):13–21, 2000.
101. Wilder E: *The Gynecological Manual*. American Physical Therapy Association, Section on Women's Health, 2000.
102. Wilson E, Payton O, Donegan-Shoaf L, et al: Muscle energy technique in patients with acute low back pain: a pilot clinical trial. *J Orthop Sports Phys Ther* 33(9):502–512, 2003.
103. Wu JM, Stinnett S, Jackson RA, et al: Prevalence and incidence of urinary incontinence in a diverse population of women with noncancerous gynecologic conditions. *Female Pelvic Med Reconstr Surg* 16:284–289, 2010.
104. Yamanishi T, Mizuno T, Watanabe M, et al: Randomized, placebo controlled study of electrical stimulation with pelvic floor muscle training for severe urinary incontinence after radical prostatectomy. *J Urol* 184:2007–2012, 2010.
105. Zivkovic V, Lazovic M, Vlajkovic M, et al: Diaphragmatic breathing exercises and pelvic floor retraining in children with dysfunctional voiding. *Eur J Phys Rehabil Med* 48(3):413–421, 2012.
106. Zondervan KT, Yudkin PL, Vessey MP, et al: Prevalence and incidence of chronic pelvic pain in primary care. *Br J Obstet Gynaecol* 106:1149–1155, 1999.

REVIEW QUESTIONS

Multiple Choice

1. What is the recommended number of Kegel exercises one should perform in a day?
   a. 10 to 20
   b. 30 to 80
   c. 50 to 100
   d. 200 to 300
2. Which of the following are possible causes of coccygodynia?
   a. Coccygeal malalignment
   b. Levator ani syndrome
   c. Myofascial trigger points of the coccygeal muscle
   d. All of the above
3. What is the most appropriate position to prescribe for Kegel exercises for a patient with a pelvic floor strength of 3/5?
   a. Modified standing
   b. Supine
   c. Prone
   d. Hook lying
4. All of the following muscles are part of the urogenital triangle in the superficial layer of muscles in the pelvic floor except:
   a. Bulbocavernosus.
   b. Bulbospongiosus.
   c. Iliococcygeus.
   d. Superficial transverse perineal.
5. The pelvic diaphragm consists of which of the following muscles?
   a. Pubococcygeus, iliococcygeus, coccygeus, superficial transverse perineal
   b. Levator ani, coccygeus, obturator internus, piriformis
   c. Pubococcygeus, iliococcygeus, coccygeus
   d. Levator ani, superficial transverse perineal, bulbocavernosus

6. Which combination of tonic and phasic fibers make up the pelvic floor musculature?
   a. 70% tonic, 30% phasic
   b. 30% tonic, 70% phasic
   c. 60% tonic, 40% phasic
   d. 40% tonic, 60% phasic
7. Which of the following describes an involuntary loss of urine with an increase in intraabdominal pressure?
   a. Functional urinary incontinence
   b. Urge urinary incontinence
   c. Overflow incontinence
   d. Mixed urinary incontinence
8. Which of the following signs and symptoms should alert the PTA to refer the patient back to his or her physician immediately?
   a. Numbness in the perineum
   b. Fever
   c. Urinary incontinence
   d. Constipation
9. All of the following positions for performing Kegel exercises are appropriate for a patient with a pelvic floor strength of 2/5 or less except:
   a. Inverted
   b. Modified standing
   c. Hook lying
   d. Prone
10. Which of the following positions for performing Kegel exercises would be most appropriate for a patient with a pelvic floor strength of 4/5?
    a. Hook lying
    b. Modified standing
    c. Squatting
    d. Supine
11. The PTA should consider a possible pelvic floor dysfunction for a patient with which of the following conditions?
    a. Piriformis syndrome
    b. Sacroiliac joint dysfunction
    c. LBP
    d. All of the above
12. Which of the following is the best physical therapy intervention for urinary incontinence?
    a. Pelvic floor strengthening
    b. Vaginal weights
    c. Surface EMG
    d. Electrical stimulation
13. Which of the following describes the involuntary loss of urine immediately after voiding, usually after leaving or rising from the toilet?
    a. Stress urinary incontinence
    b. Urgency urinary incontinence
    c. Nocturnal enuresis
    d. Postmicturition dribble
14. For patients in which of the following stages of POP would physical therapy intervention be most appropriate?
    a. 1 to 2
    b. 2 to 3
    c. 3 to 4
    d. Physical therapy intervention does not help and should not be considered for treating POP.
15. Constipation is most likely caused by which of the following:
    a. Pelvic floor dyssynergia
    b. Chronic pelvic pain
    c. IC
    d. Pelvic floor weakness

Short Answer

16. What are the four functions of the pelvic floor?
17. What muscles make up the pelvic diaphragm?
18. What are the five main categories of pelvic floor dysfunction?
19. Define the acronym PERFECT as it is used for the pelvic floor.
20. What exercise should the PTA ensure that the patient with a hypertonic pelvic floor can perform?

Fill in the Blank

21. A prolapse of the lower anterior vaginal wall involving the urethra only is called a ____________.
22. A prolapse of the lower posterior vaginal wall involving the rectum is called a ____________.
23. A prolapse where the most distal portion of prolapse protrudes >1 cm below the hymen but no farther than 2 cm less than the total vaginal length is measured as a grade ____ on the Pelvic Organ Prolapse Quantification classification system.
24. A bladder condition that usually consists of symptoms including recurring pelvic pain, pressure, or discomfort in the bladder and pelvic region, and urinary frequency and urgency is called ____________.
25. The ____________ score is used for pelvic floor strength and endurance assessment.

True/False

26. Pelvic floor strengthening is appropriate for all pelvic floor dysfunctions.
27. The majority of the pelvic floor is innervated by the pudendal nerve.
28. Coccygodynia can be caused by trigger points or muscle spasms of the levator ani muscle group.
29. Dyspareunia is pain with menstruation.
30. According to current studies, the minimum repetitions of Kegel exercises a patient should do per day to maintain pelvic floor function is 300.

Part VI

Topics in Orthopedics

This section on special topics includes a chapter on orthopedic pharmacology that presents key elements, terms, and definitions related to antiinflammatory and antibiotic agents to provide the student physical therapist assistant (PTA) and practicing clinician with a cursory introduction to the basics of orthopedic pharmacology. New to the fourth edition is a chapter on musculoskeletal imaging. Although musculoskeletal imaging is not part of the job of a PTA, the PTA should have an adequate understanding of the basics of imaging and indications for referral to the appropriate medical professional who can order images.

Orthopedic physical therapy interventions involving the PTA do not divest interest in or responsibility for the care of the whole patient. Knowledge concerning neurovascular anatomy and healing of various organ systems of the body is essential in the delivery of physical therapy procedures. An appreciation of antibacterial medications and antiinflammatory agents aids the PTA in understanding the complexity and interdependence of medications and orthopedic health care.

Chapter 28 is presented to broaden the focus of specific PTA education and expose the student to concepts of prophylactic antibacterial medications used to treat orthopedic infections, classifications of antibiotic medications and related organisms, and nonsteroidal antiinflammatory drugs (NSAIDs) and corticosteroids related to acute and chronic pain and inflammation. In the day-to-day delivery of physical therapy, the PTA encounters many orthopedic conditions requiring medications to target specific bacterial organisms and antiinflammatory agents to control pain and swelling. A basic understanding of drug administration routes and bioavailability as well as the use of NSAIDs versus the use of corticosteroids allows the student and clinician to enhance patient care more efficiently and effectively.

A practicing PTA may commonly see a patient who has had a significant setback in the rehabilitation process. This setback may be due to an acute traumatic reason but can also occur as a result of repetitive microtrauma. Multiple musculoskeletal problems can require imaging at one time or another to understand the condition better, rule out a potentially more serious problem, or allow peace of mind after a perplexing injury that does not seem to be responding in an appropriate or timely manner. Chapter 29 introduces the student and clinician to the basics of imaging, which may allow the PTA one day to suggest more easily further diagnostic testing to the supervising therapist or physician.

Chapter 28

Concepts of Orthopedic Pharmacology

LaDonna S. Hale

CHAPTER OUTLINE

LEARNING OBJECTIVES

1. Discuss pharmacokinetic concepts, including absorption, distribution, metabolism, excretion half-life, and duration of action, and their relationship and significance to rehabilitation therapies.
2. Discuss pharmacodynamic concepts, including the dose-response relationship, therapeutic window, adverse drug reactions, toxicity, tolerance, withdrawal, and addiction.
3. List the general principles of safe medication use and the role of the physical therapist assistant in optimizing patient safety.
4. Discuss general principles of treatment and prevention of orthopedic infection, including why such infections are difficult to treat and the importance of antibiotic compliance.
5. Discuss the analgesics best suited for different types of pain.
6. Discuss how opioids work differently from antiinflammatory analgesics in the treatment of pain.
7. Discuss common side effects and precautions associated with opioids, acetaminophen, nonsteroidal antiinflammatory drugs, cyclooxygenase-2 inhibitors, and corticosteroids.
8. Discuss the risk of acetaminophen overdoses during pain management.

KEY TERMS

Absorption
Adverse drug reaction (ADR)
Analgesic
Duration of action
Half-life
Neuropathic pain
Nociceptive pain
Pharmacodynamics
Pharmacokinetics

BASIC PRINCIPLES OF PHARMACOLOGY AND SAFE MEDICATION USE

Knowledge concerning the interaction between medications and the treatment and maintenance of orthopedic health is essential for the safe and effective application of rehabilitation interventions. This chapter aids the student and practicing physical therapist assistant (PTA) in providing optimal care through an introduction to key concepts of orthopedic pharmacology. Infections, pain and inflammation, and osteoporosis can significantly affect recovery and optimal application of physical therapy.

PHARMACOKINETICS

The term ***pharmacokinetics*** is used to describe what the body does to a medication. The four pharmacokinetic phases are (1) **absorption**, (2) distribution, (3) metabolism, and (4) excretion.[6]

> **Important Concepts**
>
> The term *pharmacokinetics* is used to describe what the body does to a medication. The four pharmacokinetic phases are (1) absorption, (2) distribution, (3) metabolism, and (4) excretion.

Absorption describes how the medication moves from its site of administration into the systemic circulation (into the bloodstream). Common routes of administration are listed in Table 28-1. Most medications must move from the site of administration into the systemic circulation to be effective. Others, such as topical creams or inhalers, may provide therapeutic benefits through a localized effect. Although systemic absorption may not be necessary for effectiveness of topically applied medications, it can occur and result in side effects. For example, long-term use of high-dose inhaled corticosteroids to treat asthma has

TABLE 28-1 Common Routes of Administration

Route	Description	Example Medications
Oral (PO)	Swallowed; uses the gastrointestinal tract	Most commonly used route of administration in U.S.; tablets, capsules, oral liquids
Sublingual (SL)	Under the tongue; medication rapidly absorbs into systemic circulation	Nitroglycerin tablets for chest pain
Rectal	Administered through the rectum; some absorb into systemic circulation, others provide a local laxative effect	Glycerin suppositories (laxatives); promethazine (Phenergan) for nausea
Inhalation	Into the lungs	Bronchodilators for asthma, such as albuterol inhalers; corticosteroids for asthma such as flunisolide (AeroBid) inhalers
Intranasal	Into the nose; some absorb into systemic circulation, others provide a local effect	Systemic absorption required for effectiveness: calcitonin (Miacalcin) nasal spray for osteoporosis Localized effect: intranasal decongestants (Afrin)
Intravenous (IV)	Directly into the veins; most rapid onset of action	Common route of administration in hospitals; morphine, antibiotics
Intramuscular (IM)	Into the muscle	Some vaccinations; penicillin G benzathine
Subcutaneous (SQ, SC, SubCut)	Into the subcutaneous layer of skin	Insulin; teriparatide (Fortéo) for osteoporosis
Intraarticular	Into the joint space; causes a localized effect within the joint; some systemic absorption may occur	Triamcinolone; methylprednisolone; hyaluronic acid (Orthovisc, Hyalgan) for osteoarthritis
Epidural	Into the epidural space (within the spinal column but outside the dura mater)	Fentanyl; lidocaine; corticosteroids
Transdermal (TD)	Medication patches whereby the medication moves through the skin into systemic circulation	Patches including nicotine, nitroglycerin, clonidine, contraceptives, fentanyl, and lidocaine
Topical	Creams and ointments applied to the skin with an expected localized effect; systemic absorption may or may not occur	Creams and ointments including Ben-Gay cream, capsaicin (Zostrix), hydrocortisone

been shown to result in enough systemic absorption to increase the risk of developing osteoporosis.[11,14]

The rate and extent of drug absorption through the skin can be dramatically increased by application of heat; heat-generating modalities (e.g., heating pads, ultrasound, infrared lamps, warm hydrotherapy) should not be applied near transdermal medication patches. Electromagnetic (e.g., ultraviolet radiation, lasers, diathermy) and electrical current modalities (e.g., transcutaneous electrical nerve stimulation) also should not be used near medication patches because many patches have metallic backings that conduct electrical currents, leading to significant heat generation and burns.[2]

Important Concepts

Application of heat can dramatically increase the rate and extent of drug absorption through the skin; heat-generating and electromagnetic modalities should not be applied near transdermal medication patches.

Distribution describes movement of the medication from the bloodstream into various areas of the body such as the central nervous system (CNS), breast milk, and adipose (fat) tissue. This concept can be helpful in understanding medication actions and side effects. For example, opioid pain relievers act on the CNS to relieve pain; an opioid is most effective if it can easily distribute into the CNS. Only antibiotics with good distribution into bone tissue would be effective in treating osteomyelitis.

Medications are cleared from the body through metabolism, excretion, or both. Metabolism is the biotransformation or chemical alteration of the medication. The by-product of drug metabolism is called a *metabolite*. Through metabolism, some medications are inactivated, whereas others remain active (active metabolite) but are more water soluble for easier elimination by the kidneys. Generally, metabolism occurs in the liver, but it can occur through enzymatic processes in the kidneys, lungs, and bloodstream. Differences in drug response, side effects, and safe dose can be greatly affected by genetic differences in drug metabolism.[20]

Excretion describes elimination of the medication without prior metabolism (excreted unchanged) or, more commonly, elimination of the metabolites. Generally, excretion occurs through the kidneys (renal excretion, urine), but it also occurs through the gastrointestinal tract (feces), lungs (breath), and skin (sweat).

The rate at which a drug is cleared from the body is referred to as ***half-life.*** Technically speaking, half-life is the amount of time it takes to reduce the concentration of the drug in the body by half. Drug half-lives can range from seconds to days. Anything that slows a drug's clearance lengthens its half-life. Liver metabolism and renal clearance are slower in older adults (>70 years old) compared with younger adults and likewise for persons with acute or chronic liver or kidney disease.[6] The most common type of clinically significant drug-drug interaction occurs when the presence of one drug slows the metabolism of a second drug.[20] When drug clearance is decreased for any reason and the daily dose is not also decreased, drug accumulation and toxicity can occur.

A medication's **duration of action** (the length of time it is active in the body) is related to its half-life. Drugs with a long half-life have a long duration of action. Medications with a short duration of action usually require multiple daily administrations, three or four times daily, whereas medications with longer durations of action may require dosing only once or twice daily. One way medications can overcome a short duration of action is if they are formulated as a sustained-release product. A sustained-release product is usually in tablet or capsule form and is specially designed to dissolve very slowly in the intestines. By dissolving gradually over 12 or 24 hours, its effects last longer. In general, sustained-release products should not be chewed, crushed, or broken open. Doing so can destroy the product's sustained-release properties, causing the entire dosage to be released at once.

PHARMACODYNAMICS

The term ***pharmacodynamics*** is used to describe what the medication does to the body. It is a study of the relationship between the amount of drug in the body and the response observed.[6] Pharmacodynamics include a wide variety of principles, such as the dose-response relationship, therapeutic window, adverse reactions, and toxicity.

The dose-response relationship describes the relationship between the amount of drug in the body and its expected effectiveness and likelihood and severity of side effects (e.g., the higher the dose, the more side effects seen). This relationship is closely tied to the concept of therapeutic window. A drug's therapeutic window may be described as wide or narrow. The window is defined as the minimum drug concentration needed for the drug to show effectiveness, without causing toxicity in the patient. Penicillins and most cephalosporin antibiotics have wide therapeutic windows. Drugs with narrow therapeutic windows include the anticoagulant warfarin (commonly used after orthopedic surgeries) and antiseizure medications (commonly used to treat phantom pain after amputation or diabetic **neuropathic pain**).

The term ***adverse drug reaction (ADR)*** describes any unintended effect of the medication including an exaggerated medication response; another term for this is *side effect*. An example of an exaggerated response is extreme hypotension after receiving a medication for high blood pressure. Certain ADRs may be particularly problematic in orthopedic patients, including medications that may reduce safety or increase fall risk (e.g., orthostatic hypotension, dizziness, blurred vision, hypoglycemia, ataxia, gait abnormalities) or medications that affect cognitive function.

Important Concepts

Certain medication-related side effects may reduce safety by increasing fall risk and causing cardiovascular side effects.

Many medications cause cardiovascular side effects that may complicate exertional activity by increasing heart rate (tachycardia) or blood pressure (hypertension), by blunting the expected exercise-induced increase in heart rate, or by reducing heart rate (bradycardia). The term *toxicity* is often used interchangeably with ADR or side effect, but it is most accurate to reserve this term for situations where the serum concentrations have exceeded normal levels.

Tolerance occurs when the reaction to a drug diminishes over time. Tolerance can occur to both the benefits of a medication (making it less effective over time) and the ADRs (making it better tolerated over time).[3] Withdrawal symptoms indicate physical dependency and are expected to occur with certain medications when used over a prolonged period. Withdrawal symptoms are generally the opposite of the pharmacologic effects of the medication. For example, one withdrawal symptom of a medication used to reduce blood pressure would be hypertension.

Psychological dependency, also called *addiction,* occurs with certain medications such as opioid **analgesics,** amphetamines, and benzodiazepine sleep aids as well as other substances with abuse potential, including cocaine, heroin, alcohol, caffeine, and nicotine. Withdrawal symptoms contribute to the development of addiction in that the patient continues to use the substance to avoid the unpleasantness of the withdrawal symptoms; however, having withdrawal symptoms alone does not meet the definition of addiction. It is important to understand the difference between physical and psychological dependency.[3] Psychological dependency and addiction involve strong cravings and desires for the drug that overwhelm daily life. There is a loss of control over use of the drug, and use continues despite the negative impact on quality of life.[3,5] Drug addiction is most strongly associated with medications that rapidly distribute into the CNS causing high levels of euphoria and dysregulation of the neurotransmitters involved in the body's natural reward and pleasure centers.

PRINCIPLES OF SAFE MEDICATION USE

Although PTAs are not involved in the decision-making process regarding prescription and over-the-counter (OTC) medication use, having a general understanding of commonly used medications and knowing where to look for more information can help the PTA identify medication-related problems that should be brought to the attention of the prescriber or other health care team members. PTAs often spend more time with patients during therapy sessions than a prescriber spends with the patient during a typical office visit. This time may provide opportunities to identify problems with compliance, lack of medication knowledge, ADRs, and lack of drug effectiveness. Various drug information resources exist that can be helpful in providing information, such as mechanism of action, dosing, therapeutic uses, and ADRs. Table 28-2 lists helpful

TABLE 28-2 Helpful Drug Information Resources

Reference	Description
Epocrates; Skyscape; Medscape; Micromedex	Free online websites and free app downloads for mobile devices. Source of general drug and disease information; some have information on drug costs.
Drugs.com	Free online website. Source of general drug information, a drug-drug interaction checker, and pill identifier.
Drug Information Handbook (Publisher: Lexi-Comp, updated annually)	For purchase in paperback and download for mobile devices. Source of comprehensive drug information.
Drug Facts and Comparisons (Publisher: Facts and Comparisons)	For purchase in hardbound and download for mobile devices. Source of comprehensive and very detailed drug information.

drug information resources. Although such resources exist, the PTA must be cautious about providing specific information to the patient that would be considered outside the PTA's scope of practice.

The following general principles of safe medication use can be provided to all patients:

- Keep a current list of all medications including prescription, OTC, and herbal
- Keep medications in their original containers
- Never take someone else's medication
- Take medications exactly as directed
- Do not start or stop medications without consulting the prescriber
- Report any new symptoms to the prescriber
- Don't chew, crush, or break any capsules or tablets unless instructed
- When measuring liquid medications, use only the measuring device provided
- Be knowledgeable about the medications
- Ask questions when things are unclear[9]

Important Concepts

The following general principles of safe medication use can be provided to all patients:

- Keep a current list of all medications including prescription, OTC, and herbal
- Keep medications in their original containers
- Never take someone else's medication
- Take medications exactly as directed
- Do not start or stop medications without consulting the prescriber
- Report any new symptoms to the prescriber
- Don't chew, crush, or break any capsules or tablets unless instructed
- When measuring liquid medications, use only the measuring device provided
- Be knowledgeable about the medications
- Ask questions when things are unclear

TABLE 28-3 Common Antibiotics Used to Treat and Prevent Orthopedic Infections*

Drug Class	Specific Antibiotics
Penicillins	• Amoxicillin (Amoxil) oral • Dicloxacillin (Dynapen) oral • Nafcillin (Nafcil, Unipen) injection • Oxacillin (Prostaphlin) injection, oral • Penicillin (various brands) injection, oral
Cephalosporins	• Cefaclor (Ceclor) oral • Cefadroxil (Duricef) oral • Cefazolin (Ancef, Kefzol) injection • Cefixime (Suprax) oral • Cefpodoxime (Vantin) oral • Cetazidime (Fortaz) injection • Ceftriaxone (Rocephin) injection • Cephalexin (Keflex) oral
Tetracyclines	• Doxycycline (Vibramycin) oral • Minocycline (Minocin) oral • Tetracycline (Sumycin) oral
Antifolate (sulfonamides)	• Sulfamethoxazole/trimethoprim (Bactrim, Septra) oral
Quinolones	• Ciprofloxacin (Cipro) injection, oral • Levofloxacin (Levaquin) injection, oral • Ofloxacin (Floxin) injection, oral
Miscellaneous	• Clindamycin (Cleocin) injection, oral • Gentamicin (Garamycin) injection • Vancomycin (Vancocin) injection

*This is not an all-inclusive list of antibiotics.

MEDICATIONS TO TREAT AND PREVENT ORTHOPEDIC INFECTIONS

Antibiotic use in the treatment and prevention of orthopedic related infections is common. Antibiotics are medications with the ability to kill or inhibit growth of bacteria. Common examples of antibiotics used in the hospital and outpatient orthopedic settings are listed in Table 28-3. Orthopedic infections can result in slowed recovery, permanent joint damage, amputation, nonunion in cases of fracture, removal of implanted hardware, and death as a result of sepsis. When selecting appropriate antibiotics, the type of documented or suspected bacterial pathogens, the ability of the drug to distribute adequately to the site of infection, patient allergy history, side effects, and cost are taken into consideration. Because the risk of infection after orthopedic surgeries is high, antibiotics are routinely administered before the procedure to reduce the risk of infection-related complications. The use of antibiotics to prevent an infection is referred to as *prophylaxis*.

Compliance with the prescribed antibiotic regimen is essential to reduce the risk of bacterial resistance and to improve outcomes. Patients taking oral antibiotics should take the medication exactly as instructed for the full course of therapy. It is common for patients to stop taking their antibiotic when they start to feel better (e.g., fever resolves, pain at the site of infection is reduced). Stopping the antibiotic too early can allow the infection to return or increase the risk of developing bacterial resistance to that antibiotic. To ensure optimal oral absorption, dosing instructions should be followed carefully. For example, some antibiotics should be taken on an empty stomach, defined as at least 1 hour before or 2 hours after a meal; others should be taken with meals to avoid stomach upset; others should not be taken within 2 hours of calcium-containing antacids or milk.

Another important concept regarding antibiotic compliance is around-the-clock dosing. To achieve steady blood levels of the antibiotic at the site of infection, antibiotics should be dosed at regularly spaced intervals throughout the day. For example, an antibiotic ordered to be taken three times daily should not be taken at breakfast, lunch, and supper, but rather divided evenly throughout the day every 8 hours. When the concentration of antibiotic falls below the minimum level needed to kill or inhibit bacterial growth, the weaker pathogen strains will be affected, leaving the strong pathogens to replicate and grow in numbers. Bacterial resistance can quickly result. Skipping doses creates a similar problem.

The PTA can improve outcomes by discussing with the patient the importance of following antibiotic instructions carefully and completing the full course of therapy as prescribed and referring noncompliance issues to the appropriate health care provider. Antibiotic compliance is important for all orthopedic patients but is especially important for patients with reduced peripheral circulation (e.g., patients with peripheral vascular disease and diabetes). Delivery of antibiotics to the site of infection may be particularly reduced in these populations. The PTA can also help prevent the spread of infection through thorough hand washing and adequately cleaning rehabilitation equipment between patients.

MEDICATIONS TO TREAT PAIN AND INFLAMMATION

Effective treatment of pain and inflammation not only reduces suffering but also speeds healing after injury. Patients experiencing inadequately treated pain often have compromised mobility, restricted activities of daily living, disturbed sleep, and reduced quality of life. As a result, they may be unable to participate in beneficial physical therapy to the fullest potential.

Pain is often undertreated. Pain management is heavily associated with biases related to socioeconomic status, race, culture, age, and gender. Some prescribers do not understand treatment of different types of pain; pain is not always considered to be a treatment priority; and there are misperceptions regarding the risk of opioid addiction and side effects.

The Joint Commission has emphasized pain treatment as a responsibility of health care providers and a patient's right by requiring routine pain assessment as the "fifth vital sign." It is recommended that regular assessment and documentation of pain severity, functional ability, progress toward achieving therapeutic goals, and presence of ADRs occur in children and adults.[5,21]

An analgesic is any medication that reduces pain. There are three broad categories of oral and intravenous analgesics: (1) opioids, (2) acetaminophen, and (3) antiinflammatory agents. Appropriate analgesics are chosen based on the type of pain (acute/chronic, nociceptive/neuropathic, inflammatory/noninflammatory), level of pain, side effects, and cost.

Important Concepts

There are three broad categories of oral and intravenous analgesics: (1) opioids, (2) acetaminophen, and (3) antiinflammatory agents. Appropriate analgesics are chosen based on the type of pain, level of pain, side effects, and cost.

TYPES OF PAIN

Nociceptive pain results from actual tissue damage. Nociceptive pain may be inflammatory or noninflammatory or both. Examples include osteoarthritis, bone pain, muscle sprains, and postsurgical pain. This type of pain responds well to opioid analgesics, acetaminophen, and antiinflammatory agents. Nociceptive pain specifically caused by inflammation is referred to as *inflammatory pain*. As expected, inflammatory pain responds best to the antiinflammatory agents, including corticosteroids, nonsteroidal antiinflammatory drugs (NSAIDs), and cyclooxygenase (COX)-2 inhibitors. Examples of inflammatory pain include rheumatoid arthritis, muscle aches and sprains, and bursitis.

Neuropathic pain results from damage to or dysfunction of nerves. Examples include nerve compression, fibromyalgias, diabetic neuropathy, postherpetic neuralgia, spinal cord injuries, and phantom pain after amputation. Neuropathic pain is relatively resistant to opioids, acetaminophen, and antiinflammatory agents, although these medications may be helpful in certain cases. The most effective medication to treat neuropathic pain varies depending on the patient. Medications that tend to be most effective in treating neuropathic pain are medications that slow or block nerve conduction. Antidepressants such as duloxetine (Cymbalta), amitriptyline (Elavil), desipramine (Norpramin), and venlafaxine (Effexor) are commonly used, as are anticonvulsants such as pregabalin (Lyrica), gabapentin (Neurontin), and carbamazepine (Tegretol). Effective topical products include lidocaine (Lidoderm) patch and capsaicin (Zostrix) cream.[12,18,19] The opioid analgesic tramadol (Ultram) is also often used to treat neuropathic pain because it is an opioid analgesic with additional antidepressantlike properties on nerve conduction.

Acute pain occurs after injury to the body and generally disappears when the injury heals. Chronic pain continues past the normal time of expected healing, which is assumed to be about 3 months.[5,10] Persistent pain, whether acute or chronic, generally responds better to around-the-clock dosing rather than on-demand dosing (also called *prn dosing* or *as-needed dosing*). Many types of inflammatory pain and neuropathic pain are chronic rather than acute. Opioids, acetaminophen, and NSAIDs have quick onset of action, within minutes to hours, whereas drugs for neuropathic pain, such as antidepressants and anticonvulsants, generally are not effective for several weeks.

Ideally, when treating persistent chronic pain, patients are prescribed medications with a long duration of action or sustained-release products or both to prevent the need for frequent daily administration. Patients may take a shorter acting analgesic or immediate-release product for breakthrough pain. *Breakthrough pain* is pain that occurs despite the use of regularly scheduled pain medications.[5]

OPIOID ANALGESICS

All opioid analgesics are chemically related to opium. Commonly used prescription opioid medications include morphine, oxycodone, hydrocodone, and codeine. See Appendix A for others. Opioid analgesics work within the CNS to block the transmission of pain and create a feeling of euphoria. Although pain is relieved, the underlying disease process or cause of the pain is not altered. Opioids are the most powerful medications available for treatment of nociceptive pain; they are also effective for some patients with neuropathic pain. Intravenous opioids are more commonly used for inpatient settings for moderate to severe acute pain. Oral agents can be used for mild, moderate, or severe acute or chronic pain in any setting. Opioids are sometimes administered epidurally to provide highly effective pain control directly on the spinal cord. Fentanyl (Duragesic) is available as a transdermal patch that provides control of severe, chronic pain.

Side effects of opioid analgesics include nausea and vomiting (take with food to minimize risk), allergic reactions, sedation, drowsiness, dizziness, constipation, hypotension and orthostatic hypotension, slowed heart rate, slowed respiration, impaired judgment, physical dependence, and addiction.[13] Several of these side effects reduce the patient's safety and may increase risk of falls and injury. Constipation caused by long-term opioid use is extremely common but can be treated and prevented with OTC stool softeners and mild laxatives including senna, docusate (Colace), and bisacodyl (Dulcolax) tablets.

Health care providers and patients may overestimate the risk of developing addiction when managing pain with opioids. This misperception can lead to inadequate pain control through underprescribing or underdosing and patients skipping doses or "taking as little as possible." The actual risk of developing opioid addiction following long-term use for medical management of pain is difficult to assess but has been estimated at approximately 0.2% (2 in 1000) for persons with no prior history of substance abuse, and 3.3% (33 in 1000) for the general population.[7]

> **Important Concepts**
>
> Health care providers and patients may overestimate the risk of developing addiction when managing pain with opioids. This misperception can lead to inadequate pain control through underprescribing or underdosing.

Tolerance and physical dependency are likely to occur with long-term use and are not equivalent to addiction. Although certain behaviors may seem like warning signs of addiction, the PTA should not make assumptions. Behaviors such as aggressively complaining about pain, occasionally taking more than prescribed, drug hoarding during periods of reduced pain, openly acquiring similar drugs from other medical resources, reporting unintended psychiatric effects, and resistance to changes in therapy are not signs of addiction. These behaviors are equally likely to occur in nonaddicted patients experiencing tolerance, an increase in pain level, poorly controlled pain, and anxiety related to a return of pain.[17] Prescribers must balance the legitimate medical need for opioids in patients with chronic pain with the possibility of addiction and abuse.[5]

ACETAMINOPHEN

Acetaminophen is the most commonly used OTC fever reducer and analgesic. It is effective for various noninflammatory, mild to moderate, acute, and chronic types of pain, including headaches, toothaches, sinus pain, back pain, and osteoarthritis. Its mechanism of action is unclear but likely involves inhibition of prostaglandins and COX and some CNS activity.[1] Although acetaminophen affects prostaglandins and COX, it does not have strong antiinflammatory properties and is not an NSAID.

Many oral opioids also contain acetaminophen. Acetaminophen tablets come in regular strength (325 mg per tablet) and extra strength (500 mg per tablet). Per OTC package instructions, the typical adult dose is two tablets every 4 to 6 hours for regular strength tablets, not to exceed 10 tablets (3250 mg) in a 24-hour period. The typical adult dose for extra-strength tablets is two tablets every 6 hours, not to exceed 6 tablets (3000 mg) in a 24-hour period.[13]

Acetaminophen has a strong record of safety when used at normal doses in healthy people. Compared with NSAIDs, acetaminophen is the safest OTC analgesic in patients with a history of gastrointestinal bleeding, congestive heart failure, and hypertension and in patients taking the oral anticoagulant warfarin (Coumadin). The major health concern with long-term acetaminophen use is hepatotoxicity (liver toxicity). An analysis of various national databases estimated that acetaminophen overdoses cause 56,000 emergency department visits, 26,000 hospitalizations, and 460 deaths annually in the United States, and the number of fatalities is increasing rapidly.[15] In 2009, the U.S. Food and Drug Administration convened a special meeting to discuss how to address this growing public health problem.[16]

The cause of liver toxicity involves the metabolism of acetaminophen. When used at normal dosages, most acetaminophen is metabolized into a nontoxic metabolite, and only 5% is metabolized into a liver toxic metabolite. Under normal circumstances, the body is able to detoxify this metabolite quickly, and no liver damage occurs. When used in excessive dosages or in the presence of preexisting liver impairment, the body cannot detoxify quickly enough.[6]

Patients taking acetaminophen on a long-term basis should be asked about alcohol use. Package instructions state: "If you consume three or more alcoholic drinks per day, ask your doctor whether you should take acetaminophen or other pain relievers/fever reducers."[13] The reason for this warning is that chronic alcohol use changes the metabolism of acetaminophen, resulting in a higher percentage of toxic metabolite production. Again, the body cannot detoxify quickly enough, and the risk of liver damage increases.

To minimize the risk of liver toxicity, dosages should not exceed 3250 mg/day for most healthy adults. This maximum "safe" dose may be too high for frail older adults, persons with chronic alcohol use, and patients with impaired liver function. These individuals should consult their prescriber to determine a safe acetaminophen dosage.[16]

More than 100 prescription and OTC products contain acetaminophen, including cough and cold products and some sleep aids (e.g., Tylenol PM). Persons prescribed opioids containing acetaminophen must be cautioned to check the labels of all prescription analgesics and OTC products to avoid accidental overdose. Some prescription analgesics use the abbreviation APAP (*N*-acetyl-para-aminophenol) on the label rather than acetaminophen; although this may save space on prescription labels, it can be confusing. For example, a prescription bottle labeled as "hydrocodone/APAP" contains hydrocodone and acetaminophen.

Important Concepts

More than 100 prescription and OTC products contain acetaminophen, including cough and cold products and some sleep aids. To minimize the risk of liver toxicity, the dosage for most healthy adults should not exceed 3250 mg/day.

NONSTEROIDAL ANTIINFLAMMATORY DRUGS

Four OTC NSAIDs are available: aspirin, ibuprofen, naproxen, and ketoprofen. Others are available by prescription only. Two NSAIDs are available in injection form, ketorolac and ibuprofen. OTC NSAIDs are very commonly used as fever reducers and analgesics. NSAIDs are effective for a variety of noninflammatory, mild to moderate, acute, and chronic types of pain, including headaches, back pain, and osteoarthritis, and are especially effective for inflammatory pain, including rheumatoid arthritis, carpal tunnel syndrome, acute gout, lateral and medial epicondylitis (tennis elbow and golf elbow), and bursitis.[4,6] NSAIDs can be found in various OTC products, including cough and cold products and some sleep aids (e.g., Advil PM). A few prescription opioid analgesics contain ibuprofen or aspirin (see Appendix A).

Aspirin is an NSAID, although it is often described separately because its therapeutic uses and side-effect profile are different from other NSAIDs. Aspirin should not be used in children because it can cause a rare, potentially fatal illness of childhood known as *Reye syndrome*. Aspirin has strong antiplatelet effects and is used in low dosages, 81 to 325 mg/day, to prevent ischemic strokes. Higher dosages (650 mg/dose) are required to achieve analgesic benefits.[13]

The mechanism of action of NSAIDs involves inhibition of prostaglandins and COX-1 and COX-2. Because of side effects, NSAIDs are not appropriate for all patients. NSAIDs should be avoided in patients with hypertension that is difficult to control, congestive heart failure, kidney disease, stomach ulcers, bleeding disorders, and alcoholism and in patients taking anticoagulants (e.g., warfarin).[6,13]

CYCLOOXYGENASE-2 INHIBITORS

Celecoxib (Celebrex) is the only COX-2 inhibitor on the market at the present time. Available by prescription only, celecoxib is used to treat the same types of pain as NSAIDs but with a lower risk of certain side effects. Similar to NSAIDs, celecoxib inhibits the production of prostaglandins by inhibiting the COX enzyme; however, it inhibits COX-2, but not COX-1. Inhibition of COX-2 results in the same antiinflammatory benefits as NSAIDs and side effects related to fluid accumulation (avoid in patients with hypertension, congestive heart failure, and kidney disease). Because celecoxib does not inhibit COX-1 to a large degree, it has fewer bleeding-related and stomach-related side effects, and it is safer than other NSAIDs in patients at risk for gastrointestinal bleeding, including patients older than 65 years of age, patients with bleeding disorders, patients with alcoholism, and patients taking anticoagulants.[4] Because of potential cross-sensitivity, persons allergic to sulfonamide antibiotics (e.g., sulfamethoxazole/trimethoprim [Bactrim and Septra]) should not be prescribed celecoxib.

CORTICOSTEROIDS

Corticosteroids (also called *glucocorticoids*) are produced naturally by the adrenal cortex and are involved in regulating metabolism of carbohydrates, proteins, and fats; inflammation; immune function; wound healing; and many other body systems. When used medically, corticosteroids have powerful antiinflammatory and immunosuppressant effects, making them useful in treating conditions such as rheumatoid arthritis, osteoarthritis, carpal tunnel syndrome, acute gout, lateral and medial epicondylitis, bursitis, and systemic lupus erythematosus. Corticosteroids may be administered orally, intravenously, or intraarticularly (into the joint). Commonly used corticosteroids are listed in Appendix A.

Intraarticular injections of corticosteroids (mainly methylprednisolone and triamcinolone) can provide excellent pain relief for joints with the advantage of local drug delivery and possibly fewer systemic side effects. After injection, the patient should minimize activity and stress on the joint for several days. Pain generally begins to decrease within 24 to 72 hours after injection, with maximum benefits in about 1 week. The analgesic and antiinflammatory benefits from a single injection may last 4 to 8 weeks.[6] The most commonly injected joint is the knee. Other joints may include the shoulder, wrist, temporomandibular joint, ankle, and elbow. Even localized drug delivery results in some systemic absorption.[8] Side effects from intraarticular administration are similar to side effects seen with oral and intravenous administration but are less frequent and include local side effects, such as osteonecrosis (loss of blood supply to the bone, resulting in tissue death), tendon rupture, and skin atrophy at the injection site.[6,8]

Because corticosteroids have such widespread effects on body systems, the side effects are broad and often significant, limiting their use. Corticosteroids can increase the risk for developing osteoporosis (loss of bone density). Calcium and vitamin supplementation are suggested for patients taking long-term systemic corticosteroids (>3 months); depending on the patient's bone mineral density and other risk factors, medications to treat or prevent osteoporosis may also be prescribed. Most commonly, these medications include bisphosphonates once weekly or once monthly (e.g., alendronate [Fosamax], risedronate [Actonel], ibandronate [Boniva]).

Corticosteroids can increase blood glucose (sugar) levels, especially in patients with diabetes or at high risk of diabetes. Because of their effects on metabolism of carbohydrates, proteins, and fats, high-dose corticosteroids can cause muscle myopathy, manifested as muscle weakness and abnormal fat distribution to the abdomen (potbelly), face (moon face), and upper back (buffalo hump). Other side effects of corticosteroids include edema, cataracts, glaucoma, stomach ulcers, insomnia, risk of infection, mood changes, and serious psychiatric disturbance.[6,8,13]

SUMMARY

Persons receiving rehabilitation therapy frequently take prescription and OTC medications to treat infection, pain, inflammation, and various other medical conditions. The PTA is not expected to be intimately familiar with the hundreds of commonly used medications on the market; however, knowledge of the medications discussed in this chapter is particularly applicable to the orthopedic setting. It is important to be aware of the potential impact that medications can have on rehabilitation and to understand the general principles of safe medication use. Because PTAs spend a significant amount of one-on-one time with patients, they can be important patient advocates in detecting medication-related problems, including noncompliance, lack of effectiveness, and side effects. The PTA can get assistance in clarifying potential medication issues from numerous easily accessible drug information resources as well as other members of the health care team.

GLOSSARY

Absorption: Manner in which a medication moves from its site of administration into the systemic circulation (into the bloodstream).

Adverse drug reaction (ADR): Any unintended effect of a medication including an exaggerated response; also termed *side effect.*

Analgesic: Any medication that reduces pain.

Duration of action: Length of time a drug is active in the body.

Half-life: Rate at which a drug is cleared from the body. Technical definition is the amount of time it takes to reduce the drug's blood concentration by half.

Neuropathic pain: Pain resulting from damage to or dysfunction of nerves.

Nociceptive pain: Pain resulting from tissue damage.

Pharmacodynamics: What a medication does to the body.

Pharmacokinetics: What the body does to a medication.

REFERENCES

1. Anderson BJ: Paracetamol (acetaminophen): mechanisms of action. *Paediatr Anaesth* 18:915–921, 2008.
2. Ball AM, Smith KM: Optimizing transdermal drug therapy. *Am J Health Syst Pharm* 65:1337–1346, 2008.
3. Ballantyne JC, LaForge KS: Opioid dependence and addiction during opioid treatment of chronic pain. *Pain* 129:235–255, 2007.
4. Chen YF, Jobanputra P, Barton P, et al: Cyclooxygenase-2 selective non-steroidal anti-inflammatory drugs (etodolac, meloxicam, celecoxib, rofecoxib, etoricoxib, valdecoxib and lumiracoxib) for osteoarthritis and rheumatoid arthritis: a systematic review and economic evaluation. *Health Technol Assess* 12:1–278, iii, 2008.
5. Chou R, Fanciullo GJ, Fine PG, et al: Clinical guidelines for the use of chronic opioid therapy in chronic noncancer pain. *J Pain* 10:113–130, 2009.
6. DiPiro JT, Talbert RL, Yee GC, et al: *Pharmacotherapy: A Pathophysiologic Approach*, ed 8, New York, 2011, McGraw-Hill.
7. Fishbain DA, Cole B, Lewis J, et al: What percentage of chronic nonmalignant pain patients exposed to chronic opioid analgesic therapy develop abuse/addiction and/or aberrant drug-related behaviors? A structured evidence-based review. *Pain Med* 9:444–459, 2008.
8. Habib GS: Systemic effects of intra-articular corticosteroids. *Clin Rheumatol* 28:749–756, 2009.
9. Institute for Safe Medication Practices (ISMP): *General advice on safe medication use* (website). www.ismp.org/consumers/brochure.asp. Accessed September 5, 2013.
10. International Association for the Study of Pain, Subcommittee on Taxonomy: Classification of chronic pain. Descriptions of chronic pain syndromes and definitions of pain terms. *Pain Suppl* 3:S1–S22, 6, 1986.
11. Israel E, Banerjee TR, Fitzmaurice GM, et al: Effects of inhaled glucocorticoids on bone density in premenopausal women. *N Engl J Med* 345:941–947, 2001.
12. Kroenke K, Krebs EE, Bair MJ: Pharmacotherapy of chronic pain: a synthesis of recommendations from systematic reviews. *Gen Hosp Psychiatry* 31:206–219, 2009.
13. Lacy CF, Armstrong LL, Goldman MP, et al: *Drug Information Handbook*, ed 22, Hudson, Ohio, 2013, Lexi-Comp Inc, pp *2013–2014*.
14. Lipworth BJ: Systemic adverse effects of inhaled corticosteroid therapy: a systematic review and meta-analysis. *Arch Intern Med* 159:941–955, 1999.
15. Nourjah P, Ahmad SR, Karwoski C, et al: Estimates of acetaminophen (Paracetomal)-associated overdoses in the United States. *Pharmacoepidemiol Drug Saf* 15:298–405, 2006.
16. Food and Drug Administration, HHS: Organ-specific warnings; internal analgesic, antipyretic, and antirheumatic drug products for over-the counter human use; final monograph. Final rule. *Fed Regist* 74(81):19385–19409, 2009.
17. Portenoy RK: Opioid therapy for chronic nonmalignant pain: current status. In Fields HL, Liebeskind JC, editors: *Progress in Pain Research and Management*, vol 1, *Pharmacological Approaches to the Treatment of Chronic Pain: New Concepts and Critical Issues*, Seattle, 1994, IASP Publications, pp 247–287.
18. Saarto T, Wiffen PJ: Antidepressants for neuropathic pain. *Cochrane Database Syst Rev* (4):CD005454, 2007.
19. Wiffen PJ, Collins S, McQuay HJ, et al: Anticonvulsant drugs for acute and chronic pain. *Cochrane Database Syst Rev* (3):CD001133, 2005.
20. Wilkinson GR: Drug metabolism and variability among patients in drug response. *N Engl J Med* 352:2211–2221, 2005.
21. World Health Organization: *Persisting Pain in Children: WHO Guidelines on the Pharmacological Treatment of Persisting Pain in Children with Medical Illnesses*, Geneva, Switzerland, 2012, World Health Organization Press.

REVIEW QUESTIONS

Multiple Choice

1. What is the maximum amount of acetaminophen that a healthy adult patient should take in a 24-hour period?
   a. 1500 mg
   b. 2050 mg
   c. 3250 mg
   d. 4000 mg
2. Which of the following pain relievers has little to no antiinflammatory activity?
   a. Acetaminophen
   b. Corticosteroids
   c. COX-2 inhibitors
   d. NSAIDs
3. Which of the following medications is likely to be most effective in treating neuropathic pain?
   a. Acetaminophen
   b. Antidepressants
   c. Corticosteroids
   d. NSAIDs
4. Which medications are likely to cause blood glucose control issues in a person with diabetes?
   a. Anticonvulsants
   b. Antidepressants
   c. Corticosteroids
   d. Opioid analgesics
5. Which of the following best defines "duration of action"?
   a. Length of time a drug remains active in the body
   b. Length of time for a drug to distribute into the CNS
   c. Rate at which a drug is absorbed into the systemic circulation
   d. Rate at which a drug is cleared from the body
6. Which of the following may increase drug absorption from a patch?
   a. Application of heat
   b. Application of ice
   c. Keeping an extremity immobilized
   d. Performing mild stretching exercises
7. In certain persons, COX-2 inhibitors may be prescribed instead of NSAIDs because COX-2 inhibitors have a much lower risk of:
   a. Blood sugar complications.
   b. CNS side effects.
   c. Gastrointestinal bleeding.
   d. Liver toxicity.
8. Calcium and vitamin D supplementation is recommended to reduce the risk of osteoporosis in persons taking long-term:
   a. Acetaminophen.
   b. Corticosteroids.
   c. COX-2 inhibitors.
   d. NSAIDs.
9. Adverse effects of opioids include:
   a. Addiction potential.
   b. Constipation.
   c. Orthostatic hypotension.
   d. Sedation.
   e. All of the above
10. Pain that occurs despite the use of regularly scheduled pain medications is known as:
    a. Breakthrough pain.
    b. Inflammatory pain.
    c. Neuropathic pain.
    d. Nociceptive pain.
11. A patient has been using Lortab (hydrocodone/acetaminophen) regularly for the last 6 months for chronic low-back pain. He says the medication used to cause a significant amount of sedation, but now it does not. This is known as:
    a. Abuse.
    b. Addiction.
    c. Tolerance.
    d. Withdrawal.
12. Examples of nociceptive pain include all of the following except:
    a. Bursitis.
    b. Diabetic neuropathy.
    c. Muscle sprains.
    d. Osteoarthritis.
13. Which of the following patient statements might suggest a potential problem regarding appropriate antibiotic use?
    a. "I take my antibiotic every 8 hours, spread as evenly as possible around the clock."
    b. "I was supposed to take the antibiotic for 10 days, but it worked in just 3 days, so I stopped taking it."
    c. "I'm supposed to take my antibiotic once a day on an empty stomach, so I always wait at least 2 hours after a meal."
    d. "I'm very careful not to skip doses."
14. The fentanyl (Duragesic) medication patch is used to treat chronic severe pain. This route of administration is known as:
    a. Subcutaneous.
    b. Sublingual.
    c. Topical.
    d. Transdermal.
15. Which of the following medications is the most effective (most powerful) for nociceptive pain?
    a. Acetaminophen
    b. Corticosteroids
    c. NSAIDs
    d. Opioid analgesics

Short Answer

16. Name several ways in which medications are removed or cleared from the body.
17. What are three common routes of drug administration?
18. Why are acetaminophen overdoses so common in the United States, and how can a PTA help prevent them?
19. What are some common ADRs that increase risk of falls in older adults?
20. What types of problems may occur as the result of orthopedic infections?

Fill in the Blank

21. The main toxicity concern with overuse of acetaminophen or when acetaminophen is combined with alcohol is the risk of ______________ toxicity.

22. After intraarticular injection of corticosteroids, the analgesic and antiinflammatory benefits may last for up to _______ weeks.
23. The four-letter abbreviation _________ that stands for *N*-acetyl-para-aminophenol is often used on prescription bottles that contain acetaminophen.
24. Patients taking long-term opioid analgesics almost always experience __________, and tolerance does not develop to this side effect.
25. Regular strength acetaminophen contains _______ mg per tablet, and the extra-strength product contains _______ mg per tablet.

True/False

26. Health care providers and patients often overestimate the risk of addiction potential when opioids are used for pain management.
27. Some patches have metallic backings that can conduct electrical currents, leading to significant burns if electromagnetic therapy is applied.
28. All opioid medications distribute into the CNS and can cause CNS side effects in some patients.
29. In general, sustained-release tablets and capsules should not be chewed, crushed, or broken open.
30. Behaviors such as aggressively complaining about pain, occasionally taking more than prescribed, drug hoarding during periods of reduced pain, and reporting unintended psychiatric effects are positive signs of drug addiction.

Chapter 29

Musculoskeletal Imaging

Terry Malone, Charles Hazle

CHAPTER OUTLINE

LEARNING OBJECTIVES

1. Describe the primary concepts for the application and use of plain film radiography.
2. Discuss the basic approach to looking at or reading radiographic images.
3. Describe the primary concepts for the application and use of computed tomography.
4. Describe the primary concepts for the application and use of diagnostic ultrasound.
5. Discuss the basic principles of specialized imaging techniques commonly seen in patient care.
6. Discuss the recommended approach to responding to patient queries associated with imaging.

KEY TERMS

Arthrography
Computed tomography (CT)
Diagnostic ultrasound
Ionizing radiation
Magnetic resonance imaging (MRI)
Plain film radiography
Positron emission tomography
Venography

This chapter provides basic information on imaging processes and modalities. Imaging ideally is used to confirm the clinical diagnosis derived through a thorough examination, which includes a complete history and selected manual tests and measures. The clinician appropriately selects specific imaging modalities to elucidate and confirm the existing data as the continuing evaluation process evolves. Imaging may be used excessively or as the sole basis for a clinical diagnosis; however, the data collected from the clinical examination are usually as valuable as the imaging data. The role of the physical therapist assistant (PTA) in this process is to be able to answer basic questions from clients related to the imaging process—not to interpret or make recommendations.

PLAIN FILM IMAGING

Also known as projectional radiography, plain film imaging is the classic technique of creating a two-dimensional "picture" of a body part using **ionizing radiation**. The radiation used penetrates the body part and is absorbed based on the tissue density. The radiation goes through a "tube" exiting as a beam of ions and then through the body part and projects onto the film or receptor plate. Most plain radiography today is digital, and the receptor plate provides an immediate digital display, which can be saved and manipulated via computer software. Actual hard copy films are declining in use because of the many benefits of digital imaging. This digital approach also enables decreased levels of radiation. Fig. 29-1 shows a digital radiography unit.

This process usually requires a sequence of images to enable triangulation and delineation of the location of possible areas of concern within the body part. A single projection is two-dimensional, and a second projection (typically done at a 90° angle to the first) is required to begin this process. A third projection sometimes may be required to show a tissue in profile because of bony overlap or to attain a view more likely to reveal pathologies. Figs. 29-2, 29-3, and 29-4 show various projections of the shoulder that reveal different anatomic relationships. The final result is two or three images that are labeled according to the techniques used during the acquisition. The initial classification is projection orientation (anterior to posterior, posterior to anterior, or lateral [from the side]). A description of the extremity position may be provided when appropriate (i.e., internal rotation, external rotation, flexion). When the letter "L" or "R" is on the image, it indicates that the image is of the left or right extremity—not the position in relationship to the extremity.

Important Concepts

Plain films are the most common first-line images and are nearly always done as a series—with at least two at right angles to allow triangulation.

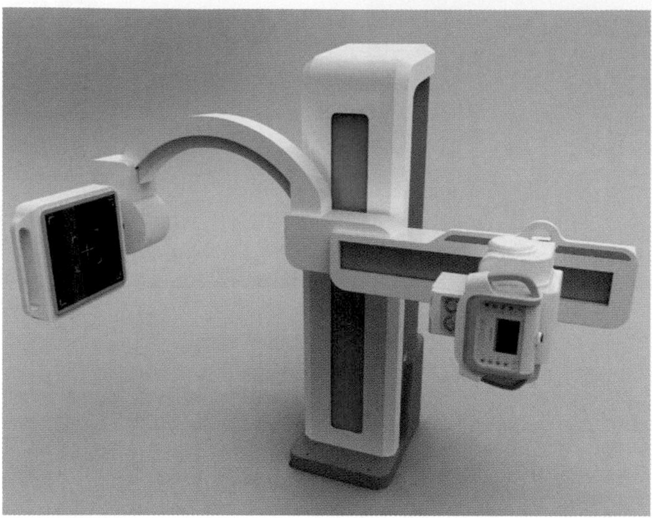

FIG 29-1 Digital radiography unit.

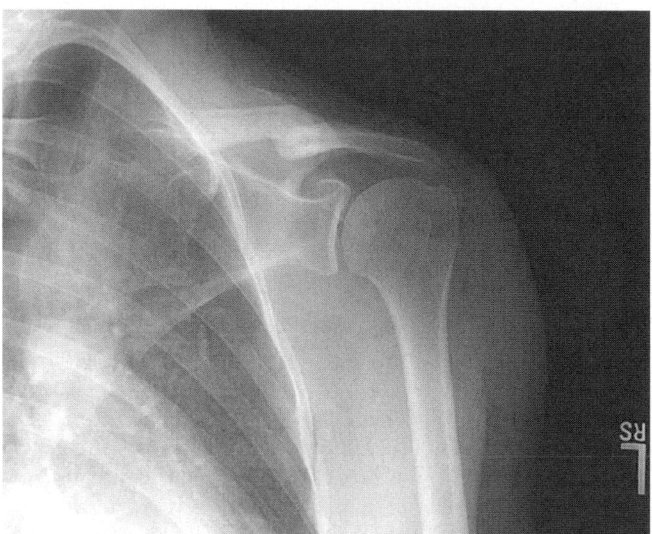

FIG 29-2 Shoulder anterior-posterior radiograph. Notice the relationship of the humeral head to the glenoid fossa. Also note the prominence of the greater tuberosity at the lateral aspect of the humeral head as the humerus is placed in external rotation. The letter "L" indicates the patient's left shoulder. The other letters indicate the initials of the technician who completed the procedure.

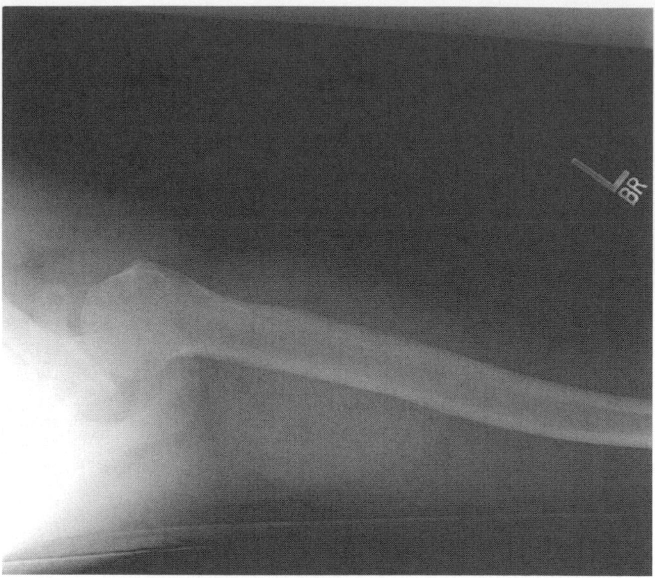

FIG 29-3 Shoulder radiograph, axillary view. In this axillary view, the relationship of the humeral head to the glenoid fossa is viewed from another perspective. The patient is supine, and the projection is from an inferior angle.

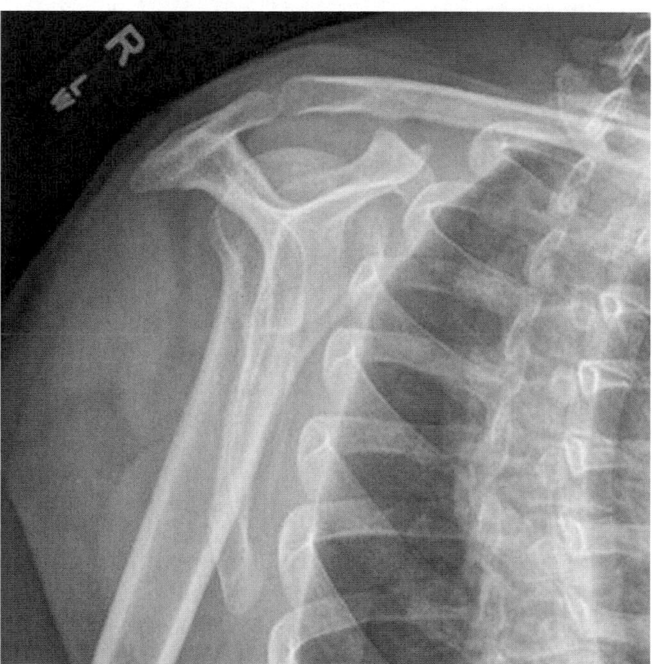

FIG 29-4 Shoulder radiograph, transthoracic (or "Y") view. In this lateral view, observe how the humeral head is superimposed on the "Y" of the scapula formed by the scapular body, coracoid process, and acromion.

The strengths of radiography include low cost, ability to be performed quickly and efficiently, and frequently giving adequate delineation for care or outlining additional imaging needs. It works well to identify fractures with disruptions of the outer, cortical bone that can be clearly seen. Limitations of radiography include often inadequate visualization when overlapping layers of bone are present and very incomplete information related to soft tissues. Figs. 29-5, 29-6, 29-7, and 29-8 demonstrate long bone fractures and the types of fractures frequently encountered and described by the nature of the fracture line and fragments—transverse, oblique, spiral, and comminuted. Figs. 29-9 and 29-10 demonstrate displacement of fracture fragments, which may have a significant impact on the care offered and the outcome. Because radiographs are generated through the use of ionizing radiation, it is possible that it can contribute to the risk of cell mutations and cancer. Radiologists attempt to minimize these risks by obtaining only the films (views) required to enable clinical decision making and treatment planning.

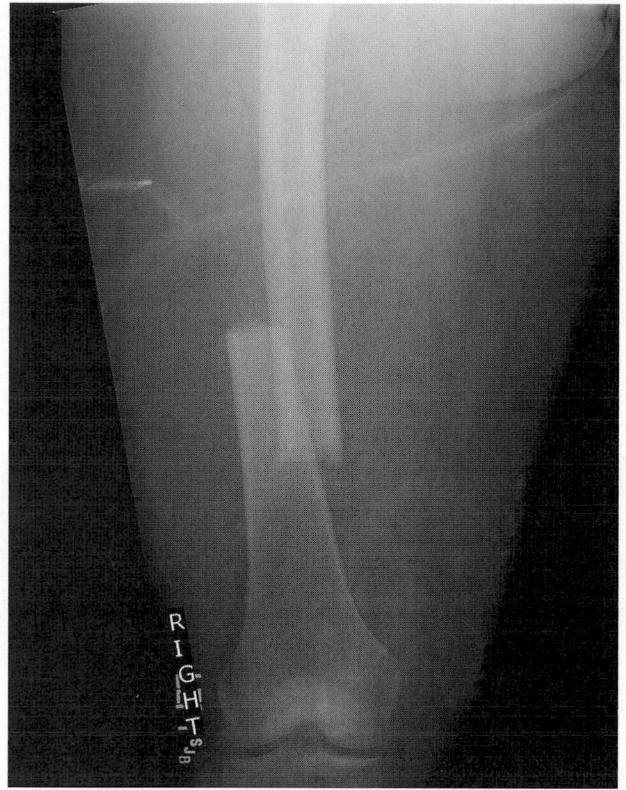

FIG 29-5 Femur transverse fracture. Observe the straight horizontal fracture line through the shaft of the femur.

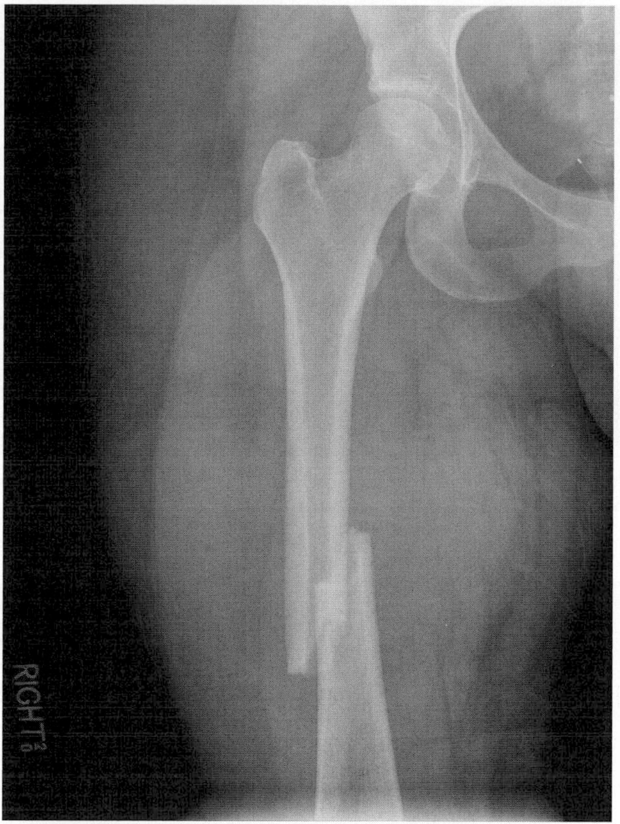

FIG 29-6 Femur oblique fracture. In contrast to the transverse fracture shown in Fig 29-5, note how the fracture line is now obliquely oriented.

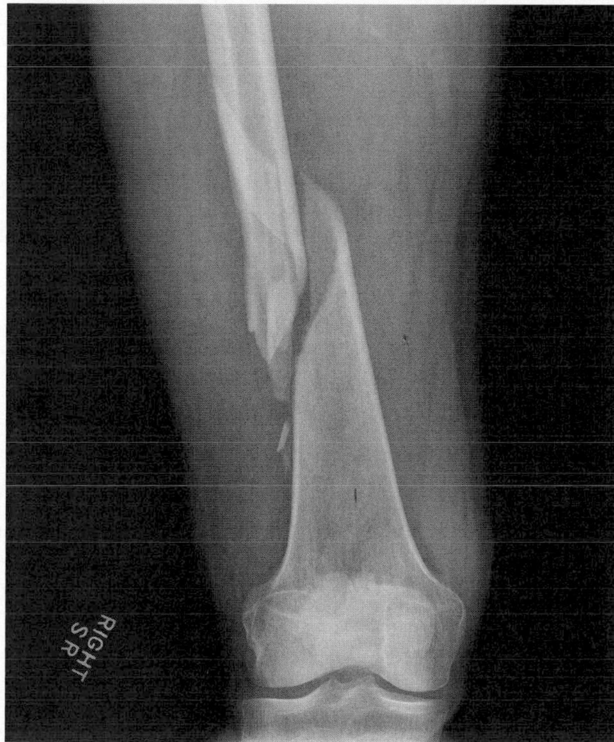

FIG 29-7 Femur spiral fracture. Although with superimposition, note the spiral orientation of the fracture line through the femur.

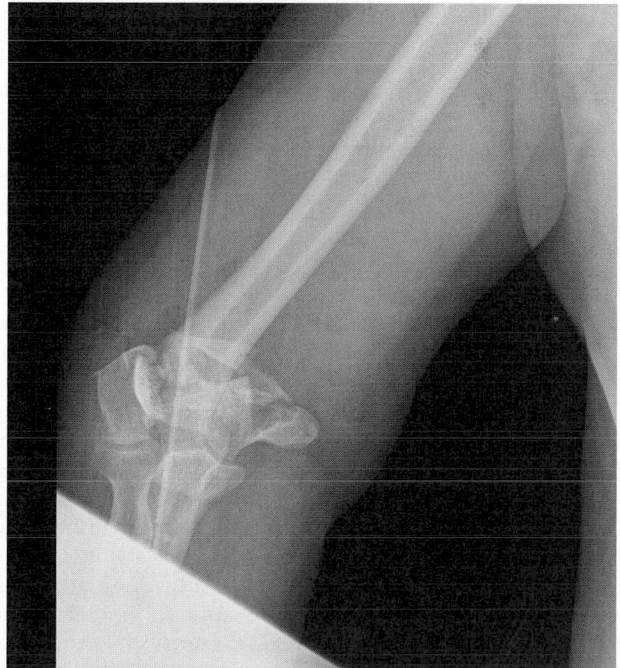

FIG 29-8 Distal humerus comminuted fracture. Note the many small bone fragments.

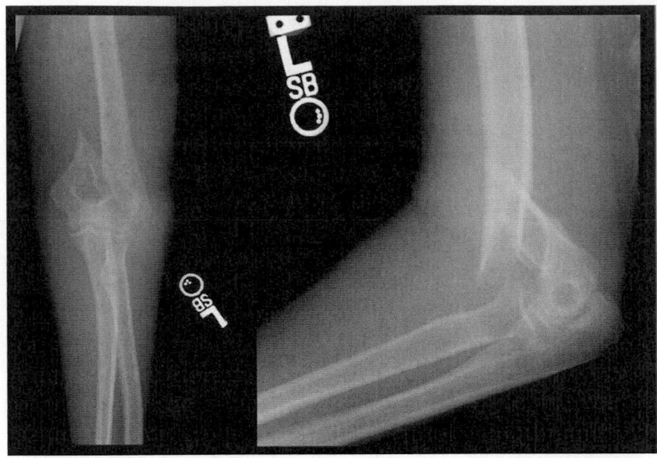

FIG 29-9 Distal humerus displaced fracture. Observe the separation and angulation of the fracture fragments.

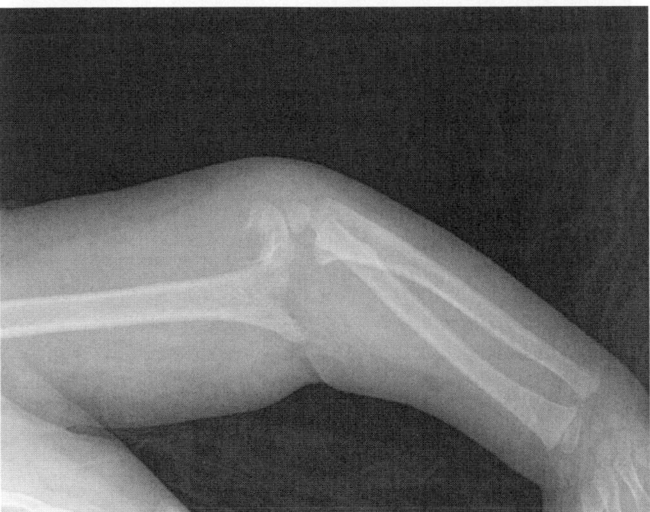

FIG 29-10 Salter-Harris type 1 fracture in a skeletally immature individual. There is a significant risk of growth disturbance when fracture occurs through a growth plate, particularly when accompanied by displacement of the fracture fragments.

COMPUTED TOMOGRAPHY

Computed tomography (CT) is an adaptation of **plain film radiography** that links sequential plain films enabling a computer to assemble a cross-sectional picture of internal structures. This technology has been greatly advanced through the use of a continuous rotational scanning process, which increases the speed of acquisition and decreases the exposure to radiation required for imaging. Also, the number of slices that can be developed has dramatically increased as computer technologies continue to enhance the generation of images and variety of final applications. These include being able to assemble the captured images and recreate three-dimensional models of internal structures. Another strength of CT is the definition of cortical (surface) bone, which frequently enables surgical planning or determines if conservative management can be used. Most commonly used CT scanners do not isolate soft tissues well and are most valuable in bony

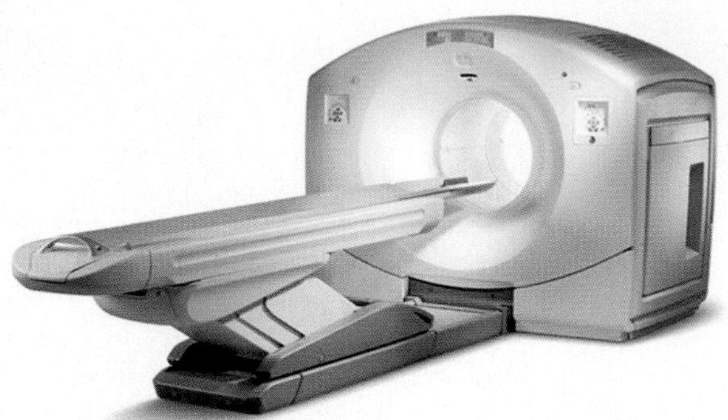

FIG 29-11 Computed tomography unit.

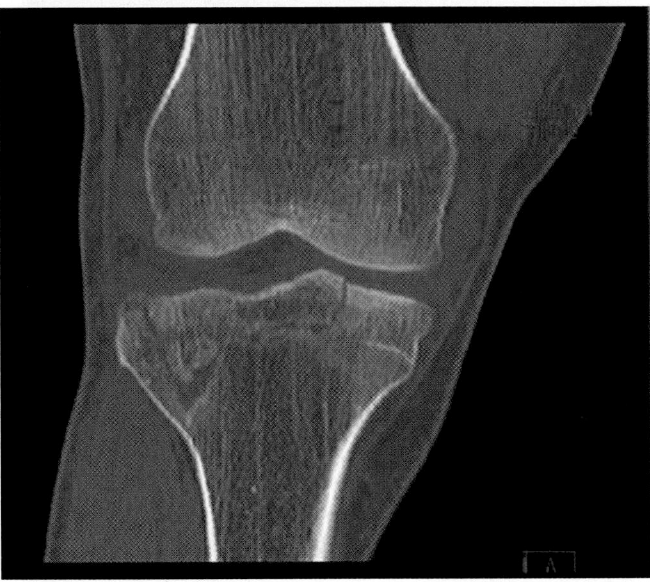

FIG 29-12 Computed tomography of a tibial plateau fracture. Where the bony anatomy is complex, computed tomography can reveal details of bone not visualized on radiography.

delineation. Fig. 29-11 shows a CT scanning unit. Fig. 29-12 is a coronal plane reconstruction from a typical CT image set, and Fig. 29-13 shows a three-dimensional reconstruction of the foot and ankle.

Important Concepts

CT is the modality of choice for bone edges and is often used to help establish definitive treatment—conservative or surgical planning.

CT scanning exposes the patient to significant radiation, and this is most dangerous when the patient is young. Table 29-1 lists the levels of exposure presented by different modalities and includes comparisons with typical background radiation from natural sources.

The American College of Radiology developed Appropriateness Criteria for selecting the images needed and defining the best approach, which have enabled better agreement of imaging modalities to be used for improved diagnostic value, while decreasing unwanted exposures to

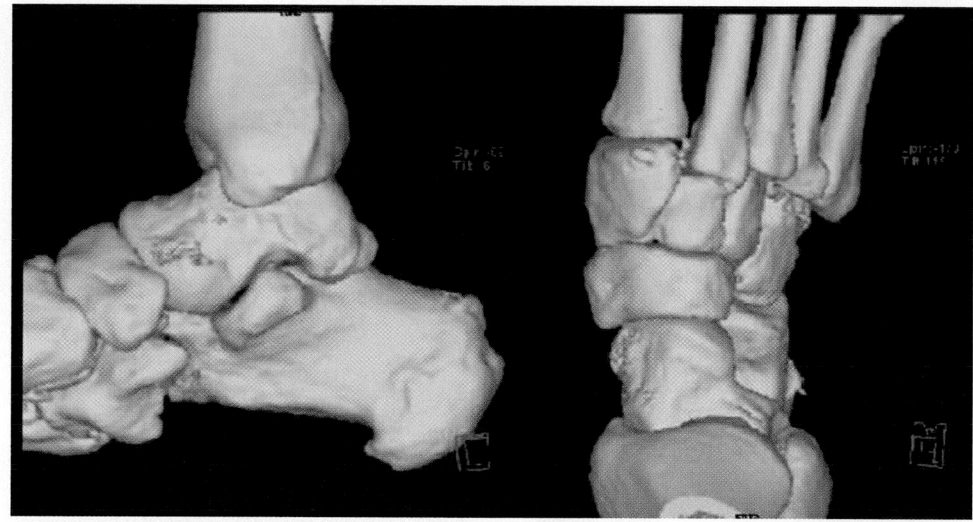

FIG 29-13 Three-dimensional computed tomography provides a striking reproduction of the bony anatomy.

TABLE 29-1 Comparison of Radiation Exposure Values

Procedure	Dose (mSv)	Equivalent Background Exposure
Cross country flight	0.03	3 days
Chest radiograph	0.1	10 days
Spine radiograph	1.5	6 months
Dental intraoral radiograph	0.005	1 day
Abdominal CT scan	10	3 years
Spine CT	6	2 years
Mammography	0.4	7 weeks
MRI	0	Unchanged
Ultrasound	0	Unchanged

CT, computed tomography; *MRI,* magnetic resonance imaging.

From Radiology Society of North America and American College of Radiology (website). http://www.radiologyinfo.org/en/safety/?pg=sfty_xray. Accessed October 21, 2013.

radiation. These selection criteria are based on clinical evidence while still considering the individual circumstances of the patient, which is best accomplished by the patient's physician. Details of imaging modality selection are best deferred to the physician supervising the patient's care.

MAGNETIC RESONANCE IMAGING

Magnetic resonance imaging (MRI) has evolved rapidly during the past 25 years related to enhanced computer applications and advanced higher strength magnets. With stronger magnets and software manipulations available, MRI is able to contrast bony and soft tissues within the body. The best explanation for patients about the MRI procedure may be to say: "You are placed in a magnetic field and different tissues in your body will be impacted differently. We then pass radio waves through the body that allow the computer to create specific images of tissues. You will hear a thumping sound during the process. All you have to do is lie still." MRI enables soft tissues to be seen well along with some aspects of bony tissues. MRI does not require radiation, and computer software shows tissues differently enabling better decisions for treatment interventions. Fig. 29-14 shows an MRI unit. Figs 29-15, 29-16, and 29-17 show examples of images, including a normal cervical spine (Fig. 29-15), a normal brain (Fig. 29-16), and a tear of the posterior portion of a knee meniscus (Fig. 29-17).

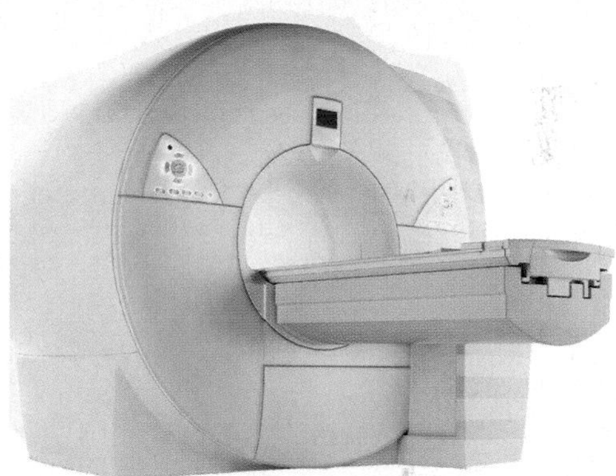

FIG 29-14 Magnetic resonance imaging unit.

A drawback that is not specific to MRI is that some clinicians inordinately weight MRI results to dictate treatment, rather than adequately considering all clinical data. An example of this problem is the use of MRI in patients with spinal conditions: A high percentage of asymptomatic persons show MRI abnormalities, especially older subjects when looking for disk pathology.[2] Some "degenerative" changes in the spine are typical of development over the life span and are often not directly associated with the presence of pain.[1] The primary strength of MRI is delineation of soft tissue and bony structure, and its main drawback is cost. A second drawback is the use of this modality when metal is in the body. Safety

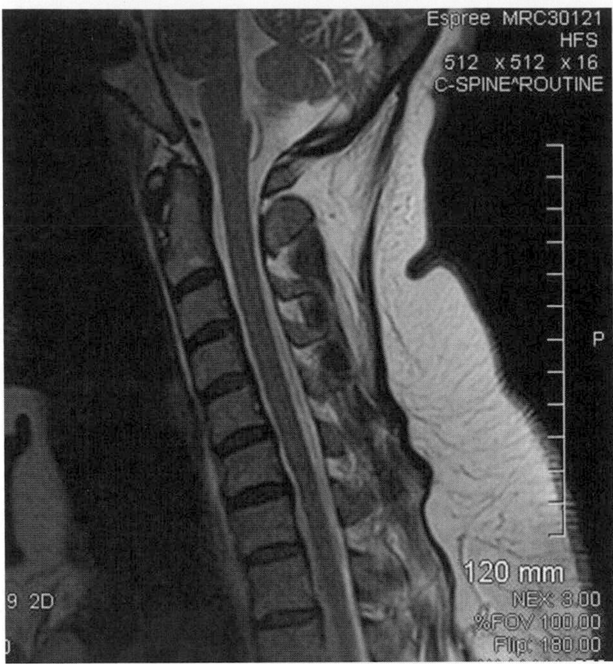

FIG 29-15 Magnetic resonance imaging of the cervical spine. Details of the bony and soft tissues are revealed in great detail in this sagittal slice of the cervical spine.

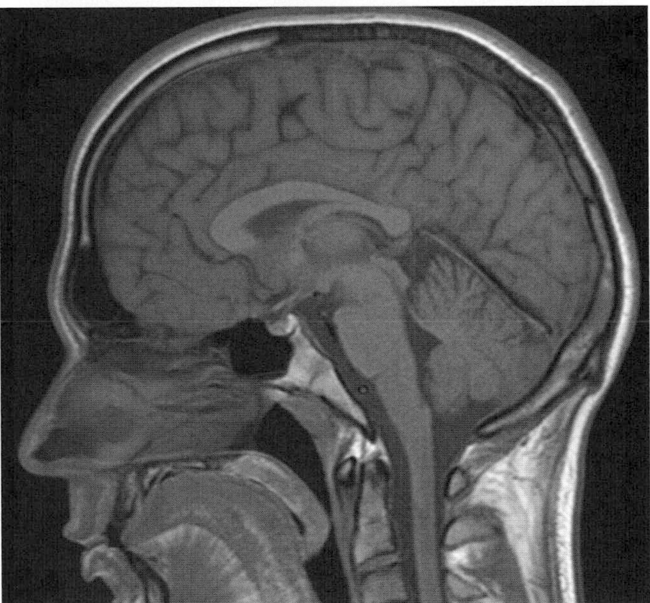

FIG 29-16 Magnetic resonance imaging of the brain demonstrates the soft tissue, including neural tissue, very well.

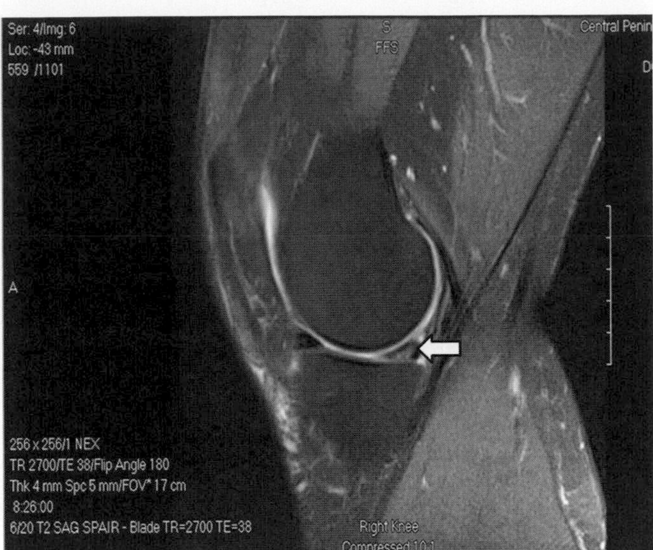

FIG 29-17 Magnetic resonance imaging of a meniscus tear. A common application of magnetic resonance imaging is to demonstrate disruptions of the musculoskeletal tissues, such as a meniscus tear as seen here.

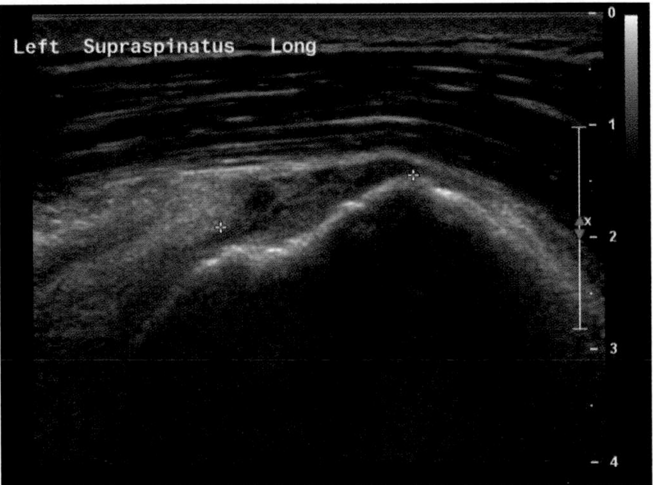

FIG 29-18 Ultrasound image of a rotator cuff tear. Note the darkened (hypoechoic) area between the two markers, indicative of a rotator cuff tear.

precautions require rigorous screening and considerations when any metal is present, including tattoos. It is anticipated that flexibility with MRI techniques will enable increased use especially as contrast media and newer computer software programs enhance tissue delineation.

Important Concepts

MRI continues to expand in its uses through additional computer algorithms, making previously underappreciated structures well defined.

DIAGNOSTIC ULTRASOUND

Ultrasound is a modality that passes sound waves into the body and records the rebounded energy. It enables assessments of tissues without radiation and can be used efficiently for certain structures. Often, the best structures are superficial and involve higher contrast, such as bone and well-aligned soft tissue such as tendon or a specific internal organ. Ultrasound can be used in real time to show muscle activation patterns during rehabilitation. Fig. 29-18 shows a **diagnostic ultrasound** at the shoulder defining a rotator cuff tear. A challenge for ultrasound to gain more widespread use is that it is user dependent, and significant experience is required to become a refined user.

Important Concepts

Although diagnostic ultrasound has many appealing qualities, it is more user dependent than other modalities and may remain less accepted.

SPECIAL STUDIES

Positron emission tomography is an imaging technique that uses radioactive tracer that is injected into the patient's bloodstream to enable the functions of the body to be studied. It is computer coordinated similar to classic tomography and enables clinicians to determine metabolic activity levels often to isolate metastatic lesions.

Arthrography used to be performed commonly to assess internal structures within joints. A radiopaque dye would be injected to "coat" specific structures, such as the meniscus of the knee or labrum of the shoulder, which would then be seen in outline on a plain film radiograph. This modality essentially has been replaced by refinements in MRI.

In **venography,** radiopaque dye is injected into the bloodstream to allow a plain film radiograph to outline blood supply. It may outline a thrombus (clot) or other vessel alteration. This modality is invasive and is not used commonly.

SUMMARY

The PTA is not often directly involved with diagnostic imaging. However, patients commonly have questions related to what they have heard or what they are soon to experience. Patients may appreciate having general explanations of the modalities, but care should be taken to avoid saying too much related to possible reasons for the imaging. Patients may hear what they hear and not be listening well. A very good rule is to default to "That's a great question for 'X' (physical therapist) or 'Y' (physician)."

Important Concepts

Your role as a PTA makes the provision of information related to imaging quite difficult. Be certain to discuss with the physical therapist the best approach for providing these data for all patients.

GLOSSARY

Arthrography: Specialized imaging that is typically accomplished by taking a series of radiographs after a radiopaque contrast medium is injected into a joint. The arthrogram is the radiographs taken while the opaque medium coats internal joint structure.

Computed tomography (CT): Tomography is the radiographic technique of obtaining slices or sections of a body part. CT refers to linking of a computer to enable all the slices to be combined to enable enhanced presentations of the scanned body part.

Diagnostic ultrasound: Sound waves are passed into the body, and their reflected response is recorded, allowing images of internal structures to be generated in real time. No ionizing radiation is used, which makes this modality attractive.

Ionizing radiation: Typically described as x-rays, ionizing radiation refers to electromagnetic waves of energy capable of causing ion formation in the body. Humans are exposed to a certain amount of ambient radiation each day. The amount of radiation absorbed from different imaging modalities can be described related to these values.

Magnetic resonance imaging (MRI): A computerized process that uses a strong magnetic field and radiowaves to image the tissues of the body. The computer program allows pictures or images to be created that delineate different tissues well throughout the body in detail. It does not use ionizing radiation and is deemed much safer for ongoing use. Also known as *nuclear magnetic resonance imaging.*

Plain film radiography: The creation of two-dimensional images of a body part by exposing it to x-ray radiation. The resulting image is directly related to the amount and density of tissue—how much is absorbed by the body as the radiation passes through the body part. Also known as *projectional radiography.*

Positron emission tomography: An imaging process in which a radioactive tracer is entered into the body and the scanning process yields three-dimensional assessments of specific structures—especially structures related to metabolic activity.

Venography: Specialized imaging that is typically accomplished by taking a series of radiographs as or after a dye (contrast agent) is infused to the vein or bone marrow. It allows assessment of veins for patency (being open or blocked).

REFERENCES

1. Endean A, Palmer KT, Coggon D: Potential of magnetic resonance imaging findings to refine case definition for mechanical low back pain in epidemiological studies: a systematic review. *Spine (Phila Pa 1976)* 36(2):160–169, 2011.
2. Radiology Society of North America and American College of Radiology (website): http://www.radiologyinfo.org/en/safety/?pg=sfty_xray. Accessed October 21, 2013.
3. Saal JS: General principles of diagnostic testing as related to painful lumbar spine disorders: a critical appraisal of current diagnostic techniques. *Spine (Phila Pa 1976)* 27(22):2538–2545, discussion 2546, 2002.

REVIEW QUESTIONS

Multiple Choice

1. Plain film imaging is created by:
   a. A radio wave being absorbed differentially by tissues.
   b. Ionizing radiation being absorbed differentially by tissues.
   c. A sound wave being absorbed differentially by tissues.
   d. Digital waves being absorbed differentially by tissues.

2. Typically what is the minimum number of projections that must be done with plain films to delineate a location of concern?
   a. One
   b. Two
   c. Three
   d. Four
3. Plain films frequently give the required information to enable management of:
   a. Cartilaginous defects.
   b. Bone contusions.
   c. Ligament sprains.
   d. Bony fractures.
4. A growth disturbance may occur in long bone fractures when the fracture includes the:
   a. Epiphysis.
   b. Cortex.
   c. Meniscus.
   d. Ligamentous insertion.
5. When a fracture is described as oblique (on a plain film), the fracture often appears:
   a. Transverse to the body.
   b. Angled much like a diagonal.
   c. Compressed.
   d. As many fragments.
6. Humeral fractures often include:
   a. Multiple fragments.
   b. An accompanying clavicle fracture.
   c. An accompanying scapular fracture.
   d. Multiple forearm fractures.
7. CT is a computer process of linked sequential __________ to create cross-sectional images.
   a. Plain films
   b. Parallel ultrasound films
   c. Positron emissions
   d. STIR films
8. CT is best used to delineate:
   a. Ligament injury.
   b. Marrow changes.
   c. Cortical bone.
   d. Meniscal injury.
9. An abdominal CT scan provides radiation exposure that approximates how much ambient radiation exposure (what you get walking around at sea level)?
   a. 3 days
   b. 30 days
   c. 3 months
   d. 3 years
10. Full-body MRI provides radiation exposure that approximates how much ambient radiation exposure (what you get walking around at sea level)?
    a. None
    b. 3 days
    c. 30 days
    d. 3 months
11. The greatest asset of MRI is that it can:
    a. Delineate dense and soft tissues.
    b. Enable depiction of tissues through ionizing radiation.
    c. Create definitive images for spinal management decisions.
    d. Best define how bone and metal are joined after an implant.
12. MRI should be used when:
    a. Plain films have defined a fracture.
    b. CT has indicated a cortical fracture.
    c. Ultrasound has not shown a fracture.
    d. Other imaging is inconclusive or soft tissue injury is suspected.
13. The primary weakness of MRI is that it is:
    a. Rarely helpful.
    b. Often not conclusive.
    c. Costly and often overly used with some conditions.
    d. Difficult for patients to endure.
14. Ultrasound is most commonly used to assess:
    a. High contrast structures.
    b. Bone fractures.
    c. Ligamentous insertions.
    d. Nerves.
15. Positron emission tomography is often used to isolate:
    a. Articular cartilage–joint surface injuries.
    b. Metabolic hot spots.
    c. Meniscal lesions of the knee.
    d. A blood clot or thrombus within a vessel.

Short Answer

16. What is the primary concern of CT use in children?
17. What does the "L" or "R" stand for on a plain film?
18. How well do MRI findings in the spine correlate to actual problems in older patients?
19. Explain why MRI would be used if the physician suspects a knee meniscus injury.
20. Discuss whether ultrasound of the shoulder could identify a rotator cuff tear.

Fill in the Blank

21. Humeral compression fractures often occur because the patient ________________.
22. Venography involves a radiopaque dye injected into the bloodstream to enable ______________ to outline blood supply.
23. The only imaging modality that enables evaluation of neural tissues is ______________.
24. When multiple cortical fragments are present and bony anatomy is complex, ___________ is often the modality of choice.
25. A major issue with ultrasound is that it is _________ dependent.

True/False

26. MRI is always the best modality for bony issues.
27. Ligaments can be evaluated by CT scan well.
28. Plain films are not done digitally because hard copies are required.
29. CT scans can be done quickly using modern equipment.
30. Using the American College of Radiology Appropriateness Criteria facilitates proper selection of an imaging modality.

Appendices

Appendix A

Commonly Used Medications in Orthopedics

Ladonna S. Hale

This is not an all inclusive list. Please consult an appropriate drug information resource for full information regarding therapeutic uses, side effects, and precautions.[1,2]

Type of Medication	Generic Name	Trade Name	Important Rehabilitation Information
Nonsteroidal antiinflammatory drugs (NSAIDs): Treat mild to moderate acute or chronic pain and inflammation	Aspirin	Bayer, Anacin, and others	• Available over-the-counter. • Not appropriate for all patients and should not be used by children or for pain or inflammation treatment by adults with difficult to control hypertension, congestive heart failure, kidney disease, stomach ulcers, bleeding disorders, and alcoholism and patients prescribed warfarin. • Important side effects: rash, increased risk of bleeding, stomach upset, and stomach ulcers. • Low dosages (81-325 mg/day) are used for antiplatelet benefits.
	Diclofenac	Cataflam, Voltaren	• Ibuprofen, naproxen, and ketoprofen are available over-the-counter. Ketorolac and ibuprofen are also available in injection form. NSAIDs are not appropriate for all patients and should not be used by patients with difficult to control hypertension, congestive heart failure, kidney disease, stomach ulcers, bleeding disorders, and alcoholism and patients prescribed warfarin. • Important side effects: rash, increased risk of bleeding, stomach upset, and stomach ulcers.
	Etodolac	Lodine	
	Fenoprofen	Nalfon	
	Ibuprofen	Advil, Motrin, and others	
	Indomethacin	Indocin	
	Ketoprofen	Orudis	
	Ketorolac	Toradol	
	Meloxicam	Mobic	
	Nabumetone	Relafen	
	Naproxen	Aleve, Anaprox, Naprosyn, and others	
	Oxaprozin	Daypro	
	Piroxicam	Feldene	
	Sulindac	Clinoril	
	Tolmetin	Tolectin	

Continued

Type of Medication	Generic Name	Trade Name	Important Rehabilitation Information
Selective COX-2 inhibitor: Treat mild to moderate acute or chronic pain and inflammation	Celecoxib	Celebrex	• Celecoxib is not appropriate for all patients and should not be used by patients with difficult to control hypertension, congestive heart failure, or kidney disease. • Safer than NSAIDs in patients with stomach ulcers, bleeding disorders, and alcoholism and patients prescribed warfarin. • Should not be taken by patients allergic to sulfonamide antibiotics.
Nonnarcotic analgesic: Treat mild to moderate, acute or chronic noninflammatory pain	Acetaminophen	Tylenol and others	• Available over-the-counter. • Does not treat inflammatory-type pain. • Generally considered safe for most patients; the most problematic side effect is liver toxicity. • Accidental overdoses are common. To reduce the risk of liver failure, adult dosages should not exceed 3250 mg/day. • Should not be used by persons who chronically consume alcohol.
Opioid analgesics and combination products: Treat mild to severe, acute or chronic pain	Codeine + acetaminophen	Tylenol #3 and others	• Opioid selection is based on level and intensity of pain. • Physical dependence can occur with chronic use; however, physical dependence does not indicate addiction. • Possibility of addiction exists. • Important side effects: stomach upset, rash, sedation, drowsiness, dizziness, constipation, low blood pressure, orthostatic hypotension, slowed respirations, and impaired judgment. Tolerance develops to most of these side effects except constipation. • Many opioids contain acetaminophen (see acetaminophen section for additional precautions)
	Hydrocodone + acetaminophen	Lortab, Lorcet, Vicodin, and others	
	Hydromorphone	Dilaudid	
	Fentanyl	Duragesic patch	
	Methadone	Dolophine	
	Meperidine	Demerol	
	Morphine	MS Contin, Oramorph, Roxanol, and others	
	Oxycodone	OxyContin	
	Oxycodone + acetaminophen	Percocet, Tylox, and others	
	Oxymorphone	Opana	
	Pentazocine + aspirin	Talwin	
	Propoxyphene	Darvon	
	Propoxyphene + acetaminophen	Darvocet	
	Tramadol	Ultram	
Bisphosphonates: Treat and prevent osteoporosis	Alendronate	Fosamax	• Osteoporosis treatment will not be effective without adequate calcium and vitamin D intake. • Oral bisphosphonates may be prescribed orally once daily, weekly, or monthly. Injection bisphosphonates may be administered annually. • Important patient instructions: Tablets should be taken on an empty stomach with a full glass of water. Patient must remain upright for at least 30 minutes after the dose. • Important side effects: bone and muscle pain, heartburn, and esophageal ulcers when patient instructions are not followed.
	Risedronate	Actonel	
	Ibandronate	Boniva	
	Zoledronic acid	Reclast	

Type of Medication	Generic Name	Trade Name	Important Rehabilitation Information
Other osteoporosis medications: Treat and prevent osteoporosis	Raloxifene	Evista	• Estrogen agonist/antagonist. • Generally used in female patients only.
	Calcitonin	Miacalcin	• Calcitonin hormone. • Administered daily as a nasal spray.
	Teriparatide	Fortéo	• Recombinant human parathyroid hormone. • Injected subcutaneously daily. • FDA approved for short-term use only (<2 years)
Corticosteroids/ glucocorticoids: Suppress and reduce inflammation	Betamethasone Cortisone Dexamethasone Fludrocortisone Hydrocortisone Methylprednisolone Prednisolone Prednisone Triamcinolone	Celestone and others Decadron Florinef various Solu-Medrol Prelone and others Deltasone Kenalog and others	• Most are available oral and/or injection. • Betamethasone, dexamethasone, prednisone, and triamcinolone may be administered intraarticularly and intradermally. • Betamethasone and triamcinolone may be administered intrasynovially. • Important side effects: increased risk of osteoporosis and infection; high blood glucose level; muscle weakness; abnormal fat distribution to abdomen, face, and upper back; edema; cataracts; glaucoma; stomach ulcers; high blood pressure; impaired wound healing; insomnia; mood changes; and even serious psychiatric disturbances. • Important side effects of intraarticular injection include: same as those just listed plus osteonecrosis, tendon rupture, and skin atrophy at injection site.

COX-2, Cyclooxygenase-2; *FDA,* U.S. Food and Drug Administration.

REFERENCES

1. DiPiro JT, Talbert RL, Yee GC, et al: *Pharmacotherapy: a pathophysiologic approach,* ed 8, New York, 2011, McGraw-Hill.
2. Lacy CF, Armstrong LL, Goldman MP, et al: *Drug information handbook 2013-2014,* ed 22, Hudson, OH, 2013, Lexi-Comp.

Appendix **B**

Reference Ranges for Commonly Used Tests

Amy Hassen, Jaime C. Paz

For the reference ranges that follow, individual laboratories in respective facilities may have different reference ranges based on their testing procedures and standards. Likely variances are specified.

The laboratory tests are categorized into their more commonly associated diagnostic category. However, there is overlap with certain tests into other diagnostic categories not specified in the tables. For example, the metabolic panel covers the endocrine and renal systems. The specific indication for the use of a test is ultimately determined by the physician.

Additionally, any laboratory value that falls outside of reference range should result in consultation with the supervising physical therapist and medical team to decide on the appropriateness of proceeding with physical therapy intervention.

Metabolic Panel Test(s)	Reference Range
Blood glucose	65-110 mg/100 mL†
Glycosylated hemoglobin (GHb, GHB, HbA_{1c})	<7% of total hemoglobin in well-controlled diabetes; 4%-5.9% in nondiabetic adults/children*
Calcium (Ca^{2+})	9-11 mg/100 mL†
Chloride (Cl^-)	95-105 mEq/L†
Osmolality	285-295 mOsm/L†
Sodium (Na^+)	135-145 mEq/L†
Potassium (K^+)	3.5-5 mEq/L†
Blood urea nitrogen (BUN)	10-20 mg/dL†
Creatinine (Cr)	Men: 0.6-1.2 mg/dL Women: 0.5-1.1 mg/dL*

Hematologic Panel Test(s)	Reference Range
Erythrocyte count (RBC count)	Male: 4.7-6.1 million/μL Female: 4.2-5.4 million/μL*
Hematocrit (Hct)	Male: 42%-50% Female: 40%-48%†
Hemoglobin, total (Hb)	Male: 13-16 g/100 mL Female: 12.0-14 g/100 mL†
Leukocyte (white blood cell) count, total (WBC count)	5,000-10,000/μL†
Erythrocyte sedimentation rate	Male: 0-9 mm/hr Female: 0-20 mm/hr†
Erythropoietin (EPO)	0-19 mU/mL§
Ferritin	Male: 16-300 ng/mL Female: 4-161 ng/mL†
Folic acid (red cells)	140-628 ng/mL‖
Iron (Fe^{2+})	56-150 μg/dL†
Iron-binding capacity, total (TIBC)	150-225 μg/dL†
Mean corpuscular hemoglobin (MCH)	27-32 pg per cell†
Mean corpuscular hemoglobin concentration (MCHC)	33-38 g/dL†
Mean corpuscular volume (MCV)	80-94 fL†

Coagulation Profile Test(s)	Reference Range
Fibrin D-dimers	≤250 ng/mL D-dimer units (DDU)[#]
International normalized ratio (PT/INR) Ratio = Patient value/reference value	0.9-1.1 (ratio)*
Prothrombin time (PT)	11-12.5 seconds*
Partial thromboplastin time (PTT)	60-70 seconds*
Activated partial thromboplastin time (APTT)	30-40 seconds*
Platelet count (Plt)	200,000-350,000/μL[†]

Cardiac Panel Test(s)	Reference Range
Creatine phosphokinase (CPK)	Men: 55-170 U/L Women: 30-135 U/L*
Creatine kinase MB (CK-M)	0%*
Troponin T (cTnT)	<0.2 pg/L*
Troponin I (cTnI)	<0.03 pg/L*
Brain natriuretic peptide (BNP)	<100 pg/mL*
High sensitivity C-reactive protein (hs-CRP)	<1.0 mg/L = low risk for developing heart disease 1.0-3.0 mg/L = average risk for developing heart disease >3.0 mg/L = high risk for developing heart disease[‡]

Arterial Blood Gases Test(s)	Reference Range
pH	7.35-7.45[†]
Oxygen, partial pressure (Po_2)	75-100 mm Hg[†]
Carbon dioxide, partial pressure (Pco_2)	35-45 mm Hg[†]
Bicarbonate (total)	21-28 mEq/L*

Liver Panel Test(s)	Reference Range
Alanine aminotransferase (ALT)	7-55 U/L[¶]
Alkaline phosphatase (ALP)	45-115 U/L[¶]
Aspartate aminotransferase (AST)	8-48 U/L[¶]
Gamma-glutamyl transpeptidase (GGT)	9-48 U/L[¶]
Bilirubin (total)	0.1-1.0 mg/100 mL[†]

*Boissonnault WG: *Primary care for the physical therapist: examination and triage*, ed 2, St Louis, 2011, Saunders.
[†]Bottomley J: *Quick reference dictionary for physical therapy*, Thorofare, NJ, 2013, Slack Incorporated.
[‡]C-reactive protein. Medline Plus (website). http://www.nlm.nih.gov/medlineplus/ency/article/003356.htm. Updated March 22, 2013. Accessed May 10, 2013.
[§]Erythropoietin test. Medline Plus (website). http://www.nlm.nih.gov/medlineplus/ency/article/003683.htm. Updated March 22, 2013. Accessed May 10, 2013.
[‖]Ghadban R: Folate (folic acid). Medscape Reference (website). http://emedicine.medscape.com/article/2085523-overview. Updated August 27, 2013. Accessed May 10, 2013.
[¶]Liver Function Tests. Mayo Clinic (website). http://www.mayoclinic.com/health/liver-function-tests/MY00093/DSECTION=results. Published September 26, 2012. Accessed May 10, 2013.
[#]Test ID: DDI. Mayo Clinic (website). http://www.mayomedicallaboratories.com/test-catalog/Clinical+and+Interpretive/9290. Accessed May 10, 2013.

Appendix C

Units of Measurement and Terminology for the Description of Exercise and Sport Performance

Amy Hassen, Jaime C. Paz

UNITS FOR QUANTIFYING HUMAN EXERCISE[2]

Mass: kilogram (kg)
Distance: meter (m)
Time: second (s)
Force: newton (N)
Work: joule (J)
Power: watt (w)
Velocity: meters per second ($m \cdot s^{-1}$)
Torque: newton-meter ($N \cdot m$)
Acceleration: meters per second^2 ($m \cdot s^{-2}$)
Angle: radian (rad)
Angular velocity: radians per second ($rad \cdot s^{-1}$)
Amount of substance: mole (mol)
Volume: liter (L)

TERMINOLOGY

Concentric action: Shortening of the muscle occurs as it generates tension and contracts against resistance.[1]

Eccentric action: Lengthening of the muscle occurs as it generates tension and contracts to control motion against a resistance.[1]

Endurance: The ability to perform low-intensity, repetitive, or sustained activities over a prolonged period of time without fatigue.

Energy: The capability of producing force, performing work, or generating heat (SI unit: joule).[2]

Exercise: Any and all activity involving generation of force by the activated muscle(s). Exercise can be quantified mechanically as force, torque, work, power, or velocity of progression.[2]

Exercise intensity: A specific level of muscular activity that can be quantified in terms of power (energy expenditure or work performed per unit of time), the opposing force (e.g., by free weight of weight stack), isometric force sustained, or velocity of progression.[2]

Force: That which changes or tends to change the state of rest or motion in matter. A muscle generates force in a muscle action (SI unit: newton).[2]

Free weight: An object of known mass, not attached to a supporting or guiding structure, which is used for physical conditioning and competitive lifting.[2]

Isokinetic: Active resistive movement that is performed at a constant speed (that is controlled by a preset rate-limiting device).[1]

Isometric: Tension develops in the muscle without any length change.[1]

Mass: The quantity of matter of an object that is reflected in its inertia (SI unit: kilogram).[2]

Muscle action: Interaction of muscle force and the external forces (body parts, gravity, objects).[2]

Power: The rate of performing work; the product of force and velocity.[1,2]

Strength: The maximal force or torque a muscle or muscle group can generate at a specified or determined velocity.[2]

Torque: The effectiveness of a force to overcome the rotational inertia of an object. The product of force and the perpendicular distance from the line of action of the force to the axis of rotation (SI unit: newton-meter).[2]

Weight: The force exerted by gravity on an object (SI unit: newton; traditional unit: kilogram of weight) (Note: mass = weight/acceleration due to gravity).[2]

Work: Force expressed through a displacement but with no limitation on time (SI unit: joule; note: 1 newton × 1 meter = 1 joule).[2]

REFERENCES

1. Kisner C, Colby LA: *Therapeutic exercise: foundations and techniques*, ed 6, Philadelphia, 2012, FA Davis.
2. Komi PV, editor: *Strength and power in sport: the encyclopaedia of sports medicine*, ed 2, Malden, MA, 2003, Blackwell Science.

Appendix D

Fracture Eponyms

Amy Hassen, Jaime C. Paz

This appendix provides a descriptive list of commonly encountered terms associated with fractures. Eponyms are labels that provide two kinds of information: the pattern of a complex injury or pathologic problem and the name of an individual who has been closely identified with that problem.

Aviator's astragalus: Implies a variety of fractures of the talus that include compression fractures of the neck, fractures of the body, or fractures with dislocations.[3,4]

Barton fracture: Displaced articular lip fracture of the distal radius; may be associated with carpal subluxation. Fracture configuration may be in a dorsal or volar direction. Dorsal fracture is the most common fracture-dislocation.[4-5]

Bennett fracture: Intraarticular avulsion fracture subluxation of the base of the first metacarpal. A small triangular fragment of the volar lip remains attached to the trapezium and trapezoid, while the metacarpal shaft displaces proximally secondary to a muscle pull.[3]

Bennett fracture, reverse: Intraarticular fracture subluxation of the fourth or fifth metacarpals.[3]

Boot-top fracture: A fracture of the distal third of the tibia and fibula that is caused by a fall while on skis attached to boots.[3]

Boxer's fracture: Fracture of the neck of the fifth metacarpal with dorsal angulation. Metacarpal head often displaces volarly.[3]

Bumper fracture: Compression fracture of the lateral tibial plateau that is often associated with a medial collateral ligament avulsion fracture of the knee.[3]

Burst fracture: Comminuted fracture of the vertebral body from axial load, usually with anterior and posterior displacement of the fragments. May occur in the cervical, thoracic, or lumbar spine.[3,4]

Chance fracture: A flexion distraction injury resulting in compression of the vertebral body. There may be ligamentous or disk disruption, or both, posteriorly. There may also be a transverse disruption of the spinous process, neural arch, and vertebral body.[3]

Chauffeur's fracture (Hutchinson fracture): Intraarticular fracture of the radial styloid initially attributed to the starting crank of an engine being forcibly reversed by a backfire. Ulnar deviation and supination are the forces involved in creating this fracture.[3-5]

Chisel fracture: Incomplete radial head intraarticular fracture that may extend 1 cm distally.[3]

Chopart fracture and dislocation: Fracture or dislocation involving Chopart joints (talonavicular and calcaneocuboid) of the foot.[3,4]

Clay-shoveler's (coal-shoveler's) fracture: Injury initially attributed to workers digging heavy clay; it has since been seen in power lifters. It is a traction fracture of the lower cervical or upper thoracic spine (most common at C7) that is due to an excessive pull of the trapezius and rhomboid muscles during heavy work.)[1,3]

Colles fracture: General term for nonarticular fractures of the distal radius with dorsal displacement of the distal fragment and volar angulation; with or without an ulnar styloid fracture.[3,4]

Cotton fractures: Trimalleolar ankle fracture with fractures of both malleoli and the posterior lip of the tibia.[3,4]

Dashboard fracture: Fracture of the posterior rim of the acetabulum caused by impact of the knee that results in impact of the femoral head against the acetabulum. Often associated with a posterior cruciate ligament injury, a femoral shaft fracture, or a patellar fracture.[3]

deQuervain fracture: Fracture of the scaphoid with volar dislocation of a scaphoid fragment and the lunate.[3]

Descot fracture: Fracture of the posterior tibia (third malleolus).[3]

Die-punch fracture: Intraarticular fracture of the distal radius secondary to impaction from the lunate. Results from axial loading from a closed fist punch.[3]

Dupuytren fracture: Fracture of the distal fibula, above the lateral malleolus, with rupture of the distal tibiofibular ligaments and the deltoid ligament (or a medial malleolus fracture).[3]

Duverney fracture: Fracture of the iliac wing without disruption of the pelvic ring.[3,4]

Essex-Lopresti fracture: Fracture of the radial head with associated dislocation of the distal radioulnar joint. Radial head is generally comminuted and displaced. Typically results from a fall on an outstretched hand (FOOSH) injury.[1,3,4]

Galeazzi fracture: Fracture of the radius and dislocation of the distal ulna.[2]

Gosselin fracture: Distal tibia V-shaped fracture that extends into the tibial plafond.[3]

Greenstick fracture: Incomplete fracture in a bone in a child, with a portion of the cortex and periosteum remaining intact on the compression side of the fracture.[3,4]

Hangman's fracture: Fracture through the pedicles or lamina of the second cervical vertebra (axis) occurring from a distraction/extension force.[3]

Hill-Sachs fracture: Posterolateral humeral head compression fracture caused by anterior glenohumeral dislocation and impaction of the humeral head against the anterior glenoid rim.[3,4]

Hoffa fracture: Coronal fracture of the medial femoral condyle.[3]

Holstein-Lewis fracture: Fracture of the distal third of the humerus with entrapment of the radial nerve.[3,4]

Hutchinson fracture: See *Chauffeur's fracture*.

Jefferson fracture: Comminuted fracture of the ring of the atlas caused by axial compressive forces. Fractures usually occur anterior and posterior to the lateral facet joints.[1,3,4]

Jones fracture: Fracture of the base of the fifth metatarsal.[2,4]

Kocher fracture: Intraarticular fracture of the capitellum of the humerus.[3]

Laugier fracture: Fracture of the trochlea of the humerus.[3]

Lisfranc fracture-dislocation: Fracture or dislocation involving Lisfranc (tarsometatarsal) joint of the foot. Typically the second to the fifth joints are involved.[3,4]

Maisonneuve fracture: Fracture of the proximal fibula caused by external rotation. This injury may occur with a syndesmosis rupture, medial malleolus fracture, rupture of the deltoid ligament, or rupture of the posterior tibiofibular ligament.[3-5]

Malgaigne fracture: Unstable pelvic fracture with vertical fractures anterior and posterior to the hip joint. Associated dislocation of the sacroiliac joint or pubic symphysis or both may also be present.[3,4]

March fracture: Stress fracture of a metatarsal.[2]

Midnight fracture: Fracture of the proximal phalanx of the fifth toe.[3]

Monteggia fracture: Fracture of the proximal third of the ulna with associated anterior dislocation of the radial head (or radial head or neck fracture).[1,4]

Nightstick fracture: Isolated fracture of the ulna secondary to direct trauma (without disruption to the interosseous membrane or either radioulnar joint).[3,4]

Paratrooper fracture: Fracture of the distal shafts of the tibia and fibula.[3]

Piedmont fracture: Oblique fracture of the distal radius without distal radioulnar joint disruption.[3]

Pilon fracture: Comminuted distal tibia intraarticular fracture with a long oblique component that is due to axial loading and impaction of the talus into the tibial plafond.[3]

Posada fracture: Transcondylar humeral fracture with displacement of the anterior distal fragment and posterior dislocation of the radius and ulna.[3,4]

Pott fracture: Misnomer that is used to describe bimalleolar fractures of the ankle. This term was originally used to describe an abduction injury at the ankle that resulted in a distal fibular fracture and disruption of the medial deltoid ligament at the ankle.[3]

Rolando fracture: A comminuted Y-shaped or T-shaped intraarticular fracture of the thumb metacarpal with resultant disruption in the articular surface of the first metacarpal.[3]

Segond fracture: Avulsion fracture of the lateral tibial condyle from the bony insertion of the iliotibial band. It is frequently associated with anterior cruciate ligament and meniscal injuries.[3,4]

Shepherd fracture: Fracture of the lateral tubercle of the posterior talar process. This fracture may simulate an os trigonum.[3,4]

Ski boot fracture: See *Boot-top fracture*.

Ski-pole fracture: Fracture of the base of the first metacarpal, which may be intraarticular.[3]

Smith fracture: Fracture of the distal radius with palmar displacement of the distal fragment; also referred to as a *reverse Colles fracture*, a *reverse Barton fracture*, or a *Goyrand fracture*. The palmar displacement of the fragment may also be referred to as a *"garden spade" deformity*.[3-5]

Sprinter's fracture: Avulsion fracture of the anterior-superior or anterior-inferior spine of the ilium secondary to a sudden muscle pull.[3]

Stieda fracture: Avulsion fracture of the medial femoral condyle at the origin of the medial collateral ligament.[3,4]

Straddle fracture: Bilateral fractures of the superior and inferior pubic rami.[3,4]

Teardrop fracture: Flexion fracture or dislocation of the cervical spine with associated triangular anterior fragment of the involved vertebrae. Posterior instability is implied with posterior displacement of the vertebral body causing spinal cord damage. Hyperextension may also cause a teardrop fracture.[3,4]

Tillaux-Kleiger fracture: Fracture of the lateral half of the distal tibial ephiphysis during differential closure of the growth plate. The medial part of the tibial physis has already fused. Occurs in adolescents between 12 and 14 years old.[3,4]

Torus fracture: Impaction fracture of childhood as the bone buckles instead of fracturing completely. The lower forearm of young children tends to be most often injured.[4,5]

Wagstaffe-LeFort fracture: Avulsion of the distal fibula at the anterior-inferior tibiofibular ligament attachment site.[3]

Walther's fracture: Transverse ischioacetabular fracture that passes through the ischiopubic junction, the acetabular cavity, and the ischial spine.[3]

Wilson fracture: Volar plate fraction of the middle phalanx of a finger.[3]

REFERENCES

1. Dutton M: *Orthopaedic examination, evaluation, and intervention*, ed 3, New York, 2012, McGraw-Hill Medical.
2. Magee DJ: *Orthopedic physical assessment*, ed 5, St Louis, 2008, Saunders.
3. McKinnis LN: *Fundamentals of musculoskeletal imaging*, ed 3, Philadelphia, 2010, FA Davis.
4. Singh AP: Popular fracture names. *Bone and Spine* (website). http://boneandspine.com/popular-fracture-names/. Accessed April 5, 2013.
5. Wheeless CR III: Trauma and fractures menu. *Wheeless' textbook of orthopaedics* (website). http://www.wheelessonline.com/ortho/trauma_fractures_index. Updated March 26, 2013. Accessed April 17, 2015.

Appendix E

Major Movements of the Body and the Muscles Acting on the Joints Causing the Movement

Amy Hassen, Jaime C. Paz

MUSCLES ACTING AT THE JOINTS CAUSING MOVEMENT

Specific muscle activation depends on the patient's posture and skeletal alignment, along with the starting position of the joint.

Joint	Joint Movement	Description	Muscles
Neck	Cervical flexion*	Chin moves toward the chest	Sternocleidomastoid Longus colli Scalenes
	Cervical extension*	Chin moves away from the chest	Rectus capitis lateralis major and minor Rectus capitis posterior major Obliquus capitis superior Semispinalis capitis Semispinalis cervicis Splenius capitus and cervicis Levator scapulae Sternocleidomastoid Upper trapezius Longissimus capitis
	Cervical rotation†	Head rotates from side to side	**To the contralateral side:** Sternocleidomastoid Upper trapezius Scalenes **To the ipsilateral side:** Obliquus capitis superior and inferior Longissimus capitis Splenius capitus and cervicis Rectus capitis posterior Levator scapulae
	Lateral bending† (flexion) of the cervical spine	Ear moves toward the shoulder	Levator scapulae Longissimus capitis Semispinalis cervicis Splenius capitis cervicis Longus colli Rectus capitis posterior major Upper trapezius Sternocleidomastoid Scalenes

Continued

Joint	Joint Movement	Description	Muscles
Shoulder	Shoulder elevation	Shoulder shrug	Levator scapulae Upper trapezius Rhomboids
	Shoulder depression	Shoulders move downward	Latissimus dorsi Pectoralis major
	Scapular elevation	Scapula moves upward	Serratus anterior Middle trapezius Levator scapulae Rhomboid (major and minor)
	Scapular depression	Scapula moves downward	Levator scapulae
	Scapular abduction (protraction)	Scapulas move further apart	Serratus anterior
	Scapular adduction (retraction)	Scapulas move closer together	Levator scapulae Trapezius (upper and middle)
	Upward rotation of the scapula	Left (from rear) scapula rotates clockwise, and right scapula rotates counterclockwise	Serratus anterior Trapezius
	Downward rotation of the scapula	Right (from rear) scapula rotates clockwise, and left scapula rotates counterclockwise	Rhomboids (major and minor) Levator scapulae
	Shoulder adduction	Arms move sideways inward toward the body	Latissimus dorsi Teres major and minor Subscapularis
	Shoulder abduction	Arms move sideways away from the body	Deltoid (middle) Supraspinatus Serratus anterior Infraspinatus Subscapularis Biceps brachii
	Shoulder flexion	Arms straight up in front of the body	Deltoid (anterior and middle) Pectoralis major Biceps brachii
	Shoulder extension	Arms move from straight up in front of body to anatomic position	Pectoralis major (sternal) Latissimus dorsi Teres major Deltoid (posterior)
	Medial rotation of the shoulder	Humerus rotates inward at the shoulder	Latissimus dorsi Teres major Pectoralis major Supraspinatus Subscapularis
	Lateral rotation of the shoulder	Humerus rotates outward at the shoulder	Infraspinatus Supraspinatus Teres minor
	Horizontal shoulder adduction	With arm straight at shoulder height to the side, move arm toward the midline	Pectoralis major
	Horizontal shoulder abduction	With arm straight at shoulder height at the midline, move arm toward the side of the body	Deltoid (posterior) Infraspinatus
Elbow	Elbow flexion	Bend elbow, making angle smaller	Biceps brachii Brachialis Brachioradialis Pronator teres
	Elbow extension	Straighten elbow, making angle larger	Triceps brachii Anconeus
Forearm	Supination of radioulnar joint	Palm is turned upward	Biceps brachii Brachioradialis Supinator Extensor carpi radialis
	Pronation of radioulnar joint	Palm is turned downward	Pronator teres Brachioradialis Extensor carpi radialis Pronator quadratus

Joint	Joint Movement	Description	Muscles
Wrist	Wrist flexion	Wrist bends toward volar surface of forearm, making angle between the hand and the forearm	Flexor carpi radialis Flexor carpi ulnaris Palmaris longus Flexor digitorum superficialis Abductor pollicis longus Extensor pollicis brevis
	Wrist extension	Wrist bends toward the dorsal surface of the forearm, making angle between the hand and the forearm	Extensor carpi radialis Extensor carpi ulnaris Extensor digitorum Abductor pollicis longus Extensor pollicis brevis Extensor pollicis longus
Spine	Lumbar flexion*	With hips locked, bend forward at the lumbar vertebrae	External oblique Internal oblique Rectus abdominis
	Lumbar extension*	With hips locked, bend backward at the lumbar vertebrae	Longissimus Iliocostalis Multifidus
	Lumbar rotation†	Trunk twists to the side	External oblique (to the contralateral side) Internal oblique (to the ipsilateral side)
	Lateral bending† (flexion) of the trunk	Trunk moves side to side (no movement at the hip)	External oblique Internal oblique Erector spinae Psoas major
Hip	Hip flexion	Bend at the hip, which reduces angle	Iliacus Psoas major Pectineus Rectus femoris Sartorius Tensor fasciae latae Adductor brevis Adductor longus
	Hip extension	Straighten at the hip, which increases angle	Hamstrings Gluteus maximus Adductor magnus
	Hip abduction	Leg moves away from the body at the hip	Gluteus medius Gluteus minimus Gluteus maximus Tensor fasciae latae Rectus femoris Sartorius
	Hip adduction	Leg moves toward the body at the hip	Gracilis Pectineus Adductor longus Adductor brevis Gluteus maximus Hamstrings
	Medial (internal) rotation of the hip	Leg rotates inward at the hip	Gluteus minimus Gluteus medius Hamstrings Pectineus Piriformis (when hip is in flexion) Adductor brevis Tensor fasciae latae
	Lateral (external) rotation of the hip	Leg rotates outward at the hip	Rectus femoris Iliacus Psoas major Sartorius Hamstrings Gluteus maximus Gluteus medius Gluteus minimus Piriformis (when hip is in extension) Obturator internus and externus Quadratus femoris Gemellus superior and inferior

Continued

Joint	Joint Movement	Description	Muscles
Knee	Knee flexion	Bend at the knee, making angle smaller	Biceps femoris Semitendinosus Semimembranosus Sartorius Gracilis Popliteus Gastrocnemius
	Knee extension	Straighten the knee, making angle larger	Vastus lateralis Vastus intermedius Vastus medialis Rectus femoris Tensor fasciae latae
	Medial (internal) rotation of the knee	Knee turns inward (knee must be bent)	Semitendinosus Semimembranosus Gracilis Popliteus
	Lateral (external) rotation of the knee	Knee turns outward (knee must be bent)	Biceps femoris Tensor fasciae latae
Ankle	Inversion (supination) of the ankle	Sole of foot turns inward	Tibialis anterior Tibialis posterior Flexor digitorum longus Flexor hallucis longus Gastrocnemius Soleus
	Eversion (pronation) of the ankle	Sole of foot turns outward	Peroneus longus Peroneus brevis Peroneus tertius Extensor digitorum longus
	Dorsiflexion of the ankle	Toes move toward shin	Tibialis anterior Extensor digitorum longus Peroneus tertius Extensor hallucis longus
	Plantar flexion of the ankle	Toes move away from the shin	Gastrocnemius Soleus Peroneus longus Peroneus brevis Tibialis posterior Flexor digitorum longus Flexor hallucis longus

*Muscles listed are active bilaterally to create motion.
†Muscles listed are active unilaterally to create motion.

REFERENCES

Levangie PK, Norkin CC: *Joint structure & function: a comprehensive analysis*, Philadelphia, 2011, FA Davis.
Oatis CA: *Kinesiology: the mechanics & pathomechanics of human movement*, ed 2, Baltimore, 2009, Lippincott Williams & Wilkins.
Reese NB: *Muscle and sensory testing*, ed 3, St Louis, 2012, Saunders.

ANALYSIS OF BASIC WEIGHT TRAINING EXERCISES*

CHIN-UP

Exercise description: Using a horizontal bar suspended above the head, grasp the bar with the palms shoulder width apart and facing the body. Pull the body vertically upward until the chin passes the bar, and then return downward in a controlled manner to the initial hanging position.

*A more detailed description of the proper lifting technique for these basic weight training exercises can be found in most weight training textbooks (e.g., Nyland J: *Clinical decisions in therapeutic exercise: planning and implementation*, Upper Saddle River, NJ, 2005, Prentice Hall; Sandler D: *Fundamental weight training*, Champaign, IL, 2010, Human Kinetics). Further information on structural kinesiology and the analysis of other weight training exercises can be found in Floyd RT: *Manual of structural kinesiology*, ed 18, Boston, 2011, McGraw-Hill.

Segment Movement	Joint Movement	Primary Muscles Involved	Phase of Isotonic Contraction
Upward motion	Elbow flexion	Biceps brachii Brachialis Brachioradialis	Concentric
	Shoulder extension	Latissimus dorsi Teres major Deltoid (posterior)	Concentric
	Scapula adduction	Trapezius Rhomboids Levator scapulae	Concentric
	Shoulder depression	Trapezius Pectoralis minor	Concentric
Downward motion	Elbow extension	Biceps brachii Brachialis Brachioradialis	Eccentric
	Shoulder flexion	Latissimus dorsi Teres major Deltoid (posterior)	Eccentric
	Scapula abduction	Trapezius Rhomboids Levator scapulae	Eccentric
	Shoulder elevation	Trapezius Pectoralis	Eccentric

LATISSIMUS PULL-DOWN

Exercise description: Gasp the bar suspended over the head with palms facing away from the body. Pull the bar down to the top of the chest (in front of the head), and then return upward in a controlled manner to the initial position.

Segment Movement	Joint Movement	Primary Muscles Involved	Phase of Isotonic Contraction
Downward motion	Elbow flexion	Biceps brachii Brachialis Brachioradialis	Concentric
	Shoulder adduction	Latissimus dorsi Teres major Pectoralis minor	Concentric
	Scapular adduction	Trapezius Rhomboids Levator scapulae	Concentric
	Shoulder depression	Trapezius Pectoralis minor	Concentric
Upward motion	Elbow extension	Biceps brachii Brachialis Brachioradialis	Eccentric
	Shoulder abduction	Latissimus dorsi Teres major Pectoralis	Eccentric
	Scapular abduction	Trapezius Rhomboids Levator scapulae	Eccentric
	Shoulder elevation	Trapezius Pectoralis	Eccentric

BENT KNEE SIT-UP

Exercise description: While lying on your back with knees bent, arms across the chest, and feet on the floor, curl upward until the elbows touch the thighs, and then return downward in a controlled manner to the initial supine position.

Segment Movement	Joint Movement	Primary Muscles Involved	Phase of Isotonic Contraction
Upward motion	Lumbar flexion	Rectus abdominis External oblique Internal oblique	Concentric
Downward motion	Lumbar extension	Rectus abdominis External oblique Internal oblique	Eccentric

SQUAT

Exercise description: With a bar across the shoulders behind the head, bend at the knees and waist, moving downward to a position where the thighs are parallel with the floor, and then return upward in a controlled manner to the standing position.

Segment Movement	Joint Movement	Primary Muscles Involved	Phase of Isotonic Contraction
Downward motion	Hip flexion	Gluteus maximus Biceps femoris Semitendinosus Semimembranosus	Eccentric
	Knee flexion	Rectus femoris Vastus lateralis Vastus medialis Vastus intermedius	Eccentric
	Ankle dorsiflexion	Gastrocnemius Soleus	Eccentric
Upward motion	Hip extension	Gluteus maximus Biceps femoris Semitendinosus Semimembranosus	Concentric
	Knee extension	Rectus femoris Vastus lateralis Vastus medialis Vastus intermedius	Concentric
	Ankle plantar flexion	Gastrocnemius Soleus	Concentric

LEG PRESS

Exercise description: Using a leg press machine, position the feet about shoulder width apart. Push the foot pad forward until the knees are extended, and then return backward in a controlled manner to the initial position.

Segment Movement	Joint Movement	Primary Muscles Involved	Phase of Isotonic Contraction
Forward motion	Hip extension	Gluteus maximus Biceps femoris Semitendinosus Semimembranosus	Concentric
	Knee extension	Rectus femoris Vastus lateralis Vastus medialis Vastus intermedius	Concentric
Backward motion	Hip flexion	Gluteus maximus Biceps femoris Semitendinosus Semimembranosus	Eccentric
	Knee flexion	Rectus femoris Vastus lateralis Vastus medialis Vastus intermedius	Eccentric

BENCH PRESS

Exercise description: While lying on your back, grasp the bar with hands shoulder width apart and palms facing toward the feet. Lower the bar in a controlled manner to a position across the chest, and then push the bar upward to the initial position.

Segment Movement	Joint Movement	Primary Muscles Involved	Phase of Isotonic Contraction
Downward motion	Elbow flexion	Triceps brachii	Eccentric
	Shoulder extension	Pectoralis Deltoid (anterior)	Eccentric
	Scapular adduction	Serratus anterior Pectoralis	Eccentric

Segment Movement	Joint Movement	Primary Muscles Involved	Phase of Isotonic Contraction
Upward motion	Elbow extension	Triceps brachii	Concentric
	Shoulder flexion	Pectoralis Deltoid (anterior)	Concentric
	Scapular abduction	Serratus anterior Pectoralis	Concentric

SHOULDER PRESS

Exercise description: Grasp the bar at chest height with hands shoulder width apart and palms facing forward. Push the bar upward until the elbows are extended, and then lower the bar in a controlled manner to the initial position.

Segment Movement	Joint Movement	Primary Muscles Involved	Phase of Isotonic Contraction
Upward motion	Elbow extension	Triceps brachii	Concentric
	Shoulder flexion	Pectoralis Deltoid (anterior)	Concentric
	Shoulder elevation	Trapezius Rhomboids Levator scapulae	Concentric
Downward motion	Elbow flexion	Triceps brachii	Eccentric
	Shoulder extension	Pectoralis Deltoid (anterior)	Eccentric
	Shoulder depression	Trapezius Rhomboids Levator scapulae	Eccentric

ARM CURL

Exercise description: While standing holding the bar with palms facing forward, curl the bar upward while bending at the elbow until the bar reaches shoulder height, and then lower the bar in a controlled manner to the initial position.

Segment Movement	Joint Movement	Primary Muscles Involved	Phase of Isotonic Contraction
Upward motion	Elbow flexion	Biceps brachii Brachialis Brachioradialis	Concentric
Downward motion	Elbow extension	Biceps brachii Brachialis Brachioradialis	Eccentric

TRICEPS PUSH-DOWN

Exercise description: Stand holding a bar attached to a cable column with the elbows bent to approximately 90°, push the bar downward until the elbows are extended, and then raise the bar in a controlled manner to the initial position.

Segment Movement	Joint Movement	Primary Muscles Involved	Phase of Isotonic Contraction
Downward motion	Elbow extension	Triceps brachii	Concentric
Upward motion	Elbow flexion	Triceps brachii	Eccentric

LEG CURL

Exercise description: While lying prone on the bench with your heels hooked under the pad, curl the weight forward until the pad reaches the buttocks, and then lower the weight backward in a controlled manner to the initial position.

Segment Movement	Joint Movement	Primary Muscles Involved	Phase of Isotonic Contraction
Forward motion	Knee flexion	Biceps femoris Semitendinosus Semimembranosus	Concentric
Backward motion	Knee extension	Biceps femoris Semitendinosus Semimembranosus	Eccentric

KNEE EXTENSION

Exercise description: While sitting on the bench with your feet hooked under the pad, extend the weight upward until the knees are extended, and then lower the weight in a controlled manner to the initial position.

Segment Movement	Joint Movement	Primary Muscles Involved	Phase of Isotonic Contraction
Upward motion	Knee extension	Rectus femoris Vastus lateralis Vastus medialis Vastus intermedius	Concentric
Downward motion	Knee flexion	Rectus femoris Vastus lateralis Vastus medialis Vastus intermedius	Eccentric

HEEL RAISE

Exercise description: While standing with a bar supported on your shoulders, raise your body upward until you are standing on your toes, and then lower your body in a controlled manner to the initial position.

Segment Movement	Joint Movement	Primary Muscles Involved	Phase of Isotonic Contraction
Upward motion	Plantar flexion	Gastrocnemius soleus	Concentric
Downward motion	Dorsiflexion	Gastrocnemius soleus	Eccentric

Index

Note: Page numbers followed by "b" indicate boxes; "f" figures: "t" tables.

D

G

N

Q

R